Lecture Notes in C<

Commenced Publication in 197
Founding and Former Series Edi.
Gerhard Goos, Juris Hartmanis, and Jan van Leeuwen

Editorial Board

David Hutchison
  Lancaster University, UK
Takeo Kanade
  Carnegie Mellon University, Pittsburgh, PA, USA
Josef Kittler
  University of Surrey, Guildford, UK
Jon M. Kleinberg
  Cornell University, Ithaca, NY, USA
Alfred Kobsa
  University of California, Irvine, CA, USA
Friedemann Mattern
  ETH Zurich, Switzerland
John C. Mitchell
  Stanford University, CA, USA
Moni Naor
  Weizmann Institute of Science, Rehovot, Israel
Oscar Nierstrasz
  University of Bern, Switzerland
C. Pandu Rangan
  Indian Institute of Technology, Madras, India
Bernhard Steffen
  University of Dortmund, Germany
Madhu Sudan
  Massachusetts Institute of Technology, MA, USA
Demetri Terzopoulos
  University of California, Los Angeles, CA, USA
Doug Tygar
  University of California, Berkeley, CA, USA
Gerhard Weikum
  Max-Planck Institute of Computer Science, Saarbruecken, Germany

Dimitris Metaxas   Leon Axel
Gabor Fichtinger   Gábor Székely (Eds.)

Medical Image Computing and Computer-Assisted Intervention – MICCAI 2008

11th International Conference
New York, NY, USA, September 6-10, 2008
Proceedings, Part I

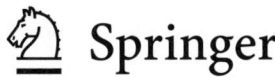 Springer

Volume Editors

Dimitris Metaxas
Rutgers University, Division of Computer and Information Sciences
110 Frelinghuysen Road, Piscataway, NJ 08854-8019, USA
E-mail: dnm@cs.rutgers.edu

Leon Axel
New York University, Department of Radiology
650 First Avenue, New York, NY 10016, USA
E-mail: leon.axel@med.nyu.edu

Gabor Fichtinger
Queen's University, School of Computing
Kingston, Ontario K7L 3N6, Canada
E-mail: gabor@cs.queensu.ca

Gábor Székely
ETH Zürich, Institut für Bildverarbeitung
ETF C 117, Sternwartstr. 7, 8092 Zürich, Switzerland
E-mail: gabor.szekely@vision.ee.ethz.ch

Library of Congress Control Number: 2008934321

CR Subject Classification (1998): I.5, I.4, I.3.5-8, I.2.9-10, J.3, J.6

LNCS Sublibrary: SL 6 – Image Processing, Computer Vision, Pattern Recognition, and Graphics

ISSN   0302-9743
ISBN-10 3-540-85987-X Springer Berlin Heidelberg New York
ISBN-13 978-3-540-85987-1 Springer Berlin Heidelberg New York

This work is subject to copyright. All rights are reserved, whether the whole or part of the material is concerned, specifically the rights of translation, reprinting, re-use of illustrations, recitation, broadcasting, reproduction on microfilms or in any other way, and storage in data banks. Duplication of this publication or parts thereof is permitted only under the provisions of the German Copyright Law of September 9, 1965, in its current version, and permission for use must always be obtained from Springer. Violations are liable to prosecution under the German Copyright Law.

Springer is a part of Springer Science+Business Media

springer.com

© Springer-Verlag Berlin Heidelberg 2008
Printed in Germany

Typesetting: Camera-ready by author, data conversion by Scientific Publishing Services, Chennai, India
Printed on acid-free paper   SPIN: 12521654   06/3180   5 4 3 2 1 0

Preface

The 11th International Conference on Medical Imaging and Computer Assisted Intervention, MICCAI 2008, was held at the Helen and Martin Kimmel Center of New York University, New York City, USA on September 6–10, 2008.

MICCAI is the premier international conference in this domain, with in-depth papers on the multidisciplinary fields of biomedical image computing and analysis, computer assisted intervention and medical robotics. The conference brings together biological scientists, clinicians, computer scientists, engineers, mathematicians, physicists and other interested researchers and offers them a forum to exchange ideas in these exciting and rapidly growing fields.

The conference is both very selective and very attractive: this year we received a record number of 700 submissions from 34 countries and 6 continents, from which 258 papers were selected for publication, which corresponds to a success rate of approximately 36%. Some interesting facts about the distribution of submitted and accepted papers are shown graphically at the end of this preface.

The paper selection process this year was based on the following procedure, which included the introduction of several novelties over previous years.

1. A Program Committee (PC) of 49 members was recruited by the Program Chairs, to get the necessary body of expertise and geographical coverage. All PC members agreed in advance to participate in the final paper selection process.

2. Key words grouped in 7 categories were used to describe the content of the submissions and the expertise of the reviewers.

3. Each submitted paper was assigned to 2 Program Committee members (a primary and a secondary) whose responsibility was to assign each paper to 3 external experts (outside of the Program Committee membership), who provided scores and detailed reports in a double blind procedure.

4. Each primary PC member together with their secondary PC member had to ensure there were no missing reviews. Once they received all three reviews, a novel author *rebuttal* phase was introduced in which the authors could respond to the anonymous reviews, if they did not agree with the reviewer's/reviewers' comments.

5. The Program Committee members provided a set of scores and summary reports for the whole set of papers for which they were responsible (typically 16 papers per PC member). They did this by using the external reviews, the author rebuttal and their own reading of the papers. A summary report by the Primary and Secondary Program Committee members was then written for each paper. Based on the summary report, approximately 36% of the papers were recommended for acceptance.

6. During a two-day meeting at Rutgers University, New Jersey, USA, with all the Program Committee members present, all papers were examined carefully, and special emphasis was placed on borderline papers and oral papers. A

top list of about 120 papers was scrutinized to provide the Program Chairs with a recommended list of 37 podium presentations (approximately 5% of the submitted papers). This recommendation had a reasonable number of oral sessions and spread of content and was adopted by the Program Chairs. The final set of accepted papers has been published in these LNCS proceedings.

7. To increase the time allocated to the 221 excellent accepted poster papers, it was decided in consultation with the MICCAI Society Board to replace the oral poster teasers by continuous video teasers run on large screens during the lunch breaks.

Due to the many submitted papers and the single paper program track, the selection procedure was very selective, and many good papers remained among the 442 rejected. We received 5 factual complaints from the authors of rejected papers. The Program Chairs, in consultation with the relevant Program Committee members who handled the papers and the reviewers, checked carefully that no mistake had been made during the selection procedure. In a few cases, an additional review was requested from an independent Program Committee member. In the end, all the original decisions were maintained and in all cases additional information was provided to the authors to better explain the final decision.

Six MICCAI Young Scientist Awards were presented by the MICCAI Society on the last day of the conference. During the two-day meeting at Rutgers the Program Committee members nominated 18 eligible papers with the highest normalized scores and potential high impact and grouped them into the 6 main categories of the conference. A subgroup of the Program Committee had to vote to elect one paper out of 3 in each category taking into account the paper's presentation at the conference.

The 2008 MedIA-MICCAI Prize was offered by Elsevier to the first author of an outstanding article in the special issue of the Medical Image Analysis Journal dedicated to the previous conference MICCAI 2007. The selection was organized by the guest-editors of this special issue.

Two new awards were also introduced at this year's MICCAI. The first is a new MICCAI Society *"Enduring Impact Award"* sponsored by Philips. This award was given to a paper that was previously published at MICCAI and has proven to have an enduring impact on the field of medical image analysis and computer assisted interventions.

The second was the MICCAI 2008 *"Significant Researcher Award"* sponsored by the organizers of MICCAI 2008 and based on the recommendation of a committee. This award was given to a researcher whose research theme has had a very significant following and impact on one or more of the MICCAI research areas, as well as on other related fields.

We would like to thank the MICCAI Society for providing valuable input and support for the conference and especially Janet Wallace (Robarts Research Institute) for all her efforts and work on making the MICCAI organization a success. We also wish to acknowledge the work of a number of people for their help in putting this conference together. We would like to thank wholeheartedly the

General Chairs, the Program Committee members and the numerous external expert reviewers (who are listed on the next page) for their exceptional work. We would like to thank James Stewart for his support and help related to the MICCAI paper submission and decision making software.

We would also especially like to thank the following people from Rutgers University: Charles McGrew and Rob Toth for providing the necessary software support; Naomi Weinberger, Regina Ribaudo, Maryann Holtsclaw, and Skip Carter for making the final PC meeting possible; the team at the Computational Biomedicine, Biomedicine, Imaging and Modeling Center (CBIM) and especially Zhen Qian for the web support and for liaising with the rest of the organizing committee.

We thank our two invited keynote speakers, Prof. Elliot R. McVeigh, Chairman of the Department of Biomedical Engineering at Johns Hopkins University School of Medicine, and Prof. John Condeelis from the Department of Anatomy and Structural Biology at the Albert Einstein College of Medicine, whose excellent presentations were a highlight of the conference.

We also note our thanks on page XV to our sponsors, without whose financial assistance the event would have been a far lesser one.

It was our pleasure to welcome the MICCAI 2008 attendees to the NYU Kimmel Center in New York City. The world's most dynamic and cosmopolitan city was a popular choice that also attracted an increased number of physicians and a record number of associated workshops and tutorials.

We look forward to welcoming you to MICCAI 2009, to be held 20-24 September in London, UK, and MICCAI 2010, scheduled to be held in Beijing, China.

September 2008

Dimitris Metaxas
Leon Axel
Gabor Fichtinger
Gabor Szekely

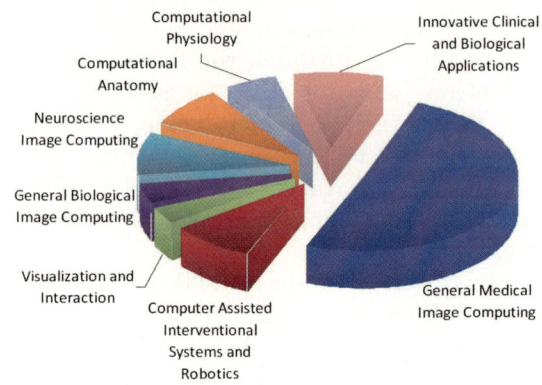
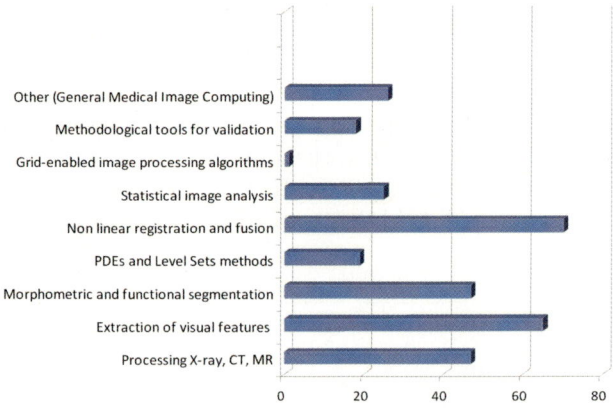
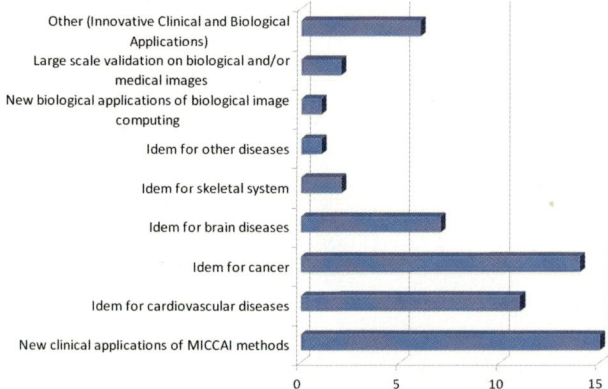

Fig. 1. View at a glance of MICCAI 2008 accepted submissions based on the declared primary keyword. A total of 258 full papers were presented.

MedIA-MICCAI Prizes

MedIA-MICCAI Prizes 2007

Two prizes were awarded by Elsevier during MICCAI 2007 to the first authors of two outstanding articles of the special issue of the Medical Image Analysis journal (volume 11, issue 5, October 2007) dedicated to the previous MICCAI 2006 conference:

- The first prize was awarded to Kilian M. Pohl (USD 700) for the article entitled: Using the Logarithm of Odds to Define a Vector Space on Probabilistic Atlases, co-authored by: Kilian M. Pohl, John Fisher, Sylvain Bouix, Martha Shenton, Robert W. McCarley, W. Eric L. Grimson, Ron Kikinis and William M. Wells. *Medical Image Analysis 11 (2007) 465–477.*
- The second prize was awarded to Masahiko Nakamoto (USD 300) for the article entitled: Recovery of Respiratory Motion and Deformation of the Liver Using Laparoscopic Freehand 3D Ultrasound System, co-authored by: Masahiko Nakamoto, Hiroaki Hirayama, Yoshinobu Sato, Kozo Konishi, Yoshihiro Kakeji, Makoto Hashizume and Shinichi Tamura. *Medical Image Analysis 11 (2007) 429–442.*

MICCAI Young Scientist Awards 2007

MICCAI Young Scientist Awards 2007 selection process:

We selected the 21 highest score papers of which the first author was a graduate student. The papers were categorized into one of 7 prize categories (3 papers/category). A sub-set from the program committee voted on the ranking of the 3 papers. The oral or poster presentations were attended before the final decision was made.

- Prize 1: Computational Anatomy
  - Winner:
    * Effects of Registration Regularization and Atlas Sharpness on Segmentation Accuracy, **Boon Thye Thomas Yeo**, Mert T. Sabuncu, Rahul Desikan, Bruce Fischl, Polina Golland, CSAIL MIT, Boston School of Medicine, Athinoula A. Martinos Center for Biomedical Imaging, USA.
  - Runners-up:
    * Localized Shape Variations for Classifying Wall Motion in Echocardiograms, **KY Esther Leung**, Johan G. Bosch, Erasmus MC, NL.
    * Automated Segmentation of the Liver from 3D CT Images Using Probabilistic Atlas and Multi-level Statistical Shape Models, **Toshiyuki Okada**, Ryuji Shimada, Yoshinobu Sato, Masatoshi Hort, Keita Yokota, Masahiko Nakamoto, Yen-Wei Chen, Hironobu Nakamura, Shinichi Tamura. Division of Image Analysis, Department of Radiology, Osaka University and College of Information Science and Engineering, Ritsumeikan Universty, Japan.
- Prize 2: Computational Physiology
  - Winner:
    * Modelling Intravasation of Liquid Distension Media in Surgical Simulators, **Stephan Tuchschmid**, M. Bajka, D. Szezerba, B. Lloyd, G. Szekely, M. Harders, Computer Vision Laboratory, ETH Zurich and Clinic of Gynecology, University Hospital Zurich, Switzerland.
  - Runners-up:
    * Towards Tracking Breast Cancer Across Medical Images Using Subject-Specific Biomechanical Models, **Vijay Rajagopal**, Angela Lee, Jae-Hoon Chung, Ruth Warren, Ralph P. Highnam, Poul M.F. Nielsen, Martyn P. Nash, Bioengineering Institute, U. Auckland NZ and Dept. of Radiology, Addenbrooke's Hospital, Cambridge, UK and Highnam Associates Ltd., NZ.
    * Real-Time Nonlinear Finite Element Analysis for Surgical Simulation Using Graphics Processing Units, **Zeike A. Taylor**, Mario Cheng, Sebastien Ourselin, BioMedIA Lab, CSIRO ICT Centre, Brisbane, Australia and CMIC UCL, London, UK.

- Prize 3: Innovative Clinical and Biological Applications
  - Winner:
    * Quantification of Blood Flow from Rotational Angiography, **Irina Waechter**, J. Bredno, D.C. Barratt, J. Weese, D.J. Hawkes, University College London, UK and Philips Research Aachen, Germany.
  - Runners-up:
    * Needle Insertion Force Modeling Using Ultrasound Displacement Measurement, **Ehsan Dehghan**, Xu Wen, Reza Zahiri-Azar, Maud Marchal, Septimui E. Salucusean, Dept ECE, U. British Columbia, Canada, TINC-GMCAO Laboratory, Grenoble, France.
    * Functional Near Infrared Spectroscopy in Novice and Expert Surgeons - a Manifold Embedding Approach, **Daniel R Leff**, Felipe Orihuela-Espina, Louis Atallah, Ara Darzi, Guang-Zhong Yang, Imperial College London, UK.
- Prize 4: Visualization and Interaction
  - Winner:
    * Simulation and Fully Automatic Multimodal Registration of Medical Ultrasound, **Wolfgang Wein**, Ali Kharmene, Dirk-Andre Clevert, Oliver Kutter, Nassir Navab, Siemens Corporate Research Princeton USA and CAMP, Technische Universität München, Germany and University Hospital Munich-Grosshadern, Germany.
  - Runners-up:
    * Three-Dimensional Ultrasound Mosaicing, **Christian Wachinger**, Wolfgang Wein, Nassir Navab, CAMP, Technische Universität München, Germany and Siemens Corporate Research, Princetown, USA.
    * pq-space Based Non-photorealistic Rendering for Augmented Reality, **Mirna Lerotic**, Adrian J. Chung, George Mylona, Guang-Zhong Yang, Imperial College London, UK.
- Prize 5: Biological and Neuroscience Image Computing
  - Winner:
    * Cell Population Tracking and Lineage Construction with Spatiotemporal Context, **Kang Li**, Mei Chen, Takeo Kanade, Carnegie Mellon University, Intel Research, Pittsburgh, USA.
  - Runners-up:
    * In-utero Three Dimension High Resolution Fetal Brain Diffusion Tensor Imaging, **Shuzhou Jiang**, H. Xue, S. Counsell, M. Anjari, J. Allsop, M. Rutherford, D. Rueckert, J.V. Hajnal, Imperial College London, UK.
    * Contributions to 3D Diffeomorphic Atlas Estimation: Application to Brain Images, **Matias Bossa**, Monica Hernandez, Salvador Olmos, University of Zaragoza, Spain.
- Prize 6: Computer Assisted Intervention Systems and Robotics
  - Winner:
    * Cardiolock: An Active Cardiac Stabilizer - First In Vivo Experiments Using a New Robotized Device, **Wael Bachta**, Pierre Renaud, Edouard Laroche, Jacques Gangloff, Antonello Forgione, LSIIT Strasbourg and LGeCo INSA Strasbourg and University Hospital of Strasbourg, France.

- Runners-up:
  * Automatic Target and Trajectory Identification for Deep Brain Stimulation (DBS) Procedures, **Ting Guo**, Andrew G. Parrent, Terry M. Peters, Robarts Research Institute, U. Western Ontario, The London Health Sciences Centre, Dept. Neurosurgery, London, Ontario, Canada.
  * Closed-Loop Control in Fused MR-TRUS Image-Guided Prostate Biopsy, **Sheng Xu**, Jochen Kruecker, Peter Guion, Neil Glossop, Ziv Neeman, Peter Choyke, Anurag K. Singh, Bradford J. Wood, Philips Research North America Briarcliff, NIH Bethesda USA and Traxtal Inc. Toronto, Canada.
- Prize 7: Medical Image Computing
  - Winner:
    * Multivariate Normalization with Symmetric Diffeomorphisms for Multivariate Studies, **Brian B. Avants**, J.T. Duda, H. Zhang, J.C. Gee, University of Pennsylvania, USA.
  - Runners-up:
    * A Hierarchical Unsupervised Clustering Scheme for Detection of Prostate Cancer from Magnetic Resonance Spectroscopy (MRS), **Pallavi Tiwari**, Anant Madabhushi, Mark Rosen, Rutgers University and University of Pennsylvania, USA.
    * Non-parametric Diffeomorphic Image Registration with the Demons Algorithm, **Tom Vercauteren**, Xavier Pennec, Aymeric Perchant, Nicholas Ayache, INRIA Sophia-Antipolis and Mauna Kea Technologies, Paris, France.

Previous Years' Winners of MedIA-MICCAI Prize Awards

- In 2006, the prize was offered to T. Vercauteren, first author of the article:

T. Vercauteren, A. Perchant, X. Pennec, G. Malandain and N. Ayache, "Mosaicing of Confocal Microscopic In Vivo Soft Tissue Video Sequences".

- In 2005, the prize was offered to D. Burschka and M. Jackowski who are the first authors of the articles:

D. Burschka, M. Li, M. Ishii, R.H. Taylor, G.D. Hager, "Scale Invariant Registration of Monucular Endoscopic Images to CT-Scans for Sinus Surgery".

M. Jackowski, C.Y. Kao, M. Qiu, R.T. Constable, L.H. Staib, "White Matter Tractography by Anisotropic Wavefront Evolution and Diffusion Tensor Imaging".

Organization

Executive Committee

General Chair   Dimitris Metaxas (Rutgers University, USA)
General Co-chair   Leon Axel (NYUMC, USA)
General Co-chair   Brian Davies (Imperial College, UK)
Program Chair   Dimitris Metaxas (Rutgers University, USA)
Program Chair   Leon Axel (NYUMC, USA)
Program Chair   Gabor Fichtinger (Queens, Canada)
Program Chair   Gabor Szekely (ETH, Switzerland)

Program Committee

Amir A. Amini (University of Louisville, USA)
Elsa Angelini (ENST, France)
Christian Barrillot (IRISA, France)
Margit Betke (Boston University, USA)
Wolfgang Birkfellner (University of Vienna, Austria)
Ela Claridge (University of Birmingham, UK)
Stephane Cotin (INRIA, France)
James Duncan (Yale, USA)
Randy Ellis (Queen's University, Canada)
Jim Gee (University of Pennsylvania, USA)
Guido Gerig (University of North Carolina, USA)
Polina Golland (MIT, USA)
Matthias Harders (ETH, Switzerland)
Nobuhiko Hata (Harvard / BWH, USA)
David Hawkes (University College London, UK)
Tianzi Jiang (The Chinese Academy of Sciences, China)
Ioannis Kakadiaris (University of Houston, USA)
Peter Kazanzides (Johns Hopkins, USA)
Erwin Keeve (CAESAR, Germany)
Joachim Kettenbach (University of Vienna, Austria)
Chandra Khambhamettu (University of Delaware, USA)
Ali Khamene (Siemens Corporate Research, USA)
Vartan Kurtcuoglu (ETH, Switzerland)
Andrew Laine (Columbia University, USA)
Alan Liu (National Capital Area Medical Simulation Center, USA)
Yanxi Liu (Pennsylvania State University, USA)
Gregoire Malandain (INRIA, France)
Edoardo Mazza (ETH, Switzerland)

Michael Miga (Vanderbilt University, USA)
Kensaku Mori (Nagoya University, Japan)
Nassir Navab (Univeristy of Munich, Germany)
Poul Nielsen (University of Auckland, New Zealand)
Sebastien Ourselin (University College London, UK)
Nikos Paragios (Ecole Centrale Paris, France)
Terry Peters (Robarts Research Inst., Canada)
Jens Rittscher (GE Global Research, USA)
Rich Robb (Mayo Clinic, USA)
Ichiro Sakuma (University of Tokyo, Japan)
Tim Salcudean (University of British Columbia, Canada)
Yoshinobu Sato (University of Osaka, Japan)
Dinggang Shen (University of Pennsylvania, USA)
Marc Thiriet (INRIA, France)
Jocelyne Troccaz (TIMC-IMAG, Grenoble, France)
Baba Vemuri (University of Florida, USA)
Simon Warfield (Harvard University, USA)
Sandy Wells (Harvard / BWH, USA)
Carl-Fredrik Westin (Harvard / BWH, USA)
Guang Zhong Yang (Imperial College, UK)
Alistair Young (University of Auckland, New Zealand)

MICCAI Board

Nicholas Ayache, INRIA, Sophia Antipolis, France
Kevin Cleary, Georgetown University, Washington DC, USA
James Duncan, Yale University, New Haven, Connecticut, USA
Gabor Fichtinger, Queen's University, Kingston, Ontario, Canada
Guido Gerig, University of Utah, Salt Lake City, Utah, USA
Anthony Maeder, University of Western Sydney, Australia
Dimitris Metaxas, Rutgers University, Piscataway Campus, New Jersey, USA
Nassir Navab, Technische Universität, München, Germany
Alison Noble, University of Oxford, Oxford, UK
Sebastien Ourselin, University College London, UK
Terry Peters, Robarts Research Institute, London, Ontario, Canada
Richard Robb, Mayo Clinic College of Medicine, Rochester, Minnesota, USA
Ichiro Sakuma, University of Tokyo, Japan
Guang-Zhong Yang, Imperial College, London, UK

MICCAI Society

Executive Officers

President   James Duncan
Executive Director   Richard Robb

Executive Secretary   Nicholas Ayache
Treasurer   Terry Peters
Elections Officer (Honorary Board member) Karl Heinz Hoehne
Awards Coordinator   Alison Noble

Society Staff

Membership Coordinator   Gabor Szekely
Publication Coordinator   Nobuhiko Hata
Communications Coordinator   Kirby Vosburgh
Industry Relations Coordinator Tina Kapur
Society Secretariat   Janette Wallace

Local Planning Committee

Sponsors and Exhibitors   Jens Rittscher
                               Kevin Zhou
                               Ioannis Pavlidis
                               Janette Wallace
Tutorials and Workshops   Andrew Laine
                               Elsa Angelini
                               Elisa Konofagou
                               Anant Madabhushi
Conference Manager   Janette Wallace
Conference Coordinator   Johanne Guillemette
                               Jackie Williams
Web/Technical Proceedings Support Zhen Qian

MICCAI 2008 Sponsors

Northern Digital, Inc.
Medtronic, Inc.
Siemens Corporate Research
Philips
GE

Sponsoring Institutions

Rutgers University
New York University
Robarts Research Institute

Reviewers

Abdelmunim, Hossam
Abolmaesumi, Purang
Aboofazeli, Mohammad
Abugharbieh, Rafeef
Acar, Burak
Acosta, Eric
Acosta Tamayo, Oscar
Adam, Clayton
Ahn, Bummo
Aja-Fernndez, Santiago
Akselrod-Ballin, Ayelet
Al-Diri, Bashir
Alexander, Andrew
Alexander, Daniel
Ali, Asem
Aljabar, Paul
Allassonnire, Stphanie
Alterovitz, Ron
Amini, Amir
An, Jungha
Angelini, Elsa
Angelopoulou, Elli
Aouadi, Souha
Archip, Neculai
Arganda-Carreras, Ignacio
Arridge, Simon R.
Atkinson, David
Aubert-Broche, Berengere
August, Jonas
Avants, Brian
Awate, Suyash
Azar, Fred S.
Bach Cuadra, Meritxell
Baillet, Sylvain
Banks, Scott
Barbu, Adrian
Bardinet, Eric
Barillot, Christian
Barmpoutis, Angelos
Barra, Vincent
Bartz, Dirk
Basdogan, Cagatay
Batchelor, Philip
Bathula, Deepti R.
Bazin, Pierre-Louis
Beek, Maarten
Beichel, Reinhard
Bello, Musodiq
Bello, Fernando
Bengtsson, Ewert
Berlinger, Kajetan
Betke, Margrit
Bhattacharya, Mousumi
Bhotika, Rahul
Bhuiyan, Alauddin
Bichlmeier, Christoph
Birkfellner, Wolfgang
Bischof, Horst
Blanc-Fraud, Laure
Blezek, Daniel
Bloch, Isabelle
Blum, Tobias
Blume, Moritz
Boctor, Emad
Boettger, Thomas
Bond, Sarah
Bosch, Johan
Bouix, Sylvain
Bouman, Charles
Bourgeat, Pierrick
Bove, Michael
Boykov, Yuri
Bresson, Xavier
Brown, Matthew
Brun, Caroline
Brunner, Gerd
Buckley, David
Buehler, Katja
Bullitt, Elizabeth
Burschka, Darius
Butson, Christopher
Cahill, Nathan
Camp, Jon
Capel, David
Cardenas, Valerie
Carmichael, Owen
Castano Moraga, Carlos Alberto
Cates, Joshua

Cattin, Philippe C.
Cebral, Juan
Chakravarty, M. Mallar
Chaney, Edward
Chang, Ruey-feng
Charpiat, Guillaume
Chefd'hotel, Christophe
Chen, Jian
Chendeb, Safwan
Chinzei, Kiyoyuki
Christensen, Gary
Chua, Joselito
Chung, Albert C.S.
Ciofolo, Cybele
Ciuciu, Philippe
Claridge, Ela
Clarysse, Patrick
Cleary, Kevin
Clerc, Maureen
Clouchoux, Cdric
Cody Hazlett, Heather
Cohen, Laurent
Collins, D. Louis
Colliot, Olivier
Comaniciu, Dorin
Comas, Olivier
Commowick, Olivier
Cong, Wenxiang
Cook, Philip
Cootes, Tim
Corso, Jason
Cotin, Stephane
Coulon, Olivier
Cowan, Brett
Crum, William
Curtis, Maurice
Dam, Erik
Davatzikos, Christos
David, Olivier
Davis, Brad
Dawant, Benoit
de Bruijne, Marleen
De Buck, Stijn
De Craene, Mathieu
de Luis Garcia, Rodrigo

Debayle, Johan
Deguchi, Daisuke
Dehghan, Ehsan
Delingette, Herv
Demirci, Stefanie
Deng, Xiang
Denney, Tom
Deriche, Rachid
Desbarats, Pascal
Descoteaux, Maxime
Desvignes, Michel
Devarajan, Venkat
Dey, Joyoni
Dhawan, Atam
DiBella, Edward
Dijkstra, Jouke
DiMaio, Simon
Doignon, Christophe
Doorly, Denis
Dorval, Thierry
Douiri, Abdel
Dowsey, Andrew
Duan, Ye
Duan, Qi
Dubois, Patrick
Duchesne, Simon
Duncan, James S
Dupont, Pierre
Durrleman, Stanley
Edmunds, Timothy
Edwards, Philip
Eggers, Georg
Ehtiati, Tina
El-Baz, Ayman
Elgort, Daniel
Elhawary, Haytham
Ellis, Randy
Elter, Matthias
El-Zehiry, Noha
Engel, Karin
Ennis, Daniel
Ertel, Dirk
Essa, Irfan
Ewers, Michael
Fahey, Frederic

Fahmi, Rachid
Fan, Yong
Farag, Aly
Fei, Jin
Fenster, Aaron
Fetita, Catalin
Feuerstein, Marco
Figl, Michael
Fillard, Pierre
Finlay, Patrick
Fischer, Gregory
Fischer, Bernd
Fleig, Oliver
Fletcher, P. Thomas
Florin, Charles
Folkesson, Jenny
Forest, Clement
Formaggia, Luca
Freysinger, Wolfgang
Fripp, Jurgen
Fritscher, Karl
Funka-Lea, Gareth
Gangloff, Jacques
Gao, Gang
Ge, Weina
Gee, Andrew
Gee, James
Geng, Xiujuan
Gerig, Guido
Gibaud, Bernard
Gilland, David
Gillies, Duncan
Gilson, Wesley
Glocker, Ben
Gobbi, David
Goh, Alvina
Goksel, Orcun
Golland, Polina
Gong, Qiyong
Goodlett, Casey
Goris, Michael
Grady, Leo
Grange, Sebastien
Grau, Vicente
Gribbestad, Ingrid

Groher, Martin
Grova, Christophe
Gu, Lixu
Guehring, Jens
Guerrero, Julian
Guetter, Christoph
Guo, Hongyu
Hadjidemetriou, Stathis
Haker, Steven
Hall, Matt
Hamarneh, Ghassan
Hanson, Dennis
Harders, Matthias
Hartley, Richard
Hastenteufel, Mark
Hastreiter, Peter
Hata, Nobuhiko
Hawkes, David
Haynor, David
He, Renjie
He, Huiguang
Hedjazi Moghari, Mehdi
Heibel, Tim Hauke
Heiberg, Einar
Heimann, Tobias
Hellier, Pierre
Hermosillo, Gerardo
Higgins, William
Hipwell, John
Hirsch, Sven
Hirschmller, Heiko
Histace, Aymeric
Hladuvka, Jiri
Ho, Jeff
Hodgson, Antony
Hoffmann, Kenneth
Hofhauser, Andreas
Hofmann, Ulrich
Holmes, Jeff
Holmes, David
Hong, Jaesung
Hong, Wei
Hontani, Hidekata
Hornegger, Joachim
Hotz, Ingrid

Howe, Robert
Hu, Mingxing
Huang, Heng
Huang, Xiaolei
Hughes, Mike
Hummel, Johann
Hunter, Peter
Izard, Camille
Jain, Ameet
Janke, Andrew
Jannin, Pierre
Jaramaz, Branislav
Jerebko, Anna
Jerosch-Herold, Michael
Ji, Songbai
Jian, Bing
Jiang, Yifeng
Jiang, Tianzi
Jin, Ge
John, Nigel
Johnston, Leigh
Jolly, Marie-Pierre
Jomier, Julien
Jones, Arthur
Jordan, Petr
Joshi, Anand
Joshi, Sarang
Kaban, Ata
Kakadiaris, Ioannis
Kambhamettu, Chandra
Kambhametu, Chandra
Karjalainen, Pasi
Karron, D.B.
Karssemeijer, Nico
Kaus, Michael
Kazanzides, Peter
Keeve, Erwin
Keil, Andreas
Kennedy, David
Kerckhoffs, Roy
Kerr, Andrew
Kerrien, Erwan
Khamene, Ali
Khayrul, Md. Khayrul
Khodarahmi, Iman

Kikinis, Ron
Kim, Boklye
Kindlmann, Gordon
King, Andrew
Kitasaka, Takayuki
Klinder, Tobias
Kobashi, Syoji
Konofagou, Elisa
Kontos, Despina
Krissian, Karl
Krueger, Timo
Kukuk, Markus
Kurazume, Ryo
Kurkure, Uday
Kurtcuoglu, Vartan
Kutter, Oliver
Kybic, Jan
Kyung, Ki-Uk
Lai, Shang-Hong
Laine, Andrew
Lambrou, Tryphon
Landman, Bennett
Langs, Georg
Lapeer, Rudy
Larsen, Rasmus
Lasowski, Ruxandra
Leahy, Richard
Lee, Jack
Lee, Jeongjin
Lee, Su-Lin
Lee, Noah
Leemans, Alexander
Lekadir, Karim
Lelieveldt, Boudewijn
Lenglet, Christophe
Lepore, Natasha
Lerotic, Mirna
Lesage, David
Li, Kang
Li, Rui Rachel
Li, Shuo
Li, Ming
Liang, Jianming
Liao, Hongen
Lienard, Jean

Lin, Xiang
Linguraru, Marius George
Linte, Cristian
Liu, Huafeng
Liu, Tianming
Liu, Alan
Liu, Yanxi
Lloyd, Bryn
Loeckx, Dirk
Loew, Murray
Lohmann, Gabriele
Lorenz, Cristian
Lucas, Yves
Ma, Burton
Madabhushi, Anant
Maddah, Mahnaz
Madore, Bruno
Maeder, Anthony
Maes, Frederik
Magee, John
Maier-Hein, Lena
Makram-Ebeid, Sherif
Malandain, Gregoire
Mangin, Jean-Francois
Marchal, Maud
Martel, Anne
Marti, Gaetan
Martin-Fernandez, Marcos
Masamune, Ken
Mattes, Julian
Maurer, Jr., Calvin R.
Mazza, Edoardo
McClelland, Jamie
McDannold, Nathan
McGraw, Tim
McInerney, Tim
Meas-Yedid, Vannary
Megalooikonomou, Vasileios
Meijering, Erik
Melbourne, Andrew
Melonakos, John
Menard, Cynthia
Mendonca, Paulo
Menegaz, Gloria
Merhof, Dorit

Meyer, Francois
Meyer, Chuck
Mignotte, Max
Modat, Marc
Modersitzki, Jan
Mohamed, Ashraf
Mollemans, Wouter
Moradi, Mehdi
Moratal, David
Morel, Guillaume
Mori, Kensaku
Morris, Dan
Mou, Xuanqin
Mousavi, Parvin
Mukherjee, Lopamudra
Murgasova, Maria
Murray, Lawrence
Myronenko, Andriy
Nakajima, Yoshikazu
Nakamoto, Masahiko
Nash, Martyn
Navab, Nassir
Neghadar, Mohammadreza
Nicolau, Stephane
Nielsen, Poul
Niessen, Wiro
Niethammer, Marc
Nikou, Christophoros
Noble, Alison
Noel, Peter
Nolte, Lutz
Novotny, Paul
Nowinski, Wieslaw L.
Oddou, Christian
O'Donnell, Lauren
O'Donnell, Thomas
Ogier, Arnaud
Okada, Kazunori
Okamura, Allison M.
Olabarriaga, Silvia
Olgac, Ufuk
Oliver, Arnau
Olivo-Marin, Jean-Christophe
Olmos, Salvador
Olszewski, Mark

Orkisz, Maciej
Ortmaier, Tobias
Osman, Nael
Otake, Yoshito
Ou, Wanmei
Ourselin, Sebastien
Padfield, Dirk
Padoy, Nicolas
Pai, Vinay
Palaniappan, Kannappan
Pan, Xiao-Bo
Pang, Wai-Man
Papademetris, Xenios
Papadopoulo, Tho
Paragios, Nikos
Park, Hae-Jeong
Park, Hyunjin
Passat, Nicolas
Patel, Rajni
Patriciu, Alexandru
Paulsen, Keith
Paulsen, Rasmus
Payandeh, Shahram
Pedersen, Michael
Pekar, Vladimir
Pennec, Xavier
Penney, Graeme
Periaswamy, Senthil
Pernus, Franjo
Perperidis, Dimitrios
Peter, Adrian
Peters, Terry M.
Petroudi, Styliani
Pezzementi, Zachary
Pham, Dzung
Pichon, Eric
Pieper, Steve
Pitiot, Alain
Pizer, Stephen
Platel, Bram
Pluim, Josien
Pock, Thomas
Podder, Tarun
Pohl, Kilian Maria
Poignet, Philippe

Pott, Peter
Poupon, Cyril
Prasad, Mithun
Prastawa, Marcel
Prima, Sylvain
Prince, Jerry L.
Promayon, Emmanuel
Pruemmer, Marcus
Qazi, Arish Asif
Qian, Zhen
Qian, Xiaoning
Radeva, Petia
Rajagopal, Vijayaraghavan
Rajagopalan, Srinivasan
Rajpoot, Nasir
Rajwade, Ajit
Rangarajan, Anand
Rasche, Volker
Rathi, Yogesh
Reinertsen, Ingerid
Reinhardt, Joseph
Remme, Espen
Restif, Christophe
Rettmann, Maryam
Rexilius, Jan
Rezk Salama, Christof
Ridgway, Gerard
Rietzel, Eike
Rittscher, Jens
Rivaz, Hassan
Rivera, Mariano
Robb, Richard A.
Roche, Alexis
Rodriguez y Baena, Ferdinando
Rodriguez-Florido, Miguel Angel
Rohde, Gustavo
Rohlfing, Torsten
Rohling, Robert
Rohr, Karl
Ross, James
Rougon, Nicolas
Rousseau, Francois
Roy, Arunabha
Rueckert, Daniel
Rueda, Sylvia

Ruiter, Nicole
Sabuncu, Mert
Sabuncu, Mert Rory
Sachse, Frank
Sakuma, Ichiro
Salcudean, Tim
Salvado, Olivier
Samset, Eigil
Santamaria-Pang, Alberto
Sarrut, David
Sato, Yoshinobu
Sbalzarini, Ivo
Scherrer, Benoit
Schmid, Volker
Schnabel, Julia A.
Schultz, Thomas
Schwartz, Jean-Marc
Schwarz, Tobias
Schweikard, Achim
Seger, Michael
Sermesant, Maxime
Shah, Shishir
Shakeri, Mostafa
Shams, Ramtin
Sharma, Aayush
Sharma, Cartik
Sharp, Greg
Shen, Li
Shen, Hong
Shen, Dinggang
Shi, Yonggang
Shimizu, Akinobu
Siddiqi, Kaleem
Sielhorst, Tobias
Siewerdsen, Jeffrey
Sikdar, Siddhartha
Simaan, Nabil
Singh, Vikas
Sinha, Tuhin
Skrinjar, Oskar
Smal, Ihor
Smedby, Orjan
Sofka, Michal
Song, Xubo
Song, Ting

Sorensen, Thomas Sangild
Souchon, Remi
Sparr, Gunnar
Sporring, Jon
Srivastava, Anuj
Staib, Lawrence
Stegmann, Mikkel B.
Stetten, George
Stewart, James
Stoeckel, Jonathan
Stolka, Philipp
Stoll, Jeff
Stough, Joshua
Stoyanov, Danail
Strother, Stephen
Studholme, Colin
Styles, Iain
Styner, Martin
Suarez, Eduardo
Subakan, Ozlem
Subramanian, Navneeth
Suinesiaputra, Avan
Summers, Ronald
Sun, Hui
Sundar, Hari
Szczerba, Dominik
Szewczyk, Jerome
Szilagyi, Laszlo
Tagare, Hemant
Talbot, Hugues
Tan, Shan
Tanner, Christine
Tanter, Mickael
Taron, Maxime
Tasdizen, Tolga
Tawhai, Merryn
Taylor, Zeike
Tedgui, Alain
Tek, Huseyin
Tendick, Frank
ter Haar Romeny, Bart M.
Teschner, Matthias
Tetzlaff, Ralf
Teverovskiy, Leonid
Thalmann, Daniel

Thiran, Jean-Philippe
Thiriet, Marc
Thirion, Bertrand
Thomas, Mani
Thomaz, Carlos
Tian, Tai-Peng
Tieu, Kinh
Tita, Ralf
Todd Pokropek, Andrew
Toews, Matthew
Tokuda, Junichi
Torabi, Meysam
Toro, Javier
Tosun, Duygu
Traub, Joerg
Troccaz, Jocelyne
Tsechpenakis, Gavriil
Tu, Zhuowen
Tustison, Nicholas
Twellmann, Thorsten
Tzafestas, Costas
Unal, Gozde
Urschler, Martin
Vaillant, Regis
van der Kouwe, Andre
van Ginneken, Bram
Van Leemput, Koen
van Walsum, Theo
Vannier, Michael
Vemuri, Baba
Ventikos, Yiannis
Vercauteren, Tom
Verma, Ragini
Vicini, Paolo
Vidal, Rene
Vilanova, Anna
Villard, Caroline
von Berg, Jens
Vosburgh, Kirby
Vrtovec, Tomaz
Wachinger, Christian
Wai, Lionel C.C.
Wang, Hui
Wang, Linwei
Wang, Zhizhou

Wang, Song
Wang, Defeng
Wang, Fei
Wang, Yongmei Michelle
Warfield, Simon
Washio, Toshikatsu
Wassermann, Demian
Weese, Jrgen
Wein, Wolfgang
Weiskopf, Daniel
Wells, William
West, Jay
Westin, Carl-Fredrik
Whitaker, Ross
Whitcher, Brandon
White, Mark
Wiemker, Rafael
Wiles, Andrew
Wolf, Ivo
Worz, Stefan
Wright, Graham
Wu, Guorong
Wu, Xiaodong
Wu, Zheng
Wuensche, Burkhard
Wyatt, Chris
Xia, Junyi
Xing, Ye
Xu, Dongrong
Xu, Sheng
Xue, Hui
Xue, Zhong
Yan, Kaiguo
Yan, Pingkun
Yang, Fuxing
Yang, Guang Zhong
Yaniv, Ziv
Yao, Jianhua
Yendiki, Anastasia
Yeo, Boon Thye
Yoo, Seung-Schik
Yoo, Terry
Yoshida, Hiro
Young, Alistair
Yuan, Quan

Yue, Ning
Yushkevich, Paul
Zacharaki, Evangelia
Zachow, Stefan
Zhan, Yiqiang
Zhan, Wang
Zhang, Qi
Zhang, Hui
Zhang, Heye
Zhang, Xiangwei
Zhang, Yong
Zhao, Fei
Zheng, Yuanjie
Zheng, Guoyan
Zheng, Yefeng
Zhong, Hualiang
Zhou, Jinghao
Zhou, S. Kevin
Zhu, Hongtu
Zhu, Yun
Zikic, Darko
Ziyan, Ulas
Zollei, Lilla
Zwiggelaar, Reyer

Table of Contents – Part I

Medical Image Computing

On Computing the Underlying Fiber Directions from the Diffusion Orientation Distribution Function ... 1
  Luke Bloy and Ragini Verma

Extracting Tractosemas from a Displacement Probability Field for Tractography in DW-MRI ... 9
  Angelos Barmpoutis, Baba C. Vemuri, Dena Howland, and John R. Forder

New Algorithms to Map Asymmetries of 3D Surfaces ... 17
  Benoît Combès and Sylvain Prima

A Distributed Spatio-temporal EEG/MEG Inverse Solver ... 26
  Wanmei Ou, Polina Golland, and Matti Hämäläinen

Tracking the Swimming Motions of *C. elegans* Worms with Applications in Aging Studies ... 35
  Christophe Restif and Dimitris Metaxas

Segmentation I

MR Brain Tissue Classification Using an Edge-Preserving Spatially Variant Bayesian Mixture Model ... 43
  Giorgos Sfikas, Christophoros Nikou, Nikolaos Galatsanos, and Christian Heinrich

Semi-Supervised Nasopharyngeal Carcinoma Lesion Extraction from Magnetic Resonance Images Using Online Spectral Clustering with a Learned Metric ... 51
  Wei Huang, Kap Luk Chan, Yan Gao, Jiayin Zhou, and Vincent Chong

Multi-level Classification of Emphysema in HRCT Lung Images Using Delegated Classifiers ... 59
  Mithun Prasad and Arcot Sowmya

A Discriminative Model-Constrained Graph Cuts Approach to Fully Automated Pediatric Brain Tumor Segmentation in 3-D MRI ... 67
  Michael Wels, Gustavo Carneiro, Alexander Aplas, Martin Huber, Joachim Hornegger, and Dorin Comaniciu

Prostate Cancer Probability Maps Based on Ultrasound RF Time
Series and SVM Classifiers 76
 *Mehdi Moradi, Parvin Mousavi, Robert Siemens, Eric Sauerbrei,
 Alexander Boag, and Purang Abolmaesumi*

A Bayesian Approach for Liver Analysis: Algorithm and Validation
Study 85
 *Moti Freiman, Ofer Eliassaf, Yoav Taieb, Leo Joskowicz, and
 Jacob Sosna*

Classification of Suspected Liver Metastases Using fMRI Images: A
Machine Learning Approach 93
 *Moti Freiman, Yifat Edrei, Yehonatan Sela, Yitzchak Shmidmayer,
 Eitan Gross, Leo Joskowicz, and Rinat Abramovitch*

Evaluation of a Cardiac Ultrasound Segmentation Algorithm Using a
Phantom 101
 *Yong Yue, Hemant D. Tagare, Ernest L. Madsen,
 Gary R. Frank, and Maritza A. Hobson*

Automatic Recovery of the Left Ventricular Blood Pool in Cardiac
Cine MR Images 110
 Marie-Pierre Jolly

MRI Bone Segmentation Using Deformable Models and Shape Priors ... 119
 Jérôme Schmid and Nadia Magnenat-Thalmann

Segmentation of Vessels Cluttered with Cells Using a Physics Based
Model 127
 *Stephen J. Schmugge, Steve Keller, Nhat Nguyen, Richard Souvenir,
 Toan Huynh, Mark Clemens, and Min C. Shin*

Streamline Flows for White Matter Fibre Pathway Segmentation in
Diffusion MRI 135
 *Peter Savadjiev, Jennifer S.W. Campbell, G. Bruce Pike, and
 Kaleem Siddiqi*

Toward Unsupervised Classification of Calcified Arterial Lesions 144
 *Gerd Brunner, Uday Kurkure, Deepak R. Chittajallu,
 Raja P. Yalamanchili, and Ioannis A. Kakadiaris*

Weights and Topology: A Study of the Effects of Graph Construction
on 3D Image Segmentation 153
 Leo Grady and Marie-Pierre Jolly

Level Set Based Surface Capturing in 3D Medical Images 162
 Bin Dong, Aichi Chien, Yu Mao, Jian Ye, and Stanley Osher

Automatic Detection of Calcified Coronary Plaques in Computed
Tomography Data Sets 170
  Stefan C. Saur, Hatem Alkadhi, Lotus Desbiolles,
  Gábor Székely, and Philippe C. Cattin

Comprehensive Segmentation of Cine Cardiac MR Images 178
  Maxim Fradkin, Cybèle Ciofolo, Benoit Mory, Gilion Hautvast, and
  Marcel Breeuwer

Segmentation of Pathologic Hearts in Long-Axis Late-Enhancement
MRI 186
  Cybèle Ciofolo and Maxim Fradkin

Automatic Subcortical Segmentation Using a Contextual Model 194
  Jonathan H. Morra, Zhuowen Tu, Liana G. Apostolova,
  Amity E. Green, Arthur W. Toga, and Paul M. Thompson

Lumbar Disc Localization and Labeling with a Probabilistic Model on
Both Pixel and Object Features.................................... 202
  Jason J. Corso, Raja' S. Alomari, and Vipin Chaudhary

Topology Preserving Warping of Binary Images: Application to
Atlas-Based Skull Segmentation.................................... 211
  Sylvain Faisan, Nicolas Passat, Vincent Noblet,
  Renée Chabrier, and Christophe Meyer

Robust Segmentation and Anatomical Labeling of the Airway Tree
from Thoracic CT Scans 219
  Bram van Ginneken, Wouter Baggerman, and Eva M. van Rikxoort

Spine Segmentation Using Articulated Shape Models 227
  Tobias Klinder, Robin Wolz, Cristian Lorenz, Astrid Franz, and
  Jörn Ostermann

Model-Based Segmentation of Hippocampal Subfields in Ultra-High
Resolution In Vivo MRI 235
  Koen Van Leemput, Akram Bakkour, Thomas Benner,
  Graham Wiggins, Lawrence L. Wald, Jean Augustinack,
  Bradford C. Dickerson, Polina Golland, and Bruce Fischl

Kinetic Modeling Based Probabilistic Segmentation for Molecular
Images 244
  Ahmed Saad, Ghassan Hamarneh, Torsten Möller, and Ben Smith

Automatic Delineation of Sulci and Improved Partial Volume
Classification for Accurate 3D Voxel-Based Cortical Thickness
Estimation from MR 253
  Oscar Acosta, Pierrick Bourgeat, Jurgen Fripp, Erik Bonner,
  Sébastien Ourselin, and Olivier Salvado

R-PLUS: A Riemannian Anisotropic Edge Detection Scheme for
Vascular Segmentation.. 262
  Ali Gooya, Takeyoshi Dohi, Ichiro Sakuma, and Hongen Liao

A Novel Method for Cortical Sulcal Fundi Extraction................... 270
  *Gang Li, Tianming Liu, Jingxin Nie, Lei Guo, and
  Stephen T.C. Wong*

Joint Segmentation of Thalamic Nuclei from a Population of Diffusion
Tensor MR Images.. 279
  Ulas Ziyan and Carl-Fredrik Westin

Bone Segmentation and Fracture Detection in Ultrasound Using 3D
Local Phase Features.. 287
  *Ilker Hacihaliloglu, Rafeef Abugharbieh, Antony Hodgson, and
  Robert Rohling*

Interactive Separation of Segmented Bones in CT Volumes Using
Graph Cut... 296
  *Lu Liu, David Raber, David Nopachai, Paul Commean,
  David Sinacore, Fred Prior, Robert Pless, and Tao Ju*

A Comparison of Methods for Recovering Intra-voxel White Matter
Fiber Architecture from Clinical Diffusion Imaging Scans.............. 305
  Alonso Ramirez-Manzanares, Philip A. Cook, and James C. Gee

Active Scheduling of Organ Detection and Segmentation in Whole-Body
Medical Images.. 313
  Yiqiang Zhan, Xiang Sean Zhou, Zhigang Peng, and Arun Krishnan

A New Stochastic Framework for Accurate Lung Segmentation............ 322
  *Ayman El-Ba, Georgy Gimel'farb, Robert Falk, Trevor Holland, and
  Teresa Shaffer*

Active Volume Models with Probabilistic Object Boundary Prediction
Module.. 331
  *Tian Shen, Yaoyao Zhu, Xiaolei Huang, Junzhou Huang,
  Dimitris Metaxas, and Leon Axel*

Improving Parenchyma Segmentation by Simultaneous Estimation of
Tissue Property T_1 Map and Group-Wise Registration of Inversion
Recovery MR Breast Images... 342
  *Ye Xing, Zhong Xue, Sarah Englander, Mitchell Schnall, and
  Dinggang Shen*

Atlas-Based Segmentation of the Germinal Matrix from in Utero
Clinical MRI of the Fetal Brain....................................... 351
  *Piotr A. Habas, Kio Kim, Francois Rousseau, Orit A. Glenn,
  A. James Barkovich, and Colin Studholme*

Segmenting Brain Tumors Using Pseudo–Conditional Random Fields ... 359
  *Chi-Hoon Lee, Shaojun Wang, Albert Murtha,
  Matthew R.G. Brown, and Russell Greiner*

Localized Priors for the Precise Segmentation of Individual Vertebras
from CT Volume Data.. 367
  Hong Shen, Andrew Litvin, and Christopher Alvino

Cell Spreading Analysis with Directed Edge Profile-Guided Level Set
Active Contours 376
  *Ilker Ersoy, Filiz Bunyak, Kannappan Palaniappan,
  Mingzhai Sun, and Gabor Forgacs*

Brain MR Image Segmentation Using Local and Global Intensity
Fitting Active Contours/Surfaces 384
  *Li Wang, Chunming Li, Quansen Sun, Deshen Xia, and
  Chiu-Yen Kao*

Model-Based Segmentation Using Graph Representations 393
  *Dieter Seghers, Jeroen Hermans, Dirk Loeckx, Frederik Maes,
  Dirk Vandermeulen, and Paul Suetens*

3D Brain Segmentation Using Active Appearance Models and Local
Regressors 401
  *Kolawole O. Babalola, Tim F. Cootes, Carole J. Twinning,
  Vlad Petrovic, and Chris Taylor*

Comparison and Evaluation of Segmentation Techniques for Subcortical
Structures in Brain MRI 409
  *Kolawole O. Babalola, Brian Patenaude, Paul Aljabar,
  Julia Schnabel, David Kennedy, William Crum, Stephen Smith,
  Tim F. Cootes, Mark Jenkinson, and Daniel Rueckert*

Shape and Statistics Analysis

Hierarchical Shape Statistical Model for Segmentation of Lung Fields
in Chest Radiographs... 417
  Yonghong Shi and Dinggang Shen

Sample Sufficiency and Number of Modes to Retain in Statistical Shape
Modelling 425
  *Lin Mei, Michael Figl, Daniel Rueckert, Ara Darzi, and
  Philip Edwards*

Optimal Feature Point Selection and Automatic Initialization in Active
Shape Model Search 434
  Karim Lekadir and Guang-Zhong Yang

MR-Less High Dimensional Spatial Normalization of ^{11}C PiB PET
Images on a Population of Elderly, Mild Cognitive Impaired and
Alzheimer Disease Patients 442
  *Jurgen Fripp, Pierrick Bourgeat, Parnesh Raniga, Oscar Acosta,
  Victor Villemagne, Gareth Jones, Graeme O'keefe,
  Christopher Rowe, Sébastien Ourselin, and Olivier Salvado*

Computational Atlases of Severity of White Matter Lesions in Elderly
Subjects with MRI 450
  *Stathis Hadjidemetriou, Peter Lorenzen, Norbert Schuff,
  Susanne Mueller, and Michael Weiner*

Simulation of Ground-Truth Validation Data Via Physically- and
Statistically-Based Warps 459
  Ghassan Hamarneh, Preet Jassi, and Lisa Tang

Shape Analysis with Overcomplete Spherical Wavelets 468
  *B.T. Thomas Yeo, Peng Yu, P. Ellen Grant, Bruce Fischl, and
  Polina Golland*

Particle-Based Shape Analysis of Multi-object Complexes 477
  *Joshua Cates, P. Thomas Fletcher, Martin Styner,
  Heather Cody Hazlett, and Ross Whitaker*

Multivariate Statistical Analysis of Whole Brain Structural Networks
Obtained Using Probabilistic Tractography 486
  *Emma C. Robinson, Michel Valstar, Alexander Hammers,
  Anders Ericsson, A. David Edwards, and Daniel Rueckert*

Optimized Conformal Parameterization of Cortical Surfaces Using
Shape Based Matching of Landmark Curves 494
  *Lok Ming Lui, Sheshadri Thiruvenkadam, Yalin Wang,
  Tony Chan, and Paul Thompson*

Construction of Hierarchical Multi-Organ Statistical Atlases and Their
Application to Multi-Organ Segmentation from CT Images 502
  *Toshiyuki Okada, Keita Yokota, Masatoshi Hori,
  Masahiko Nakamoto, Hironobu Nakamura, and Yoshinobu Sato*

Shape-Based Alignment of Hippocampal Subfields: Evaluation in
Postmortem MRI 510
  *Paul A. Yushkevich, Brian B. Avants, John Pluta, David Minkoff,
  John A. Detre, Murray Grossman, and James C. Gee*

Customized Design of Hearing Aids Using Statistical Shape Learning ... 518
  Gozde Unal, Delphine Nain, Greg Slabaugh, and Tong Fang

A Novel Explicit 2D+t Cyclic Shape Model Applied to
Echocardiography 527
  Ramón Casero and J. Alison Noble

Spatial Consistency in 3D Tract-Based Clustering Statistics 535
Matthan Caan, Lucas van Vliet, Charles Majoie, Eline Aukema, Kees Grimbergen, and Frans Vos

Dynamic Probabilistic Atlas of Functional Brain Regions for
Transcranial Magnetic Stimulation 543
Juha Koikkalainen, Mervi Könönen, Jari Karhu, Jarmo Ruohonen, Eini Niskanen, and Jyrki Lötjönen

Unbiased Stratification of Left Ventricles 551
Rajagopalan Srinivasan, K.S. Shriram, and Srikanth Suryanarayanan

3D Cerebral Cortical Morphometry in Autism: Increased Folding in
Children and Adolescents in Frontal, Parietal, and Temporal Lobes 559
Suyash P. Awate, Lawrence Win, Paul Yushkevich, Robert T. Schultz, and James C. Gee

Prediction of Biomechanical Parameters of the Proximal Femur Using
Statistical Appearance Models and Support Vector Regression 568
Karl Fritscher, Benedikt Schuler, Thomas Link, Felix Eckstein, Norbert Suhm, Markus Hänni, Clemens Hengg, and Rainer Schubert

Automatic Labeling of Anatomical Structures in MR FastView Images
Using a Statistical Atlas 576
Matthias Fenchel, Stefan Thesen, and Andreas Schilling

Conformal Slit Mapping and Its Applications to Brain Surface
Parameterization. 585
Yalin Wang, Xianfeng Gu, Tony F. Chan, Paul M. Thompson, and Shing-Tung Yau

Automatic Determination of Arterial Input Function for Dynamic
Contrast Enhanced MRI in Tumor Assessment 594
Jeremy Chen, Jianhua Yao, and David Thomasson

Robust Vessel Tree Modeling 602
M. Akif Gülsün and Hüseyin Tek

Exploratory Identification of Image-Based Biomarkers for Solid Mass
Pulmonary Tumors. 612
Ifeoma Nwogu and Jason J. Corso

Measuring Brain Lesion Progression with a Supervised Tissue
Classification System 620
Evangelia I. Zacharaki, Stathis Kanterakis, R. Nick Bryan, and Christos Davatzikos

Regularized Discriminative Direction for Shape Difference Analysis 628
  Luping Zhou, Richard Hartley, Lei Wang, Paulette Lieby, and Nick Barnes

LV Motion and Strain Computation from tMRI Based on Meshless Deformable Models 636
  Xiaoxu Wang, Ting Chen, Shaoting Zhang, Dimitris Metaxas, and Leon Axel

Surface-Based Texture and Morphological Analysis Detects Subtle Cortical Dysplasia 645
  Pierre Besson, Neda Bernasconi, Olivier Colliot, Alan Evans, and Andrea Bernasconi

Multi-Attribute Non-initializing Texture Reconstruction Based Active Shape Model (MANTRA)... 653
  Robert Toth, Jonathan Chappelow, Mark Rosen, Sona Pungavkar, Arjun Kalyanpur, and Anant Madabhushi

A Comprehensive Segmentation, Registration, and Cancer Detection Scheme on 3 Tesla *In Vivo* Prostate DCE-MRI 662
  Satish Viswanath, B. Nicolas Bloch, Elisabeth Genega, Neil Rofsky, Robert Lenkinski, Jonathan Chappelow, Robert Toth, and Anant Madabhushi

Modeling I

A New Method for Creating Electrophysiological Maps for DBS Surgery and Their Application to Surgical Guidance 670
  Srivatsan Pallavaram, Pierre-Francois D'Haese, Chris Kao, Hong Yu, Michael Remple, Joseph Neimat, Peter Konrad, and Benoit Dawant

Cardiac Electrophysiology Model Adjustment Using the Fusion of MR and Optical Imaging 678
  Damien Lepiller, Maxime Sermesant, Mihaela Pop, Hervé Delingette, Graham A. Wright, and Nicholas Ayache

Dynamic Model-Driven Quantitative and Visual Evaluation of the Aortic Valve from 4D CT 686
  Razvan Ioan Ionasec, Bogdan Georgescu, Eva Gassner, Sebastian Vogt, Oliver Kutter, Michael Scheuering, Nassir Navab, and Dorin Comaniciu

Interactive Simulation of Embolization Coils: Modeling and Experimental Validation 695
  Jérémie Dequidt, Maud Marchal, Christian Duriez, Erwan Kerien, and Stéphane Cotin

Modelling Anisotropic Viscoelasticity for Real-Time Soft Tissue
Simulation 703
  Zeike A. Taylor, Olivier Comas, Mario Cheng, Josh Passenger,
  David J. Hawkes, David Atkinson, and Sébastien Ourselin

Motion Tracking and Compensation

3D Ultrasound-Guided Motion Compensation System for Beating
Heart Mitral Valve Repair 711
  Shelten G. Yuen, Samuel B. Kesner, Nikolay V. Vasilyev,
  Pedro J. Del Nido, and Robert D. Howe

A Novel Algorithm for Heart Motion Analysis Based on Geometric
Constraints 720
  Mingxing Hu, Graeme Penney, Daniel Rueckert, Philip Edwards,
  Michael Figl, Philip Pratt, and David Hawkes

On-the-Fly Motion-Compensated Cone-Beam CT Using an a Priori
Motion Model 729
  Simon Rit, Jochem Wolthaus, Marcel van Herk, and Jan-Jakob Sonke

A Statistical Motion Model Based on Biomechanical Simulations for
Data Fusion during Image-Guided Prostate Interventions 737
  Yipeng Hu, Dominic Morgan, Hashim Uddin Ahmed, Doug Pendsé,
  Mahua Sahu, Clare Allen, Mark Emberton, David Hawkes, and
  Dean Barratt

Registration I

Spherical Demons: Fast Surface Registration 745
  B.T. Thomas Yeo, Mert Sabuncu, Tom Vercauteren,
  Nicholas Ayache, Bruce Fischl, and Polina Golland

Symmetric Log-Domain Diffeomorphic Registration: A Demons-based
Approach 754
  Tom Vercauteren, Xavier Pennec, Aymeric Perchant, and
  Nicholas Ayache

EEG to MRI Registration Based on Global and Local Similarities of
MRI Intensity Distributions 762
  Žiga Špiclin, Arne Hans, Frank H. Duffy, Simon K. Warfield,
  Boštjan Likar, and Franjo Pernuš

Nonrigid Registration of Dynamic Renal MR Images Using a Saliency
Based MRF Model 771
  Dwarikanath Mahapatra and Ying Sun

A Constrained Non-rigid Registration Algorithm for Use in Prostate
Image-Guided Radiotherapy 780
    William H. Greene, Sudhakar Chelikani, Kailas Purushothaman,
    Zhe Chen, Jonathan P.S. Knisely, Lawrence H. Staib,
    Xenophon Papademetris, and Jim Duncan

Miscellaneous I

Identifying Regional Cardiac Abnormalities from Myocardial Strains
Using Spatio-temporal Tensor Analysis 789
    Zhen Qian, Qingshan Liu, Dimitris N. Metaxas, and Leon Axel

Volume Reconstruction by Inverse Interpolation: Application to
Interleaved MR Motion Correction 798
    Torsten Rohlfing, Martin H. Rademacher, and Adolf Pfefferbaum

A Hybrid System for the Semantic Annotation of Sulco-Gyral Anatomy
in MRI Images 807
    Ammar Mechouche, Xavier Morandi, Christine Golbreich, and
    Bernard Gibaud

Towards Multi-Directional OCT for Speckle Noise Reduction 815
    Lukas Ramrath, Guillermo Moreno, Heike Mueller, Tim Bonin,
    Gereon Huettmann, and Achim Schweikard

Automatic Tracking of Escherichia Coli Bacteria 824
    Jun Xie, Shahid Khan, and Mubarak Shah

Automatic Image Analysis of Histopathology Specimens Using Concave
Vertex Graph 833
    Lin Yang, Oncel Tuzel, Peter Meer, and David J. Foran

Analysis of Surfaces Using Constrained Regression Models 842
    Sune Darkner, Mert R. Sabuncu, Polina Golland,
    Rasmus R. Paulsen, and Rasmus Larsen

A Global Approach for Automatic Fibroscopic Video Mosaicing in
Minimally Invasive Diagnosis 850
    Selen Atasoy, David P. Noonan, Selim Benhimane,
    Nassir Navab, and Guang-Zhong Yang

Riemannian Framework for Estimating Symmetric Positive Definite
4th Order Diffusion Tensors 858
    Aurobrata Ghosh, Maxime Descoteaux, and Rachid Deriche

Non-uniform Gradient Prescription for Precise Angular Measurements
Using DTI 866
    Nathan Yanasak, Jerry D. Allison, Qun Zhao, Tom C.-C. Hu, and
    Krishnan Dhandapani

Spatial Weighed Element Based FEM Incorporating a Priori
Information on Bioluminescence Tomography 874
　Jin Shi, Jie Tian, Min Xu, and Wei Yang

Geometric Deformable Model Driven by CoCRFs: Application to
Optical Coherence Tomography 883
　*Gabriel Tsechpenakis, Brandon Lujan, Oscar Martinez,
　Giovanni Gregori, and Philip J. Rosenfeld*

Contractile Analysis with Kriging Based on MR Myocardial Velocity
Imaging 892
　Su-Lin Lee, Andrew Huntbatch, and Guang-Zhong Yang

Averaging Centerlines: Mean Shift on Paths 900
　*Theo van Walsum, Michiel Schaap, Coert T. Metz,
　Alina G. van der Giessen, and Wiro J. Niessen*

On Classifying Disease-Induced Patterns in the Brain Using Diffusion
Tensor Images 908
　Peng Wang and Ragini Verma

Findings in Schizophrenia by Tract-Oriented DT-MRI Analysis 917
　*Mahnaz Maddah, Marek Kubicki, William M. Wells,
　Carl-Fredrik Westin, Martha E. Shenton, and W. Eric L. Grimson*

Task-Specific Functional Brain Geometry from Model Maps 925
　*Georg Langs, Dimitris Samaras, Nikos Paragios, Jean Honorio,
　Nelly Alia-Klein, Dardo Tomasi, Nora D. Volkow, and
　Rita Z. Goldstein*

Texture Classification in Lung CT Using Local Binary Patterns 934
　Lauge Sørensen, Saher B. Shaker, and Marleen de Bruijne

A Symmetry-Based Method for the Determination of Vertebral
Rotation in 3D 942
　Tomaž Vrtovec, Franjo Pernuš, and Boštjan Likar

Spatio-temporal Speckle Reduction in Ultrasound Sequences........... 951
　Noura Azzabou and Nikos Paragios

Surface-Based Structural Group Analysis of fMRI Data 959
　*Grégory Operto, Cédric Clouchoux, Rémy Bulot,
　Jean-Luc Anton, and Olivier Coulon*

Dynamic Cardiac Mapping on Patient-Specific Cardiac Models 967
　*Kevin Wilson, Gerard Guiraudon, Doug Jones, Cristian A. Linte,
　Chris Wedlake, John Moore, and Terry M. Peters*

Detection of DTI White Matter Abnormalities in Multiple Sclerosis
Patients 975
    Olivier Commowick, Pierre Fillard, Olivier Clatz, and
    Simon K. Warfield

Automatic Mitral Valve Inflow Measurements from Doppler
Echocardiography 983
    JinHyeong Park, S. Kevin Zhou, John Jackson, and
    Dorin Comaniciu

Motion Robust Magnetic Susceptibility and Field Inhomogeneity
Estimation Using Regularized Image Restoration Techniques for
fMRI 991
    Desmond Teck Beng Yeo, Jeffrey A. Fessler, and Boklye Kim

Cortical Surface Thickness as a Classifier: Boosting for Autism
Classification 999
    Vikas Singh, Lopamudra Mukherjee, and Moo K. Chung

Surface-Based Vector Analysis Using Heat Equation Interpolation:
A New Approach to Quantify Local Hippocampal Volume Changes 1008
    Hosung Kim, Pierre Besson, Olivier Colliot,
    Andrea Bernasconi, and Neda Bernasconi

Discovering Structure in the Space of Activation Profiles in fMRI 1016
    Danial Lashkari, Ed Vul, Nancy Kanwisher, and Polina Golland

Left Ventricle Tracking Using Overlap Priors 1025
    Ismail Ben Ayed, Yingli Lu, Shuo Li, and Ian Ross

Mean q-Ball Strings Obtained by Constrained Procrustes Analysis with
Point Sliding 1034
    Irina Kezele, Cyril Poupon, Muriel Perrin, Yann Cointepas,
    Vincent El Kouby, Fabrice Poupon, and Jean-François Mangin

Noninvasive Functional Imaging of Volumetric Cardiac Electrical
Activity: A Human Study on Myocardial Infarction 1042
    Linwei Wang, Ken C.L. Wong, Heye Zhang, and Pengcheng Shi

A Slicing-Based Coherence Measure for Clusters of DTI Integral
Curves 1051
    Çağatay Demiralp, Gregory Shakhnarovich, Song Zhang, and
    David H. Laidlaw

Brain Fiber Architecture, Genetics, and Intelligence: A High Angular
Resolution Diffusion Imaging (HARDI) Study 1060
    Ming-Chang Chiang, Marina Barysheva, Agatha D. Lee,
    Sarah Madsen, Andrea D. Klunder, Arthur W. Toga,
    Katie L. McMahon, Greig I. de Zubicaray, Matthew Meredith,
    Margaret J. Wright, Anuj Srivastava, Nikolay Balov, and
    Paul M. Thompson

Group Statistics of DTI Fiber Bundles Using Spatial Functions of
Tensor Measures 1068
  *Casey B. Goodlett, P. Thomas Fletcher, John H. Gilmore, and
  Guido Gerig*

Author Index 1077

Table of Contents – Part II

Miscellaneous II

Computational Pathology Analysis of Tissue Microarrays Predicts
Survival of Renal Clear Cell Carcinoma Patients 1
    Thomas J. Fuchs, Peter J. Wild, Holger Moch, and
    Joachim M. Buhmann

Optimal Acquisition Schemes in High Angular Resolution Diffusion
Weighted Imaging 9
    Vesna Prčkovska, Alard F. Roebroeck, W.L.P.M. Pullens,
    Anna Villanova, and Bart M. ter Haar Romeny

3D Dendrite Reconstruction and Spine Identification 18
    Wengang Zhou, Houqiang Li, and Xiaobo Zhou

Joint LMMSE Estimation of DWI Data for DTI Processing 27
    Antonio Tristán-Vega and Santiago Aja-Fernández

Evaluation of Rigid and Non-rigid Motion Compensation of Cardiac
Perfusion MRI 35
    Hui Xue, Jens Guehring, Latha Srinivasan, Sven Zuehlsdorff,
    Kinda Saddi, Christophe Chefdhotel, Joseph V. Hajnal, and
    Daniel Rueckert

3D Surface Matching and Registration through Shape Images 44
    Zhaoqiang Lai and Jing Hua

Volumetric Ultrasound Panorama Based on 3D SIFT 52
    Dong Ni, Yingge Qu, Xuan Yang, Yim Pan Chui, Tien-Tsin Wong,
    Simon S.M. Ho, and Pheng Ann Heng

Automatic Intra-operative Generation of Geometric Left
Atrium/Pulmonary Vein Models from Rotational X-Ray
Angiography 61
    Carsten Meyer, Robert Manzke, Jochen Peters, Olivier Ecabert,
    Reinhard Kneser, Vivek Y. Reddy, Raymond C. Chan, and
    Jürgen Weese

Efficient Computation of PDF-Based Characteristics from Diffusion
MR Signal 70
    Haz-Edine Assemlal, David Tschumperlé, and Luc Brun

Bayesian Motion Recovery Framework for Myocardial Phase-Contrast
Velocity MRI... 79
  Andrew Huntbatch, Su-Lin Lee, David Firmin, and
  Guang-Zhong Yang

The Effect of Automated Marker Detection on in Vivo Volumetric
Stent Reconstruction... 87
  Gert Schoonenberg, Pierre Lelong, Raoul Florent, Onno Wink, and
  Bart ter Haar Romeny

Patch-Based Markov Models for Event Detection in Fluorescence
Bioimaging... 95
  Thierry Pécot, Charles Kervrann, Sabine Bardin, Bruno Goud, and
  Jean Salamero

Belief Propagation for Depth Cue Fusion in Minimally Invasive
Surgery.. 104
  Benny Lo, Marco Visentini Scarzanella, Danail Stoyanov, and
  Guang-Zhong Yang

Deformable Mosaicing for Whole-Body MRI.......................... 113
  Christian Wachinger, Ben Glocker, Jochen Zeltner, Nikos Paragios,
  Nikos Komodakis, Michael Sass Hansen, and Nassir Navab

Impact of Rician Adapted Non-Local Means Filtering on HARDI...... 122
  Maxime Descoteaux, Nicolas Wiest-Daesslé, Sylvain Prima,
  Christian Barillot, and Rachid Deriche

Towards Regional Elastography of Intracranial Aneurysms.......... 131
  Simone Balocco, Oscar Camara, and Alejandro F. Frangi

Wall Motion Classification of Stress Echocardiography Based on
Combined Rest-and-Stress Data.................................... 139
  Sarina Mansor, Nicholas P. Hughes, and J. Alison Noble

Harmonic Surface Mapping with Laplace-Beltrami Eigenmaps......... 147
  Yonggang Shi, Rongjie Lai, Kyle Kern, Nancy Sicotte,
  Ivo Dinov, and Arthur W. Toga

Motion Correction in Respiratory Gated Cardiac PET/CT Using
Multi-scale Optical Flow... 155
  Mohammad Dawood, Thomas Kösters, Michael Fieseler,
  Florian Büther, Xiaoyi Jiang, Frank Wübbeling, and
  Klaus P. Schäfers

Parallelized Hybrid TGRAPPA Reconstruction for Real-Time
Interactive MRI.. 163
  Haris Saybasili, Peter Kellman, J. Andrew Derbyshire,
  Elliot R. McVeigh, and Michael A. Guttman

Rician Noise Removal by Non-Local Means Filtering for Low
Signal-to-Noise Ratio MRI: Applications to DT-MRI 171
　　Nicolas Wiest-Daesslé, Sylvain Prima, Pierrick Coupé,
　　Sean Patrick Morrissey, and Christian Barillot

Human Brain Myelination from Birth to 4.5 Years 180
　　Berengere Aubert-Broche, Vladimir Fonov, Ilana Leppert,
　　G. Bruce Pike, and D. Louis Collins

Toward a Flexible and Portable CT Scanner 188
　　Jeff Orchard and John T.W. Yeow

Adaptive Discriminant Wavelet Packet Transform and Local Binary
Patterns for Meningioma Subtype Classification 196
　　Hammad Qureshi, Olcay Sertel, Nasir Rajpoot, Roland Wilson, and
　　Metin Gurcan

Colon Unfolding Via Skeletal Subspace Deformation 205
　　Sandra Sudarsky, Bernhard Geiger, Christophe Chefd'hotel, and
　　Lutz Guendel

Entropy-Optimized Texture Models 213
　　Sebastian Zambal, Katja Bühler, and Jiří Hladůvka

Optimal Feature Selection Applied to Multispectral Fluorescence
Imaging 222
　　Tobias C. Wood, Surapa Thiemjarus, Kevin R. Koh,
　　Daniel S. Elson, and Guang-Zhong Yang

AutoGate: Fast and Automatic Doppler Gate Localization in B-Mode
Echocardiogram 230
　　JinHyeong Park, S. Kevin Zhou, Costas Simopoulos, and
　　Dorin Comaniciu

Estimation of Ground-Glass Opacity Measurement in CT Lung
Images 238
　　Yuanjie Zheng, Chandra Kambhamettu, Thomas Bauer, and
　　Karl Steiner

Bayesian Analysis of fMRI Data with ICA Based Spatial Prior 246
　　Deepti R. Bathula, Hemant D. Tagare, Lawrence H. Staib,
　　Xenophon Papademetris, Robert T. Schultz, and James S. Duncan

Spatiotemporal Decomposition in Object-Space along Reconstruction
in Emission Tomography 255
　　Xavier Hubert, Dominique Chambellan, Samuel Legoupil,
　　Régine Trébossen, Jean-Robert Deverre, and Nikos Paragios

Assessment of Reliability of Multi-site Neuroimaging Via Traveling
Phantom Study 263
    Sylvain Gouttard, Martin Styner, Marcel Prastawa,
    Joseph Piven, and Guido Gerig

Fieldmap-Free Retrospective Registration and Distortion Correction
for EPI-Based Functional Imaging 271
    Clare Poynton, Mark Jenkinson, Stephen Whalen,
    Alexandra J. Golby, and William Wells III

Physical-Space Refraction-Corrected Transmission Ultrasound
Computed Tomography Made Computationally Practical 280
    Shengying Li, Klaus Mueller, Marcel Jackowski, Donald Dione, and
    Lawrence Staib

Tag Separation in Cardiac Tagged MRI 289
    Junzhou Huang, Zhen Qian, Xiaolei Huang, Dimitris Metaxas, and
    Leon Axel

Visualization Tools for High Angular Resolution Diffusion Imaging 298
    David W. Shattuck, Ming-Chang Chiang, Marina Barysheva,
    Katie L. McMahon, Greig I. de Zubicaray, Matthew Meredith,
    Margaret J. Wright, Arthur W. Toga, and Paul M. Thompson

Human Vocal Tract Analysis by in Vivo 3D MRI during Phonation:
A Complete System for Imaging, Quantitative Modeling, and Speech
Synthesis 306
    Axel Wismueller, Johannes Behrends, Phil Hoole,
    Gerda L. Leinsinger, Maximilian F. Reiser, and
    Per-Lennart Westesson

Fast Motion Tracking of Tagged MRI Using Angle-Preserving Meshless
Registration 313
    Ting Chen, Xiaoxu Wang, Dimitris Metaxas, and Leon Axel

Comparison of EPI Distortion Correction Methods in Diffusion Tensor
MRI Using a Novel Framework 321
    Minjie Wu, Lin-Ching Chang, Lindsay Walker, Herve Lemaitre,
    Alan S. Barnett, Stefano Marenco, and Carlo Pierpaoli

Consensus-Locally Linear Embedding (C-LLE): Application to Prostate
Cancer Detection on Magnetic Resonance Spectroscopy 330
    Pallavi Tiwari, Mark Rosen, and Anant Madabhushi

Robotics and Interventions

Automatic Guidance of an Ultrasound Probe by Visual Servoing Based
on B-Mode Image Moments 339
    Rafik Mebarki, Alexandre Krupa, and Christophe Collewet

Gaze-Contingent 3D Control for Focused Energy Ablation in Robotic
Assisted Surgery 347
  Danail Stoyanov, George P. Mylonas, and Guang-Zhong Yang

MR Navigated Breast Surgery: Method and Initial Clinical
Experience 356
  Timothy Carter, Christine Tanner, Nicolas Beechey-Newman,
  Dean Barratt, and David Hawkes

Soft Tissue Tracking for Minimally Invasive Surgery: Learning Local
Deformation Online 364
  Peter Mountney and Guang-Zhong Yang

Combination of Intraoperative 5-Aminolevulinic Acid-Induced
Fluorescence and 3-D MR Imaging for Guidance of Robotic Laser
Ablation for Precision Neurosurgery 373
  Hongen Liao, Koji Shimaya, Kaimeng Wang, Takashi Maruyama,
  Masafumi Noguchi, Yoshihiro Muragaki, Etsuko Kobayashi,
  Hiroshi Iseki, and Ichiro Sakuma

Statistical Analysis

Discovering Modes of an Image Population through Mixture
Modeling 381
  Mert R. Sabuncu, Serdar K. Balci, and Polina Golland

Sparse Approximation of Currents for Statistics on Curves and
Surfaces 390
  Stanley Durrleman, Xavier Pennec, Alain Trouvé, and
  Nicholas Ayache

Probabilistic Anatomo-Functional Parcellation of the Cortex: How
Many Regions? 399
  Alan Tucholka, Bertrand Thirion, Matthieu Perrot, Philippe Pinel,
  Jean-François Mangin, and Jean-Baptiste Poline

Models of Normal Variation and Local Contrasts in Hippocampal
Anatomy 407
  Xinyang Liu, Washington Mio, Yonggang Shi, Ivo Dinov,
  Xiuwen Liu, Natasha Lepore, Franco Lepore, Madeleine Fortin,
  Patrice Voss, Maryse Lassonde, and Paul M. Thompson

Label Space: A Coupled Multi-shape Representation 416
  James Malcolm, Yogesh Rathi, Martha E. Shenton, and
  Allen Tannenbaum

Segmentation II

An Atlas-Based Segmentation Propagation Framework Using Locally
Affine Registration – Application to Automatic Whole Heart
Segmentation 425
  *Xiahai Zhuang, Kawal Rhode, Simon Arridge, Reza Razavi,
  Derek Hill, David Hawkes, and Sebastien Ourselin*

Atlas-Based Auto-segmentation of Head and Neck CT Images 434
  *Xiao Han, Mischa S. Hoogeman, Peter C. Levendag,
  Lyndon S. Hibbard, David N. Teguh, Peter Voet,
  Andrew C. Cowen, and Theresa K. Wolf*

Spectral Clustering as a Diagnostic Tool in Cross-Sectional MR Studies:
An Application to Mild Dementia 442
  Paul Aljabar, Daniel Rueckert, and William R. Crum

Bidirectional Segmentation of Three-Dimensional Cardiac MR Images
Using a Subject-Specific Dynamical Model 450
  *Yun Zhu, Xenophon Papademetris, Albert J. Sinusas, and
  James S. Duncan*

Intervention

Ablation Monitoring with Elastography: 2D *In-vivo* and 3D *Ex-vivo*
Studies 458
  *Hassan Rivaz, Ioana Fleming, Lia Assumpcao, Gabor Fichtinger,
  Ulrike Hamper, Michael Choti, Gregory Hager, and Emad Boctor*

Dynamic View Expansion for Enhanced Navigation in Natural Orifice
Transluminal Endoscopic Surgery 467
  *Mirna Lerotic, Adrian J. Chung, James Clark,
  Salman Valibeik, and Guang-Zhong Yang*

Robotic System for Transapical Aortic Valve Replacement with MRI
Guidance 476
  Ming Li, Dumitru Mazilu, and Keith A. Horvath

Image Thickness Correction for Navigation with 3D Intra-cardiac
Ultrasound Catheter 485
  Hua Zhong, Takeo Kanade, and David Schwartzman

Quantification of Edematic Effects in Prostate Brachytherapy
Interventions 493
  *Mohamed Hefny, Purang Abolmaesumi, Zahra Karimaghaloo,
  David G. Gobbi, Randy Ellis, and Gabor Fichtinger*

A Robot Assisted Hip Fracture Reduction with a Navigation System ... 501
  Sanghyun Joung, Hirokazu Kamon, Hongen Liao, Junichiro Iwaki,
  Touji Nakazawa, Mamoru Mitsuishi, Yoshikazu Nakajima,
  Tsuyoshi Koyama, Nobuhiko Sugano, Yuki Maeda, Masahiko Bessho,
  Satoru Ohashi, Takuya Matsumoto, Isao Ohnishi, and Ichiro Sakuma

MRI Compatibility of Robot Actuation Techniques – A Comparative
Study 509
  Gregory S. Fischer, Axel Krieger, Iulian Iordachita, Csaba Csoma,
  Louis L. Whitcomb, and Gabor Fichtinger

Robust Image-Based IVUS Pullbacks Gating 518
  Carlo Gatta, Oriol Pujol, Oriol Rodriguez Leor,
  Josepa Mauri Ferre, and Petia Radeva

Real-Time 3D Reconstruction for Collision Avoidance in Interventional
Environments 526
  Alexander Ladikos, Selim Benhimane, and Nassir Navab

Improvement of Accuracy of Marker-Free Bronchoscope Tracking Using
Electromagnetic Tracker Based on Bronchial Branch Information...... 535
  Kensaku Mori, Daisuke Deguchi, Takayuki Kitasaka,
  Yasuhito Suenaga, Yosihnori Hasegawa, Kazuyoshi Imaizumi, and
  Hirotsugu Takabatake

Cooperative Robot Assistant for Retinal Microsurgery 543
  Ioana Fleming, Marcin Balicki, John Koo, Iulian Iordachita,
  Ben Mitchell, James Handa, Gregory Hager, and Russell Taylor

An Ultrasound-Guided Organ Biopsy Simulation with 6DOF Haptic
Feedback 551
  Dong Ni, Wing-Yin Chan, Jing Qin, Yingge Qu, Yim-Pan Chui,
  Simon S.M. Ho, and Pheng-Ann Heng

Simulations of Needle Insertion by Using a Eulerian Hydrocode FEM
and the Experimental Validations 560
  Hiroyuki Kataoka, Shigeho Noda, Hideo Yokota, Shu Takagi,
  Ryutaro Himeno, and Shigenobu Okazawa

Preoperative Surgery Planning for Percutaneous Hepatic Microwave
Ablation 569
  Weiming Zhai, Jing Xu, Yannan Zhao, Yixu Song, Lin Sheng, and
  Peifa Jia

Long Bone X-Ray Image Stitching Using Camera Augmented Mobile
C-Arm 578
  Lejing Wang, Joerg Traub, Sandro Michael Heining,
  Selim Benhimane, Ekkehard Euler, Rainer Graumann, and
  Nassir Navab

Intraoperative Navigation of an Optically Tracked Surgical Robot 587
  Jordi Cornellà, Ole Jakob Elle, Wajid Ali, and Eigil Samset

Modelling Dynamic Fronto-Parietal Behaviour During Minimally
Invasive Surgery – A Markovian Trip Distribution Approach........... 595
  *Daniel Richard Leff, Felipe Orihuela-Espina, Julian Leong,
  Ara Darzi, and Guang-Zhong Yang*

Detecting Informative Frames from Wireless Capsule Endoscopic Video
Using Color and Texture Features................................. 603
  *Md. Khayrul Bashar, Kensaku Mori, Yasuhito Suenaga,
  Takayuki Kitasaka, and Yoshito Mekada*

How Does the Camera Assistant Decide the Zooming Ratio of
Laparoscopic Images? – Analysis and Implementation 611
  *Atsushi Nishikawa, Hiroaki Nakagoe, Kazuhiro Taniguchi,
  Yasuo Yamada, Mitsugu Sekimoto, Shuji Takiguchi,
  Morito Monden, and Fumio Miyazaki*

Precision Radiotherapy for Small Animal Research 619
  *Mohammad Matinfar, Iulian Iordachita, Eric Ford,
  John Wong, and Peter Kazanzides*

Modeling and Online Recognition of Surgical Phases Using Hidden
Markov Models 627
  Tobias Blum, Nicolas Padoy, Hubertus Feußner, and Nassir Navab

Prostate Brachytherapy Seed Localization with Gaussian Blurring and
Camera Self-calibration 636
  Junghoon Lee, Xiaofeng Liu, Jerry L. Prince, and Gabor Fichtinger

Virtual Reality-Enhanced Ultrasound Guidance for Atrial Ablation: *In
vitro* Epicardial Study 644
  *Cristian A. Linte, Andrew Wiles, John Moore, Chris Wedlake, and
  Terry M. Peters*

Fast Marker Based C-Arm Pose Estimation 652
  Bernhard Kainz, Markus Grabner, and Matthias Rüther

Needle Insertion Study Using Ultrasound-Based 2D Motion Tracking ... 660
  Ehsan Dehghan and Septimiu E. Salcudean

3D Dynamic Roadmapping for Abdominal Catheterizations 668
  *Frederik Bender, Martin Groher, Ali Khamene, Wolfgang Wein,
  Tim Hauke Heibel, and Nassir Navab*

Gaze-Contingent Motor Channelling and Haptic Constraints for
Minimally Invasive Robotic Surgery 676
  *George P. Mylonas, Ka-Wai Kwok, Ara Darzi, and
  Guang-Zhong Yang*

Efficient 3D Tracking for Motion Compensation in Beating Heart
Surgery 684
  Rogério Richa, Philippe Poignet, and Chao Liu

Path Planning and Workspace Determination for Robot-Assisted
Insertion of Steerable Electrode Arrays for Cochlear Implant Surgery ... 692
  Jian Zhang, Wei Wei, Spiros Manolidis, J. Thomas Roland Jr., and
  Nabil Simaan

Software Strategy for Robotic Transperineal Prostate Therapy in
Closed-Bore MRI 701
  Junichi Tokuda, Gregory S. Fischer, Csaba Csoma,
  Simon P. DiMaio, David G. Gobbi, Gabor Fichtinger,
  Clare M. Tempany, and Nobuhiko Hata

Real-Time Simulation of 4D Lung Tumor Radiotherapy Using a
Breathing Model 710
  Anand P. Santhanam, Twyla Willoughby, Amish Shah,
  Sanford Meeks, Jannick P. Rolland, and Patrick Kupelian

Construction of a Statistical Surgical Plan Atlas for Automated 3D
Planning of Femoral Component in Total Hip Arthroplasty 718
  Masahiko Nakamoto, Itaru Otomaru, Masaki Takao,
  Nobuhiko Sugano, Yoshiyuki Kagiyama, Hideki Yoshikawa,
  Yukio Tada, and Yoshinobu Sato

Modeling II

Constitutive Modeling of Human Liver Based on in Vivo
Measurements 726
  Edoardo Mazza, Patrick Grau, Marc Hollenstein, and Michael Bajka

Real-Time Simulation of Medical Ultrasound from CT Images 734
  Ramtin Shams, Richard Hartley, and Nassir Navab

Real-Time Nonlinear FEM with Neural Network for Simulating Soft
Organ Model Deformation 742
  Ken'ichi Morooka, Xian Chen, Ryo Kurazume, Seiichi Uchida,
  Kenji Hara, Yumi Iwashita, and Makoto Hashizume

Modelling Childbirth: Comparing Athlete and Non-athlete Pelvic Floor
Mechanics 750
  Xinshan Li, Jennifer A. Kruger, Jae-Hoon Chung,
  Martyn P. Nash, and Poul M.F. Nielsen

Modelling Mammographic Compression of the Breast 758
  Jae-Hoon Chung, Vijay Rajagopal, Poul M.F. Nielsen, and
  Martyn P. Nash

Cardiac Medial Modeling and Time-Course Heart Wall Thickness
Analysis 766
  Hui Sun, Brian B. Avants, Alejandro F. Frangi, Federico Sukno,
  James C. Gee, and Paul A. Yushkevich

Identification of Atherosclerotic Lesion-Prone Sites through
Patient-Specific Simulation of Low-Density Lipoprotein
Accumulation 774
  Ufuk Olgac, Vartan Kurtcuoglu, Stefan C. Saur, and
  Dimos Poulikakos

Exploring the Use of Proper Orthogonal Decomposition for Enhancing
Blood Flow Images Via Computational Fluid Dynamics 782
  Robert McGregor, Dominik Szczerba, Martin von Siebenthal,
  Krishnamurthy Muralidhar, and Gábor Székely

Fast Virtual Stenting with Deformable Meshes: Application to
Intracranial Aneurysms 790
  Ignacio Larrabide, Alessandro Radaelli, and Alejandro Frangi

Dynamic Thermal Modeling of the Normal and Tumorous Breast under
Elastic Deformation 798
  Li Jiang, Wang Zhan, and Murray H. Loew

Real-Time Liver Motion Compensation for MRgFUS 806
  James C. Ross, Rekha Tranquebar, and Dattesh Shanbhag

Passive Ventricular Mechanics Modelling Using MRI of Structure and
Function 814
  Vicky Y. Wang, Hoi Ieng Lam, Daniel B. Ennis,
  Alistair A. Young, and Martyn P. Nash

Registration II

Fast Musculoskeletal Registration Based on Shape Matching 822
  Benjamin Gilles and Dinesh K. Pai

Physically-Based Validation of Deformable Medical Image
Registration 830
  Huai-Ping Lee, Ming C. Lin, and Mark Foskey

Adaptive Boundary Conditions for Physically Based Follow-Up Breast
MR Image Registration 839
  Liesbet Roose, Dirk Loeckx, Wouter Mollemans, Frederik Maes, and
  Paul Suetens

An Incremental Method for Registering Electroanatomic Mapping Data to Surface Mesh Models of the Left Atrium............................ 847
Aditya B. Koolwal, Federico Barbagli, Christopher R. Carlson, and David H. Liang

Fast, Adaptive Expectation-Maximization Alignment for Cryo-EM 855
Hemant D. Tagare, Frederick Sigworth, and Andrew Barthel

Weight Preserving Image Registration for Monitoring Disease Progression in Lung CT 863
Vladlena Gorbunova, Pechin Lo, Haseem Ashraf, Asger Dirksen, Mads Nielsen, and Marleen de Bruijne

Localization of Pelvic Anatomical Coordinate System Using US/Atlas Registration for Total Hip Replacement 871
Pezhman Foroughi, Danny Song, Gouthami Chintalapani, Russell H. Taylor, and Gabor Fichtinger

GPU Accelerated Non-rigid Registration for the Evaluation of Cardiac Function 880
Bo Li, Alistair A. Young, and Brett R. Cowan

Non-rigid Image Registration with $S\alpha S$ Filters 888
Shu Liao and Albert C.S. Chung

Symmetric Nonrigid Image Registration: Application to Average Brain Templates Construction.. 897
Vincent Noblet, Christian Heinrich, Fabrice Heitz, and Jean-Paul Armspach

Diffusion Tensor Image Registration Using Tensor Geometry and Orientation Features 905
Jinzhong Yang, Dinggang Shen, Christos Davatzikos, and Ragini Verma

A Tensor-Based Morphometry Study of Genetic Influences on Brain Structure Using a New Fluid Registration Method 914
Caroline Brun, Natasha Leporé, Xavier Pennec, Yi-Yu Chou, Agatha D. Lee, Marina Barysheva, Grieg de Zubicaray, Matthew Meredith, Katie McMahon, Margaret J. Wright, Arthur W. Toga, and Paul M. Thompson

Effective Incorporation of Spatial Information in a Mutual Information Based 3D-2D Registration of a CT Volume to X-Ray Images 922
Guoyan Zheng

A Nonrigid Image Registration Framework for Identification of Tissue Mechanical Parameters 930
Petr Jordan, Simona Socrate, Todd E. Zickler, and Robert D. Howe

A Local Mutual Information Guided Denoising Technique and Its
Application to Self-calibrated Partially Parallel Imaging 939
    Weihong Guo and Feng Huang

Influence of Organ Motion and Contrast Enhancement on Image
Registration 948
    Andrew Melbourne, David Atkinson, and David Hawkes

Anatomy-Preserving Nonlinear Registration of Deep Brain ROIs Using
Confidence-Based Block-Matching 956
    Manik Bhattacharjee, Alain Pitiot, Alexis Roche,
    Didier Dormont, and Eric Bardinet

The Zernike Expansion – An Example of a Merit Function for 2D/3D
Registration Based on Orthogonal Functions 964
    Shuo Dong, Joachim Kettenbach, Isabella Hinterleitner,
    Helmar Bergmann, and Wolfgang Birkfellner

Registration of 4D Time-Series of Cardiac Images with Multichannel
Diffeomorphic Demons 972
    Jean-Marc Peyrat, Hervé Delingette, Maxime Sermesant,
    Xavier Pennec, Chenyang Xu, and Nicholas Ayache

An Active Contour-Based Atlas Registration Model Applied to
Automatic Subthalamic Nucleus Targeting on MRI: Method and
Validation 980
    Valérie Duay, Xavier Bresson, Javier Sanchez Castro, Claudio Pollo,
    Meritxell Bach Cuadra, and Jean-Philippe Thiran

Location Registration and Recognition (LRR) for Longitudinal
Evaluation of Corresponding Regions in CT Volumes 989
    Michal Sofka and Charles V. Stewart

Reducing Motion Artifacts in 3d Breast Ultrasound Using Non-linear
Registration 998
    Tobias Boehler and Heinz-Otto Peitgen

Semi-automatic Reference Standard Construction for Quantitative
Evaluation of Lung CT Registration 1006
    Keelin Murphy, Bram van Ginneken, Josien P.W. Pluim,
    Stefan Klein, and Marius Staring

Automatic Deformable Diffusion Tensor Registration for Fiber
Population Analysis 1014
    Mustafa Okan Irfanoglu, Raghu Machiraju, Steffen Sammet,
    Carlo Pierpaoli, and Michael Knopp

Deformable Ultrasound Registration without Reconstruction 1023
    Rupert Brooks, D. Louis Collins, Xavier Morandi, and Tal Arbel

A Theoretical Comparison of Different Target Registration Error
Estimators 1032
    Mehdi Hedjazi Moghari, Burton Ma, and Purang Abolmaesumi

Robust Brain Registration Using Adaptive Probabilistic Atlas 1041
    Jaime Ide, Rong Chen, Dinggang Shen, and Edward H. Herskovits

Using Curve-Fitting of Curvilinear Features for Assessing Registration
of Clinical Neuropathology with in Vivo MRI 1050
    Philippe Laissue, Chris Kenwright, Ali Hojjat, and Alan Colchester

A Maximal Mass Confinement Principle for Rigid and Locally Rigid
Image Registration 1058
    Julian Mattes, Johannes Gall, and Alfredo Lopez

Segmentation III

Fully Bayesian Joint Model for MR Brain Scan Tissue and Structure
Segmentation 1066
    Benoit Scherrer, Florence Forbes, Catherine Garbay, and
    Michel Dojat

Detection of Deformable Objects in 3D Images Using Markov-Chain
Monte Carlo and Spherical Harmonics 1075
    Khaled Khairy, Emmanuel Reynaud, and Ernst Stelzer

A Variational Level Set Approach to Segmentation and Bias Correction
of Images with Intensity Inhomogeneity 1083
    Chunming Li, Rui Huang, Zhaohua Ding, Chris Gatenby,
    Dimitris Metaxas, and John Gore

Markov Dependence Tree-Based Segmentation of Deep Brain
Structures 1092
    Jue Wu and Albert C.S. Chung

Author Index 1101

On Computing the Underlying Fiber Directions from the Diffusion Orientation Distribution Function[*]

Luke Bloy[1] and Ragini Verma[2]

[1] Department of Bioengineering, University of Pennsylvania, USA
lbloy@seas.upenn.edu
[2] Department of Radiology, University of Pennsylvania, USA

Abstract. In this work, a novel method for determining the principal directions (maxima) of the diffusion orientation distribution function(ODF) is proposed. We represent the ODF as a symmetric high-order Cartesian tensor restricted to the unit sphere and show that the extrema of the ODF are solutions to a system of polynomial equations whose coefficients are polynomial functions of the tensor elements. In addition to demonstrating the ability of our methods to identify the principal directions in real data, we show that this method correctly identifies the principal directions under a range of noise levels. We also propose the use of the principal curvatures of the graph of the ODF function as a measure of the degree of diffusion anisotropy in that direction. We present simulated results illustrating the relationship between the mean principal curvature, measured at the maxima, and the fractional anisotropy of the underlying diffusion tensor.

1 Introduction

Diffusion tensor imaging (DTI) has in the past decade developed into the method of choice for investigating and characterizing white matter neural architecture non-invasively. The development of DTI has led to a number of applications in which white matter connectivity has been evaluated in both healthy and diseased populations [1,2]. Additionally, measures derived from the diffusion tensor have been widely used to characterize regional anisotropy (FA), mean diffusivity (ADC) and orientation[3]. Despite DTI's growing foothold in the imaging community, it's inability to model voxels of complex white matter, i.e. multiple fibers with different orientations, different partial volume fractions, and its dependence on a Gaussian model of diffusion within a fiber tract, has prompted the development of high angular resolution diffusion imaging (HARDI) to address these concerns.

A number of approaches have been put forth to analyze HARDI data, including the spherical harmonic decomposition of the apparent diffusion coefficient

---

[*] This work was supported by the National Institute of Health via grant R01-MH-079938.

(ADC) profile, the treatment of the ADC profile as a generalized tensor, q-ball imaging (QBI)[4] and persistent angular structure MRI[5]. Various scalar measures have been proposed to describe the ADC profile, including generalized anisotropy[6] and the fractional multifiber index[7]. However the maxima of the ADC profile do not necessarily coincide with the underlying fiber directions[8], making the extraction of orientation information difficult.

The correspondence between the peaks of the diffusion orientation distribution function(ODF), which describes the probability a water molecule will diffuse along a given direction, and the principal directions(PDs) of the underlying fibers, has been established experimentally[9]. For this reason a major focus within the QBI community has been directed at developing methods to compute the ODF and its maxima. A number of methods exist to compute the maxima of the ODF, such as finite difference method [10], spherical Newton's method [11] and Powell's method [5]. With the exception of the finite difference method, whose accuracy is limited to the mesh size, these methods are numerical minimization problems and thus care must be taken to avoid small local maxima, and to ensure convergence.

We present a methodology that determines the PDs of the ODF for a given voxel by computing the stationary points of the ODF. Stationary points of a function $f(u,v)$ are points where $\frac{\partial f}{\partial u} = 0$, $\frac{\partial f}{\partial v} = 0$. Each of these stationary points is then classified based on the curvature of the graph of the ODF at that point. We designate points with a curvature greater than that of a sphere with unit area, as PDs of the ODF. Figure 1, shows the graphs of representative ODFs with 1, 2 and 3 underlying fibers. Similar to the peak anisotropy described in [12], we propose the use of the mean curvature(H) at the PDs as a measure of the degree of anisotropy of the underlying fiber parallel to that direction. We present simulation results that show our method of computing the maxima is robust to noise, as well demonstrating the relationship between H and the fractional anisotropy(FA) of underlying the underlying fiber representation. Lastly we apply our method to human data to illustrate it's ability to capture the underlying directionality of fibers in fiber crossings.

2 Methods

Following the ODF calculation from the HARDI data, we expand the ODF in the real spherical harmonics, and make use of the relationship between spherical harmonics on the unit sphere and symmetric high-order Cartesian tensors to find a tensor representation of the ODF. The details of this process are discussed in section 2.1. Subsequently, we find the stationary points of the ODF, by solving a system of polynomial equations whose coefficients are given by the tensor representation of the ODF (section 2.2). The curvatures of each of these stationary points are then calculated (section 2.3) and the stationary point is classified, based on the curvature.

Notation. As the ODF is a real valued symmetric function, we use the real spherical harmonic basis of even order, as described in [13], to represent it.

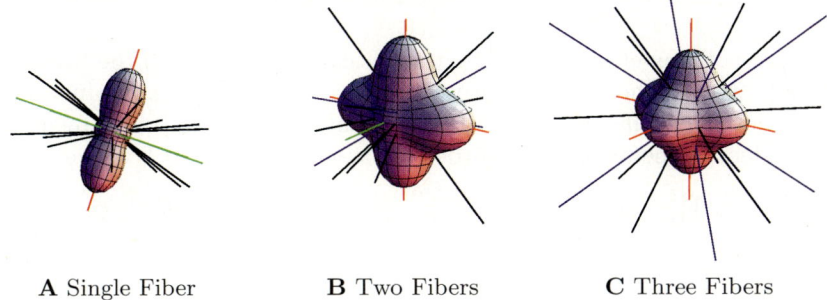

Fig. 1. Diffusion ODF reconstructions for simulated fiber populations. Reconstructions were performed with a tensor of rank 4. All fibers were modeled, using equation 6, with equal FA values (∼ 0.85), and equal volume fractions. Red lines are the detected principal directions, green lines are secondary local maxima, blue lines are local minima and black lines are saddle points. **A**: shows a single fiber, **B**: shows two fibers oriented at right angles to one another and **C**: shows 3 fibers oriented along 3 orthogonal directions.

Namely,

$$R_j = \begin{cases} \frac{1}{\sqrt{2}}(Y_l^m + (-1)^m Y_l^{-m}) & m > 0 \\ Y_l^m & m = 0 \\ \frac{i}{\sqrt{2}}((-1)^m Y_l^m - Y_l^{-m}) & m < 0 \end{cases} \quad (1)$$

where $j = \frac{(l^2+m+2)}{2} + m$, l is even and $-l \leq m \leq l$. Also in a slight abuse of notation, we will move freely between 2 equivalent expressions for the tensor product. If f is a real homogeneous polynomial of order m, then

$$f(\boldsymbol{x}) = A\boldsymbol{x}^m = \sum_{i_1,\dots,i_m=1}^{3} A_{i_1,\dots,i_m} x_{i_1} \dots x_{i_m} = \sum_{k=1}^{N} \mu_k A_k \prod_{p=1}^{m} x_{k(p)}$$

where N is the number of independent elements of A, A_k is the kth independent element of A, μ_k is the multiplicity of the element and $x_{k(p)}$ is the component of $\boldsymbol{x}$ corresponding to the pth index of the kth independent element of A.

2.1 Expressing the ODF as a Cartesian Tensor

The ODF ($\Psi(\boldsymbol{u})$) is a real valued antipodally symmetric function and thus can be expanded in the spherical harmonic basis described in equation 1. The expansion of the ODF is related to the expansion of the HARDI signal by the following relation [14,15].

$$\Psi(\boldsymbol{u}) = \sum_{j=1}^{N} 2\pi P_l(0) c_j R_j(\boldsymbol{u}) = \sum_{j=1}^{N} \psi_j R_j(\boldsymbol{u}) \quad (2)$$

where $P_l(0)$ is the Legendre polynomial of order l, $\psi_j = 2\pi P_l(0) c_j$ are the coefficients of the ODF in the R_j basis, c_j are the coefficients of the diffusion signal in the R_j basis, and R_j are the real spherical harmonic basis functions (RSH) of equation 1.

In [13], Descoteaux et al. showed that spherical harmonics and the Cartesian tensors restricted to the unit sphere were each a basis of the same functional space and that the coefficients of the RSH expansion, $\psi = \{\psi_k\}$ were related to the independent elements of a high-order diffusion T by $\psi = MT$ where

$$M = \begin{pmatrix} \mu_1 \int_\Omega \prod_{p=1}^l g_1(p) R_1(\theta,\phi) d\Omega & \cdots & \mu_N \int_\Omega \prod_{p=1}^l g_N(p) R_1(\theta,\phi) d\Omega \\ \vdots & \ddots & \vdots \\ \mu_1 \int_\Omega \prod_{p=1}^l g_1(p) R_N(\theta,\phi) d\Omega & \cdots & \mu_N \int_\Omega \prod_{p=1}^l g_N(p) R_N(\theta,\phi) d\Omega \end{pmatrix}$$

where M is a change of basis matrix and is invertible. From this and equation 2 we can represent each of the N independent elements of T as,

$$T_k = \sum_i M_{i,k}^{-1} \psi_i = 2\pi P_l(0) \sum_i M_{i,k}^{-1} c_i \qquad (3)$$

Thus the $\Psi(\boldsymbol{u}) = T\boldsymbol{u}^l$, where T is a Cartesian tensor of rank l (a rank l fully-symmetric tensor has $(l^2 + 3l + 2)/2 = N$ unique components).

2.2 Finding Stationary Points

We define the tensor product Tx^{m-1} as a vector in $\mathbb{R}^3$, whose ith component is given by $\sum_{i_2,\ldots,i_l=1}^3 T_{i_1,i_2,\ldots,i_l} u_{i_2} \ldots u_{i_m}$. Using this definition, the method of Lagrange multipliers and the fact the T is a fully symmetric tensor, the problem of finding the stationary points of $\Psi(\boldsymbol{u}) = T\boldsymbol{u}^l$ reduces to solving the following set of homogeneous polynomial equations.

$$Tx^{l-1} = \lambda x \quad \text{s.t.} \quad x^t x = 1 \qquad (4)$$

Qi [16] called a real scalar λ and a real vector u a Z-eigenvalue and a Z-eigenvector respectively if they were solutions to equation 4. Qi showed that for a given solution, x, the corresponding λ is given by $Tx^l = \Psi(x)$.

Equation 4 describes a system of homogeneous polynomial equations in 4 unknowns (x_1,x_2,x_3 and λ). We proceed by reducing equation 4 to a system of 2 variables then use the resultant of the 2 variable system to solve the system.

In practice one looks for solutions of one of three forms, $x = (1,0,0)$, $x = (t,1,0)/|(t,1,0)|$ and $x = (u,v,1)/|(u,v,1)|$, where t is the solution to an lth degree polynomial equation and where u and v are solutions to a system of 2 polynomial equations. Note that the coefficients of these polynomial equations are polynomials of the independent elements of T, and when viewed as polynomial functions of those elements, can be computed *a priori*, for a given l.

2.3 Calculating Principal Curvatures

Once the set of stationary points has been found we can calculate the corresponding curvatures, and classify each stationary point. To do this we define the surface corresponding to the graph of the ODF as

$$S = \{\Psi(\theta,\phi)(\sin(\theta)\cos(\phi), \sin(\theta)\sin(\phi), \cos(\theta)) \mid \theta \in (0,\pi), \phi \in (0,2\pi)\}$$

S is clearly a closed, orientable surface in $\mathbb{R}^3$. We choose the inward normal as our orientation, to more easily facilitate comparisons to the sphere. At a given stationary point, $p = (\theta,\phi)$, with Z-eigenvalue $\lambda = \Psi(\theta,\phi)$, we compute the Gaussian curvature (K), the mean curvature (H) and both principal curvatures (k_1, k_2) using the following equations.

$$K = \frac{eg - f^2}{EG - F^2}; H = \frac{1}{2}\frac{eG - 2fF + gE}{EG - F^2}; k_1 = H + \sqrt{H^2 - K}; k_2 = H - \sqrt{H^2 - K}$$

with $e = \lambda - \Psi_{\theta\theta}(\theta,\phi)$, $g = \lambda\sin\theta^2 - \Psi_{\phi\phi}(\theta,\phi)$, $f = -\Psi_{\theta\phi}(\theta,\phi)$ and $E = \lambda^2$, $G = \lambda^2\sin\theta^2$, $F = 0$ and $\Psi_{\circ\circ}$ is a second order partial derivative.[17]

We can now classify p as either a principal direction (PD), secondary maxima, minima or saddle according to the following rule.

$$\text{Class of } p = \begin{cases} \text{Principal Direction} & k_1 > 4\pi, k_2 > 4\pi \\ \text{Secondary Maxima} & k_1 > k_2, 0 < k_2 < 4\pi \\ \text{Minima} & k_1 < 0, k_2 < 0 \\ \text{Saddle} & k_1 > 0, k_2 < 0 \end{cases} \quad (5)$$

Thus PDs are points where the surface, in a local neighborhood, is more convex than the sphere with unit area (the ODF of an isotropic diffusion process). If the surface is convex yet shallower than that of the sphere, we classify it as a secondary maxima. Figure 1 shows labeled ODFs for cases with 1, 2 and 3 fibers. Once the PDs have been determined we associate with each the mean curvature (H), as a measure which we relate to the FA(Figure 3).

3 Results and Discussion

Simulated Data Generation. In order to evaluate our method of calculating the principal direction, we generated HARDI signal profiles using the multi-tensor model.

$$S(\boldsymbol{u}_i) = \sum_{k=1}^{n} \frac{1}{n} e^{-b\boldsymbol{u}_i \boldsymbol{D_k} \boldsymbol{u}_i} + \text{noise} \quad (6)$$

where $i = 1, \ldots, 64$ and $\boldsymbol{u}_i$ is the gradient direction used to acquire the ith diffusion weighted signal, n is the number of fibers and $\boldsymbol{D_k}$ is the diffusion tensor of the kth fiber. In our simulations, we typically use diffusion tensors with eigenvalues $(200, 200, 1700)$mm^2/sec at different orientations, and a b value equal to 3000×10^{-6}sec/mm^2. We computed the ODF using the RSH expansion of S according to equation 2. In both our simulations and real data results, we fit the ODF with a rank 4 diffusion tensor.

Experiments. Our first experiment was to examine the robustness of our method in the presence of noise. To this end, we generated 50 diffusion weighted

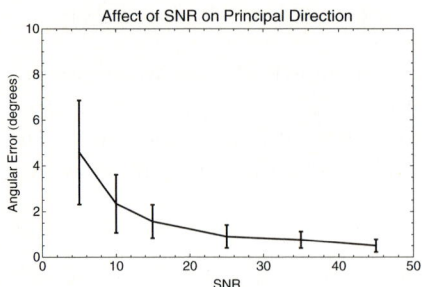 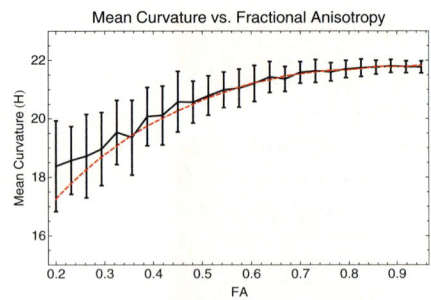

Fig. 2. Angular difference between principal direction, calculated with our method, and the principal eigenvector of the underlying tensors as a function of signal to noise ratio (SNR)

Fig. 3. Relationship between the fractional anisotropy(FA) of generating diffusion tensor and the mean principal curvature, generated without noise (dashed red line) and with SNR of 35 (solid black line)

signals, using equation 6 and a single tensor model, at six signal to noise ratios(SNRs) ranging from 5 to 45. The angle between the PD, determined using our method, and the principal eigenvector of the underlying tensor was calculated, as was the number of PDs detected. As can be seen in figure 2, even at a low SNR of 10 the mean angular error is below 5° degrees while at an SNR of 35 it drops to roughly 1° degree. As would be expected the standard deviation of the angular error decreases as the SNR increases. At a typically achievable SNR of 35 [18], our method achieves a mean accuracy of 0.7° degrees with a standard deviation of less then 0.4°. As a point of comparison a finite difference method with 1281 mesh points has a maximal accuracy of 4° degrees[10]. We found that at an SNR of 10, our method correctly identified the number of PDs in 65% of the ODFs. This rate increased to 95% at SNR of 15 and 100% at SNRs $>= 20$.

Next we were interested in understanding the relationship between the FA of an underlying fiber and curvatures of the ODF at the principal direction of the fiber. We generated 50 diffusion weighted signals using a single tensor model and equation 6 with an SNR of 35, and a mean diffusivity of $700mm^2/sec$, at a number of FA values ranging from 0.2 to 0.95. For each we calculated the principal direction using our method and the mean curvature (H) of the ODF surface at that direction and compared it to the FA value. Figure 3 shows these results (solid black line), as well as the results in the absence of noise (dashed red line). These results illustrate the non-linear, monotonically increasing, relationship between FA and H. Another notable feature of figure 3 is that the standard deviation of the mean curvature decreases as the FA increases, illustrating that noise has a more pronounced effect on isotropic diffusion processes.

Finally we applied our method to diffusion weighted images acquired of healthy volunteer. Six $b = 0$ images and 64 diffusion weighted images ($b = 1000 \times 10^{-6} sec/mm^2$) were acquired. The ODF and the PDs were computed at each voxel. Figure 4 shows a representative coronal slice of RGB image, representing the principal eigenvector of the diffusion tensor, obtained through a

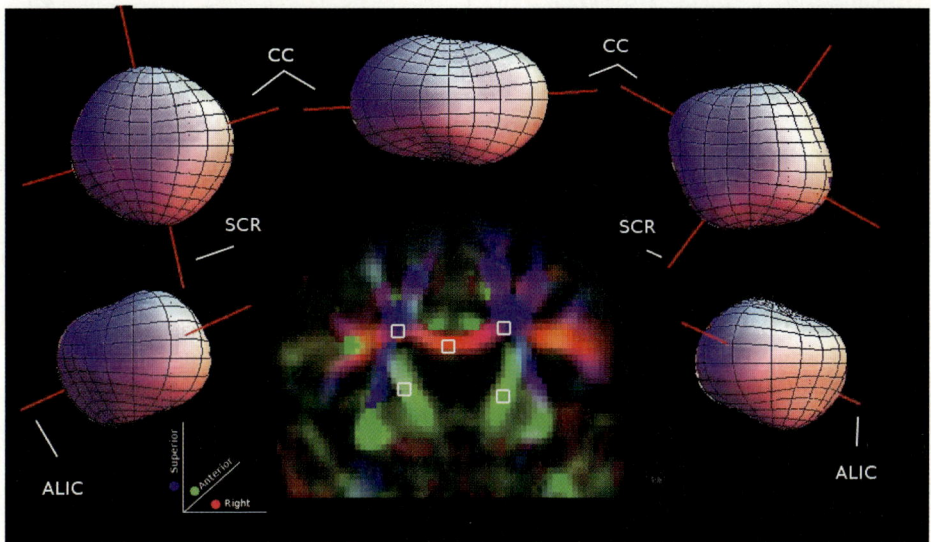

Fig. 4. Graphs showing the surface of a number of ODFs and the calculated PDs are displayed surrounding a RGB image representing the principal eigenvector of diffusion tensor. The corpus callosum (CC), the superior corona radiata (SCR) and the anterior limb of the internal capsule (ALIC) are all clearly visible as PDs of the respective graphs.

traditional DTI analysis. The surrounding graphs show the surface of the ODF along with the calculated PDs. The corpus callosum (CC), the superior corona radiata(SCR) and the anterior limb of the internal capsule (ALIC) are denoted on the graphs. Of particular importance is the ability of our method in accurately determining and distinguishing the underlying directions of the CC and the SCR in the voxels containing both.

4 Future Work

We feel that the methodology presented in this work offers a number of interesting avenues for further research. Of particularly interest is the investigation of the role that the rank of the tensor approximation has on both the accuracy of determining PDs and on the ability to distinguish two PDs that are separated by a small angle.

References

1. Wakana, S., Jiang, H., Nagae-Poetscher, L.M., van Zijl, P.C.M., Mori, S.: Fiber Tract-based Atlas of Human White Matter Anatomy. Radiology 230(1), 77–87 (2004)

2. Jellison, B.J., Field, A.S., Medow, J., Lazar, M., Salamat, M.S., Alexander, A.L.: Diffusion tensor imaging of cerebral white matter: a pictorial review of physics, fiber tract anatomy, and tumor imaging patterns. AJNR Am. J. Neuroradiol. 25(3), 356–369 (2004)
3. Basser, P.J., Pierpaoli, C.: A simplified method to measure the diffusion tensor from seven MR images. Magnetic Resonance In Medicine 39(6), 928–934 (1998)
4. Tuch, D.S.: Q-ball imaging. Magnetic Resonance in Medicine 52(6), 1358–1372 (2004)
5. Jansons, K.M., Alexander, D.C.: Persistent angular structure: new insights from diffusion magnetic resonance imaging data. Inverse Problems 19(5), 1031–1046 (2003)
6. Özarslan, E., Vemuri, B.C., Mareci, T.H.: Generalized scalar measures for diffusion MRI using trace, variance, and entropy. Magnetic Resonance in Medicine 53(4), 866–876 (2005)
7. Frank, L.R.: Characterization of anisotropy in high angular resolution diffusion-weighted MRI. Magnetic Resonance in Medicine 47(6), 1083–1099 (2002)
8. Zhan, W., Yang, Y.: How accurately can the diffusion profiles indicate multiple fiber orientations? a study on general fiber crossings in diffusion MRI. Journal of Magnetic Resonance 183(2), 193–202 (2006)
9. Perrin, M., Poupon, C., Rieul, B., Leroux, P., Constantinesco, A., Mangin, J.F., Lebihan, D.: Validation of q-ball imaging with a diffusion fibre-crossing phantom on a clinical scanner. Philos. Trans. R. Soc. Lond. B. Biol. Sci. 360(1457), 881–891 (2005)
10. Descoteaux, M.: High Angular Resolution Diffusion MRI: from Local Estimation to Segmentation and Tractography. PhD thesis, INRIA Sophia Antipolis (2008)
11. Tournier, J.D., Calamante, F., Gadian, D.G., Connelly, A.: Direct estimation of the fiber orientation density function from diffusion-weighted MRI data using spherical deconvolution. NeuroImage 23(3), 1176–1185 (2004)
12. Seunarine, K., Cook, P., Hall, M., Embleton, K., Parker, G., Alexander, D.: Exploiting peak anisotropy for tracking through complex structures. In: IEEE 11th International Conference on Computer Vision, 2007. ICCV 2007, pp. 1–8 (2007)
13. Descoteaux, M., Angelino, E., Fitzgibbons, S., Deriche, R.: Apparent diffusion coefficients from high angular resolution diffusion imaging: Estimation and applications. Magnetic Resonance in Medicine 56(2), 395–410 (2006)
14. Hess, C.P., Mukherjee, P., Han, E.T., Xu, D., Vigneron, D.B.: Q-ball reconstruction of multimodal fiber orientations using the spherical harmonic basis. Magnetic Resonance in Medicine 56(1), 104–117 (2006)
15. Descoteaux, M., Angelino, E., Fitzgibbons, S., Deriche, R.: Regularized, fast, and robust analytical q-ball imaging. Magnetic Resonance in Medicine 58(3), 497–510 (2007)
16. Qi, L.: Eigenvalues of a real supersymmetric tensor. Journal of Symbolic Computation 40(6), 1302–1324 (2005)
17. do Carmo, M.P.: Differential Geometry of Curves and Surfaces. Prentice-Hall Inc., Englewood Cliffs (1976)
18. Alexander, D.C.: Multiple-fiber reconstruction algorithms for diffusion MRI. Ann. N. Y. Acad. Sci. 1064, 113–133 (2005)

Extracting Tractosemas from a Displacement Probability Field for Tractography in DW-MRI[*]

Angelos Barmpoutis[1], Baba C. Vemuri[1,**], Dena Howland[2], and John R. Forder[3]

[1] CISE Department, University of Florida
{abarmpou,vemuri}@cise.ufl.edu
[2] Neuroscience Department, University of Florida
howland@mbi.ufl.edu
[3] Dept. of Radiology, Biomedical Engineering, U. of Florida
jforder@mbi.ufl.edu

Abstract. In this paper we present a novel method for estimating a field of asymmetric spherical functions, dubbed *tractosemas*, given the intra-voxel displacement probability information. The peaks of tractosemas correspond to directions of distinct fibers, which can have either symmetric or asymmetric local fiber structure. This is in contrast to the existing methods that estimate fiber orientation distributions which are naturally symmetric and therefore cannot model asymmetries such as splaying fibers. We propose a method for extracting tractosemas from a given field of displacement probability iso-surfaces via a diffusion process. The diffusion is performed by minimizing a kernel convolution integral, which leads to an update formula expressed in the convenient form of a discrete kernel convolution. The kernel expresses the probability of diffusion between two neighboring spherical functions and we model it by the product of Gaussian and von Mises distributions. The model is validated via experiments on synthetic and real diffusion-weighted magnetic resonance (DW-MRI) datasets from a rat hippocampus and spinal cord.

1 Introduction

The estimation of neuronal fiber orientations from diffusion-weighted MR images (DW-MRI) and the reconstruction of complex structures such as splaying and decussating fibers are problems whose solutions contribute toward achieving tractography in regions of the brain such as the optic chiasm, the hippocampus, the brain stem and others.

The local orientation of a single fiber bundle can be estimated easily from diffusion tensor images (DTI). In DTI datasets, a 2nd-order tensor has been commonly employed to approximate the local diffusivity [1]. However, it is known that 2nd-order tensors fail to approximate more complex fiber structures such as crossings, splaying and kissing structures [2].

---

[*] This research was funded in part by NIH EB007082, NIH NINDS RO1NS050699-04 and the Department of Veterans Affairs. Authors thank Dr. Timothy M. Shepherd and Mr. Min-Sig Hwang for data acquisition.
[**] Corresponding author.

More than one distinct fiber tract structure within a voxel can be estimated by employing more sophisticated models for reconstruction of the diffusion-weighted MR signal. Some of the models that have been proposed in literature include discrete [3] and continuous [4] mixture of Gaussians, higher-order tensors [5], and the spherical harmonic transformation [6]. After reconstruction of the signal, one has to compute its Fourier transform in order to obtain the displacement probability whose peaks correspond to distinct fiber orientations. The displacement probability profiles can also be computed by transforming the diffusivity profiles using the diffusion orientation transform (DOT) [7]. Multiple fiber orientations can also be estimated by reconstructing the orientation distribution function (ODF) [8] using the so called Q-ball imaging [9]. Most of the above techniques ([1,3,8,4]) can be expressed as a special case of a more generalized method in which the DW-MR signal can be expressed as the convolution over the sphere of a fiber bundle response function with the ODF [10,11]. In this spherical deconvolution approach there is no limitation regarding the number of the distinct fiber populations in the estimated ODF.

The result produced by all the above models is in the form of a spherical function representing either an ODF or an iso-surface of the displacement probability profile. In both cases the estimated spherical function characterizes the intra-voxel fiber structure without taking into consideration any inter-voxel information. As a result, the computed function is always anti-podally symmetric and therefore it can only model either single fiber tracts or symmetric crossings of multiple fiber tracts. However, it is well known that neural fiber tracts can also form asymmetric local structures such as in sprouting fibers [2]. *To date there are no existing methods in literature for estimating locally asymmetric fiber orientation functions* and one has to resort to an existing fiber tracking procedure that can accommodate for multiple fibers at a voxel [12,13,2], in order to infer the presence of a sprouting or anti-symmetric crossing structures.

In this paper we present a novel method for estimating an intra-voxel asymmetric spherical function that can model complex local fiber structures using inter-voxel information. The peaks of the estimated spherical function correspond to directions that point to distinct local fiber tracts and are appropriately dubbed *tractosemas*. Tractosema is a pointer/sign used here for neural tracts and has its roots in the Greek word sēma (sign). In our work here, we extract a field of tractosemas from a given field of ODFs or displacement probabilities by following asymmetric and orientation depended diffusion of spherical functions. The kernel that controls the diffusion process between two elements (in our case spherical functions) is defined as a function over the spatial location ($\Re^3$) and the domain (S^2 unit sphere) of the two elements, which leads us to the space $(\Re^3 \times S^2) \times (\Re^3 \times S^2)$. We construct the diffusion kernel as a tensor product of the von Mises and Gaussian probability distributions and by using it we derive an update formula for the field of tractosemas which is expressed in the form of a discrete kernel convolution.

The main contribution of this paper is that the tractosemas can depict complex asymmetric fiber structures without the need for fiber tracking. To the best of our knowledge, it is the first method that estimates a field of asymmetric spherical functions for modeling splaying fibers and other asymmetric as well as symmetric structures. Furthermore, the estimated field of tractosemas can be used as input by any existing fiber tracking algorithm for finding fiber junctions and branches without the need for multiple seeds (a common requirement in many existing methods [12,14,15,2]). Finally, the experimental results demonstrate the robustness and accuracy of our model in estimating fiber orientations in the presence of varying amount of noise as demonstrated via simulation experiments with realistic MR data synthesis [16].

2 Estimation of Tractosemas from DW-MRI

In this section we present our method on extracting tractosemas from a given field of displacement probability iso-surfaces.

2.1 Displacement Probability Estimation

The water molecule displacement probability is given by the Fourier integral

$$P(r_0 \mathbf{r}) = \int \frac{S(\mathbf{q})}{S_0} e^{-2\pi i \mathbf{q}^T \mathbf{r} r_0} d\mathbf{q} \tag{1}$$

where $\mathbf{q}$ is the reciprocal space vector, $S(q)$ is the DW-MRI signal value associated with vector $\mathbf{q}$, S_0 the zero gradient signal and $\mathbf{r}$ and r_0 is the direction and magnitude respectively of the displacement vector [17]. There are several existing methods for computing $P(r_0\mathbf{r})$ in which we either first reconstruct the signal $S(\mathbf{q})$ and then evaluate Eq. 1 [4], or we directly estimate the displacement probability from given diffusion-weighted MR data [7,18]. Also, one may obtain an alternative representation called the fiber orientation distribution (from the Q-Ball images) from which one can find the optimal fiber orientations [13,19].

In order to estimate the orientations of the underlying distinct fiber bundles a spherical function $p(\mathbf{r})$ is extracted from the volume of $P(r_0\mathbf{r})$ by either fixing r_0 [7] or by integrating over r_0 [3]. Then the orientations that correspond to the maxima of $p(\mathbf{r})$ are estimated and are used either for neural fiber tracking or further analysis [20,13,21].

$S(\mathbf{q})$ is naturally modeled by an anti-podally symmetric function and therefore its Fourier transform exhibits antipodal symmetry as well. As a result the estimated probability iso-surface $p(\mathbf{r})$ in a single voxel can not model asymmetric local neural structures such as splaying fibers. Using inter-voxel information it is possible to estimate tractosemas – which are spherical functions that are not necessarily symmetric – by diffusing a field of probability iso-surfaces. The peaks of tractosemas point to directions of distinct fiber tracts and we can extract them by employing the method presented in the following section.

2.2 Extracting Tractosemas by Diffusing Probability ISO-Surfaces

After having estimated the displacement probability $p_\mathbf{x}(\mathbf{r}) \; \forall \mathbf{x} \in \Re^3$, where $\mathbf{x}$ is the lattice index, we use the obtained spherical function field in the following diffusion process. In this process the spherical functions are updated iteratively by diffusing the displacement probability field. In general, diffusion can be seen as a smoothing process which can be performed by minimizing a smoothness measure. In our case, we minimize the following function with respect to $p_\mathbf{x}(\mathbf{r})$.

$$E(p_\mathbf{x}(\mathbf{r})) = \int_{\Re^3} \int_{S^2} K(\mathbf{x},\mathbf{y},\mathbf{r},\mathbf{v}) dist(p_\mathbf{x}(\mathbf{r}), p_\mathbf{y}(\mathbf{v})) d\mathbf{v} d\mathbf{y} \qquad (2)$$

Eq. 2 is expressed in the form of a kernel integration, where $dist(.)$ can be any norm or "edge-stopping" function [22], the kernel $K(.)$ is a function of $\mathbf{x},\mathbf{y},\mathbf{r},\mathbf{v}$, and the integration is over all vectors $\mathbf{y}$ and unit vectors $\mathbf{v}$. In our particular application, the kernel is a probability function expressing the probability of diffusion between the elements $p_\mathbf{x}(\mathbf{r})$ and $p_\mathbf{y}(\mathbf{v})$. The kernel we seek should exhibit the following properties: a) the probability of diffusion between locations $\mathbf{x}$ and $\mathbf{y}$ decreases with their distance, b) the probability of diffusion between orientations $\mathbf{r}$ and $\mathbf{v}$ decreases with the angle between them, and c) the probability of diffusion is larger at the locations along the maxima of $p_\mathbf{x}(\mathbf{r})$. These properties are satisfied by single peaked distributions. One such function used here is,

$$K(\mathbf{x},\mathbf{y},\mathbf{r},\mathbf{v}) = K_{dist}(\|\mathbf{y}-\mathbf{x}\|) K_{orient}(\mathbf{r}\cdot\mathbf{v}) K_{fiber}(\mathbf{r}\cdot(\mathbf{y}-\mathbf{x})/\|\mathbf{y}-\mathbf{x}\|)). \qquad (3)$$

The first property mentioned above is imposed by defining K_{dist} using a multivariate Gaussian distribution.

$$K_{dist}(\|\mathbf{y}-\mathbf{x}\|) = \frac{1}{(2\pi\sigma)^{3/2}} e^{-\frac{\|\mathbf{y}-\mathbf{x}\|^2}{2\sigma^3}} \qquad (4)$$

The most natural way to impose the last two properties is to employ the single peaked von Mises distribution for both K_{orient} and K_{fiber}, given by,

$$K_{orient}(cos(\phi)) = K_{fiber}(cos(\phi)) = \frac{\kappa e^{\kappa cos(\phi)}}{4\pi sinh(\kappa)} \qquad (5)$$

where ϕ is the angle between $\mathbf{r}$ and $\mathbf{v}$, and the angle between $\mathbf{r}$ and $(\mathbf{y}-\mathbf{x})$ in K_{orient} and K_{fiber} respectively. The distribution parameters σ and κ in Eq. 4 and 5 respectively control the sharpness of the kernel.

Having a discrete lattice of probabilities $p_\mathbf{x}(\mathbf{r})$ the integral over $\Re^3$ in Eq. 2 becomes summation over the lattice. Furthermore, since the Gaussian part of the kernel takes its largest values in the region around its center (at location $\mathbf{x}$), we can define a set $N(\mathbf{x})$ that contains the lattice indices in the neighborhood of $\mathbf{x}$. Furthermore, we discretize the space of unit vectors by using a 4th order subdivision of the icosahedral tessellation of the unit sphere. By using the above discretization, Eq. 2 can be written in the following form

$$E(p_\mathbf{x}(\mathbf{r})) = \sum_{\mathbf{y}\in N(\mathbf{x})} \sum_{\mathbf{v}\in S} K(\mathbf{x},\mathbf{y},\mathbf{r},\mathbf{v}) dist(p_\mathbf{x}(\mathbf{r}), p_\mathbf{y}(\mathbf{v})) \qquad (6)$$

By setting for simplicity $dist(a,b) = (a-b)^2$ and taking the derivative of Eq. 6 with respect to $p_\mathbf{x}(\mathbf{r})$ and setting it equal to zero, we derive the following update formula for the field of spherical functions (tractosemas)

$$p'_\mathbf{x}(\mathbf{r}) = \sum_{\mathbf{y}\in N(\mathbf{x})} \sum_{\mathbf{v}\in S} K(\mathbf{x},\mathbf{y},\mathbf{r},\mathbf{v}) p_\mathbf{y}(\mathbf{v}) \qquad (7)$$

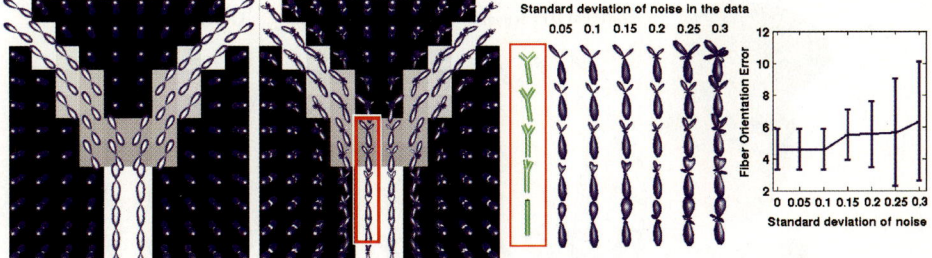

Fig. 1. Synthetic data example: a) Simulated data, b) The field of computed tractosemas, c) Tractosemas in ROI under varying noise, d) Plot of fiber orientation errors

Eq. 7 is expressed in the form of a discrete kernel convolution and it is applied iteratively to all indices **x** and vectors **r** on the discretized S^2. This method produces very efficient implementations since only kernel multiplications are involved in the evaluation of Eq. 7, which is a fully parallelizable process. Furthermore, only few iterations (2 to 3) are required to observe visually the diffused asymmetric tractosemas. Finally, choosing a different *dist* (e.g. L1 norm), would lead to more anisotropic solutions, something we are currently investigating.

3 Experimental Results

In the experiments presented in this section, we tested the performance of our method using simulated diffusion-weighted MR signal and real HARDI data sets from an isolated rat hippocampus and an excised rat spinal cord.

For the validation of tractosemas we synthesized a dataset representing splaying fiber bundles, whose orientations were taken to be tangent to two ellipsoids centered at the two lower corners of the image. The data set was of size $16 \times 16 \times 16$ and was generated by simulating the diffusion-weighted MR signal using the realistic simulation model in [16] (b-value=$1250 s/mm^2$, 81 gradient directions). After that, we estimated the displacement probability field (Fig. 1a) from the simulated signal by using the method in [18] (one can also use any other method).

The above obtained field of probability functions was then input to our proposed method for extracting tractosemas ($\sigma = 1, \kappa = 10$, 3 iterations). Fig. 1b shows the field of tractosemas computed by our technique. By observing the figure, we can see that our method estimated correctly single fiber distributions in the lower part of the image and splaying fibers in the central region of the field, which demonstrates the effectiveness of our technique. Note the smooth transition from single fiber to splaying structure in the ROI, and the expected anti-aliasing effect observed in the voxels close to the splaying fibers.

Furthermore, to quantitatively test the performance of our method in estimating fiber orientations we added varying amounts of Riccian noise (SNR between 20:1 and 3.3:1) to the data. We applied our method to these noise corrupted data sets and then computed the estimated fiber orientation errors. Figure 1d

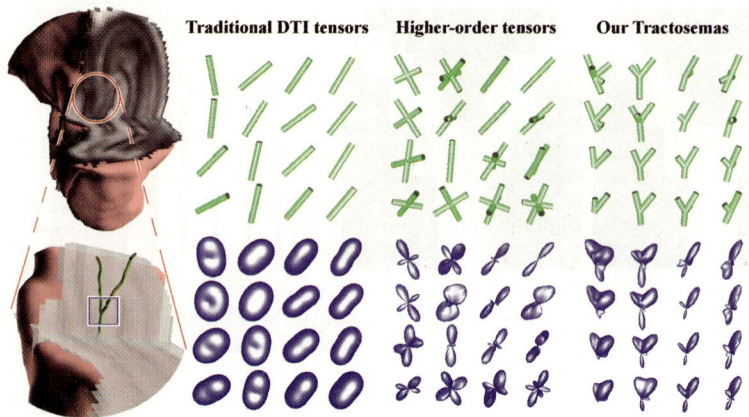

Fig. 2. Real hippocampal data. Left: The data set shown in 3D (top) and the region of interest shown enlarged (bottom). The rest of the plates depict the displacement probability profiles (bottom) and the orientations corresponding to their maxima shown as tubes (top) obtained by using: a) DTI, b) fourth order tensors, and c) Tractosemas.

depicts a plot of the mean and the standard deviation of the angle error between computed and ground truth orientations (in degrees). These results validate the accuracy of our model and demonstrate its robustness to noise.

The proposed method was also applied to a real DW-MRI from an isolated rat hippocampus (Fig. 2 left). The dataset consists of 22 images acquired using a pulsed gradient spin echo pulse sequence with TR=1.5 s, TE= 28.3 ms, G= 415 mT/m, δ= 2.4 ms, Δ= 17.8 ms, T_δ= 17 ms and $b \simeq 1250 s/mm^2$.

Figure 2 shows a region of interest (ROI) in the hippocampus containing mixture of CA3 stratum pyramidale, stratum lucidum and part of the hilus. The rest of the images in this figure show a comparison of the estimated local fiber structures using a) Diffusion tensors (order-2 DTs), b) fourth order tensors, and c) tractosemas. In the DT field we can observe two dominant orientations one pointing to the upper left and the other to the upper right corner of the ROI, however, the structure at the junction is lost. The junction was recovered using the fourth order tensors however, they depict the two aforementioned fiber orientations as symmetric structures. The complicated junction structure is correctly captured in the estimated field of tractosemas with asymmetric structures that depict splaying fibers. Fig. 3 depicts fiber tracks estimated from the hippocampal data set by following the peaks of tractosemas. The capability of tractosemas in capturing various structures is demonstrated on the left of this figure.

Finally, we extracted tractosemas from 2 control and 3 injured rat's spinal cord datasets (21 diffusion-weighted images, $b \simeq 1125 s/mm^2$). Fig. 4 shows the Cornu Posterius region in one of the control (left) and one of the injured (center) spinal cords. A variety of different fiber structures are shown (single bundles, crossings, branchings). In order to compare the estimated structures

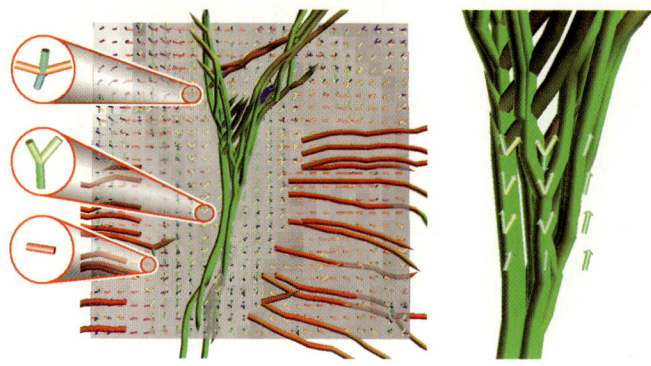

Fig. 3. The field of tractosemas estimated from the hippocampal data set. Left: Three zoomed voxels depicting the variability in the estimated structures. Right: The fiber sprouting with the estimated tractosemas superimposed.

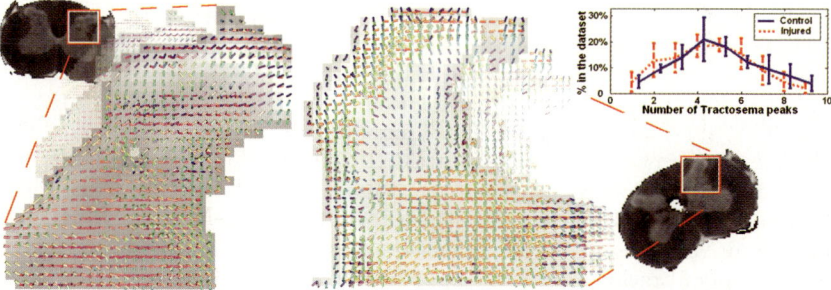

Fig. 4. Tractosemas extracted from a control (left) and an injured (center) rat's spinal cord dataset. Right: comparison of the number of peaks in the estimated tractosemas.

we plotted the average percentage of tractosemas with 1,2,3... peaks found in all control and injured sets. As it was expected, we observe a decrease in the number of peaks in the injured cords due to loss in connectivity as a result of the injury.

4 Discussion

The key difference between the proposed tractosemas and the fiber orientation distributions is that the first one is asymmetric, while the latter is symmetric. The peaks of tractosema correspond to directions that if we follow we will find the body of a distinct fiber bundle. This capability of tractosemas is due to the intervoxel information taken into consideration during the spherical function diffusion process. Finally, tractosemas are less sensitive to noise in the DW-MRI data than the displacement probability or the fiber orientation distribution. This property is evident since large amount of noise is removed by minimizing the proposed regularization term.

References

1. Basser, P.J., Mattiello, J., Lebihan, D.: Estimation of the Effective Self-Diffusion Tensor from the NMR Spin Echo. J. Magn. Reson. B 103, 247–254 (1994)
2. Basser, P.J., et al.: In vivo fiber tractography using dt-MRI data. Magnetic Resonance in Medicine 44(4), 625–632 (2000)
3. Tuch, D.S., et al.: Diffusion MRI of complex neural architecture. Neuron (40), 885–895 (2003)
4. Jian, B., Vemuri, B.C.: Multi-fiber reconstruction from diffusion MRI using mixture of Wisharts and sparse deconvolution. In: Karssemeijer, N., Lelieveldt, B. (eds.) IPMI 2007. LNCS, vol. 4584, pp. 384–395. Springer, Heidelberg (2007)
5. Ozarslan, E., Mareci, T.H.: Generalized diffusion tensor imaging and analytical relationships between DTI and HARDI. MRM 50(5), 955–965 (2003)
6. Frank, L.R.: Characterization of anisotropy in high angular resolution diffusion-weighted MRI. Magn. Reson. Med. 47(6), 1083–1099 (2002)
7. Özarslan, E., et al.: Resolution of complex tissue microarchitecture using the diffusion orientation transform (DOT). NeuroImage 31, 1086–1103 (2006)
8. Angelino, E., Fitzgibbons, S., Deriche, R.: Regularized, fast and robust analytical q-ball imaging. Magnetic Resonance in Medicine (to appear, 2007)
9. Tuch, D.: Q-ball imaging. Magn. Reson. Med. 52, 1358–1372 (2004)
10. Tournier, J., et al.: Direct estimation of the fiber orientation density function from DW-MRI data using spherical deconvolution. NeuroImage 23(3), 1176–1185 (2004)
11. Jian, B., et al.: A unified computational framework for deconvolution to reconstruct multiple fibers from diffusion weighted MRI. TMI 26(11), 1464–1471 (2007)
12. Melonakos, J., Pichon, E., Angenent, S., Tannenbaum, A.: Finsler active contours. Pattern Analysis and Machine Intelligence 30(3), 412–423 (2008)
13. Deriche, R., Descoteaux, M.: Splitting tracking through crossing fibers: Multidirectional q-ball tracking. In: ISBI, pp. 756–759 (2007)
14. Friman, O., Farneback, G., Westin, C.F.: A Bayesian approach for stochastic white matter tractography. TMI 25(8), 965–978 (2006)
15. McGraw, et al.: DTI denoising and neuronal fiber tracking. Med. IA 8, 95–111 (2004)
16. Söderman, et al: Restricted diffusion in cylindrical geometry. JMR 117 (1995)
17. Callaghan, P.T.: Principles of Nuclear Magnetic Resonance Microscopy. Clarendon Press, Oxford (1991)
18. Barmpoutis, A., et al.: Fast displacement probability profile approximation from HARDI using 4th-order tensors. In: ISBI, pp. 911–914 (2008)
19. Anderson, A.W.: Measurement of fiber orientation distributions using high angular resolution diffusion imaging. Magn. Reson. Med. 54(5), 1194–1206 (2005)
20. Maddah, M., et al.: Probabilistic clustering and quantitative analysis of white matter fiber tracts. In: Karssemeijer, N., Lelieveldt, B. (eds.) IPMI 2007. LNCS, vol. 4584, pp. 372–383. Springer, Heidelberg (2007)
21. Zhang, F., et al.: Probabilistic white matter fiber tracking using particle filtering. In: Ayache, N., Ourselin, S., Maeder, A. (eds.) MICCAI 2007, Part I. LNCS, vol. 4791, pp. 144–151. Springer, Heidelberg (2007)
22. Black, M.J., et al.: Robust anisotropic diffusion. IEEE T.I.P. 7(3), 421–432 (1998)

New Algorithms to Map Asymmetries of 3D Surfaces

Benoît Combès and Sylvain Prima

INSERM, U746, F-35042 Rennes, France
INRIA, VisAGeS Project-Team, F-35042 Rennes, France
University of Rennes I, CNRS, UMR 6074, IRISA, F-35042 Rennes, France
{bcombes,sprima}@irisa.fr
http://www.irisa.fr/visages

Abstract. In this paper, we propose a set of new generic automated processing tools to characterise the local asymmetries of anatomical structures (represented by surfaces) at an individual level, and within/between populations. The building bricks of this toolbox are: 1) a new algorithm for robust, accurate, and fast estimation of the symmetry plane of grossly symmetrical surfaces, and 2) a new algorithm for the fast, dense, nonlinear matching of surfaces. This last algorithm is used both to compute dense individual asymmetry maps on surfaces, and to register these maps to a common template for population studies. We show these two algorithms to be mathematically well-grounded, and provide some validation experiments. Then we propose a pipeline for the statistical evaluation of local asymmetries within and between populations. Finally we present some results on real data.

1 Introduction

Improved characterisation of asymmetries should help understanding the brain in normal and pathological conditions. The development of techniques for 3D imaging (especially MRI), and of processing tools for the automated analysis of grey level images has allowed the systematic study of these asymmetries [5,6]. However, artefacts in MR images, such as noise and intensity inhomogeneities, have severe confounding effects on subsequent asymmetry analyses. An alternative approach to characterise asymmetries is to segment the structure of interest first (using manual/semi-automated/automated techniques dealing with image artefacts), and then to analyse the segmented structure, by studying its boundary surface.

To our knowledge, there are only few methods allowing the automated pointwise mapping of surface asymmetries. A first approach consists in registering a template, perfectly symmetrical surface, to the surface of interest in a nonlinear way. The difference between the two displacement vectors needed to map bilateral points of the template with points of the surface is used to quantify the local asymmetry at these points [7]. A second approach normalises the surface of interest in a reference frame using several manually selected bilateral landmarks. In this reference frame, using a cylindrical coordinate system, the residual difference of radial coordinates between points of the surface having identical height and opposite azimuthal coordinates is used to quantify the local asymmetry at these points [8]. In our opinion, these methods suffer from two main limitations. First, they assume that a template (in the first approach) or a reference coordinate system (in the second) are available, which limits their application to specific problems. Second, and most importantly, the resulting mappings are *extrinsic*, as they are based on these precomputed data, and thus potentially biased by the chosen reference system.

In this paper, we propose a set of new generic automated processing tools to characterise the local asymmetries of anatomical structures (represented by surfaces) at an individual level, and within/between populations. The building bricks of this toolbox are: 1) a new algorithm for robust, accurate, and fast estimation of the symmetry plane of grossly symmetrical surfaces (Section 2), and 2) a new algorithm for the dense, non-linear matching of surfaces (Section 3). This last algorithm is used both to compute dense individual *intrinsic* asymmetry maps on surfaces, and to register these maps to a common template for population studies. We show these two algorithms to be mathematically well-grounded, and provide some validation experiments. Then we propose a pipeline for the statistical evaluation of local asymmetries within and between populations (Section 4). Finally we present some results on real data: computation of individual asymmetry maps on brain cortex, caudate nuclei and ventricles, and statistical comparison of facial asymmetry between males and females (Section 5). We conclude and give some perspectives in Section 6.

2 Symmetry Plane Computation as a ML Estimation

In this section the surface under study is represented by a cloud of points noted O. For an ideal bilateral surface having a perfect symmetry, there exists a plane P superposing each point x with its counterpart in the other side of the surface, which writes $O = S_P(O)$. However, we only deal with grossly symmetrical surfaces and thus, the cloud $S_P(O)$ is viewed as a noised version of O. In practice, we define the probability function of the data points $y_j \in S_P(O)$ as a mixture density (dependent on the unknown plane P) using the points $x_i \in O$ as follows:

$$p(y_j; P) = \sum_{x_i \in O} p(y_j, x_i; P) = \sum_{x_i \in O} A_{i,j} p(y_j | x_i; P) \qquad (1)$$

There are as many mixture components as there are points in O. Intuitively, the unknown mixture component $A_{i,j}$ conveys the affinity between the points y_j and x_i. Note that $\sum_i A_{i,j} = 1$. If we consider all the data points y_j to be independent, then the likelihood of the cloud $S_P(O)$ can be written as:

$$L(P) = \prod_{y_j \in S_P(O)} \sum_{x_i \in O} A_{i,j} p(y_j | x_i; P) \qquad (2)$$

We then define the optimal plane $\tilde{P}$ using the maximum likelihood principle. Considering the conditional densities $p(y_j|x_i; P)$ as Gaussian with variance σ^2, we use the Expectation-Maximisation (EM) algorithm to estimate P. If we note $x_j = S_P(y_j) \in O$ for the sake of simplicity, the EM algorithm can be shown to yield the very simple following iterative scheme:

> **Init**: Initialise $\tilde{P}$
> **E-step**: $\forall i,j$, $\tilde{A}_{i,j} = \dfrac{\exp(-||x_j - S_{\tilde{P}}(x_i)||^2/(2\sigma^2))}{\sum_k \exp(-||x_j - S_{\tilde{P}}(x_k)||^2/(2\sigma^2))}$
> **M-step**: $\tilde{P} = \arg\min_P \sum_{(x_i,x_j) \in O^2} \tilde{A}_{i,j}||x_j - S_P(x_i)||^2$
> **Check**: If $\tilde{P}$ has changed go to E-step else finish

The M-step has a closed-form solution and the algorithm can be shown to converge to a local maximum of the likelihood function. Further implementation choices, details on how to deal with outliers, and complete evaluation of the algorithm can be found elsewhere [9].

3 Dense Non-linear Matching as a MAP Estimation

Numerous algorithms have been proposed to estimate non-linear transformations between 3D surfaces. One of the most successful techniques [11] to have been proposed for this purpose was inspired by the ICP algorithm [10]. It consists in 1) defining a spherical neighbourhood around each point of the *moving* surface, 2) matching each point within this neighbourhood with its closest point on the *reference* surface, 3) estimating the optimal rigid-body transformation using these correspondences, and 4) smoothing this set of pointwise rigid-body transformations to get locally affine transformations. This algorithm suffers from two major problems: 1) there is no proof of its convergence, and 2) the linear part (3 × 3 matrix) of the final pointwise affine transformation is computed by weighted averaging of the rotation matrices "entrywise", which is not optimal.

In the following, we propose a new algorithm to deal with these two problems. As Feldmar & Ayache, we estimate one affine transformation for each point of the moving surface, but without using its neighbours. Instead, we add a spatial constraint on the estimated transformation, so that it is close to the transformations estimated at neighbouring points. This is performed using a probabilistic interpretation of the dense non-linear matching, which is viewed as a maximum *a posteriori* (MAP) estimation problem.

We consider two surfaces $X = \{x_i, i = 1, \ldots, L\}$ and $Z = \{z_k, k = 1, \ldots, M\}$. The problem is 1) to match each point x_i in X with a point $y_i = z_j$ in Z, and 2) to compute the affine transformation T_i relating x_i with y_i. Let us name $Y = \{y_i, i = 1, \ldots, L\}$ and $T = \{T_i, i = 1, \ldots, L\}$. We consider each point $x_i \in X$ (resp. each $T_i \in T$) as the realisation of a random variable $\mathbf{X_i}$ (resp. $\mathbf{T_i}$). We name $\mathbf{X}$ and $\mathbf{T}$ the two related sets of random variables. Then we suppose that $\mathbf{X_i}$, $\mathbf{T_i}$ and y_i relate to each other following: $\mathbf{X_i} = \mathbf{T_i}(y_i) + \epsilon$, where $\epsilon \sim \mathcal{N}(0, \sigma^2)$ as in Section 2. If we assume that the random variables $\mathbf{X_i}$ are independent then we can write the conditional probability of $\mathbf{X}$ given $\mathbf{T}$ (which is also the likelihood of the data X) as:

$$l(\mathbf{X}=X|\mathbf{T}=T;Y) = \frac{1}{(2\pi)^{3L/2}\sigma^{3L}} \exp \sum_{i=1,\ldots,L} -\frac{||x_i - T_i(y_i)||^2}{2\sigma^2}$$

It is not possible to compute the transformations T_i in a unique way without additional constraints. Given that neighbouring points must have similar T_i, we consider that $\mathbf{T}$ is a Markov random field, with a Gibbs p.d.f. defined as (A_i and t_i being the linear and translation components of T_i):

$$P(\mathbf{T}=T) = \frac{1}{Z} \exp(-\sum_{(i,j) \in C_2(X)} (\alpha ||A_i - A_j||_F^2 + \beta ||t_i - t_j||_F^2))$$

where Z is a normalisation constant, $||.||_F$ is the Frobenius norm, α, β are positive numbers, and $C_2(X)$ is the set of second-order cliques of X. In practice, the cliques are determined using a mesh: $(i,j) \in C_2 \Leftrightarrow$ there exists an edge between points x_i and x_j. Following Bayes rule, we then have $P(\mathbf{T}|\mathbf{X}) \propto l(\mathbf{X}|\mathbf{T};Y)P(\mathbf{T})$.

The optimal set of transformations $T = \{T_i, i \in 1, \ldots, L\}$ is then defined as the one maximising this posterior probability. This optimisation can be performed using the ICM algorithm [12], which consists in considering sequentially each $T_i \in T$ and maximising the posterior for T_i while keeping the other transformations fixed. This algorithm converges monotonically to a (at least local) maximum of the criterion, and boils down to:

Step 0: Initialise $\tilde{T}$
Step 1: $\forall i \ \tilde{T}_i = \arg\min_{T_i} ||x_i - A_i y_i - t_i||^2 + \sum_{j \in V_i} \left(\alpha ||A_i - \tilde{A}_j||_F^2 + \beta ||t_i - \tilde{t}_j||^2 \right)$
Step 2: If $\tilde{T}$ has changed go to Step 1 else finish

---

where V_i contains the indices of neighbours of point x_i in X. It can be shown that Step 1 has a unique solution (provided $\alpha > 0$ and $\beta \geq 0$) that is given by the following closed form solution (with $N_i = \text{card}(V_i)$):

$$\begin{cases} \tilde{A}_i = \left[\frac{\beta}{1+\beta N_i}(N_i x_i - \sum_{j \in V_i} \tilde{t}_j) y_i^T + \alpha \sum_{j \in V_i} \tilde{A}_j\right] \left[\frac{\beta N_i}{1+\beta N_i} y_i y_i^T + \alpha N_i I_3\right]^{-1} \\ \tilde{t}_i = \frac{1}{1+\beta N_i}(x_i - \tilde{A}_i y_i + \beta \sum_{j \in V_i} \tilde{t}_j) \end{cases}$$

This solution assumes that the set of correspondences Y is known, which is not the case. In practice, the set Y can be seen as a parameter of the conditional p.d.f. of $\mathbf{X}|\mathbf{T}$, and can be estimated within the ICM using the ML principle, which yields the following final iterative algorithm, that can also be shown to converge monotonically to a local minimum of $P(\mathbf{T}|\mathbf{X})$:

Step 0: Initialise $\tilde{T}$
Step 1: $\tilde{Y} = \arg\max_Y l(\mathbf{X}=X|\mathbf{T}=\tilde{T};Y)$
Step 2: $\tilde{T} = \arg\max_T P(\mathbf{T}=T|\mathbf{X}=X;\tilde{Y})$
Step 3: If $\tilde{T}$ has changed go to Step 1 else finish

Step 1 is simply solved by: $\tilde{Y} = \{\tilde{y}_i = \arg\min_{z_k \in Z} ||x_i - \tilde{T}_i(z_k)||$ for $i = 1, \ldots, L\}$. Step 2 is solved thanks to the iterative algorithm previously described. The overall algorithm has a very intuitive interpretation, as it simply boils down to the iterative estimation of the optimal correspondences between the two surfaces and the local affine transformations best superposing the two surfaces given the correspondences. In practice, the initial $\tilde{T}$ is chosen as the similarity transformation best superposing X and Z [10]. Moreover, we tackle outliers at the end of Step 1 by detecting points x_i for which y_i is a border point of Z or has a normal too different from that at x_i. The data attachment term is then set to 0 in Step 2 for these terms, whose $\tilde{T}_i$ is then estimated using only the regularisation term. A simpler, degenerate model, consists in choosing T_i as a pure translation. The comparative merits of the two models are still to be evaluated.

Note that the proposed algorithm is close to the one recently proposed by Amberg et al. [13]. However, our Markovian interpretation allows to solve Step 2 with the ICM algorithm. This provides advantages in terms of computational time and implementation easiness compared to the solution proposed by Amberg et al., which implies inversion of a sparse square matrix of size $(4\,\text{card}(X))^2$. The same can be said about many other competing algorithms, for instance those using thin plane splines as a regulariser [14,15] which are inadequate for many applications with large point sets. On the contrary, our algorithm has an average run time of 4 min on a standard PC for surfaces with 100,000 points.

4 Asymmetry Mapping

4.1 Pipeline

Using the tools presented in Sections 2 and 3, we propose the following pipeline for statistical analysis of asymmetry on surfaces $X_1, \ldots, X_n$:

- Step 1: Estimation of the symmetry plane P_k of X_k $\forall k = 1, \ldots, n$
- Step 2: Non-linear registration of X_k with $S_{P_k}(X_k)$: each point x_i in X_k is matched with a point y_i in $S_{P_k}(X_k)$; $x_i - y_i$ quantifies the asymmetry at point x_i (*individual* asymmetry mapping)
- Step 3: Non-linear registration of X_k with a template surface T: each point t_i in T is matched with a point x_i in X_k; the asymmetry measure at point x_i is then projected to point t_i on the template (*normalised* asymmetry mapping)
- Step 4: Statistical tests (within/between populations) at each point of T (t-test, Hotelling's test, *etc.*) with/without correction for multiple comparisons.

Steps 1-2-3 are displayed on Fig. 1. Once the vector $x_i - y_i$ is computed, it is possible to compute its signed (or unsigned) norm which makes the projection on the template easier and the display visually appealing. The sign is computed using the dot product between $x_i - y_i$ and the normal at x_i (computed using a mesh for instance). The template T is chosen as one of the images in the dataset and made symmetrical after its symmetry plane is estimated.

4.2 Validation of the Individual and Normalised Mappings

We evaluate the accuracy of the non-linear registration for individual and normalised asymmetry mapping on synthetic and real data. The parameters of the two algorithms (symmetry plane estimation and registration) are $\sigma = 0.5$ and $\alpha = \beta = 20$ (initial value) to 0.5 (final value) using a decreasing scale factor of 1.2. We consider 15 surfaces (laser scans of human faces). We manually define 10 homologous landmarks on each surface. These landmarks are chosen to be either pairs of bilateral or mid-facial points. Three experiments are devised:

- We register the 15 surfaces to the template T, compute the mean error between the homologous landmarks, and average these errors over the 15 surfaces.
- We compute the symmetry plane of each surface, flip the surface with respect to the plane, register the two surfaces, compute the mean error between the homologous landmarks, and average these errors over the 15 surfaces.
- We choose one of the 15 surfaces, make it symmetrical after computing its symmetry plane, add unilateral deformations and remove a given quantity of adjacent points (to generate occlusions). We map the unsigned asymmetries of the surface and project them to the template (Fig. 2). We also map the asymmetries of the surface using the approach of Ólafsdóttir et al. (performing the registration task with our tool for fair comparison) [7].

The conclusions are twofold. First, the mean error in the first experiment ($2.63\text{mm} \pm 0.59\text{mm}$) is larger than the error in the second ($0.67\text{mm} \pm 0.13\text{mm}$),

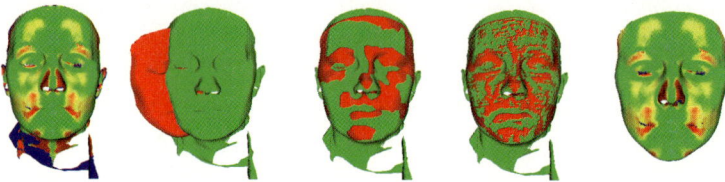

Fig. 1. Individual and normalised asymmetry mapping. From left to right: individual asymmetry mapping; surface and template before registration; surface and template after similarity-based registration; surface and template after non-linear registration; normalised asymmetry mapping on the template.

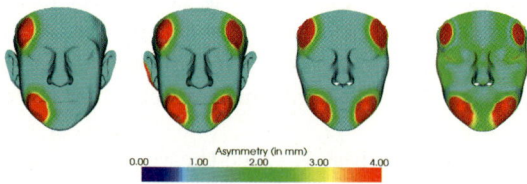

Fig. 2. Evaluation of the asymmetry mapping / comparison with another method. From left to right: a deformation field is applied to a perfectly symmetrical face; estimated asymmetry map by our method; normalised asymmetry map on the template; template-based asymmetry map as estimated by another method [7].

which is intuitive and simply suggests that two halves of a given face are more similar than two different faces. It must be noted that the measured errors include the imprecision of the manual delineation of the landmarks. Second, our algorithm has a mean accuracy of 0.6mm ± 0.5mm when recovering ground truth asymmetries, and proves to be superior to the competitive algorithm [7]. This is not surprising, as in this last method the individual asymmetry mapping is based on the registration of the two sides of the surface with the template, which is less precise than registering the two sides of the same surface together.

5 Results

We illustrate our method on different applications. First, we segment the brain cortex (300,000 points, `brainvisa.info`), the caudate nuclei and the ventricles (10,000 points, `itksnap.org`) from the T1-weighted MRI of a healthy subject, and we compute individual asymmetry maps (Fig. 3). Second, we perform the statistical analysis of face asymmetry within and between 15 healthy males and 15 females (Fig. 4) using laser scans (80,000 points, `fastscan3d.com`).

Interestingly, we recover the well-known *Yakovlevian torque* of the cortex (opposite asymmetry of the occipital and frontal lobes), hypothesized to be linked to language. Registering the two hemispheres is a difficult task and other non-linear techniques [16] will be tested for comparison with ours in future works. Mapping asymmetry of caudate nuclei is also of interest, as *e.g.* anomalies of left-right volume differences have been shown to predict attention-deficit hyperactivity disorders in children [17]. Similarly, asymmetry of lateral ventricles in utero has

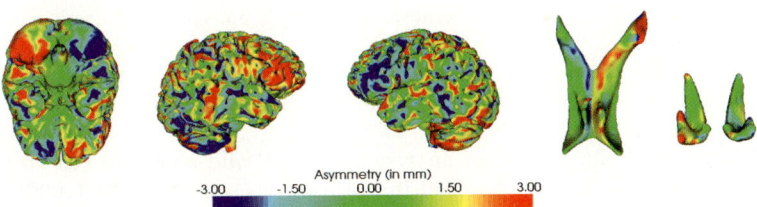

Fig. 3. Individual asymmetry mapping on a given subject. Left to right: brain cortex, lateral ventricles and caudate nuclei. Different views.

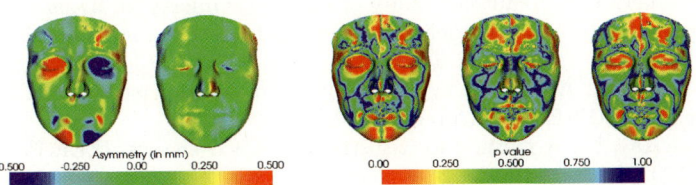

Fig. 4. Statistical analysis of asymmetry. Left to right: mean signed asymmetry maps on men/women, uncorrected p-value maps (using *t*-tests) of statistically significant asymmetry among men, among women, and comparison between men and women.

been hypothesized to be indicative of cerebral pathology [18]. At last, preliminary results on facial data suggest that the women are more symmetrical than men. Recent works also suggest that subtle facial dysmorphologies/asymmetries, could be present in schizophrenia [19].

6 Conclusion

We have presented a set of tools for the pointwise asymmetry mapping of 3D surfaces and statistical analysis of these asymmetries within and between populations. We have proved our methods to be theoretically well-grounded, provided some validation experiments, and shown them to be superior to a competitive state-of-the-art method. Further work will consist in testing other operators on the asymmetry vector field to emphasize other types of asymmetries (*e.g.* shrinking/expanding regions compared to contralateral areas). Comparisons with other techniques [6] based on grey value images will also be performed.

References

1. Toga, A., Thompson, P.: Mapping brain asymmetry. Nature Reviews Neuroscience 4(1), 37–48 (2003)
2. Holloway, R.L., et al.: Brain endocast asymmetry in pongids and hominids: some preliminary findings on the paleontology of cerebral dominance. Am. J. Phys. Anthropol. 58(1), 101–110 (1982)
3. Gannon, P.J., et al.: Asymmetry of chimpanzee planum temporale: humanlike pattern of Wernicke's brain language area homolog. Science 279(5348), 220–222 (1998)
4. Crow, T.: Cerebral asymmetry and the lateralization of language: core deficits in schizophrenia as pointers to the genetic predisposition. Current Opinion in Psychiatry 17(2), 97–106 (2004)
5. Good, C., et al.: Cerebral asymmetry and the effects of sex and handedness on brain structure: a voxel-based morphometric analysis of 465 normal adult human brains. NeuroImage 14(3), 685–700 (2001)
6. Thirion, J.-P., et al.: Statistical analysis of normal and abnormal dissymmetry in volumetric medical images. Medical Image Analysis 4(2), 111–121 (2000)
7. Ólafsdóttir, H., et al.: A point-wise quantification of asymmetry using deformation fields: application to the study of the Crouzon mouse model. In: Ayache, N., Ourselin, S., Maeder, A. (eds.) MICCAI 2007, Part II. LNCS, vol. 4792, pp. 452–459. Springer, Heidelberg (2007)
8. Liu, Y., Palmer, J.: A quantified study of facial asymmetry in 3D faces. In: IEEE Workshop on Analysis and Modeling of Faces and Gestures, pp. 222–229 (October 2003)
9. Combès, B., et al.: Automatic symmetry plane estimation of bilateral objects in point clouds. In: IEEE CVPR (June 2008)
10. Besl, P., McKay, N.: A method for registration of 3-D shapes. IEEE PAMI 14(2), 239–256 (1992)
11. Feldmar, J., Ayache, N.: Rigid, affine and locally affine registration of free-form surfaces. Int. J. Comput. Vision 18(2), 99–119 (1996)
12. Besag, J.: On the statistical analysis of dirty pictures. Journal of the Royal Statistical Society B-48(3), 259–302 (1986)

13. Amberg, B., et al.: Optimal step nonrigid ICP algorithms for surface registration. In: IEEE CVPR, pp. 1–8 (June 2007)
14. Chui, H., Rangarajan, A.: A new point matching algorithm for non-rigid registration. Computer Vision and Image Understanding 89(2-3), 114–141 (2003)
15. Jian, B., Vemuri, B.: A robust algorithm for point set registration using mixture of Gaussians. In: IEEE ICCV, pp. 1246–1251 (October 2005)
16. Bansal, et al.: ROC-based assessments of 3D cortical surface-matching algorithms. NeuroImage 24(1), 150–162 (2002)
17. Achiron, R., et al.: Cerebral lateral ventricular asymmetry: is this a normal ultrasonographic finding in the fetal brain? Obstet. Gynecol. 89(2), 233–237 (1997)
18. Castellanos, F.X., et al.: Quantitative morphology of the caudate nucleus in attention deficit hyperactivity disorder. Am. J. Psychiatry 151(12), 1791–1796 (1994)
19. Hennessy, R., et al.: Facial shape and asymmetry by three-dimensional laser surface scanning covary with cognition in a sexually dimorphic manner. J. Neuropsychiatry Clin. Neurosci. 18(1), 73–80 (2006)

A Distributed Spatio-temporal EEG/MEG Inverse Solver

Wanmei Ou[1], Polina Golland[1], and Matti Hämäläinen[2]

[1] Computer Science and Artificial Intelligence Laboratory, MIT, USA
[2] Athinoula A. Martinos Center for Biomedical Imaging, MGH, USA
wanmei@csail.mit.edu

Abstract. We propose a novel $\ell_1\ell_2$-norm inverse solver for estimating the sources of EEG/MEG signals. Based on the standard ℓ_1-norm inverse solver, the proposed sparse distributed inverse solver integrates the ℓ_1-norm spatial model with a temporal model of the source signals in order to avoid unstable activation patterns and "spiky" reconstructed signals often produced by the original solvers. The joint spatio-temporal model leads to a cost function with an $\ell_1\ell_2$-norm regularizer whose minimization can be reduced to a convex second-order cone programming problem and efficiently solved using the interior-point method. Validation with simulated and real MEG data shows that the proposed solver yields source time course estimates qualitatively similar to those obtained through dipole fitting, but without the need to specify the number of dipole sources in advance. Furthermore, the $\ell_1\ell_2$-norm solver achieves fewer false positives and a better representation of the source locations than the conventional ℓ_2 minimum-norm estimates.

1 Introduction

Localizing activated regions from Electroencephalography (EEG) or Magnetoencephalography (MEG) data involves solving an ill-posed inverse problem. This paper introduces an integrated spatio-temporal regularizer to overcome the instabilities in the standard sparse solutions.

There are two main types of inverse solvers in EEG/MEG applications: discrete parametric solvers, also known as dipole fitting [13], and distributed inverse solvers [7,17]. The standard dipole fitting algorithms estimate the location, orientation, and amplitudes of a fixed number of current dipoles. While dipole fitting often provides robust estimates for activation signals, localization is challenging when several sources are active. The quality of the results degrades substantially when the assumed number of dipoles differs from the true number [9].

In contrast, distributed solvers discretize the source space into locations on the cortical surface or in the brain volume without fixing the number of current dipoles. The solution is computed by minimizing a cost function that depends on all sources in the source space. The widely used minimum norm estimate (MNE) [7] recovers a source distribution with minimum overall energy (ℓ_2-norm) that produces data consistent with the measurements. Although MNE leads to a linear inverse operator, its solutions are often too diffuse to be biologically plausible, especially in early sensory activations. Other regularizers based on a norm penalty were proposed to model sparsity in such applications. Among them, the minimum current estimate (MCE) (ℓ_1-norm) is the most popular [17].

One of the drawbacks of the conventional MCE is its sensitivity to noise. Similar to other distributed solvers, the conventional MCE is computed at each time point separately. The solver's sensitivity to noise causes the estimated activations to "jump" among neighboring spatial locations from one time instant to another. Equivalently, the time course at a particular location can show substantially "spiky" discontinuities. To address this problem, the vector-based spatio-temporal minimum ℓ_1-norm solver (VESTAL) [10] projects the point-wise ℓ_1-norm estimates onto a set of temporal basis functions estimated from the data. Some other wavelet-based methods perform reconstruction of the coefficients of each basis function separately [6,16].

Similar to MCE, we employ the ℓ_1-norm regularizer to encourage spatial sparsity. Furthermore, we incorporate a temporal model of the source signals into the regularizer. Specifically, we assume that the source signals are linear combinations of *multiple* temporal basis functions, and apply the distributed inverse solver to the coefficients of all basis functions simultaneously, in contrast to the two-step approach proposed in [10]. This combined spatio-temporal regularizer is at the core of our $\ell_1\ell_2$-norm inverse solver, and it is motivated by a previously demonstrated method in farfield narrowband sensor array applications [12]. We construct the temporal basis functions through singular-value decomposition (SVD) of the measurements, since it compactly represents the signal subspace. Although we focus on the EEG/MEG application, the proposed framework is applicable to computed tomography reconstruction, with modifications on the spatial model so as to encourage piece-wise constant solutions (i.e., ℓ_1-norm on spatial derivatives of the source).

To summarize, the proposed solver imposes ℓ_1-norm regularization in the spatial domain and ℓ_2-norm regularization in the temporal domain. The resulting inverse problem can be formulated as a second-order cone programming (SOCP) problem and solved efficiently using the interior-point method [1]. Thanks to the integrated spatio-temporal model, our method achieves accurate reconstruction results and outperforms other solvers including MNE [7], MCE [17], and VESTAL [10].

2 Method

Under the *quasi-static* approximation of Maxwell's equations, the observed EEG/MEG signal $\mathbf{y}(t)$ at time t is a linear function of the current sources $\mathbf{s}(t)$:

$$\mathbf{y}(t) = \mathbf{A}\mathbf{s}(t) + \mathbf{e}(t), \tag{1}$$

where $\mathbf{A}$ is the $N \times M$ lead-field matrix. $\mathbf{e}(t) \sim \mathcal{N}(\mathbf{0}, \Sigma)$ is the measurement noise, where the noise covariance Σ can be estimated from the pre-stimulus data. $\mathbf{s}(t)$, $N \times 1$, and $\mathbf{y}(t)$, $M \times 1$, are vectors in the source space and the signal space, respectively. The number of sources N ($\sim 10^3 - 10^4$) is much larger than the number of measurements M ($\sim 10^2$), leading to an infinite number of solutions satisfying Eq. (1) even for $\mathbf{e}(t) = \mathbf{0}$. Without loss of generality, we can apply spatial whitening based on the estimated noise covariance Σ to both the data and the lead-field matrix, leading to $\mathbf{e}(t) \sim \mathcal{N}(\mathbf{0}, \mathbf{I})$ in the derivations.

Spatio-Temporal Model. The quasi-static assumption allows inverse estimation for each time instant independently. However, this often results in highly variable source time courses. To mitigate this problem, we utilize the knowledge of the temporal properties of the source signals to further constrain the solution. To this end, we express the data model in Eq. (1) for all time instants:

$$\mathbf{Y} = \mathbf{A}\mathbf{S} + \mathbf{E}, \tag{2}$$

where $\mathbf{Y} = [\mathbf{y}(1), \mathbf{y}(2), \cdots, \mathbf{y}(T)]$ is an $M \times T$ matrix that contains EEG/MEG measurements for all T temporal samples, and $\mathbf{S}$ is an $N \times T$ matrix that represents the source signals. Noise $\mathbf{E}$ is assumed to be independent in time.

The underlying source signals vary smoothly but with sharp changes at certain deflections [9]. To model the time-varying frequency content of the signals, we assume that the source signals are linear combinations of multiple orthonormal temporal basis functions $\mathbf{V} = [\mathbf{v}_1, \mathbf{v}_2, \cdots, \mathbf{v}_K]$ that collectively capture the temporal properties of the source signals. $\mathbf{v}_k$, $T \times 1$, denotes the kth basis function. We can therefore transform the problem into a much lower dimensional space of projection coefficients $\widetilde{\mathbf{Y}} = \mathbf{A}\widetilde{\mathbf{S}} + \widetilde{\mathbf{E}}$, where $\widetilde{\mathbf{Y}} = \mathbf{Y}\mathbf{V}$, $\widetilde{\mathbf{S}} = \mathbf{S}\mathbf{V}$, and $\widetilde{\mathbf{E}} = \mathbf{E}\mathbf{V}$. The (n,k) element of $\widetilde{\mathbf{S}}$, $\widetilde{s}_{nk}$, indicates the kth coefficient for the source signal at location n. Denoting the kth column of $\widetilde{\mathbf{E}}$ by $\widetilde{\mathbf{e}}_k$, the temporal independence assumption of $\mathbf{E}$ and orthonormality of $\mathbf{V}$ imply that $\widetilde{\mathbf{e}}_k \sim \mathcal{N}(\mathbf{0}; \mathbf{I})$, and that $\widetilde{\mathbf{e}}_k$ and $\widetilde{\mathbf{e}}_{k'}$ are independent for $k \neq k'$.

To compute the inverse solutions for all K basis functions simultaneously, we use the signal magnitude in the subspace spanned by $\mathbf{V}$, $\sqrt{\sum_{k=1}^{K} \widetilde{s}_{nk}^2}$, as an indicator of the activation status at location n. In other words, we apply ℓ_2-norm regularization to the K coefficients for each source location. Because we choose to work with orthonormal basis functions, the ℓ_2-norm of the reconstructed source signal in the temporal domain is equal to the ℓ_2-norm in the transformed domain. However, we find it more intuitive to present the model in the transformed domain. Furthermore, if two bases span the same subspace, the reconstruction results using these bases are guaranteed to be identical.

With the ℓ_1-norm regularization in the spatial domain and the ℓ_2-norm regularization in the temporal domain, we incorporate the integrated spatio-temporal $\ell_1\ell_2$-norm regularizer

$$|\widetilde{\mathbf{S}}|_{\ell_1}^{\ell_2} = \sum_{n=1}^{N} \sqrt{\sum_{k=1}^{K} \widetilde{s}_{nk}^2} \tag{3}$$

into the estimation problem:

$$\widetilde{\mathbf{S}}^* = \arg\min_{\widetilde{\mathbf{S}}} \sum_{k=1}^{K} \|\widetilde{\mathbf{y}}_k - \mathbf{A}\widetilde{\mathbf{s}}_k\|_{\ell_2}^2 + \lambda |\widetilde{\mathbf{S}}|_{\ell_1}^{\ell_2}, \tag{4}$$

where $\widetilde{\mathbf{s}}_k$ and $\widetilde{\mathbf{y}}_k$ are the kth column vectors in $\widetilde{\mathbf{S}}$ and $\widetilde{\mathbf{Y}}$. λ controls the regularization strength; $\|\mathbf{x}\|_{\ell_2} = \sqrt{\mathbf{x}^T\mathbf{x}}$. Since the ℓ_2-norm does not encourage sparsity, many coefficients for an active location are usually non-zero in the estimates. The reconstructed source signals are then obtained as linear combinations of the basis functions: $\mathbf{S}^* = \widetilde{\mathbf{S}}^* \mathbf{V}^T$. Here we focus on fixed-orientation source models, but the model can also be easily extended to the free-orientation formulation as proposed in [4,11].

The above derivations are independent of the selected basis $\mathbf{V}$, but a compact representation of the signals can substantially reduce computation. We choose to use the K largest SVD components of the measurements, which can often compactly capture the time-varying frequency content and differences in source signals from different regions.

From $\ell_1\ell_2$-Norm Regularizer to SOCP. We cannot directly apply gradient based methods to the optimization problem specified by Eq. (4) since the $\ell_1\ell_2$-norm penalty term is not differentiable at zero. However, Eq. (4) can be reduced to the second-order cone programming (SOCP) problem [1]:

$$<\widetilde{\mathbf{S}}^*, q^*, z^*, \mathbf{w}^*, \mathbf{r}^*> = \arg\min_{<\widetilde{\mathbf{S}}, q, z, \mathbf{w}, \mathbf{r}>} (q + \lambda z) \quad (5)$$

$$\text{s.t.} \quad \|\widetilde{\mathbf{y}}_k - \mathbf{A}\widetilde{\mathbf{s}}_k\|_{\ell_2}^2 \leq w_k \quad \forall\, k = 1, \cdots, K \quad (6)$$

$$\sum_{k=1}^{K} w_k \leq q; \quad \sqrt{\sum_{k=1}^{K} \widetilde{s}_{nk}^2} \leq r_n \quad \forall\, n = 1, \cdots, N; \quad \sum_{n=1}^{N} r_n \leq z \quad (7)$$

The conversion introduces new variables, q, z, $\{w_k\}_{k=1}^{K}$, and $\{r_n\}_{n=1}^{N}$. w_k is an upper bound on the discrepancy between the measurements and the signals induced by the estimated sources along $\mathbf{v}_k$. q is an upper bound on all w_k's. r_n is an upper bound on the activation strength for location n. z is an upper bound on the ℓ_1-norm of the activation strength of all N locations. At the minimum, the inequality constraints in Eq. (6-7) are satisfied with equality; otherwise, the objective function can be further reduced.

SOCP is a convex optimization problem. Linear programs and quadratically constrained quadratic programs are subsets of the SOCP problems. Furthermore, the SOCP problem is a special case of a semi-definite program, and therefore SOCP can be solved efficiently using the interior-point method [1].

3 Results

Due to the lack of ground truth in real experiments, we first study the behavior of the method and its sensitivity to noise and parameter settings using simulated data. We then compare the method to standard inverse solvers using real MEG data from a somatosensory study.

3.1 Simulation Studies

To simulate MEG measurements, we created active vertices A, B, and C (Fig. 1 top) on the cortical sheet at source spacing of 20 mm, with current source orientation along the normal to the cortex. The simulated time courses (black, Fig. 1 bottom) exhibit temporal characteristics similar to those of the auditory evoked

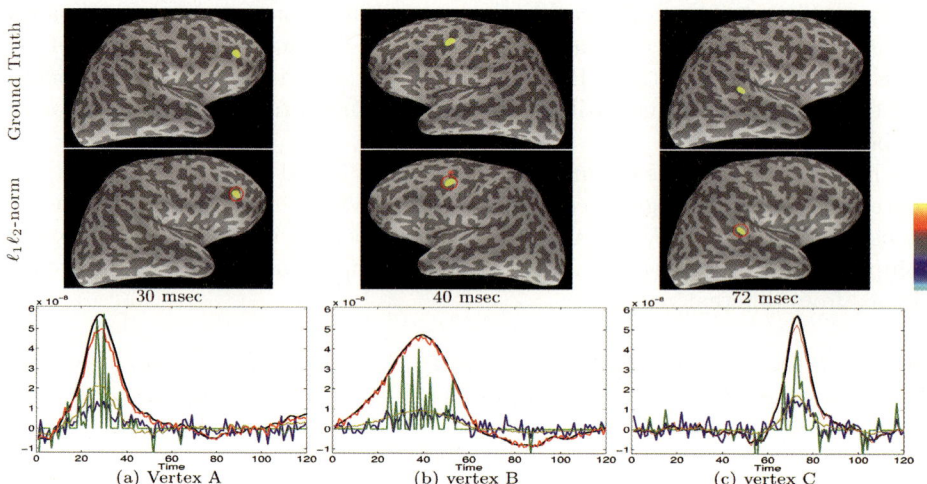

Fig. 1. Simulated study. Top: ground truth activation maps at peak response time for three sources. Middle: spatial maps estimated using $\ell_1\ell_2$-norm inverse solver for the same time points. Bottom: time courses from the three active vertices: ground truth (black), MNE (blue), MCE (green), VESTAL (yellow), and $\ell_1\ell_2$-norm (red).

responses, but with additional temporal translation and scaling. The source signals at vertices A and B show activation during overlapping time intervals, which makes the inverse problem difficult. For the forward calculations, we employed the sensor configuration of the 306-channel MEG system used in our real studies and added Gaussian noise to the signals. The resulting signals have an SNR of 3 dB, within the typically SNR range of real MEG data.

Fig. 1 shows the inverse solutions at three time frames obtained by the proposed method using three basis functions and $\lambda = 10^9$. These parameters were selected based on validation experiments presented later in this section. The red curves in Fig. 1 correspond to source signals estimated by the method. The resulting spatial maps and source time courses match well with the ground truth.

Comparison with MNE, MCE, and VESTAL. We compared the proposed method with the standard MNE, MCE, and VESTAL (Fig. 1 bottom). The estimates from the standard MNE are smaller and more diffuse when compared with the simulated signals. The estimated time courses from MCE exhibit "spiky" discontinuities due to the solver's sensitivity to noise. Projecting MCE results into the signal subspace spanned by **V** (VESTAL) removes the discontinuities, but the estimation accuracy is significantly worse than that of $\ell_1\ell_2$-norm since the two-step procedure cannot fully compensate for the errors in the original MCE solutions.

Sensitivity to Noise, Basis Selection, and Regularization. To examine the sensitivity of the method to noise and basis selection, we computed inverse solutions for 100 independently generated data sets for each noise setting (SNR 1-8 dB) and basis selection cutoff (K=1-6). Fig. 2a shows the relative mean

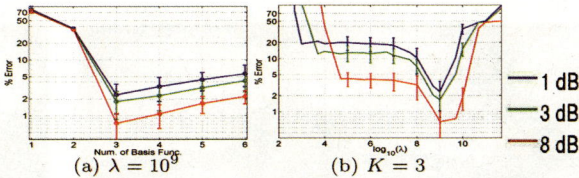

Fig. 2. Relative mean squares error for different values of basis size K and regularization parameter λ under three different SNR settings. The error bars close to the bottom of the figures appear large due to the logarithmic scale.

squares error[1] of the $\ell_1\ell_2$-norm inverse solutions. The method achieves the best performance for $K=3$ basis functions. If the chosen number of basis functions is too high, some basis functions represent noise, resulting in slight degradation of the result quality as reflected by the gentle slope on the logarithmic scale. Including too few basis functions leads to significant signal loss: the solver fails to recover the missing signals.

We also investigated the method's sensitivity to the value of the regularization parameter λ. Large λ corresponds to a high penalty on the strength of the current sources; small λ emphasizes the data fidelity term. Due to whitening, the first term in Eq. (4) is on the order of MK ($M \sim 10^2$). For an activated vertex in our experiment, $\widetilde{s}_{nk}$ is on the order of 10^{-8}. Hence, $|\widetilde{\mathbf{S}}|_{\ell_1}^{\ell_2}$ is approximately $10^{-7}K$. Therefore, $\lambda = 10^9$ balances between the data fidelity and the regularization terms in Eq. (4). Fig. 2b confirms that λ around 10^9 provides the most accurate reconstruction results. The regularization shows no effect for $\lambda < 10^3$; when $\lambda > 10^{10}$, the data fidelity term is effectively ignored in the optimization process. For $\lambda = 10^9$, the standard deviation of the 100 simulated data sets is less than 1%. In the experiments using real MEG data, we set $\lambda = 10^9$.

3.2 Real MEG Experiments

We compared the performance of the proposed solver to MNE and dipole fitting using real MEG data from median-nerve stimulation experiments. The measurements were acquired using a 306-channel Neuromag VectorView MEG system. Anatomical images, collected with a 1.5 T scanner, were used to construct the source space and the forward model [3,8].

In this study, the median nerve was stimulated at the left wrist according to an event-related protocol, with a random inter-stimulus-interval ranging from 1.5 to 2 seconds. A 200-msec baseline before the stimulus was used to estimate the noise covariance matrix. The average signal, computed from approximately 300 trials, was used as the input to the inverse solver.

The median-nerve stimulation activates a complex cortical network [9]. The first activation of the contralateral primary somatosensory cortex (cSI) peaks around

---

[1] Defined as $\dfrac{\|\text{reconstructed signals} - \text{ground truth signals}\|_{\ell_2}^2}{\|\text{ground truth signals}\|_{\ell_2}^2}$.

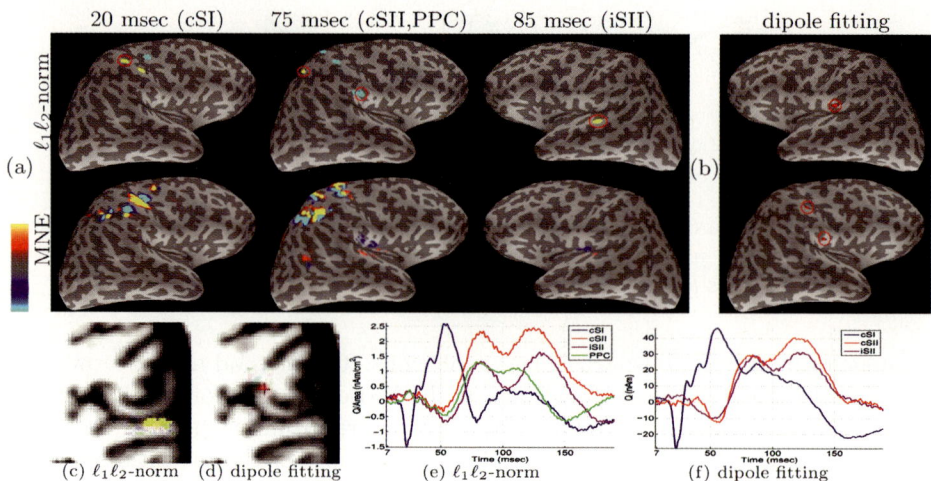

Fig. 3. Real MEG study. (a) Significance statistics of the $\ell_1\ell_2$-norm inverse solver and MNE for the median-nerve experiment. Hot/cold colors correspond to outward/inward current flow. The most active areas in the $\ell_1\ell_2$-norm solutions are highlined. (b) Dipole fitting with three sources. (c-d) Zoomed-in coronal slices for the detected iSII activations. (e-f) Reconstructed time courses for the highlined areas in (a-b).

20 msec and continues over 100 msec; then the secondary somatosensory cortex (SII) activates bilaterally between 70 and 200 msec. The posterior parietal cortex (PPC), located on the wall of the post-central sulcus, activates at 70-110 msec.

Employing six basis functions, which explain 80% variance of the data, is sufficient to capture the responses. We adopted a standard multi-resolution scheme, corresponding to source spacing of 20 and 10 mm. The efficient interior-point optimizer [15] allows us to estimate statistical significance of the resulting activations via permutation testing [14]. We controlled the false discovery rate (FDR) [5] at 0.05, computed from 5000 permutations (run time of 60 seconds per permutation). We also compared our results to MNE and dipole fitting computed using standard software packages [8,18]. In practice, experts often interpret MNE through its statistics, the dynamic statistical parameter maps (dSPM) [2], with thresholds adjusted by an expert. For the purpose of comparison, we selected the threshold for dSPM so that all four regions of interest, cSI, cSII, iSII, and PPC, were included in the dSPM.

Fig. 3a presents the activation maps obtained using $\ell_1\ell_2$-norm and MNE for one subject in the study. At 20 msec, the $\ell_1\ell_2$-norm pinpoints cSI on the postal wall of the central sulcus. MNE produces a more diffuse solution leading to false positives in the post-central sulcus. At 75 msec, both MNE and $\ell_1\ell_2$-norm capture signals from cSII. $\ell_1\ell_2$-norm successfully localizes PPC at the post-central sulcus; the location of PPC is ambiguous in the MNE results. The $\ell_1\ell_2$-norm detects iSII, but places it at the superior temporal lobe instead of the inferior parietal lobe. As shown in the volumetric display (Fig. 3cd), these two regions are very close, making the inverse problem particularly challenging. MNE also detects weak iSII signals; the location is ambiguously spread between the iSII region and the superior temporal lobe.

Dipole fitting results, shown in Fig. 3b, did not correctly localize PPC in this experiment because PPC is very close to cSI. The locations for cSI and cSII estimated by our solver match with the dipole fitting results. The correct localization of iSII using dipole fitting required manual intervention in selecting appropriate channels, in contrast to the automatic $\ell_1\ell_2$-norm solver.

Our method yields stable time courses that capture the main deflections precisely (Fig. 3e). The reconstructed time courses are similar to those estimated through dipole fitting (Fig. 3f), except for the cSI activation between 70 and 150 msec. This is due to the PPC activation missed by dipole fitting. This comparison demonstrates the ability of the $\ell_1\ell_2$-norm regularization to achieve high-quality reconstructions of source signals.

4 Conclusions

The proposed model takes advantage of the relatively smooth nature of the underlying EEG/MEG source signals via an ℓ_2-norm regularizer on the projection coefficients of the temporal basis functions. The $\ell_1\ell_2$-norm inverse solver is formulated as an SOCP problem. Performing reconstruction in the signal subspace while jointly considering the coefficients for all selected basis functions leads to stable estimates with a reduced number of false positives as confirmed by our experiments using simulated and real MEG data.

Acknowledgments. We thank Dr. Dmitry Malioutov for stimulating discussion. This work was supported in part by NIH NIBIB NAMIC U54-EB005149, NSF JHU ERC CISST, NIH NCRR mBIRN U24-RR021382, NIH NCRR NAC P41-RR13218, NIH NCRR P41-RR14075 grants, and the NSF CAREER Award 0642971. Wanmei Ou is partially supported by the NSF graduate fellowship.

References

1. Alizadeh, F., Goldfarb, D.: Second-order cone programming. Technical Report. RRR Report number 51-2001, RUTCOR, Rutgers University (2001)
2. Dale, A.M., Sereno, M.: Improved localization of cortical activity by combining EEG and MEG with MRI cortical surface reconstruction: a linear approach. J. Cogn. Neurosci. 5, 162–176 (1993)
3. Dale, A.M., et al.: Cortical surface-based analysis: I. Segmentation and surface reconstruction. NeuroImage 9, 179–194 (1999)
4. Ding, L., He, B.: Sparse source imaging in electroencephalography with accurate field modeling. Human Brain Mapping (in press)
5. Genovese, C.R., et al.: Thresholding of statistical maps in functional neuroimaging using the false discovery rate. NeuroImage 15, 870–878 (2002)
6. Geva, A.B.: Bioelectric sources estimation using spatio-temporal matching pursuit. Applied Sig. Proc. 5, 195–208 (1998)

7. Hämäläinen, M.S., et al.: Magnetoencephalography - theory, instrumentation, and applications to noninvasive studies of the working human brain. Reviews of Modern Physics 65, 413–497 (1993)
8. Hämäläinen, M.S.: MNE software user's guide. NMR Center, Mass General Hospital
9. Hari, R., Forss, N.: Magnetoencephalography in the study of human somatosensory cortical processing. Philos. Trans. R. Soc. Lond. B 354, 1145–1154 (1999)
10. Huang, M.X., et al.: Vector-based spatial-temporal minimum L1-norm solution for MEG. NeuroImage 31, 1025–1037 (2006)
11. Lin, F.-H., et al.: Distributed current estimates using cortical orientation constraints. Human Brain Mapping 27, 1–13 (2006)
12. Malioutov, M., et al.: A sparse signal reconstruction perspective for source localization with sensor arrays. IEEE Trans. Sig. Proc. 53, 3010–3022 (2005)
13. Mosher, J.C., et al.: Multiple dipole modeling and localization from spatiotemporal MEG data. IEEE Trans. Biomed. Engr. 39, 541–557 (1992)
14. Pantazis, D., et al.: A comparison of random field theory and permutation methods for the statistical analysis of MEG data. NeuroImage 25, 383–394 (2005)
15. Sturm, J.F., et al.: Self-Dual-Minimization (SeDuMi): solver for optimization problems over symmetric cones, http://sedumi.mcmaster.ca/
16. Trujillo-Barreto, N., et al.: Bayesian M/EEG source reconstruction with spatiotemporal priors. NeuroImage 39, 318–335 (2008)
17. Uutela, K., et al.: Visualization of magnetoencephalographic data using minimum current estimates. NeuroImage 10, 173–180 (1999)
18. Source modeling software (xfit), Elekta-Neuromag Oy, Helsinki, Finland

Tracking the Swimming Motions of *C. elegans* Worms with Applications in Aging Studies

Christophe Restif and Dimitris Metaxas

Rutgers, the State University of New Jersey
christophe.restif@centraliens.net

Abstract. Quantitative analysis of the swimming motions of *C. elegans* worms are of critical importance for many gene-related studies on aging. However no automated methods are currently in use. We present a novel training-based method that automatically tracks and segments multiple swimming worms, in challenging imaging conditions. The position of each worm is predicted by comparing its latest motion with a set of previous observations, and then adjusted laterally and longitudinally to fit the image. After segmentation, a variety of measures can be used to assess the evolution of swimming patterns over time, allowing a quantitative comparison of worm populations over their lifetime. The complete software is being evaluated for mass processing in biology laboratories.

1 Introduction

The nematodes *C. elegans*, short for *Caenorhabditis elegans*, have been the focus of numerous studies in the biology of aging [1]. Their motion patterns can be studied to analyze the evolution of their strength and coordination, when crawling on solid surfaces and swimming in liquid. To assess the influence of stochastic and genetic factors in aging, quantitative individual-based studies are needed, over the complete life-span of large populations of worms, based on non-invasive measures [2]. Optical microscopy is a promising tool, and many computer vision methods have been published to study the worm crawling motion [3,4,5]. Yet to the best of our knowledge, no satisfactory equivalent for swimming motion is in use. In this article we present a complete automated tool to track swimming worms on videos in challenging conditions, extract measures from the segmentation, and use them to compare individuals or mutant populations.

Tracking multiple swimming worms is a challenging computer vision task, and significantly different from crawling worms. Although optical microscopy is a method well adapted to the biological constraints of worm imaging, the images produced are not optimal for segmentation and tracking. Videos typically show a dozen worms, about four pixel wide, all with similar appearances and behaviors (see Fig. 1). The worms frequently overlap, and they need to be tracked robustly. Generic segmentation methods adapted to tracking, such as dynamic graph cuts [6] or level sets [7], are not robust enough in those conditions. Also, the following features restrict the use of explicit motion models. As invertebrate, swimming worms can show a large variety of body shapes, and change over only

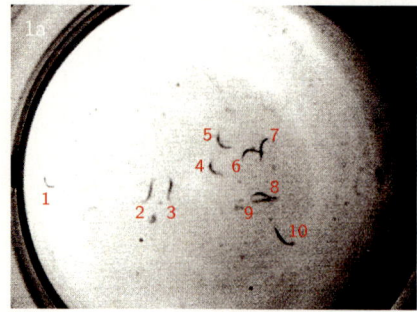 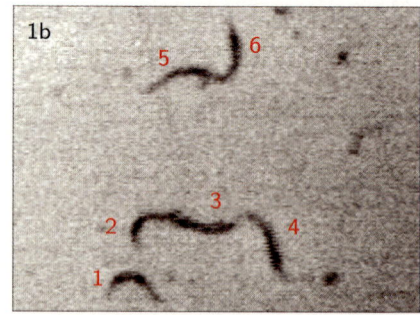

Fig. 1. A: typical frame showing ten worms. Notice the variations of background intensity and texture, the variations of worm appearances, and the partial overlaps. b: close-up of another frame showing six overlapping worms.

a few frames. They are evolving in three dimensions and imaged from above. As a result their length can visually change suddenly as a result of a body bend. Finally, in large-scale studies, the motion patterns vary significantly over time and over individuals, from vigorous and flexible to stiff and uncoordinated. Such motion patterns are to be the output of the tracking, and the use of explicit specific worm motion models for tracking [3,8] would induce a high bias.

In contrast, crawling worms move in two dimensions. They can be in contact but less frequently overlap. They also exhibit very different motions. From frame to frame, most of their body keeps the same location, only the head and tail move; and they do not show the high-frequency body bending, informally described as alternate I-C and S-Z shapes, typical of swimming. Also, as their motions are slower and more limited in space, they can be imaged at higher resolution and with better contrast. Hence, intensity thresholding and binary morphological operations can be enough for segmentation [4, 5, 3], but cannot be used in our context. The work closest to ours is [9], which addresses the tracking swimming motion. Yet it is a semi-automated tool, requiring manual input on each video on worms and background, and not fast enough for large-scale processing.

We present a complete automated tracking and segmentation method, for an unlimited number of worms. For tracking, we use the most relevant exemplars from the training set to predict each worm's position on the next frame, and adjust the prediction with segmentation methods based on standard motion detection techniques and worm-specific appearances. We model a worm as a central body line and body borders, so that subsequent measures such as the frequencies of head bending, body shapes, or total body curvature, are straightforward to compute after the segmentation. Statistics on worm populations are then computed and can be used for further phenotype analysis.

2 Method

Worm model. We model the central body line of a worm w at time t as an open polygon with n vertices $B^w(t) = \{B_i^w(t)\}_{1 \leq i \leq n}$, and use a constant width

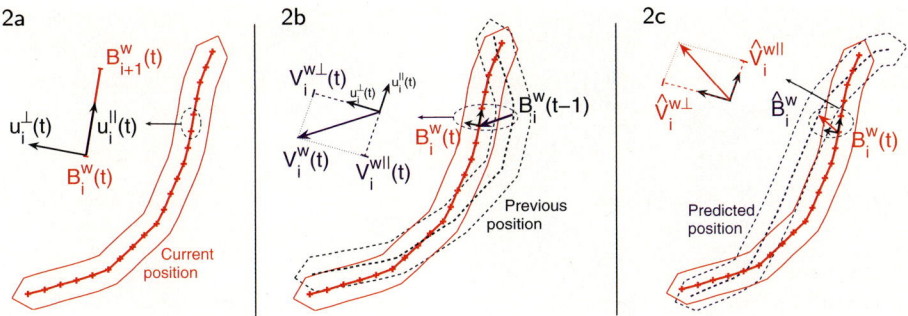

Fig. 2. Worm model for tracking prediction. 2a: Base vectors $u_i^{\|}(t)$ and $u_i^{\perp}(t)$ at vertex $B_i^w(t)$. 2b: velocity $V_i^w(t)$ and its decomposition $V_i^{w\|}(t)$ and $V_i^{w\perp}(t)$ from Eq. (2). 2c: predicted position computed with $\hat{V}_i^{w\|}(t+1)$ and $\hat{V}_i^{w\perp}(t+1)$ from Eq. (4).

of 2 pixels around $B^w(t)$ to delineate the worm body. At each vertex $B_i^w(t)$, we define the local base vectors $(u_i^{\|}(t), u_i^{\perp}(t))$ as the unit vectors parallel and perpendicular to the edge $(B_i^w(t), B_{i+1}^w(t))$, dropping the w in the notation for clarity, as illustrated in Fig. 2a, and define for the last vertex $(u_n^{\|}(t), u_n^{\perp}(t)) = (u_{n-1}^{\|}(t), u_{n-1}^{\perp}(t))$. This model follows from the morphology of the worms, which are symmetric along their central body lines; their flexibility are reflected by the evolution of the relative angles between consecutive vertices. With the local bases used, movements along $u_i^{\|}(t)$ corresponds to body stretching and compressions, and along $u_n^{\perp}(t)$, to body side-bendings. When body lengths vary and vertices are added or removed during segmentation, we resample $B^w(t)$ to $n = 100$ regularly-spaced vertices. From frame $t-1$ to frame t, we define the velocity of each vertex i of worm w and decompose it in the local base as (see Fig. 2b.):

$$V_i^w(t) = B_i^w(t) - B_i^w(t-1) = V_i^{w\|}(t) \cdot u_i^{\|}(t) + V_i^{w\perp}(t) \cdot u_i^{\perp}(t) \quad (1)$$

We then define the $2n$-dimensional *velocity vector* of worm w at time t as:

$$V^w(t) = \left(V_1^{w\|}(t), \cdots, V_n^{w\|}(t), V_1^{w\perp}(t), \cdots, V_n^{w\perp}(t) \right) \quad (2)$$

Given a worm w segmented at times $t = 1 \ldots t_0$, we compute the worm's position on the next frame $t_0 + 1$ in two steps. First, we predict its position by predicting its next velocity vector, noting those predictions $\hat{B}^w(t_0 + 1)$ and $\hat{V}^w(t_0 + 1)$. Then we adjust $\hat{B}^w(t_0 + 1)$ to the contents of frame $t_0 + 1$, and obtain the final segmentation $B^w(t_0 + 1)$.

Tracking prediction. The swimming motion of worms consists of high-frequency body bends, where a worm takes alternative S, I, Z, C, and O shapes, reflected in $V^{w\perp}$, and lower-frequency body stretching and contracting, reflected in $V^{w\|}$. Although V^w exhibits oscillatory patterns over time, strictly speaking it is non-periodic. Modeling its evolutions on the long term with a periodic function is not

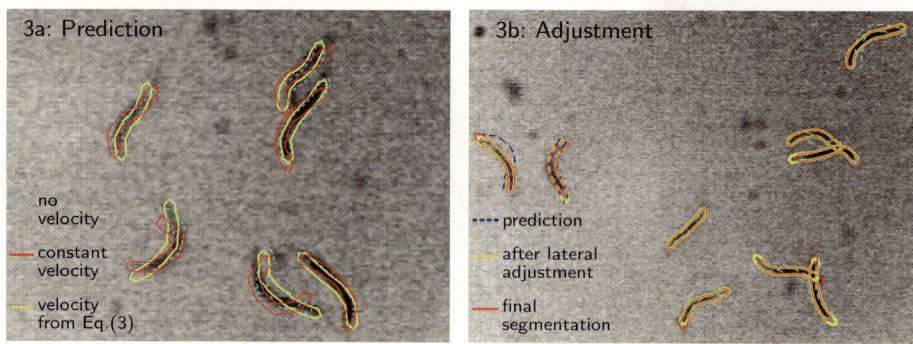

Fig. 3. Prediction and adjustment of the segmented worms. 3a: comparison of three models for the predicted position; in dotted blue, $\hat{V}^w(t_0+1) = 0$; in red, $\hat{V}^w(t_0+1) = V^w(t_0)$; in yellow, $\hat{V}^w(t_0+1)_i$ from Eq. (3). 3b: adjustments; in dotted blue, the predicted position from Eq. (4); in red: the result of the lateral adjustment by gradient ascent; in yellow: the final result after longitudinal adjustment.

reliable. Instead we use a non-parametric model for the short-term evolutions of V^w, making use of its regularity. $V^w(t_0)$ is compared to all previous observations $V^w(t)$, for $1 \leq t \leq t_0 - 1$, using the L^2 distance. Intuitively, the closer $V^w(t_0)$ is to a particular $V^w(t)$, the closer the prediction $\hat{V}^w(t_0+1)$ will be to $V^w(t+1)$. Instead of selecting only the closest vector $V^w(t)$, we use all the previous observations. $\hat{V}^w(t_0+1)$ is defined as a weighted average of the successors $V^w(t+1)$. Let $d^w(t) = \|V^w(t) - V^w(t_0)\|$ using L^2 norm, the predicted velocity vector is defined as: (the starting value $t = 0$ is explained in the following paragraph)

$$\hat{V}^w(t_0+1) = \frac{\sum_{t=0}^{t_0-1} e^{-d^w(t)} \cdot V^w(t+1)}{\sum_{t=0}^{t_0-1} e^{-d^w(t)}} \quad (3)$$

This approach shares similarities with particle filtering. However, we use all the previous observations of a worm's velocity vector as samples, as opposed to a probability-based random selection. To account for the noise in this model, we have included two terms in the computation of the average: $V^w(0) = V^w(1) = 0$. In case none of the previous velocity vectors are close to $V^w(t_0)$, the zero vector $V^w(1)$ included in Eq. (3) lowers the predicted velocity. This keeps the predicted position closer to the previous position: in effect, this reduces the significance of the prediction in case the model is not adapted. Noting the components of the predicted velocity vector $\hat{V}^w(t_0+1)$ as $\hat{V}_i^{w\|}(t_0+1)$ and $\hat{V}_i^{w\perp}(t_0+1)$, as done in Eq. (2), the predicted position of vertex i is:

$$\hat{B}_i^w(t_0+1) = B_i^w(t_0) + \hat{V}_i^{w\|}(t_0+1) \cdot u_i^\|(t_0) + \hat{V}_i^{w\perp}(t_0+1) \cdot u_i^\perp(t_0) \quad (4)$$

as illustrated in Fig. 2c. Examples of predictions are shown in red in Fig. 3a, with two alternative models shown in blue and green, respectively $\hat{V}^w(t_0+1) = 0$ and $\hat{V}^w(t_0+1) = V^w(t_0)$. This predicted body position now has to be adjusted to the frame $t_0 + 1$.

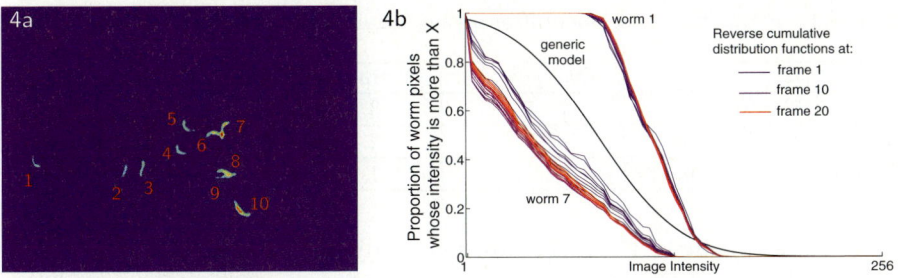

Fig. 4. Image preprocessing and worm appearances. 4a: result of the pre-processing in Eq. (5) on the image shown in Fig. 1a, using the generic appearance function. 4b: evolutions of the appearance of two worms. In black, the generic appearance function used for the first frame, computed from the training data. From blue to red: the reverse cumulative mass functions of intensities for two worms, shown for 20 successive frames.

Tracking adjustment. To overcome the image quality issues described in the introduction, images are pre-processed as follows. For each pixel (x, y) on 40 consecutive images, the median $m(x, y)$ and the standard deviation $\sigma(x, y)$ of the intensity distribution are computed. Thus for each image I, two maps are defined: the difference to the median $I - m$ and the standard deviation σ. The latter is very robust to the flickering intensity noise affecting the background, and only enhances pixels where worms are moving, have moved or will move, but is common for the 40 consecutive images. The former map is less robust to noise, but is image-specific, and enhances pixels where worms are currently moving. A third map is computed, to account for each worm's specific appearance $\mathcal{A}^w(i)$, which is defined as the proportion of pixels in worm w whose intensities are less than i. Intuitively, the darker a pixel, the more likely it is to belong to a worm, yet that likeliness depends on the worm (compare worms 1 and 7 in Fig. 1). Initially, a generic appearance function is used for all worms, shown in black in Fig. 4b; it is defined as the reverse cumulative function of a Gaussian, whose mean and standard deviation are computed from the training set using the histograms of manually segmented worms. Then, the reverse cumulative histogram of each worm is computed and incremented at each frame, and normalized accordingly, as illustrated for two worms in Fig. 4b in colors. This third map $\mathcal{A}^w(I(x, y))$ is multiplied with the other two to define the pre-processed image $\hat{I}^w(x, y)$:

$$\hat{I}^w(x, y) = \sigma(x, y) \times (I(x, y) - m(x, y)) \times \mathcal{A}^w(I(x, y)) \qquad (5)$$

To initialize the tracking, the first frame is pre-processed using the generic appearance function, as shown on Fig. 4a. A greedy line-growing method is then used on this image to fit the central body lines of worms, until all the regions of a value higher than a training-based threshold can be used to segment worms 4 pixel wide and at least 20 pixel long. In successive frames, once each worm's position is predicted using Eq. 4, only a subpart of the frame is pre-processed, 20 pixels around the predicted position, using Eq. 5 with the relevant $\mathcal{A}^w(i)$ function. The adjustment of the predicted position $\hat{B}^w$ on this pre-processed map is

Table 1. Evaluation of segmentation results against ground truth on 400 worms

Model	True positive	Average distance	Lost in tracking
$\hat{V}^w(t_0+1) = 0$	77.4 %	3.4 pixels	17 %
$\hat{V}^w(t_0+1) = V^w(t_0)$	84.7 %	2.5 pixels	12 %
$\hat{V}^w(t_0+1)$ from $Eq.$ (3)	92.4 %	1.1 pixels	4 %

performed in two steps. First, the position is adjusted laterally: each vertex $\hat{B}_i^w$ is moved along its local base vector $u_i^\perp$ by gradient ascent on $\hat{I}^w(x,y)$. Then, longitudinally, the length of the worm is adjusted to fit $\hat{I}^w(x,y)$. Extreme vertices 1 and n are removed until they stand on regions of $\hat{I}^w$ above a threshold defined from the training set, and new vertices are added at the extremities with the same greedy line-growing method as during initialization. The two steps of the adjustment are shown in Fig. 3b.

Measures. As the result of the segmentation, the central body line of a worm, defined as an open polygon, can be used to measure various features related to the worm's configuration and coordination. Here we focus on three of the measures. Let $\alpha_i^w(t)$ be the relative signed angle between the edges $(B_{i-1}^w(t), B_i^w(t))$ and $(B_i^w(t), B_{i+1}^w(t))$, measured between $-\pi$ and π. We define the head, the tail, and the absolute curvatures of worm w at time t as follows:

$$\mathcal{HC}^w(t) = \sum_{i=2}^{n/2} \alpha_i^w(t) \ , \quad \mathcal{TC}^w(t) = \sum_{i=n/2}^{n-1} \alpha_i^w(t) \ , \quad \mathcal{AC}^w(t) = \sum_{i=2}^{n-1} |\alpha_i^w(t)| \quad (6)$$

The terms 'head' and 'tail' are convenient to refer to each end of a worm, yet there is no guarantee that they correspond to the actual head and tail of the worm. Their evolution over time can still be used to estimate the number of actual head and tail bends. $\mathcal{HC}^w$ is positive when the head is turned to the left, and negative for the right. As a worm bends it head from side to side, $\mathcal{HC}^w$ oscillates between positive and negative values. The number of these oscillations over time is used to compute the average frequency of head bending over the entire video. The frequency of tail bending is defined similarly, and the higher of these two frequencies is considered as the actual worm head bend frequency. The absolute curvature $\mathcal{AC}^w$ indicates the vigor of a worm's motion. Although it oscillates over time, its distribution over the entire video sequence indicates the amplitude of bending achieved by the worm, and how much time it spent in each curvature. Results are presented below.

3 Results and Discussion

In the data set we used, images are either 640×480 or 700×520, and the frame rate is either 24 or 30 frames per second. The tracking and segmentation results were evaluated using a testing set of 400 manually segmented worms. We measured the true positive rate, the average distance between central body lines,

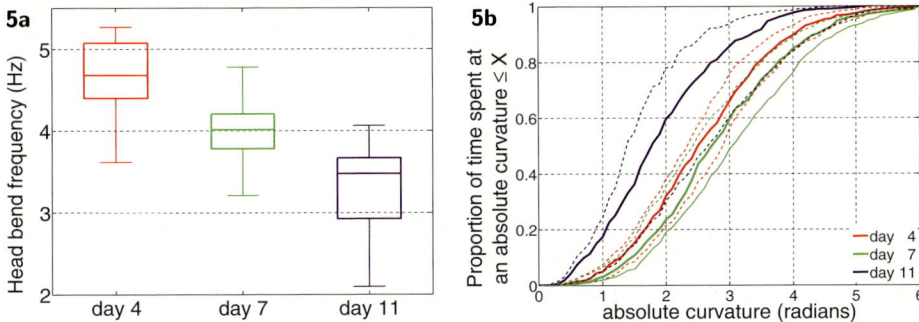

Fig. 5. Evolution of the swimming patterns of a population of mutant worms over their lifetime. 5a: head bend frequency. In each plot, the central line shows the median value of the population, the top and bottom of the box show the lower and upped quartiles, and the external lines show the extent of the remaining values. 5b: Cumulative distribution functions of the absolute curvature. For each color, the central thick line shows the median value, and the top and bottom dotted lines show the lower and upper quartiles. See page 40 for details on the measures' definition.

and the proportion of worms lost during tracking. We compared the method presented in the previous section with two other models: $\hat{V}^w(t_0+1) = 0$ (assuming no velocity) and $\hat{V}^w(t_0+1) = V^w(t_0)$ (assuming constant velocity). Results are listed in Table 1. Our method improves all three results significantly. It is to be noted that because of the imaging conditions, the manual labeling uncertainty is about one pixel around the worms' borders. Thus, the average distance to the ground truth obtained with our method, 1.1 pixels, is very accurate given the image resolution. A frame with 10 worms is segmented in 1.2 seconds on average, on a dual 3-GHz PC running Matlab 2006, which brings the complete processing of a 900-frame video under 20 minutes, and allows large-scale processing. The main current limitation of our method is that the worms to be tracked are fixed by the results of the line-growing method on the first frame.

Finally, we used our program to assess quantitatively the evolution of swimming patterns as worms age. Five different mutant worm populations were imaged at three stages of their adult lives, at day 4, 7, and 11. As a result, 30 videos, each showing 10 worms over 900 frames, were produced and processed with our program. After tracking and segmentation, the measures described above were generated. Two examples of resulting graphs for one mutant population are shown in Fig. 5. The head bend frequencies are shown to decrease gradually for all individuals. Also, the range of frequencies at day 11 is wider than at younger ages, suggesting that individuals of that mutant population age differently, some keeping more active than others. Fig. 5b shows the proportion of time spent at certain absolute curvatures. It appears that worms have similar trends on day 4 and 7, while on day 11, they spend less time at higher curvatures, showing an increase of body stiffness. The same remark on the wider range of values at day 11 applies, indicating that stiffness affects some individuals more than others at that age. Although these trends were observed qualitatively by the biologists providing the data, our program allowed the automatic generation and display of quantitative results. Similar graphs were generated to compare individual worms, the same worms at different ages, and different mutant populations. Further analysis of those results is a subject for studies on the biology of aging, and is beyond the scope of this article.

4 Conclusion

We presented an automated method to track and segment the swimming motions of C. elegans worms under challenging imaging conditions, which have not been addressed despite their significance for research, in particular on the biology of aging. The method is based on a two-step processing. First each worm's position is predicted, by comparing its latest motion to a set of previous observations. Then this prediction is adjusted, sideways and longitudinally, so that the segmented worm fits a region of high intensity variations, indicating motion, and intensity similar to its previous intensity distributions. Based on this segmentation, quantitative measures are defined to analyze the evolution of the vigor and swimming patterns of worms. Such analysis is possible at the level of an individual worm, of a population, and across populations. The complete software is currently being used by biologists for research on the aging of C.elegans.

The authors gratefully thank Prof. Monica Driscoll and her team, in particular Dr Carolina Ibañez-Ventoso and Mehul Vora, for providing the data and for their useful comments. This work is funded by NIH grant number 4-22567.

References

1. Kenyon, C.: Environmental factors and gene activities that influence life span. In: Caenorhabditis elegans, vol. II. Cold Spring Harbor Laboratory Press (1997)
2. Herndon, L.A., Schmeissner, P.J., Dudaronek, J.M., Brown, P.A., Listner, K.M., Sakano, Y., Paupard, M.C., Hall, D.H., Driscoll, M.: Stochastic and genetic factors influence tissue-specific decline in ageing C. elegans. Nature 419, 808–814 (2002)
3. Fontaine, E., Barr, A.H., Burdick, J.W.: Model-based tracking of multiple worms and fish. In: ICCV Workshop on Dynamical Vision, Rio, Brazil (October 2007)
4. Geng, W., Cosman, P., Berry, C.C., Feng, Z., Schafer, W.R.: Automatic tracking, feature extraction and classification of C. elegans phenotypes. IEEE Trans. on Biomedical Engineering 10(51), 1811–1820 (2004)
5. Roussel, N., Morton, C.A., Finger, F.P., Roysam, B.: A computational model for C. elegans locomotory behavior: Application to multiworm tracking. IEEE Trans. on Biomedical Engineering 54(10), 1786–1797 (2007)
6. Kohli, P., Torr, P.H.: Dynamic graph cuts for efficient inference in Markov Random Fields. IEEE Pattern Analysis and Machine Intelligence 29(12), 2079–2088 (2007)
7. Cremers, D., Osher, S., Soatto, S.: Kernel density estimation and intrinsic alignment for shape priors in level set segmentation. Int. J. Comp. Vis. 69(3), 335–351 (2006)
8. Brackenbury, J.: Swimming kinematics and wake elements in a worm-like insect: the larva of the midge Chironomus plumosus. Journal of Zoology 260, 195–201 (2003)
9. Tsechpenakis, G., Bianchi, L., Driscoll, M., Metaxas, D.: Tracking C. elegans populations in fluid environments for the study of different locomotory behaviors. In: Microscopic Image Analysis with Applications in Biology, Piscataway, NJ (September 2007)

MR Brain Tissue Classification Using an Edge-Preserving Spatially Variant Bayesian Mixture Model

G. Sfikas[1,3], C. Nikou[1], N. Galatsanos[2], and C. Heinrich[3]

[1] University of Ioannina, Department of Computer Science, 45110 Ioannina, Greece
[2] University of Patras, Department of ECE, 26500 Rio, Greece
[3] LSIIT-University of Strasbourg, 67412 Illkirch cedex, France

Abstract. In this paper, a spatially constrained mixture model for the segmentation of MR brain images is presented. The novelty of this work is an edge-preserving smoothness prior which is imposed on the probabilities of the voxel labels. This prior incorporates a line process, which is modeled as a Bernoulli random variable, in order to preserve edges between tissues. The main difference with other, state of the art methods imposing priors, is that the constraint is imposed on the probabilities of the voxel labels and not onto the labels themselves. Inference of the proposed Bayesian model is obtained using variational methodology and the model parameters are computed in closed form. Numerical experiments are presented where the proposed model is favorably compared to state of the art brain segmentation methods as well as to a spatially varying Gaussian mixture model.

1 Introduction

The segmentation of 3D brain magnetic resonance (MR) images into the three main tissues, namely, white matter (WM), gray matter (GM) and cerebro-spinal fluid (CSF) is of great importance in most neuroimaging applications. Although many research studies have been presented in this area, MRI brain segmentation still remains a challenging issue due to specific difficulties of MRI, such as intensity inhomogeneity, partial volume effect and acquisition noise. A first approach to the problem relied on the expectation-maximization (EM) algorithm [1,2] which led to an important category of methods resorting to Gaussian mixture models (GMM). Among them, many studies incorporate prior information (e.g. anatomical atlases) on tissue topology [3,4,5,6] or constrain the segmentation to be spatially smooth and take into account edge discontinuities (e.g. using Markov random field (MRF) priors) [7,8,9,10,11,12,13,14,15].

Modeling the probability density function (pdf) of pixel or voxel attributes with a GMM [16] is a natural way to cluster data because it automatically provides a grouping based on the components of the mixture that generated them. Furthermore, the likelihood of a GMM is a rigorous metric for clustering performance. The parameters of the GMM can be estimated very efficiently through maximum likelihood (ML) estimation using the Expectation-Maximization (EM) algorithm [16].

The prior knowledge that adjacent pixels most likely belong to the same cluster is not used in standard GMM. To overcome this shortcoming, spatial smoothness constraints may be imposed, generally applying an MRF prior, like the spatially varying Gaussian mixture model (SVGMM) in [17]. However, this model enforces smoothness between pixels belonging to different classes. Since the seminal work in [18], *line processes* were also introduced in several applications, other than brain tissue classification, to respond to this drawback, see for instance [19] and [20] for image restoration and superresolution respectively.

In this paper we propose a new, Bayesian, spatially varying Gaussian mixture model for the classification of brain images to the three tissue types (WM, GM, CSF). The main contribution of the model is that it takes into account not only that adjacent voxels are more probable to belong to the same class but it also prohibits smoothing across boundary voxels. Motivated by the studies in brain image segmentation incorporating MRF-based prior knowledge [5,7,8,9,10,11,12,13,14,15] we impose proper hyperpriors to simultaneously address local smoothing and edge preservation. The main difference with other, state of the art methods imposing MRF-type priors, is that the constraint is imposed on the probabilities of the voxel labels (generally known in mixture modeling as *contextual mixing proportions*) and not onto the labels themselves. By these means, closed form solutions are provided for the model parameters through variational inference.

2 The Bayesian Edge Preserving Spatially Varying GMM

The K-kernel spatially varying GMM differs from the standard GMM in the definition of the mixing proportions. More precisely, in the SVGMM, each voxel x^n, $n = 1, ..., N$ has a distinct vector of mixing proportions denoted by π_j^n, $j = 1, ..., K$. We call these parameters *contextual mixing proportions* to distinguish them from the mixing proportions of a standard GMM. Hence, the probability of a distinct voxel is expressed by:

$$f(x^n; \pi, \mu, \Lambda) = \sum_{j=1}^{K} \pi_j^n \mathcal{N}(x^n; \mu_j, \Lambda_j) \tag{1}$$

where $0 \leq \pi_j^n \leq 1$, $\sum_{j=1}^{K} \pi_j^n = 1$ for $j = 1, 2, ..., K$ and $n = 1, 2, ..., N$, μ_j are the Gaussian kernel means and Λ_j are the Gaussian kernel precision (inverse covariance) matrices.

We now assume that the voxels $X = \{x^1, x^2, ..., x^N\}$ are independent and generated by the graphical model shown in figure 1.

Note that a set $Z = \{z_j^n\}_{n=1..N, j=1..K}$ of $N \times K$ latent variables is introduced, in order to make inference tractable for the model. The Z variables are distributed multinomially:

$$p(Z|\Pi) = \prod_{j=1}^{K} \prod_{n=1}^{N} (\pi_j^n)^{z_j^n} \tag{2}$$

where each z^n is a binary vector, with $z_j^n = 1$ if datum n is generated by the j-th kernel and $z_j^n = 0$ otherwise.

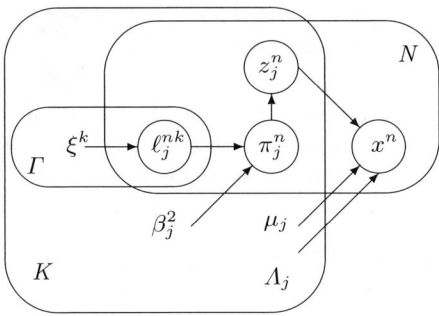

Fig. 1. Graphical model for the edge preserving spatially variant Gaussian mixture model. Superscript $n \in [1, N]$ denotes voxel index, subscript $j \in [1, K]$ denotes kernel (segment) index and $\Gamma \in [1, 26]$ describes the neighbourhood direction type.

Considering the set of *contextual mixing proportions* Π as random variables and assuming a proper prior, we can incorporate the intuitive fact that neighbouring voxels are more likely to share the same class label. We impose an edge preserving Gaussian prior on Π:

$$p(\Pi|\ell;\beta) = \prod_{j=1}^{K} \prod_{n=1}^{N} \prod_{k=1}^{\Gamma} \mathcal{N}(\pi_j^n | \pi_j^k; \beta_j^2)^{\ell^{nk}} \quad (3)$$

where ℓ^{nk} is a binary random variable we call *line-process*. If $\ell^{nk} = 1$, then there is a link on the random field between the voxel indexed n and its k-th *possible* neighbour (we denote by π^k the k-th neighbour of specific voxel n). Otherwise, if $\ell^{nk} = 0$ there is no link between them, signifying the presence of an edge. We assume that two voxels can be possible neighbours when they are vertically, horizontally or diagonally adjacent with regard to their spatial location in the three-dimensional mesh, implying $\Gamma = 26$ neighbours per voxel.

Parameters $\beta = \{\beta_1^2, \beta_2^2, ..., \beta_K^2\}$ control the spatial smoothness of the *contextual mixing proportions*. The prior in eq. (3) implies that

$$\pi_j^n - \pi_j^k \sim \mathcal{N}(0, \beta_j^2), \quad \forall k \in [1, \Gamma] \mid \ell^{nk} = 1$$

reflecting the fact that the *contextual mixing proportions* which implicitly control voxel class membership, are similar for neighbouring voxels except in case there exists an edge.

We now regard the *line process* variables ℓ^{nk} as Bernoulli distributed random variables, governed by a parameter set $\xi = \{\xi^1, \xi^2, ..., \xi^\Gamma\}$:

$$p(\ell|\xi) = \prod_{n=1}^{N} \prod_{k=1}^{\Gamma} p(\ell^{nk}|\xi^k) = \prod_{n=1}^{N} \prod_{k=1}^{\Gamma} {\xi^k}^{\ell^{nk}} (1 - \xi^k)^{(1-\ell^{nk})} \quad (4)$$

The Beta distribution is the conjugate for the Bernoulli pdf, therefore, we impose it on the ξ parameters:

$$p(\xi; \alpha_{\xi 0}, \beta_{\xi 0}) = \prod_{k=1}^{\Gamma} \frac{\Gamma(\alpha_{\xi k 0} + \beta_{\xi k 0})}{\Gamma(\alpha_{\xi k 0})\Gamma(\beta_{\xi k 0})} \xi^{k(\alpha_{\xi k 0}-1)}(1-\xi^k)^{(\beta_{\xi k 0}-1)} \quad (5)$$

The main advantage of the model in fig. 1 is that (i) it takes into account that neighboring voxels are more probably generated by the same Gaussian pdf and (ii) it does not smooth adjacent voxels separated by an edge.

3 MAP Estimation Using Variational Inference

To perform segmentation, the evidence with respect to model parameters has to be optimized:
$$\underset{\mu, \Lambda, \Pi, \beta}{\operatorname{argmax}} \ln p(X, \Pi; \mu, \Lambda, \beta)$$

This MAP solution cannot be computed directly, or even estimated using the EM algorithm, due to the Π prior distribution complexity. Therefore, we resort to variational inference [16]. This leads to an iterative scheme with one step for the computation of the stochastic parameters Z, ℓ, ξ and Π and one step for the deterministic parameters μ, Λ and β. Due to lack of space we present here the final expressions.

The expected values of the stochastic parameter are

$$<z_j^n> = \tilde{\pi}_j^n, \quad <l^{nk}> = \tilde{\xi}^{nk}, \quad <\ln \xi_k> = \psi(\alpha_{\xi k}) - \psi(\alpha_{\xi k} + \beta_{\xi k}),$$

$$<\ln(1-\xi_k)> = \psi(\beta_{\xi k}) - \psi(\alpha_{\xi k} + \beta_{\xi k}),$$

where $\psi(\cdot)$ is the digamma function and the expectations (denoted by a tilde) being as follows, with $sig(x) = (1 + e^{-x})^{-1}$:

$$\tilde{\pi}_j^n = \frac{\pi_j^n \mathcal{N}(x^n; \mu_j, \Lambda_j)}{\sum_{l=1}^{K} \pi_l^n \mathcal{N}(x^n; \mu_l, \Lambda_l)},$$

$$\tilde{\xi}^{nk} = sig\left(\sum_{j=1}^{K} \ln \mathcal{N}(\pi_j^k | \pi_j^n; \beta_j^2) + <\ln \xi_k> - <\ln(1-\xi_k)>\right),$$

$$\tilde{\alpha}_{\xi k} = \alpha_{\xi 0} + \sum_{n=1}^{N} <l^{nk}>, \quad \tilde{\beta}_{\xi k} = \beta_{\xi 0} + \sum_{n=1}^{N} <1 - l^{nk}>.$$

The *contextual mixing proportions* π_j^n are computed as the roots of a quadratic equation:
$$a_j^n \left(\pi_j^n\right)^2 + b_j^n \left(\pi_j^n\right) + c_j^n = 0 \quad (6)$$

with coefficients:

$$a_j^n = -\sum_{k=1}^{\Gamma} <l^{nk}>, \quad b_j^n = \sum_{k=1}^{\Gamma} <l^{nk}> \pi_j^k, \quad c_j^n = \frac{<z_j^n> \beta_j^2}{2}.$$

The form of the coefficients guarantees that there is always a non negative solution. The solutions of eq. (6) however will not in general satisfy the constraint $\sum_{j=1}^{K} \pi_j^n = 1, \pi_j \geq 0, \forall j \in [1..K]$ so we project the corresponding π^n vectors $\forall n \in [1..N]$ onto the constraints subspace; this is done using the quadratic programming algorithm described in [21].

Furthermore, the deterministic parameters are also obtained in closed form:

$$\tilde{\mu}_j = \frac{\sum_{n=1}^{N} <z_j^n> x^n}{\sum_{n=1}^{N} <z_j^n>}, \quad \tilde{\Lambda}_j^{-1} = \frac{\sum_{n=1}^{N} <z_j^n> (x^n - \mu_j)(x^n - \mu_j)^T}{\sum_{n=1}^{N} <z_j^n>} \quad (7)$$

$$\tilde{\beta}_j^2 = \frac{\sum_{n=1}^{N} \sum_{k=1}^{\Gamma} <l^{nk}> (\pi_j^n - \pi_j^k)^2}{\sum_{n=1}^{N} \sum_{k=1}^{\Gamma} <l^{nk}>} \quad (8)$$

The above update equations, for both the stochastic and deterministic parameters, are considered for the full range of each of the indices, namely n, j and k and are computed iteratively until convergence [22] of the variational lower bound.

4 Experimental Results

We have evaluated the proposed model on simulated images with known ground truth from the BrainWeb database [23],[24] using the voxel intensities as features.

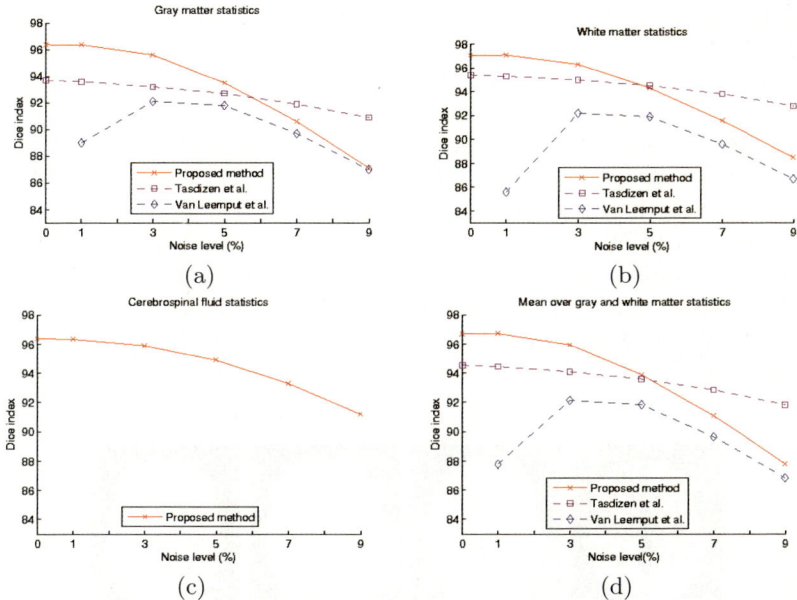

Fig. 2. Dice metric as a function of noise level for data without bias field. (a) Gray matter, (b) white matter, (c) CSF, (d) mean over gray and white matter. The dashed lines plot the results for the same images as presented in [5] and [10]. Results are not provided by the respective publications for the case in (c).

Table 1. Mean values for the Dice metric as a function of noise level over the three tissue types. The compared methods are the proposed method (Bayes-SVGMM), the non edge preserving spatially varying GMM (SVGMM) proposed in [17] and a standard GMM.

Noise (%)	Bayes-SVGMM	SVGMM	GMM
0	96.6	96.5	77.2
1	96.6	96.5	89.8
3	96.0	95.9	95.3
5	94.2	94.2	94.1
7	91.8	91.7	90.8
9	88.9	88.8	86.8

Prior to segmentation, we have preprocessed each volume so that only WM, GM and CSF are included (fig. 2). Hence, we set the number of kernels in our model to $K = 3$. The hyperparameter values of the Beta prior distribution were set to $\alpha_{\xi k0} = \beta_{\xi k0} = 1$, $\forall k$, making the prior uninformative as the data size $N \gg 1$.

The algorithm was applied to a simulated T1-weighted data without any bias field and with intensity noise levels between 0% and 9%. The noise percentages were defined with respect to the mean intensity of each tissue class. We have compared our segmentation results with two of the state of the art methods of Van Leemput et al. [10] and Tasdizen et al. [5]. In both of these studies, the Dice metric was used for evaluation. Therefore we present our results using this performance measure. Figure 2 summarizes the Dice metrics for the compared methods. In that figure, the curves for the state-of-the-art methods are reproduced from the respective publications [10,5]. As it can be observed, in all cases, our method provides better segmentations with respect to the method in [10]. Also, for low level noise the Dice metric of the proposed method is higher with respect to the method proposed in [5]. On the other hand, the method of Tasdizen et al. [5] performs better for noise levels of 7% and 9%. However, our method takes no more than 50 minutes to run on a 2.7 GHz standard PC whereas the method in [5] requires at least *six* hours runtime for convergence.

We have also compared our Bayesian model to a standard GMM as well as to the spatially varying GMM (SVGMM) proposed in [17]. In all cases, our model performed better than both methods. Both of the spatially varying models

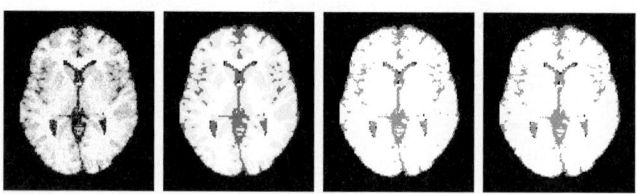

Fig. 3. Axial slices of a 3D segmentation example. From left to right: original MR slice with (9%) noise, ground truth, segmentation using a GMM, and the proposed method.

provided Dice metrics significantly better than the standard GMM. Moreover, the difference between our model and the SVGMM [17] is small but consistently in favor of our method. These differences are underpinned in table 1. A representative segmentation example is presented in figure 3.

5 Conclusion

We have presented a framework for segmenting the brain anatomy from 3D MRI. The proposed method relies on a Bayesian finite mixture model with a Gauss-Markov random field prior on the probabilities of the pixel labels. Also, the model incorporates a probabilistic line process for edge preservation. The quantitative evaluation reveals that the method not only improves the standard GMM and refines the SVGMM [17] but also performs at least at the same level as other state-of-the-art methods. A perspective of this study is the extension of the model to include more brain tissues and to integrate bias field correction into the segmentation procedure.

References

1. Kapur, T., Grimson, W.E.L., Wells III, W.M., Kikinis, R.: Segmentation of brain tissue from magnetic resonance images. Medical Image Analysis 1, 109–127 (1996)
2. Wells III, W., Grimson, W., Kikinis, R., Jolesz, F.: Adaptive segmentation of MRI data. IEEE Transactions on Medical Imaging 15, 429–442 (1996)
3. Marroquin, J., Vemuri, B., Botello, S., Calderon, F., Fernandez-Bouzas, A.: An accurate and efficient Bayesian method for automatic segmentation of brain MRI. IEEE Transactions on Medical Imaging 21, 934–945 (2002)
4. Prastawa, M., Gilmore, J., Lin, W., Gerig, G.: Automatic segmentation of neonatal brain MRI. In: Barillot, C., Haynor, D.R., Hellier, P. (eds.) MICCAI 2004. LNCS, vol. 3216, pp. 10–17. Springer, Heidelberg (2004)
5. Tasdizen, T., Awate, S., Whitaker, R., Foster, N.: MRI tissue classification with neighborhood statistics: a nonparametric entropy-minimizing approach. In: Duncan, J.S., Gerig, G. (eds.) MICCAI 2005. LNCS, vol. 3750, pp. 517–525. Springer, Heidelberg (2005)
6. Pohl, K., Bouix, S., Nakamura, M., Rohfling, T., McCarley, R., Kikinis, R., Grimson, L., Shenton, M., Wells, W.: A hierarchical algorithm for MR brain image parcellation. IEEE Transactions on Medical Imaging 26, 1201–1212 (2007)
7. Niessen, W.J., Vincken, K.L., Weickert, J., Viergever, M.A.: Three dimensional MR brain segmentation. In: Proceedings of the 6th International Conference on Computer Vision (ICCV 1998), pp. 53–58 (1998)
8. Laidlaw, D.H., Fleischer, K.W., Barr, A.H.: Partial-volume Bayesian classification of material mixtures in MR volume data using voxel histograms. IEEE Transactions on Medical Imaging 17(1), 74–86 (1998)
9. Kapur, T., Grimson, W.E.L., Kikinis, R., Wells III, W.M.: Enhanced spatial priors for segmentation of magnetic resonance imagery. In: Wells, W.M., Colchester, A.C.F., Delp, S.L. (eds.) MICCAI 1998. LNCS, vol. 1496, pp. 457–468. Springer, Heidelberg (1998)

10. Van Leemput, K., Maes, F., Vandermeulen, D., Suetens, P.: Automated model-based tissue classification of MR images of the brain. IEEE Transactions on Medical Imaging 18, 897–908 (1999)
11. Van Leemput, K., Maes, F., Vandermeulen, D., Colchester, A., Suetens, P.: Automated segmentation of multiple sclerosis lesions by model outlier detection. IEEE Transactions on Medical Imaging 20, 677–688 (2001)
12. Greenspan, H., Ruf, A., Goldberger, J.: Constrained Gaussian mixture model framework for automatic segmentation of MR brain images. IEEE Transactions on Medical Imaging 25, 1233–1245 (2006)
13. Peng, Z., Wee, W., Lee, J.H.: Automatic segmentation of MR brain images using spatial-varying Gaussian mixture and Markov random field approach. In: Proceedings of the Computer Vision and Pattern Recognition Workshop (CVPRW 2006) (2006)
14. Awate, S.P., Tasdizen, T., Foster, N., Whitaker, R.: Adaptive Markov modeling for mutual information based, unsupervised MRI brain tissue classification. Medical Image Analysis 10, 726–739 (2006)
15. Awate, S.P., Zhang, H., Gee, J.C.: A fuzzy, nonparametric segmentation framework for DTI and MRI analysis: With applications to DTI tract extraction. IEEE Transactions on Medical Imaging 26, 1525–1536 (2007)
16. Bishop, C.M.: Pattern Recognition and Machine Learning. Springer, Heidelberg (2006)
17. Nikou, C., Galatsanos, N., Likas, A.: A class-adaptive spatially variant mixture model for image segmentation. IEEE Transactions on Image Processing 16(4), 1121–1130 (2007)
18. Geman, S., Geman, D.: Stochastic relaxation, Gibbs distribution and the Bayesian restoration of images. IEEE Transactions on Pattern Analysis and Machine Intelligence 24(6), 721–741 (1984)
19. Molina, R., Mateos, J., Katsaggelos, A., Vega, M.: Bayesian multichannel image restoration using compound Gauss-Markov random fields. IEEE Transactions on Image Processing 12, 1642–1654 (2003)
20. Kanemura, A., Maeda, S., Ishii, S.: Hyperparameter estimation in Bayesian image superresolution with a compound Markov random field prior. In: Proceedings of the IEEE International Workshop on Machine Learning for Signal Processing (MLSP 2007), Thessaloniki, Greece (2007)
21. Blekas, K., Likas, A., Galatsanos, N., Lagaris, I.: A spatially constrained mixture model for image segmentation. IEEE Transactions on Neural Networks 16(2), 494–498 (2005)
22. Boyd, S., Vandenberghe, L.: Convex Optimization. Cambridge University Press, Cambridge (2004)
23. Collins, D., Zijdenbos, A., Kollokian, V., Sled, J., Kabani, N., Holmes, C., Evans, A.: Design and construction of a realistic digital brain phantom. IEEE Transactions on Medical Imaging 17(3), 463–468 (1998)
24. Kwan, R., Evans, A., Pike, G.: MRI simulation-based evaluation of image-processing and classification methods. IEEE Transactions on Medical Imaging 18, 1085–1097 (1999)

Semi-supervised Nasopharyngeal Carcinoma Lesion Extraction from Magnetic Resonance Images Using Online Spectral Clustering with a Learned Metric

Wei Huang[1], Kap Luk Chan[1], Yan Gao[1], Jiayin Zhou[2], and Vincent Chong[2]

[1] School of Electrical and Electronics Engineering, Nanyang Technological University, Singapore
[2] School of Medicine, National University of Singapore, Singapore

Abstract. In this paper, we consider the extraction of nasopharyngeal carcinoma lesion from MR images as a region segmentation problem. We propose a semi-supervised segmentation approach to segment the lesion in two steps. First, a metric is learned in a supervised fashion, which maximizes the separation between two groups of pixels (tumor or non-tumor) with minimal user interaction. Second, the learned metric is used to complete extraction of tumor region in an unsupervised fashion. Several experiments were conducted to evaluate the performance of similar methods with learned metrics for grouping or classifying pixels to form the tumor region. It is observed that the spectral clustering-based method performs well and the performance is comparable or marginally better than the discriminative SVM-based method.

1 Introduction

Nasopharyngeal carcinoma (NPC) lesion is an oral cancer developed in nasopharynx, which is different from other tumors in its occurrence, cause and clinical behavior [1]. Extracting NPC lesion region from Magnetic Resonance (MR) images for volumetric analysis is important to its treatment planning and prognosis. In order to help clinicians reduce the heavy workload of inspecting numerous MR images and delineating lesion manually, various segmentation methods have been proposed during the last decade or so [2], [3], [4], [5]. Most MR images segmentation methods can be categorized into *contour-based methods* and *region-based methods*. In contour-based methods [2], [3], active contours have been popularly used to evolve an deformable curve to the boundary of tumor. The evolving curve is driven by internal or external forces and additional constraints depending on characteristics of MR images. Although these methods require minimal user interaction to draw an initial contour inside or outside tumor regions, they require users to specify and adjust numerous parameters. For example, in the method proposed by Li et al. [3], there are totally 6 parameters with respect to various energy functional terms, constraints, etc. These parameters need to be adjusted properly for different MR images in order to ensure correct convergence of the evolving curves.

Region-based methods consider the tumor segmentation problem as a region segmentation problem. In order to discern tumor region from other non-tumor tissue regions, image pixels are classified into different tissue classes or clustered into different groups according to certain similarity criteria [4],[5]. Finding a proper metric encoding the notion of similarity is often of great importance to these methods. Since MR images data often have large varying statistical properties across scans, either making an assumption about the metrics beforehand or learning metrics based on training images and applying it to other MR scans may not match the characteristics of the two sets of images well. Therefore, it is necessary to learn different metrics for different MR images.

In this paper, we focus on learning of a metric that can be used for separating tumor regions from non-tumor regions in MR images based on *spectral clustering* [6],[7] in a semi-supervised fashion. The paper is organized as follows. In section 2, we learn a metric to measure the pairwise similarity of pixels by a supervised spectral clustering algorithm. In section 3, we elaborate how to make use of the out-of-sample extension algorithm to complete MR image segmentation. In section 4, we report several experiments and demonstrate the performance of our method and compare it with results of other similar methods. In section 5, we give the conclusion of this work.

2 Metrics Learning for NPC Lesion Extraction

2.1 A Spatially Weighted Metric

We construct a metric that reflects the pairwise similarity $d(\mathbf{x}_i, \mathbf{x}_j)$ between i-*th* and j-*th* pixel in a MR image as follows.

$$d(\mathbf{x}_i, \mathbf{x}_j) = K(\mathbf{x}_i, \mathbf{x}_j) \cdot G(\mathbf{x}_i, \mathbf{x}_j)$$
$$= \exp\left(-\frac{\|p_i - p_j\|^2}{\sigma_p^2}\right) \cdot \exp\left(-(s_i - s_j)^T \mathbf{A} (s_i - s_j)\right) \quad (1)$$

where, σ_p is a scalar and $\mathbf{A}$ is a full matrix; p_i is the spatial location of i-*th* pixel, and s_i is the feature vector based on low-level image features of i-*th* pixel. Obviously, the term $K(\mathbf{x}_i, \mathbf{x}_j)$ of Eq. (1) is a Gaussian RBF (Radial Basis Function) with a spatial localization emphasis that decreases with the increase of the distance between i-*th* and j-*th* pixel increases. Therefore, two spatially nearby pixels will have more influence on the measure of similarity than two pixels that are far apart. Our metric is different from those used in previous related works. For *N-cuts* [8], Shi et al. did not include the explicit form of the term $\mathbf{K}$ in their metric and assumed the matrix $\mathbf{A}$ as a diagonal matrix, ignoring the correlation among features. For *Ng-Jordan-Weiss* [6], they only utilized the term $\mathbf{K}$ in their metric, but p_i is a vector in a *d*-dimensional space.

To ensure Eq.(1) be a metric, it should meet the requirements of non-negativity and triangle inequality. Therefore, the matrix $\mathbf{A}$ must be positive semi-definite,

Table 1. Algorithm of metric learning with spectral clustering

Input:	a set of n points $S = \{s_1, s_2, \ldots, s_n\}$ in $\mathbf{R}^d$.
Algorithm:	
1.	Initialize parameters in our metric: $\mathbf{A}$ and σ_p^2.
2.	Calculate the pairwise similarity $d(\mathbf{x}_i, \mathbf{x}_j)$ in Eq.(1) for each data pair. Use these computed $d(\mathbf{x}_i, \mathbf{x}_j)$ as elements to construct an affinity matrix $\mathbf{D} \in \mathbf{R}^{n \times n}$ for all n points in S.
3.	Form a new diagonal matrix $\mathbf{C}$, whose (i,i) element is the sum of the i-th row of $\mathbf{D}$.
4.	Construct a matrix $\mathbf{L} = \mathbf{C}^{-1/2} \cdot \mathbf{D} \cdot \mathbf{C}^{-1/2}$, and find the k largest eigenvalues and their corresponding eigenvectors.
5.	Form a new matrix $\mathbf{X} \in \mathbf{R}^{n \times k}$ by stacking the k extracted eigenvectors in columns.
6.	Solving $\mathbf{A}$ and σ_p^2. Form an optimization problem in *Frobenius norm*: $$\min J(\mathbf{A}, \sigma_p^2) = \frac{1}{2} \left\| \mathbf{X}\mathbf{X}^T - \mathbf{X}_{part}\mathbf{X}_{part}^T \right\|_F^2 \quad (2)$$ $$s.t. \mathbf{A} \succeq \mathbf{0}$$ where, $\mathbf{X}_{part} = \mathbf{C}^{-1/2}\mathbf{E}(\mathbf{E}^T\mathbf{C}\mathbf{E})^{-1/2}\mathbf{B}$. $\mathbf{E}$ is an indicator matrix of data set partitions and $\mathbf{B}$ is an arbitrary orthogonal matrix. Applying $\mathbf{A} \succeq \mathbf{0}$ as a constraint to the optimization problem and find optimal solutions of $\mathbf{A}$ and σ_p^2 through gradient descent algorithm.
Output:	Learned parameters $\mathbf{A}$ and σ_p^2 of the metric.

i.e. $\mathbf{A} \succeq \mathbf{0}$. The aim of metric learning is to find proper parameters of the metric, so that data from different groups can be well separated. The task of learning such a metric involves finding proper $\mathbf{A}$ and σ_p^2 in our case. Hence, parameters in the metric is determined algorithmically, not empirically.

2.2 Metric Learning with Spectral Clustering

Spectral clustering [6] is often considered as an approximate solution to the *graph-cut* problem [9], which achieves partitioning of images by cutting weak links between graph nodes to separate images into various segments. Our metric learning method is performed with a spectral clustering algorithm [6]. The procedure of our metric learning algorithm based on that in [7] is presented in Table 1.

The original metric learning algorithm with spectral clustering is for the Gaussian width σ^2 of a simple Gaussian RBF metric in [7]. Since the metric in Eq.(1) is more complicated, simply applying the learning algorithm in [7] is unreasonable, and $\mathbf{A}$ in Eq.(1) has its own constraint to be satisfied, viz. $\mathbf{A} \succeq \mathbf{0}$. Therefore, we take this constraint into consideration when learning parameters of the metric via a minimization of function in Eq.(2). Through a gradient decent algorithm with constraint in Eq.(2), optimum solutions for parameters in Eq.(1) are found. Hence, a learned metric is obtained.

2.3 User Interaction

In this work, we allow clinicians to draw their own *Region of Interests* (ROI), in which they assume NPC lesion will be enclosed. The ROI can be in any arbitrary shape and the enclosure does not have to be very close to the lesion's boundary. The reason for us to do so is to utilize the prior knowledge about NPC lesion used by clinicians. By using such a ROI, we can also avoid the influence of tissues with numerous capillary vessels (e.g. nasal cavity), which share similar visual properties as NPC lesion regions after patients are injected with contrast agents for lesion enhancement. Points inside the enclosed region are sampled as positive training samples and points outside are sampled as negative training samples for constructing input S in Table 1. In our implementations, positive samples often share similar intensities and are chosen from the center area of ROI. However, negative samples are usually highly variable in intensity and more difficult to sample. A simple random sampling strategy can result in under-representation of some sub-populations (stratums) of negative points, making negative samples less representative. It will bias our learning and deteriorate the final segmentation results. Therefore, we apply *stratified random sampling* strategy [10] in sampling negative points. The optimal stratum allocation scheme used is *Neyman allocation* [10], which allocates relatively large number of negative samples if one stratum contains a larger fraction of points with largely varying intensities.

3 Tumor Segmentation through Unsupervised Out-of-Sample Extension

The second step of our method is to perform MR image segmentation by spectral clustering on pixels other than those sampled for metric learning in the previous step. The main computational burden of spectral clustering is from the eigen-decomposition of the matrix $\mathbf{L}$ of size $n \times n$, where n is the total number of pixels in a MR image. In the previous metric learning step, this is not a problem as the number of points in the labeled training sample set S are still small. If spectral clustering is used to group all points in MR images, the size of matrix $\mathbf{L}$ will become extremely large and causes problems in eigen-decomposition. For this reason, we apply the *out-of-sample extension method* [11] in our problem. The aim of this method is to map points into the spectral domain directly using a mapping function. Therefore, the main computational burden of eigen-decomposition can be avoided.

For remaining points, the similarity is calculated with respect to each sample in the training set S via the learned metric. In our work, since we use prior knowledge to enclose the NPC lesion region inside ROI, the points outside the ROI should not be considered. Hence, we have a similarity matrix $\mathbf{D}$ of size (number of remaining samples in ROI) × (number of samples in S). Although the size of this matrix is smaller than if considering all remaining points in MR images, it is still not practical to apply eigen-decomposition directly. After normalization, the affinity matrix $\mathbf{D}$ is given by

$$\mathbf{D}_{ij} = \frac{\mathbf{D}_{ij}}{\sqrt{\sum_{x \in S} \mathbf{D}_{ix} \sum_{x' \in S} \mathbf{D}_{jx'}}} \qquad (3)$$

The spectral embedding of remaining points in ROI can be computed from

$$\mathbf{X}_{mapped} = \mathbf{D} \cdot \mathbf{X} \cdot \mathbf{V}^{-1} \qquad (4)$$

where, $\mathbf{X}$ and $\mathbf{V}$ are the matrices of eigenvectors and eigenvalues obtained from the training data set S, respectively. After obtaining $\mathbf{X}_{mapped}$, we can use some clustering algorithms, such as the *K-means* algorithm ($k = 2$, for tumor or non-tumor group), to extract the NPC lesion region unsupervisedly therein.

4 Experiments and Discussion

Our method has been evaluated with 6 pairs of MR images from 6 patients, which are acquired from a $1.5T$ MR scanner (Signa, GE Medical Systems) from different patients. The feature vector s in Eq. (1) is composed of normalized intensities from T1 Weighted (T1W) (or T2 Weighted T2W) images and their corresponding Contrast Enhanced T1 Weighted (CET1W) images with fat suppression. The reason to do so is to follow the way in which clinicians manually trace NPC lesion in their practice by utilizing both T1W (or T2W) and CET1W images. We simulate the variation among radiologists by creating 4 slightly different ROIs in each pair of MR scans (from a patient) for a total of 6 patients. We further generated 4 sample sets for each ROI to test algorithm stability. Hence, we have 96 sets of training data sampled from all the MR images, and we ran 96 times of the methods to obtain a total of 96 segmentation results for each method.

To demonstrate the performance of our method over other existing similar region-based methods, we conducted several experiments and set up a statistical test for quantitative analysis of results. Besides our method, there are three other methods for comparison, including binary-class *Support Vector Machine* (SVM), *Support Vector Data Description* (SVDD) [12] of one-class SVM, and a baseline method in which one performs the same steps as in our method but without metric learning (Baseline). For SVM, we utilized Gaussian RBF kernel and *radius-margin bound* method [13] for its parameter learning. For baseline method, $\mathbf{A}$ and σ_p are set as an identity matrix and 0.1, respectively. For SVDD, a Gaussian RBF kernel with width 0.5 and a 0.1 rejection ratio are applied.

We evaluated the NPC extraction results based on two criteria with respect to NPC ground truth manually delineated by our radiologist, and they are *Positive Predictive Value* (PPV) [14] and *sensitivity*. PPV is used to evaluate the proportion of correctly extracted NPC regions. The definition of PPV is $PPV = \frac{TPs}{TPs+FPs}$ [14], where TPs is the number of *True Positives* (tumor points correctly detected) and FPs is the number of *False Positives* (non-tumor points wrongly detected as tumor points). Sensitivity is defined as $sensitivity = \frac{TPs}{RS}$, in which RS is the NPC ground truth. PPV can be biased by under-segmentation, in which the segmentation result is a tiny portion of NPC caused by small TPs and $FPs \simeq 0$.

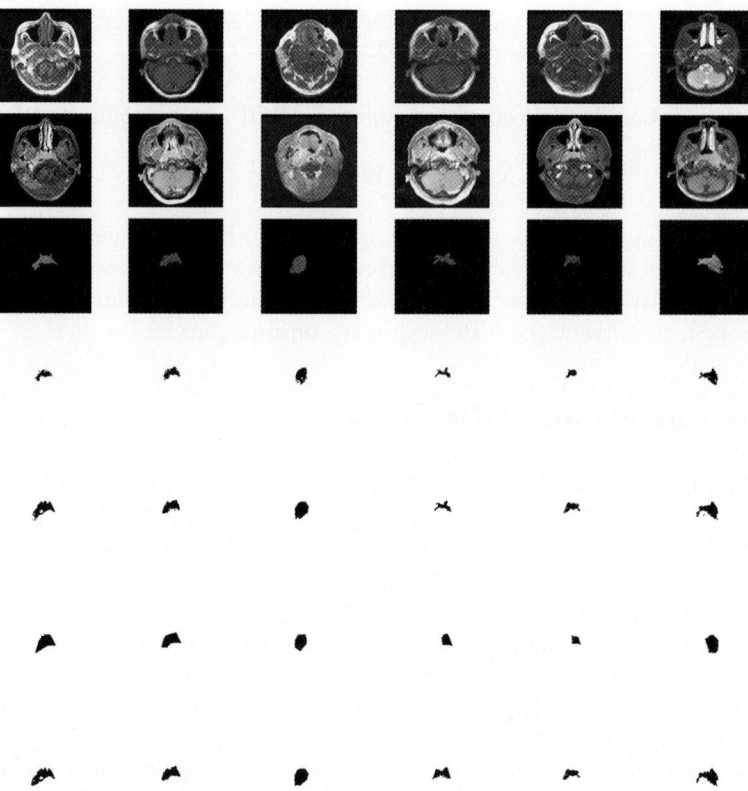

Fig. 1. (Rows from up to down) T1W (or T2W) MR images, CET1W MR images with fat suppression, NPC lesion ground truth manually traced by our radiologist, NPC extraction results by SVDD, NPC extraction results by SVM, NPC extraction results by Base line, NPC extraction results by our method.

Sensitivity can also be biased by over-segmentation, in which TPs is large due to overlapping of NPC ground truth with large segmented region. Thus, in order to have a more objective assessment, we adopt both measures for quantitative analysis. Some NPC extraction results based on the same training data and ROIs are shown in Figure 1. All extraction results have been post-processed by morphological opening and closing operations with a disk-shaped structuring element of radius 1 to remove isolated points, holes and thin line structures in identified NPC regions. We can easily see that SVM and our method achieve the most similar results compared to the ground truth. For SVDD, it tends to extract a small portion of the ground truth, since it only uses positive samples. The high whisker of SVDD PPV box in Figure 2 and the low whisker of SVDD sensitivity box in Figure 3 also substantiate this observation. For the baseline method, the ranges between upper quartiles and lower quartiles of both PPV and sensitivity boxes are large, which shows that predefined parameters work well for some sets, but not for others. For SVM and our method, a detailed statistical test is applied to further discern which

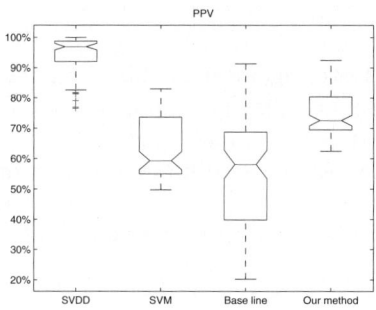 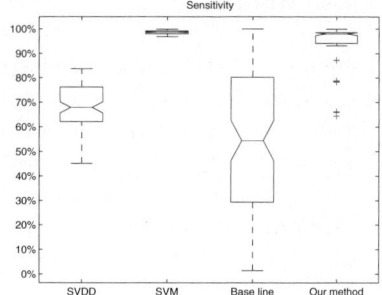

Fig. 2. PPV of four methods   **Fig. 3.** Sensitivity of four methods

Table 2. Multiple comparison test results of PPV and sensitivity of SVM and our method

	Method 1	Method 2	Mean diff	Estimated mean diff	95% Confidence int.
PPV	SVM	Our method	-14.97%	-10.64%	-6.31%
Sensitivity	SVM	Our method	-2.22%	3.81%	9.83%

method has a superior performance over another from statistical point of view. We design a test of *analysis of variance* (ANOVA) followed by post-hoc *multiple comparison test* [10]. After performing two one-way ANOVA tests for results of PPV and sensitivity from SVM and our method respectively, the *p-values* are 0, which casts serious doubt on the null hypothesis that SVM and our method are with the same PPV and sensitivity means. Therefore, two more post-hoc multiple comparison tests are applied to test which method has superior statistical PPV and sensitivity means. Results of multiple comparison test for comparisons between the two methods are in listed in Table 2. The last three columns of the table indicate the mean difference being compared (mean of Method 1 minus mean of Method 2), the estimated mean difference and a 95% confidence interval for the mean difference, respectively. From the entries in the table, we can see that, the estimated mean of our method is 10.64% higher than SVM for PPV measure, but 3.81% lower than SVM for sensitivity measure. For the comparison of two methods by PPV, a 95% confidence interval for the mean difference is $[-14.97\%, -6.31\%]$. This result gives a strong indication that for over 95% sets of data, our method achieve better results than SVM based on PPV measure from statistical viewpoint. For the comparison of two methods by sensitivity, a 95% confidence interval for the mean difference is $[-2.22\%, 9.83\%]$. From this we can see that, SVM performs better than our method for some sets of data, but not for others. Therefore, based on the conclusions derived from statistical analysis of the two measures, our method can achieve comparable or marginally better performance than SVM for the majority of data from the statistical perspective with due consideration of non-linearity in the PPV measure.

5 Conclusion

In this paper, a semi-supervised spectral clustering method based on metric learning is proposed for the extraction of nasopharyngeal carcinoma lesion from MR images. We conducted several experiments to evaluate our methods and compared it with other similar methods. Experiments results show the superiority of adopting metric learning in our method. Also, our method achieves comparable or marginally better performance than discriminative SVM-based method according to our statistical analysis.

References

1. Chang, E., Adami, H.: The enigmatic epidemiology of nasopharyngeal carcinoma. Cancer Epidemiology Biomarkers and Prevention 15, 1765–1777 (2006)
2. Xu, C., Prince, J.: Snake, shape, and gradient vector flow. IEEE TIP 7, 359–369 (1998)
3. Li, C., Kao, C., Gore, J., Ding, Z.: Implicit active contours driven by local binary fitting energy. In: IEEE CVPR, pp. 1–7 (2007)
4. Bullmore, E., Brammer, M., Rouleau, G., Everitt, B., Simmons, A.: Computerized brain tissue classification of magnetic resonance images: a new approach to the problem of partial volume artifact. Neuroimage 2, 133–147 (1995)
5. Kapur, T., Grimson, W., Kikinis, R., Wells, W.: Enhanced spatial priors for segmentation of magnetic resonance imagery. In: Wells, W.M., Colchester, A.C.F., Delp, S.L. (eds.) MICCAI 1998. LNCS, vol. 1496, pp. 457–468. Springer, Heidelberg (1998)
6. Ng, A., Jordan, M., Weiss, Y.: On spectral clustering: analysis and an algorithm. In: NIPS, pp. 64–72 (2002)
7. Bach, F., Jordan, M.: Learning spectral clustering, with application to speech separation. JMLR 7, 1963–2001 (2006)
8. Shi, J., Malik, J.: Normalized cuts and image segmentation. IEEE TPAMI 22, 888–905 (2000)
9. Boykov, Y., Veksler, O., Zabih, R.: Fast approximate energy minimization via graph cuts. IEEE TPAMI 23, 1222–1239 (2001)
10. Rice, J.: Mathematical Statistics and Data Analysis, 2nd edn. (2007)
11. Bengio, Y., Paiement, J., Vincent, P., Delalleau, O., Roux, N., Ouimet, M.: Out-of-sample extension for lle, isomap, mds, eigenmaps, and spectral clustering. In: NIPS, pp. 857–863 (2003)
12. Tax, D., Duin, R.: Support vector data desription. Machine learning 54, 45–66 (2004)
13. Chapelle, O., Vapnik, V., Bousquet, O., Mukherjee, S.: Choosing multiple parameters for support vector machines. Machine learning 46, 131–159 (2002)
14. Gunnarsson, R., Lanke, J.: The predictive value of microbiologic diagnostic tests if asymptomatic carriers are present. Statistics in medicine 21, 1773–1785 (2002)

Multi-level Classification of Emphysema in HRCT Lung Images Using Delegated Classifiers

Mithun Prasad[1] and Arcot Sowmya[2]

[1] Cedars-Sinai Medical Center,
8700 Beverly Blvd.
Los Angeles, CA 90048
[2] School of Computer Science and Engineering,
University of New South Wales,
Sydney, NSW, 2052, Australia
mithunp@cse.unsw.edu.au, sowmya@cse.unsw.edu.au

Abstract. Emphysema is a common chronic respiratory disorder characterized by the destruction of lung tissue. It is a progressive disease where the early stages are characterized by diffuse appearance of small air spaces and later stages exhibit large air spaces called bullae. A bullous region is a sharply demarcated region of emphysema. In this paper, we show that an automated texture-based system based on delegated classifiers is capable of achieving multiple levels of emphysema extraction in High Resolution Computed Tomography (HRCT) images. The key idea of delegation is that a cautious classifier makes predictions that meet a minimum level of confidence, and delegates the difficult or uncertain predictions to a more specialized classifier. In this paper, we design a two-step scenario where a first classifier chooses the examples to classify on and delegates the more difficult examples to a second classifier. We compare this technique to well known emphysema classification techniques and ensemble methods such as bagging and boosting. Comparison of the results shows that the techniques presented here are more accurate. From a medical standpoint, the classifiers built at different iterations appear to show an interesting correlation with different levels of emphysema.

Keywords: CT, emphysema, texture, delegated classifiers.

1 Introduction

High Resolution Computer Tomography (HRCT) is a valuable imaging modality for assessing diffuse lung diseases and in particular, emphysema. The automated analysis of HRCT scans poses difficult problems, because the radiographic patterns observed are often varied and subtle. Emphysema diagnosis by radiologists is often based on visual recognition of imaging patterns augmented by anatomical knowledge. Emphysema is a common chronic respiratory disorder characterised by the destruction of lung tissue and is often reflected as areas of low attenuation in CT images [1].

Emphysema regions are typically small in the early stages, but become larger and involve the lung more diffusely over time. Large air spaces called bullae may

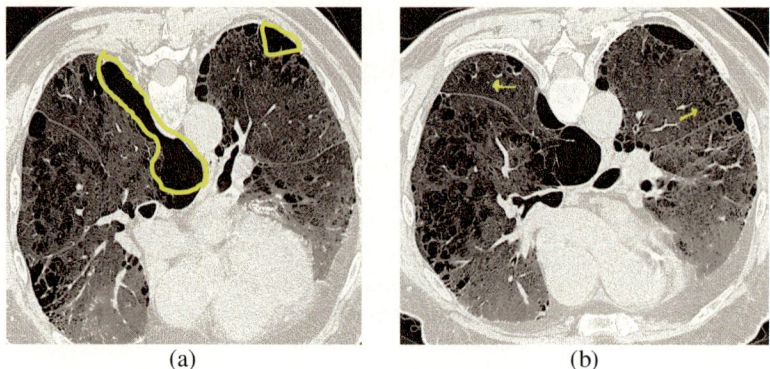

Fig. 1. 1(a) A typical HRCT scan containing bullous emphysema. 1(b). A typical HRCT scan containing diffuse regions of emphysema.

develop, particularly in the later stages. Bullous emphysema is histologically defined as the presence of emphysematous areas with complete destruction of lung tissue. Classification of bullae is useful to evaluate patients as candidates for surgery. Figure 1 visually presents examples of bullous and diffuse regions of emphysema.

The techniques utilized in this paper are intended to automate the recognition process and assist radiologists in the diagnosis of emphysema by providing accurate measures of severity across each HRCT scan. This is achieved by using the idea of delegated classifiers. In automated emphysema detection in lung images, a common technique called "Density Mask" is applied simply to threshold the image [1]. However, a fixed threshold yields unsatisfactory results when the degree of emphysema is low. Computerised techniques for classifying emphysema have been explored [2-4] using texture and machine learning approaches with reports of reasonable accuracy. However, very few techniques that distinguish the type of emphsyema have been reported [4].

The proposed system is based on delegated classifiers [5]. Delegation can be summarized by the motto: *let others do the things you cannot do well*. We use the notion of a cautious classifier which only classifies the examples for which its predictions have high confidence, leaving the other examples to another classifier. Delegated classifiers have been successfully developed and tested on "artificial" datasets from the UCI repository [5]. However, application of delegated classifiers to vision problems has not been addressed to our knowledge. In this work, we also show that delegation is capable of classifying different levels of diagnosis automatically. The levels range from the larger set of diffuse and bullous regions, to bullous regions only.

2 Methods

2.1 Texture Feature Extraction

In this work, textural features are used to characterize emphysema. We extract textural features using two main steps: automatic segmentation of the lungs and feature extraction. The lungs in the image are initially located and extracted. A suite of classical image processing techniques is used to segment lung regions using in house software [6]. This is quite a straightforward approach where the different morphological operations performed to segment lung regions include dilation, erosion and thresholding. The percentage area occupied by lung regions in the whole image is used to decide whether the image is of interest. A percentage value of less than 6 is considered unacceptable.

In our application, feature extraction is primarily based on texture as emphysema is a finding that can be well characterized by texture. A feature vector is defined as a set of textural parameters calculated on a small neighborhood of 12x12 pixels surrounding each image point belonging to the lung region. Window sizes less than 12x12 do not provide uniformity of disease patterns and window sizes larger than 12x12 are computationally expensive. The textural parameters used in the experiments are based on the following methods:

1. moments of gray level histogram of a local area
2. gray level co-occurrence matrix method (GLCMM)
3. gray level run length matrix method (GLRLMM)
4. gray level difference method (GLDM)

The GLCMM, one of the well known texture analysis methods, estimates image properties related to second-order statistics. Each entry (i,j) in GLCM corresponds to the number of occurrences of the pair of gray levels i and j at a distance d apart at an angle θ in original image. The configurations of the co-occurrence matrix used in our experiments include $1 \leq d \leq 2$ and $0 \leq \theta \leq 90$, ± 45 since these values are sufficient to cover uniformity of disease features. The GLRLMM is based on computing the number of gray level runs of various lengths in different directions. Each element of the GLRLM (i,j) specifies the estimated number of times a picture contains a run of length j, for gray level i, in the direction of angle θ. Three grey level run length matrices, where $0 \leq \theta \leq 360$ in steps of 45, are used in our experiments. The full range of θ provides greater uniformity among the various disease features used in our experiments. GLDM is concerned with the spatial gray-level distribution and spatial dependence among the gray levels in a local area. The features extracted from the methods are displayed in Table 1; some features have multiple values, as discussed above.

Table 1. Textural Features

Moments of Histogram	GLCMM	GLRLM	GLDM
Mean	Energy	Short Emphasis	Mean
SD	Entropy	Long run emphasis	Contrast
Variance	Homogeneity	Gray level uniformity	Entropy
Energy	Contrast	Primitive length uniformity	SD
Entropy		Primitive percentage	Variance

2.2 Delegation

The idea of delegation revolves around two main issues [5]. Firstly, one needs to determine a threshold or a rule to decide when to apply the first classifier and when to delegate to the second one. Secondly, one needs to determine good techniques to generate classifiers that perform better than the first one for the examples that the first one has delegated. We use a probabilistic classifier to estimate the reliability. The second issue is addressed by specializing the second classifier on examples for which the first classifier behaves worst. This is achieved by training the second classifier on solely the examples rejected by the first classifier. There are two main advantages of delegation fold. Firstly, since the first classifier is holding part of the examples, the second classifier has fewer examples for training. This results in a more efficient process than other ensemble techniques. Secondly, the resulting overall classifier is a decision list whose decisions can be traced and understood, unlike in comparable techiques.

2.2.1 Cautious Classifier

In many application areas, a classifier that abstains from making a prediction when it is not sure of being able to make the right decision is preferable over a greedy classifier that always makes a classification. A cautious classifier is one that gives predictions for the subset of inputs for which it is more confident (that may still be right or wrong) but abstains for the rest of its inputs. In other words, a cautious classifier is a partial function.

Any classifier that can reliably estimate class probabilities or the reliability of each prediction, can be converted to a cautious classifier. For a classifier f we can consider the associated functions $f_{CLASS}(e)$, $f_{CONF}(e)$ and $f_{PROBc}(e)$ (for each class c from a total of C classes). The function $f_{CLASS}(e)$ returns the class assigned by classifier f to example e, $f_{PROBc}(e)$ returns the probability of class c for example e, and $f_{CONF}(e)$ returns the highest probability among all classes for example e. Unless stated otherwise, we assume that $f_{CLASS}(e) = \arg\max_c f_{PROBc}(e)$ and $f_{CONF}(e) = \max_c \{f_{PROBc}(e)\}$.

Given these definitions, a cautious classifier f can be obtained from a soft classifier using a confidence threshold.

Decision Rule for a cautious classifier with threshold τ:

If $f_{CONF}(e) > \tau$ then predict $f_{CLASS}(e)$ else abstain

A soft classifier will be converted into a good cautious classifier if the reliabilities are well estimated, as achieved by, for instance, a good class probability estimator, or, for binary problems, a good ranker. It is the idea of completing the cautious classifiers that leads to the concept of *delegation*. If a cautious classifier f^1 decides that it is not competent to classify an example with good confidence, but wants to complete the work, then it can delegate the example to another classifier. If we had this second classifier, denoted by f^2, and a confidence threshold τ, then the delegating rule is as follows:

Decision Rule for a delegating classifier with threshold τ:

If $f^1_{CONF}(e) > \tau$ then predict $f^1_{CLASS}(e)$ else predict $f^2_{CLASS}(e)$

A common way to obtain classifier f^2 is to train it only on the training examples for which f^1 has low confidence. In this way, the second classifier will be specialized for these examples. More formally, given a training set Tr, a soft classifier f and a confidence threshold τ, we divide this set into two data sets $Tr_f^> = \{e \in Tr : f_{CONF}(e) > \tau\}$ and $Tr_f^\leq = Tr - Tr_f^>$. In other words, we can refer to $Tr_f^>$ as the "retained" or "high confidence" examples and $Tr_f^\leq$ as the "delegated" or "low-confidence" examples. In this work, we use the same threshold for training and for prediction. The approach taken here is that a classifier retains a fixed percentage of the examples. For instance, we may stipulate that the first classifier should retain 70% of the most highly ranked examples, delegating the rest to the second classifier. This technique is known as *Global Absolute Percentage*. In the case of imbalanced datasets, a technique known as *Stratified Absolute Percentage* may be used, where the decision rule can be modified to incorporate a different threshold τ_c for each class c as shown below. In the case of stratified absolute percentage, if we denote Tr_c as the examples in Tr of class c, the retained examples in this case are:

$$Tr_f^> = \{e \in Tr_c : c = f_{CONF}(e) \wedge f_{CLASS}(e) > \tau_c\}$$

<u>Decision Rule for a delegating classifier with threshold</u> $\tau_1, \tau_2, ..., \tau_c$:

If $f^1_{CONF}(e) > \tau_c$ then predict $f^1_{CLASS}(e)$ else predict $f^2_{CLASS}(e)$ where $c = f^1_{CLASS}(e)$

3 Experimental Results and Discussion

The accuracy measure is used to evaluate the performance of our algorithm. Accuracy is defined as the percentage of correctly classified examples (which includes both positive and negative examples). The emphysema regions were manually characterized in consultation with a board-certified radiologist. In the experiments, we use naive Bayesian classifier to perform classification at both levels in the delegated framework. Naive Bayes estimates the probability of class membership based on Bayes rule [7]. The delegated classifier was trained on 13 HRCT scans (chosen randomly from 8 subjects) and evaluated on a separate labelled test set comprising 60 HRCT scans (randomly chosen from 9 subjects), and the visual results are presented in Figure 2. It can be seen in 2(d) that the second classifier identifies more regions of emphysema than the first one precisely on the low-confidence examples delegated by the first classifier. This is the key to the overall improvement achieved by the delegated classifier. It is also worth noting that the low confidence examples in the HRCT scans correspond to diffuse regions of emphysema. The output of the "density mask" algorithm (Figure 2(b)) shows that a lot of noise is picked up along with the emphysema regions.

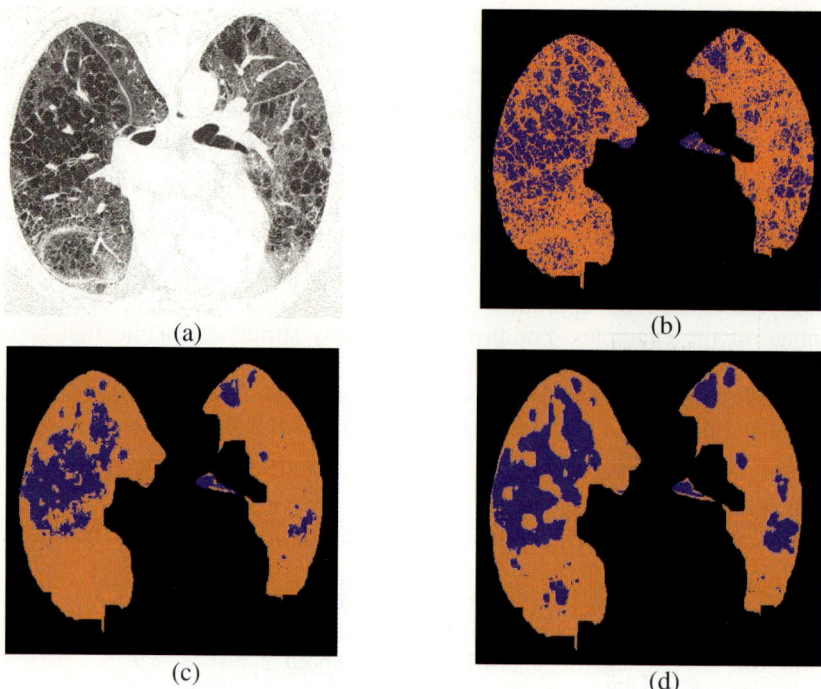

Fig. 2. 2(a) contains the original image where the dark regions correspond to emphysema. 2(b) is the output of "Density Mask" where the blue regions are emphysema. 2(c) and 2(d) correspond to the output of the first classifier and the overall classifier in the delegated framework respectively. The first classifier identifies mostly the "more confident" or the bullous regions whereas very diffuse regions of emphysema can be classified using the second classifier in the delegated framework.

Additionally, Table 2 demonstrates that accuracy is not very sensitive to the percentage of examples retained, although it seems that 60% is a good compromise. Lower percentages would mean most of the work is left to the second classifier, which is then very similar to the first one and not specialized sufficiently to improve the results. A high retention lowers the influence of the second classifier and may perhaps lead to its overfitting. However, the model appears to be robust in the sense that, with different configurations, the mean accuracy is never worse than for a single classifier (0%).

Table 2. Performance of delegated classifiers with different global absolute percentage (GAP) and stratified absolute percentage (SAP)

	0%	10%	20%	30%	40%	50%	60%	70%	80%
GAP	89	93	93	93	93	92	93	93	93
SAF	89	92	93	91	93	92	93	92	92

In addition, comparison was also performed on other well known techniques that have been explored for emphysema detection as can be seen in Table 3. The accuracy is higher for the delegated classifier (global absolute percentage of 20% used). Intuitively, the delegation forces the classifier to focus on the weak examples using a new decision rule. The "Density mask" identifies a large amount of emphysema that is mostly "not correct" as shown in figure 2.

Table 3. Comparison of average accuracy of the delegated classifier with well known emphysema classification techniques

	Average Accuracy
Density Mask	95
Seeded K-means	88
ICA – C4.5	84
ICA – Naive Bayes	84
Error Backpropagation	84
Support vector machine	86
Delegated classifier, GAP of 20%	94

Finally, we compare delegating (GAP of 20%) with two ensemble techniques, namely boosting and bagging [8], using naive Bayes as the base classifiers. As can be seen in Table 4, the delegated classifier is better than the ensemble methods in terms of average accuracy. Delegated classifiers are more efficient than classical ensemble methods, because each subsequent classifier is learned using fewer examples than the previous one. In the delegated framework, predictions of classifiers are not combined. Each instance is classified by a single classifier. This does not degrade the comprehensibility of the model as ensembles do. Additionally, comparison of the results in Table 4 was made using a mixed-effects linear model [9] and we found a significant difference between our method and the other techniques ($p<0.001$).

Table 4. Comparison between delegation and ensemble techniques. Bagging and boosting were performed with 10 and 20 iterations.

	Average Accuracy
Bagging – 10	87
Boosting – 10	88
Bagging – 20	86
Boosting – 20	89
Delegated classifier, GAP of 20%	94

4 Conclusions

In this paper, an approach to perform multi-level diagnosis of emphysema detection based on delegated classifiers has been presented. Delegation only makes predictions that meet a minimum level of confidence and delegates to another classifier otherwise. Results have been compared against "density mask", a standard approach used for emphysema detection in medical image analysis. In general, the density mask method has been known to mark more pixels as emphysematous than warranted, and it has been speculated that many marked pixels do not represent true emphysema. The results of the method proposed here appear to confirm this. Other well known computerized techniques used for classification of emphysema have also been used for comparison and the results show that by using a specialized classifier, classification accuracy can be improved. A system that is capable of differentiating the appearance of emphysema regions has been successfully reported in this paper, which would help experts in the medical setting to analyze the progressive nature of the disease. In the future, we plan to investigate the use of different base classifiers at each delegation stage. At different levels of the delegation chain, different classifiers can be used. We also plan to investigate the utility of delegated classifiers in multi-class classification tasks within the HRCT setting.

Acknowledgement

This research was partially supported by the Australian Research Council through a Linkage grant (2002-2004), with Medical Imaging Australasia as clinical and Philips Medical Systems as industrial partners.

References

1. Kinsella, M., Mueller, N.L., Abboud, R.T., Morrison, N.J., DyBuncio, A.: Quantification of emphysema by computed tomography using a density mask program and correlation with pulmonary function tests 97, 315–321 (1990)
2. Friman, O., Borga, M., Lundberg, M., Tylén, U., Knutsson, H.: Recognizing emphysema - A Neural Network Approach. In: Proceedings of 16th International Conference on Pattern Recognition (August 2002)
3. Prasad, M., Sowmya, A., Koch, I.: Feature Subset Selection using ICA for classifying Emphysema in HRCT images. In: Proc. of international conference on intelligent sensors, sensor networks and information processing, Melbourne, Australia (2004)
4. Prasad, M., Sowmya, A., Wilson, P.: Multi-level Classification of Emphysema in HRCT lung images. Pattern Analysis and Applications Journal (in press, 2007)
5. Ferri, C., Flach, P., Hernandez-Orallo, J.: Delegating classifiers. In: Proceedings of 21th International Conference on Machine Learning, pp. 106–110. Omni press, Alberta (2004)
6. Chiu, P.T., Sowmya, A.: Lung Boundary Detection and Low Level feature extraction and analysis from HRCT images. In: VISIM: Information Retrieval and Exploration of Large Medical Image Collections (October 2001)
7. Mitchell, T.: Machine Learning. McGraw Hill, New York (1997)
8. Freund, Y., Schapire, R.E.: A short introduction to boosting. Journal of Japanese Society for Artificial Intelligence 14(5), 771–780 (1999)
9. Laird, N.M., Ware, J.H.: Random Effects Models for Longitudinal Data. Biometrics 38, 963–974 (1982)

A Discriminative Model-Constrained Graph Cuts Approach to Fully Automated Pediatric Brain Tumor Segmentation in 3-D MRI

Michael Wels[1,4], Gustavo Carneiro[2], Alexander Aplas[3], Martin Huber[4], Joachim Hornegger[1], and Dorin Comaniciu[2]

[1] Chair of Pattern Recognition, University Erlangen-Nuremberg, Germany
michael.wels@informatik.uni-erlangen.de
[2] Siemens Corporate Research, IDS, Princeton, NJ, USA
[3] Institute of Radiology, University Medical Center, Erlangen, Germany
[4] Siemens, CT SE SCR 2, Erlangen, Germany

Abstract. In this paper we present a fully automated approach to the segmentation of pediatric brain tumors in multi-spectral 3-D magnetic resonance images. It is a top-down segmentation approach based on a Markov random field (MRF) model that combines probabilistic boosting trees (PBT) and lower-level segmentation via graph cuts. The PBT algorithm provides a strong discriminative observation model that classifies tumor appearance while a spatial prior takes into account the pair-wise homogeneity in terms of classification labels and multi-spectral voxel intensities. The discriminative model relies not only on observed local intensities but also on surrounding context for detecting candidate regions for pathology. A mathematically sound formulation for integrating the two approaches into a unified statistical framework is given. The proposed method is applied to the challenging task of detection and delineation of pediatric brain tumors. This segmentation task is characterized by a high non-uniformity of both the pathology and the surrounding non-pathologic brain tissue. A quantitative evaluation illustrates the robustness of the proposed method. Despite dealing with more complicated cases of *pediatric brain tumors* the results obtained are mostly better than those reported for current state-of-the-art approaches to 3-D MR brain tumor segmentation in adult patients. The entire processing of one multi-spectral data set does not require any user interaction, and takes less time than previously proposed methods.

1 Introduction

Detection and delineation of pathology, such as cancerous tissue, within multi-spectral brain magnetic resonance (MR) volume sequences is an important problem in medical image analysis. For example, a precise and reliable segmentation of brain tumors present in the childlike brain is regarded critical when aiming for the automatic extraction of diagnostically relevant quantitative or more abstract findings. This may include the volume of the tumor or its relative location. Once these findings are obtained they can be used both for guiding computer-aided

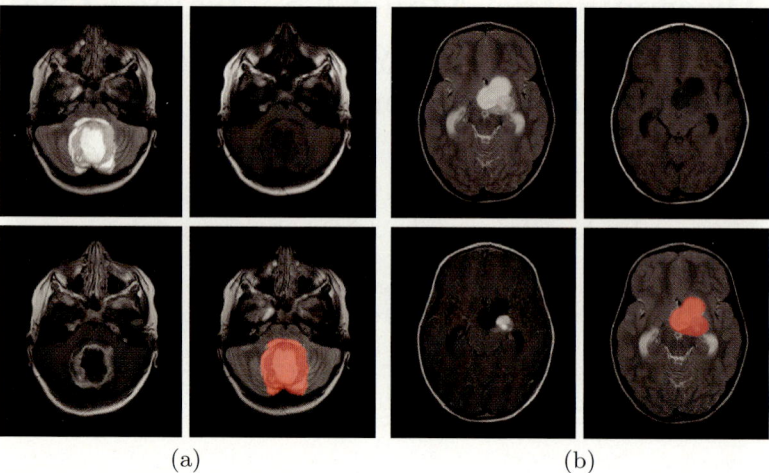

Fig. 1. Two different cases of pediatric brain tumors exhibiting heterogeneous shape and appearance. Columns (a) and (b) show axial slices of the typically acquired pulse sequences (row-wise from left to right: T2-weighted, T1-weighted, and T1-weighted after contrast enhancement) and the expert annotated ground-truth overlaid to the T2-weighted pulse sequence. Please view in color.

diagnosis and therapy planning as well as for traditional decision making. However, the manual labeling of volumetric data is usually time consuming, which has the potential to delay clinical workflow, such that there is a need for fully automatic segmentation tools in this particular context. Furthermore, manual annotations may vary significantly among experts as a result of individual experience and interpretation.

As multi-spectral 3-D magnetic resonance imaging (MRI) is the method of choice for the examination of neurological pathology such as brain cancer in pediatric patients, automatic approaches first have to be capable of dealing with the characteristic artifacts of this imaging modality: Rician noise, partial volume effects, and intra-/inter-scan intensity inhomogeneities. Second and more importantly, they have to be robust enough to handle the heterogeneous shape and appearance of pediatric brain tumors in different patients (see Fig. 1).

In this paper, we propose a fully automatic solution based on a novel top-down segmentation scheme that uses a statistical model of the pathology appearance as a constraint for a sub-sequent optimization problem. The statistical model is provided by a machine learning technique that is able to work with high-dimensional feature vectors allowing to encode characteristic voxel contexts. The optimization problem itself is stated as a search for an MAP estimate of the most-likely binary image segmentation, which permits efficient computation of a solution by means of a max-flow/min-cut optimization procedure and is optimal in terms of Bayesian classification theory.

Approaches in the field of MR brain tumor segmentation rarely rely on pure data-driven approaches due to the complexity in terms of tumor shape and appearance of the segmentation task. The vast majority of methods make use of domain knowledge using different types of representation and combine it with low-level imaging techniques. Fletcher-Heath et al. [1] use unsupervised fuzzy clustering followed by 3-D connected components with an intermediate step incorporating knowledge about the usual distribution of cerebral spinal fluid and location of the ventricular system. Gering et al. [2] use trained parametric statistical models for intensity distributions of non-pathologic brain tissue to detect model outliers on the voxel level that are considered tumor voxels in a multi-layer Markov random field framework. In a similar manner Prastawa et al. [3] detect outliers based on refined intensity distributions for healthy brain tissue initially derived from a registered probabilistic atlas, which introduces structural domain knowledge. Registration is also used in combination with voxel intensities in the adaptive template-moderated classification algorithm by [4]. More recent approaches try to enrich low level segmentation techniques, like level set evolution [5] or hierarchical clustering [6], by using supervised machine learning on higher dimensional feature sets associated with each image voxel. These feature sets are capable of representing a more general variety of domain knowledge on different levels of abstraction. In a similar manner we make use of the recently proposed technique of probabilistic boosting trees (PBT) [7] for supervised learning, which has proven its robustness and its capability for efficient training and classification in numerous applications [8,9]. The probability estimates provided by PBT are then used to constrain the highly efficient computation of minimum cuts [10] for image segmentation based on a Markov random field (MRF) prior model. It takes into account both coherence of classification labels as well as multi-spectral intensity similarities within voxel neighborhoods.

To the best of our knowledge, this is the first paper giving an integrated formulation for combining PBT classification and computation of minimum cuts. Opposed to [6,5] there is no involvement of a time consuming bias field correction step in data pre-processing. In the case of [6] this seems to be done by FAST [11], which relies on an HMRF-EM segmentation approach. In the presence of abnormal tissue types this requires the determination of the number of different intensity regions expected within each scan. Furthermore, the inherent low level segmentation might bias the final segmentation result. In contrast we build discriminative models, i.e. PBTs, whose generalization capabilities are strong enough to implicitly handle those intra-patient intensity non-uniformities. Moreover, we apply our method to the more complicated task of segmenting pediatric brain tumors where not only pathology underlies significant variation in shape and appearance but also the non-pathological "background", which is caused by ongoing myelination of white matter during maturation [12].

2 Discriminative Model-Constrained Graph Cuts Segmentation

Our segmentation method relies on the integrated formulation of an objective function that is subject to optimization via the efficient graph cuts algorithm

[10]. In the following we derive this objective function from the general MAP framework for image segmentation.

In general, the problem of segmenting an image can be stated as the search for an MAP estimate of the most likely class labels given appropriate prior and observation models in terms of probability density functions. Let $\mathcal{S} = \{1, 2, \ldots, N\}$, $N \in \mathbb{N}$, be a set of indices to image voxels. At each index $s \in \mathcal{S}$ there are two random variables: $y_s \in \mathcal{Y} = \{+1, -1\}$ and $\boldsymbol{x}_s \in \mathcal{X} = \mathbb{R}^M$, $M \in \mathbb{N}$. The former, y_s, denotes the unobservable binary segmentation of voxel s into fore- and background, whereas the latter, $\boldsymbol{x}_s$, states the observable vector of associated features that are assumed to be causally linked to the underlying class labels $y \in \mathcal{Y}$ by a unified observation model defined by a probability density function $p(\boldsymbol{x}|y)$ for $\boldsymbol{x} \in \mathcal{X}$. The emergence of the class labels themselves is described by a prior model $p(y)$. The segmentation task at hand can now be stated as the search for an MAP estimate

$$\boldsymbol{Y}^* = \operatorname*{argmax}_{\boldsymbol{Y}} p(\boldsymbol{Y}|\boldsymbol{X}) \tag{1}$$

where $p(\boldsymbol{Y}|\boldsymbol{X})$ is the joint posterior probability over the image domain $\mathcal{S}$ with $\boldsymbol{Y} = (y_s)_{s \in \mathcal{S}}$ and $\boldsymbol{X} = (\boldsymbol{x}_s)_{s \in \mathcal{S}}$. Using the Bayes rule, and assuming a uniform distribution $p(\boldsymbol{X})$, we have:

$$\boldsymbol{Y}^* = \operatorname*{argmax}_{\boldsymbol{Y}} \ln p(\boldsymbol{X}|\boldsymbol{Y}) + \ln p(\boldsymbol{Y}). \tag{2}$$

To concretize this optimization problem a region-specific probability term and an appropriate prior need to be identified. In our method $p(\boldsymbol{X}|\boldsymbol{Y})$ is provided by a PBT classifier. The machine learning technique of PBT recursively groups boosted ensembles of weak classifiers to a tree structure during learning from expert annotated data. Training a PBT resembles inducing a multivariate binary regression tree as the final strong classifier

$$H(\boldsymbol{x}) = \sum_{t=1}^{T} h_t(\boldsymbol{x}) \tag{3}$$

generated within each inner node for a feature vector $\boldsymbol{x}$ through a combination of real-valued contributions $h_t(\boldsymbol{x})$ of $T \in \mathbb{N}$ weak classifiers asymptotically approaches the additive logistic regression model [13]

$$H(\boldsymbol{x}) \approx \frac{1}{2} \ln \frac{p(y=+1|\boldsymbol{x})}{p(y=-1|\boldsymbol{x})}. \tag{4}$$

Accordingly, at each inner node v of the resulting PBT there are current approximations of the posterior probability $\tilde{p}_v(y|\boldsymbol{x})$. During classification those values are used to guide tree traversing and combined propagation of posteriors in order to get a final approximation $\tilde{p}(y|\boldsymbol{x})$ of the true posterior probability $p(y|\boldsymbol{x})$ at the tree's root node.

As mentioned above, assuming $\boldsymbol{X}$ to be distributed uniformly, and also to be independently and identically distributed, we have $p(\boldsymbol{x}|y) \propto p(y|\boldsymbol{x})$ and therefore $p(\boldsymbol{X}|\boldsymbol{Y}) \approx \prod_{s \in \mathcal{S}} \tilde{p}(y_s|\boldsymbol{x}_s)$ in (2).

The feature vectors $\boldsymbol{x}$ used for PBT classification consist of individual multispectral intensities, inter-spectrality intensity gradients, and 2-D Haar-like features [14,15] computed on an intra-axial 2-D context surrounding the voxel of interest. The Haar-like features are derived from a subset of the extended set of Haar-like feature prototypes by [16] and are represented only implicitly in memory by so-called (Rotated) Integral Images. This allows for fast re-computation of the features with respect to a given voxel when they are actually assessed. We decided on 2-D Haar-like features in contrast to the full set of 3-D Haars because of their lower computational cost and memory requirements. Also, as we intend to capture a discriminative representation of the full context, and not only of local edge characteristics at the central voxel, Haar-like feature values are computed according to the given prototypes on every valid origin and scale within the chosen voxel context.

For the prior distribution we assume a Markov random field prior model

$$p(\boldsymbol{Y}) \propto \exp(-U(\boldsymbol{Y}|\frac{1}{\lambda})) \quad (5)$$

formulated, according to the Hammersly-Clifford Theorem, as a Gibbs distribution with energy function

$$U(\boldsymbol{Y}|\frac{1}{\lambda}) = \frac{1}{\lambda} \sum_{s \in \mathcal{S}} \sum_{t \in \mathcal{N}_s} V_{st}(y_s, y_t) \quad (6)$$

where $\frac{1}{\lambda}$ with $\lambda \in\ ]0.0, +\infty[$ controls the relative influence of the spatial prior over the observation model and $\mathcal{N}_s$ states the neighborhood of voxel s. Inspired by [17] the interaction potentials are

$$V_{st}(y_s, y_t) = \exp\left(-\frac{1}{2}\sum_{l=1}^{L}\frac{(i_{s_l} - i_{t_l})^2}{\sigma_l^2}\right) \cdot \frac{\delta(y_s, y_t)}{dist(s,t)} \quad (7)$$

where vectors $(i_{s_1}, \ldots, i_{s_L})$ and $(i_{t_1}, \ldots, i_{t_L})$ denote the observed intensities at voxels s and t taken from $L \in \mathbb{N}$ aligned input pulse sequences and

$$\delta(y_s, y_t) = \begin{cases} 1 & \text{if } y_s \neq y_t \\ 0 & \text{otherwise} \end{cases}. \quad (8)$$

The function $dist(s,t)$ denotes the physical distance between voxels s and t, which varies when working on image volumes with anisotropic voxel spacing. The model emphasizes homogeneous segmentations among neighboring voxels but weights penalties for heterogeneity according to intensity similarities of the voxels involved.

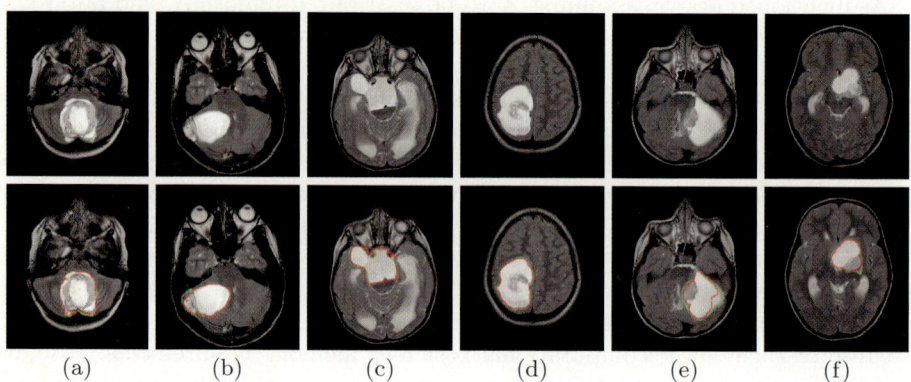

Fig. 2. Segmentation results obtained by leave-one-patient-out cross validation. The first row shows selected slices of the T2-weighted pulse sequences of the six available patient data sets. The second row shows the associated segmentation results (red) and the ground-truth segmentation (green) overlaid on the T2-weighted pulse sequence. Please view in color.

With the equality

$$\boldsymbol{Y}^* = \underset{\boldsymbol{Y}}{\mathrm{argmax}} \sum_{s \in \mathcal{S}} \ln \tilde{p}(y_s | \boldsymbol{x}_s) - \frac{1}{\lambda} \sum_{s \in \mathcal{S}} \sum_{t \in \mathcal{N}_s} V_{st}(y_s, y_t) =$$

$$\underset{\boldsymbol{Y}}{\mathrm{argmin}} \, \lambda \cdot \left(\sum_{s \in \mathcal{S}} - \ln \tilde{p}(y_s | \boldsymbol{x}_s) \right) + \sum_{s \in \mathcal{S}} \sum_{t \in \mathcal{N}_s} V_{st}(y_s, y_t) \quad (9)$$

the initial maximization problem can be transformed into a minimization problem that is in a suitable form for optimization by the graph cuts algorithm [10]. Note that the reciprocal of the regularization parameter in (6) can equivalently be used to weight the influence of the observation model over the prior model. Given (9), setting up the graph and defining the edge capacities for the associated max-flow/min-cut problem instance is straightforward. Details can be found in [17] with the difference that we do not use additional hard constraints to predetermine individual class labels of certain voxels.[1]

3 Experimental Setting and Results

For quantitative evaluation of the proposed method there were six multi-spectral expert annotated data sets of pediatric patients aged from 1 year and 5 months to

---

[1] In order to compensate for PBT misclassifications due to cerebral spinal fluid/cyst intensity ambiguities, $\tilde{p}(y_s | \boldsymbol{x}_s)$ in (9) is weighted by the likelihood of the observed multi-spectral intensities at voxel s given y. The PDFs for that are estimated during segmentation via histograms by understanding the hard voxel classification for $\tilde{p}(\boldsymbol{y}_s = 1 | \boldsymbol{x}_s) > 0.5$ as intermediate segmentation that is close to the final result.

15 years and 10 months available—among them four pilocytic astrocytomas, one pilomyxoid astrocytoma, and one anaplastic astroblastoma. Each scan consists of three 3-D images acquired at different pulse sequences (T2-weighted, T1-weighted, and T1-weighted after contrast enhancement). The resolution is $512 \times 512 \times 20$ with a voxel spacing of 0.45mm×0.45mm×6.0mm. Where necessary due to patient movement during image acquisition the pulse sequences were co-aligned by means of the MedINRIA affine registration tool (www-sop.inria.fr/asclepios/software/MedINRIA). All the sequences were further pre-processed by the following pipeline: skull stripping by the Brain Extraction Tool (BET) [18], gradient anisotropic diffusion filtering (www.itk.org), and inter-scan intensity standardization by Dynamic Histogram Warping (DHW) [19]. Note that all of the pre-processing steps involved, including co-alignment, can be performed fully automatically without any user interaction.

The PBT voxel classifiers built were restricted to a maximum depth of 10 with 10 weak classifiers per tree node. The 2-D voxel context considered was of size 11×11 on volumes down-sampled to a voxel spacing of 2.0mm×2.0mm×6.0mm. The graph cuts optimization, using Vladimir Kolmogorov's publicly available implementation [10], is carried out on the original image resolution with $\mathcal{N}_s$ defined to be a standard 6-neighborhood on the 3-D image lattice. The standard deviation $(\sigma_1, \ldots, \sigma_L)$ for the interaction potentials in (7) was estimated offline as "camera noise" within manually delineated homogeneous regions throughout the patient volumes. A leave-one-out cross validation on the patient data sets and their accompanying PBT models yielded best average segmentation scores in terms of the Jaccard coefficient $(TP/(TP+FP+FN)$ where TP, FP, and FN denote the number of true positive, false positive, and false negative voxels, respectively) for $\lambda \in [0.1, 0.5]$ such that finally $\lambda = 0.2$ was chosen for computing the results depicted in Fig. 2. In order to remove small regions of false positive voxels only the largest connected component of the graph cuts result is considered to be the final segmentation. With Jaccard coefficients of 0.78 ± 0.17 the segmentation results are better than those published by [5] (0.60) and, except for one case, in a similar range as those of [6] (0.86) who all work with adult patient data sets and partly on four pulse sequences [6]. However, comparability of results is limited because of different characteristics between the data sets used by the mentioned scientists, e.g., pediatric patients versus adult patients, additional usage of more expressive pulse sequences, presence of necrotic tissue within the tumors, restriction to a certain histological type of tumor, etc.

It takes about 1–2 minutes to process one of the multi-spectral MRI volumes in a non-optimized C++ implementation of our segmentation method on a Fujitsu Siemens Computers notebook equipped with an Intel Pentium M 2.0 GHz processor and 2 GB of memory. With the same hardware as above training one classifier takes about 4 hours. Preprocessing the images takes about 3 minutes so a total amount of 5 minutes is needed for the processing of one patient data set. In terms of total processing time our method is therefore faster than the method of [6] who claim to be fastest among current approaches to fully automatic MRI brain tumor segmentation.

4 Conclusions

The contribution of this paper is two-fold: starting from the well-known MAP framework for image segmentation we have derived a constrained minimization problem suitable for max-flow/min-cut optimization that incorporates an observation model provided by a discriminative PBT classifier into the process of segmentation. Secondly, we successfully applied the method to the difficult problem of fully automatic pediatric brain tumor segmentation in multi-spectral 3-D MRI. The experimental results obtained are mostly better than those recently published for fully automatic brain tumor segmentation in adult patients.

As the proposed method relies on the observed intensities as a very strong indicator for tumor appearance it is to some extent sensitive to symptoms affecting this feature. In the case of a hydrocephalus where circulation of CSF has nearly come to a still stand it is virtually impossible to distinguish voxels within the cystic portion of the tumor from voxels within the ventricular system from solely the intensities. This may cause the method to generate false positives and false negatives (see Fig. 2 (e)) in some cases.

In the future we will consider an extended use of prior knowledge to overcome this issue. This knowledge would have to cover not only direct tumor characteristics like shape and location, but also indirect characteristics of the surrounding non-pathological brain tissue. The goal is to detect, to segment, and to identify most types of pathological tissue that occur within pediatric brain tumors.

Acknowledgements. This work has been partially funded by the EU project Health-e-Child (IST 2004-027749). We would like to thank A. Rossi from G. Gaslini Children's Research Hospital in Genoa, Italy, for providing the MRI data used in our experiments.

References

1. Fletcher-Heath, L., Hall, L.O., Goldgof, D.B., Murtagh, F.R.: Automatic segmentation of non-enhancing brain tumors in magnetic resonance images. Artif. Intell. Med. 21(1–3), 43–63 (2001)
2. Gering, D.T., Grimson, W.E.L., Kikinis, R.: Recognizing deviations from normalcy for brain tumor segmentation. In: Int. Conf. Med. Image Comput. and Comp.-Assist. Interv., Tokyo, Japan, pp. 388–395 (September 2002)
3. Prastawa, M., Bullitt, E., Ho, S., Gerig, G.: A brain tumor segmentation framework based on outlier detection. Med. Image Anal. 8(3), 275–283 (2004)
4. Kaus, M.R., Warfield, S.K., Nabavi, A., Black, P.M., Jolesz, F.A., Kikinis, R.: Automated segmentation of MR images of brain tumors. Radiology 218, 586–591 (2001)
5. Cobzas, D., Birkbeck, N., Schmidt, M., Jagersand, M., Murtha, A.: 3D variational brain tumor segmentation using a high dimensional feature set. In: Proceedings of the Mathematical Methods in Biomedical Image Analysis (MMBIA) Workshop. 11th IEEE Int. Conf. Comp. Vis., Rio de Janeiro, Brazil, pp. 1–8 (October 2007)

6. Corso, J.J., Yuille, A., Sicotte, N.L., Toga, A.: Detection and segmentation of pathological structures by the extended graph-shifts algorithm. In: Int. Conf. Med. Image Comput. and Comp.-Assist. Interv., Brisbane, Australia, October 2007, pp. 985–993 (2007)
7. Tu, Z.: Probabilistic boosting-tree: Learning discriminative models for classification, recognition, and clustering. In: IEEE Int. Conf. Comp. Vis., Beijing, China, October 2005, pp. 1589–1596 (2005)
8. Tu, Z., Zhou, X., Comaniciu, D., Bogoni, L.: A learning based approach for 3D segmentation and colon detagging. In: Europ. Conf. Comp. Vis., Graz, Austria, pp. 436–448 (May 2006)
9. Carneiro, G., Georgescu, B., Good, S., Comaniciu, D.: Automatic fetal measurements in ultrasound using constrained probabilistic boosting tree. In: Int. Conf. Med. Image Comput. and Comp.-Assist. Interv., Brisbane, Australia (October 2007)
10. Boykov, Y., Kolmogorov, V.: An experimental comparison of min-cut/max-flow algorithms for energy minimization in vision. IEEE T. Pattern Anal. 26(9), 1124–1137 (2004)
11. Zhang, Y., Brady, M., Smith, S.: Segmentation of brain MR images through a hidden Markov random field model and the expectation-maximization algorithm. IEEE T. Med. Imag. 20(1), 45–57 (2001)
12. Murgasova, M., Dyet, L., Edwards, A.D., Rutherford, M.A., Hajnal, J.V., Rueckert, D.: Segmentation of brain MRI in young children. In: Int. Conf. Med. Image Comput. and Comp.-Assist. Interv., Copenhagen, Denmark, pp. 687–694 (October 2006)
13. Friedman, J., Hastie, T., Tibshirani, R.: Additive logistic regression: a statistical view of boosting. Ann. Stat. 28(2), 337–407 (1998)
14. Oren, M., Papageorgiou, C., Sinha, P., Osuna, E., Poggio, T.: Pedestrian detection using wavelet templates. In: IEEE Comp. Soc. Conf. Comp. Vis. and Pat. Recog., San Juan, Puerto Rico, pp. 193–199 (June 1997)
15. Viola, P., Jones, M.: Robust real-time object detection. In: 2nd International Workshop on Statistical Learning and Computational Theories of Vision, Vancouver, Canada, pp. 1–25 (July 2001)
16. Lienhart, R., Kuranov, A., Pisarevsky, V.: Empirical analysis of detection cascades of boosted classifiers for rapid object detection. In: Michaelis, B., Krell, G. (eds.) DAGM 2003. LNCS, vol. 2781, pp. 297–304. Springer, Heidelberg (2003)
17. Boykov, Y., Funka-Lea, G.: Graph cuts and efficient N-D image segmentation. Int. J. Comput. Vision 70(2), 109–131 (2006)
18. Smith, S.M.: Fast robust automated brain extraction. Hum. Brain Mapp. 17(3), 143–155 (2002)
19. Cox, I.J., Hingorani, S.L.: Dynamic histogram warping of image pairs for constant image brightness. In: IEEE Int. Conf. on Image Proc., Washington, D.C., USA, vol. II, pp. 366–369 (October 1995)

Prostate Cancer Probability Maps Based on Ultrasound RF Time Series and SVM Classifiers

Mehdi Moradi[1], Parvin Mousavi[1], Robert Siemens[2], Eric Sauerbrei[3], Alexander Boag[4], and Purang Abolmaesumi[1]

[1] School of Computing
[2] Department of Urology
[3] Department of Diagnostic Radiology
[4] Department of Pathology and Molecular Medicine,
Queen's University, Kingston, ON, Canada
purang@cs.queensu.ca

Abstract. We describe a very efficient method based on ultrasound RF time series analysis and support vector machine classification for generating probabilistic prostate cancer colormaps to augment the biopsy process. To form the RF time series, we continuously record ultrasound RF echoes backscattered from tissue while the imaging probe and the tissue are stationary in position. In an *in-vitro* study involving 30 prostate specimens, we show that the features extracted from RF time series are significantly more accurate and sensitive compared to two other established categories of ultrasound-based tissue typing methods. The method results in an area under ROC curve of 0.95 in 10-fold cross-validation.

1 Introduction

Prostate cancer accounted for 29% of cancer cases among American men and terminated the lives of 31,350 North Americans in 2007 [1]. The common clinical diagnosis method for the disease is histopathologic analysis of biopsy samples acquired under ultrasound guidance. However, most prostate tumors lack visually distinct appearances on medical images. Therefore, pathologically significant cases of cancer can be missed during biopsy, resulting in false negative or repeated trials. The goal of our research is to augment the ultrasound images with tissue typing information that can be used for targeting during biopsy.

There is a wealth of literature on ultrasound-based diagnosis of prostate cancer [2]. Texture features of B-scan images and spectral features (Lizzi-Feleppa features [3]) extracted from calibrated average spectrum of RF signals have been used along with numerous classification approaches for tissue typing [4]. Also, elastography, an automatic method for measuring the elasticity of tissue, has shown promising results in diagnosis of the disease [5]. However, the aforementioned approaches have not gained wide-spread clinical acceptance due to a variety of reasons including limited accuracy and overheads such as the need for calibration or tissue compression imposed on the clinical routine.

Recently, a new paradigm in tissue typing has been proposed by our group [6,7]. The core of the idea is that if a specific location in tissue undergoes continuous interaction with ultrasound, the time series of echoes from that location would carry "tissue typing" information. In other words, although variations in the intensity of a spatial sample of RF echo over time are partly due to different sources of noise, they depend on the tissue type as well. We have used RF time series for tissue typing in animal tissues [7] and have also employed them along with neural network classifiers for detection of prostate cancer on a small size dataset [6]. This paper is the first report of a major clinical *in-vitro* study involving 30 patients in which the performance of RF time series features has been evaluated. We report quantitative comparisons between the RF time series features, and Lizzi-Feleppa (LF) and texture features. We describe a classification approach based on an extended version of Support Vector Machines (SVM) [8] that provides posterior class probabilities for classified regions of interest (ROIs). Using these probability values, we generate cancer probability maps. Finally, we study the effects of imaging depth and acoustic power on the tissue typing capabilities of RF time series.

The paper is organized as follows: Section 2 provides the details about our data collection, feature extraction and selection techniques, and SVM-based classification and color-map generation; Section 3 provides the classification results and colormaps; Section 4 analyzes the effects of different parameters on RF time series features; and, Section 5 summarizes and concludes the paper.

2 Method

2.1 Data Collection

We have performed an extensive process of ultrasound and histopathology data collection from patients who chose prostatectomy as their treatment option at a local hospital. Data was collected from 30 patients. Extracted prostate specimens were suspended in a water bath, and were scanned along transverse planes that were 4 mm apart. The ultrasound RF data was collected using a Sonix RP (Ultrasonix Inc., Richmond, BC, Canada) ultrasound machine. A transrectal probe (BPSL9-5/55/10) was used with the central frequency set to 6.6 MHz. To form the RF time series, we continuously acquired 112 frames of RF data, at the rate of 22 frames per second (fps) from each cross-section of the tissue. Therefore, the length of RF time series in our analysis was 112 for each tissue cross-section. The maximum imaging depth was set to 4.5 cm. The RF sampling rate was 20 MHz and the number of bits per RF sample was 16.

After ultrasound data acquisition, the prostate specimens were dissected along the scanned cross-sections. The first cross-section was marked with two parallel needles that were visible in ultrasound images as two lines and defined a plane. The consequent parallel cuts were made at 4 mm intervals. Histopathological analysis of whole mount slides were acquired and used as the gold standard. The process of registering the histopathology maps to the RF frames was performed manually. Due to the elevation beam width of ultrasound signals and also inevitable errors caused by the low precision cutting process in the pathology lab, the accurate match between tumor boundaries in ultrasound and histopathology images was challenging. Therefore, only a limited number of ROIs from cross-sections for which a high level of confidence of registration could be achieved were selected. This process amounted to 1478 normal and 856 cancerous ROIs selected from 46 cross-sections. It should be noted that although only 46 of the cross-sections could be used in the training process, the developed methodology was used to generate cancer colormaps on all acquired cross-sections.

The ROI dimension was $1\ mm \times 3.5\ mm$. This included four segments of RF lines, each of length 96 samples. Our investigations show that RF time series features extracted from ROIs even as small as $1\ mm^2$ are effective for tissue typing. However, the frequency spectrum of the RF segments extracted for Lizzi-Feleppa method can not be evaluated in very short RF segments.

2.2 Features

RF time series features (S1-S6,FD). To create RF time series, we continuously recorded RF echo signals backscattered from tissue, while the imaging probe and the tissue were fixed in position. Samples of RF signals collected over time from a fixed spot of tissue formed one RF time series.

Spectral features of the RF time series (S1-S6): Each RF time series is a discrete signal of length 112 in our dataset. After removing the mean, and zero-padding of the length of the time series to 128, we used the FFT algorithm to estimate the frequency spectrum corresponding to each spatial RF sample in an ROI and then, averaged each component of the spectrum over the ROI. We normalized the average spectrum to values in [0-1] interval. The first four RF time series features (S1, S2, S3 and S4) were the average value of the normalized spectrum in four quarters of the frequency range. In other words, they summarized the low, mid-low, mid-high, and high frequency components of the signal, respectively. We also fit a regression line to values of the spectrum (versus normalized frequency). The intercept (S5) and the slope (S6) of this line were used as two more features [6].

Fractal dimension (FD) of RF time series: It has been shown that the fractal dimension of the RF time series computed based on Higuchi's algorithm [9] contains tissue typing information [7]. We computed the FD ($K_{max} = 16$) of all the time series within an ROI and averaged them to get one feature per ROI.

Lizzi-Feleppa features (LF1,LF2,LF3). Lizzi, Feleppa and their colleagues have shown that the intercept extrapolated to zero frequency (LF1), the average slope (LF2), and midband value (LF3) of a line fitted to the mid-band portion of the calibrated frequency spectrum of segments of RF A-lines, can be used as the signature of cancerous and normal tissue types in prostate [3]. We closely followed the methodology described in [3]. The calibration data for Lizzi-Feleppa method was acquired from the surface of a flat glass plate in a water bath at the transducer focal zone, with minimum amplifier gain and flat TGC. The values of slope and midband value were corrected for an assumed linear attenuation coefficient of 0.5 $dB/MHz-cm$. Feleppa et al. have averaged the spectral frequency on 10 RF segments. However, in our study, increasing the number of RF line segments from 4 to 8 (which doubles the ROI size from 3.5 mm^2 to 7 mm^2) had no significant effect on the efficiency of LF features (compare the results in Table 1 for ROI sizes of 3.5 and 7 mm^2).

Texture features. We used 12 texture features from the B-scan equivalents of the collected RF frames [4]. They included four statistical moments of the pixel intensities (mean, std, skewness and kurtosis), and eight features from the co-occurrence matrices: correlation, energy, contrast, and homogeneity computed for co-occurrence distance of $l = 1$ and separately for 0° and 90° directions.

2.3 SVM Classifier and Posterior Class Probabilities

Support vector machines use a kernel function to map the input data to a higher dimension space where a hyperplane can separate the data into different classes. The process of training a SVM classifier is equivalent to finding this optimal hyperplane in a way that minimizes the error on the training dataset and maximizes the perpendicular distance between the decision boundary and the closest data points in classes [10]. In a two class case, if the training dataset consists of N feature vectors $\{x_1, ..., x_N\}$ with class labels $y_i \in \{1, -1\}$, then the SVM training problem is equivalent to finding W and b such that [10]:

$$1/2 \times W^T W + C \sum_{i=1}^{N} \xi_i \qquad (1)$$

is minimized subject to:

$$y_i(W^T \phi(x_i) + b) \geq 1 - \xi_i \quad , \quad i = 1, ..., N \qquad (2)$$

where $\xi_i \geq 0$ are the so-called slack variables that allow for misclassification of noisy data points, and parameter $C > 0$ controls the trade-off between the slack variable penalty and the margin [10]. The function $\phi(x)$ maps the data to a higher dimensional space. This new space is defined by its kernel function: $K(x_i, x_j) = \phi(x_i)^T \phi(x_j)$. The above problem can be formulated as a quadratic optimization process. The details of the solution and its implementation can be found in [11]. We used the Gaussian Radial Basis Function (RBF) kernel:

$$K(x_i, x_j) = e^{-\gamma \|x_i - x_j\|^2} \qquad (3)$$

This was firstly due to the fact that RBF kernel has only one parameter (γ) to adjust. Also, we found SVM classifiers based on RBF kernel more accurate than linear, sigmoid, and polynomial kernels in case of our problem.

The SVM is merely a decision machine: If $f(x_n) = W^T \phi(x_n) + b > 0$, then the class label for x_n is $y_n = 1$. In other words, SVM does not provide posterior class probabilities ($P(class|input)$). In order to generate probability colormaps and also Receiver Operating Characteristic (ROC) curves based on SVM classification, one needs posterior probabilities of normal and cancer classes:

$$P_{can}(x_n) = p(y = 1|f(x_n)) \qquad (4)$$

where $P_{can}(x_n)$ stands for probability of x_n being cancerous and $P_{nor}(x_n) = 1 - P_{can}(x_n)$. Platt [12] has extended SVM for probability estimates by training an SVM and then finding the parameters of a sigmoid function of form:

$$P = (y_n = 1|f(x_n)) = \frac{1}{1 + exp(Af(x_n) + B)} \qquad (5)$$

to map the values of $f(x_n)$ to posterior probabilities. The values of parameters A and B are fit using a maximum likelihood estimation from the training set [12]. We used class probabilities generated with this method for creating the probabilistic cancer maps and also as decision thresholds for ROC curve building.

We used the publicly available C++ implementation of the SVM algorithms known as LIBSVM [11]. The entire dataset was normalized prior to training by setting the maximum value of each feature to 1 and the minimum to 0. For parameter selection (C and γ), we exhaustively searched the parameter space $1 \leq C \leq 100, 1 \leq \gamma \leq 100$ with steps of length 1. For each set of parameters, 10-fold cross-validation was performed: we trained the SVM using 90% of the data samples, classified the remaining 10%, and repeated the procedure for all 10 portions of the data. The computational expense of this exhaustive search was feasible on our parallel computing server (Sun Microsystems, Sun Fire V890).

2.4 Feature Selection

We separately performed exhaustive searches to find the best subset of texture, LF and time series features to maximize their tissue typing accuracy. These three best subsets were combined and subjected to an additional exhaustive search to find a feature vector to generate probabilistic cancer colormaps. This two stage method of feature selection was not guaranteed to provide the highest possible accuracy. An exhaustive search over all 22 features combined could have resulted in a better performing subset. However, it required examining $\sum_{n=0}^{22} C_n^{22} = 2^{22}$ subsets which was computationally infeasible. Feature space reduction based on Principle Component Analysis (PCA) was an alternative solution. We chose the two-stage method because: 1) the two-stage method enabled us to compare the performance of the three approaches of tissue typing; 2) the PCA-based features did not exceed the accuracy of the subset found in our two-stage search (regardless of the number of principle components included).

3 Results

Performance of different groups of features: We found the optimal parameters (C and γ) of the RBF-based SVM classifier separately for each group of features and used them during feature selection (see Table 1 for parameter values).

Exhaustive search for the best subset within each of the three categories of features resulted in a two-dimensional feature vector among texture features (Mean and correlation at 0°), a two-dimensional feature vector among Lizzi-Feleppa features (LF1,LF3), and a six-dimensional feature vector (S2,S3,S4,S5,S6,FD) among the proposed time series features. As Table 1 demonstrates, while texture and LF features show a similar performance, time series features significantly outperform both of them with accuracy of 82.5 ± 1.6% (compared to 74.4 ± 2.7% and 75.9 ± 1.3%). More importantly, the time series approach is the only one to provide a high sensitivity. There was no advantage in increasing the size of ROIs from 3.5 to 7 mm^2 (compare the two right columns of Table 1).

To acquire the best combination of features for cancer probability colormaps, we combined the selections of features from the three groups into a 10-dimensional feature vector and performed the exhaustive search on them. The seven dimensional subset (Mean,S2,S4,S6,FD,LF1,LF3) was found as the optimal subset considering its performance and dimension. As the last row of Table 1 reports, an accuracy of 92.1% with sensitivity of 88.3% and specificity of 94.1% was achieved with this selection of features. The area under the ROC curve acquired using this subset of features with 10-fold cross-validation was 0.95.

Table 1. Comparison of feature groups on the corresponding optimal SVM classifiers

Feature Group	SVM parameters	results for 3.5 mm^2 ROI size	results for 7 mm^2 ROI size
Best subset of Texture features (Mean and correlation at 0°)	RBF $C = 50$ $\gamma = 94$	Acc: 74.4 ± 2.7% Sen: 49.0 ± 5.1% Spe: 89.2 ± 2.6%	75.4 ± 3.4% 51.7 ± 7.1% 89.1 ± 3.9%
Best subset of Lizzi-Feleppa features (LF1,LF3)	RBF $C = 50$ $\gamma = 97$	Acc: 75.9 ± 1.3% Sen: 57.7 ± 3.8% Spe: 84.9 ± 3.0%	72.3 ± 2.8% 52.8 ± 6.3% 82.1 ± 3.7%
Best subset of Time series features (S2,S3,S4,S5,S6,FD)	RBF $C = 37$ $\gamma = 25$	Acc: 82.5 ± 1.6% Sen: 79.6 ± 2.4% Spe: 83.4 ± 3.8%	79.7 ± 3.4% 75.5 ± 5.2% 82.1 ± 3.9%
Best subset of the combination of the three groups above: (Mean,S2,S4,S6,FD,LF1,LF3)	RBF $C = 55$ $\gamma = 7$	Acc: 92.1 ± 1.8% Sen: 88.3 ± 1.2% Spe: 94.1 ± 2.1%	90.1 ± 2.6% 84.5 ± 5.1% 93.2 ± 3.3%

Probabilistic cancer colormaps: Prior to the generation of each colormap, the SVM was trained on all the training data except for the ROIs originating from the patient under study. Figure 1 demonstrates two of the colormaps acquired using the described seven-dimensional feature vector and the SVM-based probabilistic outcomes. The colormaps were generated by tissue typing of the entire peripheral zone of the prostate of patients. The colored ROIs in the colormaps were those with $P_c > 0.4$ (See Section 2.3). The choice of the threshold was rather subjective, however, we found that with the threshold of $P_c > 0.4$, the visualized maps demonstrated all the major tumors in the dataset without a significant number of false positive detections.

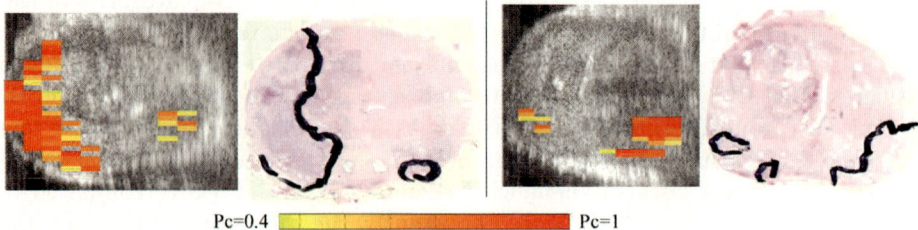

Fig. 1. Cancer probability maps along with the closest matching histopathology slide. The probe is in touch with the left side of the gland.

Quantitative validation: Colormaps can be viewed as qualitative measures of the performance of the technique. To quantitatively validate the authenticity of the technic, we performed patient-based classification experiments. In these experiments, the test data consisted only of the ROIs for which the pathological condition was confidently known. For each patient, we trained the SVM based on ROIs from all other patients and tested it on ROIs from the patient in question. With threshold probability of cancer set to $P_c = 0.4$, an average accuracy of 79% with sensitivity of 81% and specificity of 77% were achieved (area under ROC curve = 0.85). We noticed that when only texture and LF features were used, the patient-based accuracy dropped to 75% and more importantly, the sensitivity was only 68% (area under ROC curve: 0.79). In other words, the time series features are significant contributors to sensitivity of the colormaps.

4 Discussions

The effect of tissue depth: Our analysis showed that tissue typing based on RF time series features is more accurate in areas that are closer to the ultrasound probe. We witnessed a meaningful drop in the accuracy of our tissue classification (based on RF time series features) for ROIs that are more than 3 cm away from the probe (Figure 2). With the only focal point set at 2 cm, the ultrasound beams diverge increasingly at deeper areas of the tissue. Furthermore, the effects of amplifier noise are more prevalent in deeper areas. Therefore, data from the deeper areas suffer from an increasing level of noise[1]. The tissue typing information is carried in time series variations, and the increasing levels of destructive noise in deeper areas of the tissue decreases the signal to noise ratio (SNR) in the received RF time series. From the clinical point of view, the depth-dependent accuracy of the approach does not pose a significant challenge. The reason is that the most cancer-prone area of the prostate gland is the peripheral zone which is also the target of inspection during biopsy.

The effect of ultrasound power: A reduction in the acoustic transmit power of the ultrasound probe also reduces the SNR in the RF time series. The ultrasound

---

[1] Noise is measured as $\sum_{i=1}^{i=112}(x_i - \bar{x})^2$ where $\bar{x}$ is the mean of the RF time series and x_i's are the samples of the RF time series; the length of the time series is 112.

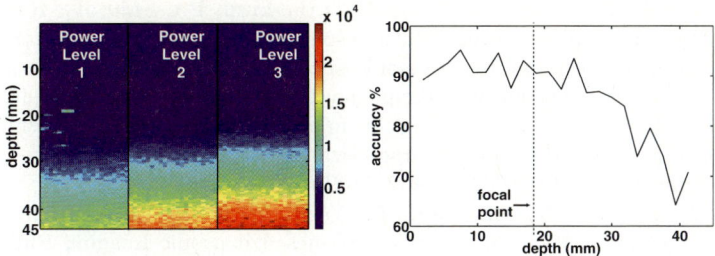

Fig. 2. Right: The accuracy of tissue typing based on time series *vs.* depth. Left: Noise at different depths for three transducer power settings ($0dB$, $-2dB$ and $-6dB$).

machine is normally operated at its highest acoustic power level to maximize the contrast and SNR. A $2dB$ reduction in the output power resulted in a drop of accuracy from $82.5 \pm 1.6\%$ to $80.4 \pm 3.1\%$. A $6dB$ power reduction caused a drop in the accuracy of the method to $70.1 \pm 3.9\%$. Figure 2 demonstrates a visual comparison of the noise levels at the three studied power settings.

5 Conclusions

The results show that the RF time series features are powerful tissue typing parameters. They are significantly more accurate and sensitive than RF spectral features [3] and also B-scan texture features. These two approaches complement the RF time series method resulting in a very effective feature vector that provides an area under ROC curve of 0.95 in 10-fold cross-validation. Based on this hybrid feature vector and an extension to the SVM classification approach [12], we created colormaps that accurately highlighted areas of tissue with high risk of cancer on ultrasound images.

The analysis of RF time series is computationally expensive compared to the analysis of single RF or B-scan frames. However, our implementations show that the feature values can be extracted from a $1\ cm^2$ area, in less than a second on a single CPU computer. The proposed method involves very limited overhead to the routine clinical examination. Nevertheless, the radiologist needs to keep a hand steady for about 3-5 seconds while the RF time series are acquired. We are planning *in-vivo* studies that will determine the effectiveness of the method in clinical practice and analyze the effects of potential hand movements. Also, we are currently performing phantom studies that will measure the sensitivity of RF time series features to changes in elasticity and scatterer size.

References

1. Jemal, A., Siegel, R., Ward, E., Murray, T., Xu, J., Thun, M.: Cancer statistics, 2007. CA: A Cancer Journal for Clinicians (57), 43–66 (2007)
2. Moradi, M., Mousavi, P., Abolmaesumi, P.: Computer-aided diagnosis of prostate cancer with emphasis on ultrasound-based approaches: A review. Ultrasound in Medicine and Biology 33(7), 1010–1028 (2007)

3. Feleppa, E.J., Kalisz, A., Sokil-Melgar, J.B., Lizzi, F.L., Liu, T., Rosado, A.L., Shao, M.C., Fair, W.R., Wang, Y., Cookson, M.S., Reuter, V.E., Heston, W.D.W.: Typing of prostate tissue by ultrasonic spectrum analysis. IEEE Transactions on Ultrasonics, Ferroelectrics, and Frequency Control 43(4), 609–619 (1996)
4. Scheipers, U., Ermert, H., Garcia-Schurmann, H.J.S.M., Senge, T., Philippou, S.: Ultrasonic multifeature tissue characterization for prostate diagnosis. Ultrasound in Medicine and Biology 20(8), 1137–1149 (2003)
5. Ophir, J., Cespedes, I., Ponnekanti, H., Yazdi, Y., Li, X.: Elastography: a method for imaging the elasticity in biological tissues. Ultrasonic Imaging 13(2), 111–134 (1991)
6. Moradi, M., Mousavi, P., Siemens, D.R., Sauerbrei, E.E., Isotalo, P., Boag, A., Abolmaesumi, P.: Discrete Fourier analysis of ultrasound RF time series for detection of prostate cancer. In: IEEE EMBC, pp. 1339–1342 (2007)
7. Moradi, M., Mousavi, P., Abolmaesumi, P.: Tissue characterization using fractal dimension of high frequency ultrasound RF time series. In: Ayache, N., Ourselin, S., Maeder, A. (eds.) MICCAI 2007, Part II. LNCS, vol. 4792, pp. 900–908. Springer, Heidelberg (2007)
8. Vapnik, V.N.: The Nature of Statistical Learning Theory. Springer, New York (1995)
9. Higuchi, T.: Approach to an irregular time series on the basis of the fractal theory. Physica D: Nonlinear Phenomena 31(2), 277–283 (1988)
10. Bishop, C.M.: Pattern Recognition and Machine Learning. Springer Science, New York (2006)
11. Fan, R.E., Chen, P.H., Lin, C.J.: Working set selection using the second order information for training SVM. Machine Learning Research 6, 1889–1918 (2005)
12. Platt, J.C.: Probabilistic outputs for support vector machines and comparison to regularized likelihood methods. In: Advances in Large Margin Classifier. MIT Press, Cambridge (2000)

A Bayesian Approach for Liver Analysis: Algorithm and Validation Study

M. Freiman[1], O. Eliassaf[1], Y. Taieb[1], L. Joskowicz[1], and J. Sosna[2]

[1] School of Eng. and Computer Science, The Hebrew Univ. of Jerusalem, Israel
[2] Dept. of Radiology, School of Medicine, Hadassah Hebrew Univ. Medical Center, Jerusalem, Israel
freiman@cs.huji.ac.il

Abstract. We present a new method for the simultaneous, nearly automatic segmentation of liver contours, vessels, and metastatic lesions from abdominal CTA scans. The method repeatedly applies multi-resolution, multi-class smoothed Bayesian classification followed by morphological adjustment and active contours refinement. It uses multi-class and voxel neighborhood information to compute an accurate intensity distribution function for each class. The method requires only one or two user-defined voxel seeds, with no manual adjustment of internal parameters. A retrospective study on two validated clinical datasets totaling 56 CTAs was performed. We obtained correlations of 0.98 and 0.99 with a manual ground truth liver volume estimation for the first and second databases, and a total score of 67.87 for the second database. These results suggest that our method is accurate, efficient, and robust to seed selection compared to manually generated ground truth segmentation and to other semi-automatic segmentation methods.

1 Introduction

Liver structure analysis from abdominal CTA scans is a key task in many clinical applications. The analysis includes liver contour and volume estimation, blood vessels identification, and, when present, tumor detection and characterization. Clinical applications include hepatomegaly and liver cirrhosis assessment, hepatic volumetry, hepatic transplantation planning, liver regeneration after hepatectomy, evaluation and planning for resection liver surgery, and monitoring of liver metastases, among many others. To be of practical clinical use, the liver analysis must be accurate, robust, fast, and nearly automatic, so that the radiologist can perform it routinely without the assistance of a technician.

Nearly automatic CT-based liver analysis is known to be a very challenging task. The main difficulties include the ambiguity of the liver boundary, the complexity of the liver surface, the presence of surrounding organs, the contrast variability between liver parenchyma and vessels, the different tumor sizes and shapes, and the presence of many small metastases. In addition, liver analysis often requires the simultaneous identification and visualization of liver contours, blood vessels, and tumors, each with their own features and characteristics.

Over the past decade, researchers have developed a variety of methods for semi-automatic and automatic segmentation and visualization of liver structures. Most of these methods segment only one structure (liver contours [1,2,3,4,5] or vessels [6]), or segment one structure at a time, usually starting with the liver surface, followed by the vessels and the metastatic lesions. The individual structure segmentation uses various techniques, such as intensity thresholding, region growing, and level-sets based methods. For example, [7,8] use adaptive binary thresholding to separately segment the liver surface, vessels, and tumors, followed by a deformable model refinement for each. Since it does not use voxel neighborhood information, it may yield noisy or erroneous liver surface segmentations, especially when large tumors are present, as they bias the intensity distribution function. Peitgen et al. [9] describe an edge-based segmentation method for the liver contour and an interactive region-growing method for the vessels and tumors. Since it requires many seeds per CT slice, it is of limited clinical use.

A key observation is that by considering each liver structure individually, the intrinsic relations between the liver parenchyma, vessels, and tumors are lost. This makes the classification more sensitive and error-prone. As an alternative, we propose a simultaneous multi-class segmentation method.

In this paper, we present a new method for the simultaneous segmentation of liver contours, vessels, and metastatic lesions from abdominal CTA scans. The method repeatedly applies multi-resolution, multi-class smoothed Bayesian classification followed by morphological adjustment and active contours refinement. The method requires only one or two seeds (in case of presence of large tumors) for initialization, with no manual adjustment of internal parameters. By using the multi-class and voxel neighborhood information, it significantly improves the discrimination quality of the intensity distribution function for each class. The multi-resolution iterative approach allows the segmentation of the entire liver surface without prior shape information and/or significant user interaction.

The main contribution of the proposed method is the integration of both intensity-based statistical method with geometrical active contours method, into an iterative, multi-scale framework which produced a nearly automatic method for the fully detailed analysis of the liver. Our method yield an accurate and robust results on two clinically validated datasets totaling 56 CTA studies, and achieved a very high score compared to other semi-automatic methods presented in the MICCAI grand-challenge [10].

2 Method

Our method consists four steps: 1) multi-class intensity model generation; 2) smoothed Bayesian classification; 3) adaptive morphological adjustment, and; 4) geodesic active contours refinement. The steps are performed in sequence and repeatedly applied to the image until no further changes occur. After each iteration, the internal parameters of the multi-class intensity model are updated before they are used in the smoothed Bayesian classification step. This coupling is designed to overcome a biased classification due to ambiguous liver boundaries

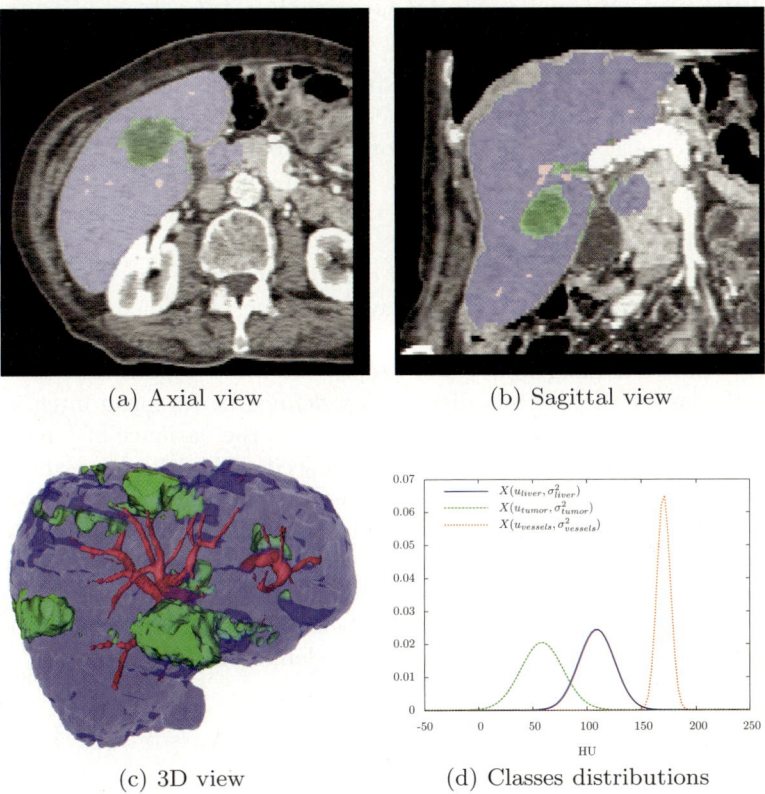

Fig. 1. Example of a segmented liver dataset. (a)-(b) 2D views of the segmentation: liver (blue), vessels (red), and tumors (green). (c) 3D visualization. (d) Gaussian distributions of the liver, tumor and vessels classes. The horizontal axis shows Hounsfield unit values; the vertical axis shows the class probabilities.

and biased seed selection. The classification updates the classes models by first computing the mean and variance of the liver and tumor classes from the current liver and tumor regions, and then updates the other classes by computing their mean and variance parameters. The morphological adjustment and the active contours refinement are then applied on the resulting classes to find the new liver and tumors regions. The iterations are necessary to fine-tune the intensity model to improve the classification and to minimize the influence of the initial voxel seed selection. Fig. 1(a)-1(c) illustrates the results of our multi-class segmentation.

To speed up the segmentation and make it more robust and accurate, we use a multi-resolution approach. The first few iterations are performed on a downsampled CTA dataset to obtain a rough contour segmentation. Subsequent iterations are performed on the original CTA dataset until no further improvements can be made. We describe each step in detail next.

2.1 Multi-class Intensity Model Generation

The first step is the construction of an intensity model that differentiates between the liver parenchyma, the liver inner vessels, the metastatic lesions, and the remaining organs and tissues, which are interpreted as background. The main challenges are the ambiguous boundary between the liver parenchyma and the outside organs (e.g the kidney), the ambiguous boundary between liver parenchyma and the liver vessels, and the similarity between lesions intensity values and other background values.

To overcome these difficulties, we first classify the voxels into two main classes, liver and lesions, according to their graylevel value. A refined five-class model is then built for each main class. The central class is the main class (e.g. liver or tumor); the remaining four classes represent other organs and tissues. We model each class with a normal distribution defined by its mean intensity value and variance. In the first iteration, the mean and the variance of a rectangular neighborhood around one manually selected seed inside the liver and, optionally, an additional seed inside a tumor (when the tumor is large) are computed and interpreted as the parameters of the liver and tumor classes. In subsequent iterations, the segmented region from the previous iteration is used to compute the mean and the variance of the liver and tumor classes. The remaining four classes model organs near and far (above/below) the liver and tumor values.

Formally, the liver and tumor classes are defined as: X_{liver}, X_{tumor} and the other four classes, X_i are modeled as:

$$X_{central} \sim N(\mu_{central}, \sigma_{central}^2) \qquad X_i \sim N(\mu_i, \sigma_i^2) \qquad (1)$$

for each i, $i \in \{near-low, near-high, far-low, far-high\}$, where $central$ is the liver or tumor class. The means of these classes defined as:

$$\mu_{near-high} = \mu_{central} + k_{near} \times \sigma_{central}$$
$$\mu_{near-low} = \mu_{central} - k_{near} \times \sigma_{central}$$
$$\mu_{far-high} = \mu_{central} + k_{far} \times \sigma_{central}$$
$$\mu_{far-low} = \mu_{central} - k_{far} \times \sigma_{central} \qquad (2)$$

where the factors k_{near} and k_{far} are determined from Chebyshev's inequality:

$$Pr(|X_i - \mu_{central}|) \geq k\sigma_{central}) \leq \frac{1}{k^2} \qquad (3)$$

This inequality ensures that at least $(1 - \frac{1}{k^2}) \times 100\%$ of the values are within k standard deviations from the mean. By setting $k_{near} = 2.2$ and $k_{far} = 4$, we ensure that at least 80% of the main class voxels will be classified as belonging to the main class, and at least 70% of the voxels that belong to the $near$ classes will be classified as $near$, even if the normal distribution assumption is incorrect. This ensures that each voxel from the ambiguous class boundary has a high probability of being both in the $central$ and $near$ classes. Its final classification is then determined from its relation to neighboring voxels. Initially, we set $\sigma_i = \sigma_{central}$ for all classes. Fig. 1(d) shows an example of the Gaussian model of the liver, tumor, and vessels classes, and their overlapping boundaries.

2.2 Voxel Classification

This step uniquely classifies each voxel according to its intensity value and its neighboring voxels [11]. Neighborhood information is important since voxel intensity values are correlated. First, we use Bayes rule to compute the probability $C_{(j,i)}$ of a voxel V_j with intensity value v_j to belong to class c_i, where $i \in \{central, near-low, near-high, far-low, far-high\}$:

$$Pr(v_j|c_i) \propto Pr(c_i|v_j)Pr(c_i) \qquad (4)$$

where $Pr(c_i|v_j)$ is obtained from the intensity model (Sec. 2.1). Since $Pr(c_i)$ is usually unavailable, we use a uniform distribution. The resulting five maps quantify the membership probability of each voxel to each class.

Next, we incorporate the neighborhood information to the classification process by smoothing the probability maps $C_{(j,i)}$ for each class i separately using an anisotropic diffusion equation [12]. The anisotropic smoothing process smoothes small peeks in the membership probability maps considered as mis-classifications while preserving sharp edges between different objects.

Finally, we apply the Maximum Posterior (MAP) rule:

$$C_{(j,final)} = \underset{c_i}{\operatorname{argmax}} Pr(v_j|c_i) \qquad (5)$$

to set the final membership of each voxel to the class with the highest probability that the voxel belongs to it. The binary segmentation image is generated by selecting only the voxels that belong to the central class.

This step is applied twice, once for the liver class, and another for the tumor class. The results are combined by taking into account only the tumor voxels inside the liver. Since the vessels appear as bright regions inside the liver, the estimation of the vessels class is based on the $X_{near-high}$ and $X_{far-high}$ distributions for voxels inside the liver.

2.3 Adaptive Morphological Adjustment

The third step is the identification of the liver region. The previous classification yields most of the liver region, with additional disconnected regions outside the liver, and holes inside the liver. The regions outside the liver correspond to anatomical structures with intensity values similar to the liver, such as the kidney and the spleen. The holes correspond to small tumors and artery and portal veins inside the liver whose intensity values are distinctly different from the liver intensity values because of the imaging contrast agent. To obtain the correct liver segmentation, the disconnected regions must be eliminated, and the holes inside the liver must be filled. This is done with adaptive morphological operations.

We first remove the disconnected regions outside the liver by identifying the largest connected component in the labeled image. Next, the holes inside the liver are classified as tumor or vessels according to the intensity model in Sec. 2.1. Finally, we adjust the liver boundary with an adaptive morphological opening operator. To overcome the inter-patient variablity of the liver size, the radiuses of the morphological operators are linearly depend on the estimated liver volume.

2.4 Active Contours Refinement

The classification and the morphological adjustment may miss parts of the liver volume. In addition, the liver boundaries may be imprecise in several regions. To correct this, we repeatedly apply a fine-tuning active contours segmentation [13]. The active contours segmentation drives the initial surface according to a feature map generated from the original image. To provide a good feature image to the active contours module, we generate a new image with a windowing function:

$$I'(x) = \begin{cases} \mu_{liver} + \sigma_{liver} & \text{if } I(x) > \mu_{liver} + \sigma_{liver}, \\ I(x) & \text{if } \mu_{liver} - \sigma_{liver} \leq I(x) \leq \mu_{liver} + \sigma_{liver}, \\ \mu_{liver} - \sigma_{liver} & \text{if } I(x) < \mu_{liver} - \sigma_{liver}. \end{cases} \quad (6)$$

where I is the original CTA data, I' is the new image, and μ_{liver} and σ_{liver} are the liver class parameters as computed in the intensity model.

3 Experimental Results

We performed a retrospective study on two validated clinical datasets totaling 56 CTAs. Our implementation used the ITK software library [14] and the smoothed Bayesian classification module [15]. Computations were performed on an Intel Core2 Quad 2.4 GHz PC with 3GB of memory. Table 1 summarize the results.

In the first study, we compared our algorithm estimation of liver volume to a manual ground truth liver volume estimation. In 26 CTA datasets [16], liver contours were manually segmented in each slice by a dedicated technologist on a Vitrea 2 workstation (Vital Images, Plymouth, MN) to serve as the ground truth. The datasets were also segmented with our method. The liver volume was then computed directly from the segmentations and compared by linear regression analysis. The mean absolute difference between the estimated liver volumes was 5.36% (std 3.48%), which was deemed accurate for clinical use. The correlation was 0.98, which is very and better than those of other automatic methods on the same database [16]. The mean difference between initializations with different seeds using our method was 0.54% (std 0.76%), which indicates that our algorithm is highly robust to seed selection. The mean segmentation time using the manual tracing was 7:24 mins, most of it user time. The mean segmentation time using our method was 6:09 mins, most of it computation time, as only a few seconds are required from the radiologist for seed selection. The computation time was deemed reasonable for clinical use. Since we did not have access to the manual segmentation, we could not compare our segmentation to the gold standard using other measures, as we did in the second study.

In the second study, we used 30 publicly available CTA datasets with ground-truth segmentations [10]. The database is divided into two groups. The first group consists of 20 datasets and is used for training and testing; The second group consists of 10 datasets and is used to evaluate segmentation algorithms. We compared our segmentation results to the ground-truth using five metrics:

Table 1. Summary of experimental results. The first column indicates the database used. The second column shows the estimated mean (std) volume difference. The third column shows the correlation with the ground-truth manual tracing segmentation. The fourth column shows the mean (std) volume estimation variations for the different seed selections, and the last column shows the average running time of our algorithm.

Database	Volume Diff. %	Correlation	Variability %	Running time (mm:ss)
1. DB 1	5.36 (3.48)	0.98	0.54 (0.76)	6:09
2. DB 2 training	2.63 (1.64)	0.99	0.004 (0.005)	6:07
3. DB 2 test	2.78 (2.14)	-	-	6:21

1) volumetric overlap; 2) relative absolute volume difference; 3) average symmetric absolute surface distance; 4) symmetric RMS surface distance, and; 5) maximum symmetric absolute surface distance. The metrics were computed for each dataset as described in [10]. The averages for 10 test datasets (20 training datasets) were as follows: 1) volumetric overlap error 8.55% (7.81%); 2) absolute volume difference 2.78% (2.63%); 3) average symmetric surface distance 1.46mm (1.28mm); 4) Root Mean Squares (RMS) symmetric surface distance 2.94mm (2.55mm); 5) maximum symmetric surface distance 26.72mm (22.77mm). The correlation between our volume estimation and the ground truth on the training set was 0.99 (note that since the ground truth is not available for the test set, we could not compute the correlation value for it). In addition, we measured the robustness of our method to three different seeds initializations on the 20 training datasets. The absolute volume difference was 0.004%, which is negligible. These results suggest that our method is both accurate and robust to seeds selections. A total score was computed as in [10] for both training and test datasets. Our method achieved a total score of 71.8 on the training set and of 67.87 on the test set. It is ranked forth of the semi-automatic method. However, all other semi-automatic methods require significantly more user interaction and do not provide vessels and tumors segmentation in addition to the liver segmentation.

4 Conclusion

We have presented a new nearly-automatic segmentation method for liver analysis. The main advantage of our method is that it simultaneously segments the liver contour, the blood vessels, and tumors inside the liver with only one or two user-selected seeds. Experimental results from two datasets totaling 56 CTA images show that our method is accurate, efficient, and robust to seed selection when compared to manually generated ground truth segmentation. In the future, we plan develop an integrated software package for the visualization and quantitative analysis of the liver to support diagnosis and surgical planning. Project homepage including movies and code is at: http://www.cs.huji.ac.il/~freiman/LiverSeg.

References

1. Okada, T., Shimada, R., Sato, Y., Hori, M., Yokota, K., Nakamoto, M., Chen, Y.W., Nakamura, H., Tamura, S.: Automated segmentation of the liver from 3D CT images using probabilistic atlas and multi-level statistical shape model. In: Ayache, N., Ourselin, S., Maeder, A. (eds.) MICCAI 2007, Part I. LNCS, vol. 4791, pp. 86–93. Springer, Heidelberg (2007)
2. Heimann, T., Wolf, I., Meinzer, H.: Active shape models for a fully automated 3D segmentation of the liver - an evaluation on clinical data. In: Larsen, R., Nielsen, M., Sporring, J. (eds.) MICCAI 2006. LNCS, vol. 4191, pp. 41–48. Springer, Heidelberg (2006)
3. Pohle, R., Toennies, K.: Segmentation of medical images using adaptive region growing. SPIE Med. Imaging 4322, 1337–1346 (2001)
4. Schenk, A., Prause, G., Peitgen, H.: Efficient semiautomatic segmentation of 3D objects in medical images. In: Delp, S.L., DiGoia, A.M., Jaramaz, B. (eds.) MICCAI 2000. LNCS, vol. 1935, pp. 186–195. Springer, Heidelberg (2000)
5. Chen, T., Metaxas, D.: A hybrid framework for 3D medical image segmentation. Med. Image Analysis 9(6), 547–565 (2005)
6. Fetita, C., Lucidarme, O., Preteux, F., Grenier, P.: CT hepatic venography: 3D vascular segmentation for preoperative evaluation. In: Duncan, J.S., Gerig, G. (eds.) MICCAI 2005. LNCS, vol. 3750, pp. 830–837. Springer, Heidelberg (2005)
7. Gao, L., Heath, D., Kuszyk, B., Fishman, E.: Automatic liver segmentation technique for 3D visualization of CT data. Radiology 201(2), 359–364 (1996)
8. Soler, L., Delingette, H., Malandain, G., Montagnat, J., Ayache, N., Koehl, C., Dourthe, O., Malassagne, B., Smith, M., Mutter, D., Marescaux, J.: Fully automatic anatomical, pathological, and functional segmentation from CT scans for hepatic surgery. Comp. Aided Surgery 6(3), 131–142 (2001)
9. Bourquain, H., Schenk, A., Link, F., Preim, B., Prause, G., Peitgen, H.: Hepavision2a software assistant for preoperative planning in living related liver transplantation and oncologic liver surgery. In: Proc. of the 16th Conf. on Comp. Assisted Radiology and Surgery (CARS 2002), pp. 341–346 (2002)
10. Ginneken, B., Heimann, T., Styner, M.: 3D segmentation in the clinic: A grand challenge. In: Heimann, T., Styner, M., van Ginneken, B. (eds.) 3D Segmentation in the Clinic: A Grand Challenge, pp. 7–15 (2007), http://www.sliver07.org
11. Teo, P., Sapiro, G., Wandell, B.: Anisotropic smoothing of posterior probabilities. In: Proc. of the 1997 Int. Conf. on Image Processing (ICIP 1997), pp. 675–678 (1997)
12. Perona, P., Malik, J.: Scale-space and edge detection using anisotropic diffusion. IEEE Trans. Patt. Analysis Mach. Intelligence 12(7), 629–639 (1990)
13. Caselles, V., Kimmel, R., Sapiro, G.: Geodesic active contours. Int. J. on Comp. Vision 22(1), 61–97 (1997)
14. Ibanez, L., Schroeder, W., Ng, L., Cates, J.: The ITK Software Guide. Kitware, Inc. ISBN 1-930934-15-7 (2005), http://www.itk.org/ItkSoftwareGuide.pdf
15. Melonakos, J., Krishnan, K., Tannenbaum, A.: An ITK filter for bayesian segmentation: itkbayesianclassifierimagefilter. Insight Journal (2006), http://www.insight-journal.org
16. Sosna, J., Berman, P., Azraq, Y., Libson, E.: Automated liver segmentation and volume calculation from mdct using a bayesian likelihood maximization technique: Comparison with manual tracing technique. In: 92nd Sci. Ass. and Ann. Meet. of the Radiological Society of N.A (RSNA 2006) (2006)

Classification of Suspected Liver Metastases Using fMRI Images: A Machine Learning Approach

M. Freiman[1], Y. Edrei[2,3], Y. Sela[1], Y. Shmidmayer[1], E. Gross[4], L. Joskowicz[1], and R. Abramovitch[2,3]

[1] School of Eng. and Computer Science, The Hebrew Univ. of Jerusalem, Israel
[2] The G. Savad Inst. for Gene Therapy, Hadassah Hebrew Univ. Medical Center, Jerusalem, Israel
[3] MRI/MRS lab HBRC, Hadassah Hebrew Univ. Medical Center, Jerusalem, Israel
[4] Pediatric Surgery, Hadassah Hebrew Univ. Medical Center, Jerusalem, Israel
freiman@cs.huji.ac.il

Abstract. This paper presents a machine-learning approach to the interactive classification of suspected liver metastases in fMRI images. The method uses fMRI-based statistical modeling to characterize colorectal hepatic metastases and follow their early hemodynamical changes. Changes in hepatic hemodynamics are evaluated from T_2^*-W fMRI images acquired during the breathing of air, air-CO_2, and carbogen. A classification model is build to differentiate between tumors and healthy liver tissues. To validate our method, a model was built from 29 mice datasets, and used to classify suspicious regions in 16 new datasets of healthy subjects or subjects with metastases in earlier growth phases. Our experimental results on mice yielded an accuracy of 78% with high precision (88%). This suggests that the method can provide a useful aid for early detection of liver metastases.

1 Introduction

The liver is the largest internal organ in the body, responsible for numerous metabolic, regulatory, transport, and immune functions. It is the second most commonly involved organ in metastatic disease, after the lymph nodes. The liver provides a fertile soil in which metastases can develop due to its rich, dual blood supply. In particular, hepatic metastases are a frequent complication in colorectal carcinoma patients. Since liver function tests in patients with liver metastases tend to be insensitive and non-specific, the disease is usually diagnosed at later stages of its development. Although numerous possible treatments are currently available, hepatic metastases are difficult to eradicate because they are discovered late. Early and accurate detection of these lesions has the potential of improving survival rates and reducing treatment morbidity.

A key physiological observation is that changes in liver blood supply can serve as an indicator for the presence of hepatic metastases [1]. While the blood supply of healthy liver predominantly enters from the portal vein, in patients with overt colorectal liver metastases, a higher proportion of liver blood flow is derived from the hepatic artery. Thus, monitoring hemodynamical changes can serve as the basis for the early detection of hepatic metastases.

Medical imaging has the potential to play an important role in the monitoring of the liver hemodynamical changes. Barash et al [2] have recently demonstrated the utility of functional Magnetic Resonance Imaging (fMRI) with hypercapnia and hyperoxia for monitoring changes in liver perfusion and hemodynamics without contrast agent administration. Based on these findings, Edrei et al [3] showed how to characterize colorectal hepatic metastases and how to follow their early hemodynamical changes. Unlike methods that use contrast agents [4,5], their method can detect steady state levels without making a compromise between the spatial and temporal resolutions. This opens up the possibility to detect smaller lesions at an earlier development stage. Since hemodynamical changes are subtle, relative, and spatially distributed, direct observation of these changes is difficult, unreliable, and time-consuming.

Computer-aided detection of early hemodynamical changes from fMRI images is a challenging task. Existing methods for brain fMRI analysis, such as mass-multivariate analysis [6,7] and region-based methods [8,9] cannot be applied to the liver. The analysis must cope with high inter-subject variability in the spatial locations of the metastases, their functional activation response, and the GRE (Gradient Recalled Echo) signal variations of the different tissues.

In previous work [10], we developed a method to classify manually selected and normalized rectangular regions on liver fMRI images as metastatic or healthy tissue. Our method uses a non-linear Support Vector Machine (SVM) [11] model constructed from manually selected samples of fMRI images taken at the advanced growth phase of the metastases. The drawbacks of this method are that it is operator-depended in region selection and normalization, and that it is biased to axis-aligned shapes, which are not conformal to metastases shapes.

This paper presents a machine-learning approach to the interactive classification of suspected liver metastases using fMRI images. The method uses fMRI-based statistical modeling to characterize colorectal hepatic metastases and follow their early hemodynamical changes. These changes are evaluated from T_2^*-W fMRI images acquired during the breathing of air, air-CO_2, and carbogen. A classification model is build to differentiate between tumor and healthy liver tissues. The advantages of our classification model are that its construction does not require user interaction and and manual normalization. Thus, it is user-independent, and more accurate as it is not biased to axis-aligned shapes. The proposed model allows radiologists to interactively examine suspicious locations of early metastases presence in anatomical MRI images.

2 Method

Our method follows the supervised learning paradigm. First, it builds a classification model from a training set of image datasets of confirmed healthy subjects or subjects with confirmed metastases at the advanced growth phase. The model is then used to classify suspicious regions in new datasets of healthy subjects or subjects with metastases at earlier growth phases. Each dataset is processed with the same dataset analysis method.

The input dataset consists of an anatomical MRI image (T_2W) and a set of fMRI-based maps representing hepatic hemodynamics. The fMRI images are acquired during the breathing of air, air-carbon dioxide (5% CO_2), and carbogen (95% oxygen; 5% CO_2) according to the protocol in [2], and co-registered.

2.1 Dataset Analysis

Dataset analysis consists of four steps as follows.

1. Hemodynamic activity maps computation

Two hemodynamic activity maps are derived from the fMRI images. The maps describe the mean relative change of the fMRI signal intensity induced by hypercapnia ($\Delta S_{co_2}(\boldsymbol{x})$) and hyperoxia ($\Delta S_{o_2}(\boldsymbol{x})$):

$$\Delta S_{co_2}(\boldsymbol{x}) = \frac{\bar{S}_{co_2}(\boldsymbol{x}) - \bar{S}_{air}(\boldsymbol{x})}{\bar{S}_{air}(\boldsymbol{x})} \times 100 \quad \Delta S_{o_2}(\boldsymbol{x}) = \frac{\bar{S}_{o_2}(\boldsymbol{x}) - \bar{S}_{co_2}(\boldsymbol{x})}{\bar{S}_{co_2}(\boldsymbol{x})} \times 100 \quad (1)$$

where $\boldsymbol{x}$ is the pixel coordinates and $\bar{S}$ is the mean signal value over all acquisitions for each gas inhalation. The colorectal hepatic metastases are present in regions with reduced ΔS_{o_2} positive values and reduced ΔS_{co_2} negative values.

2. Maps normalization

Normalization of the hemodynamic activity maps is necessary due to the high variability of the GRE signal from different subjects and in the same subject at different time points. First, the liver borders are determined from the anatomical MRI images and all the rest is eliminated from the maps. Next, each map is centered around a liver mean intensity of zero, with a standard deviation of 1:

$$\tilde{\Delta S}_{co_2}(\boldsymbol{x}) = \frac{\Delta S_{co_2}(\boldsymbol{x}) - \mu_{\Delta S_{co_2 hl}}}{\sigma_{\Delta S_{co_2 hl}}} \quad \tilde{\Delta S}_{o_2}(\boldsymbol{x}) = \frac{\Delta S_{o_2}(\boldsymbol{x}) - \mu_{\Delta S_{o_2 hl}}}{\sigma_{\Delta S_{o_2 hl}}} \quad (2)$$

where $\boldsymbol{x}$ is the pixel coordinates, $\mu_{\Delta S_{co_2 hl}}$ and $\mu_{\Delta S_{o_2 hl}}$ are the mean values of the healthy liver region, and σ is their corresponding standard deviation. Finally, each dataset is filtered with bilateral smoothing [12] to reduce the amount of noise while keeping the discontinuities between healthy and metastasis regions.

3. Maps adaptive partitioning

The next step is the partition of the hemodynamic activity maps into regions based on spatial proximity and hemodynamic activity values. Adaptive automatic partition of the maps is necessary since the number, location, and shape of the metastases varies from subject to subject. This is in contrast to brain fMRI, where the regions of cognitive activity are similar and known in advance. We compute the spatial partition into regions of similar hemodynamic activity

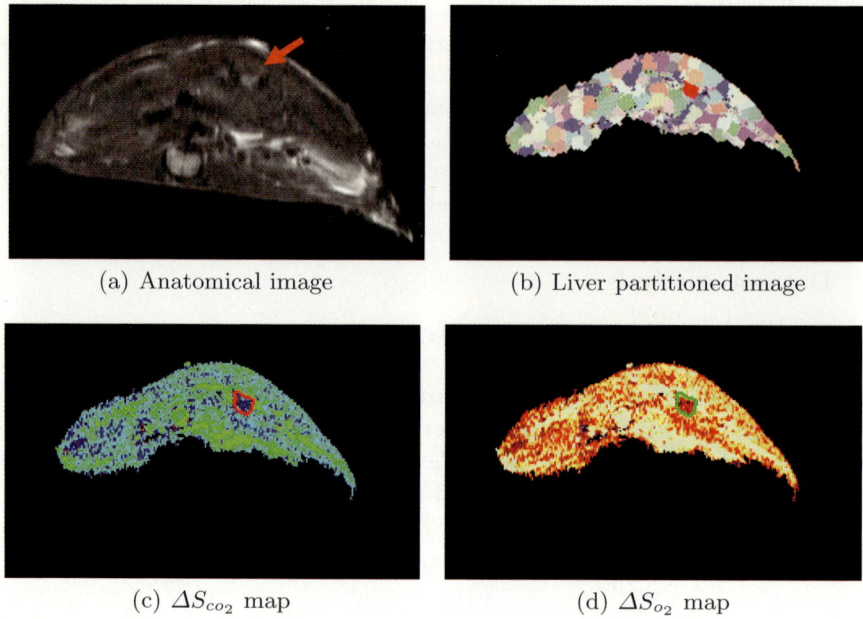

Fig. 1. Illustration of early phase hemodynamic maps partitioning: (a) anatomical MRI image (the suspected metastatic region is not yet confirmed); (b) partition map in which each region has a different color; the suspicious region is colored by red; (c)-(d) hemodynamic activity maps showing the suspicious region. Note that the hemodynamic maps are presented after normalization

by mean-shift clustering [13] of both ΔS maps. Fig. 1 shows an example of the clustering results of an early phase dataset.

4. Features extraction

Next, we compute two characteristic feature vectors for each region R_k in the partition. Since metastases have different locations, shapes, and sizes, the features vectors must be invariant to them. Since reactivity to hypercapnia and hyperoxia distinguishes between two different biological properties, we compute a separate feature vector for each map. We chose to compactly describe the regions distribution with a feature vector $\boldsymbol{f}_k$ consisting of five parameters: 1) mean; 2) standard deviation; 3) kurtosis; 4) skewness, and 5) interquartile range. This representation yields better results than using the entire histogram [10]. Fig. 2 shows two sample histograms of healthy and metastatic regions.

2.2 Model Construction

To generate the classification model of the metastases, we process the images in the training set as described above. The output is a set of regions and their feature vectors description. Each region is individually labeled by an expert radiologist as healthy/metastatic based on the anatomical MRI images.

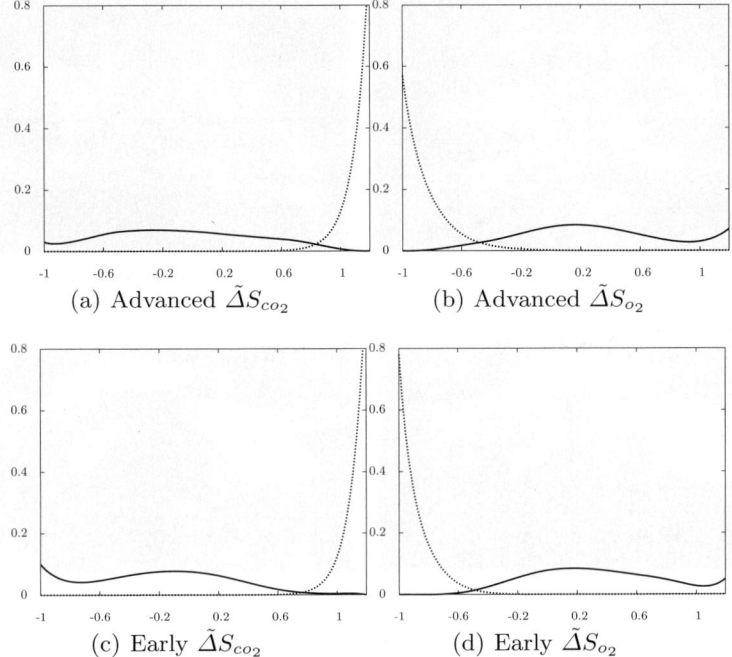

Fig. 2. Representative sample distributions of normalized hemodynamic activity maps of metastatic (dotted line) and healthy (solid line) regions: (a)-(b) advanced growth phase; (c)-(d) early growth phase

We train an SVM classification engine with the resulting set of tagged feature vector. We compute a classification model for each hemodynamic activity map separately. We use a generalized Radial Basis Function (RBF) kernel with the Earth Movers Distance (EMD) [14] as the affinity measure.

2.3 Early Classification

Once the classification model has been constructed, we use it to classify suspicious regions in new datasets of healthy subjects or subjects with metastases in earlier growth phases. The radiologist identifies a location of a suspected metastasis in the anatomical MRI. The corresponding region in the hemodynamic activity maps is then classified according to the classification model. This can be repeated for additional locations as required.

The dataset is processed following the dataset analysis method described above. The two hemodynamic activity maps are first computed and normalized. We use a truncated mean used instead of the standard mean in Eq. 2 to reduce the sensitivity to noise and to small metastases possibly present inside the liver. The maps adaptive partition is then performed on the resulting maps. The features extraction is then performed on the regions containing the locations selected by the radiologist. Since two different and independent biological

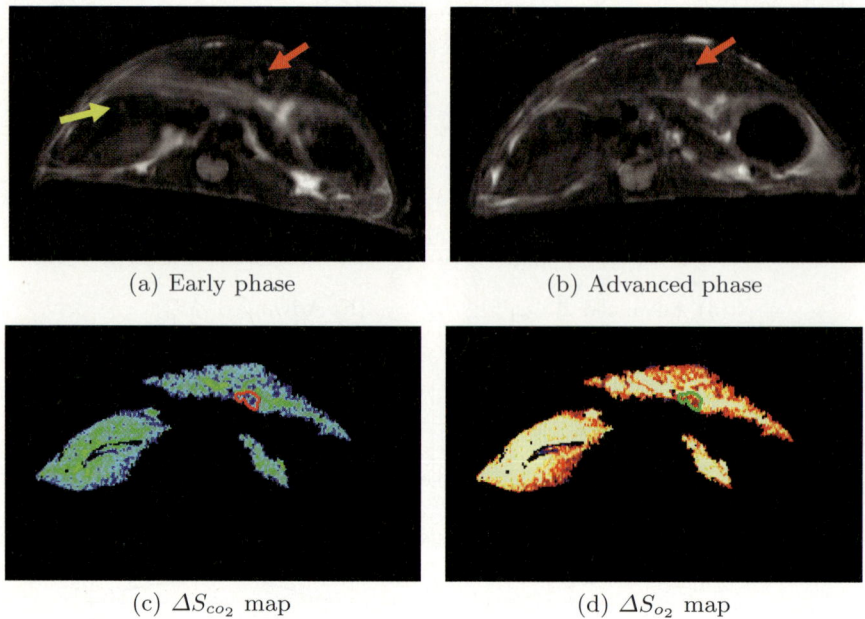

Fig. 3. Early classification example: (a) anatomical MRI image with suspected regions pointed; (b) anatomical MRI image from advanced growth phase of the same subject. Only the region pointed by the red arrow was classified as metastasis by our method, as confirmed later; (c)-(d) early phase hemodynamic activity maps. The suspected region is marked. Although the anatomical images (a-b) are not co-registered since they are acquired at different times. The correspondence between the lesions in the images was determined by an expert using their position relative to the kidneys.

processes are modeled by the two maps, we classify the hemodynamic activity maps feature vectors separately and join the results. When both are classified as metastasis, the region is considered as metastatic. Coupling the classification yielded worse results than separate treatment. Fig. 3 shows an example of the early phase confirmation. The pointed areas are the suspected regions. Note that there are no confirmed metastases in the anatomical image (Fig. 3(a)), while the corresponding hemodynamical changes are easily detectable in the hemodynamic activity maps (Fig. 3(c), 3(d)). The region pointed by the red arrow was confirmed as containing a metastasis in the advanced growth phase anatomical image (3(b)).

3 Experimental Results

We performed an animal study on CB6F1 mice that underwent splenic injection with CT-26 colon cancer cells (10^4 cells/mouse in 0.3ml) to generate metastases. Metastases progression was monitored twice a week by MRI. MRI scans were performed on a 4.7T Bruker Biospec spectrometer with a 3cm bird cage

Table 1. Summary of experimental results tabulated in a confusion matrix. The columns indicate the true class (Positive/Negative) and the rows indicate the hypothesized class (Yes/No).

	Positive	Negative
Yes	23	3
No	7	11
Total	30	14

coil. Anatomical MRI images were acquired using T_2-weighted fast SE images (TR/TE = 2000/40ms). Changes in hepatic hemodynamics were evaluated using T_2^*-weighted GRE (TR/TE=147/10ms). The images were acquired following the protocol in [2] and co-registered since the mice are fixed and immobilized under anesthesia. When metastases became large (18 days after tumor cells injection, and above), the mice were sacrificed, and their livers were taken for histology.

A classification model was generated from 25 advanced growth phase (days 14-18) datasets and 4 of healthy subjects datasets. Each dataset consist of 4-5 slices with 1-5 metastases. Since only 4 slices are available for each mouse, real 3D analysis cannot be performed. Therefore each slice was analyzed separately. The model was generated with the SVM engine implementation from [15].

To test early classification, we obtained 16 early growth phase (days 10-14) datasets, and preprocessed them as described in Sec. 2.3. An expert radiologist selected a total of 44 suspected metastases locations on the anatomical images (the metastases were not confirmed in the anatomical MRI images). The corresponding regions in the hemodynamic activity maps were then classified and confirmed later by histology or by an additional advanced growth phase anatomical MRI. Table 1 summarizes the results. The classification performance of our method was 78% accuracy, 88% precision, and of 77% recall.

4 Conclusions

We have presented a new method for the interactive classification of suspected liver metastases using fMRI images. The method uses a machine-learning approach to construct an fMRI-based statistical model to characterize colorectal hepatic metastases from a training dataset. The classification model is then used to classify suspicious regions in new datasets of healthy subjects or subjects with metastases in earlier growth phases. Our experimental results on mice yielded an accuracy of 78% with high precision (88%). This suggests that the method can provide a useful aid for early detection of metastases. We are conducting ongoing research to determine the applicability of our method to humans.

Financial support: This research was supported in part by a grant number 728/05 from the Israel Science Foundation (for RA), by the Horwitz Foundation through The Center for Complexity Science (for RA and YE).

References

1. Leveson, S., Wiggins, P., Giles, G., Parkin, A., Robinson, P.: Deranged blood flow patterns in the detection of liver metastases. Bri. J. of Surgery 72, 128–130 (1985)
2. Barash, H., Gross, E., Matot, I., Edrei, Y., Tsarfaty, G., Spira, G., Vlodavsky, I., Galun, E., Abramovitch, R.: Functional-MRI during hypercapnia and hyperoxia: a non-invasive monitoring tool for changes in liver perfusion and hemodynamics in a rat model. Radiology (243), 727–735 (2007)
3. Edrei, Y., Gross, E., Pikarsky, E., Galun, E., Abramovitch, R.: Characterization and early detection of liver metastasis by fMRI. In: The 14th Int. Soc. of Magnetic Res. in Medicine (ISMRM) Scientific Meeting (2006) (Abstract no. 1752)
4. Cuenod, C., Leconte, I., Siauve, N., Resten, A., Dromain, C., Poulet, B., Frouin, F., Clement, O., Frija, G.: Early changes in liver perfusion caused by occult metastases in rats: Detection with quantitative CT. Radiology 218(2), 556–561 (2001)
5. Totman, J., O'Gorman, R., Kane, P., Karani, J.: Comparison of the hepatic perfusion index measured with gadolinium-enhanced volumetric MRI in controls and in patients with colorectal cancer. British J. of Radiology 78(926), 105–109 (2005)
6. Mitchell, T., Hutchinson, R., Niculescu, R., Pereira, F., Wang, X., Just, M., Newman, S.: Learning to decode cognitive states from brain images. Machine Learning 57(1-2), 145–175 (2004)
7. Wang, X., Hutchinson, R., Mitchell, T.: Training fMRI classifiers to discriminate cognitive states across multiple subjects. In: Advances in Neural Inf. Processing Systems, vol. 16. MIT Press, Cambridge (2004)
8. Thirion, B., Faugeras, O.: Feature characterization in fmri data: the information bottleneck approach. Med. Image Analysis 8(4), 403–419 (2004)
9. Fan, Y., Shen, D., Davatzikos, C.: Detecting cognitive states from fmri images by machine learning and multivariate classification. In: Proc. of the Conf. on Comp. Vision and Patt. Recognition Workshop (CVPRW 2006), p. 89 (2006)
10. Freiman, M., Edrei, Y., Gross, E., Joskowicz, L., Abramovitch, R.: Liver metastases early detection using fMRI based statistical model. In: Proc. of the 5th IEEE Int. Symp. on Biomedical Imaging: From Nano to Macro (ISBI 2008) (2008)
11. Vapnik, V.: The nature of statistical learning theory. Springer, Heidelberg (1995)
12. Tomasi, C., Manduchi, R.: Bilateral filtering for gray and color images. In: Proc. of the 6th Int. Conf. on Comp. Vision (ICCV 1998), pp. 839–846 (1998)
13. Comaniciu, D., Meer, P.: Mean shift: a robust approach toward feature space analysis. IEEE Trans. Patt. Anal. and Mach. Intell. 24(5), 603–619 (2002)
14. Rubner, Y., Tomasi, C., Guibas, L.: A metric for distributions with applications to image databases. In: 6th Int. Conf. on Comp. Vision, ICCV, pp. 59–66 (1998)
15. Thorsten, J.: Making large-scale support vector machine learning practical. In: Schölkopf, B., Burges, C., Smola, A. (eds.) Advances in kernel methods: support vector learning, pp. 169–184. MIT Press, Cambridge (1999)

Evaluation of a Cardiac Ultrasound Segmentation Algorithm Using a Phantom

Yong Yue[1], Hemant D. Tagare[1,2], Ernest L. Madsen[3], Gary R. Frank[3], and Maritza A. Hobson[3]

[1] Department of Diagnostic Radiology, School of Medicine, Yale University, New Haven, CT 06511 USA*
[2] Department of Biomedical Engineering, Yale University, New Haven, CT 06520
[3] Department of Medical Physics, University of Wisconsin-Madison, Madison, WI 53706-1532, USA

Abstract. This paper evaluates the performance of a level set algorithm for segmenting the endocardium in short-axis ultrasound images. The evaluation is carried out using an anthropomorphic ultrasound phantom. Details of the phantom design, including comparison of the ultrasound parameters with in-vitro measurements, are included.

In addition to measuring segmentation accuracy, the effectiveness of the energy minimization scheme is also determined. It is argued that using the phantom along with global minimization algorithms (simulated annealing and random search) makes is possible to assess the minimization strategy.

1 Introduction

This paper has two goals: The first is to comprehensively evaluate a level set algorithm for segmenting the endocardium in B-mode short-axis cardiac ultrasound images. The second is to propose an extension of the standard evaluation methodology. The extension provides an explanation of what limits the ultimate performance of the segmentation algorithm. It does so by providing insight into the relative effectiveness of the energy function and the energy minimization strategy.

The segmentation algorithm we evaluate is a maximum-a-posteriori (M.A.P.) level-set scheme [1] using Gamma probability densities [2] using an energy minimization strategy called *tunneling descent* [3]. Tunneling descent is a deterministic technique derived from gradient descent, but is capable of escaping from poor local minima. Although tunneling descent does not guarantee a global minimum, its performance in practice is superior to gradient descent [3].

1.1 Evaluating and Explaining Accuracy

Most ultrasound segmentation algorithms are evaluated by comparison with manual segmentation [4,5,6,7]. The algorithm is considered validated if its

---
* This research was supported by the grant R01 HL077810-02 from National Heart, Lung, and Blood Institute.

performance measures are within the variation range of manual segmentation results. Although popular, evaluation with manual segmentation may suffer from observer bias and inter- and intraobserver variability.

Acknowledging the limitations of manual segmentation, some authors have attempted to access the ground truth of the ultrasound image. A number of researchers [8,9] use synthetic images which provide ground truth. Some researchers use physical phantoms [10], but the number of such studies is surprisingly low. This may be due to the difficulty of constructing a physically realistic phantom and the low interaction between the image processing and phantom design communities. Almost all of the reported cardiac-like ultrasound phantoms, are designed for tissue characterization or strain measurements [11,12,13] rather than for assessing segmentation of the boundary of the myocardium.

We evaluate the segmentation algorithm by using an anthropomorphic phantom whose geometry mimics short-axis cardiac geometry. Simulated ribs are also included in the phantom. The phantom provides an operator-free ground truth to assess the accuracy of the algorithm.

Having measured accuracy, we additionally want to know which part of the algorithm is responsible for limiting the accuracy. A segmentation algorithm can be limited in accuracy because either its energy function is a simplified approximation to the "exact" energy function (and hence ultimately not capable of accurate segmentation), or because the energy minimization is stuck at a poor local minimum.

We propose to distinguish between the two by using a global minimization algorithm. The idea is to segment the phantom images first using the algorithm, and then using a global minimizer with the same energy function. If the global minimizer segmentation differs substantially from the ground truth, then we may be suspicious of the energy function because these are the best segmentations that it is capable of. On the other hand, if the segmentations of the global minimizers are close to the ground truth but those of tunneling descent are not, then inaccuracy can be attributed to the optimization strategy.

2 Cardiac Segmentation Using Tunneling Descent

Due to lack of space, we only give a brief sketch of the segmentation algorithm here. The reader is encouraged to refer to [3] for details. The energy function J of the algorithm is the negative posterior likelihood of the image gray levels:

$$J(\phi, \beta_0, \beta_1) = \lambda_1 \left\{ \int (1 - H(\phi)) \log p_1(I \mid \alpha_1, \beta_1) dA - \int H(\phi) p_0(I \mid \alpha_0, \beta_0) dA \right\}$$
$$- \lambda_1 \log p_\beta(\beta_0, \beta_1) + \lambda_2 \int \delta_0(\phi) |\nabla \phi| dA,$$

where, ϕ is the level set function, H is Heaviside function, and δ_0 is the Dirac delta function. Further, $p_0(I \mid \alpha_0, \beta_0)$ and $p_1(I \mid \alpha_1, \beta_1)$ are Gamma distributions modeling the gray levels of ventricular cavity and myocardial tissue [2] and α_0, α_1 are the shape parameters and β_0, β_1 are the scale parameters of the Gamma

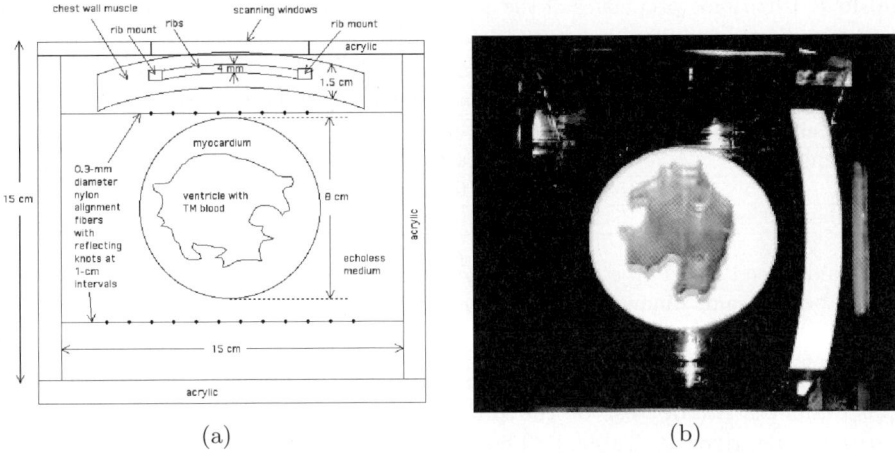

Fig. 1. Ultrasound Phantom. (a) A view of the two-dimensional phantom along the direction of translational invariance. The phantom is scanned through the scanning window at the top with the scan plane parallel to the plane of the figure. (b) The mold in the process of being cast.

distribution. The shape parameters are assumed to be known, while the scale parameters are estimated from the data, and the term $p_\beta(\beta_0, \beta_1)$ is the prior on βs. Finally, λ_1 is the external energy parameter, and λ_2 is the internal energy parameter.

Since α_0, α_1 are known, the task of the segmentation algorithm is find the ϕ, β_0, β_1 that minimize J. Minimization with respect to the βs is carried using standard gradient descent while minimization with respect to ϕ is carried out using a technique called *Tunneling Descent* (TD). Reference [3] contains a detailed description of this method including an evaluation of the sensitivity to parameters and initial conditions.

3 Ultrasound Phantom

We designed the ultrasound phantom shown in Fig. 1 for the short-axis section of the left ventricle at end diastole. Fig. 1(a) shows the design and Fig. 1(b) shows the tissue-mimicking (TM) myocardium part of the phantom during casting.

The phantom is essentially two-dimensional; it only models the short-axis cross section of the ventricle rather than the entire three dimensional shape. The phantom has two simulated ribs and two pairs of parallel fibers for aligning the scan plane of the ultrasound transducer. Each alignment fiber is a 0.3 *mm* diameter nylon fiber with a simple knot at 1 *cm* intervals along its length.

The phantom has four components: 1) a TM chest wall with simulated ribs embedded in it; 2) the TM myocardium; 3) blood; 4) a low echo TM background. All of these components are made from water, agarose, ultrafiltered whole bovine

Table 1. Ultrasonic properties of the soft-tissue mimicking materials in the phantom

TM Material	Speed (m/s)	Attenuation Coeff.		Backscatter Coeff.	
		α_0(dB cm^{-1} MHz^{-n})	n	η_0 (Sr^{-1} cm^{-1} MHZ^{-m})	m
Chest Wall	1541	0.580	1.08	1.79×10^{-6} *	3.67 *
Myocardium	1543	0.435	1.12	1.79×10^{-6}	3.67
Blood	1534	0.215	1.18	1.34×10^{-7}	3.65
Low echo background	1541	0.393	1.12	4.48×10^{-7} *	3.67 *

*Values deduced based on concentrations of glass bead scatterers relative to the same type of beads (same diameter distribution) contained in the TM myocardium.

milk, n-propanol, glass bead scatterers (7 micron diameter in blood and 22 micron diameter in the rest of the phantom [14]). Ultrasonic properties of the materials are given in Table 1. The propagation speeds and attenuation coefficients were measured by the method of [15], and the backscatter coefficients by [16].

4 Finding the Global Minimum

Recall that we intend to use global minimizers to understand what limits segmentation accuracy. In fact, we use two global minimizers: simulated annealing and random search.

4.1 Simulated Annealing (SA)

Simulated annealing (**SA**) [17,18] is a well-known minimizer which works by making random moves on the energy landscape. To minimize $J(\phi, \beta_0, \beta_1)$ the random moves correspond to perturbing the level set according to $\phi^{[n]} = \phi^{[n-1]} + \triangle\phi$. Downhill perturbations are always accepted; uphill perturbations are accepted with a probability that depends on the algorithm's "temperature" which varies according to a "schedule". We use three different temperature schedules. They all start from an initial temperature T_1 and reach a final temperature T_N in a fixed number of iterations, N. The first schedule is a linear schedule, called **SA TS1**, $T_n = T_1 - (n-1)\frac{T_1 - T_N}{N-1}$, where N is the total number of iterations. The second is a slow decay nonlinear schedule, called **SA TS2**, $T_n = a(T_1 - T_N)(1 - \arctan(\frac{n-1}{N-1}b - c)) + T_N$, where a, b, c are parameters controlling decay speed, $a = 1/(1 + \arctan(c))$ and $b = 1.5574 + c$. The third is a fast decay nonlinear schedule, called **SA TS3**, $T_n = T_1(\frac{T_N}{T_1})^{(n-1)/(N-1)}$.

4.2 Random Search (RS)

This is a heuristic algorithm developed by us. The basic idea is to maintain a set of m feasible energy minimizers which is updated at every iteration such that the new set has better minimizers than the previous set. Denoting this set

Table 2. Random research

Initialize $A^{[1]} = \{\phi_i | \phi_i = \phi^{[1]} + \triangle\phi_i,\ i = 1,\ldots,m\}$ where $\phi^{[1]}$ is a given initial level set
For n=2:N do:
 $B^{[n]} = A^{[n-1]} \bigcup \{\tilde{\phi} | \tilde{\phi} = \phi + \triangle\phi,\ \phi \in A^{[n-1]}\}$
 For every $\phi \in B^{[n]}$ calculate $\hat{\beta}_0, \hat{\beta}_1 = \arg\min_{\beta_0,\beta_1} J(\phi, \beta_0, \beta_1)$
 Sort all $\phi \in B^{[n]}$ according to their energy $J(\phi, \hat{\beta}_0, \hat{\beta}_1)$.
 Set $A^{[n]}$ to the m smallest energy ϕ's in $B^{[n-1]}$.
End do
Return the smallest energy ϕ in $A^{[N]}$.

---

in the nth iteration as $A^{[n]}$, the recipe for creating $A^{[n]}$ is as follows: all level sets in $A^{[n-1]}$ are randomly perturbed and a new set $B^{[n]}$ is created according to $B^{[n]} = A^{[n-1]} \bigcup \{\tilde{\phi} | \tilde{\phi} = \phi + \triangle\phi,\ \phi \in A^{[n-1]}\}$, where $\triangle\phi$ are the random perturbations. $B^{[n]}$ has $2m$ level sets as its elements. These are sorted according to energy and the m lowest energy level sets form $A^{[n]}$. After N iterations, the lowest energy curve in $A^{[N]}$ is taken as the global minimizer. The algorithm is initialized by setting to $A^{[1]}$ to an initial level set plus $m-1$ random perturbations of it. The pseudo-code for the algorithm is listed in Table 2.

4.3 Initialization, Random Perturbations etc.

SA and RS are both initialized at the tunneling descent segmentation. For all SA schedules, the initial and final temperatures are $T_1 = 1000$, $T_N = 1$ with a total of $N = 2000$ iterations. For SA TS2, the parameters are $a = 0.4213$, $b = 6.5574$, and $c = 5.0$. For RS, the size of the feasible solution set $A^{[n]}$ is set to $m = 100$, and the total iterations to $N = 1000$.

The level set random perturbation in both algorithms is taken to be a weighted sum of Gaussian radial basis functions. Thus, $\triangle\phi = \sum_j^{N_{rbf}} \omega_j \phi_j$, where N_{rbf} is the total number of basis functions, ω_j is the amplitude of the RBF, and $\phi_j(x) = \exp(-\frac{\|x-\mu_j\|^2}{\sigma_j^2})$, where μ_j and σ_j are the center and the standard deviation. The parameters $\omega_j, \mu_j, \sigma_j$ are generated randomly. The variances σ_j are uniformly chosen from the range $\sigma_j = 6 \sim 15$. By informal experimentation we determined that this range of σ_j gave perturbations of the speckle size in the image. We also determined that $N_{rbf} = 100$ gave sufficient basis functions for a rich perturbation.

4.4 The Best Optimizer

Typically global minimizers give the global minimum after infinite iterations. In practice, they have to be terminated after a finite number of iterations and they do not all find the same minimum at termination. For any image, we call the global minimizer that has found the lowest energy, the *best minimizer* (b.o.).

Thus, b.o.∈ {RS, SA TS1, SA TS2, SA TS3}. We use the best minimizer results for comparison with tunneling descent.

5 Experiments and Discussion

The phantom was imaged by a Phillips SONOS 7500 ultrasound system at 3.0, 5.5 and 7.5 MHz settings. The speckle size at these frequencies were 11, 9, and 8 pixels respectively. The 3.0 and 7.5 MHz images are shown in left column of Fig. 2.

All images were processed in the following way: First, the boundary of the endocardium in the image was segmented using tunneling descent. For each image, tunneling descent was deployed with three different internal energy parameters ($\lambda_2 = 40, 60, 80$), and a fixed external energy parameter ($\lambda_1 = 500$). Thus, for each image, nine segmentation experiments were performed and indexed as experiments 1 through 9 (see Table 3). After the tunneling descent segmentation, the global minimizers RS, SA TS1, TS2, and TS3 were used and the best optimizer found for each image.

The middle column of Fig. 2 shows the tunneling descent segmentation overlayed with the best optimizer segmentation. The right column shows the best optimizer segmentation overlayed with the phantom ground truth (GT).

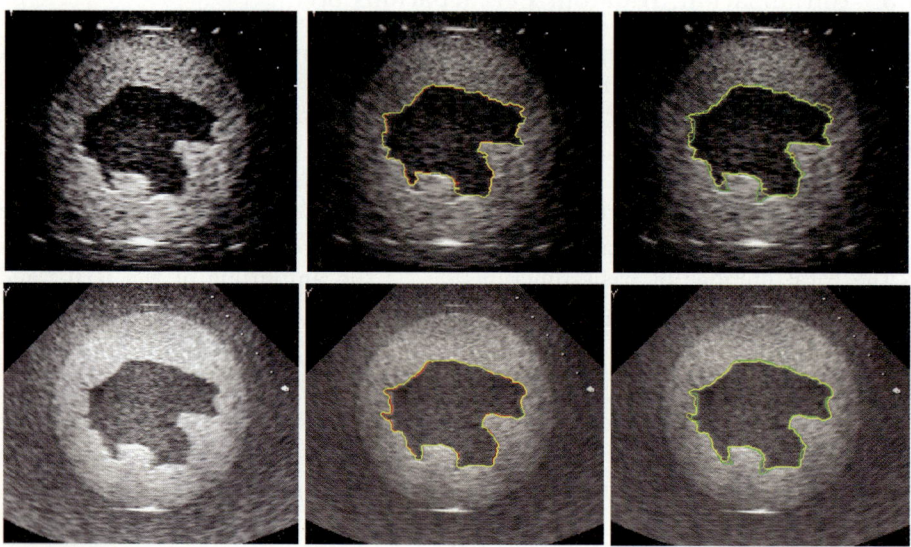

Fig. 2. Left column: ultrasound images of the phantom, acquired at 3.0 MHz(top), and 7.5 MHz (bottom). Middle column: segmentations of the best optimizers (yellow) overlaid on the segmentations of the tunneling descent (red) for the experiment 2 and and 8 (see Table 3). Right column: the segmentations of the best optimizers (yellow) overlaid on the ground truth (green).

Table 3. Evaluation of the segmentation using the ultrasound images of the phantom

	3.0 MHz			5.5 MHz			7.5 MHz		
Exp	1	2	3	4	5	6	7	8	9
λ_2^*	40	60	80	40	60	80	40	60	80
HD (GT,TD)**	10.512	10.784	10.736	15.497	15.046	14.965	9.067	9.071	8.843
MAD (GT,TD)	1.872	1.823	1.864	1.912	1.811	1.775	1.562	1.482	1.389
HD (GT,b.o.)	11.436	9.785	10.722	14.593	13.668	14.681	9.639	8.963	8.501
MAD (GT,b.o.)	2.185	1.983	2.073	1.490	1.675	1.617	1.379	1.396	1.287
ΔE(TD,b.o.)	-0.016	-0.015	-0.014	-0.015	-0.022	-0.0173	-0.013	-0.021	-0.019
HD (TD,b.o.)	5.099	3.162	4.000	5.385	3.000	2.2361	2.000	2.236	1.000
MAD (TD,b.o.)	0.718	0.557	0.464	0.928	0.554	0.549	0.601	0.512	0.415

*$\lambda_1 = 500$ for all experiments.   ** HD and MAD are measured in pixels.

The accuracy of the segmentations was evaluated by using the ground truth of the phantom. Two criteria were used for comparison: (1) The Hausdorff Distance (HD) between the segmentation and the ground truth $HD(C_1, C_2) = \max_{a \in C_1} \min_{b \in C_2} \|a - b\|$, and (2) the Mean Absolute Distance (MAD): $MAD(C_1, C_2) = 0.5 * [\frac{1}{n}\sum_{i=1}^{n} d(a_i, C_2) + \frac{1}{m}\sum_{i=1}^{m} d(b_i, C_1)]$, with $d(a_i, C_2) = \min_j \|b_j - a_i\|$. In these formulae, C_1, C_2 are the two curves being compared.

The top four rows of Table 3 show the accuracy of tunneling descent and the best optimizer in comparison to ground truth. Since the speckle size in these images is 8 ∼ 11 pixels, in all cases, tunneling descent and the best optimizer segmentations have an accuracy of one to two times the speckle size.

Next, recall from the discussion in section 1 that we are interested in not only evaluating accuracy, but also in understanding what limits the accuracy. We argued in section 1 that this could be done by comparing tunneling, the best optimizer, and the ground truth. We carried out this comparison in two ways. First, we asked whether the best optimizer minimum was significantly lower energy than the tunneling descent minimum. We did this by calculating $\Delta E(TD, b.o.) = (J(\phi_2, \beta_{0,2}, \beta_{1,2}) - J(\phi_1, \beta_{0,1}, \beta_{1,1}))/|J(\phi_2, \beta_{0,2}, \beta_{1,2})|$, where $J(\phi_2, , \beta_{0,2}, \beta_{1,2})$ is the b.o. minimum energy and $J(\phi_1, \beta_{0,1}, \beta_{1,1}))$ is the TD minimum energy. The fifth row of Table 3 shows ΔE for the nine segmentations. The numbers show that the b.o. minimum energy is smaller than the TD minimum energy by only about 2%.

Second, we compared the geometry of the segmentations found by tunneling descent and the best optimizer by calculating the Hausdorff distance and the mean absolute distance between them. The results are shown in rows six and seven of Table 3. These rows show that Hausdorff distances are less than 6 pixels and the mean absolute distances are less than 1 pixel.

It is clear from rows 5-7 that for all practical purposes, the energy minimum found by tunneling descent is as good as the minimum found by the best optimizer. In turn, this suggests that it is the energy function rather than the optimization strategy that limits the segmentation accuracy. Support for this conclusion also comes from examining the right column of Fig. 2. The figure shows very vividly that the most significant difference between the b.o. and ground truth is near sharp corners. Apparently, the energy function prevents the segmentation from entering into these sharp corners. If higher accuracy is required, the energy function will have to be modified so that some sharp corners are permitted while still constraining the rest of the segmentation curve to be smooth.

6 Conclusion

In this paper, we evaluated the accuracy of a segmentation algorithm with a phantom study. We also argued that it is important to understand the origin of any segmentation inaccuracy, and that the origin could be understood by using phantoms with global minimizers. The experiments show that TD is accurate to one to two times the speckle size, and the TD finds a minimum that is very close to the global minimum. Furthermore, the residual inaccuracy of the segmentation can be attributed to the energy function rather than the minimization scheme.

References

1. Osher, S., Paragios, N.: Geometric Level Set Methods in Imaging, Vision, and Graphics. Springer, New York (2003)
2. Tao, Z., Tagare, H., Beaty, J.: Evaluation of four probability distribution models for speckle in clinical cardiac ultrasound images. IEEE Trans. on Medical Imaging 25, 1483–1491 (2006)
3. Tao, Z., Tagare, H.: Tunneling descent for m.a.p. active contours in ultrasound segmentation. Med. Image Anal. 11, 266–281 (2007)
4. Angelini, E.D., Laine, A.F., Takuma, S., Holmes, J.W., Homma, S.: Lv volume quantification via spatiotemporal analysis of real-time 3-d echocardiography. IEEE Trans. Med. Imag. 20(6), 457–469 (2001)
5. Lin, N., Yu, W.C., Duncan, J.S.: Combinative multi-scale level set framework for echocardiographic image segmentation. Med. Image Anal. 7, 529–537 (2003)
6. Sarti, A., Corsi, C., Mazzini, E., Lamberti, C.: Maximum likelihood segmentation of ultrasound images with rayleigh distribution. IEEE Trans. Ultrason. Ferroelectr. Freq. Control 52, 947–960 (2005)
7. Dydenko, I., Jamal, F., Bernard, O., Dhooge, J., Magnin, I., Friboulet, D.: A level set framework with a shape and motion prior for segmentation and region tracking in echocardiography. Med. Image Analys. 10, 162–177 (2006)
8. Boukerroui, D., Basset, O., Baskurt, A., Gimenez, G.: A multiparametric and multiresolution segmentation algorithm of 3-d ultrasonic data. IEEE Trans. Ultrason. Ferroelectr. Freq. Control 48, 64–77 (2001)
9. Jardim, S., Figueiredo, M.: Segmentation of fetal ultrasound images. Ultrasound Med. Biol. 31, 243–250 (2005)
10. Xiao, G.F., Brady, M., Noble, J.A., Zhang, Y.Y.: Segmentation of ultrasound b-mode images with intensity inhomogeneity correction. IEEE Trans. Med. Imag. 21, 48–57 (2002)
11. Mottley, J.G., Miller, J.G.: Anisotropy of the ultrasonic attenuation in soft tissue: Measurement in vitro. J. Acoust. Soc. Am. 88(3), 1203–1210 (1990)

12. Langeland, S., D'Hooge, J., Claessens, T., Claus, P., Verdonck, P., Suetens, P., Sutherland, G.R., Bijnens, B.: R.f.-based two-dimensional cardiac strain estimation: a validation study in tissue-mimicking phantom. I.E.E.E. Trans. Ultra. Ferro. Freq. Contrl. 51(11), 1537–1546 (2004)
13. Erpelding, T.N., Hollman, K.W., O'Donnell, M.: Bubble-based acoustic radiotion force elasticity imaging. I.E.E.E. Trans. Ultra. Ferro. Freq. Contrl. 52(6), 971–979 (2005)
14. Madsen, E.L., Frank, G.R., Dong, F.: Liquid or solid ultrasonically tissue-mimicking materials with very low scatter. Ultrasound in Med. Biol. 24, 535–542 (1998)
15. Wear, K.A., Stiles, T.A., Frank, G.R., Madsen, E.L.: Interlaboratory comparison of ultrasonic backscatter coefficient measurements from 2 to 9 MHZ. J. Ultrasound in Med., 1235–1250 (2005)
16. Chen, J., Zagzebski, J., Madsen, E.L.: Tests of backscatter coefficient measurement using broadband pulses. IEEE Transactions on Ultrasonics, Ferroelectrics and Frequency Control 40, 603–607 (1993)
17. Metropolis, N., Rosenbluth, A., Rosenbluth, M., Teller, A., Teller, E.: Equations of state calculations by fast computational machine. Journal of Chemical Physics 21, 1087–1091 (1953)
18. Kirkpatrick, S., Gelatt, C., Vecchi, M.: Optimization by simulated annealing. Science 220, 671–680 (1983)

Automatic Recovery of the Left Ventricular Blood Pool in Cardiac Cine MR Images

Marie-Pierre Jolly

Siemens Corporate Research, Imaging and Visualization Dept., Princeton, NJ
marie-pierre.jolly@siemens.com

Abstract. We present a method for automatic localization and rough segmentation of the left ventricle blood pool in cardiac cine magnetic resonance images. The method first detects the whole heart using time-based Fourier analysis. It then segments the left ventricle blood pool by grouping connected components across slices using isoperimetric clustering. The system was tested on 253 datasets and failed in only 2 cases.

1 Introduction

Cardiovascular disease has become the largest cause of death in the modern world and is an important health concern. Imaging technologies such as magnetic resonance (MR) imaging allow physicians to non-invasely observe the behavior of the heart. Physicians are particularly interested in the left ventricle (LV) because it pumps oxygenated blood out to the rest of the body. Ideally, they would like to quantify the volume of the blood pool over time and estimate its ejection fraction, cardiac output, peak ejection rate, filling rate, and myocardial thickening. These quantities are easy to compute once the left ventricle is outlined in all images. Manual outlining is very cumbersome however, and most physicians limit it to the end-diastolic and end-systolic phases. This allows the system to calculate ejection fraction and cardiac output, but it is not enough information to estimate peak ejection rate or filling rate. Therefore, for complete patient care, it is very important to provide an automatic segmentation system.

This paper is concerned with the localization of the LV blood pool in the images of the 3D+T dataset (10 slices with 20 phases on the average). This is an important problem because the localized blood pool can be used to initialize a more elaborate LV segmentation algorithm. Therefore, the solution should be very robust. It is a difficult problem because MR intensities are not consistent across acquisitions and blood pixels cannot easily be identified in the images. In addition, most acquisitions cover slices beyond the LV itself to guarantee that it is seen in all phases. This means that some slices can be below the apex and contain no blood pool, and some slices can be above the mitral valve and contain the left atrium blood pool.

There has been many publications in the field of cardiac MR image segmentation. Some researchers have constructed models to help in the initialization process. Lorenzo-Valdés et al. [1] use a 4D probabilistic atlas of the heart and a 3D intensity template which they propose to register to the ED frame to localize the left and right ventricles. Mitchell et al. [2] use a hybrid active shape and appearance model and locate the heart using the Hough transform. Unfortunately, both these methods are too slow for clinical practice. In addition, models have difficulty capturing variability outside the training sets. This means that pathological cases which fall outside the standard set of shapes might not be recognized and appearance models have to be re-trained for new acquisition protocols and sequences. The solution proposed by Jolly [3] is faster, and actually used in clinical practice, but it still depends on a learned appearance represented by a Markov chain. Kaus et al. [4] combine a statistical model with coupled mesh surfaces. They originally had 169 datasets for testing but had to drop 48 of them because they exhibited breathing artifacts and through-plane motion which violated their model continuity assumption. They initialize their model by assuming that the heart is located in the center of the image which is definitely not a valid assumption.

To avoid the restriction imposed by a model, other researchers have chosen to use simple image processing techniques. These solutions however have been minimally tested [5,6] and tend to be less robust. Cocosco et al. [7] make a very restricting assumption that the coverage of the short-axis image stack should stop at the mitral valve and not go into the atrium. This is quite unreasonable as physicians tend to increase the coverage of the image stack to correct for potential motion after the acquisition of the localizer images and make sure that the LV is completely seen during all phases. Indeed, in 5 of their 32 cases, the top slice extended into the atrium and the algorithm could not separate the LV from the right ventricle (RV) without user intervention at the mitral valve. Lin et al. [8] also use simple image processing techniques and report only one failure out of 330 cases. This is the type of outstanding performance that is required for clinical practice. Unfortunately, we were not able to reproduce their results on our noisier datasets.

In this paper, we propose a new method to automatically detect and roughly segment the LV blood pool. We do not make any assumption on the quality of the acquisition or position of the heart in the images. First, the heart is localized in the images using motion information. Second, the LV blood pool is localized and roughly segmented within the heart. We tested our algorithm on 253 datasets and compared it with Argus (commercialized by Siemens Medical Solutions). Note that the goal of this work is not to segment the LV in all the images, but just to recover it in enough slices to be able to initialize a more sophisticated segmentation process.

2 Heart Localization

The first part of the algorithm consists in localizing the heart in the images and generating a region of interest to be used in the rest of the processing. We follow the recommendation from Lin et al. [8] and compute the first harmonic of the Fourier transform over time for each slice. These $H_1^s(x,y)$ images highlight

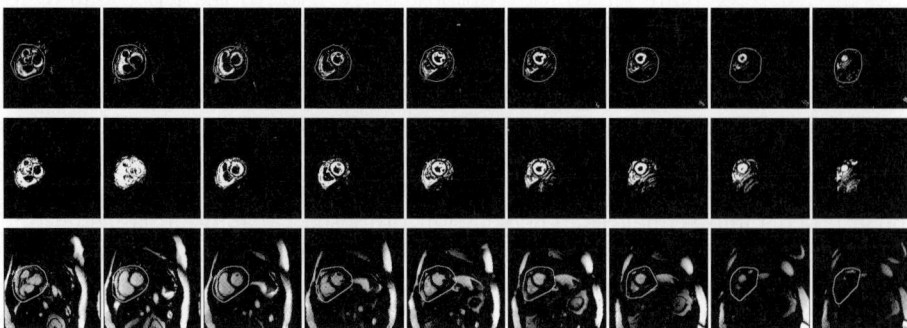

Fig. 1. Automatic heart localization: first row: first harmonic of the Fourier transform with the region extracted after 3D line fitting and distant artifact removal; second row: white connected components were kept and gray ones were discarded; third row: region of interest localizing the heart

the moving structures (cardiac chambers and great vessels). We then want to eliminate the distant moving artifacts. As in [8], a 3D line is fitted through the 2D centroids of the H_1^s images. Then, the distances weighted by the $H_1^s(x,y)$ values are histogrammed and thresholded to remove the farthest points. This procedure is repeated until the 3D centroid of the H_1^s images becomes stable.

Then, for each slice, we compute the average response $\overline{H_1^s}$ of the first harmonic. Each $H_1^s(x,y)$ image is thresholded at $2\overline{H_1^s}$ to retain only the strongly moving areas. Connected components (CC) are extracted and the next step consists of grouping them between slices to generate regions of interest that are consistent in space. To this end, the CC with largest average motion ($H_1^s(x,y)$ over all pixels) is identified in each slice and the relative motion of the other CCs is computed. In the same manner, we compute the relative size of each CC. The confidence is then defined as the relative motion times the relative size. The CCs with smallest confidence are removed one at a time until a slice containing a single CC (denoted $\hat{C}$) is identified. In the other slices, the 2D overlap between each CC and $\hat{C}$ is computed and the confidence becomes the relative size times this overlap. Connected components with a confidence lower than 0.1 are discarded. The final region of interest (ROI) is defined as the convex hull of the retained CCs in each of the slices.

Fig. 1 shows the process of heart localization on the first phase of the 9 slices of an example dataset. The first row shows the first harmonic image with the region that was extracted after 3D line fitting and distant artifact removal. The second row shows the connected components (the gray ones had low confidence and were discarded). Finally, the third row shows the detected ROI.

3 Left Ventricle Blood Pool Segmentation

In the second part of the algorithm, the system isolates the blood pool of the left ventricle inside the region of interest. The process is divided into 2 steps:

1) thresholding and connected component analysis, and 2) clustering to find the best set of connected components to describe the blood pool.

In the first step, each slice is processed one at a time. The images are thresholded inside the ROIs using Otsu's algorithm [9]. Then, the bright pixels are grouped into connected components. Here, we decided to extract 2D+T connected components for each slice rather than the 3D+T connected components proposed by Cocosco et al. [7] because the first slices of many of our datasets contained the left atrium (LA). If we had built 3D+T connected components, the bright pixels of the LV would have been connected above to the bright pixels of the LA which would have been connected below to the bright pixels of the RV, and the left and right ventricles would have been connected. With 2D+T connected components, the LV and RV are connected only in the mitral valve slice. This first steps highlights bright objects in the regions of interest, usually the LV blood pool, the RV blood pool, the aorta and other noisy regions.

In the second step, we want to group connected components between slices and identify the group that corresponds to the LV blood pool. For the grouping, we use the isoperimetric clustering algorithm proposed by Grady and Schwarz [10]. The goal of the algorithm is to partition a weighted graph by minimizing the perimeter to area ratio (i.e.: the isoperimetric ratio $h(S) = \frac{|\partial S|}{|S|}$). A graph is a pair $G = (V, E)$ with vertices $v \in V$ and edges $e \in E \subseteq V \times V$. An edge between two vertices v_i and v_j is denoted e_{ij}. In our case, the 4 largest connected components in each slice are each associated with a vertex in the graph and edges are defined between vertices in neighboring slices.

Let $A_p(v_i)$ be the area in phase p of the connected component associated with vertex v_i. Let $A^m(v_i)$ and $A^M(v_i)$ be the minimum and maximum areas over time, respectively. For each connected component, the following measures are computed:

1) Shrinking: $\mathcal{S}(v_i) = \frac{A^m(v_i)}{A^M(v_i)}$, the amount that the object contracts over time.
2) Roundness: $\mathcal{R}(v_i)$, the ratio of the smallest eigenvalue to the largest eigenvalue in 2D principal components analysis in each phase, averaged over time.
3) Connectedness: $\mathcal{C}(v_i)$, connected components when observed in each phase can be composed of multiple pieces. The relative size of each of these pieces is denoted $r_p^j(v_i), j = 1, ..., n_i$. Then, $C(v_i) = \frac{1}{P} \sum_{p=1}^{P} \sum_{j=1}^{n_i} r_p^j(v_i)$.
4) Concavity: $\mathcal{D}(v_i)$, the maximum distance (normalized between 0 and 1) between the object and its convex hull, averaged over time.

Finally, the overall confidence of a connected component is defined as $\mathcal{L}(v_i) = \frac{1}{50}\mathcal{S}(v_i)(1 - \mathcal{R}(v_i))\mathcal{C}(v_i)^{10}(1 - \mathcal{D}(v_i))^{10}$.

Edge weights, denoted $w(e_{ij})$, should indicate the similarity between vertices. The normalized area of a connected component in phase p is defined as $a_p(v_i) = \frac{A_p(v_i) - A^m(v_i)}{A^M(v_i) - A^m(v_i)}$. For each pair of connected components in neighboring slices, the following measures are computed:

1) Overlap: $\mathcal{O}(v_i, v_j)$, the intersection of the two 2D+T CCs divided by their union (if $\mathcal{O}(v_i, v_j) < 0.001$, the edge e_{ij} is discarded).

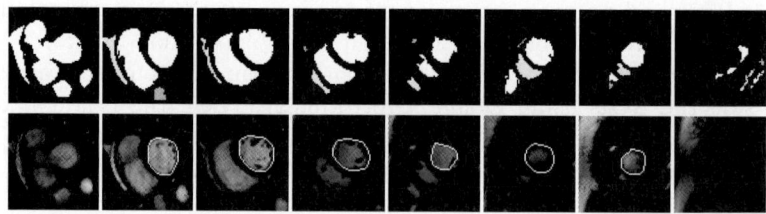

Fig. 2. Results of the LV blood pool recovery: first row: 2D+T connected components in the first phase of each slice, second row: contours for the LV blood pool cluster

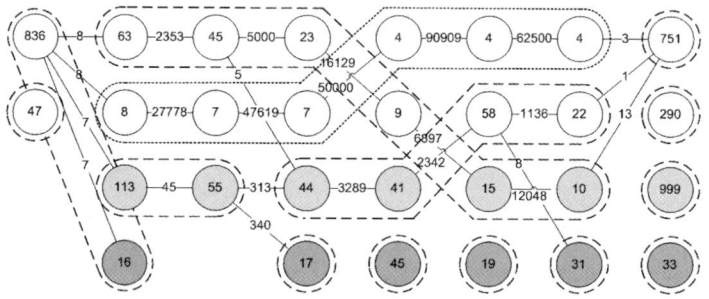

Fig. 3. Graph and isoperimetric clustering for LV blood pool recovery. The edge weights are multiplied by 10000 and the connected component confidences are multiplied by 100. Each column of vertices corresponds to a slice. The vertices and corresponding connected components in Fig. 2 have the same gray color.

2) Distance: $\mathcal{D}(v_i, v_j)$, the distance between the centers of the CCs averaged over time.
3) Resemblance of their area-time curves: $\mathcal{T}(v_i, v_j) = \frac{1}{P} \sum_p \|a_p(v_i) - a_p(v_j)\|$.
4) Difference in size: $\mathcal{S}(v_i, v_j) = \frac{1}{P} \sum_p \max(1, \frac{A_p(v_i)}{A_p(v_j)})$ where v_i is on the slice below v_j, it is expected that the components get smaller as they go down the slices closer to the apex, so $\mathcal{S}(v_i, v_j)$ should stay close to 1 for CCs in the LV blood pool.

The edge cost is then defined as $c(v_i, v_j) = \frac{\mathcal{D}(v_i, v_j)\mathcal{T}(v_i, v_j)\mathcal{S}(v_i, v_j)}{\mathcal{O}(v_i, v_j)}\mathcal{L}(v_i)\mathcal{L}(v_j)$ and the edge weight is $w(e_{ij}) = \frac{1}{c(v_i, v_j)}$.

The isoperimetric clustering algorithm is as follows. Let x be an indicator vector which takes a binary value at each vertex and encodes the partition S:

$$x_i = \begin{cases} 0 \text{ if } v_i \in S, \\ 1 \text{ if } v_i \in \overline{S}. \end{cases}$$

Then, the perimeter and area of the partition are defined as

$$|\partial S| = x^T L x \quad \text{and} \quad |S| = x^T \mathbf{1},$$

where $\mathbf{1}$ is the unit vector and L is the Laplacian matrix defined as

$$L_{ij} = \begin{cases} d_i & \text{if } i = j, \\ -w(e_{ij}) & \text{if } e_{ij} \in E, \\ 0 & \text{otherwise.} \end{cases} \quad \text{and} \quad d_i = \sum_{e_{ij}} w(e_{ij}).$$

The indicator vector is recovered by solving the linear system $Lx = 1$ which results in a real-valued solution for x. This can be converted to a binary partition by ranking the x_i's and choosing the threshold which yields the minimum value for the isoperimetric ratio $h(S)$. We choose the ground node as the center of the graph, i.e.: the vertex for which the shortest path to the farthest vertex is the smallest, which can easily be recovered using Floyd-Warshall's algorithm. This performs better to recover elongated clusters rather than the node with the largest degree as suggested in [10]. The graph is recursively partitioned until the isoperimetric ratio of the subpartitions is larger than a stopping criterion.

Once the clustering is determined, the blood pool cluster should be large and its connected components should shrink nicely over time, should be round, and should contain one main piece in each phase. The clusters are ranked in decreasing order of size, and we examine at least the first two clusters, as well as any cluster as large as the first two and any cluster of size larger than 3. We then choose the cluster $\hat{K}$ for which the function $\frac{1}{N_K^2} \sum_{v_i \in K} \mathcal{L}'(v_i)$ is minimum, where N_K is the number of vertices in cluster K and $\mathcal{L}'(v_i) = \mathcal{S}(v_i)(1 - \mathcal{R}(v_i))\mathcal{C}(v_i)^{10}$ is the confidence of a connected component. The 2D convex hulls of the connected components in $\hat{K}$ define the left ventricle blood pool.

Fig. 2 shows an example of the blood pool recovery. The first row shows the connected components and the second row shows the segmented LV blood pool. The graph that was constructed along with edge weights $w(e_{ij})$ and confidences $\mathcal{L}'(v_i)$ is shown in Fig. 3. The partitions are shown in dashed lines and the LV blood pool partition in a dotted line.

4 Experiments

We collected 253 datasets from 20 different clinical sites around the world. These datasets include both patients and volunteers and were all acquired on Siemens MR scanners. They contained between 2 and 16 slices, with an average of 10 slices and between 7 and 75 phases, with an average of 20 phases. 125 (49%) datasets started above the mitral valve plane, 7 (3%) of which were well inside the atrium and 72 (28%) datasets ended below the apex.

We ran the algorithm on all the datasets. For an average dataset of 200 images, the whole process (implemented in non-optimized C++) takes 8 seconds on a dual core laptop. By visual inspection, we consider that the algorithm succeeds if the resulting contours are around the blood pool in some slices in the dataset. We observed only 2 failures out of the 253 datasets. Both cases are shown in Fig. 4. In the first case, the strongest cluster corresponded to the aorta. In the second case, the system picked a totally wrong structure which was included in the region of interest due to some motion artifacts.

In most cases, no LV was segmented in the first and last slices. This was expected since the first slice was often above the mitral valve and the last slice

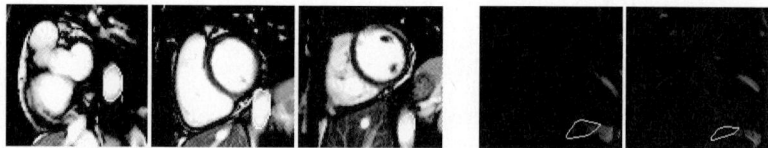

Fig. 4. The 2 failures out of 253 datasets for the blood pool segmentation algorithm

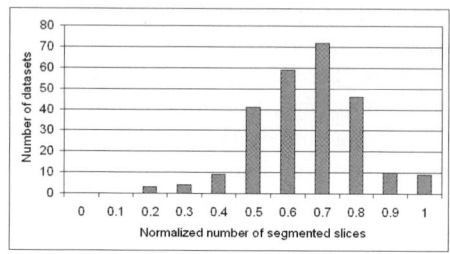

Fig. 5. Normalized number of segmented slices

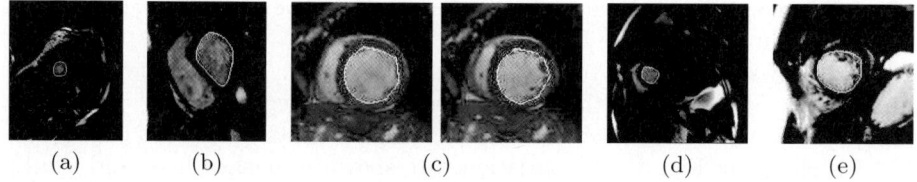

(a)   (b)   (c)   (d)   (e)

Fig. 6. Good results despite: (a) Large motion artifacts; (b) Not perfectly round LV blood pool; (c) Non contracting blood pool; (d) Heart not in the center of the image; (e) Very thin septum

was often below the apex. Fig. 5 shows the distribution of the normalized number of slices in which the LV was roughly segmented. On the average, the LV was localized in 63% of the slices. This is more than adequate to initialize a refined segmentation algorithm.

Some of the datasets were provided to us as failure cases from Argus, the commercial package from Siemens Medical Solutions (described in [3]). For 16 datasets, Argus was not able to locate the LV, and for 25 others, it identified another structure as the LV, thus causing 41 (16%) failures in total. When the system performs a fully automatic segmentation and identifies the wrong structure, the user has to redo the segmentation for the entire dataset, which can be very time consuming. This happened for 10% of the cases with Argus and for only 0.8% of the cases with our solution.

To illustrate the robustness of our method, Fig. 6 shows some examples of good results when some of the traditional assumptions are violated. In Fig. 6(a), there is a large motion artifact (streak at the bottom of the image). Fig. 6(b) shows that the LV blood pool is not always round. In Fig. 6(c) the blood pool does not contract much at ES (right) compared to ED (left). Fig. 6(d) shows that the heart is not always in the center of the image. In Fig. 6(e), the myocardium is very thin in the septum.

5 Conclusions

We have proposed a system to localize and roughly segment the left ventricular blood pool in cardiac cine MR images. In the first phase, the algorithm uses a time-based Fourier analysis to identify the moving heart. In the second phase, isoperimetric clustering is used to group 2D+T connected components and form the left ventricle blood pool. Even though the system uses simple image segmentation techniques, we have demonstrated on many different datasets that it is very robust.

At this time, we are focusing on segmenting both the endocardium (more accurately and in all slices) and the epicardium so that clinically meaningful measurements can be computed. In the near future, we will see if the same technique can be used to localize the right ventricle. Indeed, it can be seen in Figs. 2 and 3 that the other large cluster containing 6 vertices actually corresponds to the right ventricle.

Acknowledgements

We would like to thank Leo Grady at Siemens Corporate Research for his advice on the isoperimetric clustering algorithm. Also, this large study would not have been possible without the help of Carmel Hayes and Michaela Schmidt from Siemens Medical Solutions who provided all the test datasets.

References

1. Lorenzo-Valdés, M., Sanchez-Ortiz, G.I., Elkington, A.G., Mohiaddin, R.H., Rueckert, D.: Segmentation of 4D cardiac MR images using a probabilistic atlas and the EM algorithm. Medical Image Analysis 8, 255–265 (2004)
2. Mitchell, S.C., Lelieveldt, B.P.F., van der Geest, R.J., Bosch, H.G., Reiber, J.H.C., Sonka, M.: Multistage hybrid active appearance model matching: Segmentation of the left and right ventricles in cardiac mr images. IEEE Trans. Medical Imaging 20(5), 415–423 (2001)
3. Jolly, M.P.: Automatic segmentation of the left ventricle in cardiac MR and CT images. International Journal of Computer Vision 70(2), 151–163 (2006)
4. Kaus, M.R., von Berg, J., Weese, J., Niessen, W., Pekar, V.: Automated segmentation of the left ventricle in cardiac MRI. Medical Image Analysis 8, 245–254 (2004)
5. Gering, D.: Automatic segmentation of cardiac MRI. In: Ellis, R.E., Peters, T.M. (eds.) MICCAI 2003. LNCS, vol. 2878, pp. 524–532. Springer, Heidelberg (2003)
6. Phumeechanya, S., Pluempitiwiriyawej, C.: Left ventricular segmentation using double region-based snakes. In: Proc. ISBI, pp. 840–843 (2007)

7. Cocosco, C.A., Niessen, W.J., Netsch, T., Vonken, E.P.A., Viergever, M.A.: Automatic image-driven segmentation of cardiac ventricles in cine anatomical MRI. In: Proc. SPIE Applications of Digital Image Processing, vol. 5909, pp. 1–11 (1995)
8. Lin, X., Cowan, B.R., Young, A.A.: Automated detection of left ventricle in 4D MR images: Experience from a large study. In: Larsen, R., Nielsen, M., Sporring, J. (eds.) MICCAI 2006. LNCS, vol. 4190, pp. 728–735. Springer, Heidelberg (2006)
9. Otsu, N.: A threshold selection method from gray level histograms. IEEE Trans. Systems, Man and Cybernetics 9, 62–66 (1979)
10. Grady, L., Schwartz, E.L.: Isoperimetric partitioning: A new algorithm for graph partitioning. SIAM Journal on Scientific Computing 27(6), 1844–1866 (2006)

MRI Bone Segmentation Using Deformable Models and Shape Priors

Jérôme Schmid and Nadia Magnenat-Thalmann

MIRALab, University of Geneva, CH-1211 Geneva, Switzerland
{schmid,thalmann}@miralab.unige.ch

Abstract. This paper addresses the problem of automatically segmenting bone structures in low resolution clinical MRI datasets. The novel aspect of the proposed method is the combination of physically-based deformable models with shape priors. Models evolve under the influence of forces that exploit image information and prior knowledge on shape variations. The prior defines a Principal Component Analysis (PCA) of global shape variations and a Markov Random Field (MRF) of local deformations, imposing spatial restrictions in shapes evolution. For a better efficiency, various levels of details are considered and the differential equations system is solved by a fast implicit integration scheme. The result is an automatic multilevel segmentation procedure effective with low resolution images. Experiments on femur and hip bones segmentation from clinical MRI depict a promising approach (mean accuracy: 1.44 ± 1.1 mm, computation time: 2mn43s).

1 Introduction

Musculoskeletal disabilities seriously affect the majority of individuals over the age of 50. Osteoarthritis (OA) is often at origin of these disabilities, and its typical symptoms are inflammation, stiffness, pain and loss of mobility [1]. Morphological analysis [2] of (changes in) organ shapes is precious in understanding which factors (e.g., impingements) can lead to serious OA. Automatic bones segmentation can be hence used to substitute or expedite tedious manual delimitations from medical images. Moreover, bone segmentation can serve as a basis for more advanced modeling of other essential structures, such as cartilages [3] or muscles [4].

MRI is a flexible and non invasive modality. But bone segmentation can be challenging from clinical MRI images that suffer from poor image quality (imposed by time and clinical restrictions). Furthermore, bone intensity is not homogeneous in MRI due to differences in cortical and trabecular bones. This can affect some segmentation approaches (e.g., [5,6]). The use of prior knowledge considerably improves the robustness and the quality of segmentation especially when image information is missing or unreliable. Principal Component Analysis (PCA) is often used to describe the modes of variations among shapes to segment. PCA is reported in many studies on segmentation of bone [3,7,8,9] or other structures [6,10,11,12]. In Bayesian approaches, the segmentation problem is formulated as a Maximum A Posteriori (MAP) problem [6,9,12,13]. Prior knowledge is then naturally expressed as prior probabilities. Markov Random Fields (MRF) [14] express spatially varying priors and have been successfully applied to MAP-based segmentation [12,13,15]. But MAP-based methods using MRF present the inconvenient to be usually very time consuming.

Deformable models vary in type of representation (e.g., active contours [15], implicit [6,7], discrete [4,10,11,13]) and are used in segmentation techniques exploiting PCA [6,7,10,11] or MRF [13,15]. Physically-based deformable models are particularly interesting because they can be coupled with efficient computer graphics techniques (e.g., fast physically-based simulations [16,17]). The proposed approach simultaneously combines prior knowledge (PCA, MRF) and physically-based models. This novel combination confers speed and robustness to the segmentation. Unlike some MAP-PCA methods (e.g., [6]), a very fast segmentation is achieved without assuming that bone intensity is homogeneous.

In this paper, shapes are modeled as discrete deformable models by using a 2-simplex mesh representation [18]. Points of 2-simplex meshes have the nice characteristic to have the constant number of three neighbors. A shape x is represented by M 3D points: $x = \{x_1, \ldots, x_M\}$. The paper is organized as follows: shape variation modeling is first presented. Then, the segmentation method built on a multilevel forces-based implicit scheme is depicted. Finally, results of clinical MRI experiments and future work conclude this paper.

2 Shape Variation Modeling

2.1 Global Shape Statistics Based on PCA

For a given bone, N training shapes with known point correspondences are aligned with respect to a common reference frame. Based on a PCA, a statistical model of the shape variations is then built [19]. In our case, shapes are the result of a supervised segmentation procedure that fits template deformable models to corresponding images. This common approach (e.g., [10]) automatically produces a direct point correspondence. Although the correspondence may not be optimal [8,3,20], it gives satisfactory results in our experiments. An arbitrary shape x can be approximated from the computed statistics by: $x \approx T(\overline{x} + \Phi.b)$. Vector $\overline{x}$ is the mean shape, Φ is a matrix of K ($K < N$) eigenvectors, b is a shape parameters vector and T denotes the alignment transform. The eigenvectors (with eigenvalues λ_i) span the PCA subspace and express modes of variations. The degree of variation depends on the transform type and on the mesh resolution. Indeed, a PCA based on a rigid transform will capture global shape variations while an affine transform will lead to a more local description of variations. These two kinds of PCAs are denoted as rigid and affine PCA. In a similar way, shapes with a higher resolution are more adapted to express finer shapes differences.

2.2 Local Deformations Modeling Based on MRF

Let's consider $\boldsymbol{x} = \{x_1, \ldots, x_M\}$ and $\boldsymbol{Y} = \{y_1, \ldots, y_M\}$, respectively current and *true* point positions of a bone shape. Positions $\boldsymbol{x}$ are commonly the result of a procedure which exploited the PCA-based modeling. The objective is now to model the last discrepancy between current and real model. We pose $\boldsymbol{Y} = \boldsymbol{x} + \boldsymbol{\delta}$ where $\boldsymbol{\delta} = \{\delta_1, \ldots, \delta_M\}$ represent local deformations. By adapting the idea depicted in [12], the local deformations distribution is modeled by a first-order Gauss-Markov random process:

$$P(\boldsymbol{\delta}) = \frac{1}{Z_m} \exp -\frac{1}{2} \sum_{i=1}^{M} \left[\frac{1}{\eta^2} \sum_{j \in \mathcal{N}(i)} \|\delta_i - \delta_j\|^2 + \frac{1}{\sigma^2} \|\delta_i\|^2 \right] \quad (1)$$

where $\mathcal{N}(i)$ denotes the indices *neighborhood* of point i (i.e., three point indices) and Z_m designates the partition function which is a constant. Parameters η^2 and σ^2 control the smoothness and the magnitude of the deformations respectively. The term $\boldsymbol{x}$ is considered as deterministic, $\boldsymbol{Y}$ follows hence a first-order Gauss-Markov process as well. It is an unknown random process that will be inferred from observed data.

3 Segmentation Algorithm

3.1 Deformable Model Evolution

Discrete models are considered as particles with mass evolving under the Newtonian law of motion. The Newton equation relates particle position and velocity to a set of internal and external forces. The resulting time discretized differential equations system is solved by a stable implicit integration scheme [16] performing large time steps. As internal forces, we use a smoothing force [4] that penalizes strong irregularities and a PCA-based force $\boldsymbol{f}^{\text{pca}}$ (Sec. 3.3) that enforces shape constraints. External forces depend on the image intensity information (Sec. 3.2) and on current mesh point positions $\boldsymbol{x}$. They are designed to move models toward anatomical boundaries. Section 3.4 explains how the MRF modeling is exploited in a scheme involving two external forces. A step of the implicit scheme consists in evaluating forces f_i applied on each particle i at position y_i, as well as derivatives with respect to position $Df_i = \partial f_i / \partial y_i$ and velocity $Dv f_i = \partial f_i / \partial v_i$ (which is null for all the forces studied in this paper since they do not depend on velocity).

3.2 Image Force

Given the current mesh point positions $\boldsymbol{x}$, new positions $\boldsymbol{y}$ are sought in a neighborhood of $\boldsymbol{x}$ (usually along the mesh normal directions, e.g., [3,10,18]) in such a way that an energy $E_d(\boldsymbol{y}, \boldsymbol{d})$ is minimized. The image information $\boldsymbol{d}$ can include gradients, intensity neighborhoods, etc. A force $\boldsymbol{f}^{\text{im}}$ is then derived from $\boldsymbol{x}$ and the computed y. By assuming that forces are applied to particles i independently, f^{im} is modeled as a Hookean spring [18]: $f_i^{\text{im}} = \alpha^{\text{im}}(y_i - x_i)$. The coefficient α^{im} acts as a stiffness parameter. The derivative of the force is $Df_i^{\text{im}} = -\alpha^{\text{im}}\mathbf{I}$, where $\mathbf{I}$ denotes the identity matrix.

3.3 PCA-Based Force

A closest shape y is found by projecting x in the PCA space. An iterative procedure computes the adequate transformation T and appropriate constrained shape parameters $\boldsymbol{b} = b_1, \ldots, b_K$. Constraints are required to discard illegal configurations: shape parameters b_k are scaled when the Mahalanobis distance $D = \sum b_k^2/\lambda_k$ is strictly over a threshold $D_{\max}$. The threshold is calculated from the χ^2 distribution with K degrees of freedom [19]. The shape y is ultimately computed according to Sec. 2.1 formula. The same source-to-target approach is once again applied: $f_i^{\text{pca}} = \alpha^{\text{pca}}(y_i - x_i)$. However, attention must be paid on the fact that the computations of y_i and the corresponding forces are dependent on the positions of x_j, $j \neq i$. Forces and derivatives are in reality more complex. But neither instabilities nor odd behaviors were noticed in practice with the chosen approximations.

3.4 MRF-Based Force

Let's $\boldsymbol{d} = \{d_t, t \in L\}$ designates an observation field on a regular lattice defined by the image I. This field is related to the image information (Sec. 3.2). Our goal is to estimate the true (unknown) point positions $\boldsymbol{Y}^*$ by using a MAP formulation of the random process $\boldsymbol{Y}$ from the observation $\boldsymbol{d}$ [12]:

$$\boldsymbol{Y}^* = \operatorname*{argmax}_{\boldsymbol{Y}} P(\boldsymbol{Y}|\boldsymbol{d}) = \operatorname*{argmax}_{\boldsymbol{Y}} P(\boldsymbol{d}|\boldsymbol{Y})P(\boldsymbol{Y}) = \operatorname*{argmax}_{\boldsymbol{Y}} P(\boldsymbol{Y}, \boldsymbol{d}) \quad (2)$$

Commonly, $P(\boldsymbol{d}|\boldsymbol{Y})$ is assumed to follow a Gibbs distribution, i.e. $P(\boldsymbol{d}|\boldsymbol{Y})$ is proportional to $\exp -E_d(\boldsymbol{Y}, \boldsymbol{d})$. As a result, the joint distribution $P(\boldsymbol{Y}, \boldsymbol{d})$ is also a Gibbs distribution: $P(\boldsymbol{Y}, \boldsymbol{d}) = \frac{1}{Z}\exp - E(\boldsymbol{Y}, \boldsymbol{d})$. Parameter Z is assumed to be constant and independent of Y [12]. The energy is expressed as:

$$E(\boldsymbol{Y}, \boldsymbol{d}) = E_d(\boldsymbol{Y}, \boldsymbol{d}) + \beta \sum_{i=1}^{M} \left(\frac{1}{\eta^2} \sum_{j \in \mathcal{N}(i)} \|\delta_i - \delta_j\|^2 + \frac{1}{\sigma^2} \|\delta_i\|^2 \right)$$
$$= \sum_{i=1}^{M} \left[E_{d,i}(y_i, d_{y_i}) + \beta E_{m,i}(y_i, y_{\mathcal{N}(i)}) \right] = \sum_{i=1}^{M} E_i \quad (3)$$

where $\delta_i = y_i - x_i$ and d_{y_i} is the image information at y_i. The random process Y will be inferred from the image information and reference positions $\boldsymbol{x}$. The parameter β weights the regularization induced by the energy term based on spatial deformations with respect to the image-based energy term. When β is null, the procedure can be seen as a standard Maximum-Likelihood strategy that ignores geometrical considerations. To solve this MAP problem, the energy E

should be *globally* minimized which is not a trivial task. Instead, we consider E as a kind of potential energy (i.e., $f = -\nabla E$) and devise appropriate forces to be used in our framework. Each local energy E_i is derived with respect to positions y_i and y_j ($j \in \mathcal{N}(i)$), to get local contributions in forces and force derivatives. By summing up these contributions (e.g., $f_i = -\partial E_i/\partial y_i - \sum \partial E_j/\partial y_i$), forces and force derivatives can be computed on each particle in order to perform an implicit step. An analytic formulation of the energy $E_{m,i}$ derivatives can be expressed, whereas the derivative of $E_{d,i}$ cannot be explicitly formulated. Finite differences approximations may also lead to incorrect results as E_d may not vary smoothly enough. The force expression of Sec. 3.2 is thus reused to get forces and force derivatives for $E_{d,i}$ ($E_{d,i}$ is not dependent on y_j). The MAP-MRF problem resolution yields so two types of forces: f^{im} and f^{mrf} (β is then similar to a weighting parameter α^{mrf}).

3.5 Multilevel Segmentation Strategy

A Thin-Plate Splines interpolation procedure initializes generic bone shapes by using landmarks placed at specific anatomical positions. During the automatic segmentation, higher mesh resolutions are successively introduced and used in combination with previous lower resolutions. This strategy uses a bottom-up forces propagation scheme [4] between the different resolutions, which linearly combines lower with higher resolution forces. This approach yields better robustness and accuracy. At each new higher resolution introduction, three successive steps take place: (i) exploit PCA, image and smoothing forces; (ii) reduce PCA influence and keep other forces; (iii) set the current position as reference, enable MRF-based force, disable PCA and smoothing. The weight of each force is controlled by the weight factors α. Low resolution models are coupled with rigid PCA, whereas affine PCA is reserved for higher resolutions. MRF-based force is not used at the first resolution as the final result may be too far. In fact, only convergence toward a *local* minimum is ensured, so models must be close enough to the final solution.

4 Experiments and Results

An axial 3D T1 protocol (TR/TE= 4.15/1.69ms, FOV/Matrix= 35cm,256x256, resolution= 1.367x1.367x5mm) is used to acquire a large volume covering hips and thighs from a 1.5T MRI device (Philips Medical Systems). The protocol is fast (acquisition time: 3mn) but low resolution images are produced (Fig. 1). An experiment consists in segmenting hip and femur bones of both sides (Fig. 1(d)) from a volume dataset. Test datasets are not used in the training shapes construction. A set of 29 right and left female training bones is used, each training shape is available in 4 different resolutions (femur (hip) bone number of vertices: 514 (814) to 32K (52K)). A rigid PCA is performed for the lowest resolution, and affine PCAs for the remaining resolutions. 99% of the total variance is kept for each PCA. In all the experiments, we set $1/\eta^2 = 0.15$ and $1/\sigma^2 = 0.25$. The manual initialization requires the placement of 6 markers

Table 1. Mean and standard deviation of error distance with computation time

measures / dataset #	1	2	3	4	5	6
mean (mm)	1.66	1.34	1.30	1.50	1.27	1.54
std (mm)	1.25	0.82	1.15	1.20	0.95	1.22
time (s)	162	165	162	163	161	166

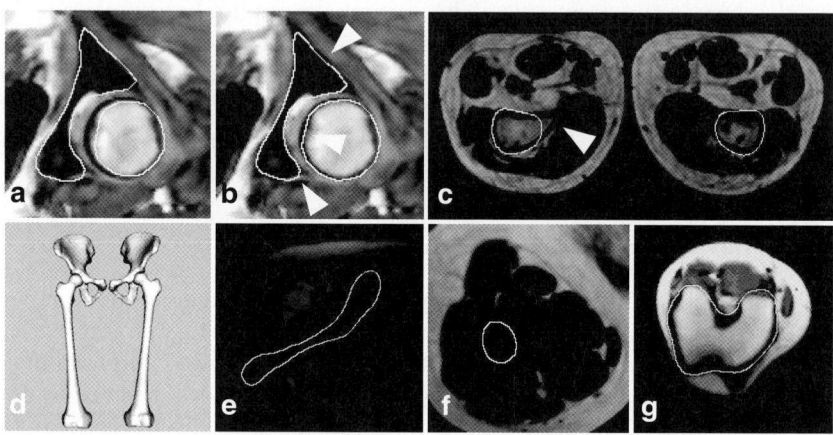

Fig. 1. Segmentation results: before (a) and after (b) usage of f^{mrf}, white arrows indicate significant improvements ($\alpha^{\mathrm{im}} = \alpha^{\mathrm{mrf}} = 0.5$). (c) Error in segmentation in case of abnormal deformation. Patient #1 has a benign osteochondrome (cartilage tumor) at the right distal femoral metaphysis (white arrow). (d) 3d reconstructed models example. (e)-(g) axial slice examples with segmentation contours.

per bone. This requires about 4-5mn in total. Segmentation error is calculated from experts contours (sometimes reduced to a series of points if contours cannot be drawn with a good confidence). Each contour point is projected on the corresponding segmented shapes and Euclidean distances are computed. Execution time of a segmentation (initialization is not counted) is monitored (used equipment: 3.40 Ghz computer with 2Gb of RAM). Table 1 reports accuracy and computation time for 6 datasets.

The average error is 1.44 ± 1.1 mm, which is close to the axial resolution (1.37 mm), and visually the segmentation looks accurate (Fig. 1). Nevertheless, a little too high standard deviation reveals some noticeable errors, essentially due to two major factors. Firstly, the poor image quality may also corrupt the gold standard manual editing, experts segmentation remains error prone. Secondly, the segmentation may fail in very noisy areas or when a bone presents a strong deviation from the training shapes. In that case, the segmentation is "over-constrained" by the priors-based forces (Fig. 1(c)). But, PCA-based forces make the process less sensitive to noise and surroundings structures (Fig. 2), the absence of PCA "regularization" creates in fact an unstable model (Fig. 2(b)). The MRF-based force efficiency is illustrated in Fig. 1(a) and 1(b), where at

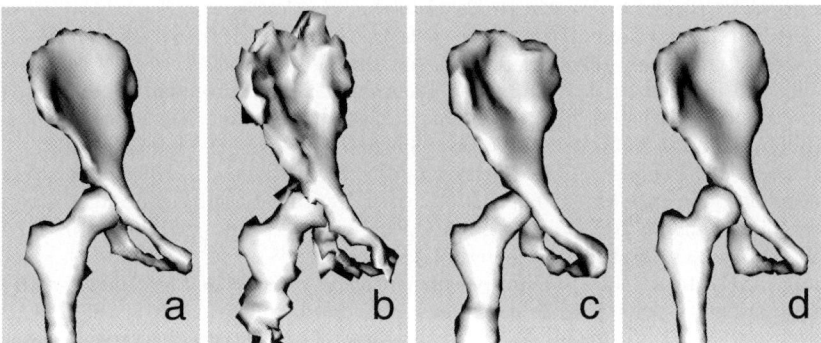

Fig. 2. PCA-based force utility: Starting from an initial model at low resolution (a) in which bones are deformed, 80 iterations are performed with different kind of forces. (b) $\alpha^{pca} = 0, \alpha^{smo} = 0, \alpha^{im} = 1$ (c) $\alpha^{pca} = 0, \alpha^{smo} = 0.5, \alpha^{im} = 0.5$ (d) $\alpha^{pca} = 0.4, \alpha^{smo} = 0.2, \alpha^{im} = 0.4$. The usage of PCA-based force clearly gives the best result.

the second mesh resolution level, the force can already capture fine details (in this ex., the error decreases from 1.94 ± 1.7 to 1.62 ± 1.5). Last but not least, time is also a strength of the method: overall time (acquisition, initialization and segmentation) takes less than 10mn. This encourages clinical use as image resolution and time constraints are not too demanding.

5 Conclusion and Future Work

The proposed method showed how prior knowledge supported by PCA and MRF brings robustness and accuracy, when they are combined with fast physically-based deformable models. Still, work remains in considering pathologies or large patient anatomical differences that are discarded by the priors-based regularization. One direction would be to add in the training shapes these differences or to balance correctly image forces with respect to other forces. Finally, the method should be adapted to higher resolution clinical datasets that cover a smaller field (i.e., focused on a joint), by tackling the issue of a more automatic initialization.

Acknowledgments. This work is supported by the 3D Anatomical Human project funded by the European Union. We would like to thank Dr. Kolo-Christophe from the Geneva University Hospital and Pascal Volino for their collaboration.

References

1. Felson, D.: Clinical Practice. Osteoarthritis of the Knee. N. Engl. J. Med. 354, 841–848 (2006)
2. Pfirrmann, C.W.A., Mengiardi, B., Dora, C., Kalberer, F., Zanetti, M., Hodler, J.: Cam and Pincer Femoroacetabular Impingement: Characteristic MR Arthrographic Findings in 50 Patients. Radiology 240(3), 778–784 (2006)

3. Fripp, J., Crozier, S., Warfield, S., Ourselin, S.: Automatic Segmentation of the Bone and Extraction of the Bone-cartilage Interface form Magnetic Resonance Images of the Knee. Phys. Med. Biol. 52, 1617–1631 (2007)
4. Gilles, B., Moccozet, L., Magnenat-Thalmann, N.: Anatomical modelling of the musculoskeletal system from MRI. In: Larsen, R., Nielsen, M., Sporring, J. (eds.) MICCAI 2006. LNCS, vol. 4190, pp. 289–296. Springer, Heidelberg (2006)
5. Lorigo, L.M., Faugeras, O.D., Grimson, W.E.L., Keriven, R., Kikinis, R.: Segmentation of Bone in Clinical Knee MRI using Texture-based Geodesic Active Contours. In: Wells, W.M., Colchester, A.C.F., Delp, S.L. (eds.) MICCAI 1998. LNCS, vol. 1496, pp. 1195–1204. Springer, Heidelberg (1998)
6. Yang, J., Duncan, J.S.: 3d image segmentation of deformable objects with joint shape-intensity prior models using level sets. Med. Image Anal. 8, 285–294 (2004)
7. Leventon, M.E., Grimson, W.E.L., Faugeras, O.: Statistical shape influence in geodesic active contours. In: Proc. IEEE Conf. Comput. Vis. Pattern Recogn., vol. 1, pp. 316–323 (2000)
8. Lamecker, H., Seebaß, M., Hege, H.C., Deuflhard, P.: A 3d statistical shape model of the pelvic bone for segmentation. In: Proc. of the SPIE, vol. 5370, pp. 1341–1351 (2004)
9. Dong, X., Gonzalez Ballester, M.A., Zheng, G.: Automatic extraction of femur contours from calibrated x-ray images using statistical information. J. Multimed. 2(5), 46–54 (2007)
10. Costa, M., Delingette, H., Novellas, S., Ayache, N.: Automatic segmentation of bladder and prostate using coupled 3d deformable models. In: Ayache, N., Ourselin, S., Maeder, A. (eds.) MICCAI 2007, Part I. LNCS, vol. 4791, pp. 252–260. Springer, Heidelberg (2007)
11. Wang, Y., Staib, L.: Physical model-based non-rigid registration incorporating statistical shape information. Med. Image Anal. 4(1), 7–20 (2000)
12. Kervrann, C., Heitz, F.: A hierarchical markov modeling approach for the segmentation and tracking of deformable shapes. Graph. Model. Image Process 60(3), 173–195 (1998)
13. Huang, R., Pavlovic, V., Metaxas, D.N.: A graphical model framework for coupling mrfs and deformable models. In: Proc. Conf. Comput. Vis. Pattern Recogn (CVPR 2004), vol. 02, pp. 739–746 (2004)
14. Geman, S., Geman, D.: Stochastic relaxation, gibbs distributions, and the bayesian restoration of images. IEEE Trans. Pattern Anal. Mach. Intell. 6, 721–741 (1984)
15. Martín-Fernández, M., Alberola-López, C.: An approach for contour detection of human kidneys from ultrasound images using markov random fields and active contours. Med. Image Anal. 9(1), 1–23 (2005)
16. Volino, P., Magnenat-Thalmann, N.: Implementing fast cloth simulation with collision response. In: Proc. Int. Conf. on Computer Graphics (CGI 2000), pp. 257–266. IEEE Computer Society, Los Alamitos (2000)
17. Nealen, A., Müller, M., Keiser, R., Boxerman, E., Carlson, M.: Physically based deformable models in computer graphics. Computer Graphics Forum 25(4), 809–836 (2006)
18. Delingette, H.: General object reconstruction based on simplex meshes. Int. J. Comput. Vis. 32(2), 111–146 (1999)
19. Cootes, T.F., Hill, A., Taylor, C.J., Haslam, J.: The use of active shape models for locating structures in medical images. In: Barrett, H.H., Gmitro, A.F. (eds.) IPMI 1993. LNCS, vol. 687, pp. 33–47. Springer, Heidelberg (1993)
20. Davies, R.H., Twining, C.J., Cootes, T.F., Waterton, J.C., Taylor, C.J.: 3d statistical shape models using direct optimisation of description length. In: Heyden, A., Sparr, G., Nielsen, M., Johansen, P. (eds.) ECCV 2002. LNCS, vol. 2352, pp. 3–20. Springer, Heidelberg (2002)

Segmentation of Vessels Cluttered with Cells Using a Physics Based Model

Stephen J. Schmugge[1], Steve Keller[3], Nhat Nguyen[1], Richard Souvenir[1], Toan Huynh[3], Mark Clemens[2], and Min C. Shin[1]

[1] Department of Computer Science, University of North Carolina at Charlotte, USA
sjschmug@uncc.edu, nhnguye1@uncc.edu, souvenir@uncc.edu, mcshin@uncc.edu
[2] Department of Biology, University of North Carolina at Charlotte, USA
mgclemen@uncc.edu
[3] Carolinas Medical Center, Charlotte,NC, USA
Steven.Keller@carolinashealthcare.org, thuynh@carolinashealthcare.org

Abstract. Segmentation of vessels in biomedical images is important as it can provide insight into analysis of vascular morphology, topology and is required for kinetic analysis of flow velocity and vessel permeability. Intravital microscopy is a powerful tool as it enables *in vivo* imaging of both vasculature and circulating cells. However, the analysis of vasculature in those images is difficult due to the presence of cells and their image gradient. In this paper, we provide a novel method of segmenting vessels with a high level of cell related clutter. A set of virtual point pairs ("vessel probes") are moved reacting to forces including Vessel Vector Flow (VVF) and Vessel Boundary Vector Flow (VBVF) forces. Incorporating the cell detection, the VVF force attracts the probes toward the vessel, while the VBVF force attracts the virtual points of the probes to localize the vessel boundary without being distracted by the image features of the cells. The vessel probes are moved according to Newtonian Physics reacting to the net of forces applied on them. We demonstrate the results on a set of five real *in vivo* images of liver vasculature cluttered by white blood cells. When compared against the ground truth prepared by the technician, the Root Mean Squared Error (RMSE) of segmentation with VVF and VBVF was 55% lower than the method without VVF and VBVF.

1 Introduction

The segmentation of vasculature in biomedical images can provide insight into analysis of vascular morphology, topology and is required for kinetic analysis of flow velocity and vessel permeability. The measurements of diameter, tortuosity, and bifurcations are often manually measured for further analysis. When the number of vessels to be analyzed is large, the automation facilitates analysis of large datasets (liver lobules can have extensive microvascular network) and decreases technician related bias.

A number of vessel segmentation algorithm has been proposed and are mostly in the domain of retina images. In this work, we developed a vessel segmentation

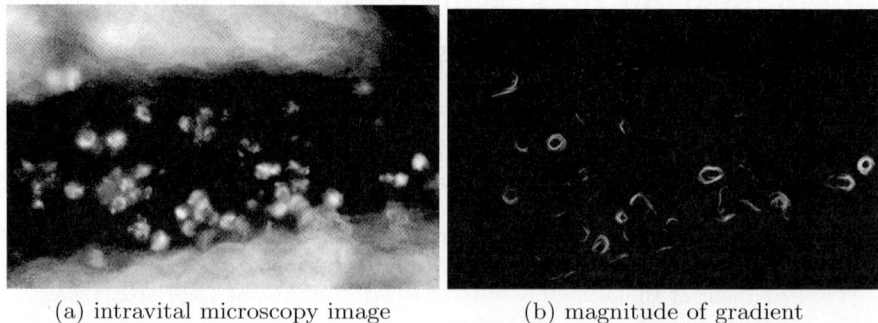

(a) intravital microscopy image (b) magnitude of gradient

Fig. 1. Vessels captured in intravital microscopy. (a) Dark area corresponds to vessels and bright, roughly circular regions inside vessels are white blood cells. Note the high level of clutter due to the traveling, rolling, and stationary cells causing a challenge in automated segmentation as the gradient magnitude is very high near cell (b).

algorithm for the images captured by an intravital microscopy (IVM). The IVM is an *in vivo* imaging method that can capture both vasculature and flowing, rolling and stationary cells inside them. Unlike the retina images, the vessels from IVM can be highly cluttered by cells (Figure 1). These clutters result in high gradient around the boundary of cells (Figure 1) and its gradient vector flow (GVF) of pixels inside vessel to point toward a cell rather than the vessel boundary (Figure 2.b). Simple removal of the static cells using cell detection does not remedy the problem because the replacement pixels also cause an unwanted gradient to form around the detected cell boundaries.

In order to robustly guide segmentation toward the boundary of vessel even in the presence of a high level of cell clutter, we segment vessels with a set of virtual point pairs called "vessel probes" by applying forces including Vessel Vector Flow (VVF) which moves the vessel probes toward the vessel area while Vessel Boundary Vector Flow (VBVF) moves the probes to localize the boundary of vessels. The probes are moved according to Newtonian physics. By incorporating cell detection, the VVF and VBVF forces are computed to minimize the effect of gradient caused by the cells. Once the probes stabilize, they are connected to delineate the vessel boundary (Figure 2.f). Our method can segment vessels even when the cells [1] and vessels [2] are static making the temporal processing ineffective. The vessel probes are randomly initialized thus the method does not require initialization. We tested the method on a set of challenging real *in vivo* images of vessels in liver of mice cluttered with white blood cells and the result is encouraging.

2 Previous Works

A number of vessel segmentation algorithms has been published over the years. Kirbas and Quek [3] provide a thorough survey of the vessel segmentation methods. Majority of the work involve segmentation in retina images. The

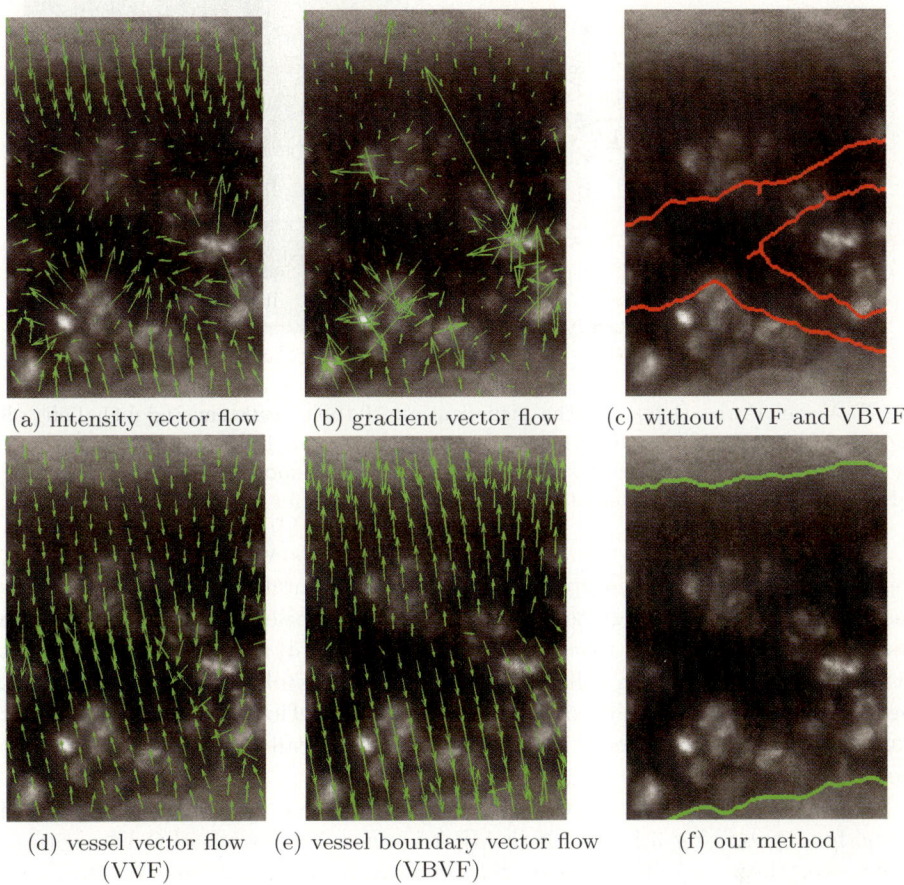

(a) intensity vector flow (b) gradient vector flow (c) without VVF and VBVF

(d) vessel vector flow (VVF) (e) vessel boundary vector flow (VBVF) (f) our method

Fig. 2. Note how the intensity vector flow (which should point toward the higher intensity is corrupted by the presence of cell (a) while the vessel vector flow points toward the center of vessels. The gradient vector flow (b) is not a reliable for pointing toward the vessel boundary. The improvement in VVF (d) and VBVF (e) directing toward the center and boundary of vessel while avoiding the noise induced by cell clutter is achieved. The final segmentation are shown in (c) and (f) and demonstrates that our method can reliably segment vessels even with a presence of cells.

segmentation in presence of clutter and pathological diseases can be problematic. Shu et al. [4] segments retina vessels in disease conditions by discarding centerlines with gradient vector fields that were inconsistent with vessels. In our work, the clutter is *inside* vessels and frequently *touching the vessel boundary* causing noise in gradient vector flow along vessel boundaries (Figure 1).

Intravital microscopy (IVM) can capture both vessels and cells resulting in new challenges. An active contour based method was used to segment the boundary of the one large blood vessel of a cremaster muscle in a video sequence [2]. A sequential frame difference forms the initialization of the snake. A multi-scale

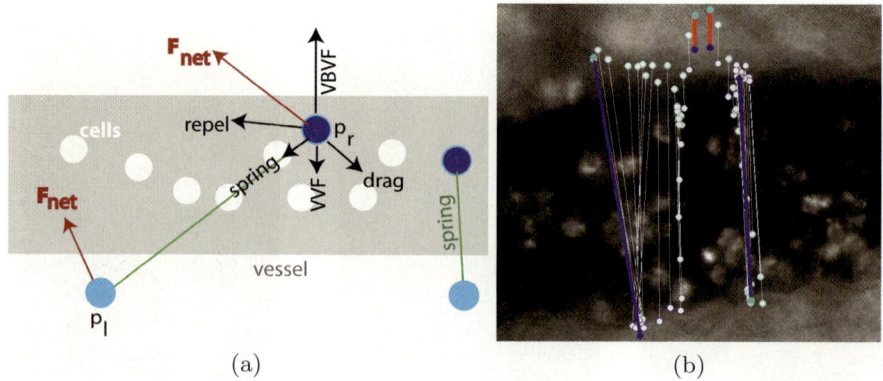

Fig. 3. Vessel Probe (left) and the visualization of their movement (right). Left: all forces are shown in black while the net force is draw in red. All forces are shown only for the left probe. Right: the iterations of the probes are shown. Probes are shown in red for initial orientation, blue at convergence, and white for all iterations in between.

approach was used to speed up the snake optimization, and gradient vector flow was used as external energy to be less resistant to noise. Also, multiple ribbon snakes [5] were used by [1] to segment the vasculature of the liver in IVM images after removing the moving cells using temporal median filtering. In our images, the vessel movement is minimal and a number of stationary cells is significant making the frame differencing ineffective for vessel localization initialization nor the removal of cells.

The 3-D vessel crawler by McIntosh and Hamarneh [6] uses a physics based model for segmenting 3-D vessels in MRA images. Points connected by springs crawl along the vessel. The crawler detects when it reaches a vessel junction and then spawns a new vessel crawler toward one of the uncrawled paths. Again, cells were not present in the vessels of images that were segmented.

3 Method

3.1 Vessel Probe

A vessel probe (p) is constructed by two virtual points, p_l and p_r, with an identical mass of m_p (Figure 3.a). The probes are moved so that center of p is inside vessel and p_l and p_r converges at the boundary of vessel. They are connected by a spring with a spring constant of K_s and the equilibrium length L which is the length of the spring at which the spring force is zero.

Initially, the virtual points of vessel probes are randomly positioned at s_l and s_r. As the same equation applies to the motion of either points, we will describe for one point and let s be a location of a virtual point. The point's velocity v and acceleration a are initialized to be zero vectors. Each virtual point responds to the net force (F_{net}) according to the Newtonian Physics.

Table 1. Forces applied on Vessel Probes. F_{net} is the sum of all forces for each virtual point.

Name	Task
Vessel Vector Flow (VVF)	moves the probe toward the vessel
Vessel Boundary Vector Flow (VBVF)	moves the virtual points to localize on the vessel boundary
Spring	keeps two virtual points connected within a reasonable length
Repel	spreads the probes to cover the vessel with a smaller number of probes
Drag	slows down the probes to converge at vessel

F_{net} is a sum of all forces applied on the probe. Forces are summarized on Table 1. Each virtual point is moved responding to F_{net} exerted for T seconds. To simplify the implementation, we make two assumptions. First, the change in the forces during T seconds due to the movement of points is not significant. Second, the direction and magnitude of force within a pixel is constant. We move each probe for T seconds by breaking T into smaller δt where F_{net} is constant (within a pixel). Note that position is calculated at a sub-pixel accuracy and the "pixel" refers to the area unit rather than a distance. The acceleration due to the force is $a_{net} = F_{net}/m_p$. At constant acceleration, the velocity after δt would be $v' = v + a_{net}\delta t$. We compute the δt using a quadratic formula, $\delta t = \frac{-2v \pm \sqrt{(2v)^2 + 8a(\hat{s}-s)}}{2a}$ where $\hat{s}$ is the intersection between the pixel boundary of s and the vector from s moved along v. The probe is moved to $s' = s + \frac{1}{2}(v'+v)\delta t$. Each probe is moved until the aggregate of δt is T. A vessel probe convergence is found when the movement is minimal.

3.2 Vessel Vector Flow Force

The cells inside vessels cause significant noise in both the gradient magnitude (Figure 1.b) and the gradient vector flow (Figure 2.b). Note that the image gradient around cell boundary is significant and often stronger rather than around vessel. Even after a median filtering (with a kernel size of 15x15), the gradient magnitude around a vessel is still relatively weak. Most of the gradient vector flow [7] points toward cells rather than a vessel boundary which will make the segmentation based on gradient vector flow difficult. We propose Vessel Vector Flow (VVF) force that will robustly attract the center of vessel probes to the center of vessel while avoiding the distraction caused by cells cluttering vessel (Figure 1).

First, we detect cells by classifying each pixel as either cell or non-cell based on the radial mean. For each pixel, we compute the means of intensity of pixels within radius ranges of [0, 7] pixels (μ_1), [8, 13] pixels (μ_2) and [13, 21] pixels (μ_3). μ_1, μ_2, and μ_3 are normalized so that their sum = 1. A pixel is classified as a cell when $\mu_1 > T_r$.

Second, we compute the direction of the vessel vector flow (q_{dir}) as a vector that will guide toward the center of vessel while avoiding the clutters caused by cells. Note that we are using the term "vector flow" as finding the vector of flow toward the higher value of a function similar to the method that computes the vector flow of *gradient* [7]. Given f to be the intensity of an image, we create an inverse of an image g so that the flow direction will guide toward a vessel area which is often darker than tissue. Then we compute the vector flow of g while minimizing the effect of cells by setting $\nabla g(x,y) = 0$ for the locations at (x,y) that has been classified as a cell pixel. To avoid the gradient near the boundary of cell, $\nabla g(x,y)$ for the locations within 5 pixels of cell pixels are also assigned the values of zero. The vector flow $q_{dir} = (u(x,y), v(x,y))$ is that minimizes

$$\xi = \int\int \mu(u_x^2 + u_y^2 + v_x^2 + v_y^2) + |\nabla g|^2 |q_{dir} - \nabla g|^2 \, dxdy$$

The normalized vector of q_{dir} ($\hat{q}_{dir}$) is used as the direction component of the VVF force (Figure 2.d). Note that they mostly point toward the center of vessel right through the cells.

Third, we compute the magnitude of VVF. We use the gravitational model to formulate the forces that attracts the probes toward the vessel while repelling from each other. In that model, the magnitude of force should be at the maximum near the convergence. The magnitude of q_{dir} is highest near the vessel boundary. We noted that the q_{dir} often converges near the center of vessels. The convergence index [8] measures the level of convergences of vectors within a window. We computed $C_{q_{dir}}$, the convergence of q_{dir}. Then, the magnitude of vector flow of $C_{q_{dir}}$ is computed as the magnitude of VVF force. The VVF force is computed by combining the magnitude and direction ($\hat{q}_{dir}$). The VVF force is visualized in Figure 2.d. Note that magnitude is generally higher near vessel center.

3.3 Vessel Boundary Vector Flow Force

The VVF attracts probes toward the vessel. We now derive Vessel *Boundary* Vector Flow (VBVF) force which will attract the points of vessel probes to the vessel boundaries. Because of the strong gradient around cell boundaries, the GVF inside a vessel often points toward cell boundaries rather than vessel boundaries (Figure 2.b). We noted the magnitude of q_{dir} is stronger near vessel boundaries. So, the vector flow of $||q_{dir}||$ is computed as the Vessel Boundary Vector Flow (**b**) (Figure 2.e).

3.4 Other Forces: Spring, Repel and Drag

First, the spring force is used to keep points on the vessel probe from drifting too far from each other when the gradient is weak. The spring force is computed as $F_s = K_s d_s$ where d_s is the displacement vector from a virtual point to the equilibrium location of spring. Second, to cover the vessel boundary with a minimum number of points, a repel force is designed to push the vessel probes from each other based on distance and orientation. The repel force exerted by probe p^i to p^j at distance d is $\frac{m_p \cdot m_p}{d^2} \boldsymbol{g}$ where $\boldsymbol{g}$ is a normalized vector from p^i to p^j. The repel force on p^i is computed as the sum of forces from all other probes. Third, for the vessel probes to converge, a drag force is applied to each point on the vessel probe. It is computed as $-K_d \boldsymbol{v}$ where K_d is the coefficient of drag.

3.5 Post Processing for Forming Continuous Vessel Boundary

After the vessel probes have converged, they are connected to form boundaries of the vessel. The probes' virtual points are connected if their orientation is nearly parallel and they are within a small distance. Then the locations along connection is fine-tuned to the greatest magnitude of Vessel Boundary Vector Flow within a small window.

4 Results

4.1 Dataset

Rats for all experimental groups were surgically prepared for intravital microscopy imaging as described in [9]. The liver is exposed and setup on an inverted fluorescence Olympus microscope. Images were captured by a DAGE-MTI SIT 66 camera at a rate of 30 frames per sec. The white blood cells were visualized using rhodamine.

4.2 Evaluation

The algorithm was tested on five real images of vessels with cell clutters. The results with and without VVF and VBVF are compared (Figure 4). For the cases without those forces, we have used intensity vector flow and GVF instead. First, the segmentation is closer to the vessel boundary and are less effected by the cells. In image 4, the gradient of the bottom left side of is just too weak.

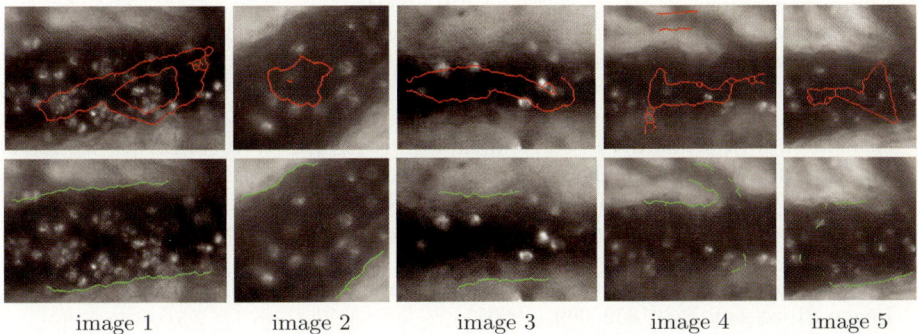

image 1   image 2   image 3   image 4   image 5

Fig. 4. Segmentation results on five real images . Top row includes results without using VVF or VBVF (using intensity vector flow and GVF instead) and the bottom row is our final results.

To quantitatively assess the performance, the ground truth of the vessel boundary of those images was prepared by a biology technician. Note that the boundary is often very weak on gradient making the absolute pixel-level accurate ground truthing difficult. For each vessel boundary pixel segmented by the algorithm, the distance to the nearest vessel boundary marked in ground truth is computed. The root mean squared error (RMSE) of the distance for all machine segmented points are computed. On average, the RMSE of our method was 55% less than the method without VVF and VBVF.

5 Conclusion

We developed a vessel segmentation algorithm that is able to segment boundaries of vessels with a significant level of clutter due to presence of cells. These cells often divert the gradient vector flow toward the cells rather than the vessel boundary. Also, a number of cells are static, making the temporal differencing ineffective. We computed two forces, Vessel Vector Flow (VVF) and Vessel Boundary Vector Flow (VBVF), that guided the vessel probes and minimized the distraction caused by cells. A set of vessel probes were randomly deployed and moved according to the net of forces. The random deployment of probes eliminated the need for initialization. Comparing against the ground truth on five real *in vivo* images, the RMSE was 55% lower with addition of VVF and VBVF.

References

1. Schmugge, S., Kamoun, W., Villalobos, J., Clemens, M., Shin, M.: Segmentation of vasculature for intravital microscopy using bridging vessel snake. In: 3rd IEEE International Symposium on Biomedical Imaging: From Nano to Macro, pp. 177–180 (April 2006)
2. Tang, J., Acton, S.T.: Vessel boundary tracking for intravital microscopy via multiscale gradient vector flow snakes. IEEE Transactions on Biomedical Engineering 51(2), 316–324 (2004)
3. Kirbas, C., Quek, F.: A review of vessel extraction techniques and algorithms. ACM Computing Surveys (CSUR) 36(2), 81–121 (2004)
4. Shu, B., Lam, Y., Yan, H.: A novel vessel segmentation algorithm for pathological retina images based on the divergence of vector fields. IEEE Transactions on Medical Imaging 27(2), 237–246 (2008)
5. Mayer, H., Laptev, I., Baumgartner, A.: Multi-scale and snakes for automatic road extraction. In: Burkhardt, H.-J., Neumann, B. (eds.) ECCV 1998. LNCS, vol. 1406, pp. 720–734. Springer, Heidelberg (1998)
6. McIntosh, C., Hamarneh, G.: Vessel crawlers: 3d physically-based deformable organisms for vasculature segmentation and analysis. In: CVPR, vol. 1, pp. 1084–1091. IEEE, Los Alamitos (2006)
7. Xu, C., Prince, J.: Snakes, shapes, and gradient vector flow. IEEE Transactions on Image Processing 7(3), 359–369 (1998)
8. Kobatake, H., Hashimoto, S.: Convergence index filter for vector fields. IEEE Transactions on Image Processing 8(8), 1029–1038 (1999)
9. Clemens, M., Zhang, J.: Regulation of sinusoidal perfusion: in vivo methodology and control by endothelins. Seminars in Liver Disease 19(4), 383–396 (1999)

Streamline Flows for White Matter Fibre Pathway Segmentation in Diffusion MRI

Peter Savadjiev[1], Jennifer S.W. Campbell[1,2], G. Bruce Pike[2], and Kaleem Siddiqi[1]

McGill University, Montréal, QC, Canada
[1] School of Computer Science & Centre For Intelligent Machines
[2] McConnell Brain Imaging Centre, Montréal Neurological Institute

Abstract. We introduce a fibre tract segmentation algorithm based on the geometric coherence of fibre orientations as indicated by a *streamline flow* model. The inference of local flow approximations motivates a pairwise consistency measure between fibre ODF maxima. We use this measure in a recursive algorithm to cluster consistent ODF maxima, leading to the segmentation of white matter pathways. The method requires minimal seeding compared to streamline tractography-based methods, and allows multiple tracts to pass through the same voxels. We illustrate the approach with a segmentation of the corpus callosum and one of the cortico-spinal tract, with each example seeded at a single voxel.

1 Introduction and Related Work

The development of algorithms for automatic white matter fibre tract segmentation in diffusion MRI is of significant interest in the community. A number of methods approach this problem by clustering individual diffusion tensors (DTs) or diffusion orientation distribution functions (ODFs), relying on Euclidean or Riemannian metrics between their shapes, e.g. [8,15,2,1] for DT data and [14,9,7] for high angular resolution diffusion (HARD) data. Whether implemented using surface evolution techniques [8,7], spectral clustering [14,15], or various Markov field models [9,2,1], these methods assume that along a white matter tract the diffusion ODFs have locally similar shape statistics. It is also often (though not always) assumed that only a single tract passes through any particular location or voxel. These two assumptions can be questioned when: 1) white matter fibre tracts cross, merge or split, 2) an individual ODF reflects multiple fibre populations, 3) partial volume effects occur along a tract, causing the tensor or ODF shape to change drastically and 4) neighbouring but distinct tract systems have regions with ODFs whose shape statistics are very similar.

A second class of automatic segmentation algorithms uses individual streamlines, obtained by a fibre tractography algorithm, followed by a clustering process. For example, Corouge *et al.* [3] define metrics between individual streamlines, such as the closest point distance, the mean distance, or the Hausdorff distance. Ding *et al.* [6] propose similar metrics. The Hausdorff distance is also used in [11], within a spectral clustering framework. All these approaches depend

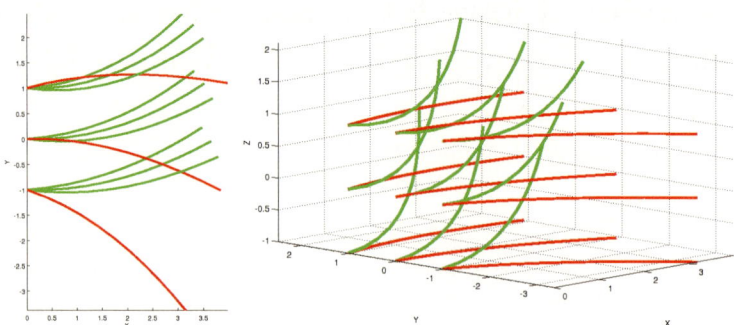

Fig. 1. Two examples of 3D streamline flows generated using equations (2) and (3), each sampled with nine streamlines. Left: An orthographic projection on the XY plane. Right: A 3D view of the flows. The flow parameters are as follows: Green: $K_T = 0.2$, $K_N = 0$, $K_B = -0.1$, $\alpha = 1.0$. Red: $K_T = -0.2$, $K_N = 0.3$, $K_B = 0$, $\alpha = 0$.

on the actual tractography algorithm used, and further, they do not explicitly utilize the differential geometry of the 3D space curves that underlie the white matter fibres.

With these limitations in mind, in this paper we model fibre tracts as streamline flows, i.e., sets of dense, approximately parallel curves (locally). Using the differential geometry of these patterns, introduced in [13], and an associated generalized helicoid model, we develop a fibre tract segmentation algorithm which is based on geometrical coherence rather than on ODF shape statistics. The approach takes as its input a volume of fibre ODF data [5]. For each fibre ODF maximum at each voxel, a best-fit local model for the underlying streamline flow is then found. Using the inferred streamline flow geometries, a pairwise consistency measure is defined between ODF maxima, leading to a recursive algorithm for clustering them in order to segment white matter fibre tracts. Because the method captures the geometry not only in the tangential (streamline) direction, but also along the normal and bi-normal directions, it requires minimal seeding when compared with methods that rely on streamline tractography (our experiments have used a single voxel seed). It also provides, as a bi-product, local curvature measures of the tracts which can be used to facilitate further analysis.

2 3D Streamline Flow Model

The streamline flow model we adopt is based on the idea of attaching a frame field to a single streamline, and then examining its "co-variation" in three basis directions [13]. This leads to three curvature functions:

$$\begin{aligned}\|\kappa_T\| &= \|\nabla_{E_T} E_T\| = \|\cos\phi \, d\theta(E_T) E_N + d\phi(E_T) E_B\|,\\ \|\kappa_N\| &= \|\nabla_{E_N} E_T\| = \|\cos\phi \, d\theta(E_N) E_N + d\phi(E_N) E_B\|,\\ \|\kappa_B\| &= \|\nabla_{E_B} E_T\| = \|\cos\phi \, d\theta(E_B) E_N + d\phi(E_B) E_B\|,\end{aligned} \qquad (1)$$

where (E_T, E_N, E_B) is the Frame Field in spherical coordinates and θ and ϕ describe the orientations of vector E_T with respect to a fixed coordinate system. A generalized helicoid model for θ, motivated by minimal surface theory, is (see [13])

$$\theta(x, y, z) = \tan^{-1}\left(\frac{K_T x + K_N y}{1 + K_N x - K_T y}\right) + K_B z. \tag{2}$$

An extended flow model which we adopt in this paper is given by (2), together with the relation

$$\phi(x, y, z) = \alpha \theta(x, y, z). \tag{3}$$

Proposition 1. *With $\phi(x, y, z) = \alpha\theta(x, y, z)$, where α is a constant, the scalar parameters K_T, K_N, K_B of the generalized helicoid model (2) and the curvatures (1) of a unique 3D streamline flow are related by:*

$$\kappa_T(0, 0, 0) = \sqrt{1 + \alpha^2}|K_T|$$
$$\kappa_N(0, 0, 0) = \sqrt{1 + \alpha^2}|K_N|$$
$$\kappa_B(0, 0, 0) = \sqrt{1 + \alpha^2}|K_B|. \tag{4}$$

Proof. Eq. (4) can be obtained by computing the gradient of $\theta(x, y, z)$ in (2) and noting that at the origin, $\nabla\theta(0, 0, 0) = (K_T, K_N, K_B)$. Similarly, given that $\phi(x, y, z) = \alpha\theta(x, y, z)$, $\nabla\phi(0, 0, 0) = (\alpha K_T, \alpha K_N, \alpha K_B)$. Since $\phi(0, 0, 0) = \theta(0, 0, 0) = 0$, this aligns the (E_T, E_N, E_B) frame at the origin with the global (x, y, z) coordinate system, so that $E_T = (1, 0, 0)$, $E_N = (0, 1, 0)$ and $E_B = (0, 0, 1)$. Eq. (4) follows from substituting the values for $E_T, E_N, E_B, \nabla\theta$ and $\nabla\phi$ into the curvature functions of (1).

3 Clustering and Fibre Segmentation through Streamline Flow Consistency

We now develop an algorithm to cluster local fibre orientations to segment fibre tracts. We take as input a dense volume of fibre ODFs extracted from the diffusion signal through a technique such as spherical deconvolution [5]. Each of these fibre ODFs is sampled along a fixed set of predefined unit-length orientations λ, and the ODF maxima are extracted, as described in Section 4.1.

3.1 Co-helicoidity

We use the generalized helicoid model as an osculating object to provide a local approximation for the streamline flow geometry in a neighborhood around each ODF maximum. We define the following consistency measure C between orientation λ at location i and orientation λ' at location j:

$$C_{\lambda, i, \lambda', j} = \frac{|\langle H_{\lambda, i}(j), (\lambda', j)\rangle| + |\langle H_{\lambda', j}(i), (\lambda, i)\rangle|}{2}. \tag{5}$$

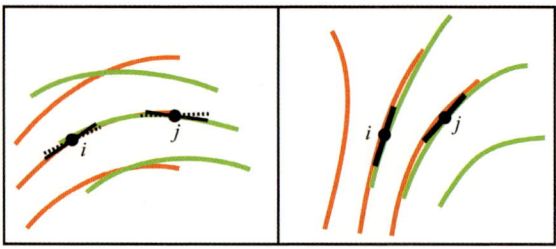

Fig. 2. Two schematic illustrations of the concept of helicoid-based consistency. Left: the orientation at location i (solid black line) is transported to location j along its inferred best-fit helicoid (orange). Similarly, the orientation at location j is transported along its helicoid (green) to location i. The transported orientations (dashed black lines) are defined as the tangents to the helicoid at the location of transport. The average angular difference between the transported and local orientations is computed as a measure of consistency. Right: a second transport example, one for which the two helicoids align perfectly at locations i and j.

Here $|.|$ denotes absolute value, and $\langle .,. \rangle$ denotes the standard dot product in $\mathbb{R}^3$. $H_{\lambda,i}(j)$ denotes the (unit) vector that results from evaluating at location j the generalized helicoid osculating object associated to orientation λ at location i. Finally, (λ, i) denotes orientation λ at location i (which is a vector of (x, y, z) coordinates).

Thus, measuring consistency between two orientations defined at two distinct locations involves transporting each orientation in turn along its osculating generalized helicoid to the location of the other orientation, evaluating the resulting angular difference, and then taking the average. Fig. 2 illustrates this concept of transport schematically. We choose this measure of consistency for its simplicity and symmetry. It is a natural extension of the ideas of co-circularity for 2D planar curves and co-helicity for 3D space curves (see [13] for a review).

3.2 ODF Clustering and Fibre Tract Segmentation

We approach the problem of fibre tract segmentation by first inferring the best-fit helicoidal osculating object for each ODF maximum at each location, as described in [13]. This operation needs to be carried out only once, offline. Then, starting at a seed voxel selected manually, for each ODF maximum at that voxel, its pairwise compatibility is computed according to (5) with all ODF maxima located within a small neighborhood centered at that voxel (we use a neighbourhood of $3 \times 3 \times 3$ voxels). If the compatibility with a maximum in the neighborhood is higher than a threshold, this maximum is added to the cluster, and the algorithm is recursively called, starting at the newly added maximum. As maxima are added to the cluster, they are marked as 'visited'. Thus, recursion stops when there are no remaining maxima that are both compatible and unmarked.

As illustrated in Fig. 2, clustering may proceed along flow streamlines as well as across them. Situations in which distinct tract systems 'kiss' each other and form a bottleneck configuration may cause the clustering to progress from one tract into the other and then backtrack along the new tract system. To prevent this, our implementation keeps track of the direction in which clustering of maxima proceeds, starting from the seed voxel, and disallows reversals in that direction. This is achieved by treating ODF maxima as vectors (which have direction), rather than simply as orientations. When a new maximum is added to the cluster, it is given a direction consistent with the direction of cluster expansion. Then, when recursion is called starting at that maximum, it proceeds only in directions consistent with the maximum direction.

4 Experiments and Results

4.1 Methods

MRI data were acquired for one healthy subject on a Siemens 3T Trio MR scanner (Siemens Medical Systems, Erlangen, Germany) using an 8-channel phased-array head coil. Diffusion encoding was achieved using a single-shot spin-echo echo planar sequence with twice-refocused balanced diffusion encoding gradients. A dataset designed for high angular resolution reconstruction was acquired with $N = 99$ diffusion encoding directions with $b = 3000$ s/mm^2, 10 T2 weighted images with $b = 0$ s/mm^2, 2 mm isotropic voxel size, 63 slices, TE = 121 ms, TR = 11.1 s, and GRAPPA parallel reconstruction with an acceleration factor of 2. The fibre ODF data was estimated using spherical deconvolution as described in [5], with a linear and regularized method performed on the diffusion ODF estimated from q-ball reconstruction. An $L = 4$ spherical harmonic basis was used, with regularization parameter $\lambda = 0.006$ [4]. The deconvolution kernel was estimated directly from the dataset being used. The maxima of the fibre ODFs, which are assumed to correspond to curve tangents, were then extracted and used in the clustering algorithm described in Section 3.2. A threshold value of 9° (chosen empirically) was used to determine whether two orientations are consistent according to (5). Voxels where the fractional anisotropy (FA) was less than 0.1 or the mean diffusivity was greater than 10^{-6} mm^2/ms were excluded.

We compare our segmentation algorithm with conventional streamline fibre tractography with a user-defined, extensive start region of interest (ROI). To do so, a streamline tractography approach robust to complex sub-voxel geometries [12] was used. The ROI was hand drawn on the entire length of the corpus callosum (CC) in the mid sagittal region of the brain. Streamlines were initiated in all voxels of the brain and those that passed through the ROI were retained. Tracking was stopped if the fractional anisotropy (FA) was less than 0.1 or the mean diffusivity was greater than 10^{-6} mm^2/ms. Tracking was seeded on a 3 × 3 × 3 grid in each start voxel.

4.2 Results

We present segmentation results for the CC and the cortico-spinal tract (CST). The algorithm of Section 3.2 was initiated in a voxel located in the CC near the mid-sagittal slice, as well as in a voxel located in the CST. For each starting voxel, a surface encompassing all voxels reached by our recursive segmentation algorithm is shown in Fig. 3. These results are anatomically plausible and demonstrate the recovery of the region common to both tract systems.

To illustrate the sense of a 3D streamline flow, in Fig. 4 we visualize the ODF maxima that are clustered together in a region where the recovered tracts overlap. Again, the recovered flows are anatomically plausible.

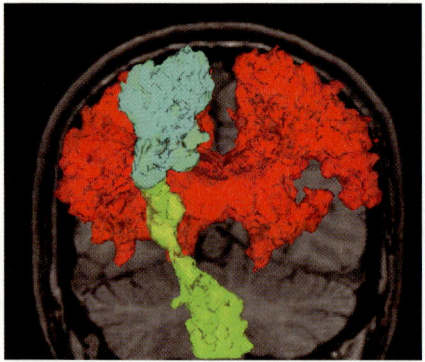

Fig. 3. A segmentation of the corpus callosum (red) and the cortico-spinal tract (green), in a coronal view (seen from the front). The blue region indicates voxels that belong to both of the segmented tracts. The anatomical slice in the background is shown to delineate the head; the recovered clusters are 3D objects and are not confined to one particular slice.

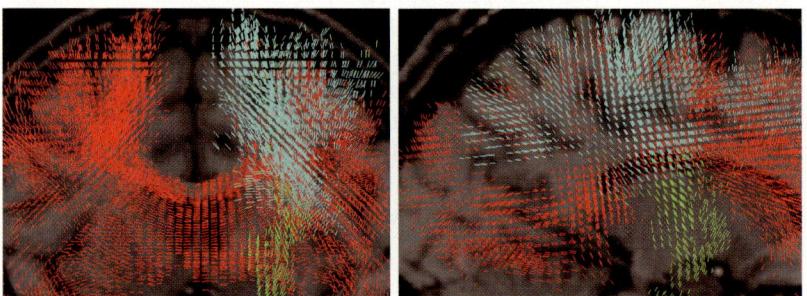

Fig. 4. A zoom-in on the region of cluster overlap as recovered by our algorithm. Left: a coronal projection (seen from behind). Right: a sagittal projection. Both figures visualize the clustered ODF maxima that belong to the corpus callosum (red), the cortico-spinal tract (green), and to *both* clusters (blue).

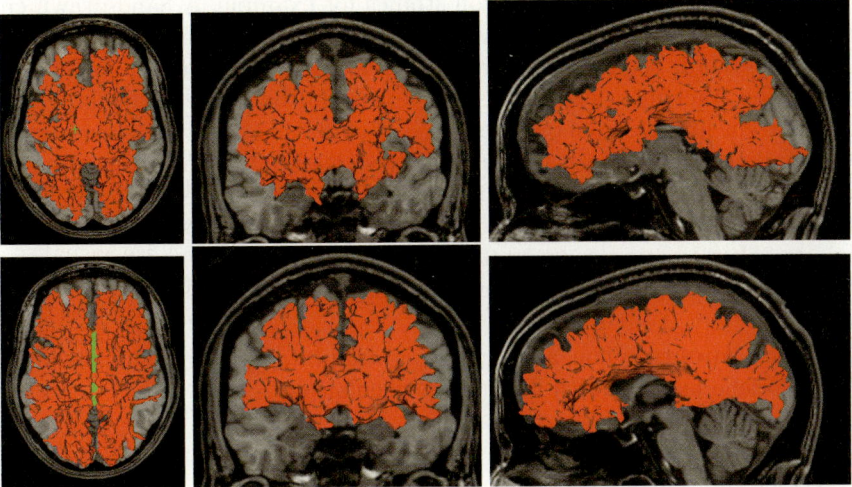

Fig. 5. Top row: corpus callosum segmentation using our method, starting at a seed voxel denoted with a crosshair (left). Bottom row: corpus callosum recovery through streamline tractography initiated in a hand-drawn region (green, left panel).

Fig. 5 compares our segmentation method with conventional streamline tractography on the CC, run as described in Section 4.1. The results are similar in that both methods recover the corona radiata and several lateral projections. However, the streamline tractography method required a hand-drawn initialization region that spans the entire CC (green ROI), whereas our segmentation method is initialized at a single voxel (marked by the green crosshair).

5 Conclusion

This article develops a fibre clustering approach based on geometric coherence with respect to a local 3D streamline flow model. The method allows ODF maxima to be clustered not only along individual streamlines, but also across them. For example, when clustering starts with a seed located in the centre of the CC, voxels near the cortex can be reached even if the direct path that connects them to the seed may not be resolvable due to partial volume effects at the crossing with the CST or the superior longitudinal fasciculus. Although the examples in this paper apply the method to fibre ODF data, it is applicable to any type of DT or HARD data. Unlike some surface evolution-based segmentation methods, multiple tracts per location can be handled.

Future work will focus on parameter selection, which is currently done empirically, as well as on a more rigorous validation, done for example through quantitative experiments on a well localized tract. It will also examine whether the segmentation results obtained from a single seed voxel are accurate enough to reduce the need for detailed protocols for the hand-drawing of ROIs [10], which would be an advantage in population studies for example. A hand-drawn cross-sectional ROI through a tract may be difficult to reproduce and may intersect nearby tracts. Our requirement for a single voxel seed located in a well-defined region of the tract may lead to less user error and better reproducibility. However, a current limitation of our method is that the propagation of support from one streamline to nearby parallel ones can also lead to false positives. We expect that the use of anatomical masks will greatly help to eliminate these. Finally, our co-helicoidity consistency measure can be incorporated as a geometric affinity metric in other existing segmentation frameworks, such as spectral clustering, and can also be used to study fibre tract shape statistics.

Acknowledgments. The authors are grateful to Maxime Descoteaux and Rachid Deriche for help with fibre ODF calculation.

References

1. Awate, S.P., Zhang, H., Gee, J.C.: A fuzzy, nonparametic segmentation framework for DTI and MRI analysis: with applications to DTI-tract extraction. IEEE Trans. Medical Imaging 26(11), 1525–1536 (2007)
2. Barmpoutis, A., Vemuri, B.C., Shepherd, T.M., Forder, J.R.: Tensor splines for interpolation and approximation of DT-MRI with applications to segmentation of isolated rat hippocampi. IEEE Trans. Medical Imaging 26(11), 1537–1546 (2007)
3. Corouge, I., Gouttard, S., Gerig, G.: Towards a shape model of white matter fiber bundles using diffusion tensor MRI. In: Proc. Intl. Symposium on Biomedical Imaging (ISBI) 2004, vol. 1, pp. 344–347 (2004)
4. Descoteaux, M., Angelino, E., Fitzgibbons, S., Deriche, R.: Regularized, fast, and robust analytical Q-Ball imaging. Magn. Res. in Medicine 58(3), 497–510 (2007)
5. Descoteaux, M., Deriche, R., Anwander, A.: Deterministic and probabilistic Q-Ball tractography: from diffusion to sharp fiber distributions. Technical Report 6273, INRIA Sophia Antipolis (July 2007)
6. Ding, Z., Gore, J.C., Anderson, A.W.: Classification and quantification of neuronal fiber pathways using diffusion tensor MRI. Magn. Res. in Medicine 49, 716–721 (2003)
7. Jonasson, L., Bresson, X., Thiran, J.-P., Wedeen, V.J., Hagmann, P.: Representing diffusion MRI in 5-D simplifies regularization and segmentation of white matter tracts. IEEE Trans. Medical Imaging 26(11), 1547–1554 (2007)
8. Lenglet, C., Rousson, M., Deriche, R.: DTI segmentation by statistical surface evolution. IEEE Trans. Medical Imaging 25(6), 685–700 (2006)
9. McGraw, T., Vemuri, B.C., Yezierski, R., Mareci, T.: Segmentation of high angular resolution diffusion MRI modeled as a field of von Mises-Fisher mixtures. In: Leonardis, A., Bischof, H., Pinz, A. (eds.) ECCV 2006. LNCS, vol. 3953, pp. 463–475. Springer, Heidelberg (2006)
10. Mori, S., Wakana, S., Nagae-Poetscher, L.M., van Zijl, P.C.M.: MRI Atlas of Human White Matter. Elsevier, Amsterdam (2005)
11. O'Donnell, L., Westin, C.F.: Automatic Tractography Segmentation Using a High-dimensional White Matter Atlas. IEEE Trans. Medical Imaging 26(11), 1562–1575 (2007)

12. Savadjiev, P., Campbell, J.S.W., Descoteaux, M., Deriche, R., Pike, G.B., Siddiqi, K.: Labeling of ambiguous sub-voxel fibre bundle configurations in high angular resolution diffusion MRI. NeuroImage 41(1), 58–68 (2008)
13. Savadjiev, P., Zucker, S.W., Siddiqi, K.: On the differential geometry of 3D flow patterns: Generalized helicoids and diffusion MRI analysis. In: Proc. IEEE Intl. Conf. on Computer Vision (ICCV 2007) (2007)
14. Wassermann, D., Descoteaux, M., Deriche, R.: Diffusion maps clustering for magnetic resonance Q-Ball imaging segmentation. Intl. Journal of Biomedical Imaging (2008); Article ID 526906, doi:10.1155/2008/526906
15. Ziyan, U., Tuch, D., Westin, C.F.: Segmentation of thalamic nuclei from DTI using spectral clustering. In: Larsen, R., Nielsen, M., Sporring, J. (eds.) MICCAI 2006. LNCS, vol. 4191, pp. 807–814. Springer, Heidelberg (2006)

Toward Unsupervised Classification of Calcified Arterial Lesions

G. Brunner, U. Kurkure, D.R. Chittajallu,
R.P. Yalamanchili, and I.A. Kakadiaris

Computational Biomedicine Lab, Depts. of Computer Science, Elec. & Comp.
Engineering, and Biomedical Engineering, Univ. of Houston, Houston, TX, USA
{gbrunner,ukurkure,drchittajallu,rpyalamanchili2,ioannisk}@uh.edu

Abstract. There is growing evidence that calcified arterial deposits play a crucial role in the pathogenesis of cardiovascular disease. This paper investigates the challenging problem of unsupervised calcified lesion classification. We propose an algorithm, *US-CALC* (UnSupervised Calcified Arterial Lesion Classification), that discriminates arterial lesions from non-arterial lesions. The proposed method first mines the characteristics of calcified lesions using a novel optimization criterion and then identifies a subset of lesion features which is optimal for classification. Second, a two stage clustering is deployed to discriminate between arterial and non-arterial lesions. A histogram intersection distance measure is incorporated to determine cluster proximity. The clustering hierarchies are carefully validated and the final clusters are determined by a new intracluster compactness measure. Experimental results indicate an average accuracy of approximately 80% on a database of electron beam CT heart scans.

1 Introduction

The National Heart Lung and Blood Institutes' 2007 disease statistics reported that in 2004, 872,000 deaths or 36% of all deaths in the United States were due to cardiovascular disease. The underlying causes of most heart attacks, and sudden cardiac deaths are inflamed, active, and growing atherosclerotic plaques believed to be vulnerable plaques. Several studies have established that the presence of calcified coronary plaque has a significant predictive value for coronary artery disease in both asymptomatic and symptomatic patients. One of the foci of modern cardiology is to identify high-risk individuals with no prior symptoms, where calcified arterial lesions could be used as biomarkers to assess a patients' risk for a cardiovascular event.

Arterial calcium can be measured by computed tomography (CT). To date, the default method is to assess the total calcium burden by various scores such as Agatston, volume or mass. These scores represent the total amount of calcified plaque in the coronary arteries [1].

The clinical standard for the initial selection of calcified arterial and non-arterial lesions is typically based on a simple threshold of contiguous pixels of at least 1 mm^2 and a CT density of at least 130 Hounsfield units (HU). However, this thresholding has the effect of selecting calcified tissues, bone, metal stents or any other metallic objects that will be included in the data. Then, the calcified areas are manually classified as arterial. From a medical point of view most of these regions are not *real* lesions. However, for ease of terminology, we refer to all selected candidate regions as lesions throughout this paper[1]. The goal of our method is to automatically separate arterial vs. non-arterial lesions.

The gold standard for clinical calcium scoring is to manually identify coronary calcifications from a thresholded scan. Although there is extensive medical literature about manual calcium scoring, surprisingly little work has been conducted from a computer science point of view. To the best of our knowledge there is no published research on unsupervised arterial lesion classification in CT heart scans. However, clustering and other unsupervised classification techniques have been widely applied for related biomedical problems. A hierarchical clustering method was proposed by Carmo et al. [2] to compute topological flow patterns for haemodynamics of the cardiovascular system. Also a hierarchical unsupervised clustering technique was introduced by Tiwari et al. [3] for the identification of cancerous areas in the prostate in Magnetic Resonance Spectroscopy data. A novel clustering method was proposed by O'Donnell and Westin [4] and was deployed to a high dimensional feature space for the purpose of finding white matter fiber correspondences across a population of five brains. However, there are certain design choices for clustering algorithms that are often not sufficiently discussed in the literature such as the initial feature space representation, clustering tendency, and validation of the clustering.

In this paper, we present an unsupervised calcified arterial lesion classification method that mines calcified lesion characteristics to cluster candidate lesions as arterial or as non-arterial. By the term non-arterial, we refer to both calcified lesions which are not located in the coronaries, and artifacts.

Our contributions are the following. First, we present a novel optimization criterion for the determination of an *optimal* lesion feature subset based on: 1) feature correlations, 2) statistical properties, and 3) clustering tendency using Hopkins statistical hypotheses testing. Second, we present a novel two stage integrated clustering schema which identifies the optimal partitioning of the lesion feature space with respect to the cophenetic correlation coefficient and a histogram intersection metric. Third, the final arterial lesion clusters are identified based on a novel intra-cluster compactness measure.

2 Methods

One of the challenges of unsupervised classification is to discriminate between object classes without actually knowing the class labels [5]. *US-CALC* proposes a holistic approach to unsupervised classification of calcified arterial lesions and explores the high dimensional vector space containing a multitude of features. The method automatically derives an *optimal* subset of features with respect

---

[1] We only distinguish between arterial and non-arterial lesions.

to an optimization criterion which is based on clustering tendency, inter-feature correlations and individual feature statistics. *US-CALC* agglomerates a nested hierarchy of calcified arterial lesions and non-lesions using two sets of orthogonal features. The detailed steps of the method are outlined below.

Algorithm. *US-CALC*
1. **Feature Extraction**
    – Compute shape, texture and statistical lesion properties
2. **Cluster Tendency and Dimensionality Reduction**
    – Perform Hopkins statistical testing
    – Compute feature correlation and statistical properties
    – Determine *optimal* feature subset
3. **First Clustering Iteration**
    – Cluster using n-dim. feature vector per lesion
4. **Second Clustering Iteration**
    – Cluster using mean and std of distances between members for every cluster
5. **Identify arterial and non-arterial lesion clusters**

Feature Extraction: Each lesion region represents a blob like structure and can be described by a set of features. Based on the appearance of lesions we decided to use a set of features that captures the shape and, the morphology of the lesions. For instance, the density across a lesion can be captured by the respective HUs. The complete set of features for each lesion consists of: *area, compactness, first and second eigenvector, eccentricity, moment features* [6], *3D coordinates of the pixel with the peak intensity in the region, mean radial lesion length, standard deviation of radial lesion length, min. and max. HU, moments 1-4 of HU values for all lesion pixels, HU range, entropy of HUs* and *15 texture features* [7]. The extracted features describe shape, texture and statistical properties of each lesion.

Clustering Tendency and Dimensionality Reduction: So far, we have created a high dimensional feature space which serves as starting point for the clustering step of *US-CALC*. The quality of the clustering is largely determined by the properties of the feature space. That raises the question: *Is there a natural structure in our feature space at all?* In order to answer that question we investigate the feature space for *clustering tendency* by testing points for randomness. In detail, we carry out an analysis that is based on checking for the *Null Hypothesis* H_0, which is to be rejected for non-random points. As a test of merit *US-CALC* incorporates the Hopkins test [8], as it has been shown to be able to robustly determine the clustering tendency in an unknown dataset [9]. The Hopkins test is based on the nearest neighbor distance, that are the distances between randomly sampled points and points from the actual distribution. In detail, let $\mathbf{X} = \{\mathbf{x}_i, i = 1, ..., N\}$, be the dataset of lesions, where N is the total number of lesions. Further, let $\mathbf{X}_s$ be a subset of $\mathbf{X}$ with M randomly selected vectors from $\mathbf{X}$, defined as $\mathbf{X}_s = \{\mathbf{x}_s, s = 1, ..., M\}, M \approx \frac{N}{10}$. Also, let $\mathbf{X}_r = \{\mathbf{x}_r, r = 1, ..., M\}$, be a set of vectors randomly distributed according to the uniform distribution. Now, we compute d_{rs} as the distance from $\mathbf{x}_r \in \mathbf{X}_r$

to its nearest vector in $\mathbf{x}_s \in \mathbf{X}_s$. Moreover, let d_{sn} be the distance from $\mathbf{x}_s$, to its nearest neighbors. We compute the actual Hopkins statistics with the lth powers of d_{rs} and d_{sn} as: $h = \frac{\sum_{r=1}^{M}(d_{rs})^l}{\sum_{r=1}^{M}(d_{rs})^l + \sum_{s=1}^{M}(d_{sn})^l}$, with $0 \leq h \leq 1$. The closer h is to one the stronger is the clustering tendency. The actual values of h are reported in Sec. 3, and indicate that the lesion feature space exhibits a strong clustering tendency. In addition to clustering tendency, feature redundancy is an important issue for any classification algorithm in general and especially for unsupervised classification methods. To that end, *US-CALC* performs a feature redundancy test resulting in an actual dimensionality reduction of the given lesion feature space. Ideally, we wish for non-overlapping and non-correlated features, as clustering techniques are more likely to generate *correct* results for that kind of vector space [5]. Hence, we introduce a criterion that identifies an *optimal* feature subset with respect to clustering tendency, feature correlation and statistical properties of each feature. Specifically, we compute the clustering tendency separately for each feature using the Hopkins test resulting in $\mathbf{h}_i$, $i = \{1, 2, ..., K\}$, with K as the number of features. Similarly, we compute the skewness and kurtosis for each feature resulting in SK_i and KU_i, for the ith feature, respectively. The choice of skewness and kurtosis is motivated by the assumption that the number of arterial calcified lesions is much smaller than the number of non-arterial lesions - which usually holds. A large skewness and/or kurtosis is an indicator of an asymmetric distribution opposed to Gaussian distributions (zero skewness). Real world datasets often tend to be non-Gaussian. Next, we compute the correlation coefficient between all features CC_{ij}, with i and j each in the range of $\{1, 2, ..., K\}$. Highly correlated features carry redundant information that can be disregarded, since those features do not provide additional discriminative power. The actual optimization criterion is to identify features that exhibit a strong clustering tendency (i.e., h close to one), a low correlation with each other, and possess a large skewness and kurtosis at the same time. Note that many feature selection algorithms are specifically developed for supervised classification tasks. In our case, we work with unlabeled data and the proposed criterion is optimal with respect to the given features and with respect to the assumptions of our proposed clustering algorithm. A detailed analysis of our findings will be addressed in a forthcoming paper. The output of this step is a feature subset $\mathbf{F}$, that reveals a strong clustering tendency while it contains as little as possible redundant information. In the next step, *US-CALC* deploys a clustering algorithm to the optimal feature subset $\mathbf{F}$.

The clustering of the lesions is performed in two steps. *US-CALC* first forms a hierarchy (see Algorithm *US-CALC* Step 3) of the lesion feature space $\mathbf{F}$, and incorporates in the second step an orthogonal set of features that is computed on the fly in step one (see Algorithm *US-CALC* Step 4). These newly computed features can be interpreted as compactness measures of the clusters that were obtained in the first clustering process. Both clustering steps undergo a strict validation check.

First Clustering Iteration: Initially, *US-CALC* partitions the lesion feature space $\mathbf{F}$ into $\{C_n; n = 1, ..., N\}$ clusters, with N denoting the number of lesions, where each cluster contains a vector that describes a single lesion. In the next step, *US-CALC* iteratively merges the initial partitions based on their feature space proximity into larger and larger clusters resulting in a nested hierarchy. This formation of a cluster hierarchy can be seen as the iterative application of a dissimilarity function to a set of possible pairs of clusters of the data matrix $\mathbf{X}$. In detail, we introduce the symmetric square $N \times N$ dissimilarity matrix $\mathcal{D}_b$, with elements d_{ij}^b. Each element represents a measure of distinction between the ith and j^{th} lesion feature vector[2]. The actual dissimilarity measure $\mathcal{H}$ can be interpreted as *closeness* or similarity of two clusters or two groups of lesion clusters. Formally, it can be written as a function: $\mathcal{H} : \mathbf{X} \times \mathbf{X} \to r \in R^+$, with r as the set of real numbers. Hence, we introduce the histogram intersection measure:

$$\mathcal{H}(\mathbf{x}_i, \mathbf{x}_j) = \sum_{i<j} min\{x_i, x_j\}. \tag{1}$$

It determines which two clusters of lesion features are most similar to each other. At this point we want to stress that the lesion feature vector is *n-dim*. Thus, we cluster high dimensional features together rather than the physical coordinates (i.e., spatial location of lesions). Now we have a way to find any two closest clusters of lesion features. In the subsequent step, we identify the next closest cluster and next closest to that. Eventually *US-CALC* obtains a hierarchy of nested clusters, where each contains a different number of lesions. In detail, *US-CALC* performs $N-1$ subsequent clustering steps resulting in a hierarchy of lesion clusters. So far we have obtained a specific partitioning of our feature space. Next, we need to ensure that we actually compute the best possible hierarchy. To that end, *US-CALC* incorporates a validation step. Let us consider the cluster hierarchy $\mathcal{T}_{ij}$ where $\mathbf{x}_i$ and $\mathbf{x}_j$ are for the first time merged in the same cluster. Further, $\mathcal{L}_{ij}$ is the proximity level where the clustering $\mathcal{T}_{ij}$ has been formed. Then, we can compute the distances between the proximity levels resulting in the cophenetic matrix $\mathcal{D}_a$[3]. Now, we can compute the cophenetic correlation coefficient CCC that measures the degree of similarity between the cophenetic matrix $\mathcal{D}_a$ and the dissimilarity matrix $\mathcal{D}_b$ obtained from the lesion features $\mathbf{X}$.

$$CCC = \frac{\frac{1}{O}\sum_{i=1}^{N-1}\sum_{j=i+1}^{N} d_{ij}^a d_{ij}^b - \mu_a \mu_b}{\sqrt{\left(\frac{1}{O}\sum_{i=1}^{N-1}\sum_{j=i+1}^{N}(d_{ij}^a)^2 - (\mu_a)^2\right)\left(\frac{1}{O}\sum_{i=1}^{N-1}\sum_{j=i+1}^{N}(d_{ij}^b)^2 - (\mu_b)^2\right)}}, \tag{2}$$

where O is a normalization factor, and, μ_a and μ_b are the respective means, $\left(\mu_a = \frac{1}{O}\sum_{i=1}^{N-1} d_{ij}^a, \mu_b = \frac{1}{O}\sum_{i=1}^{N-1} d_{ij}^b\right)$. The value of CCC is in the range of $[-1, 1]$, where values closer to 1 indicate a better agreement between the cophenetic and the proximity matrix. Hence, the CCC is a measure of how

---

[2] $\mathcal{D}_b$ fulfills all requirements of a metric.
[3] Note that $\mathcal{D}_a$ is a metric and even the ultrametric inequality holds [10].

accurately the hierarchical tree represents the dissimilarities of the original input data. The actual values of CCC are reported in Sec. 3.

Second Clustering Iteration: The second clustering step is necessary as we want to identify clusters that only contain arterial lesions. The first clustering results in an *a prior* unspecified number of clusters. However, we know that there are typically much fewer arterial lesions than non-arterial ones and we expect two categories of clusters: 1) arterial lesion clusters that are very compact with fewer members and, 2) non-arterial lesion clusters that are more scattered and typically contain many members. At this point the advantage of a two stage clustering becomes apparent. The arterial lesion clusters are more compact within than the non-arterial ones, but are not necessarily *close* to each other in terms of a vector space distance measure. Therefore, a simple one stage clustering that searches for only two clusters in the feature space would fail[4]. In the second clustering step *US-CALC* identifies dense and compact clusters of arterial lesions, given the clustering from step one. Specifically, we compute distance matrices for all members of each cluster. Note that compact clusters tend to have shorter distances between it's members on the average. The clustering procedure in step two is identical to the first one with just one exception. Instead of using the n-dim. feature vector describing each lesion, *US-CALC* only uses the mean and the standard deviation for each distance matrix. Hence the input feature space for the second clustering step is of dimension $2 \times P$, where P is the number of clusters obtained in the first clustering step. The second stage clustering results in a partitioning, too. Note, that the final clustering is also validated with the cophenetic correlation coefficient (Eq.2). In the final step *US-CALC* identifies which clusters contain arterial lesions. The most compact clusters - that are believed to be arterial lesion clusters - consists of *members* that are more *similar* to each other than to any other subgroup; such clusters show a *high mutual similarity*. As measure of compactness (intra-cluster distance) *US-CALC* incorporates:

$$\sigma_j = \left(\frac{1}{n_c} \sum_{\mathbf{x} \in C_j} ||\mathbf{x} - \mathbf{w}_j||^2 \right)^{\frac{1}{2}}, \tag{3}$$

where n_c refers to the number of clusters, and C_j denotes an individual lesion cluster with lesion members $\mathbf{x}$, and, $\mathbf{w}_j$ is the cluster representative for C_j. The final assignment of whether a lesion is arterial or not is based on the final clustering. Members of compact clusters according to Eq. 3 are labeled as arterial lesions and members of non-compact cluster are considered to be non-arterial lesions.

3 Results

Data: The heart scans have been obtained by EBCT imaging with a slice thickness of 3 mm and an x-y pixel spacing of 0.508 - 0.586 mm. We have created

---
[4] We have performed preliminary tests with k-means clustering and one stage clustering.

Table 1. Average parameters computed by *US-CALC* as described in Sec. 2

Dataset	CC	KU	SK	h	CCC Step 3	CCC Step 4
1	0.02	13.42	0.25	0.94	0.86	0.89
2	0.06	2.77	0.41	0.94	0.88	0.89
3	0.02	5.34	0.07	0.93	0.89	0.90
4	0.06	42.47	2.22	0.95	0.90	0.89

Table 2. Performance evaluation of *US-CALC* for the four datasets described in Sec. 3

Subsets	Performance measures per dataset [%]							
	DS-1		DS-2		DS-3		DS-4	
	Accuracy	f	Accuracy	f	Accuracy	f	Accuracy	f
1	80.00	80.14	83.03	84.04	80.11	80.21	80.14	80.13
2	80.00	80.00	82.35	82.05	79.64	79.67	79.73	79.69
3	77.13	77.98	84.17	84.54	75.62	75.20	81.09	81.65
4	76.61	76.97	83.07	82.27	70.55	70.42	80.13	80.06
Average	78.43	78.77	83.16	83.23	76.48	76.38	80.27	80.38

four mutually exclusive sets of arterial and non-arterial lesions. Each dataset contains between 92,296 to 102,600 lesions. In total there were more than 200 patient scans with approximately 20-35 CT image slices per scan. The number of arterial lesions per dataset was more than 1,300 (i.e., the number of non-arterial lesions is much larger). For each of the four datasets we have extracted four random subsets of non-arterial lesions that equal the number of arterial lesions.

Experiments: Upon extraction of the complete feature set, we computed the clustering tendency, the feature correlations, and the statistical properties. The optimal feature subset was determined with the values listed in Table 1. Typical selected features are the skewness and kurtosis of the HUs and the texture features described in Sec. 2. Interestingly, none of the shape features has been selected. This might be due to the similarity of shapes of the arterial and non-arterial lesions. The cophenetic correlation coefficient for **F** was approximately 0.9 for all four datasets. The value actually verifies that the clustering partitions obtained are matching *well* with the original input data. In the first clustering step the typical number of clusters was between 150 and 200.

For the actual validation of our results, manual annotations of arterial lesions were performed. Then, we compared the manually assigned labels with the actual *US-CALC* results for each of the four subsets resulting in 16 datasets. Table 2 summarizes the results for four random subsets for each of the four datasets. We report two widely used performance measures, accuracy and f-measure [11]. For the best subset *US-CALC* exhibited an accuracy of 84%.

In a second experiment, we evaluated *US-CALC* on a per patient basis. To that end, we randomly selected 10 patient scans from the four datasets. This time we included all lesions within a heart bounding box that was semi-automatically computed and visually verified. Note, that the number of arterial lesions is the same as in the first experiment. However, the number of non-arterial lesions is reduced by approximately a factor of 4. The typical total number of lesions per patient is about 300-600 per patient. Averaged over ten randomly selected patient scans *US-CALC* exhibited an accuracy of 83.15% and an f-measure of 81.61%.

4 Discussion and Concluding Remarks

We have presented a novel method for the unsupervised classification of calcified arterial lesions. The method incorporates a novel optimization criterion that reduces the feature space dimensionality and identifies an *optimal* feature subset. *US-CALC* also performs a clustering tendency step before a two stage clustering method is deployed. The second clustering step discriminates between the arterial and non-arterial lesions using a novel intra-cluster compactness measure. The results obtained are promising and provide insight into which features are *more* suitable for the characterization of the arterial lesions. The results show that the texture and statistical properties of lesion intensities were always selected over shape features. Encouraged by the performance of *US-CALC* we plan to further investigate the unsupervised feature selection method.

Acknowledgments. This work was supported in part by the Biomedical Discovery Training Program of the W.M. Keck Center for Interdisciplinary Bioscience Training of the Gulf Coast Consortia (NIH Grant No. 1 T90 DA022885 and 1 R90 DA023418), and in part by NSF Grant IIS-0431144.

References

1. Rumberger, J., Kaufman, L.: A rosetta stone for coronary calcium risk stratification: agatston, volume, and mass scores in 11,490 individuals. AJR Am. J. Roentgenol. 181(3), 743–748 (2003)
2. Carmo, B., Ng, Y., Prügel-Bennett, A., Yang, G.Z.: A data clustering and streamline reduction method for 3D MR flow vector field simplification. In: Barillot, C., Haynor, D.R., Hellier, P. (eds.) MICCAI 2004. LNCS, vol. 3216, pp. 451–458. Springer, Heidelberg (2004)
3. Tiwari, P., Madabhushi, A., Rosen, M.: A hierarchical unsupervised spectral clustering scheme for detection of prostate cancer from magnetic resonance spectroscopy MRS. In: Ayache, N., Ourselin, S., Maeder, A. (eds.) MICCAI 2007, Part II. LNCS, vol. 4792, pp. 278–286. Springer, Heidelberg (2007)
4. O'Donnell, L., Westin, C.F.: White matter tract clustering and correspondence in populations. In: Duncan, J.S., Gerig, G. (eds.) MICCAI 2005. LNCS, vol. 3749, pp. 140–147. Springer, Heidelberg (2005)
5. Jain, A., Duin, R., Mao, J.: Statistical pattern recognition: A review. IEEE Trans. Pattern Anal. Mach. Intell. 22(1), 4–37 (2000)
6. Shen, L., Rangayyan, R., Desautels, J.: Application of shape analysis to mammographic calcifications. IEEE Trans. on Medical Imaging 13(2), 263–274 (1994)

7. Laws, K.: Rapid texture identification. In: Proc. SPIE Conference on Missile Guidance, vol. 238, pp. 376–380 (1980)
8. Hopkins, B.: A new method for determining the type of distribution of plan-individuals. Annals of Botany 18, 213–226 (1954)
9. Peres, M., de Andrade-Netto, L.: A fractal fuzzy approach to clustering tendency analysis. In: Bazzan, A.L.C., Labidi, S. (eds.) SBIA 2004. LNCS (LNAI), vol. 3171, pp. 395–404. Springer, Heidelberg (2004)
10. Hartigan, J.: Representation of similarity matrices by trees. Journal of the American Statistical Association 62, 1140–1158 (1967)
11. Lewis, D., Gale, W.: A sequential algorithm for training text classifiers. In: SIGIR 1994: Proc. 17th ACM SIGIR Conf. on Research and Development in Information Retrieval, pp. 3–12. Springer, New York (1994)

Weights and Topology: A Study of the Effects of Graph Construction on 3D Image Segmentation

Leo Grady and Marie-Pierre Jolly

Siemens Corporate Research — Dept. of Imaging and Visualization
755 College Rd. East, Princeton, NJ 08540

Abstract. Graph-based algorithms have become increasingly popular for medical image segmentation. The fundamental process for each of these algorithms is to use the image content to generate a set of weights for the graph and then set conditions for an optimal partition of the graph with respect to these weights. To date, the heuristics used for generating the weighted graphs from image intensities have largely been ignored, while the primary focus of attention has been on the details of providing the partitioning conditions. In this paper we empirically study the effects of graph connectivity and weighting function on the quality of the segmentation results. To control for algorithm-specific effects, we employ both the Graph Cuts and Random Walker algorithms in our experiments.

1 Introduction

Graph-based algorithms have become well-established tools for general image segmentation problems [1,2,3]. The procedure underlying these algorithms is to: 1) Identify each pixel with a node of the graph, 2) Assign an arbitrary edge set (connectivity), 3) Use the image content to establish a set of weights on the edges, 4) Establish a partitioning criterion that may be optimized to produce a segmentation. Distinctions in the fourth step separate different graph-based segmentation algorithms. Although some attention has been paid to the first step (by associating nodes with presegmented regions), the second and third steps have been almost entirely ignored. Specifically, these steps have typically employed the same set of heuristics. Our goal in this work is to empirically study these common heuristics and determine which, if any, work best on real data.

The seeded user interface employed by many of the graph algorithms supports interactive segmentation for which the segmentation target is chosen by the user and not known *a priori* by the algorithm designer. In these cases, a small number of intensity-based edge weighting functions seem to reoccur throughout very different segmentation algorithms. Since the same weighting functions consistently reappear throughout the graph-based segmentation literature, there appears to be an unwritten assumption that the utility of these weighting functions is *independent* of the specific algorithm in use. This assumption implies that the results of testing different weighting functions with any graph-based segmentation algorithm will support valid conclusions about the weighting function that apply to all graph-based algorithms.

Edge connectivities of the image lattice have been treated similarly in the graph-based literature. In most cases, a 6-connected, 10-connected or 26-connected lattice have been employed, without much discussion of why one choice was made over another. A common feeling in the community seems to be that higher levels of connectivity do, in fact, improve the segmentation results. In rare cases, such as the Graph Cuts algorithm, this assertion is also predicted theoretically [4]. Unfortunately, the additional overhead of more edges usually results in a decrease of performance speed and therefore less-connected edge topologies are sometimes preferred.

In this work, we empirically study the effects of weighting function and graph topology on the performance of segmentation algorithms. We make the simplifying assumption that the performance effects of weighting function and graph topology are independent. Although this assumption is not likely to be strictly true, we are unaware of any claim in the literature that the weighting functions (or even weighting function parameters) should be paired with particular edge topologies. Since the assignments of weightings/topologies reoccur between different graph-based segmentation algorithms, it seems to be assumed that the weighting/topology choice is independent of the specific graph-based algorithm. Although this assumption suggests that the choice of graph-based algorithm should not bias the findings on the utility of a particular weighting function or graph topology, we employ two graph-based algorithms to control for any algorithm-specific bias toward a particular weighting function or edge connectivity. In this work, we have chosen to employ the Graph Cuts [1] and Random Walker segmentation algorithms [2] to perform our tests.

2 Method

We obtained 62 3D medical datasets containing a single segmentation target that were manually segmented by a clinical practitioner. Each volume was also given manually-placed foreground and background seeds by the same clinical practitioner that provided the manual segmentation. The data contained a range of segmentation targets including tumors, lymph nodes, cysts and other lesions. The data was acquired using different Siemens computed tomography (CT) scanners, with different reconstruction kernels and the clinical input (ground truth and seeds) was given by different clinical partners. Therefore, our results should not be biased by the details of a particular acquisition protocol or clinical individual. The datasets we used for segmentation were typically cropped from larger data acquisitions and ranged in size from roughly $40 \times 40 \times 40$ to $128 \times 128 \times 128$. Most of the datasets had different numbers of voxels in each dimension (i.e., they were not cubes) and had a greater spacing between axial slices than within the slice. All of the data acquisitions were axial scans. The XY-plane was chosen to correspond to an axial slice.

Data from CT acquisitions is sometimes considered to be easier to work with, due to the reliability of the output intensities, than other imaging modalities (e.g., ultrasound, magnetic resonance). However, our purpose in this work is not to examine the absolute performance of an algorithm to the segmentation of these targets. Instead, our goal is to compare the relative segmentations obtained through the use of different weighting functions and graph topologies in otherwise controlled conditions. The choice to use this series of CT data was made primarily due to the availability of this data in sufficient quantity to produce meaningful results.

Due to the good segmentation performance and widespread usage, we chose to employ the Graph Cuts algorithm of [1] and the Random Walker segmentation algorithm of [2]. These algorithms are representative examples of the set of modern, graph-based segmentation algorithms that input foreground/background seeds and output a label for each voxel. In order to assign a label to an unseeded voxel, the Graph Cuts algorithm computes the minimum cut separating the foreground from background seeds using a max-flow/min-cut computation [5]. In contrast, the Random Walker algorithm computes the probability that a random walker initiating its walk at each voxel first arrives at a foreground seed before arriving at a background seed. If that probability is larger than 0.5, then the voxel is labeled as foreground (otherwise it is labeled as background). It was shown in [2] that these probabilities could be efficiently computed by solving a sparse system of linear equations. In these experiments, the system of linear equations was solved iteratively using the preconditioned conjugate gradient method with a Jacobi preconditioner and solved to the same level for all examples.

Evaluation of segmentation quality with respect to ground truth is a delicate problem. In this study, we chose to employ the volume overlap and the normalized volume difference [6]. The volume overlap is generally more meaningful as a metric of segmentation quality, since it takes into account the relative position of the ground truth and the computed segmentation.

2.1 Weighting Functions

Weighting functions have been used to map intensity gradients to graph weights since at least as early as the influential work of Perona and Malik on anisotropic diffusion for image smoothing [7], and earlier image reconstruction efforts [8]. When introducing anisotropic diffusion, the authors suggested two functions used to map intensity changes to diffusion constants. These two functions were subsequently studied and determined to reflect differing models of image formation [9]. Since this time, these two functions have been employed in the Normalized Cuts algorithm [10] and subsequent graph-based segmentation algorithms [1,2,3,11]. Although these functions have generally yielded good segmentation performance, we are aware of no attempt to carefully compare the quality of results obtained with these functions. Since natural images are known to contain significant structure (and medical images presumably even more), it is not unreasonable to think that one of these weighting functions better models how to convert the image inputs into graph weights. The weighting functions initially proposed in [7] but subsequently utilized throughout the segmentation literature are

$$\text{Gaussian}: w_{ij} = \frac{1}{\text{dist}(v_i, v_j)} \exp(-\beta(g(v_i) - g(v_j))^2), \quad (1)$$

$$\text{Reciprocal}: w_{ij} = \frac{1}{\text{dist}(v_i, v_j)} \frac{1}{1 + \beta(g(v_i) - g(v_j))^2}, \quad (2)$$

where $g(v_i)$ indicates the image intensity at voxel v_i and β represents a free parameter. The function $\text{dist}(\cdot)$ accounts for differences in spacing and edge length and is computed as the Euclidean distance between voxels, taking into account voxel spacing.

The algorithms under consideration contain additional information in the form of the intensity distribution at the seeds. A natural idea is to make an assumption that the

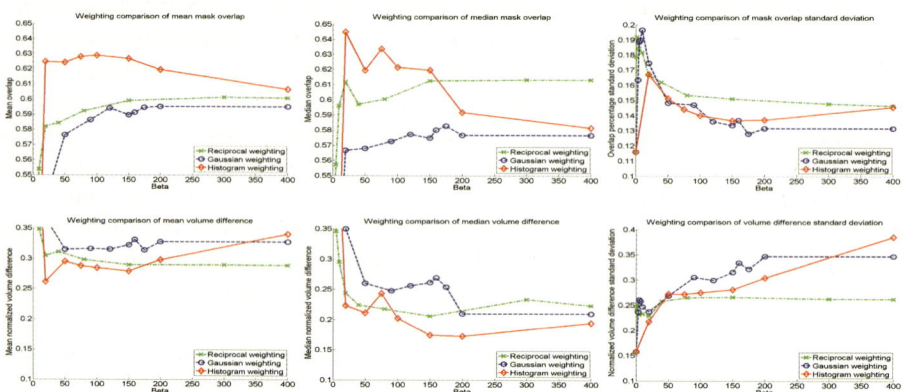

Fig. 1. Graph Cuts: Empirical comparison of weighting functions over a range of β values using the same connectivity. Marker positions indicate measured data points. Blue/dashed line with circles: Gaussian function (1), Green/dash-dot line with crosses: Reciprocal function (2), Red/solid line with diamonds: Histogram-based function (3). Top row: Comparison of mean, median and standard deviation for mask overlap measure. Bottom row: Comparison of mean, median and standard deviation for normalized volume difference.

intensities in the foreground voxels are all drawn from the same intensity distribution. This intensity distribution may be estimated using a Parzen window on the histogram of intensities contained in the foreground seeds. Given this estimation of the foreground intensities, we can look for boundaries of the foreground object with the function

$$\text{Histogram}: w_{ij} = \frac{1}{\text{dist}(v_i, v_j)} \exp(-\beta(H(g(v_i)) - H(g(v_j)))^2), \quad (3)$$

where $H(g(v_i))$ denotes the probability that image intensity $g(v_i)$ at voxel v_i is drawn from the foreground object.

For each weighting function, a range of βs was tested. In order to remove any bias for the absolute intensities of the image, the gradients were normalized by the largest gradient (in each dataset) to lie in the interval $[0, 1]$ before applying the above weighting functions. Due to numerical precision or choice of parameter, it might be possible to assign a weight to be exactly zero. To account for this possibility, a small additive constant (equal to $1e^{-6}$) was added to each weight. All experiments comparing the weighting functions were conducted using a 6-connected lattice.

2.2 Graph Topology

In 3D computer vision, the standard graph connectivities are: 6-connected, 10-connected and 26-connected. The edge set of each connectivity is defined as

$$6 - \text{connected}: \quad E = \{i, j | \ ||C(v_i) - C(v_j)|| \leq 1\}, \quad (4)$$

$$26 - \text{connected}: \quad E = \{i, j | \ ||C(v_i) - C(v_j)|| \leq \sqrt{3}\}, \quad (5)$$

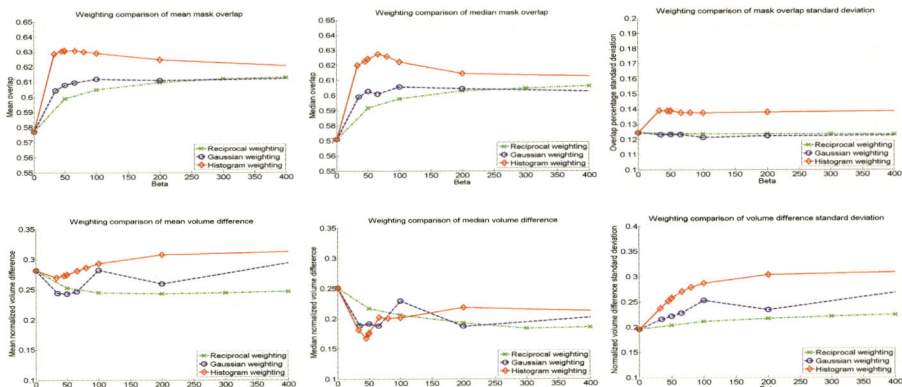

Fig. 2. Random Walker: Empirical comparison of weighting functions over a range of β values using the same connectivity. Marker positions indicate measured data points. Blue/dashed line with circles: Gaussian function (1), Green/dash-dot line with crosses: Reciprocal function (2), Red/solid line with diamonds: Histogram-based function (3). Top row: Comparison of mean, median and standard deviation for mask overlap measure. Bottom row: Comparison of mean, median and standard deviation for normalized volume difference.

where $||\cdot||$ is used to denote the standard Euclidean norm and $C(v_i)$ maps voxel v_i to its coordinates in 3D. The 10-connected case has a somewhat more complicated definition, since it gives preferential treatment to the within-slice dimensions (taken here to be the XY-plane). We may define a 10-connected lattice to be

$$10-\text{connected}: \quad E = \{i,j|\ ||C(v_i) - C(v_j)|| \leq 1\} \cup$$
$$\{i,j|\ ||C(v_i) - C(v_j)|| \leq \sqrt{2}, \forall C(v_i)_z = C(v_j)_z\}. \quad (6)$$

We make the assumption that edge connectivity and weighting function are independent design choices, i.e., if a particular connectivity improves the results, we assume that the performance increase will persist even if another weighting function is employed. Since the histogram-based weighting function (3) performed better than those based purely on image intensity (see Section 3), the same histogram-based weighting function was employed across all connectivity experiments.

3 Results

3.1 Weighting Functions

Our comparison of graph weighting functions is displayed in Figure 1 for Graph Cuts and in Figure 2 for the Random Walker algorithm. These Figures plot the mean, median and standard deviation values of the two segmentation measures across β values.

Graph Cuts responded to a different parameter range for β in the two intensity-based weighting functions than the Random Walker algorithm. For better display of Figure 1,

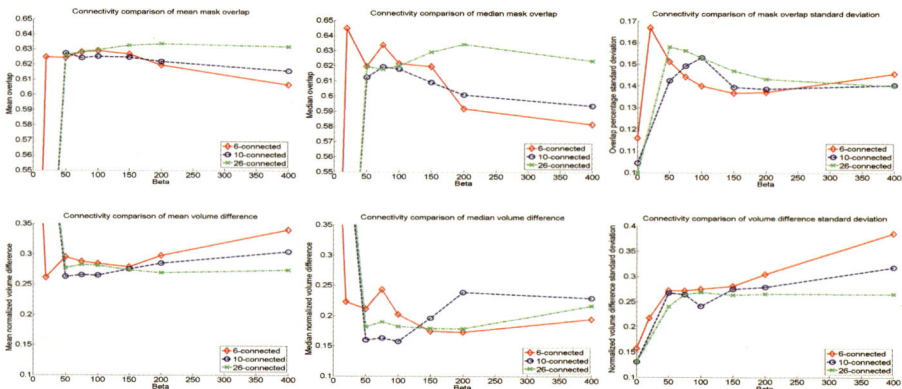

Fig. 3. Graph Cuts: Empirical comparison of graph connectivities over a range of β values using the same weighting function. Marker positions indicate measured data points. Red/solid line with diamonds: 6-connected lattice. Blue/dashed line with circles: 10-connected lattice, Green/dash-dot line with crosses: 26-connected lattice. Top row: Comparison of mean, median and standard deviation for mask overlap measure. Bottom row: Comparison of mean, median and standard deviation for normalized volume difference.

the β value used in the Gaussian function is $10\times$ the number shown on the axis, and the β value used for the Reciprocal function is $100\times$ the axis value.

Despite some differences in the behavior of both algorithms in the presence of different weighting functions, the overall behavior response is similar. Not surprisingly, the histogram-based weighting function outperforms both of the weighting functions based on intensity difference in both algorithms. However, the standard deviations of the histogram-based results were higher than the standard deviations from the intensity-based weighting functions for Random Walker, although the standard deviations across all three weighting functions were similar for Graph Cuts. All of the weighting functions appear to take a single peak at a certain β value, although the location of this peak is function-dependent. The comparison of the Gaussian and Reciprocal weighting functions, both based purely on intensity differences, is revealing. Although the Gaussian weighting function appears to be more prevalent in recent graph-based segmentation literature, the Reciprocal weighting function appears to outperform the Gaussian weighting function in two respects. For both algorithms (although more dramatically for Graph Cuts), the Reciprocal weighting function achieves an absolute higher performance with respect to both measures and a substantially lower standard deviation with respect to the volume difference measure. Additionally, the performance of the Gaussian weighting function behaves more erratically than the Reciprocal weighting function with respect to changes in β. Moreover, the peak performance of the Gaussian weighting function corresponds to a narrow range of β values, while the peak performance of the Reciprocal weighting function persists over a much broader range of β values. This finding suggests that a designer must be more selective with their choice of β when using the Gaussian weighting function than when employing the Reciprocal weighting function.

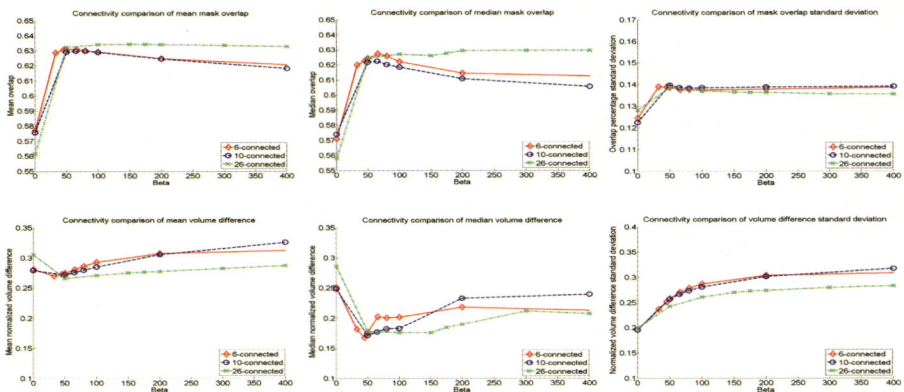

Fig. 4. Random Walker: Empirical comparison of graph connectivities over a range of β values using the same weighting function. Marker positions indicate measured data points. Red/solid line with diamonds: 6-connected lattice. Blue/dashed line with circles: 10-connected lattice, Green/dash-dot line with crosses: 26-connected lattice. Top row: Comparison of mean, median and standard deviation for mask overlap measure. Bottom row: Comparison of mean, median and standard deviation for normalized volume difference.

The intensity-based weighting functions were outperformed by the histogram-based weighting function. The form of the histogram-based function was the same as the Gaussian weighting function, except that differences in "foreground probability" were used rather than the raw intensities. It is notable that the response of the histogram-based function and the Gaussian function with respect to β followed a similar evolution, except that the histogram-based function produced consistently better performance.

3.2 Graph Topology

The segmentation performance with respect to graph topology followed a similar pattern with both graph-based algorithms. Overall, the connectivity level seemed to have a stronger effect on the Graph Cuts results than the Random Walker results.

Conventional wisdom about graph-based algorithms tends to support the notion that more edges (stronger connectivity) produce better results. Figure 4 illustrates that this notion is not necessarily correct. Of the three graph topologies, the 10-connected graph appears to exhibit inferior performance to both the 6-connected and 26-connected graphs. One explanation for this phenomenon is that the asymmetry of the 10-connected lattice (i.e., preferential treatment of the XY-plane) introduced a negative bias into its performance. One might assume that it would be appropriate to include more edges on the within-slice plane, due to anisotropic voxel spacing. However, introducing more edges within-slice further reduces the percentage of between-slice edges, which may be responsible for the negative effect.

The 26-connected lattice gave the best performance of all three graph topologies. Use of a more extensive topology leading to better performance of graph algorithms has been previously predicted in the literature for Graph Cuts [4], although the effect seems to be similar (albeit not as dramatic) for the Random Walker algorithm. Although the peak β value for the 6-connected and 10-connected lattices were roughly equal, the peak β value for the 26-connected lattice was larger. A possible explanation for this phenomenon is given by the fact that gradient normalization was performed over all edges. Since the between-slice diagonal edges present in the 26-connected lattice would be expected to be greater than the other gradients along the other edges, it is not unexpected that a larger β value would be required in the 26-connected case. This explanation suggests controlling for this phenomenon by using the same normalization for each dataset over all graph connectivities.

4 Conclusion

Graph algorithms have become very popular for 3D medical image segmentation. Although the action of each algorithm is different, the same procedures are consistently used to assign graph connectivity and edge weighting. Since these procedures persist across algorithms, there is an implicit assumption in the segmentation community that the algorithms respond similarly to the design specifications of the graph construction. In this work, differences in graph construction were controlled for algorithm-specific effects by employing both the Graph Cuts and Random Walker algorithms.

With respect to different graph weighting functions, it was found that basing the weights on differences in a probability density obtained from the foreground seeds was generally superior to weighting functions based solely on intensity gradients. This finding is not overly surprising, given that more information is being used to build the weight structure. However, it was more surprising to find that the Reciprocal weighting function, which has been employed less in recent years, outperforms the more popular Gaussian weighting function in terms of both absolute performance achieved and stability. This phenomenon was observed with both segmentation algorithms used in the study. Since the Reciprocal weighting function outperformed the Gaussian weighting function, it is possible that it would be more effective in the future to base the form of the histogram-based function on the Reciprocal weighting function.

Although different connectivities have been employed in 3D graph construction, little attention had been previously paid to the effects of topology choice. It has been previously predicted for the Graph Cuts algorithm that higher-order connectivities produce better algorithm performance [4]. Our study confirms this prediction and shows a similar response behavior for the Random Walker algorithm, but with a diminished influence of topology. Specifically, our study comparing graph construction confirms that 26-connected graphs do exhibit better performance than either 6-connected or 10-connected graphs. More surprising is that the 10-connected lattice performed worse than either the 6-connected or the 26-connected lattice. A possible explanation is that the asymmetry of the 10-connected lattice causes an unintended bias in the results.

Our experiments suggest that the best algorithm performance may be gained by using a 26-connected lattice and histogram-based weighting. If histograms are not available (or unreliable, due to small samples), the Reciprocal weighting function outperforms the Gaussian weighting function in both quality and stability.

There is much future work to be done on this topic. Three major questions remain: 1) Do these results persist with other data modalities? 2) Are better, general-purpose, graph connectivities and weighting functions possible? This paper offers the first look at empirically evaluating the effects of graph construction on algorithm performance.

References

1. Boykov, Y., Jolly, M.P.: Interactive graph cuts for optimal boundary & region segmentation of objects in N-D images. In: Proc. of ICCV 2001, pp. 105–112 (2001)
2. Grady, L.: Random walks for image segmentation. IEEE PAMI 28(11), 1768–1783 (2006)
3. Udupa, J.K., Samarasekera, S.: Fuzzy connectedness and object definition: Theory, algorithms, and applications in image segmentation. GMIP 58(3), 246–261 (1996)
4. Boykov, Y., Kolmogorov, V.: Computing geodesics and minimal surfaces via graph cuts. In: Proceedings of the International Conference on Computer Vision, vol. 1 (2003)
5. Boykov, Y., Kolmogorov, V.: An experimental comparison of min-cut/max-flow algorithms for energy minimization in vision. IEEE PAMI 26(9), 1124–1137 (2004)
6. Jolly, M.P., Grady, L.: 3D general segmentation in CT. In: Proc. of ISBI, pp. 796–799 (2008)
7. Perona, P., Malik, J.: Scale-space and edge detection using anisotropic diffusion. IEEE PAMI 12(7), 629–639 (1990)
8. Geman, S., McClure, D.: Statistical methods for tomographic image reconstruction. Proc. 46th Sess. Int. Stat. Inst. Bulletin ISI 52, 4–21 (1987)
9. Black, M.J., Sapiro, G., Marimont, D.H., Heeger, D.: Robust anisotropic diffusion. IEEE TIP 7(3), 421–432 (1998)
10. Shi, J., Malik, J.: Normalized cuts and image segmentation. IEEE PAMI, 888–905 (2000)
11. Falcão, A., Udupa, J., Samarasekera, S., Sharma, S., Elliot, B., de A. Lotufo, R.: User-steered image segmentation paradigms: Live wire and live lane. GMIP 60(4), 233–260 (1998)

Level Set Based Surface Capturing in 3D Medical Images

Bin Dong[1], Aichi Chien[2], Yu Mao[1], Jian Ye[1], and Stanley Osher[1]

[1] Department of Mathematics, University of California, Los Angeles, CA
[2] Division of Interventional Neuroradiology, David Geffen School of Medicine at UCLA, 10833 LeConte Ave, Los Angeles, CA*

Abstract. Brain aneurysm rupture has been reported to be directly related to the size of aneurysms. The current method used to determine aneurysm size is to manually measure the width of the neck and height of the dome on a computer screen. Because aneurysms usually have complicated shapes, using the size of the aneurysm neck and dome may not be accurate and may overlook important geometrical information. In this paper we present a level set based illusory surface algorithm to capture the aneurysms from the vascular tree. Since the aneurysms are described by level set functions, not only the volume but also the curvature of aneurysms can be computed for medical studies. Experiments and comparisons with models used for capturing illusory contours in 2D images are performed. This includes applications to clinical image data demonstrating the procedure of accurately capturing a middle cerebral artery aneurysm.

1 Introduction

Subarachnoid hemorrhage, primarily from brain aneurysm rupture, accounts for 5 to 10% of all stroke cases with a high fatality rate [1]. Advancements in neuroimaging technology have helped these aneurysms to be more frequently found prior to rupture. A method to determine if aneurysms are at higher risk of rupturing would be extremely valuable. Brain aneurysm rupture has been reported to be related to the size of aneurysms. It is known that the risk of rupture greatly increases as the aneurysm becomes larger [2]. Currently, methods to determine the aneurysmal size are to manually measure the size of the neck and the dome of aneurysms. However, these method may overlook important geometric information [3].

Our goal in this paper is to segment the aneurysm from the entire blood vessel with minimal human interaction. We observe from Fig. 1(d) and 1(e) that the problem can be realized as an illusory surface capturing problem, as an extension from illusory contours in 2D. Illusory contours have been intensively studied in cognitive neuroscience noting that human vision system is capable of combining nonexistent edges and making meaningful visual organization of both

---

* The research is supported by NIH GRANT, P20 MH65166; NSF GRANT, DMS-0714807.

the real and imaginary contour segments (e.g. the Kanizsa square in Fig. 1(e)). Various researchers have introduced mathematical models and techniques to mimic the human vision system in detecting and capturing perceptional contours in images [4,5,6]. These mathematical models can be used to describe the process in clinical evaluation when the location of an aneurysm needs to be identified (e.g. Fig. 1(b)). Given that our problem is to first capture and then calculate the volume and geometry of the aneurysm, representing the surface using a level set function and designing a proper surface evolution PDE is essential. In this paper, we introduce a level set and PDE based illusory surface model, inspired by the illusory contour model [6], to calculate the volume and geometry of aneurysms.

2 Method

The focus of this paper is to introduce a novel method to capture a specific part of a given surface obtained from 3D images. Therefore, we will not place emphasis on the techniques of 3D reconstruction. Interested readers can consult [7,8,9] for details on surface reconstruction. As as an example, we applied a simple thresholding method followed by fast sweeping method [10] and nonlocal means surface smoothing [9] to reconstruct the surface represented by a level set function [11], which takes positive values inside the vessel region and negative values outside (Fig. 1(a)).

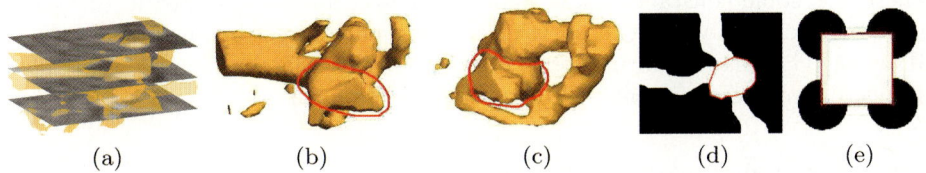

(a) (b) (c) (d) (e)

Fig. 1. (a) is an illustration of surface reconstruction using CT images. (b) and (c) are illustrations to show the location of the aneurysm (red curves) from different viewpoints. (d) is the phantom vessel image where the red curve is the illusory contour. (e) is the Kanizsa square where the red curve is the illusory contour.

2.1 Level Set Based Illusory Surface Capturing

Similar to the model introduced by Zhu et al [6] which captures illusory contours in 2D, we consider the following energy function in 3D

$$E(\phi) = \int_{\Omega} \Big(d\delta(\phi)|\nabla\phi| + \alpha H(\psi)H(\phi) + \beta\delta(\phi)|\nabla\phi| \Big) dx, \qquad (2.1)$$

where ψ is the signed distance function obtained from the previous section and $d = |\psi|$ is the corresponding unsigned distance function. The symbol ∇ is the gradient operator, $\delta(\phi)$ is the Dirac delta functional, and $H(\phi)$ is the Heaviside function. The energy term $\alpha H(\psi)$ acts as a barricade for ϕ. It forces the evolving zero level set of ϕ to stay inside of that of ψ, and it is inactive when the zero level set of ϕ is already inside ψ. As a result, the parameter α is less important than β.

From equation (2.1), the corresponding gradient flow can be written as

$$\frac{\partial \phi}{\partial t} = \delta(\phi)\nabla d \cdot \frac{\nabla \phi}{|\nabla \phi|} + \delta(\phi)d\nabla \cdot \frac{\nabla \phi}{|\nabla \phi|} - \alpha\delta(\phi)H(\psi) + \beta\delta(\phi)\nabla \cdot \frac{\nabla \phi}{|\nabla \phi|}. \quad (2.2)$$

Since the function $\delta(\phi)$ is concentrated only on the zero level set of ϕ, the PDE (2.2) only describes a motion for the zero level set of ϕ. Similar to [12], to ensure all level sets of ϕ have similar motions and to be able to solve the PDE on the entire 3D rectangular domain, we replace $\delta(\phi)$ in (2.2) by $|\nabla \phi|$ and obtain the following PDE

$$\frac{\partial \phi}{\partial t} = |\nabla \phi|\left(\nabla d \cdot \frac{\nabla \phi}{|\nabla \phi|} + d\nabla \cdot \frac{\nabla \phi}{|\nabla \phi|} - \alpha H(\psi) + \beta\nabla \cdot \frac{\nabla \phi}{|\nabla \phi|}\right). \quad (2.3)$$

Equation (2.3) is the illusory contour model proposed in [6] with a direct application in 3D. In that paper, the authors also considered the following improved model which enables the final curves to stick to sharp corners more closely

$$E(\phi) = \int_\Omega \left((1 + \nu c_{a,b}\kappa^+(\psi))d\delta(\phi)|\nabla \phi| + \alpha H(\psi)H(\phi) + \beta\delta(\phi)|\nabla \phi|\right)dx, \quad (2.4)$$

where ν is some constant, $c_{a,b}$ is some restriction function defined in (2.7) and $\kappa^+(\psi)$ is the positive part of curvature. However, a direct extension of (2.4) to 3D (using Gaussian curvature for κ) does not give satisfactory results. A detailed discussion and comparisons will be given in Section 3.1.

2.2 Modified Illusory Surface Model

Here we introduce our modified illusory surface model based on equation (2.3). We observe that the dominant force ∇d in (2.3) does not distinguish between the relatively flat regions and the sharp tip on the aneurysm (Fig. 1). Therefore, we introduce an amplification factor in front of $\nabla d \cdot \frac{\nabla \phi}{|\nabla \phi|}$ (shown in (2.5)) in order to handle problems with complicated geometry, for example the geometry with extruded bleb. It is somehow similar to [6], but instead of putting the factor in the energy as it is in (2.4), we modify (2.3). The amplification factor, denoted as $A(\psi)$, and the modified PDE are given as follows

$$\frac{\partial \phi}{\partial t} = |\nabla \phi|\left(A(\psi)\nabla d \cdot \frac{\nabla \phi}{|\nabla \phi|} + d\nabla \cdot \frac{\nabla \phi}{|\nabla \phi|} - \alpha H(\psi) + \beta\nabla \cdot \frac{\nabla \phi}{|\nabla \phi|}\right), \quad (2.5)$$

$$A(\psi) = 1 + \mu\kappa^+(\psi), \quad (2.6)$$

where μ is a constant parameter and $\kappa^+(\psi)$ is the positive part of the Gaussian curvature of ψ. By using the Gaussian curvature, we can automatically distinguish the target region (aneurysm) from the blood vessels, because both aneurysm and vessel regions have comparable values of mean curvatures, while only in the aneurysm region, especially the sharp tip (Fig. 1), is the Gaussian curvature large. Our experiments show that our model (2.5) performs better than (2.3) and (2.4), especially in the region with high Gaussian curvature. Numerical results and a discussion of our model (2.5), and the model (2.3) and (2.4) can be found in Section 3.1.

2.3 Numerical Procedure and Computations of Geometries

Since the energy functional (2.1) is not convex and, indeed, it has many local minimizers, in order to obtain a desirable solution for equation (2.3), good choices of $\phi(x, 0)$ are needed [6]. For our model (2.5), a reasonable initialization is also required. However, our model (2.5) is less restrictive on initial guesses than (2.3). This is tested and discussed in detail in the numerical section. To obtain a reasonable initial surface, we need users to select points around the area of interest and initiate the computation. We use the selected points to determine a sphere with level set function ϕ_S. Then $\phi(x, 0)$ is defined as the intersection of ϕ_S with ψ, or mathematically $\phi(x, 0) = \min\{\phi_S(x), \psi(x)\}$. In our proposed method, the selection of the points for the region of interest is the only part needs users interaction. Although automated computation is desirable, determining a pathologic region is a medical diagnosis which needs an expert's supervision. Therefore, it is reasonable to have experts' inputs and use them to initiate the computation. In the result section, we will show a clinical example of allowing the user to select as few as six points to capture the surface of a brain aneurysm.

With the initial condition described above, we employ the local level set method [13] to solve equation (2.3) and (2.5), as well as to minimize (2.4), in order to alleviate the time step restrictions and lower the complexity of our numerical computations. Generally speaking, we solve $\phi_t + c_{a,b}(\phi)V_n(\phi)|\nabla\phi| = 0$ instead of $\phi_t + V_n(\phi)|\nabla\phi| = 0$ with the restriction function $c_{a,b}$ introduced to confine all effective calculations within a narrow band of zero level set of ϕ. The restriction function $c_{a,b}$ is defined as

$$c_{a,b}(x) = \begin{cases} 1, & |x| \leq a; \\ (|x| - b)^2(2|x| + b - 3a)/(b - a)^3, & a < |x| \leq b; \\ 0, & |x| > b. \end{cases} \quad (2.7)$$

After we obtain the solution ϕ which represents the aneurysm, we calculate the volume of it by $V(\phi) = \int H(\phi)dx$, the mean curvature by $\kappa_m(\phi) = \nabla \cdot \frac{\nabla\phi}{|\nabla\phi|}$, and the Gaussian curvature [14] by $\kappa_g(\phi) = \frac{\nabla\phi^T H(\phi)\nabla\phi}{|\nabla\phi|^4}$, where

$$H(\phi) = \begin{pmatrix} \phi_{yy}\phi_{zz} - \phi_{yz}\phi_{zy} & \phi_{yz}\phi_{zx} - \phi_{yx}\phi_{zz} & \phi_{yx}\phi_{zy} - \phi_{yy}\phi_{zx} \\ \phi_{xz}\phi_{zy} - \phi_{xy}\phi_{zz} & \phi_{xx}\phi_{zz} - \phi_{xz}\phi_{zx} & \phi_{xy}\phi_{zx} - \phi_{xx}\phi_{zy} \\ \phi_{xy}\phi_{yz} - \phi_{xz}\phi_{yy} & \phi_{yx}\phi_{xz} - \phi_{xx}\phi_{yz} & \phi_{xx}\phi_{yy} - \phi_{xy}\phi_{yx} \end{pmatrix},$$

and subscripts denote the partial derivatives in Cartesian coordinates.

3 Applications in Medical Images

The algorithms are applied to brain images acquired by 3D CT angiography. The images have 512×512 in-plan spatial resolutions with each voxel size approximately $0.125mm^3$. We then extract subimages of size 54×37 for the aneurysm from the entire brain images.

3.1 Numerical Experiments and Validations

The numerical experiments were performed using MATLAB. It took approximately 90 seconds to capture the aneurysm surface using a Windows Laptop (Duo processor, 2.0GHz CPU and 2GB RAM). The numerical stopping criteria for the iteration $\phi^n \to \phi^{n+1}$ is based on $\frac{\|\phi^{n+1}-\phi^n\|_2}{\|\phi^n\|_2} <$ tolerance.

The numerical results of solving (2.3) are shown in Fig. 2, row one. Although this model has been reported with fairly good results for 2D images [6], direct application to capturing 3D surface is not satisfactory. The reason is that in [6], successful contour/surface capturing highly depends on the choice of an initial curve/surface which should cover all regions of interests. However, given that our problem is to capture a complicated surface with a few initial points, it is difficult to ensure that the assigned initial surface provides good coverage. Also, a larger initial surface will result in significant increase in the computational time. Therefore, the model (2.3) is not suited for solving our problem.

We also test the model (2.4) which was developed to improve the illusory contours at corners [6]. The results are shown in the second row of Fig. 2. This model provides some improvement at the tip of the aneurysm in comparison with the model (2.3). However, it still can not capture the entire tip which is a very

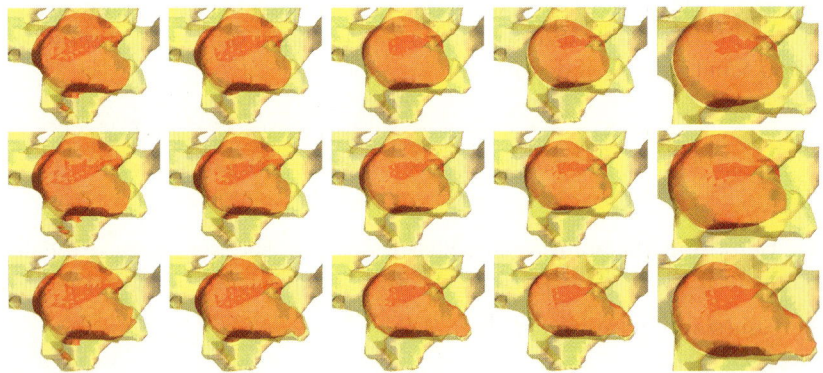

Fig. 2. Row 1-3 shows results of (2.3), (2.4) and (2.5) respectively. For the best results, parameters are $\beta = 1$ for (2.3), $(\mu, \beta) = (500, 0.05)$ for (2.4) and $(\mu, \beta) = (2000, 1)$ for (2.5). In each row, the first four figures are results at iteration=20, 100, 500 and 1000 respectively, and the last figure is the magnified view at iterations=1000. All the initial points are given as the same as the first column in Fig. 5.

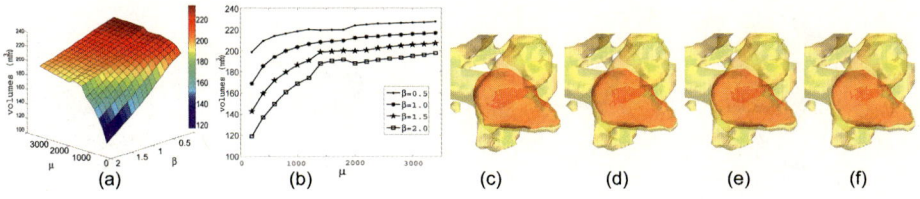

Fig. 3. (a) and (b) show the influence of (μ, β) to the captured volume. (c)-(f) show the visualization of the final surface capturing with parameters $\mu = 2000$, and $\beta = 0.5, 1, 1.5$ and 2 respectively. (d) shows the best surface capturing.

important medical feature. The reason is that fundamentally the illusory surface model (2.4) creates a boundary near the region where the concavity changes. For the aneurysm we have here, the concavity changes near the sharp tip (Fig. (2)). Therefore, (2.4) can not capture the entire aneurysm.

The results of our modified surface capturing model (2.5) are shown in the third row of Fig. 2. Using this method, we are able to capture the entire aneurysm. The reason for this significant improvement is that our modification is made directly on the force field (the factor $A(\psi)\nabla d$ in the first term of (2.5)), which guides the movement of the zero level set of ϕ towards the part of the surface with high Gaussian curvature. However, other terms in the original PDE (2.3) are kept unchanged, especially the second term $d\nabla \cdot \frac{\nabla \phi}{|\nabla \phi|}$, in contrast to the corresponding PDE of (2.4) [6].

3.2 Parameter Comparison and Geometry Computation

Since parameters β and μ in (2.5) and (2.6) can both affect the final results, we experiment on how they interact with each other and affect the quality of the captured surface and volume. Fig. 3(a) shows that the choice of β significantly changes the captured volume. In addition, the volume increases considerably with μ until it reaches 2000 (Fig. 3(b)). After that stage the captured volume does not change too much (approximately 2mm^3). In general, the larger β is, the smoother the final surface will be; however, we tend to lose the tip when β is too large, e.g. $\beta > 1$ (Fig. 3(c)-(f)). On the other hand, the larger μ is, the better the sharp tip is captured. However, the captured surface becomes rougher for large μ. Empirically, the best balance happens when $\mu = 2000$ and $\beta = 1$. Because the parameter α is less important than β (as explained at the beginning of Section 2.1) in our experiments, the parameter α is fixed to be 0.01, the constants a and b in (2.7) are 2 and 4 respectively. The captured brain aneurysm is shown in Fig. 4 with $(\mu = 2000, \beta = 1)$. Fig. 4(b) presents the volume of the aneurysm and Fig. 4(c) and 4(d) show that the area of high mean and Gaussian curvatures locates at the tip of aneurysm. It has been suggested by researchers that certain geometrical characteristics such as a bleb and tip may be associated with aneurysm rupture. Thus the information of mean curvature,

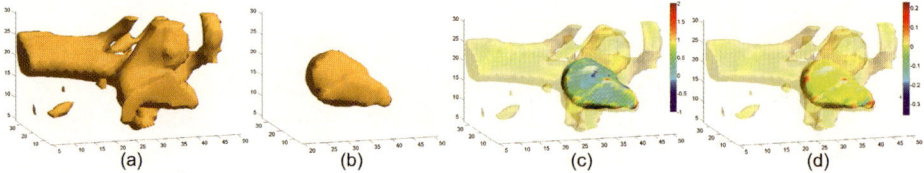

Fig. 4. (a) Is the entire structure of the arteries and aneurysm; (b) is the captured aneurysm through our illusory surface algorithm (2.5); (c) and (d) are the mean and Gaussian curvatures of the aneurysm. Both of them show that the curvatures around the tip of the aneurysm are relatively high.

which can indicate the geometry change in value, may provide a new tool to study aneurysm rupture in the future.

3.3 Validation

To further test the robustness of our algorithm, we validate the modified surface capturing model by selecting different initial points. Six sets of points indicating the target region (aneurysm) are used to initiate our algorithm. The parameters $\alpha = 0.01$, $\beta = 1$, and $\mu = 2000$ are used in the algorithm, as determined in the previous section. Results are shown in Fig. 5. The volumes captured by different initial points are $204.5 \pm 8.65 \text{mm}^3$ (mean ±standard deviation). As a result, we expect the deviation of the volume computation which can be caused by different users is only about 4% of the total aneurysm volume. Our future work will involve applying this model to different blood vessels and further confirm the accuracy and reproducibility of our algorithm.

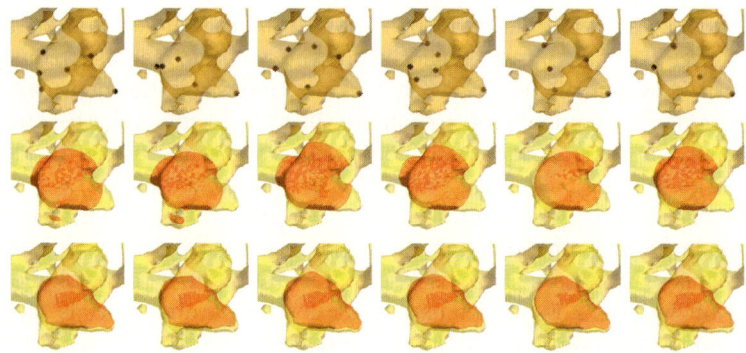

Fig. 5. The resulting volumes for the different points chosen by users from left to right are: 207.375mm^3, 205.875mm^3, 217.5mm^3, 207mm^3, 193.875mm^3 and 195.75mm^3. Top row is the given points by users. Middle row is the corresponding initial surfaces. Bottom is the corresponding final captured surfaces.

4 Conclusion

A method to quantify the volume and geometry of brain aneurysms is needed to better study how they associate with aneurysmal growth and rupture. In this paper, we introduced a level set based PDE model to capture and compute the geometry of brain aneurysm. We introduced a supervised strategy with only one parameter β and no more than six initial points determined by users to capture surfaces of aneurysms. The numerical results showed that the final surface captured the entire target region and we were able to compute the volume and curvatures for clinical studies. There is huge variation among brain aneurysms and being able to quantify the geometry of irregular shapes is especially important for studying the associations of shape with rupture. Our future work will involve applying this algorithm to diverse aneurysm shapes and improving the algorithm for different clinical purpose.

References

1. Kassell, N.F., Torner, J.C.: Aneurysmal rebleeding: a preliminary report from the Cooperative Aneurysm Study. Neurosurgery 13(5), 479–481 (1983)
2. Unruptured intracranial aneurysms–risk of rupture and risks of surgical intervention. International Study of Unruptured Intracranial Aneurysms Investigators. N. Engl. J. Med. 339(24), 1725–1733 (1998)
3. Raghavan, M.L., Ma, B., Harbaugh, R.E.: Quantified aneurysm shape and rupture risk. J. Neurosurg. 102(2), 355–362 (2005)
4. Geiger, D., Pao, H.K., Rubin, N.: Salient and Multiple illusory surfaces. In: IEEE Computer Society Conference on Conputer Vision and Pattern Recognition, San Barbara, CA (June 1998)
5. Sarti, A., Malladi, R., Sethian, J.A.: Subjective surfaces: A geometric model for boundary completion. Int. J. Comp. Vision 46(3), 201–221 (2002)
6. Zhu, W., Chan, T.F.: Capture illusory contours: A level set based approach. UCLA CAM Report 03-65 (2003)
7. Yim, P.J., Cebral, J.J., Mullick, R., Marcos, H.B., Choyke, P.L.: Vessel surface reconstruction with a tubular deformable model. IEEE Transactions on Medical Imaging 20(12), 1411–1421 (2001)
8. Chen, J., Amini, A.A.: Quantifying 3-D vascular structures in MRA images using hybrid PDE and geometric deformable models. IEEE Transactions on Medical Imaging 23(10), 1251–1262 (2004)
9. Dong, B., Ye, J., Osher, S.J., Dinov, I.: Level set based nonlocal surface restoration, CAM-Report 07-44 (2007)
10. Tsai, R., Cheng, L.-T., Osher, S.J., Zhao, H.K.: Fast sweeping method for a class of Hamilton-Jacobi equations. SIAM J. Numer. Analy. 41, 673–694 (2003)
11. Osher, S.J., Fedkiw, R.P.: The Level Set Method and Dynamic Implicit Surfaces. Springer, New York (2002)
12. Zhao, H.K., Chan, T.F., Merriman, B., Osher, S.J.: A variational level set approach to multiphase motion. J. Comput. Phys. 127, 179–195 (1996)
13. Peng, D., Merriman, B., Osher, S.J., Zhao, H.K., Kang, M.: A PDE-based fast local level set method. J. Comput. Phys. 155, 410–438 (1999)
14. Goldman, R.: Curvature formulas for implicit curves and surfaces. Computer Aided Geometric Design 22, 632–658 (2005)

Automatic Detection of Calcified Coronary Plaques in Computed Tomography Data Sets

Stefan C. Saur[1], Hatem Alkadhi[2], Lotus Desbiolles[2], Gábor Székely[1], and Philippe C. Cattin[1,3]

[1] Computer Vision Laboratory, ETH Zurich, Switzerland
saur@vision.ee.ethz.ch
[2] Institute of Diagnostic Radiology, University Hospital Zurich, Switzerland
[3] CMBE, University of Basel, Switzerland*

Abstract. The detection of calcified plaques is an essential step in the assessment of coronary heart diseases. However, manual plaque segmentation is subjected to intra- and inter-observer variability. We present a novel framework for the automatic detection of calcified coronary plaques in Computed Tomography images. In contrast to the state-of-the-art, both the native and the angio data sets are included to gain additional information about each plaque for its detection and subsequent assessment. The framework was successfully tested on 127 patients where 85.5% of the calcified and 96% of the obstructive plaques have been detected.

1 Introduction

Coronary heart diseases (CHD) are a major cause of death within the United States [1] and other western countries. Early detection and quantification of coronary plaques is therefore of high interest. Depending on the degree of stenosis and the patient's health state, several treatment options exist: a coronary artery bypass graft (CABG), a drug eluting stent, or balloon angioplasty. Computed Tomography (CT) is a frequently used modality for the detection of plaques as it shows a good correlation with the gold standard Intravascular Ultrasound [2] and is, apart from the X-ray dose, not invasive. The standard scanning protocol for plaque assessment consists of two scans: a native, low resolution scan and a higher resolution angio scan with contrast agent. The first one is mainly used for Calcium Scoring as calcified plaques are clearly visible. The latter nicely visualizes the vessel lumen and as such allows to assess the degree of a stenosis. It furthermore allows to localize and characterize soft plaques.

For the automatic detection of plaques, it is helpful to delineate the coronary arteries, i.e. determining the centerline or a full segmentation of the vessel lumen. A comprehensive overview of existing segmentation algorithms for tubular structures can be found in [3]. With the various branches of the coronary

---

* This work has been supported by the CO-ME/NCCR research network of the Swiss National Science Foundation (http://co-me.ch). The authors thank MeVis Research (Bremen, Germany) for their support.

artery tree segmented, it is possible to analyze each branch for the presence of plaques. Toumoulin et al. [4] used a level set approach to detect both the inner and outer wall of a vessel in CT data sets and were therefore able to identify calcified plaques. Rinck et al. [5] also computed the inner and outer vessel wall to assess atherosclerotic plaques in coronary arteries using shape-based segmentation. Their algorithm, however, had to be manually initialized with a seed point before and after each plaque. Išgum et al. [6] applied a heart and aorta segmentation to native data sets and used specific features to automatically detect coronary calcifications using a two-stage classification system with a k-NN classifier and a feature selection scheme. They could detect 73.8% of the calcified plaques at the expense of an average of 0.1 false positives per scan. A 'Plaque Map' for CT images that uses color-based isometric lines and a bird's eye view to support the plaque detection was introduced in [7]. However, this method is only a visual aid for the manual detection of plaques. A model-based approach to semi-automatically measure the degree of stenosis in carotid arteries was developed by Frangi et al. [8] for MR images. Adame et al. [9] combined model-based segmentation and fuzzy clustering to detect the vessel wall, lumen and lipid core boundaries in MR images. Also for MR images, Sun et al. [10] used a Fuzzy C-Means based clustering algorithm to characterize plaque constituents.

With one exception, all aforementioned methods require substantial user intervention. The approach proposed in [6] is fully automatic but only detects calcified plaques in native data sets for Calcium Scoring. In this paper, we propose a framework for the automatic detection of calcified coronary plaques. In contrast to the previous techniques, we incorporate both the angio and native data set. Using both data sets has the advantage that more information for each plaque is available, both for its detection and subsequent assessment.

2 Method

This section presents a framework for the automatic detection of coronary calcified plaques. As in general both the angio and native CT scans are acquired for the assessment of plaques, no additional scan is required for the application of the proposed method. The basic concept can be summarized as follows. In the pre-processing steps (A)+(B) the aorta is detected and the coronary tree is segmented. The third step (C) extracts putative plaque candidates using an intensity-based threshold. This results in many false positives (FP) due to noise, inhomogeneous contrast agent distribution and other CT artifacts. In step (D) the plaques in the angio data set with the highest calcification are rigidly registered to the native plaques. The last two steps (E)+(F) use a rule based approach to maximize the number of detected plaques while minimizing FP. Throughout the processing pipeline, four sets are used to represent the actual state of the detection process: (1) $\mathcal{A}$ contains the unverified angio plaque candidates, (2) $\mathcal{N}_{130}$ the unverified native plaque candidates, (3) $\mathcal{N}_{200} \subset \mathcal{N}_{130}$ is a subset of $\mathcal{N}_{130}$ and contains the highly calcified but still unverified plaques only and (4) the initially empty set $\mathcal{V}$ contains the verified plaques.

(A) Aorta Detection. A point p_{aorta} in the ascending aorta is automatically detected in the angio data set [11] and the voxels in a $7 \times 7 \times 7$ neighborhood around p_{aorta} are used to compute the mean Hounsfield (HU) intensity μ and standard deviation σ of the contrast agent. These parameters are then later used to automatically select the threshold for the plaque candidate extraction.

(B) Coronary Artery Tree. The rough estimate of the vessel's centerline is obtained with a livewire algorithm [12], using only the intensity and gradient features as costs. Seed points need to be manually placed at the orifices of the coronary arteries from the aorta and in the distal ends of the various branches. The livewire algorithm was further modified to automatically detect bifurcations to extract the branching information of the coronary artery tree. For this, the centerline starting at the currently processed distal seed point may terminate either in one of the seed points at the orifices or in an existing centerline generated by previously processed seed points. The starting and terminal points of each centerline are kept for the subsequent lumen segmentation. The vessel lumen is segmented using graph-cut (GC) [13]. For this, each detected branch is reformatted along its centerline to get a stack of cross-sectional images. GC is then applied to each cross-sectional slice using a circular shape prior [14]. The resulting segmentation mask is then transformed back into the original angio data set.

(C) Candidate extraction. Plaque candidates are extracted using an intensity threshold from both the angio and the native data set.

Angio data set. The coronary artery segmentation of the previous step is used to restrict the plaque candidates to only those within the coronary arteries. The subsequent marching cube algorithm then generates meshes of all putative plaques. The iso-surface value $(\mu + 5\sigma)$ is adaptively chosen according to the contrast agent density observed in the aorta. Each connected mesh is regarded as an angio plaque candidate a_i which is stored in the list $\mathcal{A}$. Each candidate a_i is additionally assigned an intensity score s depending on its 90%-quantile intensity I of its voxels and defined by

$$s = \begin{cases} 0 & : \quad I < \mu + 2\sigma \\ \log_{10}\left(9\frac{I-(\mu+2\sigma)}{500\text{ HU}-(\mu+2\sigma)} + 1\right) & : \quad \mu + 2\sigma \leq I < 500\text{ HU} \\ 1 & : \quad I > 500\text{ HU} \end{cases}$$

The 90%-quantile for the intensity I was chosen to avoid outliers stemming from CT artifacts. The intensity score is defined for values $I \geq \mu + 2\sigma$ to potentially include extremely weak calcified plaques. However, those are currently not extracted and processed in the proposed framework.

Native Data Set. A radiation absorption intensity threshold of $th_i = 130$ HU is applied to the native data set. To ignore most of the bones, connected components larger than 5000 mm^3 are discarded. The resulting binary image is used as a mask for the native data set and the meshes of all plaques with an iso-surface value of 130 HU are then extracted using again the marching cube algorithm.

Each connected mesh is regarded as a native plaque candidate n_i and is stored in the list $\mathcal{N}_{130}$. The same procedure is repeated but with $th_i = 200$ HU, to generate a set of higher calcified native candidates called $\mathcal{N}_{200}$.

(D) Plaque registration. Although the native and angio data sets are acquired consecutively, they are generally not well registered due to the beating heart, breathing and minor patient movement. It is therefore the aim of the rigid plaque registration to determine the rotation $\boldsymbol{R}$ and translation $\boldsymbol{T}$ between both data sets. This registration allows to take over the coronary segmentation results from the angio to the native data set such that the native candidates can also be limited to the segmented vessel regions. Furthermore, it enables to compare plaque features from both data sets with each other. To avoid misregistrations, only the very high calcified native plaques of $\mathcal{N}_{200}$ as well as the angio plaques with a score $s > 0.95$ and a volume $v > 5$ voxels are considered for registration. As due to the different scan resolutions the shape between corresponding angio and native candidates may differ, only the barycenters of their meshes are used during the two stage registration process. These barycenters are stored in the list $\mathcal{R}_\mathrm{N}$ for the native and $\mathcal{R}_\mathrm{A}$ for the angio candidates, respectively. Misregistrations might occur if a large plaque in the low resolution native data set in fact consists of multiple smaller plaques in the angio data set. To resolve this ambiguity, additional points are added to $\mathcal{R}_\mathrm{N}$ by sampling all native plaques with an extension greater than 4 mm. Starting from the barycenter, additional points are placed with a step width of $\Delta = 2$ mm in both directions along the plaque's main axis as long as they are situated within the plaque (Fig. 1a).

In the first stage of the rigid registration, an optimal translation $\boldsymbol{t}^*$ is searched. The rotation is disregarded in this phase as according to our experience it has only a minor impact on the final registration. The optimal translation $\boldsymbol{t}^*$ is obtained by first choosing an arbitrary point from $\mathcal{R}_\mathrm{A}$ as a reference a_ref. Then, for each point $p_n \in \mathcal{R}_\mathrm{N}$, the translation $\boldsymbol{t} = \boldsymbol{p_n} - \boldsymbol{a_\mathrm{ref}}$ is computed (Fig. 1b) and applied to $\mathcal{R}_\mathrm{A}$ resulting in $\mathcal{R}_{\mathrm{A}'}$ (Fig. 1c). Correspondences between angio and native candidates are established by mapping each transformed $p_{a'_i} \in \mathcal{R}_{\mathrm{A}'}$ to the point $p_{n_i} \in \mathcal{R}_\mathrm{N}$ with the smallest euclidean distance (Fig. 1c). Afterwards, the energy $E_{p_n} = E_1 + E_2 + E_3$ is computed. The first energy term $E_1 = \|\boldsymbol{t}\|$ accounts for the length of $\boldsymbol{t}$ which should be minimal as only a small heart motion between the angio and native data set is expected. The second term $E_2 = \sum_i \|\boldsymbol{p_{a'_i}} - \boldsymbol{p_{n_i}}\|$ considers the remaining distance between the angio and native barycenters of corresponding candidate pairs. The third energy term E_3 compares how similar the spatial distribution of the angio candidates is with the spatial distribution of the mapped native candidates. For this, the distance $e_{a_{ij}} = \|\boldsymbol{p_{a_i}} - \boldsymbol{p_{a_j}}\|$ of any possible combination of two different points $p_{a_i}, p_{a_j} \in \mathcal{R}_\mathrm{A}, i \neq j$ is compared with the distance $e_{n_{ij}} = \|\boldsymbol{p_{n_i}} - \boldsymbol{p_{n_j}}\|$ of the corresponding mapped native candidates. The energy E_3 is then defined as $E_3 = \frac{1}{n} \sum |e_{a_{ij}} - e_{n_{ij}}|$ where n is the total number of possible combinations.

In the second stage, the known mapping of angio-native pairs with the minimum energy E_{p_n} is taken to compute the final registration parameters $\boldsymbol{R}$ and $\boldsymbol{T}$, using the algorithm from Horn [15] which requires at least three point pairs. For fewer pairs, R is assumed to be the unity matrix. T is set to $\frac{1}{2}((p_{a_1}-p_{n_1})+(p_{a_2}-p_{n_2}))$ for two, to $p_{a_1}-p_{n_1}$ for one, and to the null vector if no plaque pair is present. The rotation R and translation T are then applied to all native candidates from $\mathcal{N}_{130}$. Those falling outside of the vessel boundaries after the registration are discarded. All matched angio-native candidate pairs are added to $\mathcal{V}$ and removed from $\mathcal{A}$ and $\mathcal{N}_{130}$, respectively.

(E) Distance rule. Several distance checks are applied to confirm the verified candidates resulting from the registration process and to search for additional pairs that were not considered by the registration process due to their low intensity. Outliers in the registration can occur if a plaque is visible in the angio data set but not in the native acquisition. Then, the corresponding plaque is mapped to a wrong - in general more distant - candidate. Therefore, all previously verified angio-native candidate pairs in $\mathcal{V}$ are re-evaluated. If the distance between the angio and native plaque is larger than 0.5 mm, the candidate pair is removed from $\mathcal{V}$ and put back to $\mathcal{A}$ or $\mathcal{N}_{130}$, respectively. Additional angio-native candidate pairs are detected by iterating through $\mathcal{A}$ and checking for each angio candidate a_i if there is a native plaque n_i within a distance of 0.5 mm. If yes, this pair is added to $\mathcal{V}$ and removed from $\mathcal{A}$ and $\mathcal{N}_{130}$.

(F) Intensity score rule. This rule considers the fact that large angio plaque candidates with high intensity values are very likely to be plaques even though a corresponding native candidate is missing. An angio candidate is added to $\mathcal{V}$ and removed from $\mathcal{A}$ if its volume is larger than 1 mm^3 and $s \geq 0.75$.

3 Results

The proposed framework was developed in C++ based on the platform MeVis-Lab (MeVis Bremen, Germany) and evaluated on 127 patients (81 males, 46 females, mean age 63.8±12.0, range 35–88). To guarantee robustness, only the first 20 patients were used for development and parameter selection. Both angio and native scans were acquired on a Dual-Source CT scanner (Somatom Definition, Siemens Medical Solutions, Forchheim, Germany) with standard protocols. The in-plane resolution ranged from 0.25–0.73 mm (512 × 512 voxels). The slice thickness/slice spacing was 0.75–1 mm/0.4–1 mm for the angio and 3 mm/1.5–3 mm for the native data sets. The number of slices varied between 115 and 392 for the angio and between 26 and 101 for the native acquisitions, respectively.

The ground truth was obtained by manual plaque segmentation by a radiologist. The type of plaque (calcified or mixed), the degree of stenosis and the proximal and distal end position of each plaque were determined. A plaque with a stenosis greater than 50% was regarded as obstructive which was observed for 54 plaques (41 calcified, 13 mixed). In total 649 calcified and 102 mixed plaques were labeled. Figure 2a shows the allocation of these plaques over the patients. Besides the 33 cases with no plaques, most patients had between 1-8 plaques.

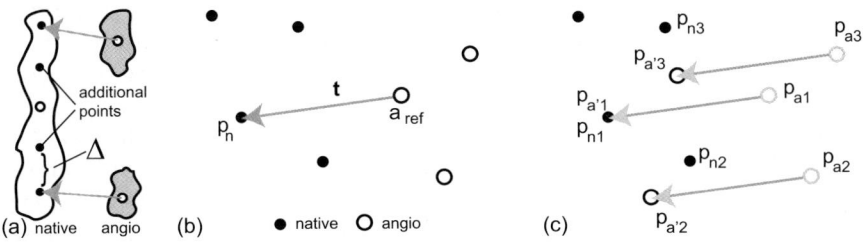

Fig. 1. Plaque registration. (a) Additional points are added for large native plaque candidates. (b) Reference point a_{ref} and translation vector t (c) Translation and mapping of angio candidates $p_{a'_i}$ to closest native candidates p_{n_i}.

Table 1. Number (percentage) of detected calcified and mixed plaques as well as the number of true (TP) and false (FP) positives, and the positive predictive value (PPV) for the candidates of the detection framework after each processing step. Some larger plaques are represented by multiple smaller candidates such that the number of TP and detected plaques is not identical.

		expert	candidate extraction	plaque registration	distance rule	intensity score rule
plaques	calcified	649	594 (91.5%)	436 (67.2%)	497 (76.6%)	560 (86.3%)
	mixed	102	85 (83.3%)	66 (64.7%)	75 (73.5%)	82 (80.4%)
candidates	TP	751	760	544	644	723
	FP	0	699	50	59	100
	PPV	100.0%	52.1%	91.6%	91.6%	87.8%

The verified plaque candidates from $\mathcal{V}$ were compared with the ground truth data to determine the number of true (TP) and false positives (FP). The number of detected labeled plaques as well as the positive predictive value $PPV = TP/(FP+TP)$ after each processing step are summarized in Table 1. The framework detected 86.3% of the calcified and 80.4% of the mixed plaques which leads to a total detection rate of 85.5% with a PPV of 87.8%. In total 109 (89 calcified, 20 mixed) plaques were missed. The mean extension $\bar{d}_e$ of the missed calcified and mixed plaques was 1.3 mm and 4.9 mm, respectively. One small obstructive calcified ($d_e = 1.2$ mm) and one obstructive mixed plaque ($d_e = 3.4$ mm) were not detected, resulting in a detection rate of 96% for the hazardous obstructive plaques. The extent of mixed plaques includes both the lipid and calcified part. Therefore, those missed plaques appear larger although only the small calcified part could not be detected. Figure 2b shows an example of detected angio-native plaque candidate pairs before the registration is applied to the native candidates.

4 Discussion and Conclusion

We presented a framework for the automatic detection of calcified coronary plaques. Through the proposed novel integration of both the native and the angio data sets into the detection process, we were able to achieve a good detection rate of 85.5%. However, a direct comparison to the method proposed by Išgum et al. [6] would not be feasible for several reasons: First of all, we encountered with 0.79 a higher average number of FP per patient. We assume that the detection rate from Išgum et al. [6] would improve if a comparable number of FP would be allowed. Further, the study population of Išgum et al. [6] consisted of women in their menopause whereas our population was a subset of a typical population scheduled for CT Coronary Angiography. Išgum et al. [6] only detected calcified coronary plaques in the native data set for Calcium Scoring, whereas our presented framework identifies the plaques both in the native and angio data set and establishes correspondences among them. Through this it will become possible to provide detailed information, i.e. both the Calcium Score and the degree of stenosis for each plaque individually.

An analysis of the FP has shown that they accumulate only in a small number of 37 patients (Fig 2a) where they mostly arose due to an inhomogeneous contrast agent distribution within the distal part of the right coronary artery. The not detected plaques were generally small and with two exceptions non-obstructive. In general, those small plaques did not have a major impact on the diagnoses as a physician mainly looks for stenoses or large plaques.

Although, many plaques could be detected by applying an intensity-based threshold, this would result in a high number of FP. Therefore, we added additional steps to verify the extracted plaque candidates. The registration step alone significantly reduced the number of FP. This is obvious as only highly calcified plaques were included. It also explains the decreased detection rate compared to the previous step. Additional criterions for the evaluation of the remaining weaker calcified plaque candidates could considerably improve the detection rate, nevertheless eventually at the expense of increased FP rate.

The good performance of the proposed approach can be mainly attributed to the fusion of the native and angio data set. This allowed to carry over the segmented vessels into the native data set and thereby reducing the FP rate.

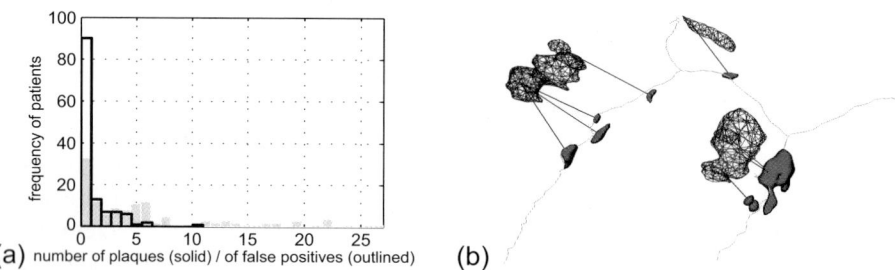

Fig. 2. (a) Histogram showing the distribution of the number of plaques per patient (solid bars) and the distribution of false positives (FP) accounted per patient (outlined bars). (b) Example of established correspondences between angio a_i (solid) and native candidates n_i (mesh) before the registration is applied to the native candidates.

Moreover, weakly calcified plaques, hardly discriminable from the contrast agent in the angio data set, could be detected. The approach still offers a wide range of possible improvements that can be easily integrated due to its modular design. In particular we are working on methods to automatically classify the detected plaques and to estimate the degree of stenosis. Furthermore, we are investigating methods to automatically label the segments of the coronary artery tree. This would allow for the fully automatic generation of a detailed medical report.

References

1. Rosamond, W., et al.: Heart Disease and Stroke Statistics–2008 Update. Circulation 117(4), 25–146 (2008)
2. Achenbach, S., et al.: Detection of Calcified and Noncalcified Coronary Atherosclerotic Plaque by Contrast-Enhanced, Submillimeter Multidetector Spiral Computed Tomography. Circulation 109(1), 14–17 (2004)
3. Kirbas, C., Quek, F.: A Review of Vessel Extraction Techniques and Algorithms. ACM Comput. Surv. 36(2), 81–121 (2004)
4. Toumoulin, C., et al.: Coronary Characterization in Multi-slice Computed Tomography. In: Comput. Cardiol., pp. 749–752 (2003)
5. Rinck, D., et al.: Shape-based Segmentation and Visualization Techniques for Evaluation of Atherosclerotic Plaques in Coronary Artery Disease. In: SPIE (2006)
6. Išgum, I., Rutten, A., Prokop, M., van Ginneken, B.: Detection of coronary calcifications from computed tomography scans for automated risk assessment of coronary artery disease. Med. Phys. 34(4), 1450–1461 (2007)
7. Komatsu, S., et al.: Detection of Coronary Plaque by Computed Tomography With a Novel Plaque Analysis System, 'Plaque Map', and Comparison With Intravascular Ultrasound and Angioscopy. Circulation 69(1), 72–77 (2005)
8. Frangi, A., Niessen, W., Nederkoorn, P., et al.: Three-Dimensional Model-Based Stenosis Quantification of the Carotid Arteries from Contrast-Enhanced MR Angiography. In: MMBIA, pp. 110–118 (2000)
9. Adame, I.M., et al.: Automatic segmentation and plaque characterization in atherosclerotic carotid artery MR images. MAGMA 16(5), 227–234 (2004)
10. Sun, B., et al.: Automatic Plaque Characterization Employing Quantitative and Multicontrast MRI. Magnetic Resonance in Medicine 59(1), 174–180 (2008)
11. Saur, S., et al.: Automatic Ascending Aorta Detection in CTA Datasets. In: Bildverarbeitung für die Medizin, pp. 323–327 (2008)
12. Barrett, W.A., Mortensen, E.N.: Interactive live-wire boundary extraction. Medical Image Analysis 1(4), 331–341 (1997)
13. Boykov, Y., Jolly, M.P.: Interactive Graph Cuts for Optimal Boundary & Region Segmentation of Objects in N-D Images. In: ICCV, vol. 1, pp. 105–112 (2001)
14. Slabaugh, G., Unal, G.: Graph cuts segmentation using an elliptical shape prior. In: ICIP, vol. 2, pp. 1222–1225 (2005)
15. Horn, B.K.P.: Closed-form solution of absolute orientation using unit quaternions. Journal of the Optical Society of America 4, 629–642 (1987)

Comprehensive Segmentation of Cine Cardiac MR Images

Maxim Fradkin[1], Cybèle Ciofolo[1], Benoit Mory[1], Gilion Hautvast[2], and Marcel Breeuwer[2]

[1] Medisys Research Lab, Philips Healthcare, Suresnes, France
[2] Healthcare Informatics, Philips Healthcare, Best, The Netherlands

Abstract. A typical Cardiac Magnetic Resonance (CMR) examination includes acquisition of a sequence of short-axis (SA) and long-axis (LA) images covering the cardiac cycle. Quantitative analysis of the heart function requires segmentation of the left ventricle (LV) SA images, while segmented LA views allow more accurate estimation of the basal slice and can be used for slice registration. Since manual segmentation of CMR images is very tedious and time-consuming, its automation is highly required. In this paper, we propose a fully automatic 2D method for segmenting LV consecutively in LA and SA images. The approach was validated on 35 patients giving mean segmentation error smaller than one pixel, both for LA and SA, and accurate LV volume measurements.

1 Introduction

A typical Cardiac Magnetic Resonance (CMR) examination includes acquisition of a sequence of short-axis (SA) and long-axis (LA) images covering the cardiac cycle. Quantitative analysis of the heart function (ejection fraction, myocardial thickness and thickening, etc.) requires segmentation of the left ventricle (LV) SA images. LA views, in addition, allow more reliable LV shape estimation, especially near the apex and the valve plane. The later can be used for the accurate and reproducible determination of the basal SA slice, which is known to be one of the major factors of interobserver variability in LV measurements [1,2]. Automatic multi-view segmentation methods, enabling to obtain highly reproducible LV measurements [3], are thus highly desirable.

Many publications propose automatic or semi-automatic methods for segmenting the LV in SA CMR images [4,5,6,7,8] or in multiple views [9,10,11], to mention a few. Since SA CMR images, acquired over multiple breath-holds, are often misregistered due to patient motion or inconsistent respiration, 3D segmentation and analysis methods require a registration preprocessing step [12,13,14,15,16]. Alternatively to image-based alignment, one can use for this purpose LV contours extracted from multiple views [17]. In contrast to [3], where LA contours had to be drawn manually to initialize SA segmentation, we propose a *fully automatic* method following similar workflow.

The paper is organized as follows: Section 2 gives a concise description of the proposed method; in Section 3 validation results are presented and discussed; conclusions are given in Section 4.

2 Method

Among 2D segmentation methods, explicit active contours [18] remain popular, since the underlying discrete contour representation is sufficient to capture the fairly smooth shape of the LV. However, this representation often produces slowly converging algorithms that are quite sensitive to initial conditions and parameterization. While there are various solutions to tackle those issues within the original framework, an interesting alternative representation using B-splines has been proposed in [19]. This continuous representation is compact and allows the semi-local control of smooth curves. Those advantages have motivated the design of our spline-based deformable template of the LV.

Most active contour methods are based on the minimization of an objective criterion and tend to be locally trapped by spurious image features during the optimization process. The *greedy optimization* framework [20] used in this paper offers a valuable compromise between computational complexity, robustness and flexibility. Not only it gives in most cases an acceptable solution by avoiding local minima, but also allows *easy incorporation of dissimilar image constraints* and *prior knowledge* (e.g., both differentiable and non-differentiable). We follow a two-stage approach: First, we robustly detect LV position on LA view(s) using standard image acquisition geometry and rigid template deformation. The precise delineation of the LV is done by deforming the template locally, through greedy optimization. Second, the segmented LA contours are used for initialization of deformable templates in the relevant SA slices, which are then adjusted using the same, as for LA, optimization paradigm.

2.1 Deformable Template Geometry

Our parametric template relies on *interpolating* splines controlled by *as few nodes as possible*. More specifically, the myocardium is modeled as a closed ribbon structure, composed of an imaginary centerline (dashed in Fig. 1) and a variable width. Both the centerline $\boldsymbol{C}(s) = [x(s), y(s)]$ and the ribbon width $w(s)$ are continuous spline interpolations of a discrete set of $\{p_k = (x_k, y_k, w_k)\}$ samples defined at each node. Among the advantages of this compact representation is the natural coupling between the endocardium and the epicardium (the inside and outside contours). We also define two enclosed regions $\mathcal{M}$ and $\mathcal{B}$, corresponding respectively to the myocardium and blood pool areas, as shown in Fig. 1.

2.2 Minimization Criterion

The optimal solution of our segmentation problem is the set of template parameters minimizing a criterion that expresses the goodness of fit between the geometrical model and the image evidence, given some *a priori* knowledge. In the remainder, I is the image and the λ_i's are scalar weights balancing the various terms. Let $\boldsymbol{p} = \{p_k = (x_k, y_k, w_k)^T, k \in [\![1, N]\!]\}$ be our parametric model. The problem can now be formalized as follows:

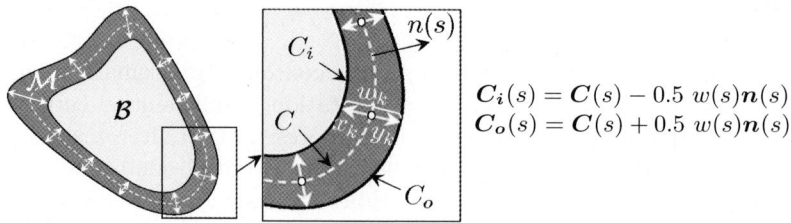

Fig. 1. Template geometry (**left**); Detailed zoom (**center**)

$$\min_{\boldsymbol{p}} \left\{ F(\boldsymbol{p}, I) = \underbrace{F_s(\boldsymbol{C}, w)}_{\text{shape}} + \underbrace{F_c(\boldsymbol{C_i}, \boldsymbol{C_o}, I)}_{\text{contour}} + \underbrace{F_r(\mathcal{M}, \mathcal{B}, I)}_{\text{region}} \right\}$$

Shape: *Shape* constraint is composed of three terms:

$$F_s(\boldsymbol{C}) = \lambda_0 F_{regularity}(\boldsymbol{C}, w) + \lambda_1 F_{smoothness}(\boldsymbol{C}) + \lambda_2 F_{similarity}(\boldsymbol{C}) \quad (1)$$

The first one regularizes template width:

$$F_{regularity}(\boldsymbol{C}, w) = \int_0^1 |w'(s)| ds$$

The *smoothness* term controls centerline curvature:

$$F_{smoothness}(\boldsymbol{C}) = \int_0^1 |\kappa(s) - \kappa_0| ds$$

where $\kappa(s)$ stands for the curvature of the centerline $\boldsymbol{C}(s)$ and κ_0 is a desired curvature, *e.g.* setting it to average curvature constrains the contour to be circular (see Sec. 2.5).

The *similarity* term constraints the template curve shape to be affinely similar with a pre-defined shape $\tilde{\boldsymbol{C}}$. It is defined as an error of the best affine transformation T between the given contour $\boldsymbol{C}$ and a pre-defined contour $\tilde{\boldsymbol{C}}$:

$$F_{similarity}(\boldsymbol{C}) = \int_0^1 |\boldsymbol{C}(s) - T(\tilde{\boldsymbol{C}}(s))|^2 ds$$

Contour: The contour term stands for the contour contrast, both local (first two terms) and global (last term):

$$F_c(\boldsymbol{C_i}, \boldsymbol{C_o}, I) = \lambda_3 \int_0^1 \nabla I(\boldsymbol{C_i}(s)).\boldsymbol{n}(s) ds - \lambda_4 \int_0^1 |\nabla I(\boldsymbol{C_o}(s)).\boldsymbol{n}(s)| ds + \lambda_5 (\overline{m} - \overline{b})$$
(2)

where ∇I is the image gradient, $n(s)$ contour's normal, $\overline{m}$ and $\overline{b}$ are the average intensities of the regions $\mathcal{M}$ and $\mathcal{B}$, respectively.

Region: The myocardium and the blood pool gray levels, except for the papillary muscles region, should be homogeneously distributed. Therefore we can define F_r using a minimal variance criterion such as:

$$F_r(\mathcal{M}, \mathcal{B}, I) = \frac{\lambda_6}{|\mathcal{M}|} \int_{\mathcal{M}} |I(x,y) - \overline{m}|^2 \, dxdy + \frac{\lambda_7}{|\mathcal{B}|} \int_{\mathcal{B}} |I(x,y) - \overline{b}|^2 \, dxdy \quad (3)$$

where region $\mathcal{M}$ (resp. $\mathcal{B}$) has average intensity $\overline{m}$ (resp. $\overline{b}$) and area $|\mathcal{M}|$ (resp. $|\mathcal{B}|$). In order to increase robustness to the expected presence of papillary muscles, which breaks the blood pool homogeneity assumption, a rather effective approach is to remove the contribution of a certain percentage (e.g., 15%) of the darkest pixels in region $\mathcal{B}$ from the variance computation.

2.3 Optimization Strategy

We use a greedy optimization scheme embedded in a coarse-to-fine approach to optimize simultaneously the nodes position and ribbon width. Due to using very few nodes and a global criterion, each optimization step influences an important portion of the model, thus allowing potential jumps over local minima. Unfortunately, casting normals with such a sparse sampling makes the solution dependent on the initial position of the nodes, hence decreasing parameterization invariance. We compensate for this drawback of the original scheme by a systematic sliding of all nodes along the centerline between each iteration.

2.4 Segmentation of Long Axis Images

Template creation and initial pose: The initial template should resemble the LV shape, so its centerline can be approximated by an ellipse which axes are aligned with the main axes of the LV; it is slightly bended inside for modeling valve shape (Fig. 2-left). For initialization of LA template, we need to define its position (p_c) and orientation ($\vec{u}$). These parameters can be first obtained in patient coordinates, and then easily transformed into the image ones. When two LA views are available, we reasonably assume (due to standard acquisition planning) that an intersection of the two LA image planes is approximately aligned with the real LA of the heart (Fig. 2-center) and therefore can be taken as $\vec{u}$ (it is taken co-oriented with the Z axis of the SA). The template origin p_c is obtained as an intersection of the axis $\vec{u}$ with the middle slice of the SA volume. When only one LA view is available, we align $\vec{u}$ with Z axis of the SA volume, and the template origin is defined as a closest $\vec{u}$ point to the center of SA volume p_o, since a typical SA acquisition is centered on LV (Fig. 2-right).

Template deformation: The deformation is done in two steps: coarse (rigid) and fine (local). At the coarse step, the initial template is affinely optimized using only two minimization terms, namely *contour* (Eq. 2) and *region* (Eq. 3), since the shape is implicitly conserved by the transformation. Note also that

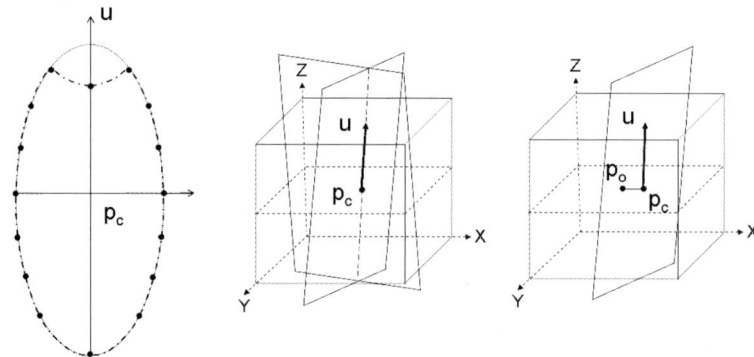

Fig. 2. LA template: centerline as an ellipse with upper bending modeling the valve (**left**); LA template initial pose using SA volume, represented as a cube, and two LA views, represented as planes (**center**); Similarly to later, LA template initial pose with SA volume and only one LA view (**right**)

in the contour term only global contrast contributes at this stage ($\lambda_3, \lambda_4 \rightarrow 0$). This step, allowing to robustly detect the LV position, is followed by a local deformation, using all three terms. In the *contour constraint*, only local contrast is now put to contribution ($\lambda_5 \rightarrow 0$), while in the *shape constraint* (Eq. 1) only *regularity* and *similarity* terms are used ($\lambda_1 \rightarrow 0$). In addition, contour resulting from the coarse step is used as $\tilde{C}$, which preserves certain contour similarity with the initial shape and in particular allows to softly constrain valve concavity.

2.5 Segmentation of Short Axis Images

Template creation and initial pose: The SA template centerline can be approximated by a circle. Thus, SA template creation is quite obvious since one only needs to define the template center and radius (Fig. 3-left). Given the LA segmentation results, the LV LA contour(s) intersections are found at each SA slice. If two LA contours are available, the template parameters are found by fitting a best circle through 4 intersection points (Fig. 3-center), while if only one contour is given, the template center is defined as the middle of the intersection segment and its radius as a half of its length (Fig. 3-right). Note that if no LA images are available, the initialization of SA templates can still be done using robust ring detection algorithm [21].

Template deformation: The SA template deformation follows the same coarse-to-fine scheme as the LA. The optimization terms used at coarse step are exactly the same as in Sec. 2.4. At the fine step, the *contour* and the *region* terms are again the same as for LA, while the *shape constraint* comprises only *regularity* and *smoothness* terms (in the later one, κ_0 is set to the average contour curvature to impose contour circularity, thus also substituting the *similarity* term).

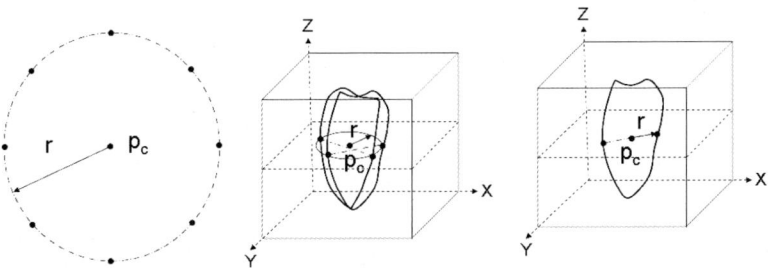

Fig. 3. SA template centerline as a circle (**left**); SA template initial pose using intersection of two LA contours with a SA volume slice (**center**); SA template initial pose using intersection of only one LA contour with a SA volume slice (**right**)

3 Validation

Data: The clinical data used for validating our method included 35 patients. SA cine CMR scans comprised 9-14 slices and 15-50 phases; all SA images were 256x256 in size, covering a field of view ranging from 360x360 mm up to 450x450 mm. For 5 patients two LA views (2 chambers (CH) and 4CH) were available, while for the remaining ones only 4CH LA views were acquired. All LA images were 256x256 in size, covering a field of view ranging from 350x350 mm up to 460x460 mm. Manual delineations, done by an expert, were available for all end-diastolic (ED) images (325 in total of SA and 40 for LA).

Results: To compare the result of our automatic segmentation method with the manually delineated contours, we measured the mean distance (ε_{mean}), the root-mean-square (RMS) distance (ε_{rms}) and the maximum distance (ε_{max}) between the resulting contours and the manual ones, using method explained in [22]. For SA images, mean positioning errors was 1.3 mm for the endocardium and 1.5 mm for the epicardium, for a pixel size ranging from 1.4 mm to 1.8 mm (see Table 1). For LA images, mean positioning errors was 1.3 mm for the endocardium and 1.1 mm for the epicardium, for a pixel size ranging from 1.3 mm to 1.8 mm. An excellent correlation was found between "manual" and "automatic" volumes ($r=0.90$, $P < 0.001$), with mean difference -10 ± 18 ml ($P = 0.002$). Note that all results were obtained with exactly the same method settings and without any user interaction. An example of segmentation results for one patient (2 LA views and 8 SA slices) is shown in Fig. 4. In our current implementation, the overall segmentation time is around 1 second per image on a 3.2 GHz PC, thus segmentation of a typical image phase (SA+LA) takes about 10 seconds.

Discussion: LA template initialization proved to be robust even using only one LA image, the same stands for the initialization of SA templates from only one LA segmentation contour. Note also that SA initialization was robust to slices misregistration, since possible initialization inaccuracies were compensated by the rigid deformation. Producing a mean positioning error inferior to one pixel for

Table 1. Endocardial and epicardial positioning errors compared to manual contours

	Endocardial contours			Epicardial contours		
	ε_{mean} (mm)	ε_{rms} (mm)	ε_{max} (mm)	ε_{mean} (mm)	ε_{rms} (mm)	ε_{max} (mm)
SA	1.27 ± 0.54	1.56 ± 0.70	3.29 ± 1.62	1.56 ± 0.85	1.93 ± 1.04	4.06 ± 2.18
LA	1.32 ± 0.41	1.69 ± 0.55	4.55 ± 1.84	1.13 ± 0.42	1.52 ± 0.67	4.01 ± 2.27

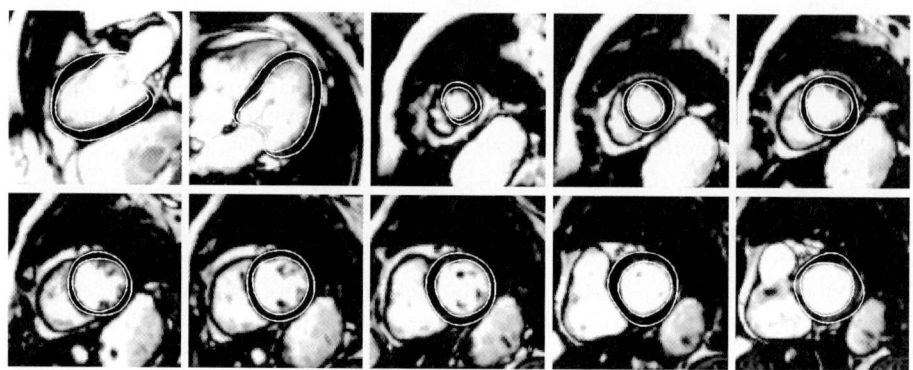

Fig. 4. LV segmentation example for one patient (from left to right, up to bottom): LA 2CH image; LA 4CH image; consecutive slices of SA volume from apex to valve

both SA and LA images, comparable with inter-expert drawing variability [11], the method proved accurate and robust. We validated the method for ED phase only, since the segmentation of the whole cardiac cycle can be then obtained using automatic contour propagation [22], shown to preserve its accuracy within acceptable ranges while being much faster than phase-by-phase segmentation.

4 Conclusion

We developed a fully automatic, robust and accurate method for segmentation of CMR SA and LA acquisitions, enabling easy introduction of prior knowledge and constraints in the optimization framework. The method was extensively validated by comparing the segmentation results with manually drawn endocardial and epicardial contours for 35 patients (325 SA slices and 40 LA images). The positioning error was inferior to one pixel for both SA and LA images and is comparable with interobserver variability. The resulting contours can be used for SA slice alignment, contour propagation and accurate LV parameter estimation.

References

1. Weaver, A., et al.: Magnitude and causes of interobserver discrepancies in CMR volumme measurements: critical importance of choice of the basal slice. Journal of Cardiovascular Magnetic Resonance 1, 82–83 (2006)

2. Anderson, J., et al.: Normal cardiac magnetic resonance measurements and interobserver discrepancies in volumes and mass using the papillary muscle inclusion method. The Open General and Internal Medicine Journal 1, 6–12 (2007)
3. van Geuns, R., et al.: Automatic quantitative left ventricular analysis of cine MR images by using threedimensional information for contour detection. Radiology 240(1), 215–221 (2006)
4. Mitchell, S.C., et al.: Multistage hybrid active appearance model matching: segmentation of left and right ventricles in cardiac MR images. IEEE Trans. Med. Imag. 20(5), 415–423 (2001)
5. Kaus, M.R., et al.: Automated segmentation of the left ventricle in cardiac MRI. Medical Image Analysis 8(3), 245–254 (2004)
6. Niessen, W.J., et al.: Geodesic deformable models for medical image analysis. IEEE Trans. Med. Imag. 17(4), 634–641 (1998)
7. Paragios, N.: A variational approach for the segmentation of the left ventricle in cardiac image analysis. Int. J. Comp. Vision 50(3), 345–362 (2002)
8. Jolly, M.P.: Automatic segmentation of the left ventricle in cardiac MR and CT images. Int. J. Comp. Vision 70(2), 151–163 (2006)
9. Lelieveldt, B., et al.: Multi-view active appearance models for consistent segmentation of multiple standard views: application to long- and short-axis cardiac MR images. In: Int. Congress Series, vol. 1256, pp. 1141–1146 (2003)
10. Lotjonen, J., et al.: Statistical shape model of atria, ventricles and epicardium from short- and long-axis MR images. Medical Image Analysis (8), 371–386 (2004)
11. van Assen, H., et al.: SPASM: A 3D-ASM for segmentation of sparse and arbitrarily oriented cardiac MRI data. Medical Image Analysis 10, 286–303 (2006)
12. Moore, J., et al.: A high resolution dynamic heart model based on averaged MRI data. In: Ellis, R.E., Peters, T.M. (eds.) MICCAI 2003. LNCS, vol. 2878, pp. 549–555. Springer, Heidelberg (2003)
13. Lotjonen, J., et al.: Correction of movement artifacts from 4-d cardiac short- and long-axis MR data. In: Barillot, C., Haynor, D.R., Hellier, P. (eds.) MICCAI 2004. LNCS, vol. 3217, pp. 405–412. Springer, Heidelberg (2004)
14. Perperidis, D., et al.: Statistical shape model of atria, ventricles and epicardium from short- and long-axis MR images. Medical Image Analysis 9(8), 441–456 (2005)
15. Hautvast, G., Cocosco, C., Kedenburg, G., Breeuwer, M.: Alignment of short axis and long axis cine cardiac MR images. In: CARS 2006, vol. 1, pp. 59–60 (2006)
16. Slomka, P.J., et al.: Automated registration of multiple single breath-hold cardiac MRI images. Intl. Soc. Mag. Reson. Med. 14, 1207 (2006)
17. Li, T., Denney, T.: Registration of short and long-axis images in cine cardiac MRI. Intl. Soc. Mag. Reson. Med. 14, 1208 (2006)
18. Kass, M., Witkin, A., Terzopoulos, D.: Snakes: active contour models. Int. J. Comp. Vision 1(4), 321–331 (1987)
19. Menet, S., Saint-Marc, P., Medioni, G.B.: BSnakes: implementation and application to stereo. In: Image Understanding Workshop, Pittsburgh, PA, pp. 720–726 (1990)
20. Williams, D.J., Shah, M.: A fast algorithm for active contours and curvature estimation. CVGIP: Image Understanding 55(1), 14–26 (1992)
21. Breeuwer, M., Hautvast, G., Mory, B., Fradkin, M.: Automatic segmentation of short-axis cine cardiac magnetic resonance. In: CARS 2008 (2008)
22. Hautvast, G., et al.: Automatic contour propagation in cine cardiac magnetic resonance images. IEEE Trans. Med. Imag. 25(11), 1472–1482 (2006)

Segmentation of Pathologic Hearts in Long-Axis Late-Enhancement MRI

Cybèle Ciofolo and Maxim Fradkin

Medisys Research Lab, Philips Healthcare, Suresnes, France
cybele.ciofolo@philips.com

Abstract. We propose a new method to segment long-axis cardiac MR images acquired with a late-enhancement protocol. Detecting the myocardium boundaries is difficult in these images because healthy myocardium appears dark while the intensity of enhanced areas ranges from gray to white, depending on the myocardial damage. In this context, geometrical template deformation, alternated with the update of a damaged tissue map, allows us to include abnormal myocardium parts in the final segmentation. The template and map are initialized using short-axis images and the deformation parameters are adapted according to the type of enhancement pattern. Good segmentation results are obtained on a database of real pathologic heart images presenting various types of abnormal myocardium tissues.

1 Introduction

Viability assessment is nowadays an unavoidable part of cardiac examinations, used for both surgery and therapy planning. In particular, the proportion of viable myocardium is a major factor in determining whether a patient may benefit from revascularization. In order to locate and quantify the extent of abnormal myocardial tissues, clinicians generally use late-enhancement cardiac magnetic resonance (LE CMR) images, which are acquired around twenty minutes after contrast agent injection. At the LE CMR acquisition time, due to the loss of membrane integrity in damaged tissues, the constrast agent accumulates in abnormal parts of the myocardium, which are consequently enhanced (become bright) while healthy myocardium remains dark, as shown in Fig. 1. Although short-axis (SA) slices are useful to have a global estimation of the damaged tissues position in the left ventricle, they are generally acquired with poor resolution along the ventricle long axis (around 5 to 10mm). Long-axis (LA) images (2 chambers and 4 chambers views) consequently bring useful additional information to viability studies, especially concerning the apical area.

Many publications and commercial products propose automatic or semi-automatic methods to segment the left ventricle in CMR images. However, most of them, involving shape and appearance models [1,2], deformable meshes [2], level sets [3,4] or graph-cuts [5] relate to functional (or cine) images, in which there is no enhanced area in the myocardium. As for late-enhancement acquisitions, in addition to semi-automatic approaches, generally used to delineate the

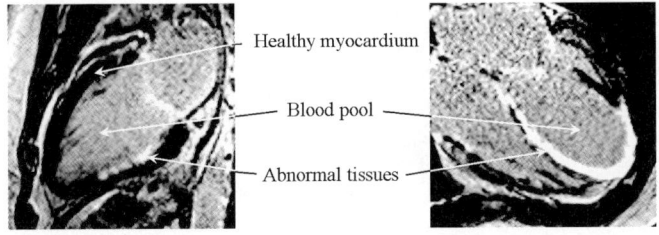

Fig. 1. Examples of long-axis late-enhancement images of pathologic hearts

myocardium contours in SA images [6,7], one automatic segmentation algorithm was published by Dikici et. al. [8] and more recently, we also proposed a new automatic approach [9]. But to the best of our knowledge, no method has yet been reported for segmenting LE LA images, which is the objective of this work.

The main difficulty with processing LE CMR data is the non-homogeneous intensity of the myocardium resulting from contrast agent accumulation in abnormal tissues, which leads to various enhanced patterns, depending on the myocardial damage. Moreover, contrary to SA images, no ring shape prior can be used to segment the myocardium in LA images. In this work, we present an iterative algorithm which alternates the deformation of a geometrical template toward the myocardium boundaries and the update of a damaged tissue map to guide the deformation. This is done automatically, except for a one-time user choice which specifies the enhancement pattern among four pre-defined ones.

This paper is organized as follows: the myocardium segmentation method is presented in Section 2 and quantitatively assessed in Section 3, then we conclude in Section 4.

2 Method

This section describes the main features of our algorithm: the deformable template representing the myocardium, the associated binary map of abnormal tissues and the iterative workflow which leads to the final segmentation.

2.1 Deformable Template

Template description. The myocardium is modelled as a closed ribbon structure with an imaginary centerline $\boldsymbol{C}(s) = (x(s), y(s))$ and a variable width $w(s)$, both of which are continuous spline interpolations of a discrete set of $\{p_k = (x_k, y_k, w_k)\}$ samples defined at each node (see Fig. 2). This compact representation provides a natural coupling between the endocardium $\boldsymbol{C_i}$ and the epicardium $\boldsymbol{C_o}$ (the inside and outside contours). We also define the two regions $\mathcal{M}$ and $\mathcal{B}$, corresponding respectively to the myocardium and blood pool, as shown in Fig. 2.

Template deformation. We aim at finding the set of parameters minimizing a criterion that expresses the match of the template and the image evidence,

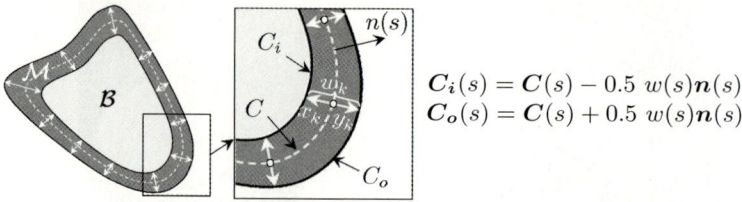

Fig. 2. Template geometry (left); Detailed zoom (center)

given some prior knowledge. Built from observations of typical cardiac images, this knowledge is translated into mathematical terms expressing shape, contour and region constraints. In the remainder, I is the image and the λ_i's are scalar weights balancing the various terms. Let $\boldsymbol{p} = \{p_k = (x_k, y_k, w_k)^T, k \in [\![1, N]\!]\}$ be our parametric model. The problem can now be formalized as follows:

$$\min_{\boldsymbol{p}} \left\{ F(\boldsymbol{p}, I) = \underbrace{F_s(\boldsymbol{C}, w)}_{\text{shape}} + \underbrace{F_c(\boldsymbol{C_i}, \boldsymbol{C_o}, I)}_{\text{contour}} + \underbrace{F_r(\mathcal{M}, \mathcal{B}, I)}_{\text{region}} \right\}$$

Shape: the first part of this term constraints the template curve shape to be affinely similar with a pre-defined shape $\tilde{\boldsymbol{C}}$. It is defined as the error of the best affine transformation T between the current contour $\boldsymbol{C}$ and a pre-defined contour $\tilde{\boldsymbol{C}}$. The second part is a regularity constraint on the template width variation:

$$F_s(\boldsymbol{C}, w) = \lambda_0 \int_0^1 |\boldsymbol{C}(s) - T(\tilde{\boldsymbol{C}}(s))|^2 ds + \lambda_1 \int_0^1 |w'(s)|^2 ds.$$

At the beginning of the segmentation, $\tilde{\boldsymbol{C}}$ is the initial template. During the segmentation process, it is updated as explained in the segmentation workflow described in Section 2.3, and set equal to the most recent template shape, which is more reliable than the initial one. One particular advantage of this similarity term is to softly constrain the valve plane shape and curvature.

Contour: The endocardium and the epicardium walls are preferred locations of image gradients, as expressed by:

$$F_c(\boldsymbol{C_i}, \boldsymbol{C_o}, I) = \lambda_2 \int_0^1 \nabla I_{in}(s) ds - \lambda_3 \int_0^1 |\nabla I_{on}(s)| ds,$$

where $\nabla I_{in} = \nabla I(\boldsymbol{C_i}(s)).\boldsymbol{n}(s)$ (respectively ∇I_{on} with $\boldsymbol{C_o}$), ∇I is the image gradient and $\boldsymbol{n}(s)$ is the outward-pointing normal to the centerline. To implement this term, we use gradient filters that express prior knowledge on the relative intensity of normal and abnormal parts of the myocardium, as explained in the *Special processing for abnormal tissues* paragraph below.

Region: The blood pool gray levels should be homogeneously distributed. Also, normal myocardium tissues are dark while abnormal ones are bright, which results in a strong global contrast with the blood pool. Therefore we have:

$$F_r(\mathcal{M}, \mathcal{B}, I) = \frac{\lambda_4}{|\mathcal{M}|} \int_{\mathcal{M}} |I(x,y) - \overline{m}| \, dx dy$$
$$+ \frac{\lambda_5}{|\mathcal{B}|} \int_{\mathcal{B}} |I(x,y) - \overline{b}| \, dx dy + \lambda_6(\overline{m} - \overline{b}),$$

where region $\mathcal{B}$ has an average intensity $\overline{b}$ and area $|\mathcal{B}|$, while the expected intensity is $\overline{m}$ for the myocardium region $\mathcal{M}$.

Special processing for abnormal tissues. As mentioned earlier, the intensities of abnormal myocardial parts differ from those of healthy regions, which implies some adaptation of the criterion terms. Abnormal areas are detected with a map of abnormal tissues that is computed and updated during the segmentation process, as explained in Section 2.2. If the detection is positive, as damaged myocardium is brighter than the surrounding organs, the gradient filters defining the expected contrast along the borders are inverted. For the same reason, the expected value inside the myocardium $\bar{m}$ (used in F_r) is the maximum value of the intensity range instead of the minimum value for healthy myocardium. Let us note that these extremal values are not *ad hoc* parameters but come from the acquisition parameters of real LE CMR images, which are tuned so that the healthy myocardium appears as dark as possible and scars as bright as possible.

Initialization. Correctly positioning the geometrical template with no prior information concerning damaged tissues is very difficult, especially if large parts of the myocardium are enhanced. For this reason, the template is initialized using the segmentation result that is automatically obtained in the SA images acquired in the same examination as the LA views [9]. The SA result consists in two 3D meshes representing the inner and outer myocardium walls in the stack of SA images. To initialize the template position, we compute the intersection between the meshes, the SA slices and the LA plane. This results in pairs of points (endocardium and epicardium) sampled along the myocardium (Fig. 3(a-b)). However, SA and LA images being acquired at different breatholds, they are slightly misaligned and the intersections can be used for initialization only. Each pair of points then defines the template width associated to a node initially positioned at the center of the pair. As the SA slices do not intersect the left ventricle apical area, an additional node is computed by extrapolation: $\mathbf{x}_{p_a} = \frac{1}{2}(\mathbf{x}_{p_0} + \mathbf{x}_{p_1}) + ((\mathbf{x}_{p_0} - \mathbf{x}_{p_2}) + (\mathbf{x}_{p_1} - \mathbf{x}_{p_3}))$, where $\mathbf{x}_{p_i}$ is the position vector of the node p_i, whose location on the template is shown in Fig. 3(c). The width associated to the extrapolated p_a node is the average width computed over all the other nodes. Finally, the centerline is interpolated from the nodes position and the nodes are equally resampled to obtain the initial template (Fig. 3(d)).

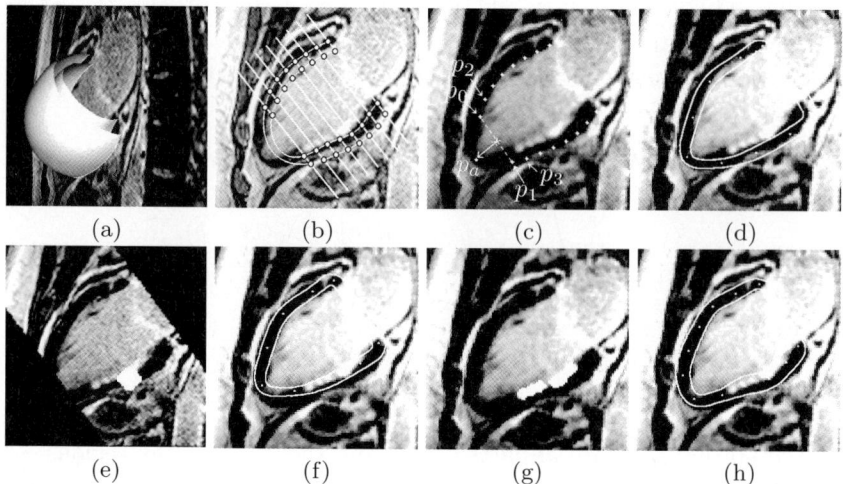

Fig. 3. (a)-(b) Intersection of SA meshes with SA slices and LA plane; (c) Initial position of the template nodes; (d) Initial template; (e) Initial map of abnormal tissues based on SA meshes, with black areas corresponding to regions not covered by the SA slices, where no information is available; (f) Coarse segmentation based on initial map; (g) Updated map of abnormal tissues; (h) Final result based on updated map

Optimization. We use a *greedy* optimization scheme [10] embedded in a coarse-to-fine approach to simultaneaously optimize the nodes position and ribbon width.

2.2 Map of Abnormal Tissues

Map description. The map of abnormal tissues is a binary 2D image with the same dimensions as the LA image, whose non-zero pixels indicate the location of likely abnormal tissues. Examples of such maps superimposed on the LA image are shown in Fig. 3(e) and Fig. 3(g).

Map initialization. The organs surrounding the myocardium constitute a textured background, which makes the detection of abnormal tissues very difficult if no prior information about the left ventricle boundaries is provided at the beginning of the segmentation process. Consequently, the 3D meshes resulting from SA segmentation are used once again. More precisely, our SA automatic algorithm detects abnormal tissues by comparison with the mean blood pool intensity and labels the corresponding vertices in the 3D meshes. Among these vertices, the closest to the LA plane are projected onto it. Simple morphological operations (closing and dilation) applied on the projected labels lead to the initial map of abnormal tissues (Fig. 3(e)).

Map update. After the first (or coarse) segmentation operation, the map is updated using the current position of the template contours. First, an area of interest is defined along the centerline. This area has to be large enough in the blood pool direction to include subendocardial scars. Then, a thresholding followed by morphological closing and dilation are done in the area of interest to obtain a new map with large "likely abnormal tissues" areas (Fig. 3(g)).

2.3 Segmentation Workflow

The segmentation is done with the following succession of operations:

1. *Fully automatic segmentation of SA views* (Result visible in Fig. 3(a));
2. *Initalization of the geometrical template position* (Fig. 3(b-d));
3. *Initial map of abnormal tissues estimation* (Fig. 3(e));
4. *Coarse deformation of the geometrical template* (Fig. 3(f)): at this stage, as the initial map may not include all abnormal tissues, the segmentation is difficult for images presenting large transmural scars (see Fig. 4(b)). A strong weight is consequently given to the shape term to avoid large deformations around damaged areas;
5. *Update of both the map of abnormal tissues and $\tilde{C}$ contour* (Fig. 3(g));
6. *Fine deformation of the geometrical template according to the updated map* (Fig. 3(h)): the map is now more reliable and the shape constraint is relaxed. Stronger and lower weights are given respectively to the homogeneity and contour terms, which allows the final contours to enclose damaged areas.

Four sets of deformation parameters are pre-defined, corresponding to the type of damaged tissues: large transmural scar, sub-endocardial scar, diffuse or small enhanced areas and no visible scar. At the beginning of the segmentation process, one single choice is required from the user to select one of these four abnormality types. This is the only user interaction that is used in this algorithm.

3 Results

We quantitatively assessed the performance of the method on a database of 20 LE CMR LA acquisitions of 256×256 pixels, with a pixel size of 1.5mm, containing various types of abnormal tissues (large white transmural scars, sub-endocardial scars, scattered white areas...). Three skilled operators provided manual contours for comparison with our segmentation algorithm.

Qualitative results. The myocardium is well segmented in all images, as shown in Fig. 4. The scar map and the decrease of the contrast constraint in the contour term during the fine segmentation phase allow the contours to enclose sub-endocardial scars (Fig. 4(a) and 4(c)). This is of critical importance to compute clinical parameters such as the transmural extent of myocardial damage, generally expressed as a percentage (25%, 50%, 75% or 100%) of the myocardium width. On the other hand, this may induce slight inaccuracies along fuzzy boundaries, especially around the papillary muscles (Fig. 4(d)) or along the valve plane. However, this does not affect the damage areas and the related clinical parameters, it is thus considered as acceptable.

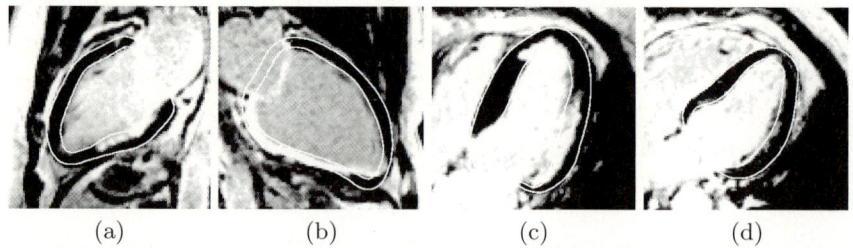

(a) (b) (c) (d)

Fig. 4. Examples of segmentation results with various enhancement patterns. (a) Subendocardial scar; (b) Large transmural scar; (c) Several sub-endocardial scars; (d) Fuzzy endocardium boundary.

Table 1. Mean distance D (in millimeters and pixels) to manual contours drawn by 3 human observers ($Ref1$ to $Ref3$) and inter-observer variability

Contour	Unit	D_{Ref1}	D_{Ref2}	D_{Ref3}	Variability
Endocardium	mm	2.4 ± 0.9	2.6 ± 0.9	2.3 ± 0.8	1.7 ± 0.7
	pixels	1.6 ± 0.6	1.7 ± 0.6	1.5 ± 0.5	1.1 ± 0.5
Epicardium	mm	2.3 ± 1.0	2.4 ± 0.9	2.4 ± 1.1	1.5 ± 0.9
	pixels	1.5 ± 0.6	1.6 ± 0.6	1.6 ± 0.7	1.0 ± 0.6

Quantitative assessment. The distance between contours segmented with our algorithm and contours drawn by each of the three experts is computed after exclusion of the valve plane area: the manual contours are drawn so that the valve plane is defined by a straight line and all the points above this line are automatically excluded from all contours. The mean distance values are summarized in Table 1, as well as the mean distance between each manual contour and the same contour drawn by the two other operators, which illustrates inter-observer variability.

The mean positioning error is around 1.5 pixels, which is a reasonable result to compute viability parameters, given that the inter-observer variability is around or higher than 1 pixel, depending on the contour. Let us note that these variability values are larger than those observed in functional (cine) images [11], showing that the segmentation of LE CMR data is particularly challenging. Also, the areas where larger errors occur correspond to areas with larger inter-observer variability, such as fuzzy boundary regions like low-contrasted scars, around the papillary muscles or regions close to the valve plane.

Finally, the LA segmentation takes 7 seconds in average with a 3.19GHz PC.

4 Conclusion

We proposed a new method to delineate myocardial contours in long-axis late-enhancement images with a minimal user interaction, using a deformable template and binary scar maps. The quantitative evaluation showed that the obtained contours are accurately positioned and are eligible to automatically compute clinical parameters, such as the transmural extent of myocardial scar following heart infarct.

Acknowledgments

We are grateful to Benoît Mory from the Medisys Research Lab of Philips Healthcare for helping us in designing the deformable template and associated optimization scheme. We also would like to thank Gilion Hautvast and Marcel Breeuwer from Philips Healthcare — The Netherlands for fruitful discussions, active participation in programming and providing us with images and manual contours.

References

1. Mitchell, S.C., et al.: Multistage hybrid active appearance model matching: segmentation of left and right ventricles in cardiac MR images. IEEE Trans. Med. Imag. 20(5), 415–423 (2001)
2. Kaus, M.R., et al.: Automated segmentation of the left ventricle in cardiac MRI. Medical Image Analysis 8(3), 245–254 (2004)
3. Niessen, W.J., et al.: Geodesic deformable models for medical image analysis. IEEE Trans. Med. Imag. 17(4), 634–641 (1998)
4. Paragios, N.: A variational approach for the segmentation of the left ventricle in cardiac image analysis. International Journal of Computer Vision 50(3), 345–362 (2002)
5. Jolly, M.P.: Automatic segmentation of the left ventricle in cardiac MR and CT images. International Journal of Computer Vision 70(2), 151–163 (2006)
6. Noble, N.M.I., et al.: The automatic identification of hibernating myocardium. In: Barillot, C., Haynor, D.R., Hellier, P. (eds.) MICCAI 2004. LNCS, vol. 3217, pp. 890–898. Springer, Heidelberg (2004)
7. Heiberg, E., et al.: Semi-automatic quantification of myocardial infarction from delayed contrast enhanced magnetic resonance imaging. Scandinavian Cardiovascular Journal 39(5), 267–275 (2005)
8. Dikici, E., et al.: Quantification of delayed enhancement MR images. In: Barillot, C., Haynor, D.R., Hellier, P. (eds.) MICCAI 2004. LNCS, vol. 3216, pp. 250–257. Springer, Heidelberg (2004)
9. Ciofolo, C., et al.: Automatic myocardium segmentation in late-enhancement MRI. In: IEEE International Symposium on Biomedical Imaging: From Nano to Macro (ISBI), pp. 225–228 (2008)
10. Williams, D.J., Shah, M.: A fast algorithm for active contours and curvature estimation. Computer Vision, Graphics and Image Processing: Image Understanding 55(1), 14–26 (1992)
11. Hautvast, G., et al.: Automatic contour propagation in cine cardiac magnetic resonance images. IEEE Trans. Med. Imag. 25(11), 1472–1482 (2006)

Automatic Subcortical Segmentation Using a Contextual Model

Jonathan H. Morra[1], Zhuowen Tu[1], Liana G. Apostolova[1,2], Amity E. Green[1,2], Arthur W. Toga[1], and Paul M. Thompson[1]

[1] Laboratory of Neuro Imaging, UCLA School of Medicine, Los Angeles, CA, USA
[2] UCLA Dept. Neurology and Alzheimer's Disease Research Center, Los Angeles, CA, USA

Abstract. Automatically segmenting subcortical structures in brain images has the potential to greatly accelerate drug trials and population studies of disease. Here we propose an automatic subcortical segmentation algorithm using the auto context model. Unlike many segmentation algorithms that separately compute a shape prior and an image appearance model, we develop a framework based on machine learning to learn a unified appearance and context model. We trained our algorithm to segment the hippocampus and tested it on 83 brain MRIs (of 35 Alzheimer's disease patients, 22 with mild cognitive impairment, and 26 normal healthy controls). Using standard distance and overlap metrics, the auto context model method significantly outperformed simpler learning-based algorithms (using AdaBoost alone) and the FreeSurfer system. In tests on a public domain dataset designed to validate segmentation [1], our new algorithm also greatly improved upon a recently-proposed hybrid discriminative/generative approach [2], which was among the top three that performed comparably in a recent head-to-head competition.

1 Introduction

Segmentation of subcortical structures on brain MRI is vital for many clinical and neuroscientific studies. In many studies of brain development or disease, subcortical structures must typically be segmented in large populations of patients and healthy controls, to quantify disease progression over time, to detect factors influencing structural change, and to measure treatment response. In brain MRI, the hippocampus and caudate nucleus are structures of great neurological interest, but are difficult to segment automatically.

3D medical image segmentation has been intensively studied. Most approaches fall into two main categories: those that design strong shape models [3,4,5] and those that rely more on strong appearance models (i.e., based on image intensities) or discriminative models [6,7]; atlas-based, shape-driven and other segmentation methods were recently compared in a caudate benchmark test [1]; despite the progress made, no approach is yet widely used due to (1) slow computation, (2) unsatisfactory results, or (3) poor generalization capability.

In object and scene understanding, it has been increasingly realized that context information plays a vital role [8]. Medical images contain complex patterns including features such as textures (homogeneous, inhomogeneous, and structured) which are also influenced by acquisition protocols. The concept of context covers intra-object consistency (different parts of the same structure) and inter-object configurations (e.g., expected symmetry of left and right hemisphere structures). Here we integrate appearance and context information in a seamless way by automatically incorporating a large number of features through iterative procedures. The resulting algorithm has almost identical testing and training procedures, and segments images rapidly by avoiding an explicit energy minimization step. We test our model for hippocampal segmentation in healthy normal subjects, individuals with Alzheimer's disease (AD), and those in a transitional state, mild cognitive impairment (MCI) and compare the results with a learning-based approach [2] and the publicly available package, FreeSurfer [3].

2 Methods

2.1 Problem

The goal of a subcortical image segmenter is to label each voxel as belonging to a specific region of interest (ROI), such as the hippocampus. Let $X \in (x_1 \ldots x_n)$ be a vector encompassing all N voxels in each manually-labeled training image and $Y \in (y_1 \ldots y_N)$ be the label for each example, with $y_i \in 1 \ldots K$ representing one of K labels (for hippocampal segmentation, this reduces to a two-class problem). According to Bayesian probability, we look for the segmentation

$$Y^* = \operatorname*{argmax}_{Y \in K} p(Y|X) = \operatorname*{argmax}_{Y \in K} p(X|Y)p(Y)$$

where $p(X|Y)$ is the likelihood and $p(Y)$ is the prior distribution on the labeling Y. However, this task is very difficult. Traditionally, many "bottom-up" computer vision approaches (such as SVMs using local features [7]) work hard on directly learning the classification $p(Y|X)$ without encoding rich shape and context information in $p(Y)$, whereas many "top-down" approaches such as deformable models, active surfaces, or atlas-deformation methods impose a strong prior distribution on the global geometry and allowed spatial relations, and learn a likelihood $p(X|Y)$ with simplified assumptions. Due to the intrinsic difficulty in learning the complex $p(X|Y)$ and $p(Y)$, and searching for the Y^* maximizing the posterior, these approaches have achieved limited success.

Instead, we attempt to model $p(Y|X)$ directly by iteratively learning the marginal distribution $p(y_i|X)$ for each voxel i. The appearance and context features are selected and fused by the learning algorithm automatically.

2.2 Auto Context Model

A traditional classifier can learn a classification model based on local image patches, which we now call

$$\mathbf{P}_k^{(0)} = (\mathbf{P}_k^{(0)}(1), ..., \mathbf{P}_k^{(0)}(n))$$

where $\mathbf{P}_k^{(0)}(i)$ is the posterior marginal for label k at each voxel i learned by a classifier (e.g., boosting or SVM). We construct a new training set

$$S_1 = \{(y_i, X(N_i), \mathbf{P}^{(0)}(N_i)), i = 1..n\},$$

where $\mathbf{P}^{(0)}(i)$ are the classification maps centered at voxel i. We train a new classifier, not only on the features from the image patch $X(N_i)$, but also on the probability patch, $\mathbf{P}^{(0)}(N_i)$, of a large number of context voxels. These voxels may be either near or very far from i. It is up to the learning algorithm to select and fuse important supporting context voxels, together with features about image appearance. For our purposes, our feature pool consisted of 18,099 features including intensity, position, and neighborhood features. Our neighborhood features were mean filters, standard deviation filters, curvature filters, and gradients of size 1x1x1 to 3x3x3, and Haar filters of various shapes from size 2x2x2 to 7x7x7. Our AdaBoost weak learners were decision stumps on both the image map and probability map. Once a new classifier is learned, the algorithm repeats the same procedure until it converges. The algorithm iteratively updates the marginal distribution to approach

$$p^{(n)}(y_i|X(N_i), \mathbf{P}^{(n-1)}(N_i)) \rightarrow p(y_i|X) = \int p(y_i, y_{-i}|X) dy_{-i}. \qquad (1)$$

In fact, even the first classifier is trained the same way as the others by giving it a probability map with a uniform distribution. Since the uniform distribution is not informative at all, the context features are not selected by the first classifier. In some applications, e.g. medical image segmentation, the positions of the anatomical structures are roughly known after registration to a standard atlas space. One then can provide a probability map of the structure (based on how often it occurs at each voxel) as the initial $\mathbf{P}^{(0)}$.

We can prove that at each iteration, ACM is decreasing the error ϵ_t. If we note that the error of one example (i), at time $t-1$ is $\mathbf{P}^{(t-1)}(i)(y_i)$ and at time t

---

Given a set of training images together with their label maps, $S = \{(Y_j, X_j), j = 1..m\}$: For each image X_j, construct probability maps $\mathbf{P}_j^{(0)}$, with a distribution (possibly uniform) on all the labels. For $t = 1, ..., T$:

- Make a training set $S_t = \{(y_{ji}, X_j(N_i), \mathbf{P}_j^{(t-1)}(N_i)), j = 1..m, i = 1..n\}$.
- Train a classifier on both image and context features extracted from $X_j(N_i)$ and $\mathbf{P}_j^{(t-1)}(N_i)$ respectively.
- Use the trained classifier to compute new classification maps $\mathbf{P}_j^{(t)}(i)$ for each training image X_j.

The algorithm outputs a sequence of trained classifiers for $p^{(n)}(y_i|X(N_i), \mathbf{P}^{(n-1)}(N_i))$

Fig. 1. The training procedures of the auto-context algorithm

is $p^t(y_i|X_i, \mathbf{P}^{(t-1)}(i))$, then we can use the log-likelihoods to formulate the error over all examples as in eqn. 2.

$$\epsilon_{t-1} = -\sum_i \log \mathbf{P}^{(t-1)}(i)(y_i), \quad \epsilon_t = -\sum_i \log p^{(t)}(y_i|X_i, \mathbf{P}^{(t-1)}(i)) \quad (2)$$

First, it is trivial to choose $p^{(t)}$ to be a uniform distribution, making $\epsilon_t = \epsilon_{t-1}$. However, boosting (or any other effective discriminative classifier) is guaranteed to choose weak learners to create $p^{(t)}$ that minimize ϵ_t and will fail if none such exists, so therefore, if AdaBoost completes, $\epsilon_t \leq \epsilon_{t-1}$.

3 Results

3.1 Caudate Segmentation

We first tested our algorithm on a recently established caudate segmentation dataset [1]. 4 datasets were provided in this grand challenge competition, 2 for training and 2 for testing. As described in the documents from the organizers: "All MRI images are scanned with an Inversion Recovery Prepped Spoiled Grass sequence on a variety of scanners (GE, Siemens, Philips, mostly 1.5 Tesla). Some datasets have been acquired in axial direction, whereas others in coronal direction. All datasets have been re-oriented to axial RAI-orientation, but have not been aligned in any fashion." Due to space limits, we refer the readers to [1] for definitions of the error metrics reported here. Results on the two test datasets were uploaded to the benchmark server; performance was measured by the benchmark test organizers. The first two rows are UNC pediatric and elderly datasets, and the third is from the Brigham Women's Hospital.

Table 1. Error metrics on the caudate segmentation by [2]; the overall score is 59.71

Case	OE	Score	VD	Score	AD	Score	RMSD	Score	MD	Score	Total
UNC Ped	40.35	74.62	-23.21	59.46	0.86	68.25	1.21	78.38	5.64	83.41	72.82
UNC Eld	38.75	75.63	-17.23	69.77	0.75	72.15	1.14	79.64	6.79	80.02	75.44
BWH PNL	41.76	73.73	-26.62	53.78	1.51	49.10	3.50	42.05	25.27	28.41	49.42
Average All	40.84	74.31	-23.93	58.30	1.22	57.89	2.53	57.45	17.33	50.62	59.71

Table 2. Error metrics for caudate segmentation by the algorithm proposed here; the overall score is 73.38

Case	OE	Score	VD	Score	AD	Score	RMSD	Score	MD	Score	Total
UNC Ped	33.42	78.98	-12.05	76.50	0.68	74.76	1.09	80.47	12.09	64.44	75.03
UNC Eld	36.79	76.86	-0.69	80.04	0.72	73.37	1.31	76.53	17.61	48.21	71.00
BWH PNL	32.07	78.50	-13.62	74.42	1.17	76.55	1.75	76.45	12.83	62.26	73.64
Average All	33.34	78.26	-10.60	76.03	0.97	75.51	1.52	77.31	13.67	59.78	73.38

Given the ground truth segmentation (A) and an automated segmentation (B), along with $d(a,b)$ defined as the Euclidean distance between 2 points, a and b, we define the following error metrics:
- Precision = $\frac{A \cap B}{B}$
- Recall = $\frac{A \cap B}{A}$
- Relative Overlap = $\frac{A \cap B}{A \cup B}$
- Similarity Index = $\frac{A \cap B}{(\frac{A+B}{2})}$
- $H_1 = \max_{a \in A}(\min_{b \in B}(d(a,b)))$
- $H_2 = \max_{b \in B}(\min_{a \in A}(d(b,a)))$
- Hausdorff = $\frac{H_1 + H_2}{2}$
- Mean = $\text{avg}_{a \in A}(\min_{b \in B}(d(a,b)))$

Fig. 2. Error metrics used to validate hippocampal segmentations. We note that the Hausdorff distance here is not the standard Hausdorff distance, but instead an alternate way to create a symmetric distance measure.

3.2 Hippocampal Segmentation

For a second test of our algorithm, we segmented the hippocampus in a dataset from a study of Alzheimer's disease (AD) which significantly affects the morphology of the hippocampus [9]. This dataset includes 3D T1-weighted MRIs of individuals in three diagnostic groups: AD, mild cognitive impairment (MCI), and healthy elderly controls. All subjects were scanned on a 1.5 Tesla Siemens scanner, with a standard high-resolution spoiled gradient echo (SPGR) pulse sequence with a TR (repetition time) of 28 ms, TE (echo time) of 6 ms, field of view of 220mm, 256x192 matrix, and slice thickness of 1.5mm. For training we used 27 brain MRIs (9 AD, 9 MCI, and 9 healthy controls), and for testing we used an independent set of 83 brain MRIs (35 AD (age 77.40 ± 6.10), 22 MCI (age 72.27 ± 6.16), and 26 healthy controls (age 65.38 ± 8.35)). Prior to any training or testing, all subjects were registered using 9-parameter linear registration to a population mean template [10]. Fig. 3 shows a typical segmentation of the hippocampus after 0, 1, 4, and 10 iterations of ACM, compared with those of FreeSurfer. Zero iterations of ACM would be equivalent to traditional AdaBoost. Second, to assess segmentation performance quantitatively, we used a variety of error metrics, defined in Fig. 2.

Table 3 summarizes the results through 10 iterations of ACM, and shows that, based on our metrics at least, it segments the hippocampus more accurately than FreeSurfer when using the standardized priors distributed with FreeSurfer. FreeSurfer tends to overestimate the size of the hippocampus as shown by the high recall, but lower precision. Our algorithm takes about 2 hours to train per iteration of ACM, but less than one minute to test (segment a new hippocampus) regardless of the number of ACM iterations, whereas FreeSurfer takes about 10-12 hours to segment a new brain. In fairness, FreeSurfer segments many hundreds of structures, but our algorithm, in this context, is only segmenting the hippocampus (although we could learn a model for any subcortical structure). Also, FreeSurfer is not given the opportunity to learn the specific nuances of this particular dataset, whereas our algorithm is trained on this dataset, which means that FreeSurfer's segmentation could improve if it was given the opportunity to create an atlas based on this dataset. However, FreeSurfer is not provided with training options, and we used it in the standard way.

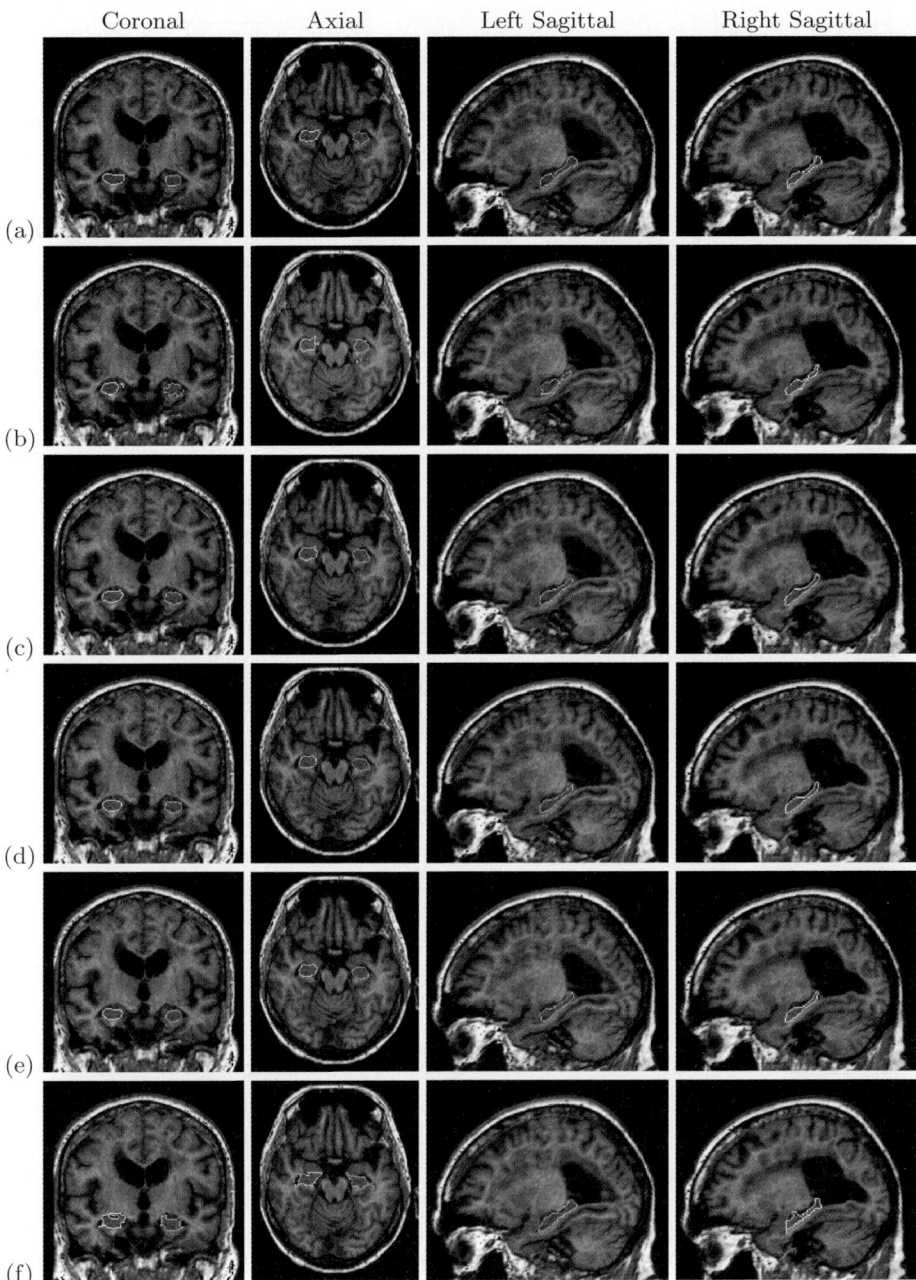

Fig. 3. Hippocampal segmentations improve with the number of ACM iterations. (a) ground truth manual segmentation by an expert (b) 0 ACM iterations (c) 1 ACM iteration (d) 4 ACM iterations (e) 10 ACM iterations (f) FreeSurfer.

Table 3. Precision, recall, relative overlap (R.O.), spatial index (S.I.), Hausdorff distance, and mean distance are reported for training and testing hippocampal segmentation after 10 iterations of ACM. FreeSurfer statistics are also reported for the same dataset for comparison. Distance measures are expressed in millimeters. A value of 1 is optimal for precision, recall, relative overlap, and similarity index; lower values are better for distance metrics.

Training	Left	Right	Testing	Left	Right	FreeSurfer	Left	Right
Precision	0.914	0.883	Precision	0.860	0.857	Precision	0.587	0.588
Recall	0.868	0.836	Recall	0.845	0.750	Recall	0.878	0.917
R.O.	0.802	0.859	R.O.	0.739	0.656	R.O.	0.543	0.558
S.I.	0.890	0.857	S.I.	0.849	0.785	S.I.	0.700	0.713
Hausdorff	2.96	3.85	Hausdorff	3.68	4.61	Hausdorff	5.44	5.04
Mean	0.00204	0.00331	Mean	0.00411	0.00370	Mean	0.432	0.271

Table 4. Percent change is calculated for precision, recall, relative overlap (R.O.), spatial index (S.I.), Hausdorff distance, and mean distance of traditional AdaBoost (ACM with 0 iterations) and ACM with 10 iterations

Training	Left	Right	Testing	Left	Right
Precision	28.90%	10.92%	Precision	36.08%	13.81%
Recall	49.35%	35.89%	Recall	42.12%	27.14%
R.O.	74.95%	42.82%	R.O.	73.85%	34.66%
S.I.	42.57%	25.54%	S.I.	43.22%	20.90%
Hausdorff	-69.53%	-45.82%	Hausdorff	-63.27%	-39.13%
Mean	-83.97%	-48.07%	Mean	-80.85%	-52.75%

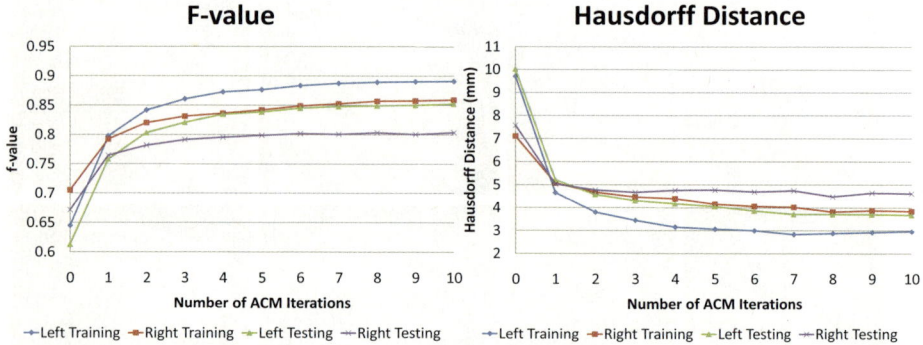

Fig. 4. Effects of varying the number of iterations of ACM on the Hausdorff distance, and the f-value, defined as the average of precision and recall. All error metrics tested in this paper improved as the number of ACM iterations increased.

To show the greatly increased power of using ACM versus just AdaBoost without ACM, Fig. 4 shows how two error metrics improve with the number of iterations of ACM. Fig. 4 shows that ACM gives a large initial improvement, which levels off after about 4 iterations, in both the training and testing datasets, which shows that the AdaBoost learners at this point are relying too much on the features based on $\mathbf{P}^{(t-1)}(N_i)$ and not adding new informative features based on $X(N_i)$. A stopping criterion can also be formulated, such as $\sum_i (\mathbf{P}^{(t)}(i) - \mathbf{P}^{(t-1)}(i))^2 < \epsilon$ (although this is not employed in this paper). Table 4 summarizes the added benefit of ACM, and shows an improvement in all metrics tested, especially the distance metrics and the relative overlap.

4 Conclusion

As shown using a variety of standard overlap metrics, ACM can improve the segmentation performance of AdaBoost for hippocampal and caudate delineation on MRI. ACM is applicable to a wide variety of imaging applications, such applications include tumor recognition and segmenting other subcortical structures; these applications will be the topic of future study. Additionally, ACM can be combined with any pattern recognition algorithm, not just AdaBoost, but AdaBoost allows easy incorporation of features based on $\mathbf{P}^{(t-1)}$.

References

1. van Ginneken, B., Heimann, T., Styner, M.: 3D Segmentation in the Clinic: A Grand Challenge. In: Proc. of MICCAI Workshop (2007)
2. Tu, Z., Narr, K., Dinov, I., Dollár, P., Thompson, P., Toga, A.: Brain anatomical structure parsing by hybrid discriminative/generative models. IEEE TMI (2008)
3. Fischl, B., et al.: Whole brain segmentation: Automated labeling of neuroanatomical structures in the human brain. Neurotechnique 33, 341–355 (2002)
4. Yang, J., Staib, L.H., Duncan, J.S.: Neighbor-constrained segmentation with level set based 3D deformable models. IEEE TMI 23(8), 940–948 (2004)
5. Pohl, K., Fisher, J., Kikinis, R., Grimson, W., Wells, W.: A Bayesian model for joint segmentation and registration. NeuroImage 31(1), 228–239 (2006)
6. Heckemann, R.A., Hajnal, J.V., Aljabar, P., Rueckert, D., Hammers, A.: Automatic anatomical brain MRI segmentation combining label propagation and decision fusion. Neuroimage 33(1), 115–126 (2006)
7. Powell, S., Magnotta, V., Johnson, H., Jammalamadaka, V., Pierson, R., Andreasen, N.: Registration and machine learning based automated segmentation of subcortical and cerebellar brain structures. NeuroImage 39(1), 238–247 (2008)
8. Oliva, A., Torralba, A.: The role of context in object recognition. Trends in Cognitive Sciences 11(12), 520–527 (2007)
9. Becker, J., Davis, S., Hayashi, K., Meltzer, C., Lopez, O., Toga, A., Thompson, P.: 3D patterns of hippocampal atrophy in mild cognitive impairment. Archives of Neurology 63(1), 97–101 (2006)
10. Collins, D., Neelin, P., Peters, T.M., Evans, A.C.: Automatic 3D intersubject registration of MR volumetric data in standardized Talairach space. J. Comput. Assist Tomogr. 18, 192–205 (1994)

Lumbar Disc Localization and Labeling with a Probabilistic Model on Both Pixel and Object Features

Jason J. Corso, Raja' S. Alomari, and Vipin Chaudhary[*]

Department of Computer Science and Engineering
University at Buffalo, State University of New York
jcorso@cse.buffalo.edu

Abstract. Repeatable, quantitative assessment of intervertebral disc pathology requires accurate localization and labeling of the lumbar region discs. To that end, we propose a two-level probabilistic model for such disc localization and labeling. Our model integrates both pixel-level information, such as appearance, and object-level information, such as relative location. Utilizing both levels of information adds robustness to the ambiguous disc intensity signature and high structure variation. Yet, we are able to do efficient (and convergent) localization and labeling with generalized expectation-maximization. We present accurate results on 20 normal cases (96%) and a promising extension to a pathology case.

1 Introduction

Past [1] and recent [2] studies have suggested a need for repeatable quantitative intervertebral disc degeneration (IDD) assessment methods. IDD is prevalent, especially in modern times—about 12 million Americans have some type of IDD—and can cause very high pain levels. One example of an IDD is herniation, where the disc, a structure that acts like a shock-absorber between vertebrae, bulges out of place causing fragments of disc material to press on the nerve roots in the spinal column. In the clinic, a radiologist diagnoses an IDD by first localizing and labeling each intervertebral disc and then identifying any pathology in a given disc based on its local geometry and appearance.

Accurate localizing and labeling is necessary for diagnosis of an IDD pathology. However, the underlying image signal is ambiguous: the intensity of a disc greatly overlaps with that of the spinal nerve fibers. Even the structure can change from case to case, with possible bending of the spinal column (scoliosis) and missing or additional vertebrae [3]. In Figure 1, we show a normal example of the lumbar region of the spinal column with the discs labeled according to the standard scheme.

In this paper, we propose a method to automate the detection and labeling of the intervertebral discs from single MR radiographs. Although we study lumbar discs, our method is directly extensible to the full spinal column. Our method is based on a two-level probabilistic model. On the

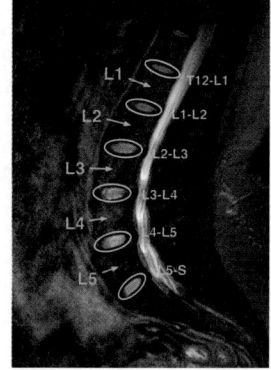

Fig. 1. Lumbar region

[*] This work was supported in part by a grant from NYSTAR.

first level, we model the local pixel-level properties of the discs, such as appearance. On the second level, we capture the object-level geometrical and contextual relationships between discs. The model parameters are estimated from previously labeled cases (supervised learning). The two-level model insulates the localization of the discs from the complex appearance variation in the underlying radiograph leading to a robust and efficient algorithm.

2 Related Work

Automatic localization and labeling of inter-vertebral discs has been a focus of the medical imaging community for over two decades, and it has largely evaded researchers due to the ambiguous disc appearance and high structural variation. Early methods, e.g., Chwialkowski et al. [4], are primarily model- or heuristic-based such as analyzing a horizontal cross-section of intensities to search for the posterior and anterior disc edge. These early models have been influential (e.g., [5]), but were generally tested on few cases and it is not known if they scale.

The recent work by Peng et al. [5] uses such a model-based approach to localize the disc position based on template convolution and an intensity profile. Output from this process is used to help automatically pick the sagittal slice from the *volume* to work with; the slice with minimum variance for peaks of the intensity profile are used. Pekar et al. [6] also develop an approach for labeling the vertebral column as part of scan geometry planning (a step beyond selecting a particular slice from an existing scan). They search for possible disc locations and then do 3D connected components to find disc centers. Masaki et al. [7] also propose a method for automated geometry planning based on intensity and a Hough transform. Five radiologists agree in 9 out of 10 cases that the automatic image plane is as good as or better than manual.

Weiss et al. [8] propose a semi-automatic technique for labeling discs. The user manually marks one disc and then the algorithm proceeds by an iterative intensity-analysis based method. The upper and lower halves of the spine are independently processed using threshold values, filters and noise suppression operators. The technique is highly dependent on imaging quality and data dependent thresholding values. Zheng et al. [9] do segmentation of lumbar vertebrae using digital videofluoroscopic images, which are more noisy than the standard MR radiographs but have a time component. They propose a method based on shape descriptors and a Hough transform (relatively high dimension); the method is validated on synthetic data and a single *in vivo* sequence.

Our proposed method is most similar to the recent work by Schmidt et al. [10]. These two works take a step away from the heuristic driven approaches and construct probabilistic models. [10] define a probabilistic graphical model based on the vertebrae. It incorporates appearance and shape information and uses the A* algorithm, which does a best-first greedy coordinate search for the solution. Their method assumes a full 3D volume, which is not a current clinical standard. In contrast, our method uses a single T2 radiograph (current clinics use multi-spectral radiographs). Their method uses comparatively opaque discriminative models, while we develop a generative probabilistic model that also incorporates appearance and object information but in a more direct, transparent manner. We structure our model in two levels to increase robustness to variation and make it plausible to do full inference using expectation-maximization.

3 Approach

3.1 Conventional Labeling Approach

Our goal is to localize each disc connected to the lumbar vertebrae. One standard probabilistic approach is to formulate a labeling problem with one label per disc and do inference by assigning the most probable label at each pixel. The brain structure labeling work of Fischl et al. [11] is an example of this standard problem formulation. Concretely, let $\Lambda = \{s = (x,y) : 0 \leq x < n, 0 \leq y < m\}$ be the image lattice and consider the image as a map from the lattice to intensities[1], $\texttt{I}\colon \Lambda \mapsto \mathbb{R}$. Define the set of disc labels $\mathcal{A} = \{1, \ldots, 6\}$ (there are six discs connected to lumbar vertebrae), and a set $\mathcal{T}$ of label variables t_i with one for each pixel $i \in \Lambda$. Then, given an image $\texttt{I}$, one seeks the maximum a posteriori estimate of the labels:

$$\mathcal{T}^* = \arg\max_{\mathcal{T}} P(\mathcal{T}|\texttt{I}) \ . \tag{1}$$

However, this inference problem is non-trivial; one typically must make an assumption of independence or rely on (opaque) discriminative models such as the randomized tree classifier as done by Schmidt et al. [10]. Both assumptions may break down due to the high degree of intensity similarity to neighboring anatomy and across discs, the large spatial variability of the discs, and pathological discs (e.g., herniation). Furthermore, it is difficult to incorporate high- or object-level information (such as the relative disc ordering) into this formulation since all of the variables are represented at the pixel level. This difficulty not only affects the robustness of modeling, but also makes it necessary to add post-processing constraints to enforce additional problem specific constraints, such as each disc being a closed elliptical region.

3.2 Two-Level Probabilistic Model

We instead propose a two-level probabilistic model that only requires conditional independence, is generative (more transparent), and adequately insulates the localization variables from the pixel intensities while at the same time modeling the exact disc geometry rather than solely pixel-level labels. Let $\mathcal{D} = \{d_1, d_2, \ldots, d_6\}$ be the set of disc variables with each $d_i = (x_i, y_i)^\mathsf{T}$ representing the disc center (they could also include disc angle, boundary, etc.). Inferring these from an image is our ultimate goal, but we avoid doing it directly due to the difficulties mentioned above. Rather, we introduce a set of auxiliary variables, called disc-label variables and denoted $\mathcal{L} = \{l_i, \forall i \in \Lambda\}$. The disc-labels make it plausible to separate the disc variables from the image intensities; i.e., the disc-label variables will capture the local pixel-level intensity models while the disc variables will capture the high-level geometric and contextual models of

---

[1] These are MR images, but we consider the pixel values as simple intensities without incorporating any special MR related model.

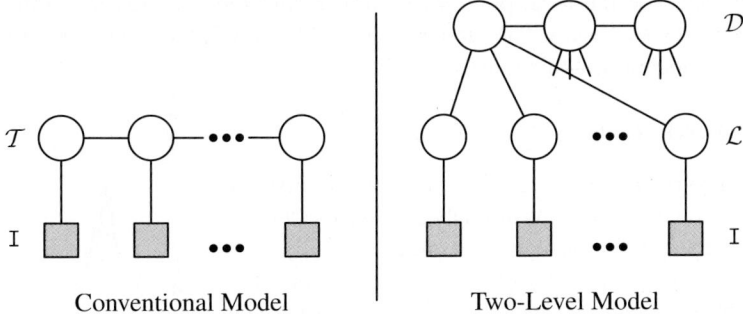

Fig. 2. Graphical models depicting the conventional probabilistic model and our proposed two-level probabilistic model. Our model (right) separates the low- or pixel-level information from the high- or object-level information adding disc localization robustness to the common intensity and structure variation. In the figure, filled squares are observed data (the image) and hollow circles are latent variables. The image and first level ($\mathcal{T}$ and $\mathcal{L}$) sit on the 2D or 3D image lattice Λ, but the high level is a single 1D chain with one node per disc.

the full set of discs. Each disc-label variable can take a value of $\{-1, +1\}$ for non-disc or disc, respectively. Note the simpler situation than above where we had a particular label for each disc. Figure 2 presents and compares the two modeling situations.

We marginalize over the possible disc-labelings since these are auxiliary variables giving the following optimization function:

$$\mathcal{D}^* = \arg\max_{\mathcal{D}} \sum_{\mathcal{L}} P(\mathcal{L}, \mathcal{D}|\mathtt{I}) = \arg\max_{\mathcal{D}} \sum_{\mathcal{L}} P(\mathcal{L}|\mathcal{D}, \mathtt{I}) P(\mathcal{D}) \ , \qquad (2)$$

where the second equality follows from the multi-level nature of the model (the disc variables are assumed independent of the intensities). Note the summation is over a very large set of possible assignments ($2^{|\Lambda|}$). We model it as a Gibbs distribution:

$$P(\mathcal{L}|\mathcal{D}, \mathtt{I}) = \frac{1}{Z[\mathcal{L}]} \exp\bigg[-\beta_1 \sum_{s \in \Lambda} U_\mathrm{I}(l_s, I(s)) \qquad \leftarrow \text{intensity} \quad (3)$$

$$- \beta_2 \sum_{s \in \Lambda} U_\mathrm{D}(l_s, \mathcal{D}) \bigg] \qquad \leftarrow \text{spatial}$$

$$P(\mathcal{D}) = \frac{1}{Z[\mathcal{D}]} \exp\bigg[-\beta_3 \sum_{d_i \in \mathcal{D}} U_\mathrm{L}(d_i) \qquad \leftarrow \text{location}$$

$$- \beta_4 \sum_{(i \sim j)} V_\mathrm{D}(d_i, d_j) \bigg] \qquad \leftarrow \text{disc-context}$$

where $\beta_k \geq 0, k = \{1, \ldots, 4\}$ are tunable parameters and $Z[\cdot]$ are the partition functions. The $(\cdot \sim \cdot)$ notation denotes the set of neighboring elements on the disc chain. Each term will be explicitly defined in the following sections.

The first level, $P(\mathcal{L}|\mathcal{D}, \mathtt{I})$, captures the probability of a particular labeling given both the underlying image and the overlying disc variables. Each potential function models a different aspect of the local pixel-level information (the aspect is mentioned on the right of each equation-line). The second level $P(\mathcal{D})$ models the high-level information about the disc locations and context.

3.3 Low Level Terms

Intensity. The potential, $U_\text{I}(l_s, \mathtt{I}(s))$, models the pixel appearance $\mathtt{I}(s)$ based on its current label l_s. We use a Gaussian for the disc pixels, motivated by empirical study of the distribution of disc pixels (figure 3), and take the negative-log of it for the potential. The parameters of the Gaussian, μ_I and σ_I^2, are learned from labeled training data (specific details in experiments section §4). We drop the normalizing term since it does not depend on the specific intensity value:

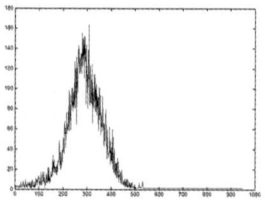

Fig. 3. Disc intensity empirical distribution

$$U_\text{I}(l_s, \mathtt{I}(s)) = \begin{cases} \frac{(\mathtt{I}(s)-\mu_I)^2}{2\sigma_I^2} & \text{if } l_s = +1 \\ -\log\left(1 - \exp\left[-\frac{(\mathtt{I}(s)-\mu_I)^2}{2\sigma_I^2}\right]\right) & \text{if } l_s = -1 \end{cases} \quad (4)$$

Since there are a (small) finite number of intensities, the second case (with the log) can be precomputed and cached without incurring great computational burden.

Spatial. The potential $U_\text{D}(l_s, \mathcal{D})$ models the spatial relationship between a disc-label and the set of discs. Intuitively, a disc-label is more likely to take value $+1$ the closer it is to the location specified by one of the discs. We compute the covariance matrix Σ_i (i.e., shape) of each disc d_i during training (roughly, the discs are elliptically shaped) and then base the spatial potential on the squared Mahalanobis distance:

$$U_\text{D}(l_s, \mathcal{D}) = l_s \cdot \min_{d_i \in \mathcal{D}} \left[(s - d_i)^\mathsf{T} \Sigma_i^{-1} (s - d_i)\right] \quad . \quad (5)$$

The potential assigns energy proportional to the distance of the closest disc, and the label variable acts as a switch: when $l_s = -1$, being far from the closest disc is lower energy than being closer to it and vice versa.

3.4 High Level Terms

Location. The potential $U_\text{L}(d_i)$ measures the distance of disc d_i to its expected location. Similar to the spatial low level term in (5), we estimate the covariance Σ_i for each disc (same as above) and, in this case, the mean location μ_i. We do the estimation offline from training data. The squared Mahalanobis distance defines the potential:

$$U_\text{L}(d_i) = (d_i - \mu_i)^\mathsf{T} \Sigma_i^{-1} (d_i - \mu_i) \quad . \quad (6)$$

Disc-Context. The potential $V_\text{D}(d_i, d_j)$ captures the high-level contextual relationship between two *neighboring* discs. Consider the discs form a chain; then the neighboring pairs are nearest neighbors on the chain. Since we include only the spatial location for each disc variable, the distance between neighboring discs is a natural measure for this potential. Inspecting the empirical distribution of these distances (figure 4) suggests a Gaussian parameterized by μ_D, σ_D^2, and its negative log for the energy. Let $e_{ij} = |d_i - d_j|_2$, then

$$V_D(d_i, d_j) = \frac{(e_{ij} - \mu_D)^2}{\sigma_D^2} \,. \tag{7}$$

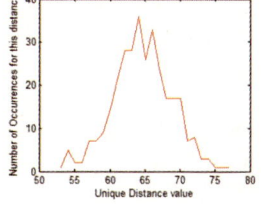

Fig. 4. Empirical distribution of disc distances

3.5 Inference Using Generalized Expectation-Maximization

We use the generalized EM (gEM) algorithm [12] to solve (2). We initialize $\mathcal{D}^0$ by setting each disc d_i in its mean location μ_i, which we've learned offline from training data. Then, we iteratively estimate the posterior over the disc-label variables, $\mathcal{L}$, and refine the disc variables by maximizing the expected log likelihood (ELL):

E-step → $$F^t(\mathcal{L}) = P\left(\mathcal{L}|\mathcal{D}^t, \mathtt{I}\right) \tag{8}$$

M-step → $$\mathcal{D}^{t+1} = \arg\max_{\mathcal{D}} \left[\log P(\mathcal{D}) + \sum_{\mathcal{L}} F^t(\mathcal{L}) \log P(\mathcal{L}, \mathtt{I}|\mathcal{D})\right] \tag{9}$$

Inference with gEM is tractable without resorting to monte carlo methods because of the underlying structure of our two-level model. Since no dependencies are defined among the disc-label variables $\mathcal{L}$, we factor them into independent local terms:

$$P(\mathcal{L}|\mathcal{D}, \mathtt{I}) = \prod_{s \in \Lambda} \frac{1}{Z[l_s]} \exp\left[-\beta_1 U_{\mathtt{I}}(l_s, I(s)) - \beta_2 U_D(l_s, \mathcal{D})\right] \,. \tag{10}$$

Thus, we directly evaluate the full posterior (8) and log terms (9) during optimization. Since the partials are not analytically available, we execute a finite differences-based gradient ascent algorithm to iteratively maximize the ELL. It is beyond the scope of this paper to go into full detail; basically, iteratively for each disc variable d_i, we evaluate the local gradient of the ELL by perturbing d_i by a set of changes $\{\delta\}$. For each perturbation, we fully evaluate (9) and change d_i by the δ yielding the maximum (if no δ increases the function, we do not change d_i). We stop when no d_i has changed.

4 Experimental Results

We use 20 pathology-free cases of clinical T2-weighted MR data for the lumbar spinal column (e.g., figure 1). The images have been acquired on a 3T Philips Medical Systems Intera Scanner with a voxel resolution of $0.5 \times 0.5 \times 4.5$ mm^3. From each case, we extract the four middle slices giving a total of 80 radiographs. We work in 2D because there is there is 5mm inter-slice space and it is standard clinical practice. We have manually annotated the images to specify each disc center as well as to label a subset

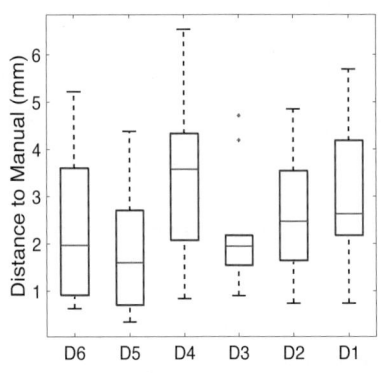

Exp.	D6	D5	D4	D3	D2	D1	Out of 48
1	0.6	0.3	6.5	0.9	0.8	3.3	45
2	1.3	0.7	4.3	1.6	2.7	2.2	47
3	2.6	2.7	3.3	1.8	0.7	2.7	47
4	5.2	0.6	0.8	1.5	1.6	0.7	46
5	0.9	1.6	4.9	2.2	3.5	4.2	44
6	3.6	4.4	3.8	4.2	4.8	5.7	45
7	1.9	1.4	1.6	2.0	2.2	1.4	48
8	2.0	1.5	2.4	1.3	3.3	2.5	48
9	0.7	1.7	2.1	2.2	2.1	2.2	47
10	4.8	4.2	3.9	4.7	4.9	5.1	45
Average	2.36	1.91	3.33	2.24	2.67	2.98	
Accuracy (mm)							96.2%

Fig. 5. Results of cross validation (CV). Every time two cases (8 images) are pulled out and training is perfomed on the other 72 images. (Left) A box-plot showing summary statistics of Euclidean distances over all testing cases in CV. The line in each box is the median, the top and bottom are the 75th and 25th percentiles, and plusses are statistical outliers. (Right) The mean Euclidean distances for each of the 10 CV experiments and the labeling results (right-most column) marking how many discs were localized inside of the correct disc. Accuracy is 96.2%.

of the disc pixels so that we could perform training of the necessary parameters for our model (intensity, spatial, etc.). We set the parameters of the model β_1 through β_4 by hand; these could be learned by various supervised parameter estimation algorithms.

We have performed a leave-two-out cross validation (CV) experiment. In each CV sub-experiment, we separate all four images from two cases to be used for testing and leave the rest (72 images in 18 cases) for training; this prevents bias since multiple slices are taken from the same case. Figure 5 summarizes the results of this experiment using two quantitative mechanisms: the Euclidean distance to the known disc center and a boolean score that is yes if the inferred label lies anywhere inside of the disc (this is scored manually). A distance of less than 3mm is within the margin of error in human labeling of the disc center. The discs are labeled from bottom to top, i.e., D1 is S-L5. Our scores are comparable or superior to [10] (depending on which variant of their algorithm is analyzed), but they use a full 3D volume and opaque discriminative models while we use a 2D image and transparent generative models. We have focused exclusively on the lumbar region while they do the full spine (our model is directly extensible).

Figure 6 shows the labeling in four test images; the first three are from our dataset and the fourth is a pathology case. The images show a green line that traces the path during disc optimization and a plus for the converged point. We can see (e.g., left-most D4) that even when initialization is far from the true disc, the two-level model is able to drive the variable to an accurate position. Although the model is not designed to handle the abnormalities presented in the fourth case (disc degeneration, bottom two), we are able to successfully localize each disc in this image too, suggesting our model could extend to the more complicated cases of abnormalities (with some enhancements). One failure we see is D3 in the left-most image; here, the disc is labeled but the model fails to accurately localize the disc center.

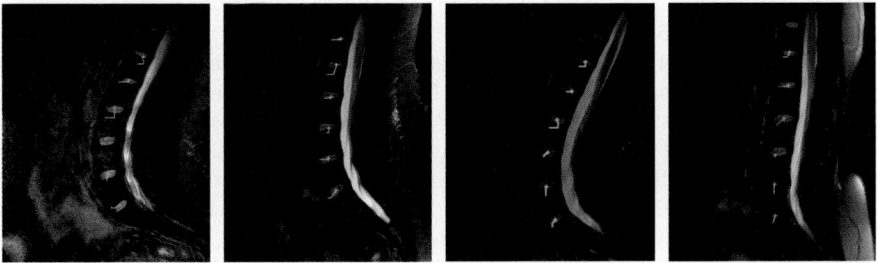

Fig. 6. Labeling results. Each image shows disc optimization path and a plus for the converged point. The right-most image is an abnormal case not in our data-set.

5 Summary and Discussion

We have proposed a two-level probabilistic model for robustly localizing and labeling intervertebral discs. The unifying model incorporates both pixel-level information (e.g., appearance) and high-level information (e.g., spatial relationship between discs) in a single coherent generative model. This two-level approach insulates the high-level inferences (about disc localization) from the pixel-level variations.

Our quantitative results show good localizing and labeling performance: about 96% labeling accuracy in a cross validation experiment. We plan to extend the size of the dataset and adapt the method to pathological cases, which is our ultimate goal. As the example in figure 6 shows, the generalization to pathological cases is possible with the straightforward potentials proposed in this paper, but will require extensions to the model. To that end, we plan to enhance the model by incorporating local texture into the low-level terms and disc orientation and shape into the high-level terms.

References

1. Jenkins, J.P., Hickey, D.S., Zhu, X.P., Machin, M., Isherwood, I.: Mr imaging of the intervertebral disc: A quantitative study. British Journal of Radiology 58(692), 705–709 (1985)
2. Antoniou, J., Mwale, F., Demers, C.N., Beaudoin, G., Goswami, T., Aebi, M., Alini, M.: Quantitative magnetic resonance imaging of enzymatically induced degraded of the nucleus pulposus of inteverbetral discs. Spine 31(14), 1547–1554 (2006)
3. Dalley, A.F., Agur, A.M.R.: Atlas of Anatomy. Lippincott Williams and Wilkins (2004)
4. Chwialkowski, M.P., Shile, P.E., Peshock, R.M., Pfeifer, D., Parkey, R.W.: Automated detection and evaluation of lumbar discs in mr images. In: Proc. of IEEE EMBS (1989)
5. Peng, Z., Zhong, J., Wee, W., Lee, J.: Automated vertebra detection and segmentation from the whole spine MR images. In: Proc. of IEEE EMBS, vol. 3 (2005)
6. Pekar, V., Bystrov, D., Heese, H.S., Dries, S.P.M., Schmidt, S., Grewer, R., Harder, C., Bergmans, R.C., Simonetti, A.W., Muisinkel, A.: Automated planning of scan geometries in spine MRI scans. In: Ayache, N., Ourselin, S., Maeder, A. (eds.) MICCAI 2007, Part I. LNCS, vol. 4791, pp. 601–608. Springer, Heidelberg (2007)
7. Masaki, T., Lee, Y., Tsai, D.Y., Sekiya, M., Kazama, K.: Automatic detectmination of the imaging plane in lumbar mri. In: Proc. of SPIE Med. Img., pp. 1252–1259 (2006)

8. Weiss, K.L., Storrs, J.M., Banto, R.B.: Automated spine survey iterative scan technique. Radiology 239(1), 255–262 (2006)
9. Zheng, Y., Nixon, M.S., Allen, R.: Automatic segmentation of lumbar vertebrae in digital videofluoroscopic imaging. IEEE Trans. on Medical Imaging 23(1), 45–52 (2004)
10. Schmidt, S., Kappes, J., Bergtholdt, M., Pekar, V., Dries, S.P., Bystrov, D., Schnorr, C.: Spine Detection and Labeling Using a Parts-Based Graphical Model. In: Karssemeijer, N., Lelieveldt, B. (eds.) IPMI 2007. LNCS, vol. 4584, pp. 122–133. Springer, Heidelberg (2007)
11. Fischl, B., Salat, D.H., Busa, E., Albert, M., Deiterich, M., Haselgrove, C., Kouwe, A.v.d., Killiany, R., Kennedy, D., Klaveness, S., Monttillo, A., Makris, N., Rosen, B., Dale, A.M.: Whole brain segmentation: Automated labeling of neuroanatomical structures in the human brain. Neuron. 33, 341–355 (2002)
12. Dempster, A.P., Laird, N.M., Rubin, D.B.: Maximum Likelihood From Incomplete Data via the EM Algorithm. Journal of the Royal Statistical Society – Series B 39(1), 1–38 (1977)

Topology Preserving Warping of Binary Images: Application to Atlas-Based Skull Segmentation

Sylvain Faisan[1], Nicolas Passat[1], Vincent Noblet[1], Renée Chabrier[2], and Christophe Meyer[3]

[1]LSIIT - UMR CNRS 7005, Strasbourg I University, France
[2]LINC - UMR CNRS 7191, Strasbourg I University, France
[3]University Hospital of Besançon, France

Abstract. Lots of works have been recently carried out in the field of non-rigid registration to ensure the estimation of one-to-one mappings. However, warping a binary image with such transformations may alter its discrete topological properties if common resampling strategies are considered. This paper proposes an original method for warping a binary image according to some continuous and bijective mapping, while preserving its discrete topological properties. Results obtained in the context of atlas-based segmentation highlight the interest of the approach. Indeed, the method has been successfully applied to the segmentation of skull structures from a database of 15 CT-scans, providing both geometrically and topologically satisfactory results.

1 Introduction

Image warping is the process of applying some geometric transformation to an image. Given an image M and a continuous deformation field h, the goal is to compute the warped image S, so that for each voxel v, $S(v) = M(h(v))$. Since $h(v)$ does not necessarily correspond with grid point, some interpolation techniques are required to evaluate $M(h(v))$.

Although several image interpolation techniques (linear, cubic) [1] have been proposed for grey-level images, no specific attention has been paid to the case of binary data. Common interpolation techniques, except the nearest neighbour interpolation, do not guarantee the resampled image S to remain a binary image. To circumvent this limitation, it is possible to use a thresholding as post-processing of interpolation to get a binary image. Unfortunately, warping a discrete image according to a continuous and bijective (*i.e.* topology-preserving) deformation field with these common interpolation techniques may fail in preserving its *discrete* topological properties. Quite surprisingly, many works have been devoted to develop registration methods providing deformation fields which preserve the continuous topology, while the topology preservation of discrete objects deformed by such fields has not yet been considered. Based on these considerations, we propose an algorithm for warping a binary image according to a topology-preserving deformation field without altering its discrete topology.

The proposed approach is inspired from concepts generally considered in the context of segmentation, where topology preservation is a crucial issue. The segmentation methods dealing with this constraint are often based on the concept of 3-D simple points [2] (*i.e.* points whose addition or removal from a binary object does not alter its topology), which can be locally characterised in constant time, leading to fast algorithms. The basic idea of the proposed method is to modify the initial image in a homotopy-preserving fashion by adding and removing simple points until converging to a solution that is as close as possible to the continuous warped image.

The paper is organised as follows. In Section 2, the proposed method is described. In Section 3, results in the context of atlas-based segmentation are presented. Conclusions and perspectives are provided in Section 4.

2 Method

The method of warping a binary image M according to a continuous and bijective deformation field h can be stated as the following constrained optimisation problem:

$$\hat{S} = arg \min_{S \sim M} d(S, M, h) \,, \qquad (1)$$

where S is a binary image constrained to be topologically equivalent to M and $d(S, M, h)$ a distance between S and the continuous warped image $M(h)$. This paper presents a method to tackle this problem. We first introduce in Sec. 2.1 the distance $d(S, M, h)$. Then, we explain in Sec. 2.2 how to constrain S to be topologically equivalent to M during the optimisation process. Finally, the optimisation strategy is detailed in Sec. 2.3. A global overview of the method is given in Alg. 1.

2.1 Cost Function

Since M and S are constrained to have the same topology, there is a one-to-one relation between connected components (CCs) of M and the ones of S. These CCs can be background CCs (BCCs) or object CCs (OCCs), each CC corresponding to a distinct label. We define $\mathcal{N}(v, S, M)$ as the CC in M which corresponds to the CC in S that encloses voxel v. The distance $d(S, M, h)$ between S and the continuous warped image $M(h)$ is considered hereafter as the cost function, and is computed as follows:

$$d(S, M, h) = \sum_{v \in S} \rho(v, S, M, h) \,, \text{ with } \rho(v, S, M, h) = \min_{v' \in \mathcal{N}(v, S, M)} \|v' - h(v)\| \,, \qquad (2)$$

where $\rho(v, S, M, h)$ is the distance between $h(v)$ and the CC of M which is associated to the CC that encloses v in S. To clarify the idea, the computation of the cost function is illustrated in a 2-D case in Fig. 1. $\rho(v, S, M, h)$ can be efficiently evaluated by computing the chamfer distance map of the CC of M (the one associated to the CC that encloses v in S) and by evaluating its value at position $h(v)$. Notice that the chamfer distance map can be computed one time for each CC.

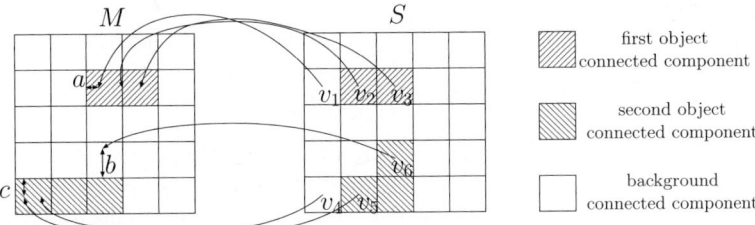

Fig. 1. Illustration of the computation of $\rho(v, S, M, h)$ for 6 pixels. M is composed of two OCCs and of one BCC. $\rho(v, S, M, h)$ is equal to 0 for v_2, v_3, and v_5 since $h(v_2)$, $h(v_3)$, and $h(v_5)$ belong to the same CC as v_2, v_3, and v_5, respectively. However, v_6 belongs to the second OCC whereas $h(v_6)$ belongs to the BCC so that $\rho(v_6, S, M, h)$ is equal to b, namely, the distance between $h(v_6)$ and the second OCC (in M). In the same way, $\rho(v_1, S, M, h) = a$ and $\rho(v_4, S, M, h) = c$.

2.2 Topology Handling

At the beginning of the method, S is initialized to M and is then modified by iterative removal/addition of simple points. The label of a simple point is changed if it decreases the cost function. When changing the label of v, it is associated unambiguously to a unique CC, since it is a simple point. To determine this CC, two images representing the labels of S are used. They are updated during the whole process with S.

The removal/addition of simple points can be not appropriated when a voxel has to be "translated". The translation can be interpreted in terms of an addition (resp. a removal) followed by a removal (resp. an addition) of simple points. However, the cost function is estimated after each label modification. Consequently, the first modification may increase the cost function, leading to refuse this operation, whereas both modifications may decrease the cost function. That is why the concept of topology-preserving translation is defined. This notion is interpreted here as the simultaneous modification of the status of a couple (v, v') of adjacent voxels such that $S(v) = 1 - S(v')$. To guarantee topology preservation, it is sufficient to check that v (resp. v') is simple for S and v' (resp. v) is simple in S' obtained from S after the modification of v (resp. v'). The translation at voxel v is performed if it actually reduces the cost function. If the point v can be translated in different ways, the translation which minimises at best the cost function is chosen.

2.3 Optimisation Strategy

The purpose of the optimisation strategy is to reach the minimal value of the cost function by iterative removal/addition of simple points or by topology-preserving translations, *i.e.*, to converge to a model topologically equivalent and - as much as possible - geometrically similar to the continuous deformed image $M \circ h$. The selection of simple points to remove/add requires a list $\mathcal{L}$ which contains all simple points of S presenting a positive cost. The cost is defined as the benefit to change the label at simple point v. More precisely, the modification of $S(v)$ enables to decrease the cost function from the cost $c(v, S, M, h)$:

$$c(v, S, M, h) = d(S, M, h) - d(S', M, h) = \rho(v, S, M, h) - \rho(v, S', M, h) , \quad (3)$$

where S' is the image obtained from S by modifying the value at v.

During the dynamical scheme, when modifying a simple point v in S to obtain a new image S', there is no need to recompute the whole list $\mathcal{L}$ since (i) $c(v', S, M, h) = c(v', S', M, h)$ for all voxels $v' \neq v$, and (ii) simple property of points can only be modified in the 26-neighbourhood of v. Consequently, the algorithm proceeds as follows until $\mathcal{L}$ is empty. The point of highest cost, denoted v_0, is removed from the list. The label of S at v_0 is then modified. This may change the simple points which are in the 26-neighbourhood of v_0: points which were not simple (resp. simple) and which become simple (resp. non-simple) must be added if they have a positive cost (resp. removed) in (resp. from) $\mathcal{L}$.

When $\rho(v, S, M, h) = 0$, the voxel v belongs to the correct CC. A cost $\rho(v, S, M, h) > 0$ can result from the fact that $h(v)$ is at the interface of objects (h being a continuous field) or from topological constraints. However, it may also result from the convergence of the method to a local minimum. To deal with this issue, we check for all voxels v verifying $\rho(v, S, M, h) > 0$ if it is possible to translate v to reduce the cost function without topology modification. It may happen that a translation generates new simple points in the neighbourhood of the involved points, enabling to keep deforming the current image S by "classical" simple point modification.

In order to avoid convergence onto local minima (resulting from geometrical or topological constraints) which can appear with large displacements, the deformation is performed in a "smooth" way by considering $N + 1$ intermediate deformation fields computed from h, namely $h^{(0)}$, $h^{(1)}$, ..., $h^{(N)}$ such that:

$$\begin{cases} h^{(0)} = Id, \ h^{(N)} = h & (i) \\ \forall j \in [0, N-1], \forall v \in S, \ \|h^{(j+1)}(v) - h^{(j)}(v)\| < 1 & (ii) \end{cases} \quad (4)$$

Constraint (ii) provides a lower bound for N: $N \geq \max_{v \in S} \|h(v) - v\|$. The deformation fields $h^{(i)}$ ($0 < i < N$) are finally defined by:

$$\forall v \in S, h^{(i)}(v) = v + \frac{i}{N}(h(v) - v) . \quad (5)$$

The optimisation scheme just described is achieved by considering sequentially $h^{(1)}$, $h^{(2)}$, ..., $h^{(N)}$. The algorithm is finally described in Alg. 1.

3 Application: Skull Segmentation from CT Scan Data

3.1 Experiments

One important application of the proposed approach concerns atlas-based segmentation [3]. Such methods rely on a binary model M of the structures of

Algorithm 1. Topology-preserving warping of binary images

Input: M (binary image to warp according to h), h (transformation field)
Output: S (warped binary image)

$S = M$
$(h^{(i)})_{i=1}^N$ = transformation fields obtained from h
for $h^* = h^{(1)}$ to $h^{(N)}$ **do**
  $\mathcal{L}$ = list of simple points with positive cost $c(v, S, M, h)$ in S
  repeat
    while $\mathcal{L} \neq \emptyset$ **do**
      v = point of highest cost in $\mathcal{L}$
      $S(v) = 1 - S(v)$ /* switch the label of v in S */
      Update $\mathcal{L}$ considering the new status of points in the neighbourhood of v
    end while
    for all voxels v verifying $\rho(v, S, M, h) > 0$ and which can be translated with v' by reducing the cost function **do**
      $(S(v), S(v')) = (1 - S(v), 1 - S(v'))$ /* perform the translation */
      Update $\mathcal{L}$ considering the new status of points in the neighbourhood of v, v'
    end for
  until $\mathcal{L} = \emptyset$
end for

interest which has been obtained from the segmentation of an image R. When searching the structures of interest in a new image I, the first step consists in estimating a deformation field h by registering R onto I. The structures of interest in I, denoted S, are then obtained by transforming M according to h. The binary image topology-preserving deformation is also of great interest since we guarantee that M and S have the same topology. In the sequel, the method is proposed for the segmentation of skull structures from CT-scan data.

The proposed strategy consists in deforming a pre-processed skull template associated to a reference CT image R. This template models the parts of the skull which have to be segmented in a geometrically and topologically correct fashion. In particular, it is composed of one connected component, and has no cavity but ten holes corresponding to the foramen magnum, the zygomatic arches, etc. (see Fig. 2). This template is actually the binary image M which has to be warped according to a 3-D deformation field h estimated by registering R onto the CT image I to be segmented.

3.2 Results

The efficiency of the method is not evaluated in terms of segmentation accuracy since it largely depends on the precision of the estimated deformation field. The goal of this experiment is to validate the proposed method (PM) and to show the benefit of the approach with comparison to other interpolation methods, namely, the nearest neighbour interpolation (M_1), and the linear interpolation followed by a thresholding with a threshold of 0.5 (M_2). These methods are compared from two points of view, a topological one and a geometrical one.

From a topological point of view, the average number of OCCs (see b_0 in Tab. 1), of holes (b_1), and of cavities (b_2=number of BCCs -1) are computed for the 15 transported segmentation maps obtained for each method. The proposed method is the only one guaranteeing topology preservation: the topology

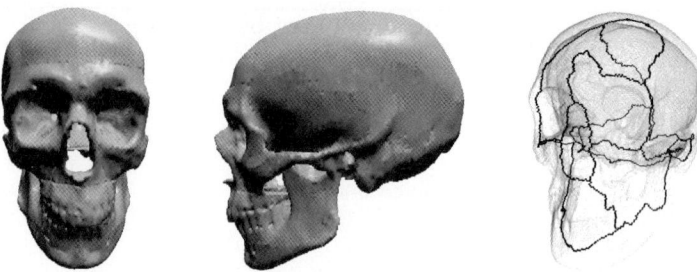

Fig. 2. Skull template used in the proposed application. Left, middle: whole template. Right: template visualised with its topological skeleton. It has to be noticed that this is a *partial* template: structures such as the vertebrae, for example, are not modelled since their segmentation is not required here.

is strongly altered by methods M_1 and M_2 (leading to connected component splitting, hole and cavity generations, etc.). For example, method M_1 generates on average a number of 150 undesired cavities in the segmentation result. To illustrate this point, Fig. 3 presents a typical result for the proposed method (right) and for the M_2 method (left).

From a geometrical point of view, the segmentation maps obtained with the proposed approach (Fig. 3, right) is satisfactory since similar to the result obtained with M_2 (the M_1 and M_2 methods provide by construction geometrically correct results). To provide quantitative comparison, the following strategy is used. As M is composed of only one OCC and one BCC, the computation of $\rho(v, S, M, h)$ is possible for each method (to compute $\rho(v, S, M, h)$ for the M_1 and M_2 approaches, voxels, for which $S(v) = 1$, are associated with the OCC, and the others correspond to the BCC). We observe firstly that the ratios of points for which $\rho(v, S, M, h) = 0$ are identical for the three methods (98.6%). Results resumed in Tab. 1 provide the ratios of the other points (namely 1.4%)

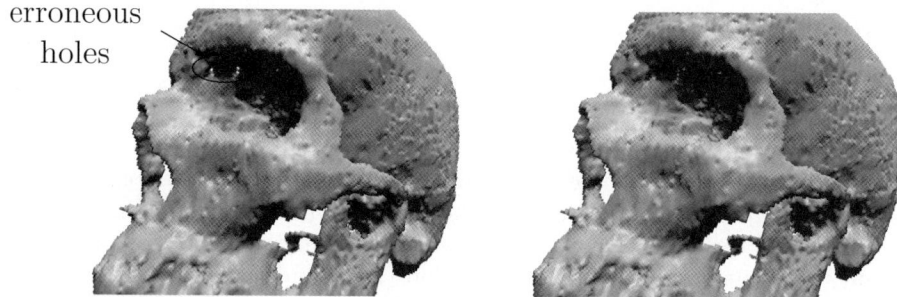

Fig. 3. Segmentation results obtained with method M_2 (left) and the proposed method (right). The topology has been altered in the left image, but preserved in the right one. Note that the surfaces are visually noisy since the *real* discrete results are visualised here without mesh generation.

Table 1. Comparison of the proposed method (PM) from a geometrical (P_i, $\bar{d}$, and $d_{\max}$) and from a topological (b_i) point of view with the nearest neighbour interpolation (M_1) and the linear interpolation with thresholding (M_2). P_i: ratio (%) of points v for which $\rho(v, S, M, h)$ is in $](i-1), i].25.10^{-2}$ mm (this ratio is computed without considering voxels for which $\rho(v, S, M, h)$ is equal to 0); $\bar{d}$: mean distance of $\rho(v, S, M, h)$; $d_{\max}$: maximal value of $\rho(v, S, M, h)$ for the 15 cases; b_0 (resp. b_1, b_2): number of object connected components (resp. holes, cavities).

	P_1	P_2	P_3	P_4	P_5	$\bar{d}$	$d_{\max}$	b_0	b_1	b_2
M_1	61.87	30.43	7.39	0.31	0.00	$3.70.10^{-3}$	0.87	1.33 ± 0.59	109 ± 51.0	150 ± 71.0
M_2	62.18	37.82	0.00	0.00	0.00	$3.44.10^{-3}$	0.50	1.06 ± 0.25	24.8 ± 8.00	7.20 ± 2.80
PM	62.19	37.77	0.04	10^{-3}	10^{-4}	$3.44.10^{-3}$	1.06	1.00 ± 0.00	10.0 ± 0.00	0.00 ± 0.00

in terms of distance. The inspection of the results shows that the three methods are relatively similar. Note that the maximal distance is a little bit higher (but still low) for the proposed method. More precisely, on the 15 considered cases, 5 segmentation maps have a unique voxel v whose value $\rho(v, S, M, h)$ is lightly greater than one (the maximal value encountered in the 15 cases for ρ is 1.06). This is due to the fact that the topology preservation induces here geometric constraints. Finally, we can conclude that the geometry is similar for the three methods, but only the proposed approach can correctly handle topology. It has to be noticed that the algorithm has also been tested with objects composed of several CCs. Results are satisfactory but not presented in this paper.

3.3 Discussion

We can notice that medical image segmentation methods [4,5,6] based on topology-preserving deformation of a binary model[1] have been proposed in the last years. They *generally* rely on simple algorithmic processes and hypotheses: (*i*) they use monotonic transformations which either remove *or* add simple points from/to a model M necessarily surrounding/surrounded by S, (*ii*) such models are proposed for structures having a non-complex topology or topologically simplified, and (*iii*) only simple deformation functions (based on grey-level values or distance maps) are considered. The deformation strategy proposed here leads to a segmentation method based on the same concepts but presenting several important improvements: the methods can use *non-trivial* topological models which evolve in a *non-monotonic* and topology-preserving fashion under the guidance of *complex* deformation functions.

4 Conclusion

A new method for warping a binary image in a discrete topology preserving fashion according to a continuous topology preserving deformation field has been proposed. Further works will consist in extending this method to label images.

---

[1] Some methods are based on *label* models, unfortunately with several approximations [7,8] resulting from still open theoretical problems on label image topology.

Such extension will require to develop a sound theoretical framework for topological modelling and deformation of such images.

The proposed method has been successfully applied to medical image segmentation. Another perspective is to consider the proposed framework for devising strategies whose behaviour may evolve during the deformation process, for example by performing in parallel segmentation and registration, as proposed in [9].

References

1. Lehmann, T., Gonner, C., Spitzer, K.: Survey: interpolation methods in medical image processing. IEEE Transactions on Medical Imaging 18(11), 1049–1075 (1999)
2. Bertrand, G., Malandain, G.: A new characterization of three-dimensional simple points. Pattern Recognition Letters 15(2), 169–175 (1994)
3. Dawant, B., Hartmann, S., Thirion, J.P., Maes, F., Vandermeulen, D., Demaerel, P.: Automatic 3-D segmentation of internal structures of the head in MR images using a combination of similarity and free-form deformations: Part I, methodology and validation on normal subjects. IEEE Transactions on Medical Imaging 18(10), 902–916 (1999)
4. Mangin, J.F., Frouin, V., Bloch, I., Régis, J., López-Krahe, J.: From 3D magnetic resonance images to structural representations of the cortex topography using topology preserving deformations. Journal of Mathematical Imaging and Vision 5(4), 297–318 (1995)
5. Dokládal, P., Lohou, C., Perroton, L., Bertrand, G.: Liver blood vessels extraction by a 3-D topological approach. In: Taylor, C., Colchester, A. (eds.) MICCAI 1999. LNCS, vol. 1679, pp. 98–105. Springer, Heidelberg (1999)
6. Passat, N., Ronse, C., Baruthio, J., Armspach, J.P., Bosc, M., Foucher, J.: Using multimodal MR data for segmentation and topology recovery of the cerebral superficial venous tree. In: Bebis, G., Boyle, R., Koracin, D., Parvin, B. (eds.) ISVC 2005. LNCS, vol. 3804, pp. 60–67. Springer, Heidelberg (2005)
7. Bazin, P.L., Pham, D.: Topology-preserving tissue classification of magnetic resonance brain images. IEEE Transactions on Medical Imaging 26(4), 487–496 (2007)
8. Miri, S., Passat, N., Armspach, J.P.: Topologically-based segmentation of brain structures from T1 MRI. In: ISMM 2007, vol. 2, pp. 33–34 (2007)
9. Faisan, S., Passat, N., Noblet, V., Chabrier, R., Armspach, J.P., Meyer, C.: Segmentation of head bones in 3-D CT images from an example. In: ISBI 2008, pp. 81–84 (2008)

Robust Segmentation and Anatomical Labeling of the Airway Tree from Thoracic CT Scans

Bram van Ginneken, Wouter Baggerman, and Eva M. van Rikxoort

Image Sciences Institute, University Medical Center Utrecht, The Netherlands

Abstract. A method for automatic extraction and labeling of the airway tree from thoracic CT scans is presented and extensively evaluated on 150 scans of clinical dose, low dose and ultra-low dose data, in inspiration and expiration from both relatively healthy and severely ill patients. The method uses adaptive thresholds while growing the airways and it is shown that this strategy leads to a substantial increase in the number, total length and number of correctly labeled airways extracted. From inspiration scans on average 170 branches are found, from expiration scans 59.

1 Introduction

Multi-slice CT scanning technology has revolutionized the in vivo study of the lungs and motivates the need for pulmonary image analysis [1]. Automated extraction and labeling of the bronchial tree from thoracic CT scans is vital to accurately quantify airway morphology which is increasingly used to measure progression and response to treatment for a variety diseases. Another important application is computer-assisted bronchoscopy.

A wide variety of methods have been developed to segment the airways [2,3,4,5,6,7,8,9,10,11]. Some of these include or focus specifically on anatomical labeling of airway segments [2,12,13]. Most methods have been evaluated on a small number of scans. Evaluation on low-dose scans is rare ([14] is an exception), as are application to expiration scans and scans with substantial pathology.

In this work, a method is proposed to segment the complete airway tree. Our approach is based on the generic tree extraction framework outlined in [4,6] and introduces several modifications and new rules for accepting segments. A key contribution is the introduction of a multi-threshold approach to increase robustness. Furthermore, a novel algorithm for anatomical labeling is presented.

Extensive results are presented from 150 scans that include clinical dose, low dose and ultra low-dose, inspiration and expiration scans and data from asymptomatic subjects as well as interstitial lung disease patients with massive pathology.

2 Method

The backbone of our algorithm is an implementation of the framework given in [4,6]. In this section we discuss the initialization, briefly review the framework, describe our rules for accepting voxels, fronts and segments, introduce the multi-threshold extension of the method and finally describe the anatomical labeling algorithm.

Initialization. The trachea and the lungs are automatically segmented with a method based on [15,16]. Central dark circular regions are searched to find a start point in the trachea, followed by region growing with multiple optimal thresholds to extract the trachea and the lungs. The lung segmentation is used to infer the scan orientation. From the trachea segmentation a seed point is determined in the axial slice that contains the center of gravity of the structure. Only growing in the basal direction is allowed.

Tree segmentation framework. The segments of the bronchial tree are obtained by wavefront propagation. The initial seed point provides the first front. At every iteration, all unprocessed voxels connected to the front that satisfy the *voxel criteria* form the new wavefront. The segment is allowed to keep growing when the front meets the *wavefront criteria*. If the new front consists of multiple parts, a segment is complete and accepted if it complies with the *segment criteria*. To avoid spurious front splittings due to noise, a large 80-connectivity value is used to detect them. New fronts are pushed on a stack and the next front from the stack is propagated. The algorithm terminates when the stack is empty. While the fronts propagate, the centerline or skeleton of the tree and the local segment diameter are computed and this information is used in several of the acceptance criteria. An important difference with [4,6] is that we use region growing to obtain the new front. To avoid diamond- or cuboid-shaped fronts, growing is restricted to within a sphere from the last calculated center point with a diameter slightly larger than the last calculated segment diameter.

Rules for accepting voxels, wavefronts and segments. Voxels are accepted when their density (in Hounsfield Units or HU) is below a threshold t, or (to be less sensitive to noise) the HU value in a $3 \times 3 \times 3$ neighborhood around the voxel is $< t$. For every new front, three checks are applied to the segment grown so far, and if they are violated the entire segment is removed. First, the segment's current radius must be smaller than 1.5 times the minimum radius found in any parent segment. This ensures that diameters of bronchi diminish. When leaking occurs, this rule is typically violated. Second, a front is not allowed to touch any other segment (segments are grown in a breadth first fashion). Third, the length of the segment should not be more than 5 times its radius. This ensures that partly grown segments are accepted before a leakage occurs that could discard a large part of an airway. A completed segment is only accepted if it meets two more requirements: The angle it makes with its parent should be $< 100°$ and the average ratio of radii of two consecutive fronts should not exceed 1.1. The latter check ensures that the segment is not widening, which typically indicates leakage.

Postprocessing. After the bronchial tree has been extracted, several postprocessing steps are performed. First all minor trailing segments (i.e. segments without descendants) are removed. Segments are considered minor if their length is smaller than 3 mm and their volume is below 25 mm^3. Next, the tree structure

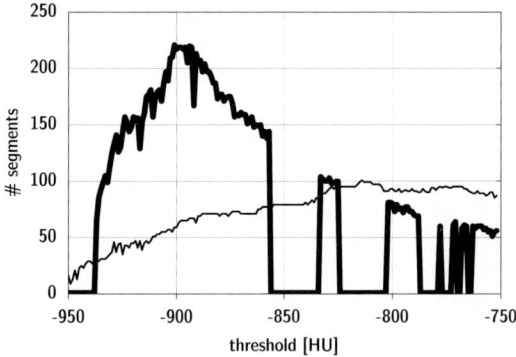

Fig. 1. The total number of segments found in the airway tree as a function of the threshold t for voxel acceptance for two scans. The thick line demonstrates that the results can be sensitive to small changes in t. For both cases, the multi-threshold method found many more segments: 289 and 181 for the thick and thin line, respectively.

is scanned for segments that have exactly one descendant, and these segments are merged. Finally, holes in the segments, primarily caused by noise, are filled. *Adaptive acceptance rules.* We have observed that with these rules for accepting wavefronts and segments, leakage into the parenchyma is virtually impossible to occur, and thus all segments found are true airways. Not all airways are found, however, and in fact it is possible that large parts of the airway tree are missed. Quite often, small changes in the value for the voxel acceptance threshold t, have a profound effect on the number and total length of detected airways. Note that it is not the case that higher values for t automatically lead to more voxels considered airways. Surely, more voxels are accepted when computing a new front when t is increased, but these fronts or these segments may subsequently be rejected by the front and segment acceptance rules. The algorithm thus manifests a complex interplay between the rules at various levels. The effect is illustrated in Fig. 1. This figure also shows that the optimal value for t varies from scan to scan. For most scans, $t = -900$ gives the best results, so this value was used in what we refer to as the single threshold method.

To overcome these limitations and obtain a more robust segmentation that includes as many peripheral airways as possible, we propose to make the process adaptive. Every segment is first grown with a high threshold $t = -750$. If rejected, the segment is regrown with a lower threshold $t + k\Delta t$ with $k = 1, \ldots, 18$ and $\Delta t = -10$. This is referred to as the multi-threshold method. It renders the extraction process adaptive: at every position in the scan the maximum number of airway voxels are selected while the front and segment rules still ensure that no leaking can occur.

Anatomical labeling. After the tree has been segmented, anatomical labels for branches up to the segmental level are automatically assigned. We use 32 distinct labels following the nomenclature from [12]. The fact that trifurcations are usually two consecutive bifurcations lead us to define five small intermediate segments that may or may not be present.

Table 1. Average number and total length (in mm) of all airways per generation, per scan, split over the three databases

| | Database 1 | | Database 2 | | Database 3 | |
| | single | multi | single | multi | single | multi |
gen.	# length	# length	# length	# length	# length	# length
1	2 97	2 99	2 92	2 96	2 88	2 88
2	4 66	4 68	4 64	4 70	4 58	4 59
3	8 102	8 100	7 85	8 103	7 88	8 90
4	14 188	16 214	7 87	13 162	11 141	14 163
5	17 251	27 378	4 50	14 179	15 206	24 298
6	14 193	35 430	2 28	8 85	14 178	32 366
7	10 140	27 330	1 17	5 54	10 130	29 294
8	5 84	18 218	1 9	2 29	7 83	21 208
9	4 62	11 143	0 3	1 10	4 57	15 153
10	2 30	7 92	0 1	0 2	3 35	10 100
11	1 13	4 55	0 0	0 0	2 16	10 61
>11	1 11	5 56	0 0	0 0	2 17	10 69
all	81 1238	166 2183	30 434	59 789	82 1096	174 1949

To assign the labels, the segment labels of 17 trees were manually assigned. The distribution of several segment characteristics were studied, and orientation, average radius, and angle with the parent segment were found most discriminative. Assuming independent normal distributions for these characteristics over the segments, we can measure a probability that a particular label should be assigned to a test segment. To assign the actual label, we look at the probability of the segment conditioned on those of its children and grand children. Labels are assigned in a recursive process, starting at the trachea, which is known from the initial seed point. At every step all unlabeled segments with a labeled parent are considered and the most probable labels are assigned.

3 Experimental Results

Experiments have been performed on three databases, each holding 50 scans from 16-slice scanners or higher, with sub-millimeter near isotropic resolution. Database 1 contains low-dose ($CTDI_{vol} \approx 3$ mGy) scans from a lung cancer screening program from asymptomatic subjects, scanned at full inspiration. Database 2 contains scans from the same subjects, now scanned at ultra-low-dose ($CTDI_{vol} \approx 1$ mGy) at end-expiration. Database 3 consists of scans from patients with interstitial lung disease with severe abnormalities present in the scans, all acquired at full inspiration and with a clinical dose ($CTDI_{vol} \approx 10$ mGy).

We applied both the single and the multi-threshold method to all 150 scans. Table 1 reports the total number of segments found and their length, per generation. Table 2 list for each lobar and segmental branch how often is was detected. Fig. 2 compares the results of the single and multi-threshold method in a

Table 2. For each of the 32 labeled segments in the bronchial tree, the percentages of extraction are listed for each database and for the single threshold method (S) and the multi-threshold method (M)

	Database 1		Database 2		Database 3	
	S	M	S	M	S	M
Trachea	100	100	100	100	100	100
RMB	98	100	100	100	92	96
RUL	96	98	98	100	92	94
RB1	96	98	68	94	82	88
RB2	92	96	72	94	84	86
RB3	94	98	80	96	86	88
BronInt	96	98	98	100	92	94
RB4+5	96	98	86	98	92	94
RB4	74	96	58	88	74	90
RB5	74	96	58	88	74	90
RB6	96	98	86	98	92	94
RLL7	96	98	72	98	82	92
RB7	94	98	62	94	80	88
RLL	94	98	62	94	80	88
RB8	84	98	34	80	62	78
RB9	84	96	40	80	58	80
RB10	84	98	36	80	60	78
LMB	98	100	100	100	92	96
LUL	96	100	94	98	92	92
LB1+2	92	98	76	96	82	92
LB1	82	96	54	88	68	88
LB2	82	96	54	88	68	88
LB3	94	98	40	86	86	88
LB4+5	94	98	90	98	84	90
LB4	80	96	42	74	74	88
LB5	80	96	42	74	74	88
LLB6	96	100	94	98	92	92
LB6	96	98	74	96	84	90
LLB	96	98	74	96	84	90
LB8	88	98	40	82	76	88
LB9	92	98	44	88	76	88
LB10	88	98	38	84	70	86
Overall average	91	98	68	92	81	90

scatterplot. Fig. 3 shows results for Database 1 (low-dose inspiration) versus the most challenging data used in this study, Database 2 (ultra-low dose expiration).

We have evaluated the accuracy of the labeling by asking two trained human observers to click points in each of the 32 segments. In a preliminary study on 36 scans we found that for the branches detected by the multi-threshold algorithm (98, 92 and 90%, for the three databases, respectively) 90% were correctly labeled. Most errors were caused by anatomical variations in the airway trees.

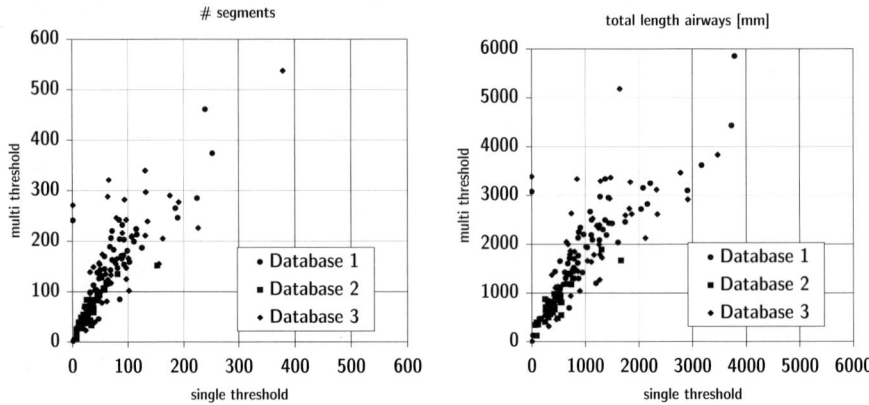

Fig. 2. Scatterplots showing number of segments (left) and total length of all airways in mm (right) found with the single and multi-threshold method. Each point represents one scan.

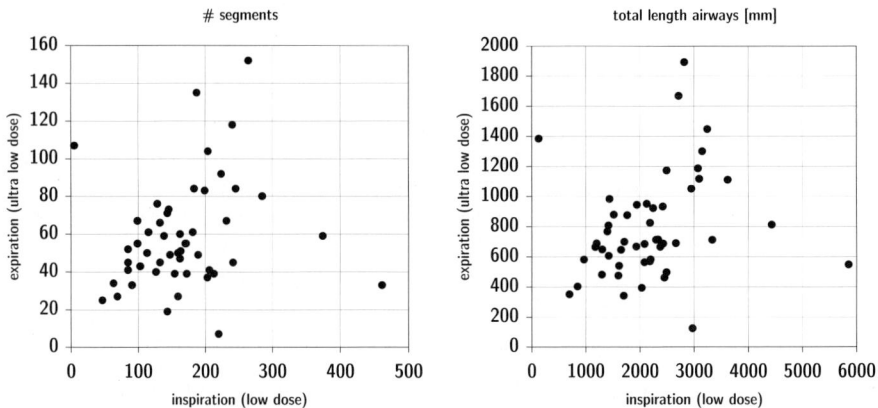

Fig. 3. Scatterplots showing number of segments (left) and total length of all airways in mm (right) found for the 50 scans in Database 1 (low dose, inspiration scans of asymptomatic subjects) versus the 50 scans in Database 2 (same subjects, scanned with ultra low dose in expiration). Each point represents one scan. Note the different scales on horizontal and vertical axis.

4 Discussion and Conclusion

The multi-threshold method effectively uses different HU thresholds for different parts of the bronchial tree. This appears very effective to avoid leakage, and thus early termination of the growth process, which we believe to be the main limitation of the single threshold strategy and previous methods that follow this approach [4,6,14]. Those methods already substantially outperform methods that do not employ the higher level rules at segmental level, like explosion control region growing. An average number of 170 airways detected in inspiration scans is impressive compared to results reported in other studies. Table 2 shows that the multi-threshold method is capable of extracting the bronchial tree up to segmental level quite robustly, and that its results are substantially better than those of the single threshold method. Both methods produce, by design, almost no false positive findings (incorrect branches). They are also fast, even the multi-threshold growing process requires only around 10 seconds on a single-core PC. The labeling takes less than two seconds.

A limitation of using variable thresholds is that the airway diameter estimation may not be consistent throughout the tree. We believe the current system should be followed by an additional step in which the airway lumen and wall are precisely determined.

In all scans we have inspected, there were very small peripheral bronchi present that were not extracted. A specific search for more distal airways and a mechanism to connect these to the tree [7,10] might improve performance even more. Note that such schemes require vastly more computation time. Another useful extension would be to use more elaborate rules for accepting voxels, fronts and segments, based on more complex image information and statistical analysis, as was recently proposed in [11].

The evaluation of the anatomical labeling is not based on the entire test set and thus preliminary. The accuracy of the procedure could be improved if the possibility of identifying the main anatomical variations in the airway tree up to segmental level were included in the labeling algorithm. Nevertheless it is clear that the majority of labels assigned by our method is correct.

Comparison of the results from Database 1 and 2 shows that the extraction of airways from expiration scans is substantially more difficult, but still generally feasible for the first few generations of the airway tree. The minor differences between Database 1 and 3 show that the proposed method is largely robust to pathology. It is also noteworthy that the total amount and length of airways extracted varies strongly from scan to scan. This makes it clear that comparing results from different methods obtained on different scans is tricky. It would be very useful to compare the different approaches on a single common database.

In conclusion, we have presented a fast, fully automatic method to extract the bronchial tree far into the periphery of the lungs and in addition label the most important branches. By locally adapting the threshold for accepting voxels as being airway, the algorithm is able to grow into airways with thin walls or absent walls at bifurcations, without leaking into the lung parenchyma. Extensive experiments have demonstrated that the method is robust and effective in finding a large number of airways up to ten generations or more.

References

1. Sluimer, I.C., Schilham, A., Prokop, M., van Ginneken, B.: Computer analysis of computed tomography scans of the lung: a survey. IEEE Trans. Med. Im. 25(4), 385–405 (2006)

2. Mori, K., Hasegawa, J., Suenaga, Y., Toriwaki, J.: Automated anatomical labeling of the bronchial branch and its application to the virtual bronchoscopy system. IEEE Trans. Med. Im. 19(2), 103–114 (2000)
3. Swift, R.D., Kiraly, A.P., Sherbondy, A.J., Austin, A.L., Hoffman, E.A., McLennan, G., Higgins, W.E.: Automatic axis generation for virtual bronchoscopic assessment of major airway obstructions. Comp. Med. Imag. & Graph 26, 103–118 (2002)
4. Schlathölter, T., Lorenz, C., Carlsen, I.C., Renisch, S., Deschamps, T.: Simultaneous segmentation and tree reconstruction of the airways for virtual bronchoscopy. In: Proc. SPIE, vol. 4684, pp. 103–113 (2002)
5. Kiraly, A.P., Helferty, J.P., Hoffman, E.A., McLennan, G., Higgins, W.E.: Three-dimensional path planning for virtual bronchoscopy. IEEE Trans Med. Im. 23(11), 1365–1379 (2004)
6. Bülow, T., Lorenz, C., Renisch, S.: A general framework for tree segmentation and reconstruction from medical volume data. In: Barillot, C., Haynor, D.R., Hellier, P. (eds.) MICCAI 2004. LNCS, vol. 3216, pp. 533–540. Springer, Heidelberg (2004)
7. Fetita, C.I., Prêteux, F., Beigelman-Aubry, C., Grenier, P.: Pulmonary airways: 3-D reconstruction from multislice CT and clinical investigation. IEEE Trans. Med. Im. 23(11), 1353–1364 (2004)
8. Tschirren, J., Hoffman, E.A., McLennan, G., Sonka, M.: Intrathoracic airway trees: segmentation and airway morphology analysis from low-dose CT scans. IEEE Trans. Med. Im. 24(12), 1529–1539 (2005)
9. Palágyi, K., Tschirren, J., Hoffman, E.A., Sonka, M.: Quantitative analysis of pulmonary airway tree structures. Comput. Biol. Med. 36(9), 974–996 (2006)
10. Higgins, W.E., Graham, M.W., Gibbs, J.D.: Robust system for human airway tree segmentation. In: Proc. SPIE, vol. 6914 (2008)
11. Lo, P., de Bruijne, M.: Voxel classification-based airway tree segmentation. In: Proc. SPIE, vol. 6914 (2008)
12. Tschirren, J., McLennan, G., Palágyi, K., Hoffman, E.A., Sonka, M.: Matching and anatomical labeling of human airway tree. IEEE Trans. Med. Im. 24, 1540–1547 (2005)
13. Bülow, T., Lorenz, C., Wiemker, R., Honko, J.: Point based methods for automatic bronchial tree matching and labeling. In: Proc. SPIE, vol. 6143 (2006)
14. Wiemker, R., Ekin, A., Opfer, R., Bülow, T., Rogalla, P.: Unsupervised extraction and quantification of the bronchial tree on ultra-low-dose vs. standard-dose CT. In: Proc. SPIE, vol. 6143 (2006)
15. Hu, S., Hoffman, E.A., Reinhardt, J.M.: Automatic lung segmentation for accurate quantitation of volumetric X-ray CT images. IEEE Trans. Med. Im. 20(6), 490–498 (2001)
16. Sluimer, I.C., Prokop, M., van Ginneken, B.: Towards automated segmentation of the pathological lung in CT. IEEE Trans. Med. Im. 24(8), 1025–1038 (2005)

Spine Segmentation Using Articulated Shape Models

Tobias Klinder[1,2], Robin Wolz[2], Cristian Lorenz[2], Astrid Franz[2], and Jörn Ostermann[1]

[1] Institut für Informationsverarbeitung, Leibniz University of Hannover, Germany
klinder@tnt.uni-hannover.de
[2] Philips Research Europe - Hamburg, Sector Medical Imaging Systems, Germany*

Abstract. Including prior shape in the form of anatomical models is a well-known approach for improving segmentation results in medical images. Currently, most approaches are focused on the modeling and segmentation of individual objects. In case of object constellations, a simultaneous segmentation of the ensemble that uses not only prior knowledge of individual shapes but also additional information about spatial relations between the objects is often beneficial. In this paper, we present a two-scale framework for the modeling and segmentation of the spine as an example for object constellations. The global spine shape is expressed as a consecution of local vertebra coordinate systems while individual vertebrae are modeled as triangulated surface meshes. Adaptation is performed by attracting the model to image features but restricting the attraction to a former learned shape. With the developed approach, we obtained a segmentation accuracy of 1.0 mm in average for ten thoracic CT images improving former results.

1 Introduction

Segmentation is still one of the main challenging problems in medical image analysis. In order to improve the segmentation results, prior knowledge is usually included in the form of anatomical models. For that purpose, complex geometrical models of various individual anatomical objects have been built supporting several medical applications, e.g., [1,2].

In case of object constellations, simultaneous multi-object segmentation is often beneficial compared to the separate segmentation of individual objects. Model-based segmentation of single objects typically leads to misadaptations in cases of no clear object boundary, similar structures in close vicinity, or pathologies. The result is thereby sensitive to model initialization. Moreover, the capture range of the segmentation is often very limited. However, by modeling not only the shape of individual objects but also the spatial relations to other objects, significant improvements can be achieved.

---

* We would like to thank Katrina Read from Philips Medical Systems, Cleveland (USA) as well as the University of Maryland Medical Center, Baltimore (USA) for all image data.

So far, little work focused on multi-object modeling and segmentation. Recently, de Bruijne et al. [3] presented a method for modeling relations between shape constellations using conditional probabilities between 2D-contours. A different way for multi-object modeling has been proposed by Boisvert et al. [4] where object relations are modeled as statistics on rigid transformations between the objects. However, both approaches have not been included to a model adaptation framework. One common way to account for multiple objects throughout the segmentation is to introduce a coupling term in the respective formulations as proposed, e.g., for coupled active contours [5] or level sets [6]. While overlapping between neighboring objects is prevented, spatial relations are not modeled.

In this paper, we present a two-scale framework for modeling object constellations with the individual parts interacting on each other throughout the entire adaptation. Although, we work exemplarily on spine segmentation in CT images, the method can be adapted to other object constellations due to its general formulation. Despite showing high contrast in CT, a separate segmentation of individual vertebrae often leads to unsatisfying results in images with low resolution or in case of pathologies. Without including knowledge about the constellation, vertebra shape models have to be positioned very close to their corresponding image structures to prevent adaptation to neighboring vertebrae having similar shape and intensity.

In Sect. 2, the principal idea of our approach is introduced. Basically, our modeling scheme is divided into two parts. A global spine model captures the constellations of objects while local vertebra models provide shape information of individual vertebrae. Patient individualization is achieved by subsequently adapting both parts with detailed formulations given in Sect. 2.1 and 2.2, respectively. Finally, spine segmentation is performed for thoracic CT images using the developed approach with results presented in Sect. 3.

2 Methods

In order to obtain a fast and robust framework, we follow a two-scale modeling scheme. On the one hand, a global model captures the object constellation by expressing the spine shape as a consecution of local vertebra coordinate systems (VCS) which have been earlier defined in [7]. On the other hand, local vertebra models provide shape information in the form of triangulated surface meshes of each individual object. For model adaptation, both parts are to be applied subsequently. By adapting the global model to the image, corresponding positions of individual objects are roughly to be found. Afterwards, local vertebra models are adapted providing the exact vertebra contour.

Adaptation for global and local model is based on the same idea. By using a physical metaphor an external energy (E_{ext}) drives the model towards image features while an internal energy (E_{int}) restricts attraction to a learned shape

$$E = E_{\text{ext}} + \alpha E_{\text{int}} . \qquad (1)$$

The parameter α controls the trade-off between both energy terms. The final position is in each case found by applying Eq. 1 iteratively.

2.1 Global Model Adaptation

Model-based adaptation is known to be dependent on careful initialization. Once adaptation is misled, it can hardly recover. Thus, a global adaptation framework moves the individual objects closer to the respective image structure. By expressing the spine as a consecution of K rigid transformations between $K+1$ VCSs, a flexible representation of the object constellation is found that provides a large to small scale approach. Note that the representation as a consecution of rigid transformations has to be expressed relative to a reference VCS.

For the definition of the respective energies, an appropriate distance measure between two rigid transformations has to be found. For that purpose, the representation of the rotation as a rotation vector is introduced. The rotation vector is defined as the product of the axis of rotation expressed as a unit vector $\mathbf{n}$ and an angle of rotation θ. With the rotation vector representation, we use the left-invariant distance definition between two rigid transformations in [4]:

$$d(T_1, T_2) = N_\omega(T_2^{-1} \circ T_1) \quad \text{with} \quad N_\omega(T)^2 = N_\omega(\{\mathbf{r},\mathbf{t}\})^2 = \|\mathbf{r}\|^2 + \|\omega \mathbf{t}\|^2 \quad (2)$$

where ω is used to weight the relative effect of rotation and translation, $\mathbf{r}$ is the rotation vector, and $\mathbf{t}$ the translation vector. As proposed in [4], the weight factor ω is set to 0.05. With this distance function, the respective energies as explained in detail below are defined as quadratic differences between a current and an 'optimal' position.

External Energy. The key idea of the global external energy is to drive each object towards its corresponding image structure. Thus, we define the feature function

$$F_i(\mathbf{x}_i) = -\mathbf{n}_i^T \nabla I(\mathbf{x}_i) \frac{g_{\max}(g_{\max} + \|\nabla I(\mathbf{x}_i)\|)}{g_{\max}^2 + \|\nabla I(\mathbf{x}_i)\|^2} \quad (3)$$

that is carried out for each mesh surface independently judging the position in the image. The feature function is indeed evaluated for each triangle of the surface mesh at the position of the triangle barycentre $\mathbf{x}_i$. The image gradient $\nabla I(\mathbf{x}_i)$ is projected onto the face normal $\mathbf{n}_i$ of each triangle and damped by $g_{\max}$. The feature values of all triangles are summed up providing one value per vertebra for the current position.

The search for new positions is performed by testing for each object various discrete locations inside a local neighborhood around a given position. For that purpose, a cartesian grid inside a bounding box around the given position is defined. In order to not only cope with translations but also rotations, the original object is rotated in discrete steps around all axes obtaining L rotation matrices $\mathbf{R}_l$. At each of the N grid positions, the feature function is evaluated for the corresponding surface mesh translated by $\mathbf{t}_n$ as well as its L rotated versions. Due to the frequent presence of local minima, this exhaustive search is preferred to other optimization strategies but will be replaced in future by stochastic optimization methods.

The transformation resulting in the highest feature strength determines the new position of the object:

$$\text{argmax}_{\mathbf{R}_l, \mathbf{t}_n} \sum_{i \in M} F_i(\mathbf{R}_l \mathbf{x}_i + \mathbf{t}_n), \quad (4)$$

where M is the number of triangles per mesh.

After finding the most promising positions for a pair of neighboring objects m and n, we can define the global external energy for the corresponding k-th transformation:

$$E_{\text{ext}_k} = d(\tilde{T}_{\text{VCS}_m}^{-1} \cdot \tilde{T}_{\text{VCS}_n}, T_k)^2 \quad (5)$$

where $\tilde{T}_{VCS_m}$ and $\tilde{T}_{VCS_n}$ are the transformations of the corresponding VCSs at the new positions to the world coordinate system. Thus, $\tilde{T}_{\text{VCS}_m}^{-1} \cdot \tilde{T}_{\text{VCS}_n}$ gives the transformation between the corresponding VCSs. The final transformation T_k between the neighboring objects will be determined by minimizing Eq. 1.

Internal Energy. Driving the model towards high image features as performed by the external energy is restricted by the internal energy to prevent false attraction. The internal energy preserves similarity of the ensemble towards an earlier learned constellation model. In this case, our spine model covers the mean spine shape as well as its variability. Since the spine is expressed as a consecution of rigid transformations that do not belong to a vector space but to a Lie Group, conventional statistics can not be applied. Instead, statistical methods applied to Riemannian manifolds are used. The following formulation is based on [4] that recently presented a statistical model of the spine expressed as a consecution of rigid transformations. However, an inclusion to an adaptation framework has so far not been presented.

Following the statistics for Riemannian manifolds, the generalization of the usual mean called the Fréchet mean is defined for a given distance as the element μ that minimizes the sum of the distances with a set of elements $x_0, \ldots, x_N$ of the same manifold $\mathcal{M}$:

$$\mu = \arg\min_{x \in \mathcal{M}} \sum_{i=0}^{N} d(x, x_i)^2. \quad (6)$$

Since the mean is given as a minimization, we use the gradient descent method performed on the summation obtaining

$$\mu_{n+1} = \text{Exp}_{\mu_n}\left(\frac{1}{N} \sum_{i=0}^{N} \text{Log}_{\mu_n}(x_i)\right). \quad (7)$$

The functions Exp and Log are respectively the exponential map and the log map associated with the distance $d(x,y)$. The exponential map projects an element of the tangent plane on the manifold $\mathcal{M}$ and the log map is the inverse function. For the calculation of exponential and log map associated with the defined distance of Eq. 2, we refer to [4].

Finally, the generalized cross covariance Σ_{xy} is the expectation in the tangent plane of the mean using the log map

$$\Sigma_{xy} = \frac{1}{N} \sum_{i=0}^{N} \text{Log}_{\mu_x}(x_i) \text{Log}_{\mu_y}(y_i)^T . \qquad (8)$$

In our case, the constellation of the spine is expressed as a multivariate vector $\mathbf{C}$ of K individual transformations $\mathbf{C} = [T_1, T_2, T_3, \ldots, T_K]^T$ obtaining for the mean and the covariance

$$\mu = \begin{pmatrix} \mu_1 \\ \mu_2 \\ \vdots \\ \mu_K \end{pmatrix} \quad \text{and} \quad \Sigma = \begin{pmatrix} \Sigma_{T_1 T_1} & \Sigma_{T_1 T_2} & \cdots & \Sigma_{T_1 T_K} \\ \Sigma_{T_2 T_1} & \Sigma_{T_2 T_2} & \cdots & \Sigma_{T_2 T_K} \\ \vdots & \vdots & & \vdots \\ \Sigma_{T_K T_1} & \Sigma_{T_K T_2} & \cdots & \Sigma_{T_K T_K} \end{pmatrix} . \qquad (9)$$

With Eq. 9, the formulation for the statistical spine model is given. In order to reduce the dimensionality of our model, principal component analysis is performed on the covariance matrix.

Now, we define the global internal energy for each transformation T_k as

$$E_{\text{int}_k} = d\left(\text{Exp}_{\mu_k}\left(\sum_{i=1}^{t} b_i \mathbf{a}_{i,k}\right), T_k\right)^2 \quad \text{with} \quad \mathbf{b} = \mathbf{A}^T (\text{Log}_{\mu} \mathbf{C}) \qquad (10)$$

where the matrix of the individual eigenvectors $\mathbf{a}_i$ is denoted as $\mathbf{A}$ and b_i is the coordinate of the weight vector $\mathbf{b}$ associated with the i-th principal component. The internal energy penalizes differences between the model and the current constellation. The closest constellation to the model is determined by projecting the given constellation $\mathbf{C}$ in the sub-space defined by the principal components.

Optimization. After calculating the respective energy terms, the final transformations T_k between the individual objects are determined by minimizing

$$E(T_k) = d(T_{\text{ext}_k}, T_k)^2 + \alpha \cdot d(T_{\text{int}_k}, T_k)^2 \qquad (11)$$

for each object separately. The transformations T_{ext_k} and T_{int_k} are obtained from the external and internal energy, respectively. The final transformation $T_{k_{\text{opt}}}$ is found using a Downhill-Simplex optimizer. As the representation of the ensemble as a consecution of rigid transformations requires a reference VCS, the vertebra with the highest feature strength is taken as the reference in each iteration.

2.2 Local Model Adaptation

After positioning the vertebra models using the global model adaptation, a local non-rigid free-form deformation similar to [8] of the individual surface meshes is carried out. Segmentation of all vertebrae is performed simultaneously with the individual shapes interacting on each other to prevent misadaptations.

External Energy. The local external energy

$$E_{\text{ext}} = \sum_{i \in T} w_i (\mathbf{e}_{\nabla \mathbf{I}}(\mathbf{x}_i + \tilde{\mathbf{c}}_i))^2 \quad \text{with} \quad w_i = \max\{0, F_i^*(\mathbf{x}_i + \tilde{\mathbf{c}}_i) - \delta \|\tilde{\mathbf{c}}_i\|^2\} \qquad (12)$$

drives each triangle barycentre $\mathbf{x}_i$ towards a detected potential anatomical surface point $\mathbf{x}_i + \tilde{\mathbf{c}}_i$. The unit vector $\mathbf{e}_{\nabla I}$ points in direction of the image gradient at the surface point $\mathbf{x}_i + \tilde{\mathbf{c}}_i$.

For each triangle barycentre $\mathbf{x}_i$, surface detection is carried out within a locally defined sampling grid along the triangle surface normal. At each candidate position $\mathbf{c}_k$, the feature function is evaluated and finally the point $\tilde{\mathbf{c}}_i$ is chosen that maximizes the objective function

$$\tilde{\mathbf{c}}_i = \mathrm{argmax}_{\mathbf{c}_k} \left\{ F_i^*(\mathbf{x}_i + \mathbf{c}_k) - \delta \|\mathbf{c}_k\|^2 \right\}. \quad (13)$$

The parameter δ controls the trade-off between feature strength and distance.

As a feature function, we apply the one already defined in Eq. 3 but with an additional factor c penalizing overlapping resulting in $F_i^* = c \cdot F_i$.

If no collision with a neighbored mesh is present, the factor c will be equal to one. In case of a collision, c becomes the smaller the deeper the detected point is inside the neighbored mesh. Note that this formulation does not prohibit collision but makes points that lie inside other meshes less attractive.

An effective implementation of the collision detection is achieved by labeling all meshes and assigning adjacent surface patches of neighboring vertebrae. Since collision detection has to be only carried out for corresponding adjacent surfaces that potentially overlap, the computational complexity is significantly reduced.

Internal Energy. As a regularization, the local internal energy

$$E_{\mathrm{int}} = \sum_{j \in V} \sum_{k \in N(j)} ((\hat{\mathbf{v}}_j - \hat{\mathbf{v}}_k) - s\mathbf{R}(\mathbf{v}_j - \mathbf{v}_k))^2 \quad (14)$$

preserves shape similarity of all adapted vertices $\mathbf{v}_j$ to the model vertices $\hat{\mathbf{v}}_j$ with $N(j)$ being the set of neighbors of vertex j. neighboring vertices are those connected by a single triangle edge. The scaling factor s and the rotational matrix $\mathbf{R}$ are determined by a closed-form point-based registration method based on a singular value decomposition prior to calculation of Eq. 14.

Optimization. In the final optimization scheme for the local model adaptation, the vertex positions of the triangular surface mesh are indeed the parameters to be varied. As only interdependencies between neighboring vertices exist and the energy terms are of a quadratic form, the conjugate gradient method is used for minimization of the final equation system with a sparsely filled matrix.

3 Results

For our model building, vertebra models were adapted to 18 thoracic CT data sets using [7]. In case of misadaptations, manual corrections were performed. From the adapted surface meshes, mean shape models of all vertebrae as well as a statistal model of rigid transformations between the VCSs was created.

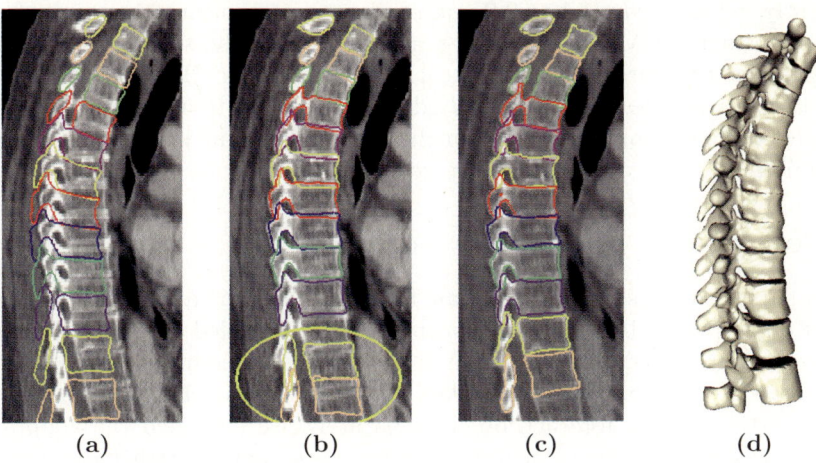

(a) (b) (c) (d)

Fig. 1. Automatically positioned models (a) are adapted using SCDM (b) and two-scale method (c). Due to the consideration of overall constellation, misadaptation of T11 and T12 could be overcome and overlapping between neigbored models could be decreased. Surface rendering of adapted meshes (d).

Table 1. Adaptation result for ten test data sets showing average ± standard deviation (maximum) of segmentation error (values in mm). For each algorithm, the result for one chosen test case is examplarily given in detail.

	Collision Detection		Two-Scale	
	Patient 6	6 Data Sets	Patient 1	10 Data Sets
SCDM	1.3±0.3 (6.9)	1.1±0.2 (5.5)	2.8±1.7 (8.9)	2.7±2.8 (9.0)
new	0.9±0.3 (6.0)	0.9±0.2 (5.4)	0.8±0.2 (5.8)	1.0±0.3 (6.5)

The new framework was applied to ten test data sets including pathologies like strong calcifications between vertebrae or scoliosis. In each case, model initialization was given by [7]. Reference segmentation was provided by manually positioning and automatically adapating the individual surface models. Misadaptations were again manually corrected. As the main contributions of our framework are the global adaptation and the collision detection during local adaptation, we compared our results to the adaptation using the shape-constrained deformable model method (SCDM) [8]. Automatic segmentation was compared to the reference by calculating for each vertex of the adapted mesh the closest point on the reference surface. One problem that could be circumvented by our framework is the misadaptation of several models to wrong neighboring vertebrae as examplarily shown in Fig. 1. In the ten test cases, this secenario occured for four patients. In the remaining six data sets, SCDM already adapted to the correct image structure. To investigate the effect of collision detection, we compared the segmentation result for these six data sets using SCDM and SCDM with collision detection but no global model. As shown in Tab. 1, the mean error could be slightly reduced from 1.1 to 0.9 mm in average. Comparing the results for all ten cases using SCDM with our two-scale framework, the segmentation results were significanty improved from 2.7 to 1.0 mm in average. However, it has to be noted that the results are slightly biased due to the fact that the creation of the reference segmentation was based on the same algorithm with additional user interaction.

4 Conclusion

In this paper, we presented a two-scale framework for the automatic segmentation of object constellations. The constellation is modeled as a consecution of local coordinate systems while the individual objects' shape is presented as a triangulated surface model. In contrast to former approaches performing only non-rigid deformation for each object separately, we extended the adaptation allowing a simultaneous segmentation of the constellation with individual objects interacting on each other. Compared to former approaches, a significant improvement of the segmentation result has been achieved while at the same time the capture range for the adaption has been increased. Furthermore, we are more robust against pathologies in spine shape with the developed approach due to the inclusion of a statistical spine shape model.

References

1. Lorenz, C., von Berg, J.: A comprehensive shape model of the heart. Medical Image Analysis 10, 657–670 (2006)
2. Blaffert, T., Barschdorf, H., von Berg, J., Dries, S., Franz, A., Klinder, T., Lorenz, C., Renisch, S., Wiemker, R.: Lung lobe modeling and segmentation with individualized surface meshes. In: Proc. SPIE Medical Imaging 2008 (to appear, 2008)
3. de Bruijne, M., Lund, M., Tanko, L., Pettersen, P., Nielsen, M.: Quantitative vertebral morphometry using neighbor-conditional shape models. In: Larsen, R., Nielsen, M., Sporring, J. (eds.) MICCAI 2006. LNCS, vol. 4190, pp. 1–8. Springer, Heidelberg (2006)
4. Boisvert, J., Pennec, X., Labelle, H., Cheriet, F., Ayache, N.: Principal spine shape deformation modes using Riemannian geometry and articulated modes. In: Perales, F.J., Fisher, R.B. (eds.) AMDO 2006. LNCS, vol. 4069, pp. 346–355. Springer, Heidelberg (2006)
5. Zimmer, C., Olivo-Marin, J.: Coupled parametric active contours. IEEE Trans. Pattern Anal. Mach. Intell. 27(11), 1838–1842 (2005)
6. Rousson, M., Khamene, A., Diallo, M., Celi, J.C., Sauer, F.: Constrained surface evolutions for prostate and bladder segmentation in ct images. In: Liu, Y., Jiang, T., Zhang, C. (eds.) CVBIA 2005. LNCS, vol. 3765, pp. 251–260. Springer, Heidelberg (2005)
7. Klinder, T., Lorenz, C., von Berg, J., Dries, S., Bülow, T., Ostermann, J.: Automated model-based rib cage segmentation and labeling in CT images. In: Ayache, N., Ourselin, S., Maeder, A. (eds.) MICCAI 2007, Part II. LNCS, vol. 4792, pp. 195–203. Springer, Heidelberg (2007)
8. Weese, J., Kaus, M., Lorenz, C., Lobregt, S., Truyen, R., Pekar, V.: Shape constrained deformable models for 3D medical image segmentation. In: Insana, M.F., Leahy, R.M. (eds.) IPMI 2001. LNCS, vol. 2082, pp. 380–387. Springer, Heidelberg (2001)

Model-Based Segmentation of Hippocampal Subfields in Ultra-High Resolution In Vivo MRI

Koen Van Leemput[1,2], Akram Bakkour[1,3], Thomas Benner[1],
Graham Wiggins[1], Lawrence L. Wald[1,4], Jean Augustinack[1],
Bradford C. Dickerson[1,3], Polina Golland[2], and Bruce Fischl[1,2,4]

[1] Athinoula A. Martinos Center for Biomedical Imaging, Department of Radiology,
MGH, Harvard Medical School, USA
[2] Computer Science and Artificial Intelligence Laboratory, MIT, USA
[3] Department of Neurology, MGH, Harvard Medical School, USA
[4] Harvard-MIT Division of Health Sciences and Technology, MIT, USA

Abstract. Recent developments in MR data acquisition technology are starting to yield images that show anatomical features of the hippocampal formation at an unprecedented level of detail, providing the basis for hippocampal subfield measurement. Because of the role of the hippocampus in human memory and its implication in a variety of disorders and conditions, the ability to reliably and efficiently quantify its subfields through in vivo neuroimaging is of great interest to both basic neuroscience and clinical research. In this paper, we propose a fully-automated method for segmenting the hippocampal subfields in ultra-high resolution MRI data. Using a Bayesian approach, we build a computational model of how images around the hippocampal area are generated, and use this model to obtain automated segmentations. We validate the proposed technique by comparing our segmentation results with corresponding manual delineations in ultra-high resolution MRI scans of five individuals.

1 Introduction

Models of brain structures generated from magnetic resonance imaging (MRI) data have grown in complexity in recent years, evolving from simple models with few classes such as gray matter, white matter and cerebrospinal fluid (CSF) [1,2,3], into more complex ones representing a multitude of neuroanatomical structures [4,5,6]. Still, while many brain structures such as the thalamus, the amygdala, or the hippocampus consist of multiple distinct, interacting subregions, they are mostly treated as a single entity because of the limited image resolution of typical structural MRI scans. Recently, however, substantial developments in MR data acquisition technology have made it possible to acquire images with remarkably higher resolution and signal-to-noise ratio than was previously attainable [7]. Such scans show many cortical and subcortical structures in unprecedented detail, and offer new opportunities for explicitly quantifying individual subregions, rather than their agglomerate, directly from in vivo MRI data.

Analyzing large imaging studies of ultra-high resolution MRI scans requires computational techniques to automatically extract information from the images.

This is technically difficult because, although the images show greater anatomical detail than traditional MRI scans, many boundaries between substructures of interest remain hard to discern. In manual delineations, the extent of specific subregions is often inferred from the extent of other, more clearly defined structures by relying on prior neuroanatomical knowledge, rather than on local intensity information alone. The success of automated methods therefore depends critically on computational models that provide prior information about the relative location, shape, and appearance of the structures of interest.

In this paper, we present an automated segmentation technique for the subfields of the hippocampus in ultra-high resolution MRI data based on state-of-the-art computational models. Although the methodology is applicable to other brain structures as well, we identified the hippocampus as our driving application because it is a necessary component in a variety of memory functions, as well as the locus of structural change in aging, Alzheimer's disease (AD), schizophrenia, and other conditions. Distinct hippocampal subregions have been shown to be implicated in different memory subsystems [8,9] and be differentially affected in aging and AD [10]. Therefore, the ability to measure, through in vivo neuroimaging, subtle changes in these subregions promises to have widespread application in both basic neuroscience and clinical research.

2 Model-Based Hippocampal Subfield Segmentation

We use a Bayesian modeling approach, in which we first build an explicit computational model of how an MRI image around the hippocampal area is generated, and subsequently use this model to obtain fully automated segmentations. The model incorporates a *prior* distribution that makes predictions about where neuroanatomical labels typically occur throughout the image, and is based on the generalization of probabilistic atlases [2,3,4,5,11] developed in [12]. The model also includes a *likelihood* distribution that predicts how a label image, where each voxel is assigned a unique neuroanatomical label, translates into an MRI image, where each voxel has an intensity.

2.1 Prior: Mesh-Based Probabilistic Atlas

Let $L = \{l_i, i = 1, \ldots, I\}$ be a label image with a total of I voxels, with $l_i \in \{1, \ldots, K\}$ denoting the one of K possible labels assigned to voxel i. Our prior models this image as being generated by the following process:

- A (irregular) tetrahedral mesh covering the image domain of interest is defined by the *reference position* of its N mesh nodes $\boldsymbol{x}^r = \{\boldsymbol{x}_n^r, n = 1, \ldots, N\}$, and by a set of label probabilities $\boldsymbol{\alpha} = \{\boldsymbol{\alpha}_n, n = 1, \ldots, N\}$. Node n is associated with a probability vector $\boldsymbol{\alpha}_n = \{\alpha_n^1, \ldots, \alpha_n^K\}$, satisfying $\alpha_n^k \geq 0$ and $\sum_k^K \alpha_n^k = 1$, that governs how frequently each label occurs around that node.
- The mesh is deformed from its reference position by sampling from a Markov random field (MRF) model regulating the position of the mesh nodes:

$$p(\boldsymbol{x}) \propto \exp\Big(-U_{\boldsymbol{x}^r}(\boldsymbol{x})\Big) = \exp\Big(-\sum_{t=1}^{T} U_{\boldsymbol{x}^r}^t(\boldsymbol{x})\Big), \quad (1)$$

where $U_{\boldsymbol{x}^r}^t(\boldsymbol{x})$ is a penalty for deforming tetrahedron t from its shape in the reference position $\boldsymbol{x}^r$, and $U_{\boldsymbol{x}^r}(\boldsymbol{x})$ is an overall deformation penalty obtained by summing the contributions of all T tetrahedra in the mesh. We use the penalty proposed in [13], which goes to infinity if the Jacobian determinant of any tetrahedron's deformation approaches zero, and therefore insures that the mesh topology is preserved.

- In the deformed mesh with position $\boldsymbol{x}$, the probability of observing label k in a pixel i with location $\boldsymbol{x}_i$ is modeled by

$$p_i(k|\boldsymbol{x}) = \sum_{n=1}^{N} \alpha_n^k \phi_n(\boldsymbol{x}_i), \quad (2)$$

where $\phi_n(\cdot)$ denotes an interpolation basis function attached to mesh node n that has a unity value at the position of the mesh node, a zero value at the outward faces of the tetrahedra connected to the node and beyond, and a linear variation across the volume of each tetrahedron. Assuming conditional independence of the labels between voxels given the mesh node locations, we obtain the probability of seeing label image L: $p(L|\boldsymbol{x}) = \prod_{i=1}^{I} p_i(l_i|\boldsymbol{x})$.

It has previously been demonstrated that the mesh's connectivity, reference position $\boldsymbol{x}^r$, and label probabilities $\boldsymbol{\alpha}$ can be learned from a set of manually labeled example images [12]. The learning involves selecting the model that maximizes the probability of observing the example label images, or, equivalently, that minimizes the number of bits needed to encode them. An example of the prior, derived from 4 manually labeled hippocampi, is shown in figure 2. Note that the image domain is non-uniformly sampled, with areas containing little information covered by larger tetrahedra.

2.2 Likelihood: Imaging Model

For the likelihood distribution, we employ a simple, often-used model according to which a Gaussian distribution with mean μ_k and variance σ_k^2 is associated with each label k. Given label image L, an intensity image $Y = \{y_i, i = 1, \ldots, I\}$ is generated by drawing the intensity in each voxel independently from the Gaussian distribution associated with its label:

$$p(Y|L, \boldsymbol{\theta}) = \prod_{i=1}^{I} p(y_i | \mu_{l_i}, \sigma_{l_i}^2) = \prod_{i=1}^{I} \frac{1}{\sqrt{2\pi\sigma_{l_i}^2}} \exp\Big(-\frac{(y_i - \mu_{l_i})^2}{2\sigma_{l_i}^2}\Big),$$

where the parameters $\boldsymbol{\theta} = \{\mu_1, \sigma_1^2, \ldots, \mu_K, \sigma_K^2\}$ are assumed to be governed by a uniform prior: $p(\boldsymbol{\theta}) \propto 1$.

2.3 Model Parameter Estimation

In a Bayesian setting, assessing the Maximum A Posteriori (MAP) parameter values $\{\widehat{\boldsymbol{x}}, \widehat{\boldsymbol{\theta}}\}$ involves maximizing

$$p(\boldsymbol{x}, \boldsymbol{\theta}|Y) \propto p(Y|\boldsymbol{x}, \boldsymbol{\theta})p(\boldsymbol{x})p(\boldsymbol{\theta}) \propto \left(\prod_{i=1}^{I} \sum_{k=1}^{K} p(y_i|\mu_k, \sigma_k^2) p_i(k|\boldsymbol{x}) \right) p(\boldsymbol{x}),$$

which is equivalent to minimizing

$$\sum_{i=1}^{I} \left(-\log \left[\sum_{k=1}^{K} p(y_i|\mu_k, \sigma_k^2) p_i(k|\boldsymbol{x}) \right] \right) - \log p(\boldsymbol{x}). \quad (3)$$

We use an EM-style majorization technique [14,15], where we calculate a statistical classification that associates each voxel with each of the neuroanatomical labels

$$W_i^k = \frac{p(y_i|\mu_k, \sigma_k^2) p_i(k|\boldsymbol{x})}{\sum_{k'} p(y_i|\mu_{k'}, \sigma_{k'}^2) p_i(k'|\boldsymbol{x})}$$

and subsequently use this classification to construct an upper bound to eq. (3) that touches it at the current parameters estimates [16]:

$$\sum_{i=1}^{I} \left(-\log \left[\prod_{k=1}^{K} \left(\frac{p(y_i|\mu_k, \sigma_k^2) p_i(k|\boldsymbol{x})}{W_i^k} \right)^{W_i^k} \right] \right) - \log p(\boldsymbol{x}). \quad (4)$$

Optimizing this upper bound w.r.t. the Gaussian distribution parameters $\boldsymbol{\theta}$, while keeping $\boldsymbol{x}$ fixed, yields the closed-form expressions

$$\mu_k = \frac{\sum_{i=1}^{I} W_i^k y_i}{\sum_{i=1}^{I} W_i^k}, \quad \sigma_k^2 = \frac{\sum_{i=1}^{I} W_i^k (y_i - \mu_k)^2}{\sum_{i=1}^{I} W_i^k}, \quad k = 1, \ldots, K.$$

With these estimates of $\boldsymbol{\theta}$, the classification and the corresponding upper bound are updated, and the estimation of $\boldsymbol{\theta}$ is repeated, until convergence. We then re-calculate the upper bound, and optimize it w.r.t. the mesh node positions $\boldsymbol{x}$, keeping $\boldsymbol{\theta}$ fixed. Optimizing $\boldsymbol{x}$ is a registration process that deforms the atlas mesh towards the current classification, similar to the schemes proposed in [5,17]. The gradient of eq. (4) with respect to $\boldsymbol{x}$ is given in analytical form through the interpolation model of eq. (2) and the deformation model of eq. (1). We perform this registration by gradient descent. Subsequently, we repeat the optimization of $\boldsymbol{\theta}$ and $\boldsymbol{x}$, each in turn, until convergence.

2.4 Image Segmentation

Once we have an estimate of the model parameters $\{\widehat{\boldsymbol{x}}, \widehat{\boldsymbol{\theta}}\}$, we can use it to obtain an approximation to the MAP anatomical labeling. Approximating $p(L|Y) = \int_{\boldsymbol{x}} \int_{\boldsymbol{\theta}} p(L|Y, \boldsymbol{x}, \boldsymbol{\theta}) p(\boldsymbol{x}, \boldsymbol{\theta}|Y) \mathrm{d}\boldsymbol{x} \mathrm{d}\boldsymbol{\theta}$ by $p(L|Y, \widehat{\boldsymbol{x}}, \widehat{\boldsymbol{\theta}}) \propto p(Y|L, \widehat{\boldsymbol{\theta}}) p(L|\widehat{\boldsymbol{x}})$, we have

$$\widehat{L} = \arg\max_{L} p(L|Y) \simeq \arg\max_{\{l_i, i=1,\ldots,I\}} \prod_i p(y_i|\widehat{\mu}_{l_i}, \widehat{\sigma}_{l_i}^2) p_i(l_i|\widehat{\boldsymbol{x}}),$$

which is obtained by assigning each voxel to the label with the highest posterior probability, i.e., $\widehat{l}_i = \arg\max_k W_i^k$.

3 Experiments

We performed experiments on ultra-high resolution MRI data collected as part of an ongoing imaging study assessing the effects of normal aging and AD on brain structure. Using a prototype custom-built 32-channel head coil with a 3.0T Siemens Trio MRI system [7], we acquired images via an optimized high-resolution MPRAGE sequence that enables 380 μm in-plane resolution (TR/TI/TE = 2530/1100/5.39 ms, FOV=448, FA = 7°, 208 slices acquired coronally, thickness = 0.8mm, acquisition time = 7.34 min). To increase the signal-to-noise ratio, 5 acquisitions were collected and motion-corrected to obtain a single resampled (to 380 μm isotropic) high contrast volume that covers the entire medial temporal lobe.

Using a protocol developed specifically for this purpose, the subfields of the right hippocampus were manually delineated in images of 5 subjects (2 younger and 3 older cognitively normal individuals). These delineations included the fimbria, presubiculum, subiculum, CA1, CA2/3, and CA4/DG fields, as well as choroid plexus, hippocampal fissure, and lateral ventricle, as shown in figure 1. Voxels outside of these structures were automatically labeled as gray matter, white matter, or CSF using an EM-based tissue classifier [2].

We restricted our automated analysis to a region of interest (ROI) around the right hippocampus only. To this end, we defined a cuboid ROI of size 100x60x160 voxels in an image of a younger normal individual not included in the study (template image). This ROI was automatically aligned to each image under study using an affine Mutual Information based registration technique [18,19], by first aligning the whole template image covering the entire brain, followed by a registration of the ROI only. Atlas meshes were then computed and applied in the area covered by this ROI in each image.

We used a 3-level multi-resolution optimization strategy, in which the image under study and the atlas mesh were subject to a gradually decreasing amount of spatial smoothing. In order to simplify the optimization process, we restricted the number of labels throughout the multi-resolution scheme to four, merging the gray matter with the presubiculum, subiculum, and CA fields, the white matter with the fimbria, the lateral ventricle with choroid plexus, and CSF with the hippocampal fissure. This restriction was then removed to obtain the final segmentation. The whole segmentation process was fully automated and took about 1.5 hours per subject on a 2.33GHz Intel Core2 processor.

We evaluated our automated segmentation results using a leave-one-out cross-validation strategy: we built an atlas mesh from the delineations in 4 subjects, and used this to segment the image of the remaining subject. We repeated this process for each of the 5 subjects, and compared the automated segmentation results with the corresponding manual delineations. Towards the tail of the hippocampus, the manual delineations no longer discerned between the different subfields, but rather lumped everything together as simply "hippocampus" (see figure 1). Since the starting point of this "catch-all" label was arbitrary chosen in each subject, with its volume ranging from 5 to 17% of the total hippocampal volume in different subjects, voxels that were labeled as such in either the automated or manual segmentation were not included in the comparisons.

For each of seven structures of interest (fimbria, CA1, CA2/3, CA4/DG, presubiculum, subiculum, and hippocampal fissure), we calculated the Dice overlap coefficient, defined as the volume of overlap between the automated and manual segmentation divided by their mean volume. Since we are ultimately interested in detecting *changes* in hippocampal subfields between different patient populations, we also evaluated how well differences in subfield volumes between subjects, as detected by the manual delineations, were reflected in the automated segmentations. To this end, we performed a linear regression on the absolute volumes detected by both methods, calculating Pearson's correlation coefficient for each structure.

4 Results

Figure 1 compares the manual and automated segmentation results qualitatively on a set of cross-sectional slices. The upper half of figure 3 shows the average Dice overlap measure for each of the structures of interest, along with the minimum and maximum across the 5 subjects. All of the larger structures, ranging in average size from 6,100 voxels for CA1 to 14,300 voxels for CA2/3, have an average Dice coefficient of around 0.7 or higher. Smaller structures such as the fimbria (on average 1,700 voxels) and the hippocampal fissure (on average 1,400 voxels) are more challenging and have a lower Dice coefficient of around 0.58 and 0.45, respectively.

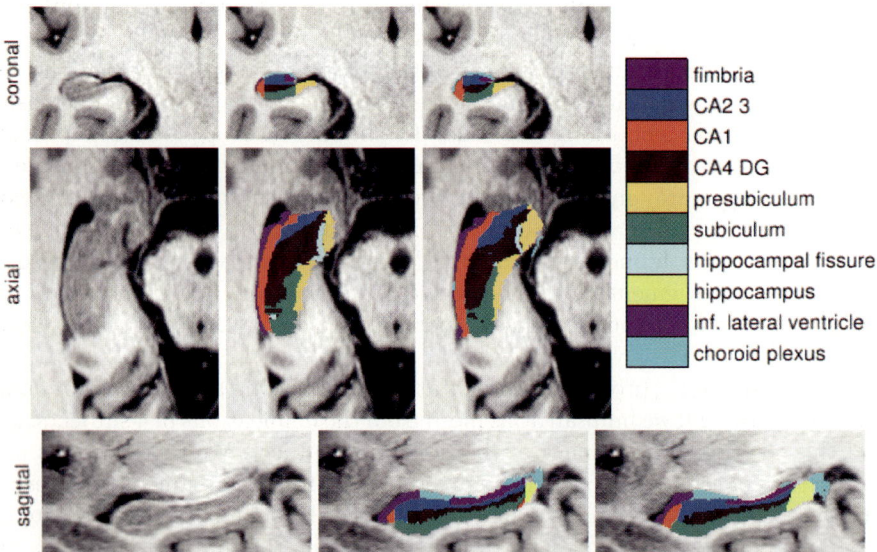

Fig. 1. From left to right: ultra-high resolution MRI data, manual delineations, and corresponding automated segmentations

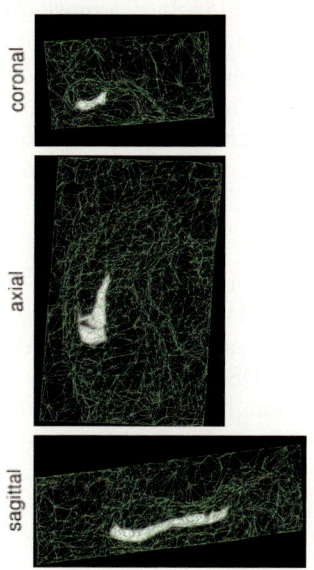
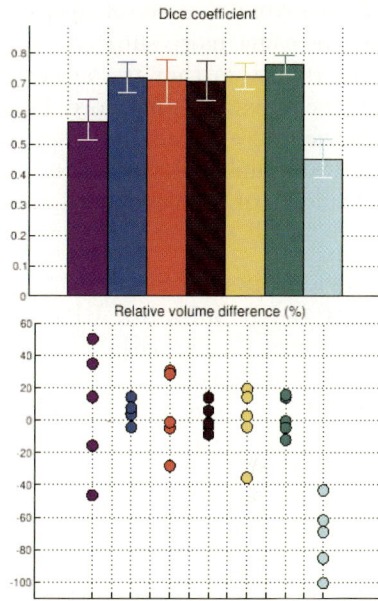

Fig. 2. Mesh-based probabilistic atlas, derived from manual delineations in 4 subjects, warped onto the 5th subject shown in figure 1. Bright and dark intensities correspond to high and low prior probability for subiculum, respectively.

Fig. 3. Dice overlap measures (top) and relative volume differences (bottom) between automated and manual segmentations. The colors are as in figure 1.

The lower half of figure 3 shows, for each structure, the volume differences between the automated and manual segmentations relative to their mean volumes. Regarding Pearson's correlation coefficient, the automatically calculated volumes of CA4/DG and CA2/3 are strongly correlated with the manual ones, with a correlation coefficient of approximately 0.98 ($p \leq 0.004$) and 0.93 ($p \leq 0.024$), respectively. CA1 and subiculum correlate to some degree (correlation coefficient of 0.73 and 0.71, p-values not significant), whereas presubiculum and fimbria do not seem to correlate at all (correlation coefficient of 0.02 and -0.18, p-values not significant). Interestingly, despite the hippocampal fissure's low Dice overlap measure, its automated measurements correlate better with the manual ones than do some structures with much higher Dice coefficients (correlation coefficient 0.85, $p \leq 0.068$). The low Dice coefficient is apparently caused by a systematic underestimation of the hippocampal fissure volume by the automated method.

5 Discussion

In this paper, we demonstrated a model-based approach to automated hippocampal subfield segmentation in ultra-high resolution MRI and presented preliminary results on a small number of subjects. Future work will include a more thorough validation, using more subjects with repeat scans and manual delineations by different raters, so that the accuracy and repeatability of our method can be placed in context. Furthermore, in order to analyze invaluable existing imaging studies that were acquired at more standard image resolutions, we also plan to develop a modified likelihood for standard resolution images that includes an explicit model of the partial volume effect [20].

Acknowledgments. Support for this research was provided in part by the NIH NCRR (P41-RR14075, R01 RR16594-01A1, NAC P41-RR13218, and the BIRN Morphometric Project BIRN002, U24 RR021382), the NIBIB (R01 EB001550, R01EB006758, NAMIC U54-EB005149), the NINDS (R01 NS052585-01, R01 NS051826) as well as the MIND Institute. Additional support was provided by The Autism & Dyslexia Project funded by the Ellison Medical Foundation.

References

1. Wells, W., et al.: Adaptive segmentation of MRI data. IEEE Transactions on Medical Imaging 15(4), 429–442 (1996)
2. Van Leemput, K., et al.: Automated model-based tissue classification of MR images of the brain. IEEE Transactions on Medical Imaging 18(10), 897–908 (1999)
3. Ashburner, J., Friston, K.: Unified segmentation. NeuroImage 26, 839–885 (2005)
4. Fischl, B., et al.: Whole brain segmentation: Automated labeling of neuroanatomical structures in the human brain. Neuron 33, 341–355 (2002)
5. Pohl, K., et al.: A Bayesian model for joint segmentation and registration. NeuroImage 31, 228–239 (2006)
6. Heckemann, R., et al.: Automatic anatomical brain MRI segmentation combining label propagation and decision fusion. NeuroImage 33(1), 115–126 (2006)
7. Wiggins, G., et al.: 32-channel 3 Tesla receive-only phased-array head coil with soccer-ball element geometry. Magn. Res. in Medicine 56(1), 216–223 (2006)
8. Zeineh, M., et al.: Dynamics of the Hippocampus During Encoding and Retrieval of Face-Name Pairs. Science 299(5606), 577–580 (2003)
9. Gabrieli, J., et al.: Separate Neural Bases of Two Fundamental Memory Processes in the Human Medial Temporal Lobe. Science 276(5310), 264 (1997)
10. Small, S., et al.: Evaluating the function of hippocampal subregions with high-resolution MRI in AD and aging. Microsc. Res. and Tech. 51(1), 101–108 (2000)
11. Shattuck, D., et al.: Construction of a 3D probabilistic atlas of human cortical structures. NeuroImage 39, 1064–1080 (2008)
12. Van Leemput, K.: Probabilistic brain atlas encoding using Bayesian inference. In: Larsen, R., Nielsen, M., Sporring, J. (eds.) MICCAI 2006. LNCS, vol. 4190, pp. 704–711. Springer, Heidelberg (2006)
13. Ashburner, et al.: Image registration using a symmetric prior–in three dimensions. Human Brain Mapping 9(4), 212–225 (2000)
14. Dempster, A.P., et al.: Maximum likelihood from incomplete data via the EM algorithm. Journal of the Royal Statistical Society 39, 1–38 (1977)
15. Stoica, P., Selén, Y.: Cyclic minimizers, majorization techniques, and the EM algorithm: A refresher. IEEE Signal Processing Magazine, 112–114 (2004)

16. Minka, T.: Expectation-Maximization as lower bound maximization. Technical report, MIT (1998)
17. D'Agostino, E., et al.: A unified framework for atlas based brain image segmentation and registration. In: Pluim, J.P.W., Likar, B., Gerritsen, F.A. (eds.) WBIR 2006. LNCS, vol. 4057, pp. 136–143. Springer, Heidelberg (2006)
18. Wells, W., et al.: Multi-modal volume registration by maximization of mutual information. Medical Image Analysis 1(1), 35–51 (1996)
19. Maes, F., et al.: Multimodality image registration by maximization of mutual information. IEEE Transactions on Medical Imaging 16(2), 187–198 (1997)
20. Van Leemput, K., et al.: A unifying framework for partial volume segmentation of brain MR images. IEEE Transactions on Medical Imaging 22(1), 105–119 (2003)

Kinetic Modeling Based Probabilistic Segmentation for Molecular Images

Ahmed Saad[1,2], Ghassan Hamarneh[1], Torsten Möller[2], and Ben Smith[1,2]

[1] Medical Image Analysis Lab
[2] Graphics, Usability, and Visualization Lab,
School of Computing Science, Simon Fraser University, Canada
{aasaad,hamarneh,torsten,brsmith}@cs.sfu.ca

Abstract. We propose a semi-supervised, kinetic modeling based segmentation technique for molecular imaging applications. It is an iterative, self-learning algorithm based on uncertainty principles, designed to alleviate low signal-to-noise ratio (SNR) and partial volume effect (PVE) problems. Synthetic fluorodeoxyglucose (FDG) and simulated Raclopride dynamic positron emission tomography (dPET) brain images with excessive noise levels are used to validate our algorithm. We show, qualitatively and quantitatively, that our algorithm outperforms state-of-the-art techniques in identifying different functional regions and recovering the kinetic parameters.

1 Introduction

Molecular imaging is a new scientific area merging concepts of molecular biology with non-invasive imaging technologies. In dPET [1], for example, radioactive tracers can act as biomarkers to track spatio-temporal molecular and cellular processes. Kinetic modeling (KM) is an essential step for molecular image quantification [2]. KM parameters of tissue perfusion, tracer transport or receptor binding are typically calculated by fitting the average time activity curves (TACs) within a region of interest (ROI) to underlying mathematical models. Manual ROI delineation of functional regions is a tedious, time-consuming, and error-prone task, that relies on subjective user assessment and is influenced by image quality. This leads to inaccuracies in KM parameter estimation.

In this paper, we focus on segmentation and KM parameter estimation from dPET as it is considered the leading technology for molecular imaging due to its high specificity and sensitivity. Nevertheless, our proposed method is applicable to other modalities whose analysis utilize KM such as dynamic contrast enhanced magnetic resonance imaging and contrast enhanced ultrasound.

Several methods had been proposed to segment dPET images into different functional regions. Barber applied factor analysis to planar dynamic Gamma camera images to identify functional regions [3]. Gou et al. applied hierarchical TAC clustering [4]. This algorithm was purely based on the TAC dynamics ignoring the spatial-domain information. Kamasak et al. simultaneously clustered and estimated each cluster's TAC directly from the sinogram data, without the need for tomographic reconstruction [5]. However, using such a projection domain based approach makes it difficult to incorporate much needed user knowledge given the low SNR. Maroy et al. extracted the dPET TACs in the organ cores, where they are least affected by motion and spillover effects [6]. This algorithm might be problematic for regions with small cores and low SNR, since a large number of TACs is needed to achieve acceptable estimates of organ kinetics. Saad et al. incorporated a KM based image prior constraint during the segmentation instead of considering only the observed TACs [7]. However, their approach did not guarantee globally optimal segmentations nor did it address PVE.

In this paper, we develop a multi-class, seed-initialized, iterative segmentation algorithm for molecular images. Random walker (RW) [8] is adopted at the core of our algorithm (Sec. 2.1) guaranteeing a global optimal segmentation in each iteration with automatically updated seeds. A KM image prior term is incorporated into RW to capture the underlaying physiological information (Sec. 2.2). An iterative, self-learning, uncertainty-based approach is developed to overcome the low SNR for image prior estimation, especially with a low number of user provided seeds (Sec. 2.3). The KM parameter fitting utilizes a confidence-weighted averaging of TACs in each region, which addresses the problem of PVE (Sec. 2.4).

2 Method

The details of our KM based RW with self-learning (RWSL-KM) method are given in the following sections.

2.1 Random Walker

As proposed in [8], the RW segmentation is formulated in a graph theoretic setting where image pixels are graph vertices v and edge weights w reflect similarity between neighboring pixels. The probability of assigning label $q \in \{1, 2, ..., Q\}$ to vertex v_i reflects the probability of a random walker starting at v_i reaching the seeds of region q out of Q possible regions. This results in a probability vector x_i^q. The set of user-labeled seeds is denoted V_L and the set of unlabeled vertices is denoted V_U. The probability of a labeled vertex $v_i \in V_L$ with label s is given by $x_i^q = 1$ if $q = s$ and 0 otherwise. Grady et al.[8] showed that an x^q that minimizes the energy functional

$$E_{total}^q(x^q) = \gamma_{reg} E_{reg}^q(x^q) + \gamma_{prior} E_{prior}^q(x^q), \quad (1)$$

can be obtained by solving the following linear system of equations

$$(\gamma_{reg} \triangle_{UU} + \gamma_{prior} \sum_{q=1}^{Q} \Lambda_U^q) x_U^q = -\gamma_{reg} \triangle_{UL} x_L^q + \gamma_{prior} \lambda_U^q \quad (2)$$

where E_{prior} and E_{reg} are the data fidelity and regularization energy terms, respectively. $\triangle_{UU}$ and $\triangle_{UL}$ are partitions from the combinatorial graph Laplacian matrix defined in [8]. λ_i^q represent the likelihood that vertex v_i belongs to class

q. Λ^q is a diagonal matrix with values λ^q along the diagonal. γ_{reg} and γ_{prior} are weighting parameters; setting their values is discussed in (Sec. 2.3). With x_i^q in hand, vertex v_i is assigned a label using argmax x_i^q.
q

We extend the classical RW formulation to deal with time-varying dPET images in the following ways:

- Each vertex v_i now represents a TAC I_i, where $I_i = [I_i^1 I_i^2 ... I_i^T]$ and T is the total number of time steps. I_i is typically sampled non-uniformly with time, with smaller sampling intervals suffering from lower SNR, which in turn is due to the lower Gamma photon counts acquired in a shorter interval.
- The similarity between two TACs I_i and I_j is measured using the weighted L_2 distance $g_{ij} = \sqrt{\sum_{t=1}^{T}(I_i^t - I_j^t)^2 z_t}$, where z_t is a weight that accounts for the non-uniform time sampling encountered in dPET. Shorter sampling intervals with lower SNR are weighted less.
- A reciprocal weighting function is used to calculate the edge weights $w_{ij} = \frac{\beta}{g_{ij}+\epsilon}$, where β is a mapping parameter and ϵ is a small number for stability.

2.2 Kinetic Modeling Based Image Prior Terms

In order to calculate the likelihood term λ_i^q in (2), we need to estimate the TAC distribution in different classes. However, higher dimensional density estimation is impractical beyond a few dimensions [9], which is the case for dPET data since a TAC at each pixel is a roughly 40 dimensional vector ($T \approx 40$ time steps). Further, there are no training images that we can use for the density estimation as different tracers lead to completely different intensity distributions. Here, we assume that the TAC classes are multivariate Gaussian distributions with the same scaled identity covariance matrix but with different means, which is the same assumption as in the widely used K-means clustering algorithm. We can now consider the distance to the class mean TAC as the inverse of the likelihood term with proper mapping, as follows

$$u_i^q = \sqrt{\sum_{t=1}^{T} \|I_i^t - \mu_q^t\|^2 z_t} \quad (3)$$

where u_i^q represents the weighted L_2 intensity difference between TAC I_i and mean TAC μ_q for class q.

As dPET tracer kinetics are often described using compartmental KM, we apply the KM process to the means μ^q for the Q classes prior to applying (3). We thus ensure that the prior terms capture the physiological phenomena under consideration and not only the observed TACs from the dPET data. Consequently, (3) becomes

$$u_{fit_i}^q = \sqrt{\sum_{t=1}^{T} \|I_i^t - \mu_{fit_q}^t\|^2 z_t} \quad (4)$$

where μ_{fit_q} is the activity TAC produced by solving a specific KM (e.g. two tissue compartmental KM) for each region mean activity μ_q [7]. The likelihood at each vertex is then estimated by

$$\lambda^q_{fit_i} = \Upsilon/(u^q_{fit_i} + \epsilon) \quad (5)$$

where Υ is a free mapping parameter. By incorporating KM TAC likelihood terms into RW, (2) becomes

$$(\gamma_{reg}\triangle_{UU} + \gamma_{prior}\sum_{q=1}^{Q}\Lambda^q_{U_{fit}})x^q_U = -\gamma_{reg}\triangle_{UL}x^q_L + \gamma_{prior}\lambda^q_{U_{fit}}. \quad (6)$$

2.3 Self-learning Using Uncertainty Principles

The main assumption underlying RW is that labels are diffused on the graph according to the similarity between TACs. On the one hand, low SNR affects the similarity calculations, which in turn affects the energy term E_{reg}. On the other hand, we can not build a good estimate for E_{prior} with the low number of seeds expected from the user. Here, we develop a self-learning technique to boost the number of vertices used in the prior estimation E_{prior}. Self-learning is a commonly used concept in semi-supervised learning, in which a classifier is first trained with a small amount of labeled data and then used to classify the unlabeled data. Then, the most confident unlabeled vertices, together with their predicted labels, are added to the training set. The classifier is re-trained and the procedure repeated [10]. To identify the most confident vertices, we use uncertainty principles from information theory. The entropy at v_i is defined as

$$h(v_i) = \sum_{q=1}^{Q} x^q_i \log_2(x^q_i). \quad (7)$$

Vertices with sufficiently high certainty or confidence will have a sufficiently low entropy, i.e. $h(v_i) < \aleph$, where $\aleph$ is a confidence threshold, and are, hence, dubbed *confident*. Nevertheless, confident vertices are not at par with user-specified seeds. Therefore, they are added to a new set $V_{confident}$, rather than to the seeds set V_L (i.e. $x^q \neq 1$ for $v_i \in V_{confident}$ whereas $x^q_L = 1$ for $v_i \in V_L$), to allow them to be relabeled as the algorithm iterates. Each region mean TAC μ_q is estimated by averaging all TACs $\forall v_i \in V_{confident} \cup V_L$ with label q.

Energy minimizing segmentation methods, RW included, are generally sensitive to the choice of weighting between spatial regularization and conformance to certain appearance or pixel intensity. In (6), such weighting balance is dictated by the weighting parameters γ_{reg} and γ_{prior}. We devise a novel, automatic iteration-dependant schedule for setting these weighting parameters. Given an initial small number of seeds, we wish to weight the E_{reg} term more to ensure that the vertices added to $V_{confident}$ will be spatial neighbors and similar to the seeds. As the algorithm iterates, we wish to weight the E_{prior} more as we will have a better estimate of the TAC distribution in different classes given the larger number of vertices added to $V_{confident}$. So (6) is modified as follows

$$(\alpha \triangle_{UU} + (1-\alpha) \sum_{q=1}^{Q} \Lambda_{U_{fit}}^{q}) x_{U}^{q} = -\alpha \triangle_{UL} x_{L}^{q} + (1-\alpha) \lambda_{U_{fit}}^{q}. \qquad (8)$$

The α scheduling can be written as $\alpha(k+1) = \zeta \alpha(k)$ where $0 < \zeta < 1$ and k is the iteration index.

2.4 Certainty Weighted Mean TAC

After the labeling process, the standard KM proceeds by *equally-weighted* averaging of all the TACs belonging to each functional region to produce μ_{final_q} [2]. Here, we propose a *certainty-weighted* averaging to calculate each region's mean TAC by utilizing the confidence of the labeling process. This compensates for the PVE by weighting pure tissue TACs differently, compared to those of mixture-tissues using the uncertainty principles. More specifically

$$\mu_{final_q} = \frac{\sum_{v_i \text{ labeled } q} \psi_i I_i}{\sum_{v_i \text{ labeled } q} \psi_i} \quad \text{where} \quad \psi_i = 1/(h(v_i) + \epsilon). \qquad (9)$$

Our RWSL-KM method is summarized in Alg.1.

Algorithm 1. Kinetic modeling based random walker with self-learning

Input: (i) dynamic molecular image data and (ii) user seeds for different classes.
Result: Segmented functional regions with their corresponding kinetic parameters.
Initialize V_L from user seeds and $V_{confident} = \{\}$.
Initialize $k = 0$ and $\alpha(k) = 1$.
repeat
    Compute the probability $x_i^q \ \forall q$ at each $v_i \in V_U$ by applying (8).
    Assign a class to v_i using $\underset{q}{\text{argmax}} \ x_i^q$.
    Update $V_{confident}$ by adding v_i to $V_{confident}$ iff $h(v_i) < \aleph$.
    Compute each region mean TAC μ_q using only $v_i \in V_{confident} \cup V_L$.
    Find KM parameters producing μ_{fit_q} closest to μ_q in the least-square sense [7].
    Update $\alpha(k+1) = \zeta \alpha(k)$ and $k = k + 1$.
until Convergence: No significant change in either μ_{fit_q} or $V_{confident}$
Compute *final* certainty-weighted region mean TAC μ_{final_q} by applying (9).

---

3 Materials and Implementation

We used synthetic and simulated dPET data with known ground truth to evaluate the proposed algorithm. For the synthetic dPET data, we generated an [18F]FDG-PET image dataset with TACs corresponding to 6 functional regions

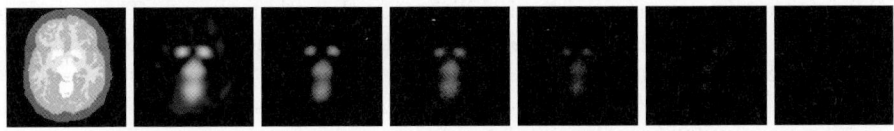

Fig. 1. From left to right: Labeled 2D Brain MRI slice. The last time step slice (highest SNR) of the synthetic dPET data blurred with a Gaussian kernel (i.e. introduces PVE) with increasing noise levels $[0, 1, 3, 5, 8, 10]\sigma$, where 0σ level has no additive noise.

($Q = 6$): background (BG), skull (SK), grey matter (GM), white matter (WM), cerebellum (CM) and putamen (PN). A two-tissue compartmental KM was used to simulate the dynamics for different regions with real kinetic parameters from the dPET clinical literature. The resulting TACs are assigned to a 2D downsampled labeled MRI image that was blurred with a Gaussian filter (full width at half maximum = 8mm). We ran 5 trials each with 5 Gaussian noise levels $[1, 3, 5, 8, 10]\sigma$. σ is used to scale the unit variance of the random noise generator to the scale of the synthetic TAC intensity at each time step. The dPET image has dimensions of 91×109 with 46 time steps: 12×10s, 10×30s, 10×120s, 10×300s and finally 4×600s with an isotropic voxel size of 2mm. Fig 1 shows the MRI slice used and the last dPET time step with different noise levels. We show the last time step as it has the highest SNR, as is typical in dPET (i.e. the preceding time frames are even noisier).

For the simulated dPET data, we used the publicly available simulated 3D+time dataset PET-SORTEO with known ground truth [11]. Ten simulated [^{11}C]Raclopride PET brain studies, accounting for inter-subject anatomical variability as well as different dPET image degradation factors, have been used. The PET-SORTEO image has dimensions of $128 \times 128 \times 63$ with 26 time steps: 6×30s, 7×60s, 5×120s and finally 8×300s with voxel size of $2.11 \times 2.11 \times 2.42$mm^3.

In order to validate our algorithm, we compare it with two of the state-of-the-art techniques in dPET segmentation: K-means with KM and a MRF-regularized version thereof [7], abbreviated KMN-KM and MRF-KM, respectively. We also compare to the original RW (with necessary extensions noted in (Sec. 2.1)) [8]. For the synthetic experiment, the comparison criterion is based on the recovery of the FDG glucose metabolic rate $K = K_1 k_3/(k_2 + k_3)$ [4]. We define the KM recovery error as

$$RE^q = \|K^q_{fit} - K^q_{true}\|^2 \qquad (10)$$

where K^q_{true} is the ground truth K used to generate the data in a functional region q. A perfect segmentation technique is the one that can recover K^q_{true} (yielding $RE^q = 0$). Each segmentation technique produces different K^q_{fit}.

The KM development is based on COMKAT [12]. The RW is partially based on the code accompanying [8]. We chose empirically the following values for the algorithm free parameters $\beta = 1$, $\Upsilon = 1$, $\alpha(0) = 1$, $\zeta = 0.9$ and $\aleph = 1.1863$ with $Q = 6$. The value of $\aleph$ corresponds to a minimum likelihood probability of 0.8 for one class and equal probabilities for the other classes. The same set of seeds was used for the initialization of different segmentation techniques: to calculate the initial means for KMN-KM and MRF-KM, and as initial seeds for RW and RWSL-KM. $|V_L|$ is 2.5% of the original image size in the 2D synthetic experiment and 0.02% in the simulated 3D experiment.

4 Results

Fig 2 qualitatively compares the four algorithms using the synthetic data with a noise level of 5σ. KMN-KM and MRF-KM result in isolated, scattered functional labels especially in the WM and GM regions. Further, the PN is underestimated as it has very similar kinetics to the CM region. Classical RW results in Voronoi regions with respect to the provided seeds due to the excessive noise (in agreement with [8]). RWSL-KM overcomes these two limitations and performs better than the other approaches. Most of the regions are sufficiently recovered especially in the PN region. Nevertheless, RWSL-KM misclassified a band around the CM as PN (green surrounding blue). Also, the area between the GM and the SK was misclassified as WM (the yellow perimeter). These misclassifications are the result of PVE. This behavior is not surprising and can further be explored by examining the uncertainty map (rightmost image in Fig 2). This image is a mapping of the negative entropy at each pixel to a grey level color: uncertain pixels appear darker. Misclassified regions with low certainty (darker) indicate that the classification of these regions is almost arbitrary. This supports our justification that the extracted mean TAC from each region should be weighted by the amount of certainty at each voxel (as in (9)) before estimating the kinetic parameters, which is the main objective of dPET analysis and not the segmentation per se.

Fig 3 shows a quantitative comparison between the different algorithms according to (10). It shows that K calculated from certainty-weighted mean TAC using RWSL-KM (RWSL-KM-CW) constantly outperforms other algorithms. Furthermore, Fig 3 shows that our method even outperforms ground truth labeling. This may seem unrealistic at first, however given that the ground truth labeling itself is a crisp (non fuzzy) labeling, TACs at the interface between functional regions will suffer from PVE and hence produce worse K estimates. This is particularly noticed in WM, CM and PN. Our certainty-weighted averaging, on the other hand, can handle the PVE well.

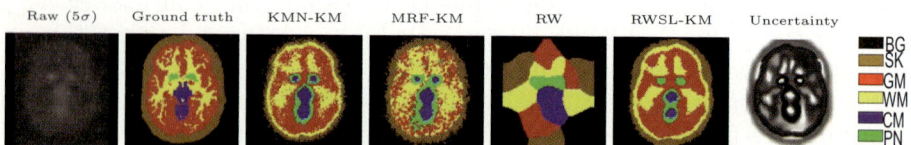

Fig. 2. Comparison between four segmentation algorithms. The rightmost figure is the negative entropy map generated by RWSL-KM (uncertain regions appear darker).

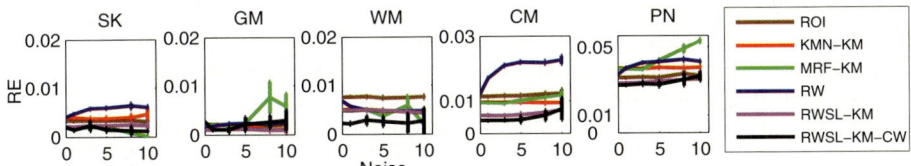

Fig. 3. Recovery error (RE) of the physiological parameters with different noise levels and multiple trials. ROI corresponds to the mean TAC extracted using the ground truth labeling. RWSL-KM-CW uses the certainty weighted mean TAC for each region. Note the different scale on the y-axis to demonstrate the differences between algorithms.

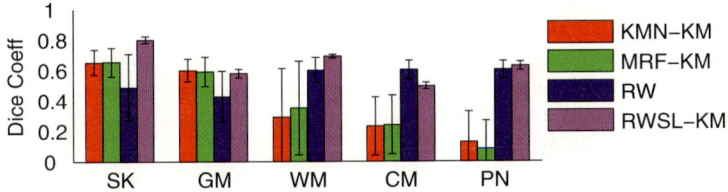

Fig. 4. Performance evaluation between the four algorithms using the Dice metric. The error bars show one standard deviation.

For the simulated dPET data, we don't have access to the generated kinetics, so we can not evaluate the algorithm according to (10). Hence, we chose the Dice coefficient to measure the overlap between a segmented region and ground truth. Note that the Dice metric doesn't take the segmentation confidence into account, so one of the features of our algorithm is unutilized. Fig 4 shows the Dice coefficient averaged over 10 patients. It shows the RWSL-KM outperforming the different algorithms except for the CM region and slightly in the GM region. This can be explained by knowing that the CM region should be devoid of the Raclopride tracer, which is the reason it is used as the reference tissue in graphical KM methods [2]. Further, RWSL-KM exhibits the lowest variability in different regions, especially in the GM region.

5 Discussion

In this paper, we developed a semi-supervised segmentation technique for molecular images incorporating spatial regularization, kinetic modeling and uncertainty principles. We showed qualitatively and quantitatively that RWSL-KM produces better results than other state-of-the-art techniques.

We intend to extend RWSL-KM by incorporating structural MRI or CT information for better localization of tracer activity. Further, we need to investigate the performance of our algorithm with real datasets from multiple modalities.

References

1. Rudin, M.: Molecular Imaging: Basic Principles and Applications in Biomedical Research. Imperial College Press (2005)
2. Morris, E.D., Endres, C.J., Schmidt, K.C., Christian, B.T.: Kinetic modeling in Positron Emission Tomography. In: Wernick, M., Aarsvold, J.N. (eds.) Emission Tomography: The Fundamentals of PET and SPECT. Academic, San Diego (2004)
3. Barber, D.C.: The use of principal components in the quantitative analysis of Gamma camera dynamic studies. Phys. Med. Biol. 25, 283–292 (1980)
4. Guo, H., Renaut, R., Chen, K., Reiman, E.: Clustering huge data sets for parametric PET imaging. Journal of Biosystems 71, 81–92 (2001)
5. Kamasak, M.E., Bayraktarb, B.: Unsupervised clustering of dynamic PET images on the projection domain. In: Proceedings of the SPIE Medical Imaging, pp. 1539–1548 (2006)
6. Maroy, R., Boisgard, R., Comtat, C., Frouin, V., Cathier, P., Duchesnay, E., Dolle, F., Nielsen, P.E., Trebossen, R., Tavitian, B.: Segmentation of Rodent whole-body dynamic PET images: An unsupervised method based on voxel dynamics. IEEE TMI 27, 342–354 (2008)
7. Saad, A., Smith, B., Hamarneh, G., Möller, T.: Simultaneous segmentation, kinetic parameter estimation, and uncertainty visualization of dynamic PET images. In: Ayache, N., Ourselin, S., Maeder, A. (eds.) MICCAI 2007, Part II. LNCS, vol. 4792, pp. 726–733. Springer, Heidelberg (2007)
8. Grady, L.: Multilabel random walker image segmentation using prior models. In: Proceedings of CVPR, pp. 763–770 (2005)
9. Scott, D.: Multivariate Density Estimation. Wiley, New York (1992)
10. Zhu, X.: Semi-supervised learning literature survey. Technical report, Department of Computer Sciences, University of Wisconsin, Madison (2005)
11. Reilhac, A., Batan, G., Michel, C., Grova, C., Tohka, J., Costes, N., Evans, A.C.: Validation of PET SORTEO: a platform for simulating realistic PET studies and development of a database of simulated PET volumes. IEEE Trans. Nucl. Sci. 52, 1321–1328 (2004)
12. Muzic, R., Cornelius, S.: COMKAT: compartment model kinetic analysis tool. JNM 42(4), 636–645 (2001)

Automatic Delineation of Sulci and Improved Partial Volume Classification for Accurate 3D Voxel-Based Cortical Thickness Estimation from MR

Oscar Acosta[1], Pierrick Bourgeat[1], Jurgen Fripp[1], Erik Bonner[1], Sébastien Ourselin[2], and Olivier Salvado[1]

[1] The Australian e-Health Research Centre, ICTC-CSIRO, Brisbane, QLD, Australia
{Oscar.Acosta,Pierrick.Bourgeat,Jurgen.Fripp,Erik.Bonner,
Olivier.Salvado}@csiro.au
[2] Centre for Medical Image Computing, University College London, UK
S.Ourselin@cs.ucl.ac.uk

Abstract. Accurate cortical thickness estimation *in-vivo* is important for the study of many neurodegenerative diseases. When using magnetic resonance images (MRI), accuracy may be hampered by artifacts such as partial volume (PV) as the cortex spans only a few voxels. In zones of opposed sulcal banks (tight sulci) the measurement can be even more difficult. The aim of this work is to propose a voxel-based cortical thickness estimation method from MR by integrating a mechanism for correcting sulci delineation after an improved partial volume classification. First, an efficient and accurate framework was developed to enhance partial volume classification with structural information. Then, the correction of sulci delineation is performed after a homotopic thinning of a cost function image. Integrated to our voxel-based cortical thickness estimation pipeline, the overall method showed a better estimate of thickness and a high reproducibility on real data ($R^2 > 0.9$). A quantitative analysis on clinical data from an Alzheimer's disease study showed significant differences between normal controls and Alzheimer's disease patients.

1 Introduction

Automatic measurement of cortical thickness from 3D magnetic resonance (MR) images can aid diagnosis and longitudinal studies of a wide variety of neurodegenerative pathologies, such as Alzheimer's disease. The approaches previously proposed in the literature can be broadly categorised as mesh-based [6] and voxel-based [1,2,3,4,5]. Operating directly on the 3D voxel grid, voxel based techniques are more computationally efficient but less robust to noise and missegmentation as they typically lack the mechanisms required to assess and correct topological errors in gray matter (GM), white matter (WM) and cerebrospinal fluid (CSF) segmentations. Tissue classification and cortical thickness measurement can be considerably affected by partial volume (PV) effect due to the finite resolution of MRI compared to the size of the considered structures. Thus, a voxel representing more than one tissue type in opposite banks of tight sulci may appear fused as CSF is not detected between the folds of gray matter. This results in erroneously high thickness estimates for these regions.

Few approaches have been proposed to estimate and cut misdetected sulci. In [2], the GM/CSF partial volume voxels between opposing banks of sulci are identified using a combination of their distance to the white matter and the classification of neighbouring voxels. This method, however, requires removal of noise and intensity inhomogeneities in a prior step. Hutton [1] uses the thickness to identify deep sulci from GM layers growing consecutively from the WM. However, no additional information is used to ensure that sulci are correctly identified and does not account for partial volume information to accurately compute the thickness. Diep [4] proposed to cut sulci using the probability of the voxel being CSF in abnormally thick areas, but it lacks a partial volume model to properly identify CSF voxels buried inside deep sulci.

Unlike these approaches, we propose a technique based on an improved partial volume (PV) classification and topological operators to better delineate the buried sulci and to accurately compute the thickness. Firstly, the proposed partial volume classification method accounts for the distance to the WM, favoring the detection of GM/CSF voxels in oposed sulcal banks. Secondly, for detecting the remaining non-classified mixed voxels in buried sulci (100% GM) we used a distance ordered homotopic thinning DOHT [16] of a sulcal function, controlled by a surface terminality criteria. Then, the resulting skeletonized surface combined with the partial volume maps are used to correct the hard segmentations for computing the thickness. After correction of WM, GM and CSF segmentations, the GM thickness is computed using the Laplacian definition [7] with a more efficient PDE implementation [8], and using the PV maps for initialisation [5] achieving subvoxel accuracy.

2 Method

2.1 Pure Tissue Segmentation

Based on the expectation maximisation segmentation (EMS) algorithm [9], we have implemented a method for segmentation of brain tissues into GM, WM and CSF which includes a polynomial based bias field correction and Markov random fields to reduce the effects of noise. The Colin atlas and associated priors are first affinely registered to the data using a robust block matching approach [10], followed by a diffeomorphic Demons non-rigid registration [11]. The registered priors are then used to initialise the EMS and enforce spatial consistency throughout the segmentation. Finally, hard segmentations are obtained after the EMS by labelling each voxel with the most probable tissue.

2.2 Partial Volume Estimation

PV along the interfaces of pure tissues is estimated by modeling the mixture of pure tissues and performing a maximum *a posteriori* classification (MAP). We improved the two-stage procedure relying on both intensity and spatial information used previously by [13,14,15]. The Euclidean distance from the WM (and its gradient) are combined with the spatial information to favour classification of GM/CSF mixed voxels in the GM, improving the delineation of the sulci. Three pure classes (GM, WM, CSF) and two mixture classes (GM/CSF, GM/WM) are considered. Thus, the labels are restricted to the set $\Gamma = \{GM, CSF, WM, CSF/GM, GM/WM\}$. Since voxels containing PV are mostly present along boundaries, we assume that each voxel contains at most two tissues [12], and PV classification is restricted to the region formed by a dilated GM (radius 4). As in [14], labels j/k indicate mixed voxels of the pure tissue types j and k. The output of the classification is an image C of labels for each voxel as $C = \{c_i : i = 1, .., N, c_i \in \Gamma\}$.

Intensity model. Pure voxels are assumed to have a Gaussian probability density function, defined by its mean (μ) and standard deviation (σ), whereas mixed voxels are modeled with a probability density function as in [12]:

$$p(x_i|c_i = j/k) = \int_0^1 \frac{1}{\sqrt{2\pi det(\Sigma(w))}} exp\left[-\frac{1}{2}(x_i - \mu(w))^T \Sigma^{-1}(x_i - \mu(w))\right] dw \quad (1)$$

where the mean and covariance matrix of the mixture are a function of the means and covariances of the pure tissue classes as $\mu(w) = w\mu_j + (1-w)\mu_k$; $\Sigma(w) = w^2 \Sigma_j + (1-w)^2 \Sigma_k$ and w represents the fraction of j within the mixed voxel.

Local spatial interaction model. To take into account dependency on the neighbouring tissue types, a Markov prior that models local spatial interaction was implemented. The labelling is performed using a Potts model. As in ([13,14,15]), we use the ICM algorithm [17] to search for the optimal labelled image as

$$\lambda_i^{n+1} = arg\ max_{\gamma \in \Gamma} \left[log\ p(x_i|\gamma) - 2\beta \sum_{q \in N_q} \frac{\delta(\lambda_q^n, \gamma)}{d(i,q)}\right] \quad (2)$$

where $d(i,q)$ is the distance between centers of voxels i and q, λ_i^n is the label at the $n-th$ update, β controls the strength of the prior (typically $\beta = 0.05$) and N_q represents the set of voxels in the 26-neighbourhood of i. Building on [13,14] who used a similar approach, we modified $\delta(\lambda_i, \lambda_q)$, λ_i and λ_q being the labels of the voxels i and q. We introduced two functions, namely f_1 and f_2 that modulate the influence of the Euclidean distance to the WM, D_{WM}. The design of $f_{1,2}$ takes advantage of local maxima where $\| \nabla D_{WM} \| \to 0$ when a voxel likely belongs to a sulci (Fig.1(c)). Thus,

$$\delta(\lambda_i, \lambda_q) = \begin{cases} f_1(D_{WM}) & if\ \lambda_i = \lambda_q\ and\ \lambda_q = GM \\ f_2(D_{WM}) & if\ they\ share\ a\ tissue\ type \\ & and\ \lambda_q = GM/CSF \\ -2, & if\ \lambda_i = \lambda_q\ and\ \lambda_q \neq GM \\ -1, & if\ they\ share\ a\ tissue\ type \\ +1, & otherwise \end{cases} \quad (3)$$

where $\qquad f_{1,2}(D_{WM}) = A.exp[-\alpha D_{WM}].exp[-k \| \nabla D_{WM} \|^2] + B \qquad (4)$

For f_1: $A = -1, \alpha = 0.1, B = -1, k = 1$ and for f_2: $A = 1, \alpha = 0.1, B = -2, k = 1$. f_1 varies between $[-1, -2]$, and tends to attenuate the influence of neighbouring GM voxels when $\| \nabla D_{WM} \|$ goes to zero. Conversely, f_2 varies between $[-2, -1]$ tending to reinforce the influence of labels GM/CSF in the neighbourhood when $\| \nabla D_{WM} \|$

tends to zero. Thus, these functions favor both reclassification of pure tissue voxels GM as GM/CSF (by f_1) and preservation of classified voxels GM/CSF (by f_2). The design of $f_{1,2}$ follows the same reasoning as for detecting plate-like structures [18]. As depicted in Fig. 1(d) the sulci are well delineated in the resulting GM partial volume maps (GMPVC).

Fractional content. Once voxels have been classified as a mixture of pure tissue, their fractional content $F_{j/k}$ between tissue j and k is computed as in [12] using the bias corrected intensity $\bar{x}_i$, and the means of the two pure tissue types μ_j and μ_k, such that:

$$F_{j/k} = U\left(\frac{\mu_j - \bar{x}_i}{\mu_j - \mu_k}\right) \qquad (5)$$

where $U(\cdot)$ is a limiter restricting the range of the fractional content to $[0,1]$. The partial volume coefficients (PVC) map of GM (and similarly for WM and CSF), is defined as GMPVC = $F_{\text{GM/WM}} \cup F_{\text{GM/CSF}}$.

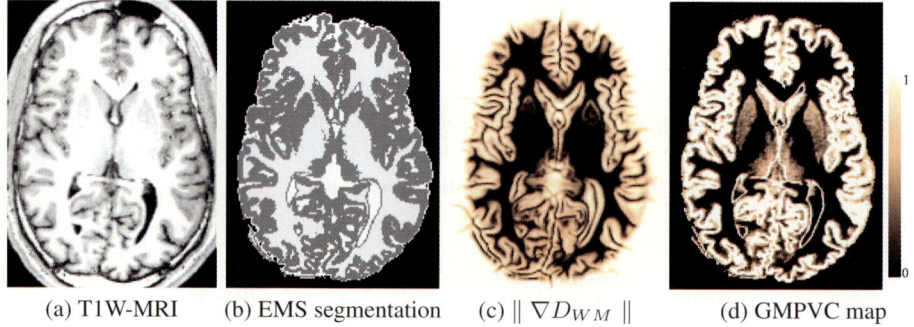

(a) T1W-MRI (b) EMS segmentation (c) $\|\nabla D_{WM}\|$ (d) GMPVC map

Fig. 1. (a) Axial cut plane of a T1-W MR Image, (b) pure tissue segmentation, (c) gradient of the Euclidean distance to the WM ($\|\nabla D_{WM}\|$), (d) GM partial volume image (GMPVC map)

2.3 Sulci Delineation and Correction of Hard Segmentation

To complete the delineation of sulci in very tight zones not detected after the partial volume classification (Fig. 2d), a procedure based on homotopic thinning is employed. Thus, the hard segmentations are corrected by the medial surface (3D skeleton) from the local minima of a sulci likelihood function, F_s, computed from the WM and CSF partial volume maps (WMPVC,CSFPVC) as

$$F_s = (1 - CSFPVC_\sigma)\|\nabla D_{WMPVC_{50}}\| \qquad (6)$$

where $D_{WMPVC_{50}}$ is the distance to the WMPVC (PVC>50%) and $CSFPVC_\sigma$ is a Gaussian convolved CSFPVC map ($\sigma = 1$). The CSFPVC shifts the local minima of F_s towards the maximum of CSF, overcoming the problem of sulci asymmetry. The thinning of F_s is performed using a two stage distance-ordered homotopic thinning (DOHT) [16]. However, rather than only using the center of maximal balls technique in the first stage, which makes the method scale-dependent, the first skeleton is completed by adding all the local minima over F_s following the direction of $\nabla D_{WMPVC_{50}}$. In the second step, voxels are recursively deleted until the medial surface is obtained.

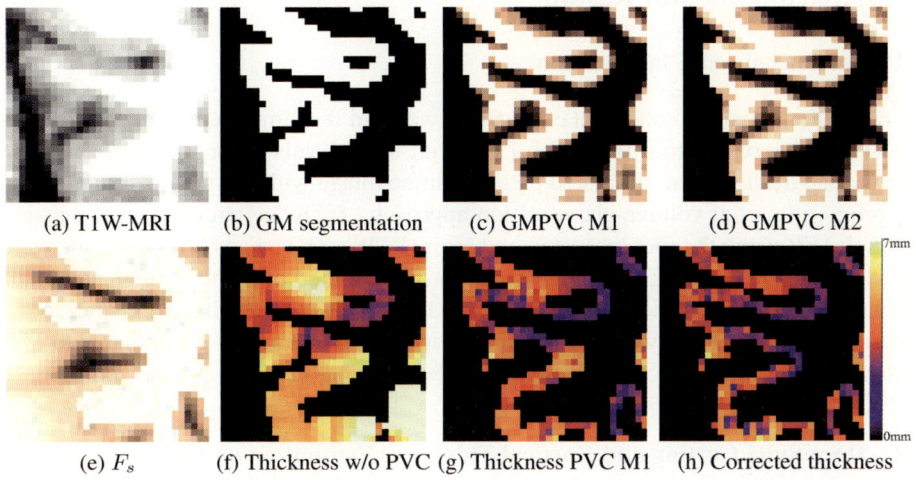

Fig. 2. (a) Deep sulci in original T1W-MRI, (b) GM hard segmentation (No PVC), (c) GMPVC map with method (M1) [13] and (d) with the proposed method (M2), (e) cost function F_s where the DOHT is performed using [16], (f-h) corresponding thickness estimation: (f) in the GM hard segmentation, without taking into account the PVC, (g) using GMPVC M1 and (h) using improved GMPVC map after correcting sulci delineation

2.4 Cortical Thickness Estimation

Cortical thickness is computed using Jones's approach [7] where Laplace's equation is solved in the GM volume (with the WM and CSF voxels adjacent to the boundaries of the GM set to fixed potentials) such that $\nabla^2 f(\mathbf{x}) = 0$.

The solution $f(\mathbf{x})$ is a scalar field which divides the cortex into a set of equipotential sublayers. The normalised gradient of the Laplace solution provides streamlines between the WM and CSF, which do not intersect, are locally perpendicular to the equipotential sublayers, and provide a unique correspondence between the two boundaries. The tangent vectors of the correspondence trajectories $\vec{T}$ correspond to the normalised gradient vector field of $f(\mathbf{x})$, regularised using a Gaussian function G_σ with $\sigma = 1$ such that $\vec{T} = G_\sigma * \frac{\nabla f}{\|\nabla f\|}$.

Whereas Jones [7] explicitly traces streamlines (Lagrangian approach), Yezzi [8] proposed a more efficient method which involves solving a pair of first order linear partial differential equations (PDE) without any explicit construction of correspondences (Eulerian approach). We implemented a hybrid Eulerian-Lagrangian approach [5], in which the PV information is used to initialise the PDE, achieving subvoxel accuracy. The PV content of each boundary voxel is combined with the direction of the tangent field, to accurately measure the position of the boundary through ray-casting. The implementation is based on a dichotomy search, with decreasing stepsize down to $\epsilon = 1/10^{-3}$ of the voxel size. In opposed sulcal banks the position of the boundary is computed as the point where the GMPVC is minimum.

3 Experiments and Results

3.1 Partial Volume Classification

To evaluate the partial volume classification, we used the simulated T1W MR 3D images ($1mm^3$ voxels) from BrainWeb [19], with noise levels ranging from 1% to 9%. The ground truth was the simulated partial volume image with 0% noise. We compared the proposed partial volume classification approach ($f(D_{WM})$) against other existing methods [13] using the root mean squared error (RMS). The means for pure tissue were derived either from the EMS segmentation or recomputed over the segmented voxels from the EMS hard segmentation (M1). Fig. 3(a) depicts the results. Compared to the other methods, the RMS was considerably reduced. On average 14% compared to M1, with the greatest differences in the GM (12.2%) and CSF (29.3%) as expected.

3.2 Deep Sulci Cutting and Cortical Thickness Estimation on Real Data

From the OASIS database [20], we extracted 20 young healthy subjects who underwent 4 scans at baseline and 4 more scans during a subsequent session after a short delay (less than 90 days). For each session, an average motion-corrected image (co-registered average of all available data) was used for our reliability test. The scans were T1W MPRAGE with isotropic $1mm^3$ resolution. By using the proposed method, we found a mean ± (std. dev.) cortical thickness over the whole brain of 2.49mm ± 0.11 for all the subjects, which is within the accepted range of cortical thickness for healthy young adults (Fig.3b). When the PV is not taken into account as in [8], the computed mean thickness was 4.69mm ± 0.11.

The sum of square of differences was computed for each ROI of the AAL template to assess the error between the two measurements (Fig. 4). The cerebellum and subcortical

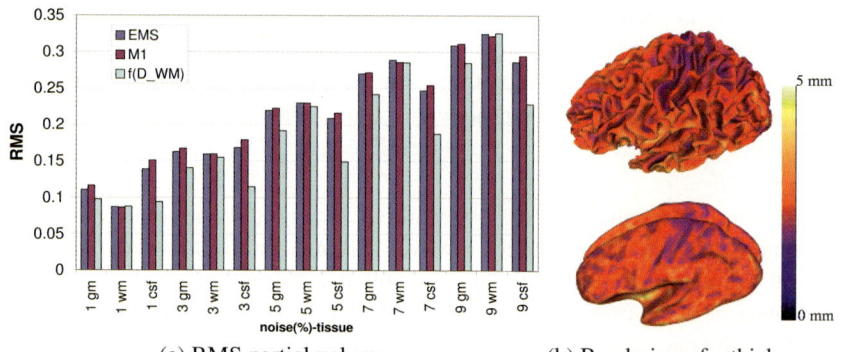

(a) RMS partial volume (b) Rendering of a thickness map.

Fig. 3. (a) RMS comparisons between different methods for computing partial volume: i) Using the means from the EMS, ii) computing the means from the hard segmentation (M1) and iii) including the distance functions $f_{1,2}(D_{WM})$ as proposed. (b) *Top:* Rendering of a thickness map for a healthy young adult shown over the WM/GM surface and *Bottom:* over a partially inflated surface.

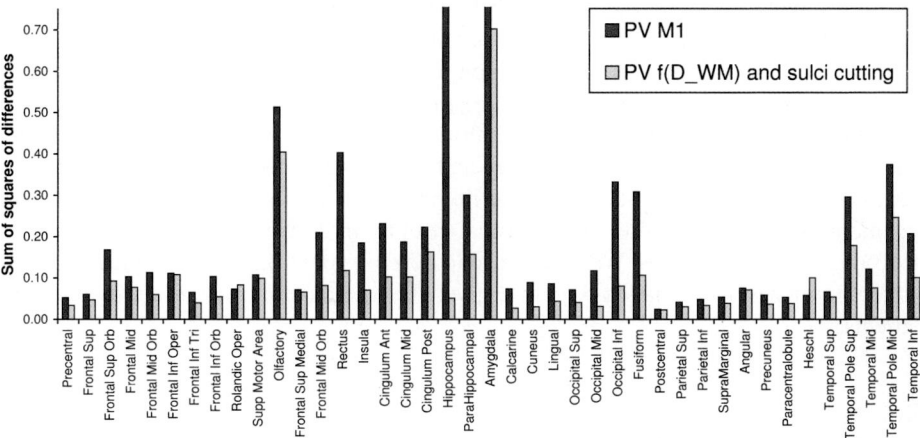

Fig. 4. Sum of square of differences of regional cortical thickness between baseline and repeat for 20 young healthy subjects

nuclei were excluded from the analysis. We found a significant reduction of error in the temporal lobe, with a drastic reduction in the hippocampal region when comparing the proposed method (Improved PVC and cut sulci) with the measure performed after partial volume classification using [13] (PVM1). The Pearson coefficient for all the regions was above 0.9, except for the olfactory (0.79) and a paired t-test did not reveal any significant differences between the 2 measurements ($p > 0.01$).

The technique was also applied to a database of 3D MPRAGE MRI from our Alzheimer's disease (AD) study (The Australian Biomarker, Imaging And Lifestyle Study-AIBL). We extracted 23 subjects: 12 healthy elderly (HE) and 11 AD patients. The mean age was 70.4 ± 7.35 for the HE and 69.5 ± 6.7 for the AD. Regional analysis showed significant differences ($p<0.001$) in the hippocampus (8.5% atrophy), parahippocampus (6.6%) and posterior cingulum (5%) and ($p<0.01$) in the temporal and frontal lobes between HE and AD. The p-values were greater when using M1 for almost all the regions indicating that the statistical significance increased using the proposed approach.

4 Discussion and Conclusions

In this work we have presented a novel voxel-based method for accurate cortical thickness estimation, which integrates a mechanism for delineating deep sulci based on partial volume classification. The main contribution lies in two points: Firstly, it introduces an improved partial volume classification method which favours labelling of mixed GM/CSF voxels. Secondly, it corrects hard segmentations (GM voxels that must be reclassified as GM/CSF) after a homotopic thinning of a sulcal function, obtained from the resulting PVC maps. Partial volume classification was improved when compared with other methods using the BrainWeb fuzzy maps as ground truth. Both fractional tissue content estimation and thinning resulted in reliable brain tissue segmentation for more accurate cortical thickness estimation. Our method showed a high reproducibility on real data, with an extremely good agreement between the baseline and repeat scan. Furthermore, a preliminary quantitative analysis on clinical data showed significant differences between healthy elderly and Alzheimer's disease patients, consistent with results previously published in the literature. In the future, we plan to use our technique on clinical data to study cortical atrophy in Alzheimer's disease and other neurodegenerative diseases. We intend also to develop voxel-based techniques for inter-subject comparisons, a challenging issue given the large anatomical variability between patients.

References

1. Hutton, C., De Vita, E., et al.: Voxel-based cortical thickness measurements in MRI. Neuroimage (2008)
2. Lohmann, G., Preul, C., Hund-Georgiadis, M.: Morphology-based cortical thickness estimation. In: Taylor, C.J., Noble, J.A. (eds.) IPMI 2003. LNCS, vol. 2732, pp. 89–100. Springer, Heidelberg (2003)
3. Srivastava, S., Maes, F., et al.: An automated 3D algorithm for neo-cortical thickness measurement. In: Ellis, R.E., Peters, T.M. (eds.) MICCAI 2003. LNCS, vol. 2879, pp. 488–495. Springer, Heidelberg (2003)
4. Diep, T.M., Bourgeat, P., Ourselin, S.: Efficient use of cerebral cortical thickness to correct brain MR segmentation. In: IEEE-ISBI 2007, Washington DC, USA, pp. 592–595. IEEE, Los Alamitos (2007)
5. Bourgeat, P., Acosta, O., et al.: Improved cortical thickness measurement from MR images using partial volume estimation. In: IEEE-ISBI 2008, Paris, France, pp. 205–208. IEEE, Los Alamitos (2008)
6. Lee, J., et al.: A novel quantitative cross-validation of different cortical surface reconstruction algorithms using MRI phantom. Neuroimage 31(2), 572–584 (2006)
7. Jones, S., Buckbinder, B., Aharon, I.: Three-dimensional mapping of cortical thickness using Laplace's equation. HBM 11(1), 12–32 (2000)
8. Yezzi, A., Prince, J.: An Eulerian PDE approach for computing tissue thickness. IEEE-TMI 22(10), 1332–1339 (2003)
9. van Leemput, K., Maes, F., et al.: Automated model-based bias field correction of MR images of the brain. IEEE-TMI 18(10), 885–896 (1999)
10. Ourselin, S., Roche, A., et al.: Reconstructing a 3D structure from serial histological sections. IVC 19(1), 25–31 (2001)
11. Vercauteren, T., Pennec, X., et al.: Non-parametric diffeomorphic image resgistration with the demons algorithm. In: Ayache, N., Ourselin, S., Maeder, A. (eds.) MICCAI 2007, Part II. LNCS, vol. 4792, pp. 319–326. Springer, Heidelberg (2007)
12. Santago, P., Gage, H.: Quantification of MR brain images by mixture density and partial volume modeling. IEEE-TMI 12(3), 566–574 (1993)
13. Shattuck, D., Sandor-Leahy, S., et al.: Magnetic resonance image tissue classification using a partial volume model. Neuroimage 13(5), 856–876 (2001)
14. Tohka, J., Zijdenbos, A., Evans, A.: Fast and robust parameter estimation for statistical partial volume models in brain MRI. NeuroImage 23(1), 84–97 (2004)

15. Kim, J., Singh, V., et al.: Automated 3D extraction and evaluation of the inner and outer cortical surfaces using a Laplacian map and partial volume effect classification. NeuroImage 27(1), 210–221 (2005)
16. Pudney, C.: Distance-Ordered Homotopic Thinning: A Skeletonization Algorithm for 3D Digital Images. CVIU 72(3), 404–413 (1998)
17. Besag, J.: On the statistical analysis of dirty pictures. J. Roy. Stat. Soc. 48, 259–302 (1986)
18. Frangi, A., Niessen, W., et al.: Multiscale Vessel Enhancement Filtering. In: Wells, W.M., Colchester, A.C.F., Delp, S.L. (eds.) MICCAI 1998. LNCS, vol. 1496, pp. 130–138. Springer, Heidelberg (1998)
19. Cocosco, C., Kollokian, V., et al.: Brainweb: Online interface to a 3D MRI simulated brain database. NeuroImage (Proc. of 3-rd Int. Conf. Func. Mapp Human Brain) 5, S425 (1997)
20. Marcus, D.S., Wang, T.H., et al.: Open access series of imaging studies (OASIS): Cross-sectional MRI data in young, middle aged, nondemented, and demented older adults. J. Cogn. Neurosci. 19, 1498–1507 (2007)

R-PLUS: A Riemannian Anisotropic Edge Detection Scheme for Vascular Segmentation

Ali Gooya[1], Takeyoshi Dohi[2], Ichiro Sakuma[1], and Hongen Liao[1,3]

[1] Graduate School of Engineering, the University of Tokyo, The University of Tokyo
[2] Graduate School of Informaiton Science and Technology, The University of Tokyo
[3] Translational Systems Biology and Medicine Initiative, The University of Tokyo
7-3-1, Hongo, Bunkyo, Tokyo, 113-8656
{gooya,ichiro,liao}@bmpe.t.u-tokyo.ac.jp

Abstract. In this paper, detection of edges in oriented fields is addressed. In some applications such as vessel segmentation because of the intrinsic orientation of the structures, edge detection is only demanded in a particular subspace. This is specially usefull when a curve evolution is chosen for segmentation since gradients in parallel to vessel orientation may stop the contour. An anisotropic edge detection scheme is generalized on a Riemannian manifold using the local structure tensor. The method is the generalization of the *PLUS* operator proposed in [8] for accurate curved edge detection. Examples are given and the comparison is made with the state-of-the-art flux maximizing flow which indicates that significant improvements in terms of leakage minimization and thiner vessel delineation is achievable using our methodology.

1 Introduction

Magnetic Resonance Angiography (MRA) is increasingly used to provide volumetric information of vascular system. Accurate assessment of MRA images requires that the vessel structures to be extracted from MRA data sets. Currently, a number of techniques have been developed for vessel segmentation based on the advanced level set evolutionary methods [11,1].

Despite of relative success from some of these methods, segmentation of long thin structures is still considered as a delicate task. Most of these techniques are edge detection based and therefore, their success mainly depends on the accuracy of the detected edges. Classic edge detection methods have shown to produce inaccurate estimation of the edges for curved surfaces (such as blood vessels). Haralick edge detection operator, $I_{\xi\xi}$, [7] defines the edge as a point where the gradient magnitude is maximized along side the image gradient orientation, but under-estimates the actual radius of the curved surfaces. Zero-crossing of Laplacian ΔI or "Marr-Hildreth" [10] edge detection gives an over estimation because of the system point spread function (PSF). Since both $I_{\xi\xi}$ and ΔI appear to be dislocated in opposite direction[9], Verbeek and van Vliet [8] proposed the *PLUS* operator which sums $I_{\xi\xi}$ and ΔI, which improves the accuracy of the edge location an order better.

As we will see the original (Euclidean) *PLUS* edge detection has a shortcoming to segment elongated thin vessels. The reason is that *PLUS* edge detector has a isotropic behaviour, meaning that it is equally sensitive to gradients in all orientations. Therefore, in a contour propagation scenario, those noisy image gradients parallel to the main orientation prevent further propagation. In fact, sensitivity is mainly needed across the planes normal to vessel local orientation. This paper proposes a Riemannian generalization of the *PLUS* operator (hereafter called *R-PLUS*) using the local structure tensor which improves the continuity of the extraced vessels. A simple form of such a tensor is given and illustrated using an example and a few TOF-MRA data sets.

1.1 Related Work

For segmentation of thin structures, Gazit *et al.*[3] proposed a combinational curve evolution method, using Haralick edge detector and Chan-Vese minimal variance functional and geodesic active contours. Our methodology is different from that model, since we utilize local structure information for edge detection, and the method does not depend on GAC or Chan-Vese model. Flux maximizing flow was introduced by Vasilevsky [2] that integrates the directions of gradient vectors into the evolution equation so that the gradient flux through the evolving curve is maximized (here after called FLUX). With respect to the authors, we show that in fact since the FLUX is basically a Marr-Hildreth kind of edge detection scheme, it usually overestimates vessel widths (particularly in thinner vessels with high isophote curvature) while using our method more accurate segmentation is achieved in lower contrast thin vessels.

2 Basic Edge Detection Schemes

Zero crossing of Laplacian ΔI was proposed by Marr-Hildreth in [10] as an edge detector. Haralick edge detector [7]finds the image locations where $|\nabla I|$ has a local maximum along the gradient. In other word, edge is defined as a point where the directional derivative of $|\nabla I|$ along side $\boldsymbol{\xi} = \frac{\nabla I}{|\nabla I|}$, i.e, $I_{\xi\xi}$ is zero:

$$\nabla |\nabla I|.\boldsymbol{\xi} = 0 \tag{1}$$

This implies that the inside the object $\nabla|\nabla I|.\boldsymbol{\xi}$ is negative and the outside positive. Both Haralick and Marr-Hildreth edge detection schemes suffer from dislocation error in identifying curved edges. Since dislocations from these schemes are in opposite directions, Verbeek et al [8] proposed zero crossing of the summation: $\Delta I + I_{\xi\xi}$ (the *PLUS* operator) for edge detection and achieved better accuracy. This corresponds to an energy functional consisting of two components: the first one minimize (maximize the norm) the outward flow of the image gradient field on the object border, and the second one minimizes the a regional integral, summing values of $\nabla|\nabla I|.\boldsymbol{\xi}$ inside the object. In the next section, these functionals are generalized on a Riemannian manifold.

3 Riemannian *PLUS* Edge Detector

Assume for a given open region D, the evolving surface is represented as the zero level of the level set function $\phi(x)$ where $\phi(x) < 0$ for inside of the object, and $\phi(x) > 0$ for outside. $H(x)$ and is representing Heaviside function such that $H(x) = 1$ if $x \geq 0$ otherwise $H(x) = 0$. Also $\delta(x) = \frac{d}{dx} H(x)$ is the Dirac delta function. Further, assume that M is the Riemannian manifold defined on D and endowed by the metric $g = \{g_{i,j}\}$ [4]. The generalization of *PLUS* operator to M is straight forward. All Euclidean gradient $\nabla(.)$ vectors are transformed to: $\nabla_g(\cdot) = g^{-1}\nabla(\cdot)$. Considering the fact that dot product under the space metric is now defined as: $<\boldsymbol{x}, \boldsymbol{y}>_g = \boldsymbol{x}^t.g.\boldsymbol{y}$ and taking care of all the quantities involved in terms of the metric g such energy functional can be written as:

$$E = \int_M \delta(\phi) \nabla_g^t I . g . \nabla_g \phi + \int_M H(-\phi) \nabla_g^t \| \nabla_g I \|_g . g . \frac{\nabla_g I}{\| \nabla_g I \|_g} \quad (2)$$

where ∇_g and $\| \cdot \|_g$ denotes the gradient and the norm on the manifold. The first term is in fact a line integral measuring the flux on the object border and the second term is the regional term. Minimization of this regional functional implies negative Riemannian dot product operator employed in the equation (1) inside the object, and maximizing the (norm) of *geodesic* flux on the border. Using co-area formula equation (2) can be written as:

$$\int_D \delta(\phi) \nabla_g^t I . g . \nabla_g \phi |g|^{1/2} dx + \int_D H(-\phi) \nabla_g^t \| \nabla_g I \|_g . g . \frac{\nabla_g I}{\| \nabla_g I \|_g} |g|^{1/2} dx \quad (3)$$

in which $|g|$ denotes the determinant of the metric. Considering the fact that $\| \nabla_g I \|_g = \| \nabla I \|_{g^{-1}}$, (3) can be simplified as:

$$E = \int_D \delta(\phi) \nabla^t I . g^{-1} . \nabla \phi |g|^{1/2} dx + \int_D H(-\phi) \nabla^t \| \nabla I \|_{g^{-1}} . g^{-1} . \frac{\nabla I}{\| \nabla I \|_{g^{-1}}} |g|^{1/2} dx \quad (4)$$

In which the gradient vectors appear in Euclidean version. It is easy to see that the Euler-Lagrangian minimizing equation of (4) is as follows :

$$\frac{\partial \phi}{\partial t} = \delta(\phi) [div(|g|^{1/2} g^{-1} \nabla I) + \nabla^t \| \nabla I \|_{g^{-1}} . g^{-1} . \frac{\nabla I}{\| \nabla I \|_{g^{-1}}} |g|^{1/2}] \quad (5)$$

Using Libnitz formula this can be rephrased as:

$$\frac{\partial \phi}{\partial t} = \delta(\phi) [div(|g|^{1/2} g^{-1} \nabla I) - 0.5 \| \nabla I \|_{g^{-1}} div(\frac{|g|^{1/2} g^{-1} \nabla I}{\| \nabla I \|_{g^{-1}}})] \quad (6)$$

Let us have a closer look at (6). The first term computes the g-Laplacian of the projected image gradient and it has high responses if ∇I has large components in parallel to main eigen vector of g^{-1}. This is an important property which should be considered in the design of the g, the metric tensor. The second term is the geodesic mean curvature of the image isolevels, and has a similar role as topological complexity minimizer, i.e., $I_{\eta\eta}$ in the Euclidean version [3]. We observe that for $g = I_d$, (the identity matrix), equation (6) reduces to $\partial\phi/\partial t = \Delta I - 0.5 I_{\eta\eta}$, i.e, the Euclidean *PLUS* operator. However, generalization using the metric tensor g allows a selective behaviour of the edge detection mechanism. All we have to do is to design an appropriate tensor that eliminates the gradient vectors in parallel with main orientation of the local structure.

4 Design of the Metric Tensor

We utilize the structural tensor to define our metric tensor. The local structure tensor at point x can be obtained using the following summation in the neighborhood of $N\{x\}$ [6]:

$$T(x) = \sum_{N\{x\}} \nabla(G_\sigma(x) * I(x))\nabla^t(G_\sigma(x) * I(x)) \qquad (7)$$

Where $G_\sigma(x)$ is a Gaussian with a standard deviation σ. Let $0 \leq \lambda_1 < \lambda_2 < \lambda_3$ and $C_i = \boldsymbol{e_i}\boldsymbol{e_i}^t, i = 1, 2, 3$ be the eigen values and their corresponding eigen components of the structure matrix T.

As mentioned in the previous section the tensor g^{-1} should maintain its main components in support of ∇I if it is normal to the local orientation, and in other way the gradients should be eliminated. In this paper we consider a simple form for g^{-1}:

$$g^{-1}(t) = \epsilon(t) C_1 + C_2 + C_3 \qquad (8)$$

Where $0 \leq \epsilon(t) \leq 1$ is a decreasing function such that: $\epsilon(0) = 1.0$ which controls the anisotropic behaviour of the tensor. This important property of time-dependency can be explained as follows: in the beginning of the evolution the tensor is isotropic, and all the directions have the same opportunity to be spanned which helps finding the vessel branchings. Anisotropy is increasing in time, and removes the noisy gradients. This behaviour mimics lowering temperature in optimization by simulated annealing and inhibits local minimums.

5 Multi-scale Computation

Multi-scale implementation of (6) can be achieved in a similar way as described in [2]. That means $div(\boldsymbol{v})$ terms are computed as the outward flux of the $\boldsymbol{v}$ on hemo-centric spheres with different radius r and then maximum is chosen over the range of scales:

$$div(\boldsymbol{v}) = \sup_r \{1/N \sum_q \boldsymbol{v}(r\boldsymbol{n_q}).\boldsymbol{n_q}\} \qquad (9)$$

Where $\boldsymbol{n_q}$ is unit outward normal vector on the sphere surface. In our implementation N, the number of the sampling points on the sphere is fixed to 24, the range of scales was 0.3, 0.54, 0.99 and 1.6 voxel and entries of $\boldsymbol{v}$ and $\boldsymbol{n}$ with non-integer index, are interpolated linearly.

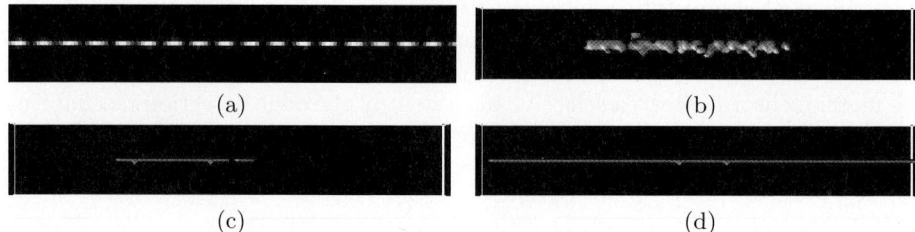

Fig. 1. Riemannian edge detection: (a) Maximum projection image, segmentations obtained from: (b) FLUX, (c) Euclidean PLUS operator ($g^{-1} = I_d$), (d) R-PLUS operator, edges across the model is not detected and a continuous tube is discovered

6 Implementation

In order to have a working contour evolution a few issues must be considered. Since we segment vessels that appear brighter than background, to allow proper vessel edge detection we only allow negative values on the second term in (6). This eliminates the edges resulting from objects with opposite brightness polarity.

A regularized version of delta function,δ_ε is utilized with the same definition as in [5], we used $\varepsilon = 0.5$. Finally smoothness is achieved using minimal surface principle curvature introduced in [?]. Therefore using the tensor metric defined in (8), vessel segmentation evolution is as follows:

$$\frac{\partial \phi}{\partial t} = \delta_\varepsilon(\phi)[\nabla.(g^{-1}\nabla I) - 0.5 \parallel \nabla I \parallel_{g^{-1}} S(\nabla.(\frac{g^{-1}\nabla I}{\parallel \nabla I \parallel_{g^{-1}}})) + \alpha \hat{k}] \quad (10)$$

Where $S(x) = x$ if $x < 0$ otherwise 0. The program is implemented using *Insight Toolkit* and mex library funcitons are called from MATLAB on a Linux system.

7 Synthetic Data Experiment

The maximum intensity projection of a synthetic image is shown in Fig.1.a. We embed a few gap-like signal drop effect along side the model and the target volume is *assumed* to be a straight rod. A Gaussian noise was generated and added with the image. Segmentation using FLUX is shown in panel (b). A few leakage can be observed and the segmented structure appears wider than MIP. Euclidean *PLUS* segmentation is shown in (c) which is insufficient to fully discover the target since it has detected the embedded gaps and contour has been trapped in between. However, *R-PLUS* has successfully passed over the signal droppings and the target has been successfully segmented (d). This is because the edges from those gaps are suppressed by projection through g^{-1}. Meanwhile in contrary to (b), a tighter edges have been obtained across the model, which is closer to the actual edge points of the model.

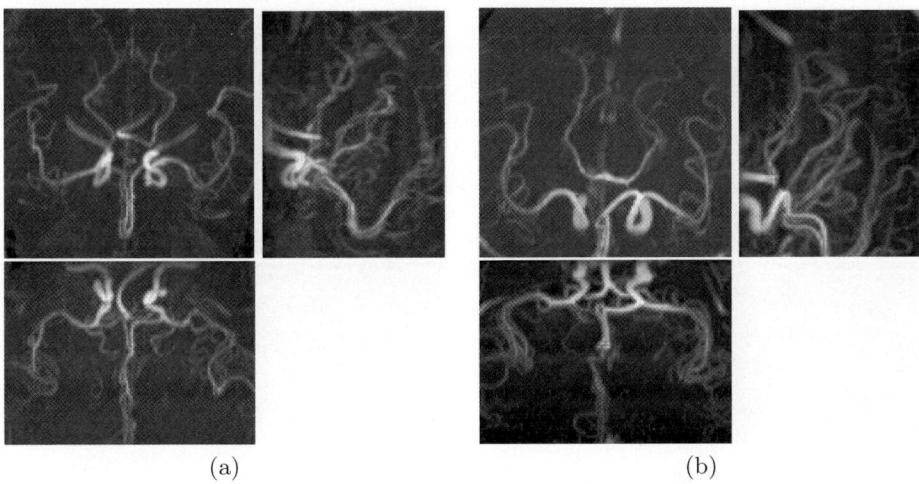

Fig. 2. MIP images of two 149×149×107 3T TOF-MRA data sets used for segmentation

8 Vessel Segmentation

The efficiency of the proposed edge detection scheme was tested on real data obtained using 3T TOF-MRA protocol. Data sets are randomly chosen from MIDAS Data Server at Kitware, Inc and was resized to a isotropic sampling matrix and then smoothed using a Gaussian smoothing filter with $\sigma = 0.3$ voxel. Segmentation was applied on a selected ROI containing most of vasculatures. Fig.2 indicates the maximum intensity projection of two data sets after smoothing. In these experiments, we set the curvature weight $\alpha = 0.025$. Segmentation result is shown in Fig.3. Initialization was achieved by thresholding the speed image (the right hand side of equation (10)) and intial seeds obtained with the most negative values. Consideration was given to include no seed points outside of vessels. After convergence of isotropic $PLUS$ ($\epsilon(t) = 1.0$) operator, which was obtained after almost 10^3 iterations, the result was feed to R-$PLUS$ ($\epsilon(t) \simeq 0.0$) and further propagation was observed. This results in detection and merging of some thinner vessels as indicated by arrows in the right column of Fig.3. The result was also compared to FLUX as shown in Fig.4. As it can be observed, vessels are not delineated in the same thickness as they appear in the MIP image (only one volume is shown), and the segmentation includes significant leakage to background area in that term. Similar results has been reported in a recent work in [11].

9 Discussion

In this paper a new Riemannian edge detection scheme was proposed based on the $PLUS$ operator introduced in [8]. Into our knowledge, this extention is new and has not been addressed yet. Also a new level set PDE was proposed for vessel

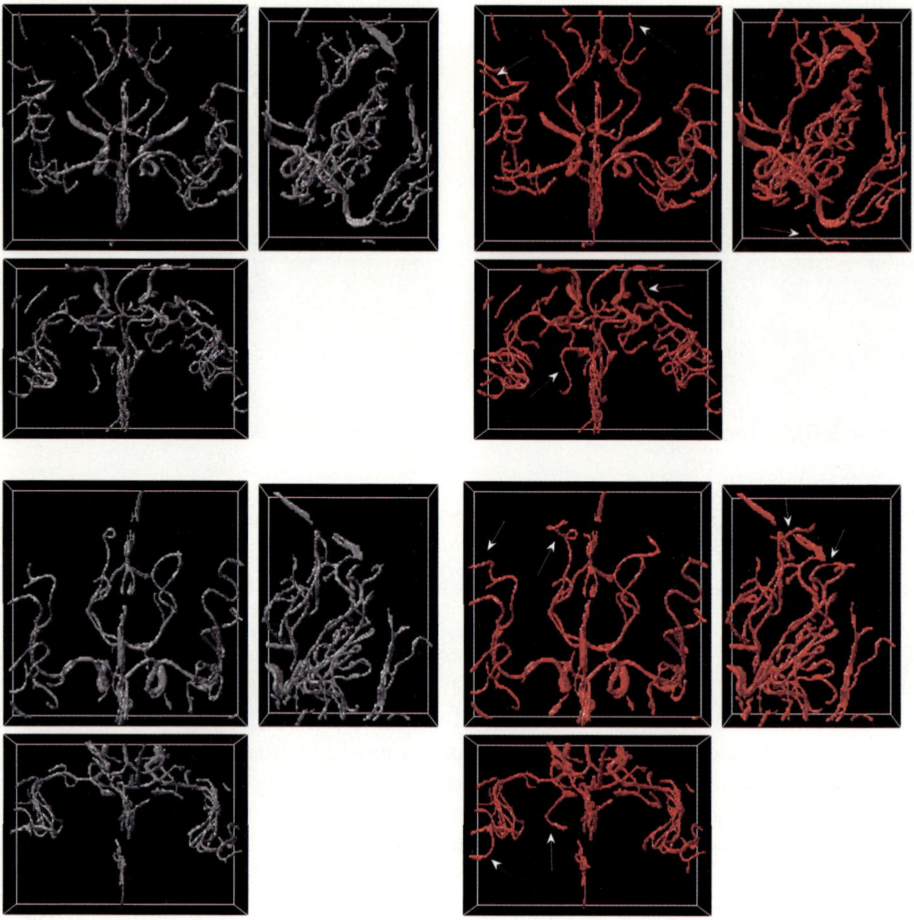

Fig. 3. Segmentations of the first (top) and second (bottom) data sets using: PLUS (left column), R-PLUS (right column). Arrows indicated some vessels that are discovered using R-PLUS.

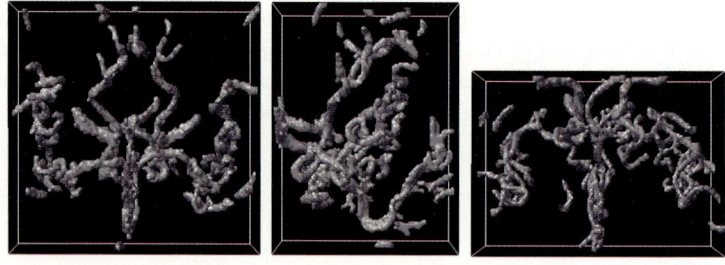

Fig. 4. Segmentation of the first data set using FLUX

segmentation. The tensor metric introduced in this work has a simple form and it can be extended into more complex forms. Yet it is effective and eliminates noisy gradient vectors. The systematic edge detection accuracy problem with similar works [3,2] was addressed and a comparison with standard FLUX method. Our results revealed that the method is able to segment more detailed structures and finer elements. Validation and comparion using other kind of data sets remains as our future research activities.

This study was supported in part by the Special Coordination Funds for Promoting Science and Technology in Japan, and Grant for Industrial Technology Research (07C46050), New Energy and Industrial Technology Development Organization, Japan (both to H. Liao); the Grant-in-Aid for Scientific Research of the Japan Society for the Promotion of Science (17100008 to T. Dohi) and (20.08051 to I.Sakuma).

References

1. Lorigo, L.M., Faugeras, O.D., Grimson, W.E.L., Kerivan, R., Kikinis, R., Nabavai, A., Westin, C.F.: CURVES: Curve evolution for vessel segmentation. Medical Image Analysis 5, 195–206 (2001)
2. Vasilevsky, A., Siddiqi, K.: Flux maximizing geometric flows. IEEE Trans. Pat. Anal. Mach. Intel. 24(12), 1565–1578 (2002)
3. Gazit, M.H., Kimmel, R., Peled, N., Goldsher, D.: Segmentation of thin structures in volumetric medical images. IEEE Trans. Image Proc. 15(2), 354–363 (2006)
4. Shah, J.: Riemannian Drums, Anisotropic Curve Evolution and Segmentation. In: Nielsen, M., Johansen, P., Fogh Olsen, O., Weickert, J. (eds.) Scale-Space 1999. LNCS, vol. 1682, pp. 129–140. Springer, Heidelberg (1999)
5. Chan, T.F., Vese, A.: Active contours without edges. IEEE Trans. Imag. Proc. 10, 266–277 (2001)
6. Weickert, J.: Coherence-enhancing diffusion filtering. Inter. Journal of Computer Vision 31, 111–127 (1999)
7. Haralick, R.: Digital step edge from zero crossing of second directional derivatives. IEEE Trans. Patt. Rec. Mach. Vis. 1(1), 58–68 (1984)
8. Verbeek, P.W., van Vliet, L.J.: On the location error of curved edges in low-pass filtered 2D and 3D images. IEEE Trans. Patt. Rec. Mach. Vis. 16(7), 726–733 (1994)
9. Bouma, H., Vilanova, A., van Vliet, L.J., Gerritsen, F.A.: Correction for the dislocation of curved surfaces caused by the PSF in 2D and 3D images. IEEE Trans. Patt. Rec. Mach. Vis. 27(9), 1501–1507 (2005)
10. Marr, D., Hildreth, E.: Theory of Edge Detection. A Computational Approach to Edge Detection. Proc. Roy. Soc. Lond. B 207, 187–217 (1980)
11. Law, M.W.K., CHung, A.C.S.: Weighted local variance-based edge detection and its application to vascular segmentation in Magnetic Resonance Angiography. IEEE Trans. Imag. Proc. 26(9), 1224–1241 (2007)

A Novel Method for Cortical Sulcal Fundi Extraction

Gang Li[1,2], Tianming Liu[1], Jingxin Nie[2], Lei Guo[2], and Stephen T.C. Wong[1]

[1] The Center for Biotechnology and Informatics, The Methodist Hospital Research Institute and Department of Radiology, The Methodist Hospital, Weill Medical College of Cornell University
[2] School of Automation, Northwestern Polytechnic University, Xian, China

Abstract. Sulcal fundi are 3D curves along the bottom of sulcal regions of the human cerebral cortex. In this paper, we propose a novel automatic method for extraction of sulcal fundi from triangulated cortical surface. Compared to existing methods, the proposed method can find accurate sulcal fundi using curvatures and curvature derivatives without manual interaction. Given a triangulated cortical surface, our method is composed of four steps: estimating curvatures and curvature derivatives for each vertex, detecting the sulcal fundi segments in each triangle, linking the sulcal fundi segments and combining of adjacent sulcal fundi, and connecting breaking sulcal fundi and smoothing using the fast marching method on the cortical surface. The proposed sulcal fundi extraction method is applied to ten normal brain inner cortical surfaces. We quantitatively validated the proposed method of sulcal fundi extraction using manually labeled sulcal fundi by experts as the ground truth.

1 Introduction

The human cerebral cortex is a highly convoluted structure composed of sulci and gyri, corresponding to the valleys and ridges on cortical surface respectively. Sulcal fundi are 3D curves along the bottom of sulcal regions of human cerebral cortex. Major sulci and gyri are common anatomical landmarks in human brains, even though the pattern of sulci and gyri geometry could be quite different across individuals [1]. Thus, major sulci have been extensively used for assisting deformable registration of MR brain images and analyzing the variation of healthy human brain, as well as differentiating the difference between normal brain and diseased ones. Since it is extremely time consuming to label sulci manually, automation has been actively investigated. Methods have been proposed for sulci or sulcal fundi extraction either on MR volumetric images [2, 4, 9] or constructed cortical surfaces [3, 5, 6, 7, 8, 9, 13]. Skeletization or thinning based methods [2, 4, 6, 8] and curve tracking based methods [3, 13] are among the most commonly used techniques for sulci or sulcal fundi extraction. However, applying skeletization or thinning based methods onto the cortical surface cannot assure that the extracted sulcal fundi are unbiased from the true sulcal fundi, as the sulcal regions might not be symmetric around sulcal fundi. On the other hand, in curve tracking based methods, start or end points of sulcal fundi have to be manually selected. Thus, computational methods for finding sulcal fundi in an automated and accurate manner are much needed.

2 Method

2.1 Overview

In this paper, we propose a novel automatic method for extraction of sulcal fundi from triangulated cortical surface. Compared to existing methods, the proposed method can automatically find the accurate sulcal fundi using curvatures and curvature derivatives. Given a constructed triangulated cortical surface, our method of sulcal fundi extraction is composed of four steps, as summarized in Figure 1. Firstly, we adopt the finite difference method to estimate the principal curvatures and directions and the curvature derivatives along the principal directions for each vertex. Then we detect the sulcal fundi segments in each triangle based on the curvatures and curvature derivatives. Afterwards, we link the sulcal fundi segments into continuous sulcal fundi curves and combine adjacent sulcal fundi curves caused by numerical estimation errors. Finally, we connect the breaking sulcal fundi curves and smooth bumping sulcal fundi by applying the fast marching method on the cortical surface.

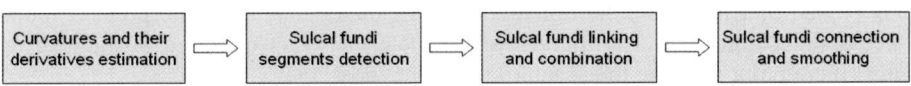

Fig. 1. Flow chart of the sulcal fundi extraction method

2.2 Estimating Curvatures and Curvature Derivatives

Curvatures and their derivatives are fundamental properties for cortical surface analysis. Herein, we adopt a robust method to estimate principal curvatures, principal directions, and curvature derivatives along principal directions as described in [10].

2.3 Detection of Sulcal Fundi Segments

To determine whether each triangle contains sulcal fundi segments or not, we adopt a similar method describe in [11], which is originally developed for ridge and valley detection on mesh and resembles to work in [16]. Given a triangulated cortical surface denote the maximum principal curvature be c_{max} (the curvature with maximum absolute value in the two principal curvatures) and the corresponding principal direction be $\mathbf{p}_{max}$. Denote $d_{max} = \partial c_{max}/\partial \mathbf{p}_{max}$ as the directional derivative of c_{max} along with $\mathbf{p}_{max}$. The criterion for sulcal fundi segment detection is formulated as:

$$c_{max} < 0, \; d_{max} = \partial c_{max}/\partial \mathbf{p}_{max} = 0, \; \partial d_{max}/\partial \mathbf{p}_{max} > 0 \qquad (1)$$

It means that sulcal fundi should be at the location where c_{max} is negative and the first order directional derivative of c_{max} vanishes (zero-crossing of d_{max}), and the second order directional derivative of c_{max} reaches positive values. Given a triangle in a cortical surface (denoting the three vertices as: $\mathbf{v}_1, \mathbf{v}_2$ and $\mathbf{v}_3$), we check whether the triangle contains sulcal fundi segments by inspecting whether the three edges contain sulcal fundi points. Without loss of generality, we use the edge formed by $\mathbf{v}_1$ and $\mathbf{v}_2$ as an instance. Firstly, we inspect c_{max} at vertices $\mathbf{v}_1$ and $\mathbf{v}_2$ to make sure:

$$c_{max}(\mathbf{v}_1) < 0 \text{ and } c_{max}(\mathbf{v}_2) < 0 \qquad (2)$$

Then, we check whether the edge contains the first order directional derivative of c_{max} vanished point with the following formula:

$$d_{max}(\mathbf{v}_1)\mathbf{p}_{max}(\mathbf{v}_1) d_{max}(\mathbf{v}_2)\mathbf{p}_{max}(\mathbf{v}_2) < 0 \qquad (3)$$

Then, to make sure that the edge contains true sulcal fundi point in theory, the maximum principal curvature decreases along the edge should satisfy:

$$d_{max}(\mathbf{v}_1)\mathbf{p}_{max}(\mathbf{v}_1)(\mathbf{v}_2-\mathbf{v}_1) < 0 \text{ or } d_{max}(\mathbf{v}_2)\mathbf{p}_{max}(\mathbf{v}_2)(\mathbf{v}_1-\mathbf{v}_2) < 0 \qquad (4)$$

Herein, we loose the conditional checks. If the edge passes the above three conditional checks, a strict sulcal fundi point is found in the edge. Otherwise, if the edge only passed the first two conditional checks, a candidate sulcal fundi point is found. Once a sulcal fundi point is found, we calculate the exact unbiased position of the sulcal fundi point with the linear interpolation method [11]:

$$\mathbf{v} = \frac{|d_{max}(\mathbf{v}_1)| \times \mathbf{v}_2 + |d_{max}(\mathbf{v}_2)| \times \mathbf{v}_1}{|d_{max}(\mathbf{v}_1)| + |d_{max}(\mathbf{v}_2)|} \qquad (5)$$

After checking the three edges in the triangle, if two of the three edges have sulcal fundi points, we connect the two points as a sulcal fundi segment; otherwise if all of the three edges contain sulcal fundi points, we connect the three vertices to the center of the triangle to form three sulcal fundi segments, which might correspond to the location of intersection of the sulcal fundi curves. Afterwards, we distinguish the segments as strict or candidate sulcal fundi segments. If a sulcal fundi point in a segment is a candidate point, we consider the segment as a candidate sulcal fundi segment, or a strict segment otherwise. Figure 2 shows an instance of sulcal fundi segments detection in a cortical surface.

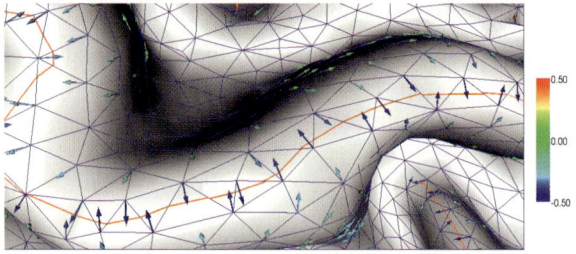

Fig. 2. An instance of sulcal fundi segment detection in a cortical surface. The orange curves represent the sulci fundi segments. The arrow at each vertex indicates the maximum principal direction and the colors of the arrows indicate the values of the maximum principal curvatures.

2.4 Linking Sulcal Fundi Segments

With the detected sulcal fundi segments, we link them into continuous sulcal fundi curves. We distinguish the sulcal fundi segments into strict and candidate segments, because we observe sometimes candidate segments can connect with strict segments to form a continuous sulcal fundi curve. If we only use strict segments, the sulcal fundi will be interrupted around candidate segments. Starting from a strict segment, a sulcal fundi curve is formed by adding adjacent segments that shares the same edge or center with the current segment. After linking we obtain a set of sulcal fundi curves. Due to the error of numerical estimation, sulcal fundi around junction regions are often interrupted. To deal with this situation, we check one ring neighborhood of each vertex. If two or more different sulcal fundi are in the neighborhood and c_{max} at the vertex is negative, we combine these sulcal fundi together.

2.5 Connection of Breaking Sulcal Fundi and Smoothing

After linking the sulcal fundi segments and combining adjacent sulcal fundi, we obtained a series of continuous sulcal fundi curves. Some sulcal fundi may be very short, which correspond to the breaking sulcal fundi or inherently short, minor sulcal fundi. Thus we have to connect breaking sulcal fundi together, however, we may not know which ones are interrupted and which ones are inherently short. To deal with this problem, we adopt the fast marching method on triangulated surface [12]. From each ending point of the extracted sulcal fundi curves, we search in a geodesic region (8mm as the geodesic threshold) to find out whether other sulcal fundi are in the region. Once other sulcal fundi curves are found, we tentatively connect the end point to the found sulcal fundi by computing the weighted geodesic path on the surface using fast marching method. As the sulcal fundi are located at regions with large negative c_{max}, we set the marching speed at vertex $\mathbf{x}$ as follows:

$$F_1(\mathbf{x}) = \begin{cases} 1.0, & \text{if } (c_{max}(\mathbf{x}) < T) \\ e^{\alpha}, & \text{if } (c_{max}(\mathbf{x}) > -T) \\ e^{\alpha|c_{max}(\mathbf{x})-T|} \end{cases} \quad (6)$$

where T is a curvature threshold parameter and α is a weighting parameter. This formula makes sure the sulcal root regions have faster marching speeds, and gyral crown regions have slower marching speeds. We set $T = -1.0$ and $\alpha = -5.0$ throughout the paper. However, the geodesic path may wrongly connect two inherent separated sulcal fundi by a gyral crown region. To avoid this situation, we inspect c_{max} on the geodesic path. Since we know c_{max} is positive at gyral crown regions, if c_{max} at a point on the path is positive, we consider the geodesic path going through gyral crown regions and regards it as a fake sulcal fundi and discard it; otherwise, we add the geodesic path as a part of the sulcus fundi to connect breaking sulcal fundi. Figure 3 (a) shows an example of connecting breaking sulcal fundi.

Due to the numerical estimation error of curvatures and their derivatives, the extracted sulcal fundi may contain some sudden bumps as show in figure 3 (b). Therefore, we have to smooth the extracted sulcal fundi to make it more practical.

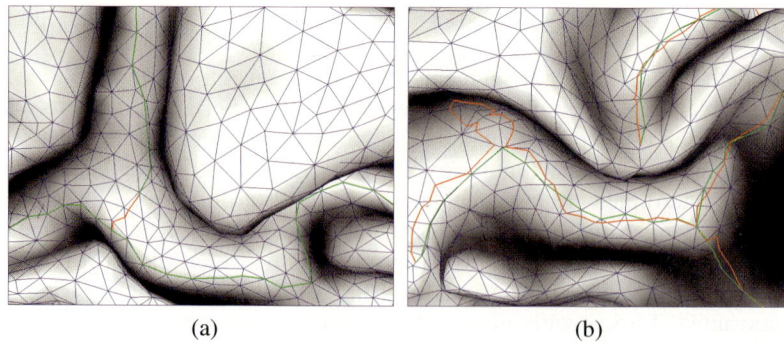

Fig. 3. Examples of connecting breaking sulcal fundi and smoothing sulcal fundi. The green curves are the original extracted sulcal fundi. In (a) the orange curve connects the breaking sulcal fundi. In (b) the orange curves are the smoothed sulcal fundi.

Meanwhile, we want to keep the smoothed sulcal fundi close to the originally extracted sulcal fundi. To handle this issue, we adopt the fast marching method to extract the weighting geodesic path from sulcal fundi starting points to the corresponding end points or junction points for smoothing and set the marching speed at each vertex as:

$$F_2(\mathbf{x}) = \beta \times F_1(\mathbf{x}) + (1-\beta) \times S(\mathbf{x}) \tag{7}$$

Where the term $S(x)$ is used to favor vertices closing the original sulcal fundi, and β is a parameter used to control the tradeoff between favoring c_{max} and favoring closeness to the original sulcal fundi. In the current implementation, $S(\mathbf{x})$ is set to be:

$$S(\mathbf{x}) = 1 - \min_{\mathbf{x}_i}(|\mathbf{x}-\mathbf{s}_i|/|\mathbf{x}-\mathbf{x}_i|) \tag{8}$$

$\mathbf{x}_i$ is the one-ring adjacent vertices of $\mathbf{x}$ while $\mathbf{s}_i$ is the sulcal fundi point on the edge formed by $\mathbf{x}$ and $\mathbf{x}_i$. If no sulcal fundus point exists in edges formed by $\mathbf{x}$, $S(\mathbf{x})$ is set to be 0. The straightforward explanation is that the closer is the current vertex to sulcal fundus point, the favorer is the current vertex in smoothing. The parameter β is set as 0.7 in the paper. Using the marching speed calculated above, we smooth the sulcal fundi by computing the weighted geodesic path between the sulcal fundi start points and the corresponding end points or junction points. Figure 3 (b) shows an example of extracted sulcal fundi before and after smoothing.

To summarize, our new method of sulcal fundi extraction consists of four steps: estimating curvatures and their derivatives, detection of sulcal fundi segments, linking sulcal fundi segments and combining adjacent sulcal fundi, and connecting breaking sulcal fundi and smoothing. Figure 4 shows an example of extracted sulcal fundi.

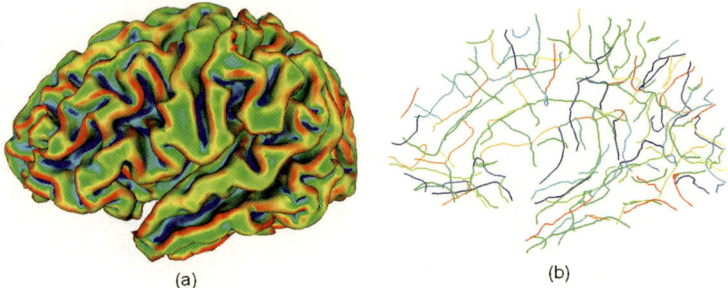

Fig. 4. An example of the extracted sulcal fundi. (a) A cortical inner surface with estimated maximum principal curvature. (b) The finally extracted sulcal fundi.

3 Evaluation and Validation

We tested the sulcal fundi detection method on the inner surface of 10 normal human brains. All the cortical surfaces are generated via the BrainVISA software [14]. In the inner surfaces of right hemispheres of the 10 subjects, after linking sulcal fundi segments as curves, we find 124.4 sulcal fundi connecting components on average with the standard derivation 6.7; after combining adjacent sulcal fundi curves, the number is reduced to 83.9 on average with the standard derivation 3.7; after connecting breaking sulcal fundi curves, the number is further reduced to 59.1 on average with the standard derivation 5.1. We have visually inspected the sulcal fundi extraction results and found no fatal errors in the 10 cases. Figure 5 shows two examples of extracted sulcal fundi on the inner surface of the right hemisphere.

To quantitatively evaluate the accuracy of sulcal fundi extraction method, we have experts manually label major sulcal fundi on the cortical inner surface of the right hemisphere of the 10 cases. We use two measurements to validate the performance. Denote the ground truth sulcal fundi as S_g and automatic extracted sulcal fundi as S_a, the two distance measurements are defined as:

$$d_{min} = \frac{1}{n} \sum_{i \in n} \min_{j \in m} |S_a(i) - S_g(j)| \qquad (9)$$

$$d_{max} = \max_{i \in n} (\min_{j \in m} |S_a(i) - S_g(j)|) \qquad (10)$$

where n and m are the total point numbers in sulcal fundi S_a and S_g respectively. d_{min} measures the average distance from all the points in S_a to the corresponding closet point in S_g. And d_{max} measures the worst maximum distance from all the points in S_a to the corresponding closet point in S_g. We use several major sulci including central, precentral, postcentral, superior frontal, superior temporal, cingulate and calcarine sulcus to validate the performance of the method. Figure 6 shows an example of several manual labeled sulcal fundi and automatically extracted sulcal fundi on a lateral surface of a subject. For the convenience of inspection, we also

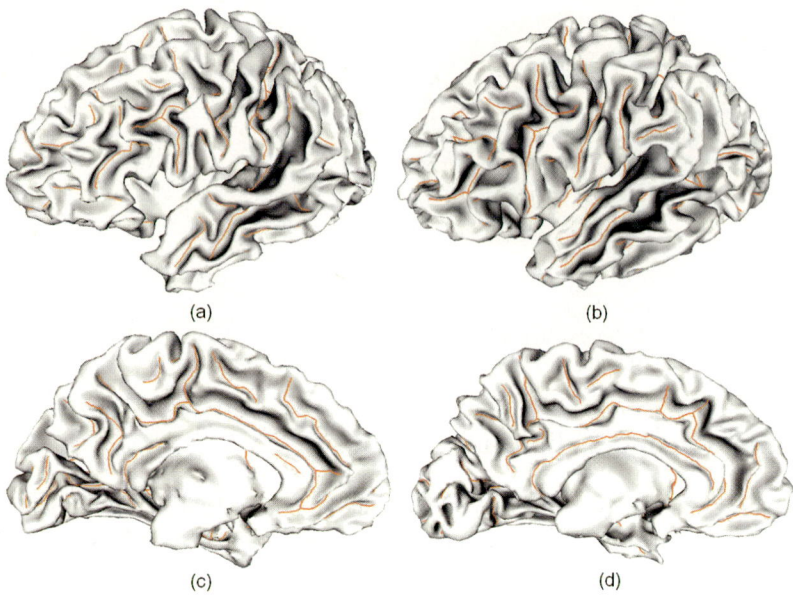

Fig. 5. Extracted sulcal fundi (orange curves) on the inner surfaces of two subjects. (a) and (b) are lateral view. (c) and (d) are medial view.

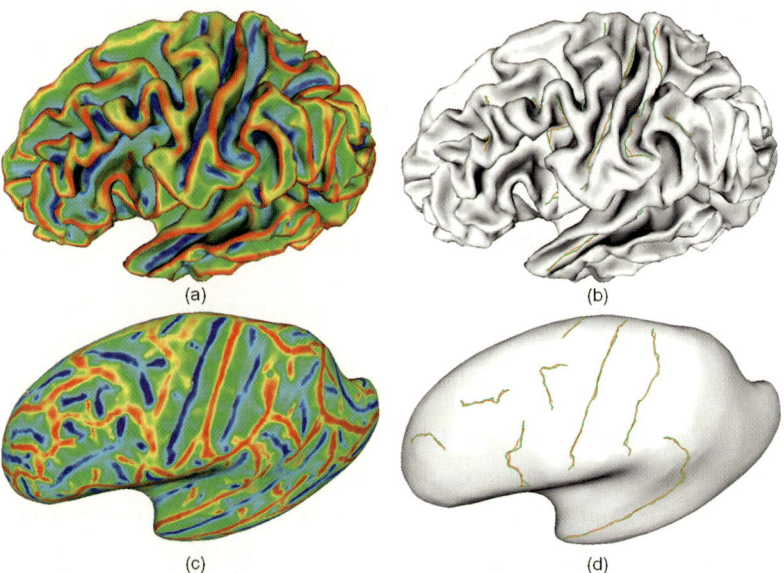

Fig. 6. An example of manual labeled and automatic extracted suclal fundi on a lateral inner surface. (a) and (c) are maximum principal curvature maps on the surface and the corresponding inflated surface. (c) and (d) are manual labeled and automatic extracted sulcal fundi overlaid on the surface and inflated surface. The green curves are automatic extracted sulcal fundi and the yellow curves are manually labeled sulcal fundi.

overlay the sulcal fundi on the inflated surface. The inflated surface is generated via a method similar to [15]. As we can see the two sulcal fundi sets are close to each other. Table 1 shows the details of average d_{min} the several sulcal fundi on the 10 subjects. The average d_{min} is consistently less than 0.7 mm and the d_{max} is consistently less than 3.2 mm, indicating the good performance of the proposed method. Currently the method is implemented using the C/C++ language. On an Intel Core2 1.86GHz machine with 2GB memory, it takes around 8 seconds extract all the sulcal fundi on the inner surface of a hemisphere.

Table 1. The d_{min} of several major sulcal fundi on the inner surfaces of the 10 subjects

Sulcus (mm)	Central	Pre-central	Post-central	Superior frontal	Superior temporal	Cingulate	Calcarine
1	0.61	0.93	0.92	0.52	0.62	0.66	0.51
2	0.66	0.74	0.49	0.60	0.60	0.73	0.56
3	0.71	0.57	0.73	0.55	0.67	0.32	0.82
4	0.81	0.57	0.51	0.41	0.64	0.30	0.46
5	0.62	0.61	0.66	0.64	0.52	0.45	0.58
6	0.71	0.35	0.78	0.70	0.65	0.62	1.16
7	0.61	0.78	0.49	0.58	0.67	0.38	0.53
8	0.57	0.64	0.69	0.42	0.63	0.35	0.44
9	0.72	0.54	0.63	0.39	0.65	0.62	0.50
10	0.78	0.62	0.49	0.90	0.61	0.48	0.46
Average	0.68	0.64	0.64	0.57	0.63	0.49	0.60

4 Conclusion

In this paper, we presented a novel automated method for accurately extracting sulcal fundi on the cortical surface of the human brain. The method has been applied to 10 normal subjects on inner surface and its performance has been evaluated using the ground truth defined by experts manually labeled sulcal fundi. The evaluation results show that the proposed method is able to extract sulcal fundi efficiently and accurately.

Acknowledgement

This study is funded by a Bioinformatics Program grant from The Methodist Hospital Research Institute to STCW.

References

1. Ono, M., Kubik, S., Abarnathey, C.: Atlas of the Cerebral Sulci. Thieme Medical Publishers (1990)
2. Lohmann, G.: Extracting line representations of sulcal and gyral patterns in MR images of the human brain. IEEE Trans. On Medical Imaging 17(6), 1040–1048 (1998)

3. Khaneja, N., Miller, M., Grenander, U.: Dynamic programming generation of curves on brain surfaces. IEEE Trans. On PAMI 20(11), 1260–1265 (1998)
4. Goualher, G.L., Procyk, E., Collins, D.L., Venugopal, R., Barillot, C., Evans, A.C.: Automated extraction and variability analysis of sulcal neuroanatomy. IEEE Trans. On Medical Imaging 18(3), 206–217 (1999)
5. Tao, X., Prince, J.L., Davatzikos, C.: Using a statistical shape model to extract sulcal curves on the outer cortex of the human brain. IEEE Trans. on Medical Imaging 21(5), 513–524 (2002)
6. Rivi'ere, D., Mangin, J.-F., Papadopoulos-Orfanos, D., Martinez, J., Frouin, V., R'egis, J.: Automatic recognition of cortical sulci of the human brain using a congregation of neural networks. Med. Image. Anal. 6, 77–92 (2002)
7. Rettmann, M.E., Han, X., Xu, C., Prince, J.L.: Automated sulcal segmentation using watersheds on the cortical surface. NeuroImage 15(2), 329–344 (2002)
8. Kao, C., Hofer, M., Sapiro, G., Stern, J., Rehm, K., Rottenberg, D.A.: A geometric method for automatic extraction of sulcal fundi. IEEE Trans. On Medical Imaging 26(4), 530–540 (2007)
9. Tu, Z., Zheng, S., Yuille, A.L., Reiss, A.L., Dutton, R.A., Lee, A.D., Galaburda, A.M., Dinov, I., Thompson, P.M., Toga, A.W.: Automated extraction of the cortical sulci based on a supervised learning approach. IEEE Trans. On Medical Imaging 26(4), 541–552 (2007)
10. Rusinkiewicz, S.: Estimating curvatures and their derivatives on triangle meshes. In: Proc. 3DPVT, pp. 486–493 (September 2004)
11. Ohtake, Y., Belyaev, A., Seidel, H.P.: Ridge-valley on meshes via implicit surface fitting. Proc. SIGGRAPH 23(3), 609–612 (2004)
12. Kimmel, R., Sethian, J.A.: Computing geodesic paths on manifolds. Proc. Natl. Acad. Sci. USA 95(15), 8431–8435 (1998)
13. Tao, X., Han, X., Rettmann, M., Prince, J., Davatzikos, C.: Statistical study on cortical sulci of human brains. In: Insana, M.F., Leahy, R.M. (eds.) IPMI 2001. LNCS, vol. 2082, pp. 475–487. Springer, Heidelberg (2001)
14. Cointepas, Y., Mangin, J.F., Garnero, L., Poline, J.B., Benali, H.: BrainVISA: Software platform for visualization and analysis of multimodality brain data. NeuroImage 13, S98 (2001)
15. Tosun, D., Rettmann, M.E., Prince, J.L.: Mapping techniques for aligning sulci across multiple brains. Med. Image. Anal. 8, 295–309 (2004)
16. Thirion, J.-P.: The extermal mesh and understanding of 3D surfaces. International Journal of Computer Vision 19, 115–128 (1996)

Joint Segmentation of Thalamic Nuclei from a Population of Diffusion Tensor MR Images

Ulas Ziyan[1] and Carl-Fredrik Westin[1,2]

[1] MIT Computer Science and Artificial Intelligence Lab, Cambridge MA, USA
[2] Laboratory of Mathematics in Imaging, Brigham and Women's Hospital, Harvard Medical School, Boston MA, USA*

Abstract. Several recent studies explored the use of unsupervised segmentation methods for segmenting thalamic nuclei from diffusion tensor images. These methods provide a plausible segmentation on individual subjects; however, they do not address the problem of consistently identifying the same functional areas in a population. The lack of correspondence between the segmented nuclei make it more difficult to use the results from the unsupervised segmentation tools for morphometry. In this paper we present a novel segmentation algorithm to automatically segment the gray matter nuclei while ensuring consistency between subjects in a population. This new algorithm, referred to as Consistency Clustering, finds correspondence between the nuclei as the segmentation is achieved through a single model for the whole population, similar to the brain atlases experts use to identify thalamic nuclei.

1 Introduction

Diffusion tensor imaging (DTI) is a relatively new imaging modality that measures free water diffusion, i.e. Brownian motion, of the endogenous water in tissue [1]. In human brain tissue, the water diffusion is not the same in all directions, since it is obstructed by structural elements such as cell membranes or myelin [1]. When this obstruction constrains the water diffusion in a coherent direction, such as within the cerebral white matter, the resulting water diffusion tensor becomes anisotropic, containing information about the directionality of the white matter connectivity. Thus, quantification of water diffusion in tissue through DTI provides a unique way to analyze white matter organization of the brain.

Unlike white matter, the tissue in gray matter is less organized in orientation. The lack of coherent orientation limits the use of DTI for gray matter analysis in some areas, such as the cerebral cortex. However, there are certain gray matter structures that exhibit coherence in diffusion direction due to the presence of coherent white matter near these structures, such as the thalamus. The thalamus

---

* The authors would like to thank Jonathan J Wisco for providing the thalamus masks and manual segmentations of the nuclei. This work was supported by NIH NIBIB NAMIC U54-EB005149, NIH NCRR NAC P41-RR13218 and R01-MH074794.

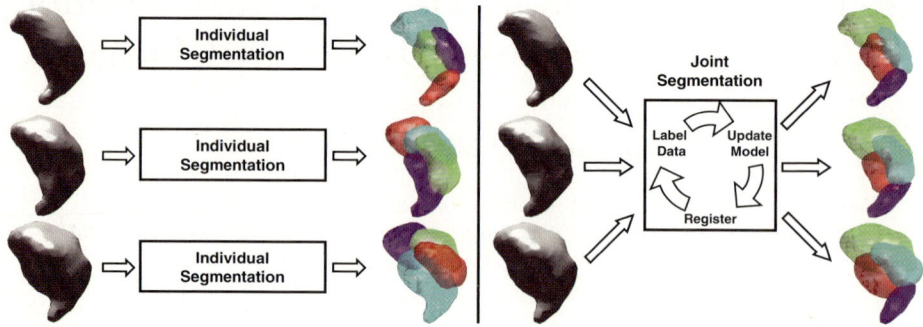

Fig. 1. Schematic description of previous thalamus segmentation algorithms [2,3,4,5] (left) as opposed to the Consistency Clustering (right)

acts as the central relay station of the brain with nearly all of the sensory tract projections reach to the cortex passing through the thalamus. Since functionally related pathways target the same region of cortex once they leave the thalamus, they result in organization of diffusivity within the thalamus. This organized diffusion can be measured in DTI, and it has been proposed that the thalamic nuclei can be distinguished by their characteristic diffusion orientation [2].

Precise identification of the thalamic nuclei is essential in a clinical setting, since many motor-control disorders are surgically corrected by applying chronic electrical stimulation to the appropriate functional area of the thalamus. Currently, these regions are detected qualitatively before the operation using generic atlases along with structural MRI [6], which does not provide adequate contrast to identify the distinct nuclei. Changes have also been reported in the thalamic nuclei during the progression of a large number of diseases, including schizophrenia [7] and Parkinson's disease [8].

Since the realization that thalamic nuclei can be resolved through DTI, several segmentation algorithms have been proposed to segment the thalamic nuclei. The earliest segmentation method, which depends on DTI data only from within the thalamus, uses the k-means clustering algorithm [2]. Later, other clustering methods have been proposed that use spectral clustering [3], level-sets [4] and the mean-shift algorithm [5]. These later methods avoid some of the weaknesses of the k-means, which includes a bias toward ellipsoidal clusters and sensitivity to initialization. Even though each of these clustering algorithms produce plausible segmentations for any given subject in a population, they do not find a correspondence between the segments acquired from different subjects.

In this paper, we present a new approach to the segmentation of thalamic nuclei. Unlike the previous methods, this new algorithm, referred to as Consistency Clustering (CC), is designed to segment multiple subjects simultaneously and find a correspondence between the segmentation results (Figure 1). CC achieves these goals by learning a thalamic model of the population under investigation, which serves as a probabilistic atlas of the thalamic nuclei. This model involves a spatial component as well as a directional component for each nuclei. CC also performs a poly-rigid registration to account for inter-subject variability. Since the segmentation of each individual subject is done according to a common model, the consistency of segmentations between subjects is ensured. This joint segmentation approach results in a segmentation for each subject and determines a correspondence between subjects. Also, the thalamic model, which is learned from a population of labeled or unlabeled data, serves as an anatomical atlas for the population under investigation.

In the following sections, we first describe the theory behind the method, and then present results from several experiments that demonstrate the feasibility of the proposed method with DTI data from 10 healthy participants.

2 Theory

In this section we formulate the problem of joint segmentation of thalamic nuclei as a maximum likelihood problem and solve it using the generalized expectation maximization algorithm [9]. The algorithm iteratively increases the joint probability of observing the set of thalami under investigation. The joint probability is measured in terms of a mixture density model that accounts for spatial distribution of the nuclei as well as the principal diffusion orientation. The inter-subject variability is also handled within the same framework by introducing a set of parameters describing a poly-rigid registration.

The DTI data is modeled with a set of parameters, $\Theta = \{\pi_c, \boldsymbol{\mu}_c, \boldsymbol{\Sigma}_c, \boldsymbol{\nu}_c, \kappa_c\} \cup \{\boldsymbol{R}_s\}$, where c is an index over clusters, i.e. $c \in \{1, 2, \ldots, C\}$ and s is an index over subjects, i.e. $s \in \{1, 2, \ldots, S\}$. Given these parameters, the likelihood of the subjects becomes:

$$\Lambda(X, V; \Theta) = \prod_{i=1}^{N} \sum_{c=1}^{C} \pi_c f_x(\boldsymbol{x}_i; \Theta) f_v(\boldsymbol{v}_i; \Theta),$$

where we assume independence between every observed sample (voxel) and also independence between the spatial location $\boldsymbol{x}_i$ and principal diffusion orientation $\boldsymbol{v}_i$. We model the spatial distribution with a Gaussian:

$$f_x(\boldsymbol{x}; \Theta) = f_x(\boldsymbol{x}; \boldsymbol{\mu}_c, \boldsymbol{\Sigma}_c) = \frac{1}{(2\pi)^{3/2} |\boldsymbol{\Sigma}_c|^{1/2}} \exp\left(-\frac{1}{2}(\boldsymbol{x} - \boldsymbol{\mu}_c)^T \boldsymbol{\Sigma}_c^{-1}(\boldsymbol{x} - \boldsymbol{\mu}_c)\right),$$

where $\boldsymbol{\mu}_c$ is the mean vector and $\boldsymbol{\Sigma}_c$ is the covariance matrix. We model the distribution of the principal diffusion directions with a von Mises-Fisher distribution:

$$f_v(\boldsymbol{v}; \Theta) = f_v(\boldsymbol{v}; \boldsymbol{\nu}_c, \kappa_c) = C(\kappa_c) exp\left(\kappa_c \boldsymbol{\nu_c}^T \boldsymbol{v}\right),$$

where $\boldsymbol{\nu}_c$ is the mean orientation and κ_c is the concentration parameter. The constant, $C(\kappa) = \kappa^{1/2}/(2\pi)^{3/2} I_{1/2}(\kappa)$, and $I_{1/2}(\kappa)$ is a modified Bessel function of the first kind and order 1/2. Under this model, we formulate our problem as a maximum likelihood estimation of the parameter set Θ:

$$\Theta^* = \arg\max_{\Theta} \Lambda(X, V; \Theta).$$

In the next sections we present the update equations for our formulation to iteratively estimate Θ^*. Detailed derivations have been omitted due to limited space.

2.1 E-Step

In the E-step, CC updates the membership probabilities for each voxel, given the estimate of the parameter set at iteration (n), $\Theta^{(n)}$:

$$p(c|\boldsymbol{x}_i, \boldsymbol{v}_i; \Theta^{(n)}) \propto \pi_c^{(n)} f_x(\boldsymbol{R}_s^{(n)} \circ \boldsymbol{x}_i; \boldsymbol{\mu}_c^{(n)}, \boldsymbol{\Sigma}_c^{(n)}) f_v(\boldsymbol{R}_s^{(n)} \circ \boldsymbol{v}_i; \boldsymbol{\nu}_c^{(n)}, \kappa_c^{(n)}),$$
$$\triangleq p_{ci}^{(n)},$$

where $p_{ci}^{(n)}$ is normalized at every iteration, so that $\sum_c p_{ci}^{(n)} = 1$ for all voxels.

2.2 M-Step

In the M-step, CC updates the parameter set Θ to maximize the expected value of the log likelihood. Ignoring constant term that does not depend on Θ, the expected value of the log likelihood is derived as:

$$\beta(X, V; \Theta) = \sum_{i=1}^{N} \sum_{c=1}^{C} p_{ci}^{(n)} \left(\log \pi_c + \log f_x(\boldsymbol{R}_s^{(n)} \circ \boldsymbol{x}_i; \Theta^{(n)}) + \log f_v(\boldsymbol{R}_s^{(n)} \circ \boldsymbol{v}_i; \Theta^{(n)}) \right) \tag{1}$$

For a given parameter set $\Theta^{(n)}$, the update equations for $\Theta^{(n+1)}$ are derived using Lagrange multipliers for the corresponding constraints and setting the derivative of (1) to zero. Let $P_c^{(n)} \triangleq \sum_{i=1}^{N} p_{ci}^{(n)}$, then the resulting update equations are:

$$\pi_c^{(n+1)} = P_c^{(n)}/N,$$

$$\boldsymbol{\mu}_c^{(n+1)} = \left(1/P_c^{(n)}\right) \times \sum_{i=1}^{N} p_{ci}^{(n)} \boldsymbol{x}_i,$$

$$\boldsymbol{\Sigma}_c^{(n+1)} = \left(1/P_c^{(n)}\right) \times \sum_{i=1}^{N} p_{ci}^{(n)} \left(\boldsymbol{x}_i - \boldsymbol{\mu}_c^{(n+1)}\right) \left(\boldsymbol{x}_i - \boldsymbol{\mu}_c^{(n+1)}\right)^T,$$

$$\boldsymbol{r}_c = \sum_{i=1}^{N} p_{ci}^{(n)} \boldsymbol{v}_i,$$

$$\bar{r}_c = \|\boldsymbol{r}_c\|/P_c^{(n)},$$

$$\boldsymbol{\nu}_c^{(n+1)} = \boldsymbol{r}_c/\|\boldsymbol{r}_c\|,$$

$$\kappa_c^{(n+1)} \approx \left(3\bar{r}_c - \bar{r}_c^3\right) / \left(1 - \bar{r}_c^2\right),$$

where the last equation is an approximation to the true parameter κ_c [10].

Registration: Registration parameters are also updated in the m-step. We parametrize the registration as one rigid transformation per cluster per subject, i.e.,

$$R_s^{(n)} \circ x_i = R_{sc}^{(n)}(x_i - \mu_{sc}^{(n)}) + \mu_{sc}^{(n)} + t_{sc}^{(n)},$$
$$R_s^{(n)} \circ v_i = R_{sc}^{(n)} v_i,$$

where $\mu_{sc}^{(n)} = \sum_{i \in s} p_{ci}^{(n-1)} x_i / \sum_{i \in s} p_{ci}^{(n-1)}$, and represents the weighted mean of the voxel locations in a given subject. Similar to other parameters, setting the derivative of (1) to zero, we get:

$$t_{sc}^{(n+1)} = \mu_c^{(n+1)} - \mu_{sc}^{(n+1)},$$

where $\mu_c^{(n+1)} = \sum_{i \in s} \sum_c p_{ci}^{(n)} x_i / \sum_{i \in s} \sum_c p_{ci}^{(n)}$. Unfortunately, the same technique does not lead into a simple analytical solution for the rotation matrices, $R_{sc}^{(n+1)}$. However, we derive a maximum likelihood optimization function and optimize the function using a numerical scheme. The resulting optimization function is:

$$R_{sc}^{(n+1)} = \arg\max_{R_{sc}} \sum_{i \in s} 2\kappa_c^{(n+1)} \nu_c^{(n+1),T} R_{sc} v_i - x_i^T R_{sc}^T \Sigma_c^{(n+1),T} R_{sc} x_i$$

s.t. $R_{sc} R_{sc}^T = I$ and $|R| = 1$.

We further parametrize R_{sc} using Euler angles so that the constraints are automatically met. Then we find optimal values for the Euler angles (and therefore R_{sc}) using a simplex search method [11].

3 Methods

3.1 Image Acquisition and Pre-processing

DTI data were acquired using a twice-refocused spin-echo EPI sequence [12] on a 3 Tesla Siemens Trio MRI scanner using an 8-channel head coil. The sequence parameters were TR/TE=8400/82 ms, b=700 s/mm^2, gmax=26 mT/m, 10 T2 images, 60 diffusion gradient directions. The resulting images had 2×2 mm in-plane resolution with a slice thickness of 2 mm with 0 mm gap.

Correction for motion and residual eddy current distortion was achieved by registering all of the scans to the first acquired non-diffusion-weighted scan for each participant. The registration used a 12 degree-of-freedom global affine transformation and a mutual information cost function [13]. Trilinear interpolation was used for the resampling. The diffusion tensor were calculated for each voxel using the formulas of [14].

The diffusion tensor volumes were normalized to MNI-space (Montreal Neurological Institute) by registering each participant's T2 volume to a skull-stripped version of the MNI 152-subject T2 template [15] and then applying the transformation to the diffusion tensor volumes with 12 degree-of-freedom global affine transformation. The tensors were reoriented using the rotational portion of the atlas transformation.

Thalamus masks were then drawn manually for each individual by a trained neuro-anatomist. The masks were drawn for each hemisphere on each individual's

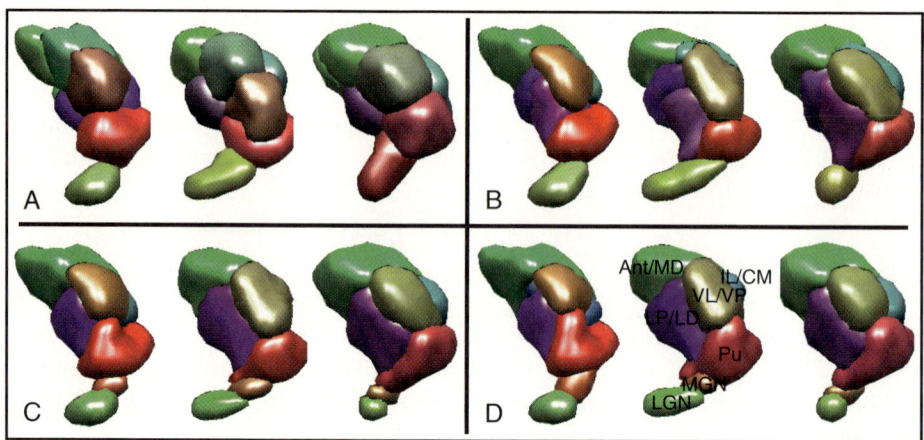

Fig. 2. Segmentation results from three subjects' left thalamic hemispheres are shown. Colors indicate the mean diffusion orientation in each cluster. (A) Segmentations obtained using k-means have an ellipsoidal bias and they do not correspond well between subjects. (B) Segmentations obtained using CC with no prior information are consistent among subjects. (C) Segmentation using CC with prior information are both consistent among subjects and match well with the expert segmentations. (D) Expert labeled thalami are shown. Note that even though the segmentations in (C) and (D) look very similar, they are not exactly the same (see Figure 3).

MNI-normalized FA map following the guidelines from [16]. Each hemisphere was further segmented into its seven nuclei on the corresponding tensor map by the neuro-anatomist following the drawings of [16].

3.2 Experiments

CC was validated on 10 normal subjects' DTI datasets. Each subject's thalami (only the left hemispheres) were segmented individually using the k-means algorithm as described in [2] and spectral clustering as described in [3] to create benchmarks. The same thalami were then segmented jointly using CC with the same (uniform) initialization used for the k-means algorithm. The joint segmentation resulted in corresponding segmentations in all subjects, whereas the k-means clustering did not (Figure 2A, B). To test the use of prior information, we repeated the joint segmentation experiment 10 times for each thalami in a leave-one-out fashion. For each joint segmentation, we fixed the voxel labels for 9 of the subjects at the expert labels (to "anchor" the model), and let the last subject's labels vary. The resulting segmentations were not only consistent among subjects (Figure 2C), but also matched well qualitatively with the expert labels (Figure 2D).

We also quantified the accuracy of the segmentation results against the expert labels using the Dice volume overlap measure [17] (Figure 3). Both spectral clustering and CC without prior information resulted in comparable volume

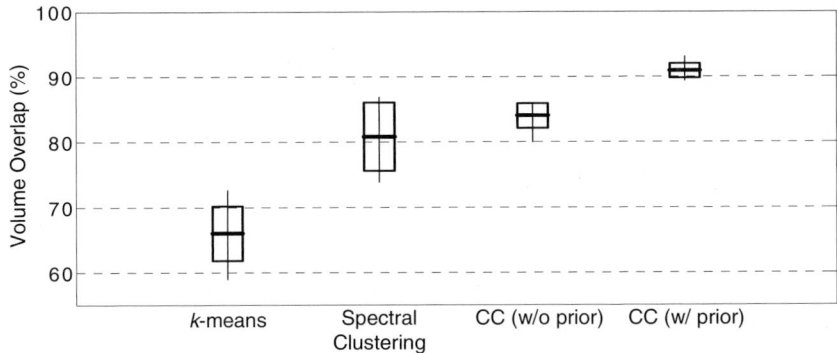

Fig. 3. Volume overlaps between the expert segmentations and segmentations obtained using k-means [2], spectral clustering [3] and Consistency Clustering (CC), without and with prior information on the expert labels, from the left hemispheres from 10 subjects. The boxes indicate one standard deviation around the mean, and the thin lines indicate the range.

overlaps, while k-means performed the worst due to its simple nature. Furthermore, CC resulted in a slightly higher average overlap and less variability around this average among subjects, indicating a better performance overall. The decrease in the variability is due to the increased consistency of segmentations between the subjects. Not surprisingly, the use of prior information improved the volume overlaps, indicating the need for prior information and the weakness of the unsupervised algorithms for replicating expert preference.

The algorithm took under 2 minutes to converge on a desktop personal computer with a non-optimized MATLAB implementation for the joint segmentation of 10 subjects. The algorithm's complexity is linear with the number of voxels for fixed number of clusters, similar to the simple k-means clustering.

4 Discussion and Conclusion

In this paper we presented a novel algorithm, called Consistency Clustering, for jointly segmenting a population of diffusion tensor images of the deep gray matter. The joint segmentation resulted not only in plausible segmentations for each subject, but also correspondence between the subjects. This is an important difference between the CC and previous algorithms proposed to segment the gray matter, since without correspondence between the segmentations of individual subjects, it is difficult to assign consistent anatomical labels to the resulting segmentations. Also, without consistent and anatomically meaningful segmentations, the quantitative morphometry becomes a challenge in the gray matter.

CC not only provided consistent segmentations for the population, but it was also able to handle prior information about the expert labels. Also, through the use of labels from other subjects in the population, the algorithm was able to produce segmentations that were both qualitatively and quantitatively very similar to the expert's preference. Therefore, CC can be used in two different ways to produce consistent segmentations in a population. The first way involves running the algorithm unsupervised on the population, and then assigning anatomical labels to the segmentations only on one of the subjects. The labels are then automatically transferred to the rest of the subjects since the correspondence problem is already solved at this stage. The second way involves labeling one or several subjects by hand, and then using these labeled subjects as prior information to label the rest of the population according to the expert preference.

Either way, CC (or a variant with an improved model for the thalamic nuclei) is a powerful tool that provides fast and consistent segmentation of the deep gray matter and has a use in a variety of applications such as in quantitative morphometry studies and pre-surgical planning.

References

1. Basser, P., Mattiello, J., Bihan, D.L.: MR diffusion tensor spectroscopy and imaging. Biophys. J. 66, 259–267 (1994)
2. Wiegell, M.R., et al.: Automatic segmentation of thalamic nuclei from diffusion tensor magnetic resonance imaging. Neuroimage 19, 391–402 (2003)
3. Ziyan, U., Tuch, D., Westin, C.F.: Segmentation of thalamic nuclei from DTI using spectral clustering. In: Larsen, R., Nielsen, M., Sporring, J. (eds.) MICCAI 2006. LNCS, vol. 4191, pp. 807–814. Springer, Heidelberg (2006)
4. Jonasson, L., et al.: A level set method for segmentation of the thalamus and its nuclei in DT-MRI. Signal Process. 87(2), 309–321 (2007)
5. Duan, Y., Li, X., Xi, Y.: Thalamus segmentation from diffusion tensor magnetic resonance imaging. Journal of Biomedical Imaging (2) (2007)
6. Guridi, J., et al.: Targeting the basal ganglia for deep brain stimulation in parkinson's disease. Neurology 55, S21–S28 (2000)
7. Portas, C., et al.: Volumetric evaluation of the thalamus in schizophrenic male patients using magnetic resonance imaging. Biol. Psych., 649–659 (1998)
8. Giroux, M.L., et al.: Medication related changes in cerebral glucose metabolism in Parkinson's disease. In: ICFMHB, p. 237 (1998)
9. Mclachlan, G.J., Krishnan, T.: The EM Algorithm and Extensions. Wiley-Interscience, Chichester (2007)
10. Banerjee, A., Dhillon, I.S., Ghosh, J., Sra, S.: Clustering on the unit hypersphere using von Mises-Fisher distributions. J. Mach. Learn. Res. 6, 1345–1382 (2005)
11. Lagarias, J.C., et al.: Convergence properties of the nelder-mead simplex method in low dimensions. SIAM Journal of Optimization 9, 112–147 (1998)
12. Reese, T.G., et al.: Reduction of eddy-current-induced distortion in diffusion MRI using a twice-refocused spin echo. MRM 49(1), 177–182 (2003)
13. Jenkinson, M., et al.: Improved optimization for the robust and accurate linear registration and motion correction of brain images. NeurImg 17, 825–841 (2002)
14. Basser, P.J., Mattiello, J., LeBihan, D.: Estimation of the effective self-diffusion tensor from the NMR spin echo. J. Magn. Reson. B 103(3), 247–254 (1994)
15. Mazziotta, J.C., et al.: A probabilistic atlas of the human brain: theory and rationale for its development. Neuroimage 2(2), 89–101 (1995)
16. Ooteman, W., Cretsinger, K.: Thalamus Tracing Guidelines, http://www.psychiatry.uiowa.edu/mhcrc/IPLpages/manual_tracing.htm
17. Dice, L.R.: Measures of the amount of ecologic association between species. Ecology 26, 297–302 (1945)

Bone Segmentation and Fracture Detection in Ultrasound Using 3D Local Phase Features

Ilker Hacihaliloglu[1], Rafeef Abugharbieh[1], Antony Hodgson[2], and Robert Rohling[1,2]

[1] Department of Electrical and Computer Engineering
[2] Department of Mechanical Engineering, University of British Columbia,
Vancouver, BC, Canada
ilkerh@ece.ubc.ca, rafeef@ece.ubc.ca, ahodgson@mech.ubc.ca,
rohling@ece.ubc.ca

Abstract. 3D ultrasound (US) is increasingly considered as a viable alternative imaging modality in computer-assisted orthopaedic surgery (CAOS) applications. Automatic bone segmentation from US images, however, remains a challenge due to speckle noise and various other artifacts inherent to US. In this paper, we present intensity invariant three dimensional (3D) local image phase features, obtained using 3D Log-Gabor filter banks, for extracting ridge-like features similar to those that occur at soft tissue/bone interfaces. Our contributions include the novel extension of 2D phase symmetry features to 3D and their use in automatic extraction of bone surfaces and fractured fragments in 3D US. We validate our technique using phantom, *in vitro,* and *in vivo* experiments. Qualitative and quantitative results demonstrate remarkably clear segmentations results of bone surfaces with a localization accuracy of better than 0.62mm and mean errors in estimating fracture displacements below 0.65mm, which will likely be of strong clinical utility.

Keywords: 3D ultrasound, local phase features, 3D Log-Gabor filters, 3D phase symmetry, bone segmentation.

1 Introduction

The two most common imaging modalities used in orthopaedic surgery are fluoroscopy (projection x-rays) and computed tomography (CT). Although both methods provide clear images of bone structures, CT normally cannot be performed intraoperatively and fluoroscopy typically produces two dimensional images only, which makes it difficult for surgeons to assess the 3D shape and position of bones and bone fragments (e.g. during reduction procedures). This is particularly important in complex fracture cases involving bones such as the distal radius, responsible for about one sixth of all fractures seen in emergency departments in the United States [1], and the pelvis [2]. Furthermore, both CT and fluoroscopy use ionizing radiation, which raises important safety concerns for both patients and surgeons.

Ultrasound (US) imaging is non-ionizing, fast, portable, inexpensive and capable of real time imaging, but, unfortunately, US images typically contain significant speckle and other artifacts which complicate image interpretation and automatic processing [3]. If anatomical structures of interest could be visualized and localized with sufficient accuracy and clarity, 3D US may in fact become a strong practical alternative imaging modality for selected applications in orthopaedic surgery, particularly for computer-assisted applications where the image can be processed to provide quantitative information on the location of bone structures.

Manual identification of bone surfaces in 2D US for orthopedic surgery application was reported in [4]. Manual processing, however, is time consuming and operator dependent, and thus limits clinical practicality. While some studies have shown some promise in automatically identifying the bone surface based on intensity and gradient information (or a combination of both) these techniques were limited to 2D US, and remained sensitive to typical image variability and choice of processing parameters [5]. Daanen et al [6] proposed a method where prior knowledge of bone appearance was incorporated. However, fractured bone surfaces do not have a continuous smooth surface and prior knowledge of fragment shape is mostly unavailable. Other approaches combined intensity and gradient-based techniques with multimodal registration of US to preoperative CT [7]. However, preoperative CT requires additional time and expense and is not always considered necessary for diagnosis or treatment, so it is only available in selected cases.

Local phase based features have been used in US image analysis, e.g. for localizing endocardial border points in echocardiography [8]. In [9], Hacihaliloglu et al proposed using phase features extracted automatically from 2D slices to identify bone boundaries in US data. However, 2D methods do not take advantage of correlations between adjacent images (i.e., along the axis perpendicular to the scan plane direction) and are therefore subject to spatial compounding errors as well as errors due to beam thickness effects. In this paper, we extend local phase based processing to 3D US volumes using 3D Log-Gabor filters. Specifically, we construct a 3D local phase symmetry measure which produces strong responses at bone surfaces and suppresses responses elsewhere. We quantitatively investigate the accuracy of our technique in localizing bone surfaces and assess the technique's ability to resolve displaced bone fragments. The current study is therefore the first to show that bone surfaces and fractures can be accurately localized using local phase features computed directly from 3D ultrasound image volumes.

2 Methods

In US images, bone surfaces typically appear blurry with non-uniform intensity and substantial shadowing beneath the surface. The thickness of the response at the leading edge ranges from 2-4 mm [3] for a typical transducer. In [3], it was shown that the actual bone surface lies between the highest gradient and the highest intensity points of this thick response. We propose that it would therefore be more appropriate to use a ridge detector, rather than an edge detector, to identify the bone surface location as the latter would produce responses on both sides of the band at the bone surface.

2.1 3D Local Phase Symmetry Feature

The purpose of ridge detection is to capture the major axis of symmetry of a feature at some specified spatial scale. Signals that have even symmetry about the origin will have real (and even) Fourier transforms, while signals that have odd symmetry will have imaginary (and odd) Fourier transforms. Signals that are neither perfectly odd nor perfectly even will have complex Fourier transforms (i.e. have both real and imaginary parts) where the resultant phase values reflects their degree of symmetry. Local phase information of a 1D signal can be obtained by convolving the signal with a pair of band-pass quadrature filters (an odd filter and an even filter). Using two filters in quadrature enables the calculation of signal amplitude and phase at a particular scale (spatial frequency) at a given spatial location. A good choice of quadrature filters is the Log-Gabor filter which can be constructed with arbitrary bandwidth. In order to obtain simultaneous localization of spatial and frequency information, analysis of the signal must be done over a narrow range (scale) of frequencies at different locations in the signal. This can be achieved by constructing a filter bank using a set of quadrature filters created from rescalings of the Log-Gabor filter. Each scaling is designed to pick out particular frequencies of the signal being analyzed. In [10] Kovesi investigated symmetry information by looking at the points where the response of the even filter dominates the response of the odd filter taking the difference of their absolute values. In this paper we extend this analysis to 3D using 3D Log-Gabor filters.

The transfer function (G) of a 3D Log-Gabor filter in the frequency domain (1) is constructed as the product of two components: a one dimensional Log Gabor function that controls the frequencies to which the filter responds and a rotational symmetric angular Gaussian function that controls the orientation selectivity of the filter [11].

$$G(\omega, \phi, \theta) = \exp(\frac{(\log(\omega/\omega_0))^2}{2(\log(\kappa/\omega_0))}) \times \exp(-\frac{\alpha(\phi_i, \theta_i)^2}{2\sigma_\alpha^2}) \quad (1)$$

Here κ determines the bandwidth of the filter in the radial direction and ω_0 is the filter's center spatial frequency. To achieve constant shape ratio filters, which are filters that are geometric scalings of a reference filter, the term κ/ω_0 must be kept constant. The angle between the direction of the filter, which is determined by the azimuth (ϕ) and elevation (θ) angles, and the position vector of a given point f in the frequency domain is given by $\alpha(\phi_i, \theta_i) = \arccos(f.v_i /\| f \|)$. $v_i = (\cos\phi_i \cos\theta_i, \cos\phi_i \sin\theta_i, \sin\phi_i)$ is a unit vector in the filter's direction. Here σ_α defines the extent of spreading in the angular direction. To get higher orientation selectivity, the angular function must become narrower.

The scaling of the radial Log Gabor function is achieved by using different wavelengths which are based on multiples of a minimum wavelength, λ_{min}, which is a user-definable parameter. The relationship between the filter scale m, and the filter center frequency ω_0 is defined as $\omega_0 = 2/\lambda_{min} \times (\delta)^{m-1}$ where $\delta=3$ is a scaling factor defined for computing the center frequencies of successive filters. After investigating convolution results of various 1D scanline profiles of a distal radius, scanned *in vivo*, with a pair of quadrature filters at different scales, selecting a single scale ($m=1$) with a large wavelength ($\lambda_{min}= 25$) gave well localized bone surface phase features. A value of $\kappa/\omega_0 = 0.25$ provided good surface localization in the presence of speckle. For the angular component, we found empirically after some experimentation with models of the human distal radius and pelvis that it was possible to get good orientation resolution while containing an adequate range of frequencies by selecting $\sigma_\alpha = 14.3°$. The filter bank used in this work uses 15 different (α) 3D filter orientations. Our local phase analysis of a 3D image volume $V(x,y,z)$ proceeds by convolving the image with the 3D Log Gabor filters. Let $M^e_{rm}(\omega,\phi_r,\theta_r) = real(G(\omega,\phi_r,\theta_r))$ and $M^o_{rm}(\omega,\phi_r,\theta_r) = imag(G(\omega,\phi_r,\theta_r))$ denote the real (even) and imaginary (odd) parts, respectively, at a scale m and orientation r, and let $\hat{H}(u,v\ t)$ be the Fourier transform of $V(x,y,z)$. We can think of the responses of each quadrature pair of filters as forming a response vector $[e_{rm}(x,y,z), o_{rm}(x,y,z)] = [\boldsymbol{F^{-1}}(\hat{H}(u,v,t) M^e_{rm}(\omega,\phi_r,\theta_r)), \boldsymbol{F^{-1}}(\hat{H}(u,v,t) M^o_{rm}(\omega,\phi_r,\theta_r))]$. Here $\boldsymbol{F^{-1}}$ denotes the inverse Fourier transform operation.

Extending Kovesi's work where 2D phase symmetry was defined as in [10], we construct a 3D phase symmetry measure, for different scales (m) and orientations (r):

$$3DPS(x,y,z) = \frac{\sum_r \sum_m \lfloor [|e_{rm}(x,y,z)| - |o_{rm}(x,y,z)|] - T_r \rfloor}{\sum_r \sum_m \sqrt{e_{rm}^2(x,y,z) - o_{rm}^2(x,y,z)} + \varepsilon} \qquad (2)$$

Here $\lfloor A \rfloor = \max(A,0)$, ε is a small number included to avoid division by zero, and T is a noise threshold calculated as a specified number (k) of standard deviations (σ) above the mean (μ) of the local energy distribution. Based on this, T is defined as: $T = \mu + k \times \sigma$ and the distribution is expected to be Rayleigh [12]. The response of the smallest scale filter is used for the calculation of μ and σ since it has the largest bandwidth and will give the strongest noise response. For different US transducers and scales, k can be tuned to provide a balance between the detected bone surface and speckle scale. The noise threshold parameter k was set to 5. Throughout our experiments the selected filter parameters were not changed.

2.2 Experimental Setup

We designed two different experiments to quantitatively evaluate the performance of the proposed 3D local phase-based bone segmentation method. The first experiment aimed at assessing the localization accuracy of our bone surface detection technique and the second at assessing the accuracy of measuring relative displacements between bone fragments, as this is a clinically relevant task for which we would like to use 3D US imaging. Acquisition was performed on a GE Voluson 730 Expert ultrasound machine (GE Healthcare, Waukesha, WI) with a 3D RSP5-12 probe. This is a mechanized probe where a linear array transducer is swept through an arc range of 20°. The reconstructed US volumes were 199×119×50 voxels (lateral×axial×elevational) with an isotropic voxel size of 0.19mm. Our algorithm was implemented in MATLAB and run on an Intel Pentium 4 PC (3.64 GHz, 2GB of RAM). A human left radius Sawbone (Sawbones Inc., Vashon, WA), an *in vitro* pig leg and *in vivo* scans of a human distal radius were used in the validation experiments. In addition to our two quantitative studies, we also present qualitative results for an *in vivo* scan of a human distal radius and for an *ex vivo* scan of a porcine tibia and fibula.

Experiment 1 Surface Localization: In order to quantify our bone localization accuracy, a stylus with a spherical tip was placed at a variety of locations on the surface of a bone or bone model. Two situations were assessed: (A) a plastic bone model (Sawbone) in a water tank, and (B) an *ex vivo* porcine specimen.

(A) Sawbone Specimen: Scans of the Sawbone model were performed inside a water tank with the long axis of the bone aligned with the axis of the linear array of the mechanized transducer. This alignment produced the clearest depiction of the bone surface. Images of the Sawbone were obtained at varying depths (shallow, middle, deep) by changing the probe position inside the water tank. Different depths produce different US resolutions in the elevation and lateral directions of the linear array. Realignment of the Sawbone was performed at each depth to ensure the bone was aligned with the probe's central slice. To test the accuracy of surface localization at different beam orientations relative to the bone surface, as might occur in clinical use, we used two different orientations for the phantom – horizontal and inclined at 20°. At each probe position, the US volume acquisition was repeated with a stylus tipped with a small spherical bead (3.0 mm in diameter) placed on the bone to provide the 'gold standard' for the true bone location. The bead was placed and scanned at 30 different locations along the bone surface for each of the 3 depth settings. To ensure that the bead was centered in the elevation direction, the position of the stylus was adjusted until the clearest surface reflection was obtained. The location of the dot-like bright intensity response which is the top of the bead tip, f, and the location of the intensity response of the bone surface obtained from the phase algorithm, b, were then extracted (Fig. 1a-c). These two measurements, b and f, were obtained in a highly automated and repeatable manner using a subpixel edge detection algorithm. To ensure that the images with and without the bead in place were otherwise identical, the Sawbone and probe were both fixed for both image acquisitions. The bone surface localization error was therefore defined as: $error = D (b f)$, where D is the bead diameter and b and f are expressed in mm. When the US beam was not perpendicular to the bead on the bone surface, the position of the underlying bone surface was compensated for using the geometry calculations shown in Figure 1c. Since mechanized 3D ultrasound probes use a set of 2D images to reconstruct a volume, the effect of the finite beam thickness is incorporated into the volume data via the reconstruction process. Compared to a single 2D image, volumetric data provides information about the bone response away from a single plane, so the analysis implicitly includes beam thickness effects.

(B) Ex Vivo Porcine Specimen: In order to investigate the effect of a soft tissue interface on our localization accuracy, we conducted an *ex vivo* experiment on a porcine tibia and fibula. First, the soft tissue was removed of the bone and the same spherical bead-tipped stylus described above was placed against the bone. The removed soft tissue was then overlaid, leaving the bead underneath the tissue and touching the bone. Again, a set of 3D scans were obtained with the bead positioned at 30 different locations along the bone surface. The error calculation proceeded in the same manner described in part (A) above.

Experiment 2 Fracture Misalignment Detection: Identification of fractures and proper assessment of fracture reduction is of special importance in orthopaedic surgery. Our second experiment was thus designed to assess the ability of the proposed local phase-based technique to detect small gaps between bone fragments from 3D US data. First, the Sawbone was broken into two parts and each part was glued to the top surface of a metal block. For tracking purposes, infrared emitting diodes (IREDs) were glued onto the surface of one of the metal blocks. This part was tracked with an optical tracking system (OPTOTRAK 3020, Northern Digital Inc., Waterloo, ON, Canada with 3D localization accuracy of 0.1 mm in the directions parallel to the front of the camera) which was used to provide the gold standard displacement measurements. The other block with the second bone fragment was kept fixed. In total, 5 fixed displacements ranging from 0.8 to 2.2 mm in the vertical (Fig.1 d) and horizontal directions were then introduced. Tests were conducted with either a thick layer of ultrasound gel or a 3 cm thick slice of bovine tissue overlaid on the bone model. In both cases, the misalignment was tracked with the OPTOTRAK with a total of 10 3D US volumes obtained for each misalignment. The displacements along the top edges of the fracture boundaries were measured on each 2D slice of the 3D phase volume in which they appeared and then averaged. This result was then compared with the known applied displacement.

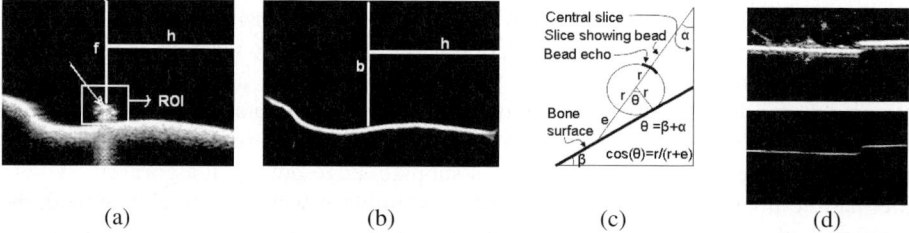

Fig. 1. Bone localization accuracy assessment (a-c: experiment 1, d: experiment 2). (a) Central slice of an US volume of a Sawbone. Arrow points to the fiducial (bead) attached to the bone. (b) Corresponding slice of 3D volume resulting from our proposed local phase processing. (c) For cases where the bead is not aligned with the central slice of the volume, the location of the bone surface can be calculated from the geometry of the angle of the plane showing the bead (α), the angle of the bone surface (β) and the radius of the bead (r). (d) Central slice of an US volume(top) obtained by scanning phantom Sawbone bone fragments after introducing a vertical displacement and corresponding slice from our proposed method (bottom).

3 Results

Experiment 1 Localization Accuracy:
(A) Sawbone Specimen: The processing time was approximately 43s for each 3D volume. For both the horizontal and inclined specimens the mean error was calculated from the measurements taken at the 30 different bead locations for each depth setting. Among the three different depth settings the middle scanning depth resulted in a mean error of 0.62mm (SD 0.24mm) and 0.53mm (SD 0.28mm) inside the bone surface response on the 3DUS volume for the horizontal and inclined specimens, respectively. Compared to the other two depth settings these values were the highest error results obtained.

(B) Bovine Specimen: For the cadaver experiment the mean localization error was 0.44mm inside the bone surface response.

Experiment 2 Fracture Misalignment Detection: The mean errors in estimating fracture displacements were -0.65mm and 0.5mm for horizontal and vertical misalignments, respectively, for the fractures imaged through bovine tissue. The error results obtained when the gel was used as an imaging medium were −0.5mm and 0.4mm respectively.

Qualitative Results: Figure 2 shows a qualitative comparison of local-phase-processed images of a human distal radius with the original 3D US volume of the same bone. The local phase images are notably clearer than the 3DUS image, and the 3D version of the local phase images is markedly smoother than the 2D version, where each slice is treated independently in the latter.

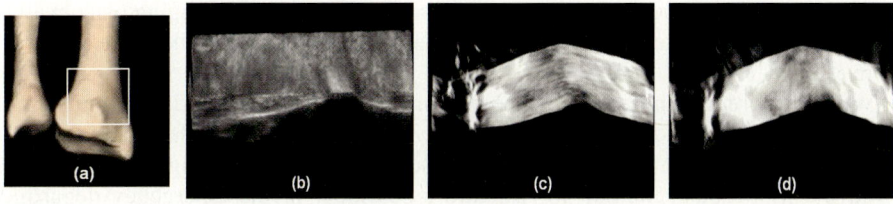

Fig. 2. Qualitative results on *in-vivo* human distal radius. (a) Area imaged. (b) Captured 3D US volume. (c) 2D phase feature image. (d) Proposed 3D phase symmetry image.

Figure 3 shows other qualitative examples where scans of an intact *ex-vivo* porcine tibia and fibula and fractured distal radius Sawbone were acquired. Note how the local phase processed images allow clear visualization of the entire bone surface and of the fracture line.

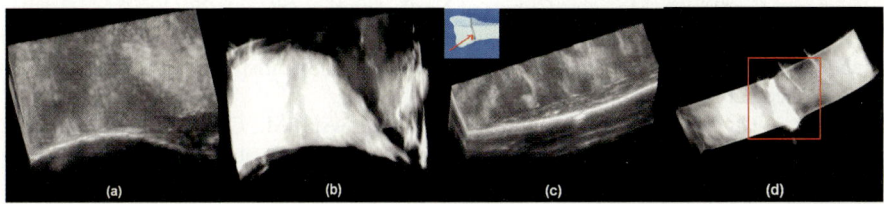

Fig. 3. Qualitative results obtained from *ex vivo* porcine tibia fibula specimen and Sawbone with soft tissue overlaid. (a) 3D US volume of intact bone. (b) Corresponding 3D phase symmetry image. (c) 3D US of a distal radius Sawbone fracture imaged with soft tissue overlaid on top. (d) 3D phase of (c) where the detected fracture is shown inside the red rectangle.

4 Discussion and Conclusions

In this paper we proposed a novel approach for accurate and fully automatic extraction of bone surfaces directly in 3D ultrasound volumes based on local phase symmetry image features that employ 3D Log-Gabor filters. Bone surface localization accuracy assessed using bone models and *ex vivo* porcine specimens showed a maximum mean error of 0.44 mm and a low standard deviation across the sampled points of only 0.16 mm; these errors were relatively independent of the depth of the soft tissue/bone interface and of the inclination of the probe relative to the bone surface. Furthermore, the 3D phase method has high localization accuracy even when the US beam is not perfectly normal to the bone surface. Horizontal and vertical displacements between model bone fragments were also accurately measured with a maximum mean error under 0.65 mm. The obtained results are encouraging for using local phase processed images in fracture assessment since the average accuracy required for such application is typically in the range of 2-4mm [13]. A comparison of *in vivo* scans of the human distal radius showed that a true 3D analysis produced a noticeably smoother image of the bone surface than previously reported 2D analysis. We expect that such 3D processing will be of special importance during the assessment of fractures where good accuracy is needed to avoid malunions. Furthermore, since there is no need to align the imaging plane with the anatomical area of interest, evaluation of the fractured area can likely be performed more rapidly.

We are currently investigating the performance of the method in volumes constructed using freehand 2D US and stitched 3D volumes where a larger region of interest can be obtained. Future work will also focus on establishing the feasibility of using the proposed technique for fracture assessment in the emergency department and for fracture reduction assessment in orthopaedic trauma applications, particularly of distal radius fractures.

References

1. Hanel, D.P., Jones, M.D., Trumble, T.E.: Wrist fractures. Orthop. Clin. North. Am. 33(1), 35–57 (2002)
2. Coppola, P.T., Coppola, M.: Emergency department evaluation and treatment of pelvic fractures. Emergency Medicine Clinics of North America 18(1), 1–27 (2000)
3. Jain, A.K., Taylor, R.H.: Understanding bone responses in B-mode ultrasound images and automatic bone surface extraction using a bayesian probabilistic framework. In: Proc. of SPIE Medical Imaging, pp. 131–142 (2004)
4. Barratt, D.C., Penney, P.G., Chan, S.K., Slomczykowski, M., Carter, T.J., Edwards, P.J., Hawkes, D.J.: Self calibrating 3D-ultrasound-based bone registration for minimally invasive orthopaedic surgery. IEEE Transactions on Medical Imaging 25, 312–323 (2006)
5. Kowal, J., Amstutz, C., Langlotz, F., Talib, H., Ballester, M.G.: Automated bone contour detection in ultrasound B-mode images for minimally invasive registration in computer assisted surgery an in vitro evaluation. The International Journal of Medical Robotics and Computer Assisted Surgery, 341–348 (2007)
6. Daanen, V., Tonetti, J., Troccaz, J.: A fully automated method for the delineation of osseous interface in ultrasound images. In: Barillot, C., Haynor, D.R., Hellier, P. (eds.) MICCAI 2004. LNCS, vol. 3216, pp. 549–557. Springer, Heidelberg (2004)
7. Amin, D.V., Kanade, T., Digioia, A.M., Jaramaz, B.: Ultrasound registration of the bone surface for surgical navigation. Journal of Computer Aided Surgery 8, 1–16 (2003)
8. Mulet-Parada, M., Noble, J.A.: 2D+T boundary detection in echocardiography. Medical Image Analysis 4(1), 21–30 (2000)

9. Hacihaliloglu, I., Abugharbieh, R., Hodgson, A.J., Rohling, R.N.: Enhancement of bone surface visualization from 3D ultrasound based on local phase information. In: Proc. IEEE Ultrasonics Symposium, pp. 21–24 (2006)
10. Kovesi, P.: Symmetry and Asymmetry from Local Phase, AI 1997. In: Tenth Australian Joint Conference on Artificial Intellegence, pp. 185–190 (1997)
11. Dosil, R., Pardo, X.M., Fernandez-Vidal, X.R.: Data driven synthesis of composite feature detectors for 3D image analysis. Journal of Image and Vision Computing, 225–238 (2006)
12. Kovesi, P.: Image Features From Phase Congruency. Videre: A Journal of Computer Vision Research (1999)
13. Phillips, R.: The accuracy of surgical navigation for othopaedic surgery. Current Orthopaedics, 180–192 (2007)

Interactive Separation of Segmented Bones in CT Volumes Using Graph Cut

Lu Liu, David Raber, David Nopachai, Paul Commean, David Sinacore,
Fred Prior, Robert Pless, and Tao Ju[*]

Washington University in St. Louis, St. Louis MO 63130, USA
taoju@cs.wustl.edu
http://www.cs.wustl.edu/~taoju

Abstract. We present a fast, interactive method for separating bones that have been collectively segmented from a CT volume. Given user-provided seed points, the method computes the separation as a multi-way cut on a weighted graph constructed from the binary, segmented volume. By properly designing and weighting the graph, we show that the resulting cut can accurately be placed at bone-interfaces using only a small number of seed points even when the data is noisy. The method has been implemented with an interactive graphical interface, and used to separate the 12 human foot bones in 10 CT volumes. The interactive tool produced compatible result with a ground-truth separation, generated by a completely manual labelling procedure, while reducing the human interaction time from a mean of 2.4 hours per volume in manual labelling down to approximately 18 minutes.

1 Introduction

Segmenting bone tissues from CT volumes is a common and important operation in various applications, including the measurement of bone mineral density (BMD). A number of different methodology have been reported for bone segmentation (see a recent survey in [1]). Due to the relatively higher tissue density of bones (especially cortical and trabecular bones) than other surrounding tissues, intensity thresholding [2,3] or edge-detection [4,5] are among the most common approaches in segmenting cortical and trabecular bones in a CT volume. A typical result of segmentation is shown in Figure 1 (b) for a CT scan of a foot in (a), segmented by edge-filtering on each transverse slice [5].

Unfortunately, the segmented CT volume using thresholding or edge detection often cannot be directly used for bone analysis, such as BMD measurement, which requires delineation of the complete boundary for each individual bone. The bones in this segmentation (Figure 1 (b)) often exhibit incomplete interiors, due to bone marrow and the lower density trabecular bone, and neighboring bones are often connected.

A number of methods can be used for filling the bone interior in a segmented CT volume, notably morphological closing followed by contour filling

[*] Corresponding author.

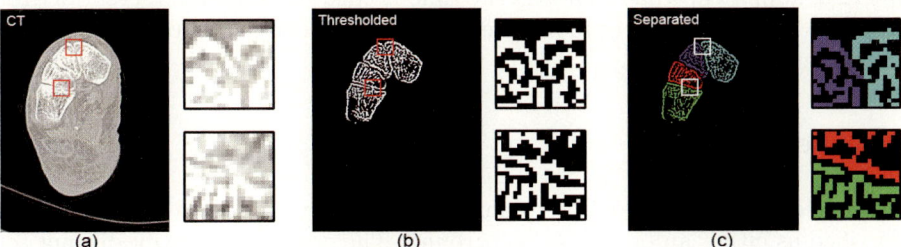

Fig. 1. Bone separation in a segmented CT volume. (a): A transverse slice of a CT volume. (b): The slice after an edge-detection-based segmentation. (c): The slice after individual bones (colored differently) are separated in the segmented volume.

[3] or connected-component analysis [2]. In contrast, methods for separating out each individual bone has been scarce at best. Westin et. al. [2] applied tensor-filtering to the grayscale CT volume before performing intensity thresholding. While the number of connections between bones are reduced using this approach, connections may still exist. Kang et. al. [3] proposed to use a special bone mask customized to the shape of the bone, such as the femoral head. However, creating masks for bones with less distinctive shapes (such as cuneiform) and large inter-subject variability can be as challenging as the separation task itself. In our experience, bone separation in the human foot where many connections exist (see Figure 1 (b)) is a labor-intensive process, even with the help of existing software that provide automated image processing capabilities such as finding connected-components. In our clinical setting, separating 12 bones in a human foot from a CT volume by going through each transverse slice and manually separate voxels belonging to different bones takes an average of 2.4 hours.

In this paper, we propose a fast, interactive method for separating segmented bones using a graph cut approach. Although graph cut algorithms have been successfully employed for interactive object/background segmentation [6] and multiple-objects labelling [7] in grayscale images, the success has largely relied on the change in image intensity or texture on the interface between the object and background or between neighboring objects. These assumptions do not hold for bones in a grayscale CT volume, which exhibit an inhomogeneous texture that is often indistinguishable from the texture at their interfaces (Figure 1 (a)). Here we show how graph cut, when applied to a segmented CT volume represented as a weighted graph, can yield accurate bone separation with a small amount of user input. The key component of this algorithm is a novel graph weighting function that captures the density of connections among neighboring voxels in a binary volume. An example result of our algorithm is shown in Figure 1 (c).

Based on the algorithm, we developed an interactive user-interface for bone separation. The tool simplifies the tedious manual process of bone-labeling on each slice to only placing one or more seed points on each bone. In our experiment with separating the 12 bones in a human foot, we observed that the use of the tool yields compatible results with our previous, completely manual labelling approach, while reducing the time needed for human intervention from 2.4 hours to approximately 18 minutes per volume. Such reduction is a significant improvement in practice.

2 The Method

We consider a segmented CT volume as a binary volume where each voxel is classified as either an object or background. The goal is to identify disjoint sets of object voxels that belong to each individual bone. Our key observation is that the connections between a bone and its neighboring tissues are usually fewer and sparser than those that constitute the bone itself (Figure 1 (b)). To identify each bone, we represent the collection of all object voxels as nodes in a graph where neighboring voxels are connected by graph edges. Given a set of seed voxels each labelled as one of the bones, we set up and solve a multi-way graph cut problem whose solution is a partitioning of the graph into multiple subsets, one for each individual bone.

In the following, we first review the multi-way graph cut problem and classical solutions to this problem. Then we present graph construction from a segmented CT volume, and in particular, two ways to improve an initial, un-weighted graph with the goal that the computed cut in the graph is likely to be placed at bone-interfaces. Finally, we present a user-interface that utilizes the algorithm for interactive bone separation.

2.1 The Multi-way Graph Cut Problem and Solutions

Here we consider a weighted undirected graph $G(V, E)$, where V is a set of nodes and E is a set of edges, each connecting two nodes in V and associated with a weight. Given a set $T \subseteq V$ of k *terminal* nodes, a *multi-way cut* is a subset of edges $C \subseteq E$ such that no path exists between any two nodes of T in the residue graph $G(V, E \setminus C)$. The multi-way cut problem aims at finding the cut C with the minimal size $|C|$, computed as the sum of edge weights in the cut. Intuitively, a multi-way cut disconnects all terminal nodes in the way that involves the least amount of change to the graph.

When $k = 2$, the 2-way cut problem can be solved by a polynomial time method, notably the Ford-Fulkerson algorithm [8]. However, the general multi-way cut problem when $k \geq 3$ is known to be NP-hard [9]. Several polynomial-time algorithms have been proposed to compute a near-minimal cut with varying approximation accuracy [9,10,11]. In our implementation, we adopt the combinatoric isolation algorithm of Dahlhaus *et. al.* [9] that computes the multiple-way cut as the union of 2-way cuts, each disconnecting one terminal node from the others. The heuristic, while simple, achieves a provable $2 - \frac{2}{k}$ approximation ratio. To compute each 2-way cut, we adopt an efficient implementation of the Ford-Fulkerson algorithm [12] that maintains a breadth-first search tree.

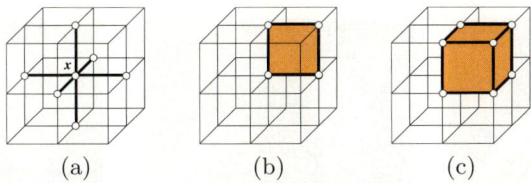

Fig. 2. (a): The 6 neighbors of a voxel x. (b): A voxel face. (c): A voxel cell.

2.2 Multi-way Graph Cut for Bone Separation

To construct the graph from a segmented CT volume, we create one node for each object voxel and connect two nodes representing neighboring object voxels by an edge. We adopt the classical 6-connectivity from digital topology [13], where each 3D voxel may have maximally 6 spatial neighbors (as illustrated in Figure 2 (a)). To apply the multi-way cut, we ask the user to provide a small number of object voxels (called seeds), each labelled as one of the k desired bones. Note that for each bone, the user may specify more than one seeds with that label (which are useful for dealing with noisy inputs, see Section 3). For each label $i \in [1, k]$, we create one terminal node t_i and connect it to all seeds with that label (Figure 3 (a)). Denoting the graph as $G(V, E)$ and the multi-way cut as C, voxels belonging to the ith bone are identified as the set of non-terminal nodes in V that are connected to t_i in the residual graph $G(V, E \setminus C)$ (Figure 3 (b)).

In order for multi-way cuts to be placed at bone-interfaces, the initial graph structure needs to be further adjusted and weighted. Below we present two specific modifications to the initial, un-weighted graph constructed above:

Seed expansion: Note that if only a single seed voxel is provided for each bone, the resulting cuts will most likely enclose just the seed itself due to the small number of edges (≤ 6) connected to a voxel. To resolve this problem without requiring the user to specify a large number of seeds, we automatically expand from a seed voxel x provided by the user to label all voxels connected to x via a path in the graph of length $\leq \alpha$ as seeds of the same label, where α is a user-defined parameter.

Edge weighting: The weighting of the graph edges directly influences the placement of the optimal cut. To ensure that each seed retains its label after the cut,

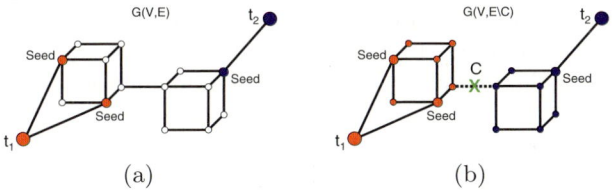

Fig. 3. (a): A graph with 3 labelled seeds (2 red and 1 blue) and 2 augmented terminals t_1, t_2. (b): Removing cut edge C partitions the graph into two labelled components.

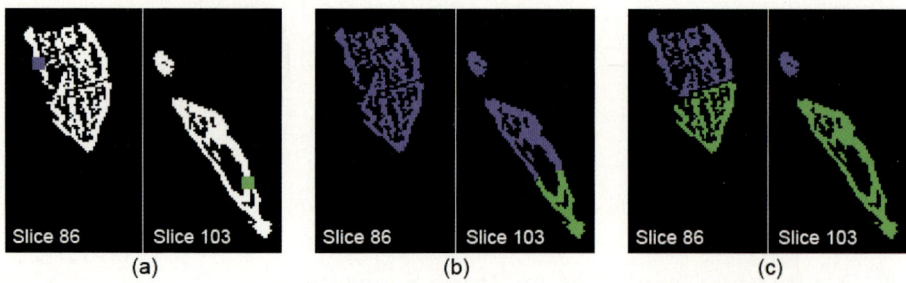

Fig. 4. The effect of edge-weighting on graph cut: (a) The input volume with two seeds on two slices. (b) Separation as a result of graph cut on a uniformly weighted graph. (c) Improved cut using non-uniform weighting that correctly separates the metatarsal 2 (green) from cuneiform 2 (blue).

edges connecting seeds and terminal nodes will be associated with an infinitely large weight. For the remaining edges in the graph that connect neighboring voxels, a straight-forward approach is to associate each edge with a same positive weight. The resulting cuts of this uniform weighting scheme essentially minimize the *number* of edges in the cut, and therefore likely to reside at the bone-interfaces when the connections between bones are few. However, we have observed that it is not uncommon for the number of connections between two bones to exceed those at a cross-section of one of the bones, causing the cut to be misplaced in the middle of that bone, as shown in Figure 4 (b).

For more robust separation, we adopt a different, non-uniform weighting scheme to prevent cuts in the middle of a bone. The key observation is that the voxels in the cortical bone usually form a contiguous, shell-like shape, while connections between bones are typically sparsely located. As a result, a weighting scheme that gives larger weights to edges that are more densely surrounded by other edges would favor the cuts between the bones. In practice, we characterized the local density of edges by the presence of voxel faces and voxel cells, as shown in Figure 2 (b,c). A voxel face is a group of 4 neighboring voxels that form a square, and a voxel cell is a group of 8 neighboring voxels that form a cube. To compute the weight at a graph edge that connects two voxels x, y, we use a simple linear sum $w_0 + w_1 * f + w_2 * c$ of the number of voxel faces, f, and voxel cells, c, that contain both voxels x, y, where w_j are pre-defined parameters. In our tests, the non-uniform weighting scheme effectively avoids cuts through the middle of cortical bones. In the example of Figure 4 (c), the improved cut correctly separates the metatarsal 2 (green) from cuneiform 2 (blue).

2.3 Interactive Tool

Using the proposed method, we have developed an interactive tool for simultaneous separation of multiple bones in a segmented CT volume (Figure 5 left). Given an input volume, the user first places one or more seeds for each bone, by

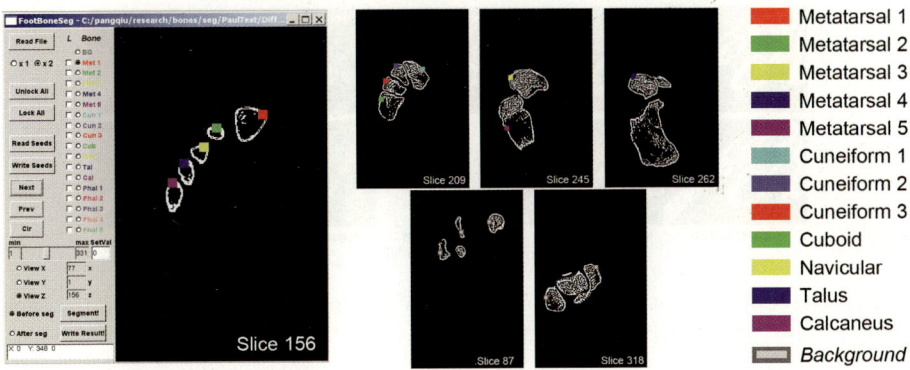

Fig. 5. The interactive tool for bone segmentation (left), where 5 seeds are placed on one transverse slice, other slices (middle) on which the user placed the seeds, and the color utilized to delineate each bone (right)

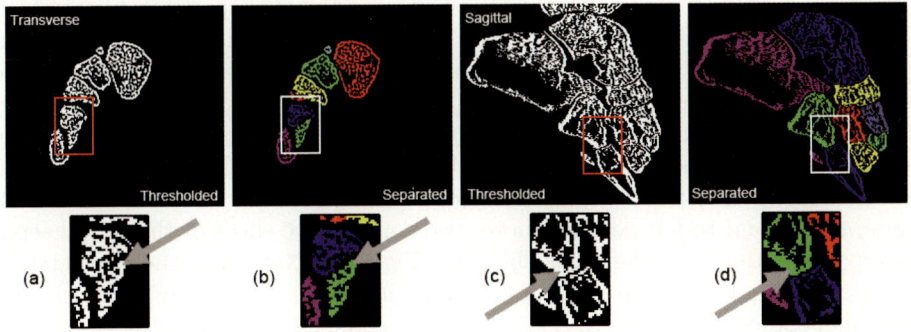

Fig. 6. A transverse slice (left) and a sagittal slice (right) before and after interactive separation using the seeds shown in Figure 5

"painting" the voxel on a 2D slice with a color associated with that bone. The tool then automatically computes a separation between the bones and displays the voxels colored by their corresponding labels (Figure 6 (b,d)). The user can further adjust the result by labelling more voxels on the input volume, and the separation will be updated using the expanded set of seeds.

3 Results and Validation

We tested the method and the graphical tool's ability to separate the 12 human mid-foot bones that have been collectively segmented from CT scans. The 12 bones and their corresponding color labels are shown on the right of Figure 5. We used parameters $\alpha = 8$ and $\{w_0, w_1, w_2\} = \{1, 4, 16\}$ for graph construction. These parameters were selected empirically using one CT volume, and used for all volumes. All tests were performed on a PC with 2GHz CPU and 2GB memory.

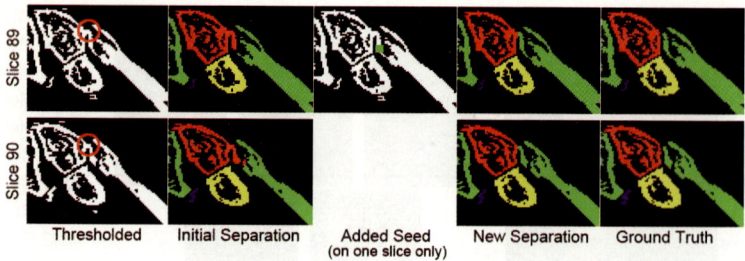

Fig. 7. The tool allows the user to interactively add new seeds when the initial separation is unsatisfactory. See Section 3.

We found that a reasonable separation of the majority of the bones can be achieved in most volumes by using only 1 seed per bone plus a number of background seeds (gray-colored in Slice 87 and 318 of Figure 5) that indicate the non-bone tissues. The top images in Figure 6 show the separation result, viewed from a transverse and a sagittal slice, using just the seeds shown in Figure 5. In the close-up views of the bone interface between metatarsal 4 (blue) and cuboid (green) at the bottom of Figure 6, the arrows on the transverse and sagittal slice point to the same voxel in 3D. While it is difficult even for a human user to determine what bone this voxel belongs to by only examining the transverse slice, the algorithm makes a correct decision by considering the full 3D connectivity.

Figure 7 demonstrates incremental improvement of separation using the tool. Here, the second-to-left column shows two consecutive slices of the initial separation computed from the seeds shown in Figure 5. Note that the cut between metatarsal 2 (green) and cuneiform 3 (red) has been incorrectly placed in the proximal end of metatarsal 2, due to a strong connection between the two bones there in the input volume and the weak connection within the cortical shell for the proximal end of metatarsal 2. After providing one more seed (middle column), the new cut is placed at the desired location (middle-right column).

The tool was tested with two users in 3 different sessions on 10 CT volumes (e.g., one of the users processed the volumes twice at different times), and the results were compared with that of a prior process where a user manually separated bone voxels on each transverse slice (Table 1). The error between an interactively separated volume, I, and the ground truth volume, M, is computed using the Dice's coefficient [14] $1 - \frac{2|I \cap M|}{|I|+|M|}$, where $|I|$ is the number of labelled voxels in I and $I \cap M$ is the number of object voxels that have the same bone label in both I and M. The maximum error among all 10 CT volumes is less than 1.5% with no more than 0.25% differences between sessions. The main source of this error arises from the fact that the separation of neighboring bones can be achieved by either removing the voxels between them (Figure 1 (c) bottom right) or labelling these voxels to be one of the bones (Figure 1 (c) top right). Such choices are automatically determined by the graph-cut algorithm in our interactive tool, but have been made subjectively by the human operator when creating the ground-truth volume.

Table 1. Accuracy of interactive separation of 12 bones in 10 CT volumes performed by 2 users in 3 different sessions (T1,T2,T3), compared to ground truth, slice-by-slice manual separation

ID	Dimension	# Object Voxels	# Seeds T1	Error T1	# Seeds T2	Error T2	# Seeds T3	Error T3	Max Diff.
1	180×352×204	478788	30	0.90%	28	0.82%	29	0.85%	0.08%
2	176×383×215	515706	28	0.78%	28	0.94%	31	0.95%	0.17%
3	169×407×176	463207	25	0.71%	27	0.72%	32	0.68%	0.04%
4	179×373×169	430627	32	0.72%	36	0.85%	44	0.77%	0.13%
5	193×450×153	598157	29	1.32%	31	1.26%	35	1.32%	0.06%
6	193×336×216	480429	40	0.99%	29	0.74%	27	0.91%	0.25%
7	160×361×214	518369	41	0.94%	29	0.99%	32	1.16%	0.22%
8	216×388×177	468017	24	0.74%	29	0.79%	27	0.75%	0.05%
9	184×379×165	807342	42	1.43%	41	1.46%	47	1.30%	0.16%
10	166×447×172	602184	46	1.04%	34	1.20%	43	1.24%	0.20%

The key advantage of the interactive tool versus manual separation is the efficiency, as the user only needs to provide < 50 seed voxels in the whole volume, in contrast to manually separating individual bones on every transverse slice. Using the tool, all 3 sessions took less than 3 hours for all 10 volumes (e.g., approximately 18 minutes per volume), while the manual labelling that generated the ground truth took approximately 1.5 to 3 hours for each volume.

4 Conclusion

We presented a graph-cut method for interactive separation of bones that have been collectively segmented from a CT volume. The core of the method is a novel construction of a weighted graph from a binary volume so that the computed multi-way cuts properly reside on the bone interfaces. The resulting tool has been shown to be effective in segmenting practical data while dramatically reducing the human labor in this process. The method can be used as a pre-process to existing approaches [2,3] that further fill the interior of individual bones.

Acknowledgement

Funding is provided by NIH grant R21DK79457 and NSF grant CCF-0702662.

References

1. Wang, L.I., Greenspan, M., Ellis, R.: Validation of bone segmentation and improved 3-D registration using contour coherency in ct data. IEEE Transactions On Medical Imaging 25(3), 324–334 (2006)

2. Westin, C.F., Warfield, S.K., Bhalerao, A., Mui, L., Richolt, J.A., Kikinis, R.: Tensor controlled local structure enhancement of ct images for bone segmentation. In: Wells, W.M., Colchester, A.C.F., Delp, S.L. (eds.) MICCAI 1998. LNCS, vol. 1496, pp. 1205–1212. Springer, Heidelberg (1998)
3. Kang, Y., Engelke, K., Kalender, W.A.: A new accurate and precise 3D segmentation method for skeletal structures in volumetric ct data. IEEE Trans. Med. Imaging 22(5), 586–598 (2003)
4. Elmooutaouakkil, A., Peyrin, F., Elkafi, J., Laval-Jeantet, A.M.: Segmentation of cancellous bone from high resolution computed tomography images: Influence on trabecular bone measurements. IEEE Trans. Med. Imaging 21(4), 354–362 (2002)
5. Commean, P.K., Ju, T., Liu, L., Sinacore, D.R., Hastings, M.K., Mueller, M.J.: Tarsal and metatarsal bone mineral density measurement using volumetric quantitative computed tomography. Journal of Digital Imaging (accepted, 2008)
6. Boykov, Y.Y., Jolly, M.P.: Interactive graph cuts for optimal boundary & region segmentation of objects in n-d images. In: ICCV 2001, p. 105 (2001)
7. Grady, L., Funka-Lea, G.: Multi-label image segmentation for medical applications based on graph-theoretic electrical potentials. In: ECCV Workshops CVAMIA and MMBIA, pp. 230–245 (2004)
8. Ford, L.R., Fulkerson, D.R.: Maximal flow through a network. Canadian Journal of Mathematics 8, 399–404 (1956)
9. Dahlhaus, E., Johnson, D.S., Papadimitriou, C.H., Seymour, P.D., Yannakakis, M.: The complexity of multiterminal cuts. SIAM J. Comput. 23(4), 864–894 (1994)
10. Călinescu, G., Karloff, H., Rabani, Y.: An improved approximation algorithm for multiway cut. In: STOC 1998: Proceedings of the thirtieth annual ACM symposium on Theory of computing, pp. 48–52 (1998)
11. Karger, D.R., Klein, P.N., Stein, C., Thorup, M., Young, N.E.: Rounding algorithms for a geometric embedding relaxation of minimum multiway cut. In: Proceedings, ACM Symposium on Theory of Computing, pp. 668–678 (1999)
12. Boykov, M.Y., Kolmogorov, M.V.: An experimental comparison of min-cut/max-flow algorithms for energy minimization in vision. IEEE Trans. Pattern Anal. Mach. Intell. 26(9), 1124–1137 (2004)
13. Kong, T.Y., Rosenfeld, A.: Digital topology: introduction and survey. Comput. Vision Graph. Image Process 48(3), 357–393 (1989)
14. van Rijsbergen, C.J.: Information Retrieval. Butterworths, London (1979)

A Comparison of Methods for Recovering Intra-voxel White Matter Fiber Architecture from Clinical Diffusion Imaging Scans

Alonso Ramirez-Manzanares, Philip A. Cook, and James C. Gee

Penn Image Computing and Science Laboratory (PICSL), Department of Radiology,
University of Pennsylvania, Philadelphia, PA, USA
{alram,cookpa,gee}@mail.med.upenn.edu

Abstract. Diffusion tensor magnetic resonance imaging is widely used to study the structure of the fiber pathways of brain white matter. However, the diffusion tensor cannot capture complex intra-voxel fiber architecture such as fiber crossings. Consequently, a number of methods have been proposed to recover intra-voxel fiber bundle orientations from high angular-resolution diffusion imaging scans, which are optimized to resolve fiber crossings. In this work we study how multi-tensor, spherical deconvolution, analytical QBall and diffusion basis function methods perform under clinical scanning conditions. Our experiments indicate that it is feasible to apply some of these methods in clinical data sets.

Keywords: DW-MRI, crossing fibers, HARDI, Multi-DT, QSpace.

1 Introduction

The most widely-used approach to study water diffusion in the human brain is diffusion tensor imaging (DTI) [1], where the diffusion tensor's (DT) main eigenvector corresponds to the axis of maximum diffusion. In white matter fiber tracts, the main eigenvector is aligned with the local average orientation of the fibers, making it possible to study patterns of brain connectivity *in-vivo*.

The chief limitation of DTI is that the DT is constrained to represent only one maximum diffusion orientation and thus it is inadequate in voxels where two or more fiber bundles cross, split or "kiss". This represents a significant problem for diffusion tractography, where we rely on local fiber-orientation estimates to reconstruct fiber pathways. According to [2], as many as one third of white-matter voxels contain more than one fiber bundle orientation. A number of methods have been developed to resolve heterogeneous intra-voxel fiber structures, [3] gives a review. In this study we focus on approaches that use data acquired at a fixed "b-value" with independent gradient directions, which is the type of data usually acquired for DTI. DTI scans use b-values of approximately 1000 s/mm^2 for optimal performance [4], and can be computed with a minimum of six gradient orientations. High angular resolution diffusion imaging (HARDI) scans typically use a relatively large set of gradient directions and higher b-values, to develop the contrast for multi-fiber reconstruction.

Recent improvements in the speed of image acquisition, combined with demand for high-quality DT data, have led to an increased adoption of DTI acquisition protocols using 30 or more gradient directions, which opens the possibility of applying HARDI methods in clinical scans. It is therefore useful to investigate how the HARDI methods perform under contemporary DTI scanning protocols. Even though most of reported methods provide some experimental validation, to the best of our knowledge there is not a reported comparison for several methods under the same conditions using a clinically realistic DTI acquisition protocol. In this paper, we compare five previously published HARDI methods under the same simulated acquisition settings for synthetic as well as for human DW-MRI data. The methods are explained in the following section.

1.1 Methods for Intra-voxel Fiber Estimation

First, we introduce the basic models for the normalized DW signal $A(\mathbf{q})$ given the diffusion wavenumber $\mathbf{q}$:

$$A(\mathbf{q}) = \int_{R^3} p(\mathbf{x}) \cos(\mathbf{q}^T \mathbf{x}) d\mathbf{x}, \tag{1}$$

$$A(\mathbf{q}) = \sum_{i=1} \alpha_i \exp(-\mathbf{q}^T \mathbf{D}_i \mathbf{q} \tau), \tag{2}$$

$$A(\mathbf{q}) = \int_{R^3} A(\mathbf{q}; \mathbf{x}_0) f(\mathbf{x}) d\mathbf{x}. \tag{3}$$

Model (1) involves the particle displacement Probability Density Function (PDF) p, (2) is the Gaussian Mixture Model (GMM) and (3) associates the Fiber Orientation Distribution (FOD) f estimated by Spherical Deconvolution (SD). DT's are denoted by $\mathbf{D}_j$ with contribution $\alpha_i \in [0,1]$, τ is the effective diffusion time and $A(\mathbf{q}; \mathbf{x}_0)$ is the DW signal for a fiber along orientation $\mathbf{x}_0$, see [3].

For our comparison study we select a set of methods from the literature: Multi-DT (MDT)[5], analytical QBall (AQBI) [6], Maximum Entropy Spherical Deconvolution (MESD) [7], Non-negativity Constrained Super-Resolved Spherical Deconvolution (SCSD) [8], and Diffusion Basis Functions (DBF) [9]. Next we briefly describe these methods (see [10] for a study of similarities among them).

1. **MDT [5].** This method assumes the GMM (2). The fitting procedure requires non-linear optimization. In [5] the DT's eigenvalues were fixed and the GMM was fitted by a multi-start gradient descent algorithm. We optimize the full diffusion tensors subject to non-negativity of the eigenvalues, using a Levenberg-Marquardt algorithm [11]. A problem for this method is the need for model selection as a pre-processing step.
2. **AQBI [6].** By using the Funk transform, a projection of p along the orientation $\mathbf{x}$ is proportional to the integral of $A(\mathbf{q})$ over the circle perpendicular to $\mathbf{x}$. We use the novel analytical reconstruction approach which introduces a regularization term based on the Laplace–Beltrami operator. This modification improves fiber orientation detection. The non-parametric nature allows

one to recover an arbitrary number of fiber orientations but makes the estimation noise sensitive.
3. **MESD [7]**. This is a generalization of the Persistent Angular Structure (PAS) method. The PAS function is parameterized by a maximum-entropy model. The PDF estimation is achieved by evaluating an integral only for a fixed radius sphere in **q** space. This representation allows one to recover high quality solutions of the angular structure of p, although the required non-linear optimization is computationally expensive.
4. **SCSD [8]**. This proposal extends previous proposals on SD which deconvolve the FOD f from model (3). This work tackles the ill-conditioned problem of classical SD approaches by constraining the non-negativity of the FOD components, which allows super-resolution: the FOD can be estimated with more parameters than measured signals.
5. **DBF [9]**. A discrete version of the GMM is proposed by fixing a tensor basis consisting of anisotropic diffusion tensors with principal directions isotropically distributed on the sphere. A dictionary of DBF is computed (one signal per basis tensor), so that $A(\mathbf{q})$ is explained as a non-negative linear combination of the DBF. The fitting procedure is based on a Basis Pursuit optimization framework which searches for the smallest possible number of DBF to represent the signal.

The rest of the paper is organized as follows. We explain the comparison framework in section 2. The results are presented in section 3 and finally we discuss the experiments and present our conclusions in Section 4.

2 Experimental Methods

To implement the various methods, we use: a) the code provided by the authors for methods MESD, SCSD, AQBl and DBF, and b) open-source implementations for method MDT in the Camino toolkit [11]. Also, we use the proposed parameters supplied with the software as described below. For AQBl we use harmonic order $l = 8$ and regularization amount $\lambda_{LB} = 0.006$; no FOD sharpening is applied. For the MESD method we use a PAS filter with radius 1.4. For SCSD we use spherical harmonic order $l_{max} = 10$, $\lambda = 1$, $\tau = 10\%$. For DBF method we use the reported 129 basis orientations. Peak detection was performed for AQBl, MESD and SCSD by using the Camino toolkit [11]. Following [8], peaks smaller than 20% of the magnitude of the largest peak were eliminated. Correspondingly, for DBF and MDT we eliminated tensors with coefficients α_i less than 20% of the largest coefficient. We provided to SCSD and DBF the same *profile signal for a single fiber bundle* $A(\mathbf{q}; \mathbf{x}_0)$, which is computed using the average DT in voxels thought to contain a single fiber bundle. In the brain data, we fitted the DT to the data set, then we calculate average eigenvalues from tensors with *linear* coefficient larger than both *spheric* and *planar* coefficients, which are defined in [12]. In the synthetic data, we generated synthetic noisy measurements from voxels containing a single diffusion tensor.

We use data from three sources in the experiments:

1. **Synthetic data - free diffusion model.** The DW-MRI signal was synthesized from the GMM (2). The DT principal eigenvalue was set to 1×10^{-3} mm^2 / s and the second and third eigenvalues were 2.22×10^{-4} mm^2 / s, so that the Fractional Anisotropy (FA) [1] is equal to 0.74 and the diffusion ratio (longitudinal/transversal) is equal to 4.5. The above values were taken from a sample of tensors observed in the brain data from a healthy volunteer (see below). The number of tensors in each voxel of synthetic data is either two or three and the crossing angle is varied between 30 and 90 degrees. A random rotation was applied to all tensors in each voxel before the data was generated, to simulate fiber bundles at different orientations.

2. **Synthetic data - restricted diffusion model.** The MDT and the DBF methods both use the GMM, so they have an advantage when data is synthesized from a GMM. We therefore perform one experiment with data generated from a Monte-Carlo (MC) simulation of diffusion within and around impermeable cylinders. For the simulation, 10^5 simulated water molecules were evenly distributed on a substrate consisting of a regular grid of impermeable, hollow cylinders of radius 5 $\times 10^{-6}$ m, separated by 13 $\times 10^{-6}$ m. The simulated MR acquisition was designed to be as similar as possible to the human brain acquisition (below): nine measurements at $b = 0$ and sixty at $b = 1000$ s/ mm^2, diffusion time $\Delta = 0.035$ s and pulse width $\delta = 0.017$ s. The algorithm for simulating the diffusion and the MRI acquisition is explained in [13] and implemented in the Camino toolkit [11]. When the diffusion tensor is fitted to this data, the FA is close to 0.74, as is used in the GMM experiments. To generate data from a fiber crossing, we rotate half of the cylinders by 90 degrees and repeat the simulation.

3. **Human brain data.** A single healthy volunteer was scanned on a Siemens Trio 3T scanner. The DWI acquisition parameters were as follows: single-shot echo-planar imaging, nine images for b=0 s/mm^2, 60 DW images with unique, isotropically distributed orientations (b=1000 s/ mm^2), TR=6700 ms, TE=85 ms, 90° flip angle, voxel dimensions equal to $2 \times 2 \times 2$ mm^3. We compute the fiber orientations using each method, first using all 60 of the diffusion weighted measurements, and then with subsets of various sizes. The purpose of this experiment is to report the method's stability if fewer than 60 measurements were acquired. In order to preserve the isotropic distribution of directions, we compute evenly-distributed subsets using the method presented in [14].

3 Results

The top part of Table 1 presents results for the synthetic signal generated with free diffusion model. The results show the following configurations of the GMM: a) a two fiber crossing with random crossing angle $60^o > \gamma_i < 90^o$, denoted as $2_{90}^{\approx}$, b) a three fiber crossing with random crossing angle $60^o > \gamma_i < 90^o$, denoted as $3_{90}^{\approx}$, and c) a two fiber crossing with crossing angle γ_i denoted as 2_{γ_i}. Sixty

Table 1. Numerical results for comparison with synthetic signals (free diffusion and cylinder restricted models). We show in bold the best results per category.

		Free Diffusion														
		SNR=10					SNR=20					SNR=30				
		$\bar{n}_-$	$\bar{n}_+$	$\bar{\epsilon}_\theta$	σ_{ϵ_θ}	$\bar{\epsilon}_\alpha$	$\bar{n}_-$	$\bar{n}_+$	$\bar{\epsilon}_\theta$	σ_{ϵ_θ}	$\bar{\epsilon}_\alpha$	$\bar{n}_-$	$\bar{n}_+$	$\bar{\epsilon}_\theta$	σ_{ϵ_θ}	$\bar{\epsilon}_\alpha$
MDT	$2\widetilde{\widetilde{90}}$	0.2		18.9	12.2	0.20	0.1		11.7	10.1	0.15	**0.0**		7.6	6.3	0.12
	$3\widetilde{\widetilde{90}}$	0.3		27.7	14.8	0.18	0.8		25.5	14.8	0.25	0.8		24.1	13.8	0.25
	2_{30}	0.5		18.2	15.6	0.28	**0.6**		14.6	11.7	**0.31**	**0.6**		13.7	10.7	**0.34**
	2_{40}	0.4		18.6	13.7	0.28	0.5		15.9	10.0	0.30	0.5		14.2	9.8	0.29
	2_{50}	0.3		20.3	12.1	0.26	0.3		16.5	10.5	0.26	0.3		13.1	7.9	0.24
	2_{60}	0.3		19.2	11.1	0.23	0.2		14.0	8.2	0.22	**0.0**		10.6	7.3	0.18
AQBI	$2\widetilde{\widetilde{90}}$	0.6	**0.0**	19.8	**11.4**	0.31	0.7	**0.0**	20.3	11.0	0.37	0.8	**0.0**	20.6	10.0	0.40
	$3\widetilde{\widetilde{90}}$	1.0	**0.0**	28.7	15.4	0.25	1.4	**0.0**	28.9	12.8	0.40	1.5	**0.0**	29.2	11.8	0.43
	2_{30}	1.0	**0.0**	11.5	**3.7**	0.50	1.0	**0.0**	12.3	2.6	0.50	1.0	**0.0**	12.9	1.9	0.50
	2_{40}	1.0	**0.0**	14.9	**5.2**	0.50	1.0	**0.0**	16.8	**3.2**	0.50	1.0	**0.0**	17.5	**2.3**	0.50
	2_{50}	1.0	**0.0**	18.5	**6.3**	0.50	1.0	**0.0**	21.0	**3.8**	0.50	1.0	**0.0**	22.0	**2.8**	0.50
	2_{60}	0.9	**0.0**	22.0	**9.3**	0.45	1.0	**0.0**	24.0	**5.5**	0.50	1.0	**0.0**	25.5	**4.1**	0.50
MESD	$2\widetilde{\widetilde{90}}$	**0.0**	0.7	21.7	12.7	0.12	**0.0**	0.4	14.5	10.5	0.10	**0.0**	0.1	10.7	8.1	0.08
	$3\widetilde{\widetilde{90}}$	**0.0**	**0.0**	26.1	14.1	**0.08**	**0.0**	**0.0**	**20.1**	**12.4**	**0.08**	0.1	**0.0**	16.5	11.7	**0.08**
	2_{30}	0.3	0.3	24.1	21.1	**0.26**	0.8	0.1	14.7	17.5	0.35	0.9	**0.0**	12.2	11.5	0.40
	2_{40}	0.2	0.5	23.6	17.0	**0.21**	0.4	0.2	19.6	17.0	0.26	0.8	**0.0**	14.9	12.1	0.38
	2_{50}	0.1	0.5	23.9	15.6	**0.17**	0.2	0.2	19.5	13.1	0.21	0.3	**0.0**	16.3	12.5	0.26
	2_{60}	**0.0**	0.6	22.5	13.5	**0.14**	0.1	0.3	17.8	11.9	0.15	0.1	0.1	13.3	9.1	0.13
SCSD	$2\widetilde{\widetilde{90}}$	0.1	**0.0**	19.1	13.8	**0.11**	**0.0**	**0.0**	12.6	11.1	**0.08**	0.1	**0.0**	8.9	7.8	**0.07**
	$3\widetilde{\widetilde{90}}$	0.2	**0.0**	26.2	**13.6**	0.10	0.2	**0.0**	22.2	13.3	0.08	0.1	**0.0**	17.0	**11.5**	0.07
	2_{30}	1.0	**0.0**	12.7	6.6	0.47	1.0	**0.0**	13.3	**1.5**	0.49	1.0	**0.0**	13.8	**0.9**	0.50
	2_{40}	0.9	**0.0**	16.0	11.4	0.45	1.0	**0.0**	15.4	4.2	0.47	1.0	**0.0**	16.4	6.9	0.48
	2_{50}	0.7	**0.0**	19.1	12.1	0.38	0.8	**0.0**	16.5	9.6	0.43	0.8	**0.0**	15.0	9.3	0.45
	2_{60}	0.2	**0.0**	20.0	12.5	0.21	0.2	**0.0**	15.7	11.5	0.20	0.2	**0.0**	12.1	8.4	0.18
DBF	$2\widetilde{\widetilde{90}}$	**0.0**	0.5	**17.9**	12.2	**0.11**	**0.0**	0.4	**11.5**	9.0	**0.08**	**0.0**	0.4	7.8	5.3	**0.07**
	$3\widetilde{\widetilde{90}}$	**0.0**	**0.0**	26.7	14.7	**0.08**	**0.0**	**0.0**	21.5	14.9	**0.06**	**0.0**	**0.0**	**16.4**	12.8	**0.06**
	2_{30}	0.6	0.1	12.6	7.0	0.31	0.7	**0.0**	**11.7**	4.1	0.35	0.7	**0.0**	**11.5**	3.9	0.36
	2_{40}	0.4	0.1	16.0	10.9	0.26	**0.3**	0.2	**13.5**	7.1	**0.24**	**0.2**	0.1	**12.0**	6.7	**0.23**
	2_{50}	0.2	0.2	**17.4**	10.6	0.20	**0.1**	0.2	**13.7**	9.0	**0.18**	**0.1**	0.3	**10.7**	6.2	**0.16**
	2_{60}	**0.0**	0.3	**18.0**	10.9	0.15	**0.0**	0.3	**12.6**	9.0	**0.13**	**0.0**	0.3	8.8	6.2	**0.10**

	MC Cylinder restricted diffusion, 2 Fibers 90°															
	SNR=10					SNR=20					SNR=30					
	$\bar{n}_-$	$\bar{n}_+$	$\bar{\epsilon}_\theta$	σ_{ϵ_θ}	$\bar{\epsilon}_\alpha$	$\bar{n}_-$	$\bar{n}_+$	$\bar{\epsilon}_\theta$	σ_{ϵ_θ}	$\bar{\epsilon}_\alpha$	$\bar{n}_-$	$\bar{n}_+$	$\bar{\epsilon}_\theta$	σ_{ϵ_θ}	$\bar{\epsilon}_\alpha$	
MDT	**0.0**		9.1	5.4	0.10	**0.0**		4.1	2.2	0.06	**0.0**		2.7	**1.4**	0.04	
AQBI	0.1	**0.0**	12.2	7.4	0.08	**0.0**	**0.0**	6.6	4.2	0.03	**0.0**	**0.0**	4.4	2.7	0.03	
MESD	**0.0**	**0.0**	8.6	4.5	**0.05**	**0.0**	**0.0**	4.2	**2.0**	**0.02**	**0.0**	**0.0**	2.8	**1.4**	**0.02**	
SCSD	**0.0**	**0.0**	11.1	5.6	0.10	**0.0**	**0.0**	6.2	3.5	0.13	**0.0**	**0.0**	4.4	2.5	0.14	
DBF	**0.0**	0.4	**8.2**	5.8	0.07	**0.0**	0.1	**3.5**	2.5	0.03	**0.0**	**0.0**	**2.1**	1.6	**0.02**	

Table 2. Comparison for human brain data, entries show how the solution changes as the number of diffusion encoding orientations (#**q**) is decreased (best values in bold)

#	MESD					SCSD					DBF				
q	$\bar{n}_-$	$\bar{n}_+$	$\bar{\epsilon}_\theta$	σ_{ϵ_θ}	$\bar{\epsilon}_\alpha$	$\bar{n}_-$	$\bar{n}_+$	$\bar{\epsilon}_\theta$	σ_{ϵ_θ}	$\bar{\epsilon}_\alpha$	$\bar{n}_-$	$\bar{n}_+$	$\bar{\epsilon}_\theta$	σ_{ϵ_θ}	$\bar{\epsilon}_\alpha$
50	**0.1**	**0.1**	**6.9**	**9.7**	**0.06**	**0.1**	**0.1**	10.0	12.9	0.07	0.2	**0.1**	8.2	14.1	0.07
40	**0.1**	**0.1**	9.8	11.7	**0.08**	**0.1**	**0.1**	16.0	15.0	0.09	0.2	**0.1**	10.8	15.2	0.09
30	**0.1**	**0.1**	12.9	13.1	**0.09**	**0.1**	0.2	16.0	14.3	0.10	0.2	0.2	13.5	15.9	0.11

voxels of synthetic data are generated for each configuration. Rician noise was added to each measurement to produce the desired signal to noise ratio (SNR) in the $b = 0$ images. For each voxel, given the ground-truth and a set of recovered orientations, we first compute the number of axon bundles not recovered, n_-; or the number of extra bundles n_+ found by the reconstruction – if the number of fiber bundles matches the true value, both of these quantities are zero. To compute the orientation error, we match the orientations returned from the methods to the ground truth, pairing directions such that the error is minimized. Thus the angle error ϵ_θ and the absolute difference of the size compartments ϵ_α are computed for each ground-truth orientation. We compute the mean value for the errors and the standard deviation for the angular error (σ_{ϵ_θ}). All of the error metrics are defined such that the smallest number (shown in bold font) is the best result. The comparison of the methods in the MC simulation experiment is shown on the bottom part of Table 1. For these experiments we generate 60 voxels of data by adding noise to the data synthesized from the single-fiber and the crossing-fiber simulations.

For human brain data we show a qualitative comparison in Figure 1 for the three most successful methods: MESD, SCSD and DBF. For the visualization of MESD and SCSD, we use the same diffusion tensors as in the DBF solution, aligned to the MESD and SCSD peaks and scaled by the strength of each peak. For the DBF visualization, tensors are scaled by the contribution of each basis

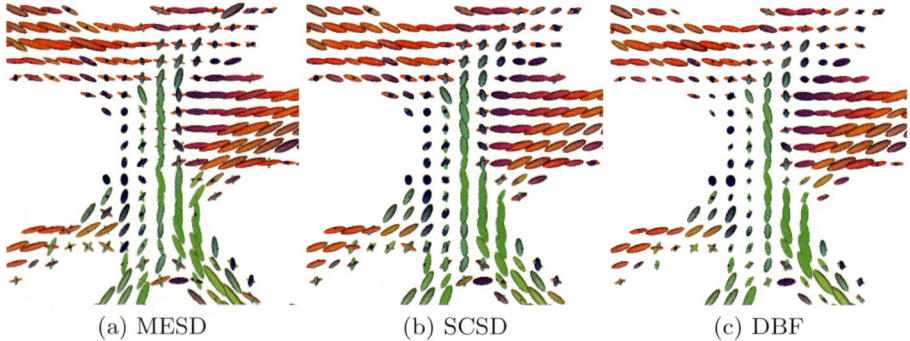

(a) MESD   (b) SCSD   (c) DBF

Fig. 1. Results for different methods in brain DW-MRI, the image shows the intersection of posterior corona radiata and tapetum-splenium of corpus callosum

function to the solution. We note that there is not a significant difference in the solutions: the mean difference error among them is $\bar{\epsilon}_\theta \approx 8.5^o$, $\bar{n}_- \approx 0.21$ and $\bar{n}_+ \approx 0.21$ for 936 voxels. The performance comparison in human data tests the consistency of the methods when there is less available DW-MRI data. The "ground truth" is the fiber orientations calculated by using all of the data (#**q** = 60) and report in Table 2 how the results differ for each as we diminish the number of diffusion encoding orientations (# **q** $\in [50, 40, 30]$). The MESD method performs most consistently with less DW-MRI data.

4 Discussion and Conclusions

For the synthetic data results in Table 1, the MDT method produces good results compared to some other methods, though here we indicate a priori the model to fit (2 or 3 DT). In real data we would have to use a separate model selection procedure, however, it appears that this method would perform well given accurate model selection.

The synthetic results also suggest that AQBl, at least in the implementation used here, cannot be successfully applied to scans acquired under our b=1000 s/ mm^2/60-direction DTI protocol. It presents high $\bar{n}_-$ values which indicate a systematic underestimation of the number of fiber bundles. For the 30 degree crossing angle all methods are detecting only one fiber in most cases, according to the high $\bar{n}_-$ values. The SCSD method also presents the smallest overestimation of the number of fiber orientations, but it is also more likely to underestimate the number of fiber bundles than MESD and DBF. The DBF method produces the smallest angular error, and performs similarly to MESD in estimating the number of fiber orientations. The relative performance of the methods is unchanged when synthesizing data from the GMM or from a MC diffusion simulation.

For the human brian data results in Table 2 and Figure 1, the MESD method is most robust when the number of diffusion encoding orientations is reduced, followed by DBF and SCSD respectively. The results for 60 diffusion encoding orientations (in Figure 1) are very similar for MESD, SCSD and DBF methods.

Regarding computation effort, MESD is the most expensive (with an average of 57 s per voxel, Java implementation), followed by SCSD (1.36 s per voxel, Matlab implementation) and DBF (0.16 s per voxel, Matlab implementation) respectively (on an AMD Opteron 2.4 GHz CPU). This study shows that it is possible to recover competitive estimations with low computational burden (i.e. by using SCSD or DBF).

The main contribution of this paper is the comparison of how multi-fiber methods perform in a realistic DTI data set. The results in synthetic data suggest that a small improvement in accuracy can be gained by using DBF, though the difference in angular error is fairly small (approximately 2 degrees). The DBF calculation is significantly faster than MESD and comparable to SCSD. MESD performs best in human brain data with fewer diffusion gradient directions, however this comes at the expense of much longer computation time.

Acknowledgments. We thank Maxime Descoteaux, Rachid Deriche and Donald Tournier for the provision of code, we also thank Kiran Seunarine and Matt Hall for help with the Camino toolkit. The authors gratefully acknowledge the NIH for support of this work through grants HD042974, HD046159, MH068066 and NS045839. This research was supported in part by CONACYT Mexico by a postdoctorate scholarship to A. Ramirez-Manzanares.

References

1. Basser, P.J., Pierpaoli, C.: Microstructural and physiological features of tissues elucidated by quantitative DT-MRI. J. Magn. Reson. B 111, 209–219 (1996)
2. Behrens, T.E.J., Berga, H.J., Jbabdi, S., Rushworth, M.F.S., Woolrich, M.W.: Probabilistic diffusion tractography with multiple fibre orientations: What can we gain? NeuroImage 34(1), 144–155 (2007)
3. Alexander, D.C.: Multiple-fibre reconstruction algorithms for diffusion MRI. Annals of the New York Academy of Sciences 1046, 113–133 (2005)
4. Alexander, D.C., Barker, G.J.: Optimal imaging parameters for fiber-orientation estimation in diffusion MRI. NeuroImage 27, 357–367 (2005)
5. Tuch, D.S., Reese, T.G., Wiegell, M.R., Makris, N., Belliveau, J.W., Wedeen, V.J.: High angular resolution diffusion imaging reveals intravoxel white matter fiber heterogeneity. Magn. Reson. Med. 48(4), 577–582 (2002)
6. Descoteaux, M., Angelino, E., Fitzgibbons, S., Deriche, R.: Regularized, fast and robust analytical Q-ball imaging. Magn. Reson. Med. 58(3), 497–510 (2007)
7. Alexander, D.C.: Maximum entropy spherical deconvolution for diffusion MRI. In: Proc. Inf. Processing Med. Imaging, Glenwood Springs, CO, USA, pp. 76–87 (2005)
8. Tournier, J.D., Calamante, F., Connelly, A.: Robust determination of the fibre orientation distribution in diffusion MRI: Non-negativity constrained super-resolved spherical deconvolution. NeuroImage 35(4), 1459–1472 (2007)
9. Ramirez-Manzanares, A., Rivera, M., Vemuri, B.C., Carney, P., Mareci, T.: Diffusion basis functions decomposition for estimating white matter intravoxel fiber geometry. IEEE Trans. Med. Imaging 26(8), 1091–1102 (2007)
10. Jian, B., Vemuri, B.C.: A unified computational framework for deconvolution to reconstruct multiple fibers from DW-MRI. IEEE Trans. Med. Imaging 26(11), 1464–1471 (2007)
11. Cook, P.A., Bai, Y., Nedjati-Gilani, S., Seunarine, K.K., Hall, M.G., Parker, G.J., Alexander, D.C.: Camino: Open-source diffusion-MRI reconstruction and processing. In: Proc. 14th Scientific Meeting of the ISMRM, Seattle, WA, USA, p. 2759 (2006)
12. Westin, C.F., Peled, S., Gudbjartsson, H., Kikinis, R., Jolesz, F.A.: Geometrical diffusion measures for MRI from tensor basis analysis. In: Proc. 5th Scientific Meeting of the ISMRM, Vancouver, Canada, p. 1742 (1997)
13. Hall, M.G., Alexander, D.C.: Finite pulse width improve fibre orientation estimates in diffusion tensor MRI. In: Proc. 14th Scientific Meeting of the ISMRM, Seattle, WA, USA, p. 1076 (2006)
14. Cook, P.A., Symms, M., Boulby, P.A., Alexander, D.C.: Optimal acquisition orders of diffusion-weighted MRI measurements. J. Magn. Reson. Imaging 25(5), 1051–1058 (2007)

Active Scheduling of Organ Detection and Segmentation in Whole-Body Medical Images

Yiqiang Zhan, Xiang Sean Zhou, Zhigang Peng, and Arun Krishnan

Siemens Medical Solutions USA, Inc., Malvern, PA 19355

Abstract. With the advance of whole-body medical imaging technologies, computer aided detection/diagnosis (CAD) is being scaled up to deal with multiple organs or anatomical structures simultaneously. Multiple tasks (organ detection/segmentation) in a CAD system are often highly dependent due to the anatomical context within a human body. In this paper, we propose a method to schedule multi-organ detection/segmentation based on information theory. The central idea is to schedule tasks in an order that each operation achieves maximum expected information gain. The scheduling rule is formulated to embed two intuitive principles: (1) a task with higher confidence tends to be scheduled earlier; (2) a task with higher predictive power for other tasks tends to be scheduled earlier. More specifically, task dependency is modeled by conditional probability; the outcome of each task is assumed to be probabilistic as well; and the scheduling criterion is based on the reduction of the summed conditional entropy over all tasks. The validation is carried out on two challenging CAD problems, multi-organ detection in whole-body CT and liver segmentation in PET-CT. Compared to unscheduled and *ad hoc* scheduled organ detection/segmentation, our scheduled execution achieves higher accuracy with faster speed.

1 Introduction

Whole-body Computed Tomography (CT), Positron Emission Tomography (PET) and Magnetic Resonance (MR) scanning is being accepted for various clinical applications across different organs, *e.g.*, assessment of cancer metastasis in lymph nodes [1] or bones [2], evaluation of the extent and distribution of polymyositis [3], and detection of ankylosing spondylitis [4]. While whole-body scans reveal comprehensive anatomical/functional information of human body, the vast amount of image data makes the detection of potential disease burdensome. Accordingly, computer aided detection/diagnosis (CAD) at a whole body level becomes more desirable to provide useful "second opinions" to radiologists. In practical clinical applications, whole-body CAD is required to detect/segment multiple organs or anatomical structures in limited time. (For simplicity, we denote organ detection/segmentation as *"task"* in the remainder of this paper.) Due to the anatomical context within a human body, the dependency between tasks can be exploited to increase the efficiency and performance of CAD systems. For example, the relatively easier task of femoral head localization in CT

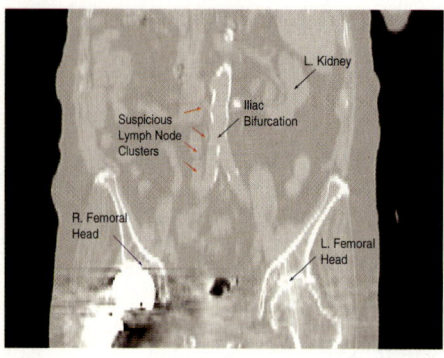 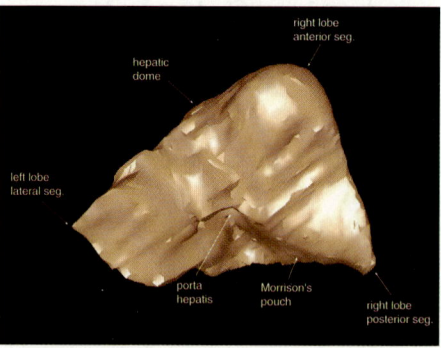

Fig. 1. (Left) A representative abdominal CT image. The blue arrow points to an artificial metal "femoral head". The red arrows point to suspicious abdominal lymph node clusters, which are often close to the iliac bifurcation of the aorta. (Right) Liver model with critical anatomical landmarks.

(bone is very bright in CT) will facilitate a quick and accurate localization of the iliac bifurcation of the aorta, which in turn greatly help the detection and identification of abdominal lymph node clusters.

One way to principally exploit such dependency is to model it as a *scheduling problem*. Due to the unique nature of human anatomy, the scheduling problem of whole-body CAD has three characteristics. *First*, the scheduling problem is highly flexible. The accuracy and speed of whole-body CAD, however, is significantly different with different schedules. *Second*, due to missing data, artifacts or diseases, the scheduler of whole-body CAD must be an *active* one. In other words, the scheduling must be adaptive to the specific patient data at the *runtime*. Refer to the previous example, in general cases, the detector of iliac bifurcation should be fired next to the "femoral head localization". However, as shown in Fig. 1, for a patient who has an *artificial* metal femoral head, the femoral head detector might not detect it correctly. In this situation, instead of firing the "iliac bifurcation detector", the scheduler should trigger the detectors of other organs, *e.g.*, kidneys, which can be localized accurately without the inference of femoral heads. *Third*, the probabilistic factors influence organ detection/segmentation in two aspects: (1) tasks are often statistically dependent, as the relative locations of organs are not deterministic; and (2) the outcome of tasks usually embeds uncertainties.

Although scheduling problems have been extensively studied in different research areas (A brief review will be presented in section 2.), the existing methods can not be directly borrowed to schedule organ detection/segmentation in whole-body CAD, due to the aforementioned unique characteristics. In this paper, we propose to study the scheduling problem of whole-body CAD from an information theoretic view. In this framework, tasks are modeled as a set of *measurements* that aim to achieve the diagnostic information from medical images. (In this paper, "task", "measurement" and "operation" share the same meaning by default.) The principle is to schedule tasks in an order that is optimal in an information-theoretic sense. More specifically, we explore the gauge of *information gain* to define the scheduling criterion. Based on this criterion, a sequential decision making process is employed to schedule tasks in whole-body CAD.

2 Related Work

In the last several decades, the topics of scheduling have been extensively studied in the areas of operation research [5] and theoretical computer science [6]. Many scheduling rules/methods were proposed to deal with scheduling problems in various applications, including manufacturing, service industries, transportation and practical computer systems, *etc.*. While earlier studies mainly focus on deterministic systems, more researchers move to flexible and stochastic systems recently. In [7], the scheduling policies for flexible systems are investigated. That paper analyzes an open processing network model with discretionary routing and showed, in general, unbalanced workload routing with priority sequencing gives better performance than a balanced one. In [8], Chou *et al.* studied a stochastic single machine problem, where the actual processing time of tasks are not known until processing is completed. They proved that when task processing times are mutually independent random variables, weighted shortest expected processing time among available jobs heuristic is asymptotically optimal for the single-machine problem. Although these scheduling problems share one or several features with that of whole-body CAD, neither of them account all the aforementioned characteristics of whole-body CAD.

3 Method

3.1 Problem Statement

From an information theoretic view, the scheduling of whole-body CAD is akin to an extensively studied topic in computer vision, *active object recognition*. Recall the previous example, the whole-body CAD aims to gain diagnostic *information* (Do the abdominal lymph node clusters exist? Where are they?) through a set of *measurements* (femoral heads localization, iliac bifurcation localization and lymph node clusters detection). It is in analogy to active object recognition, which aims to identify objects (*information*) by collecting pictures with different sensor parameters (*measurements*). Indeed, information theory has been successfully employed in active object recognition. In Denzlers *et al.*'s pioneer work[9], an information theoretic formalism is proposed to select optimal sensor parameter during iterative state estimation. The benefits of the method were demonstrated in an object recognition application using an active camera. Although this method is not an off-shelf method to schedule tasks in whole-body CAD, it inspired us to consider our problem from an information theoretic way.

A whole-body CAD system aims to obtain diagnostic information, by executing a set of organ detection/segmentation. The diagnostic information is presented by a set of variables $\{x_i\}$, *e.g.*, the locations of the organs under study.

Each task (organ detection/segmentation) in whole-body CAD actually delivers a measurement y_j to decrease the ambiguity of $\{x_i\}$. Notably, y_j usually belongs to $\{x_i\}$. In a more general sense, however, y_j can be out of $\{x_i\}$. For example, y_j can be a variable representing the center of a template with multiple organs, which is not interested by the CAD system but is helpful to organ localization.

From an information theoretic view, the optimal schedule becomes a task sequence that maximally gains diagnostic information, *i.e.*, maximally decreases the uncertainty of $\{x_i\}$.) Therefore, we model the scheduling problem as a sequential decision making process. (Although the sequential process might not obtain global optimal solution, it has run-time efficiency that is important to CAD.) At each step, the decision is: "Given the current measurements, what is the next y_j, upon measurement, gains most diagnostic information?"

3.2 Scheduling Criterion Based on Information Gain

Assume that $\{x_i\}$ are the variables of interest for a CAD system. The distribution of y_j is Ψ prior to the measurement process. After the measurement, its distribution shrinks, or *changes* in general, to Φ. According to the information theory [10], the information gain after this particular measurement of y_j is:

$$IG_{y_j} = \sum_i (H(x_i|y_j \in \Psi) - \int_{y_j \in \Psi} H(x_i|y_j \in \Phi)p(y_j)dy_j) \quad (1)$$

Here we use the expression $y_j \in \Psi$ to mean "y_j has the support Ψ" or "y_j has the distribution Ψ". And $H(x_i|y_j \in \Psi)$ and $H(x_i|y_j \in \Phi)$ are conditional entropies defined in the following form:

$$H(x_i|y_j \in \Phi) = -\int_{y_j \in \Phi} p(y_j) \int_{x_i \in X_i} H(x_i|y_j) dx_i dy_j \quad (2)$$

$$= -\int_{y_j \in \Phi} p(y_j) \int_{x_i \in X_i} p(x_i|y_j) \log p(x_i|y_j) dx_i dy_j \quad (3)$$

If y_j is taken from the set $\{x_i\}$, the first term in Eq. (1) goes away because it becomes constant for all y_j. In general, however, we can have y_j's outside of $\{x_i\}$. Then, Eq. (1) is meaningful in its complete form.

The basic principle of our IG-based scheduling rule is that a particular measurement operation $y_{j^*} \in \{y_j\}$ will be preferred over others if it delivers a maximal value for IG. The justification behind this principle is described as follows. According to Eq. (1), information gain is determined by three factors: (1) the support of y_j before measurement, Ψ, (2) the measurement uncertainty of y_j, Φ, and (3) the dependency between y_j and $\{x_i\}$, $p(x_i|y_j)$. Indeed, it is the interplay of all these three factors that determine the speed and the accuracy of multiple organ detection/segmentation. Importantly, since information gain embeds all probabilistic factors that influence the speed and performance of whole-body CAD, the IG-based scheduling method is expected to achieve better performance than *ad hoc* strategies, such as "pick the most confident operation first"

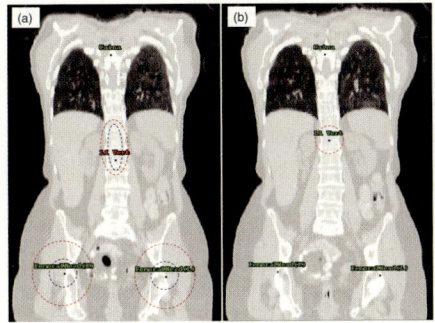
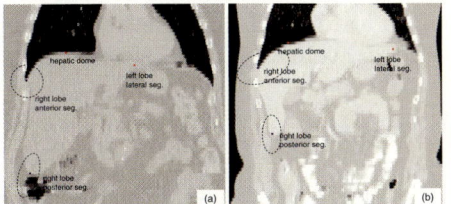

Fig. 2. An example to show the effectiveness of the proposed scheduling method in multi-organ localization. For illustration purpose, detected results are projected to the same coronal view.

Fig. 3. Active scheduling using the information gain-based scheduling method. The red and blue points denote the detected and undetected landmarks, respectively. The black dashed ellipses denote the support of the prior distribution of the landmark location before measurement. Results are projected to the same coronal view.

or "pick the task that other tasks mostly depend on". In Fig. 2, we present a rather simplified but intuitive example to show the effectiveness of the IG-based scheduling criterion. In this example, the system aims to localize four organs: carina of trachea, left femoral head, right femoral head and L1 vertebra. The dependency between different organ localization is modeled by the relative spatial locations between different organs. More specifically, the positions of the localized organs are used to estimate the positions of the remaining ones to reduce the search range of organ localizers. Let us assume the carina of trachea has been localized. As shown in Fig.2 (a), the estimated position of the L1 vertebra has the minimum support (denoted by the red dashed ellipses). If we use an *ad hoc* schedule strategy that prefers the task having the minimum support, the next organ to be localized should be the L1 vertebra. However, since the neighboring anatomical structures, *e.g.*, the L2 and the T12 vertebra, usually have similar appearance as L1, the L1 localizer has large uncertainty in the vertical direction (Gaussian-fitted uncertainty is denoted by the blue dashed ellipses in Fig.2 (a)) and gets the wrong result (denoted by the red point in Fig. 2 (a)). In other words, the "uncertain" measurement of L1 is not expected to deliver large information gain. According to our IG-based scheduling criterion, instead, the two femoral heads that have stronger "shrink" from Ψ to Φ are preferred as the next organs to be localized. (The supports of Ψ and Φ in Eq. (1) are defined by the red and blue dashed ellipses in Fig. 2 (a), respectively.) After localizing the two femoral heads, the support of the "un-measured" L1 vertebra is significantly reduced (denoted by the red dashed ellipses in Fig.2 (b)) and the localizer is able to successfully localize it (denoted by the green point in Fig. 2 (b)) without being confused by L2 or T12 vertebra.

To effectively evaluate Eq. (1), we employ a Monte-Carlo simulation method. Instead of estimating the conditional probability density function, we sample the conditional entropy using $p.d.f$s that describes detection/segmentation uncertainty and probabilistic relations between different tasks. As all of these $p.d.f$s can be learned off-line, the Monte Carlo simulation method has run-time efficiency in evaluating information gain.

4 Results

We start the validation from a relatively uniform task set, the localization of multiple organs in whole-body CT images. In this system, each organ is localized by a generic, learning-based localizer. (The learning-based localizer is a 3D extension of Viola and Jones's detection method [11] with expanded feature sets. The details of the localizer are omitted due to the limited space.) The dependency between organ localization is modeled by the spatial relations between different organs. More specifically, the positions of the localized organs are used to estimate the positions of the remaining ones to reduce the search range of organ localizers. The uncertainty of the organ localizers ($\Psi(.)$ in Eq. (1)), and the spatial relations between different organs are learned from 40 training samples. Multi-variant Gaussian distribution is used to model the estimation and localization uncertainty.

The experiment is carried out to localize of six organs (carina of trachea, L1 vertebra, left kidney, right kidney, left femoral head, right femoral head) from 18 whole-body CT scans (resolution:$0.927mm \times 0.927mm \times 2.5mm$). We compare the speed and the accuracy using three different scheduling methods: (1) Unscheduled independent organ localization, (2) *Ad hoc* scheduled organ localization (The *ad hoc* scheduling rule prefers the organ whose location is most correlated with other organs.), and (3) *IG*-based scheduled organ localization. As shown in Fig. 4 and Table 1, our method achieves the best accuracy with the fast speed.

In the second set of experiments, our scheduling method is carried onto another CAD problem: liver segmentation in PET-CT scans. To initialize the deformable model, our method detects seven anatomical landmarks as shown in Fig. 1). Here, each task is the detection of an individual landmark. Again, the

Table 1. Quantitative comparison of organ localization error

	Unscheduled organ localization		Ad hoc Scheduled organ localization		IG-based Scheduled organ localization	
	Avg. Err. (mm)	Max Err. (mm)	Avg. Err. (mm)	Max Err. (mm)	Avg. Err. (mm)	Max Err. (mm)
Trachea Carina	1.97	4.20	2.02	7.14	1.97	4.20
Femoral Head	4.47	10.40	4.67	11.08	4.60	9.96
Kidney	9.98	19.66	9.15	21.09	8.97	19.00
L1 Vertebra	**5.58**	**36.00**	**5.47**	**36.85**	**3.37**	**7.03**

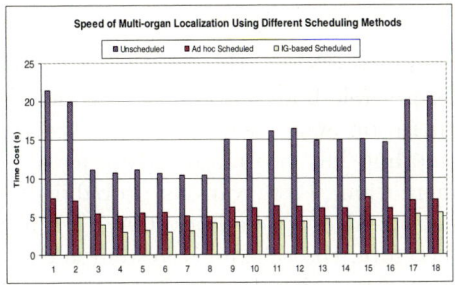 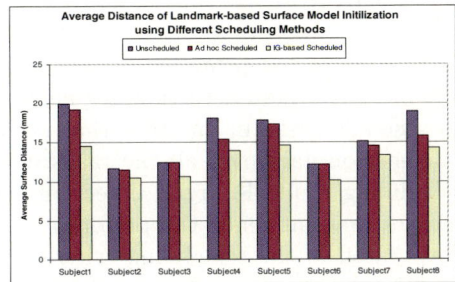

Fig. 4. Comparison of the speed of multi-organ localization using different scheduling methods (on 18 whole-body CT scans)

Fig. 5. Quantitative comparison of the landmark-based surface initialization error (on 8 PET-CT cases) using different scheduling methods

generic learning-based landmark detectors and the modeling of the dependency between different tasks are similar to the first experiment.

The experiment is carried on 40 whole-body CT scans (CT resolution: $1.36mm \times 1.36mm \times 5mm$, PET resolution: $5.3mm \times 5.3mm \times 5mm$). We found the *IG*-based scheduling method is actually adaptive to image data. As shown in Fig. 3, the relative locations between the *detected* hepatic dome and left lobe lateral seg. are different in two scans. Based on the prediction from two detected landmarks, the estimated position (prior distribution) of right lobe posterior seg. has more compact support in case 1 (Fig. 3a). "Localization of right lobe anterior seg." is thus expected to achieve less information gain in case 2 than in case 1. Therefore, while the detection order in case 1 is "...→**right lobe anterior seg.→right lobe posterior seg.**", the detection order in case 2 becomes "...→**right lobe posterior seg.→right lobe anterior seg.**". The quantitative comparison is shown in Fig. 4 and 6. Again, our method is superior to other two in terms of detection accuracy and speed.

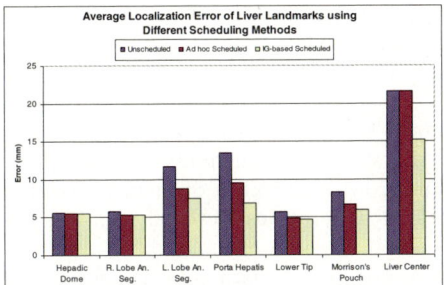 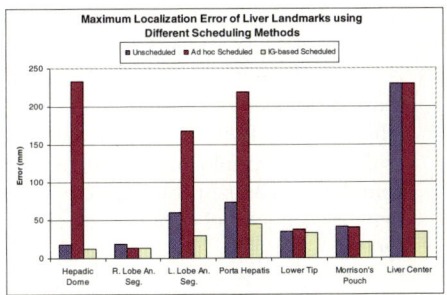

Fig. 6. Quantitative comparison of the localization of multiple liver landmarks using different scheduling methods. (Left) Average landmark detection error of 40 PET-CT cases. (Right) Maximum landmark detection error of 40 PET-CT cases.

5 Conclusions

In this paper, we proposed a rigorous formula to address the scheduling problem of multi-organ detection/segmentation in whole-body CAD. The key idea is to schedule tasks in an order that each operation achieves maximum expected information gain over all the tasks. Our method has two major advantages in scheduling multiple organ detection/segmentation. *First*, various probabilistic factors that influence the performance and speed of whole-body CAD are incorporated in the scheduling criterion. Therefore, the scheduled system is able to achieve more accurate results with less computational cost. *Second*, in our scheduling method, the *next* task is always determined based on current system status. Accordingly, the whole-body CAD is scheduled in an *active* way and thus adaptive to different patient images. Experimental results showed that our method achieves the best performance with fastest speed. Due to the generality of this framework, we plan to extend this method to CAD systems with more complicated task set.

References

1. Visvikis, D., Ell, P.J.: Impact of technology on the utilisation of positron emission tomography in lymphoma: current and future perspectives. European Journal of Nuclear Medicine and Molecular Imaging 30, S106–S116 (2002)
2. Niitsu, M., Takeda, T.: Solitary hot spots in the ribs on bone scan: value of thin-section reformatted computed tomography to exclude radiography-negative fractures. J. Comput. Assit. Tomogr. 27, 469–474 (2003)
3. O'Connell, M., Powell, T., Brennan, D., Lynch, T., McCarthy, C., Eustace, S.: Whole-body MR imaging in the diagnosis of polymyositis. AJR Am. J. Roentgenol. 179, 967–971 (2002)
4. Weber, U., Pfirrmann, C.W., Kissling, R.O., Hodler, J., Zanetti, M.: Whole body mr imaging in ankylosing spondylitis: a descriptive pilot study in patients with suspected early and active confirmed ankylosing spondylitis. BMC Musculoskeletal Disorders 8 (2007)
5. Brucker, P.: Scheduling algorithms (2004)
6. Pruhs, K., Sgall, J., Torng, E.: Handbook of Scheduling: Algorithms, Models, and Performance Analysis. CRC Press, Boca Raton (2003)
7. Nam, I.: Dynamic scheduling for a flexible processing network. Operations Research 49, 305–315 (2001)
8. Chou, M.C., Liu, H., Queyranne, M., Simchi-Levi, D.: On the asymptotic optimality of a simple on-line algorithm for the stochastic single-machine weighted completion time problem and its extensionsbrownian models of open processing networks:canonical representation of workload. Operations Research 54, 464–474 (2006)
9. Denzler, J., Brown, C.M.: Information theoretic sensor data selection for active object recognition and state estimation. IEEE Trans. PAMI 24, 145–157 (2002)
10. Cover, T., Thomas, J.: Elements of information theory (1991)

11. Viola, P., Jones, M.J.: Robust real-time face detection. International Journal of Computer Vision 57, 137–154 (2004)
12. Florin, C., Paragios, N., Funka-Lea, G., Williams, J.: Liver segmentation using sparse 3D prior models with optimal data support. IPMI (2007)
13. Zhan, Y., Shen, D.: Deformable segmentation of 3-D ultrasound prostate images using statistical texture matching method. IEEE Trans. Med. Imaging 25, 256–272 (2005)
14. Bookstein, F.: Principal warps: thin-plate splines and the decompotion of deformations. IEEE Trans. PAMI 11, 567–585 (1989)

A New Stochastic Framework for Accurate Lung Segmentation

Ayman El-Ba[1], Georgy Gimel'farb[2], Robert Falk[3], Trevor Holland[1], and Teresa Shaffer[1]

[1] Bioimaging Laboratory, Bioengineering Department, University of Louisville, Louisville, KY, USA
[2] Department of Computer Science, University of Auckland, Auckland, New Zealand
[3] Director, Medical Imaging Division, Jewish Hospital, Louisville, KY, USA

Abstract. New techniques for more accurate unsupervised segmentation of lung tissues from Low Dose Computed Tomography (LDCT) are proposed. In this paper we describe LDCT images and desired maps of regions (lung and the other chest tissues) by a joint Markov-Gibbs random field model (MGRF) of independent image signals and interdependent region labels but focus on most accurate model identification. To better specify region borders, each empirical distribution of signals is precisely approximated by a Linear Combination of Discrete Gaussians (LCDG) with positive and negative components. We modify a conventional Expectation-Maximization (EM) algorithm to deal with the LCDG and develop a sequential EM-based technique to get an initial LCDG-approximation for the modified EM algorithm. The initial segmentation based on the LCDG-models is then iteratively refined using a MGRF model with analytically estimated potentials. Experiments on real data sets confirm high accuracy of the proposed approach.

1 Introduction

Lung Cancer remains the leading cause of cancer-related deaths in the US. In 2006, there were approximately 174,470 new cases of lung cancer and 162,460 related deaths [1]. Early diagnosis of cancer can improve the effectiveness of treatment and increase the patient's chance of survival. Segmentation of the lung tissues is a crucial step for early detection and diagnosis of lung nodules. Accurate segmentation of lung tissues from LDCT images is a challenging problem because some lung tissues such as arteries, veins, bronchi, and bronchioles are very close to the chest tissues. Therefore, the segmentation cannot be based only on image signals but have to account also for spatial relationships between the region labels in order to preserve the details of the lung region.

In the literature, there are many techniques developed for lung segmentation in CT images. Sluimer et al. [2] presented a survey on computer analysis of the lungs in CT scans. This survey addressed segmentation of various pulmonary structures, registration of chest scans, and their applications. Hu et al. [3], proposed an optimal gray level thresholding technique which is used to select a threshold value based on the unique characteristics of the data set. A segmentation-by-registration scheme was proposed by Sluimer et al. [4] for automated segmentation of the pathological lung in CT. For more on lung segmentation techniques, refer, e.g., to the survey by Sluimer et al. [2].

2 Joint Markov-Gibbs Model of LDCT Lung Images

Let $\mathbf{R} = \{(i,j,z) : 1 \leq i \leq I, 1 \leq j \leq J, 1 \leq z \leq Z\}$ denote a finite arithmetic grid supporting grayscale LDCT images $\mathbf{g} : \mathbf{R} \to \mathbf{Q}$ and their region maps $\mathbf{m} : \mathbf{R} \to \mathbf{X}$. Here, $\mathbf{Q} = \{0, \ldots, Q-1\}$ and $\mathbf{X} = \{1, \ldots, X\}$ are the sets of gray levels and region labels, respectively, where Q is the number of gray levels and X is the number of image classes to separate by segmentation.

The MGRF model of images to segment is given by a joint probability distribution of LDCT images and desired region maps $P(\mathbf{g}, \mathbf{m}) = P(\mathbf{m})P(\mathbf{g}|\mathbf{m})$. Here, $P(\mathbf{m})$ is an unconditional distribution of maps and $P(\mathbf{g}|\mathbf{m})$ is a conditional distribution of images, given a map. The Bayesian MAP estimate of the map, given the image $\mathbf{g}$, $\mathbf{m}^* = \arg\max_{\mathbf{m}} L(\mathbf{g}, \mathbf{m})$ maximizes the log-likelihood function:

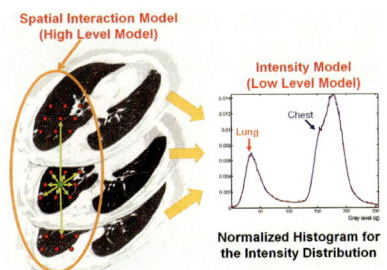

Fig. 1. Illustration of joint Markov-Gibbs model of LDCT lung images

$$L(\mathbf{g}, \mathbf{m}) = \log P(\mathbf{g}|\mathbf{m}) + \log P(\mathbf{m}) \qquad (1)$$

In this work we focus on accurate identification of the spatial interaction between the lung voxels ($P(\mathbf{m})$) and the intensity distribution for the lung tissues ($P(\mathbf{g}|\mathbf{m})$) as shown in Fig. 1.

2.1 Spatial Interaction Model of LDCT Images

Generic Markov-Gibbs model of region maps [5] that accounts for only pairwise interactions between each region label and its neighbors has generally an arbitrary interaction structure and arbitrary Gibbs potentials identified from image data. For simplicity, we restrict the interactions to the nearest voxels (26-neighborhood) and assume, by symmetry considerations, that the interactions are independent of relative region orientation, are the same for all classes, and depend only on intra- or inter-region position of each voxel pair (i.e. whether the labels are equal or not). Under these restrictions, the model is similar to the conventional auto-binomial ones [5] and differs only in that the potentials are not related to a predefined function and have analytical estimates.

The symmetric label interactions are three-fold: the closest horizontal-vertical-diagonal in the current slice (hvdc), the closest horizontal-vertical-diagonal in the upper slice (hvdu), and the closest horizontal-vertical-diagonal in the lower slice (hvdl). The potentials of each type are bi-valued because only coincidence or difference of the labels are taken into account. Let $\mathbf{V}_a = \{V_a(x,\chi) = V_{a,\text{eq}} \text{ if } x = \chi$ and $V_a(x,\chi) = V_{a,\text{ne}} \text{ if } x \neq \chi : x, \chi \in \mathbf{X}\}$ denote bi-valued Gibbs potentials describing symmetric pairwise interactions of type $a \in \mathbf{A} = \{\mathsf{hvdc}, \mathsf{hvdu}, \mathsf{hvdl}\}$ between the region labels. Let $\mathbf{N}_{\mathsf{hvdc}} = \{(1,0,0), (0,1,0), (-1,0,0), (0,-1,0)\}$, $\mathbf{N}_{\mathsf{hvdu}} = \{(0,0,1), (-1,-1,1), (-1,1,1), (1,-1,1), (1,1,1)\}$, and $\mathbf{N}_{\mathsf{hvdl}} = \{(0,0,-1), (-1,-1,-1), (-1,1,-1), (1,-1,-1), (1,1,-1)\}$ be subsets of inter-voxel offsets for the 26-neighborhood system. Then the Gibbs probability distribution of region maps is as follows:

$$P(\mathbf{m}) \propto \exp\left(\sum_{(i,j,z)\in \mathbf{R}} \sum_{a \in \mathbf{A}} \sum_{(\xi,\eta,\zeta)\in \mathbf{N}_a} V_a(m_{i,j,z}, m_{i+\xi, j+\eta, z+\zeta})\right) \quad (2)$$

To identify the MGRF model described in Eq. (2), we have to estimate the Gibbs Potentials $\mathbf{V}$. In this paper we introduce a new analytical maximum likelihood estimation for the Gibbs potentials[1].

$$V_{a,\mathrm{eq}} = \frac{X^2}{X-1}\left(f'_a(\mathbf{m}) - \frac{1}{X}\right) \quad \text{and} \quad V_{a,\mathrm{ne}} = \frac{X^2}{X-1}\left(f''_a(\mathbf{m}) - 1 + \frac{1}{X}\right) \quad (3)$$

where $f'_a(\mathbf{m})$ and $f''_a(\mathbf{m})$ denote the relative frequency of the equal and non-equal pairs of the labels in all the equivalent voxel pairs $\{((i,j,z), (i+\xi, j+\eta, z+\zeta)) : (i,j,z) \in \mathbf{R}; (i+\xi, j+\eta, z+\zeta) \in \mathbf{R}; (\xi,\eta,\zeta) \in \mathbf{N}_a\}$, respectively.

2.2 Intensity Model of LDCT Lung Images

Let $q; q \in \mathbf{Q} = \{0,1,\ldots,Q-1\}$, denote the Q-ary gray level. The discrete Gaussian is defined as the probability distribution $\Psi_\theta = (\psi(q|\theta) : q \in \mathbf{Q})$ on $\mathbf{Q}$ such that $\psi(q|\theta) = \Phi_\theta(q+0.5) - \Phi_\theta(q-0.5)$ for $q = 1,\ldots, Q-2$, $\psi(0|\theta) = \Phi_\theta(0.5)$, $\psi(Q-1|\theta) = 1 - \Phi_\theta(Q-1.5)$ where $\Phi_\theta(q)$ is the cumulative Gaussian function with a shorthand notation $\theta = (\mu, \sigma^2)$ for its mean, μ, and variance, σ^2.

We assume the number K of dominant modes, i.e. regions, objects, or classes of interest in a given LDCT images, is already known. In contrast to a conventional mixture of Gaussians and/or other simple distributions, one per region, we closely approximate the empirical gray level distribution for LDCT images with an LCDG having C_p positive and C_n negative components such that $C_\mathrm{p} \geq K$:

$$p_{\mathbf{w},\Theta}(q) = \sum_{r=1}^{C_\mathrm{p}} w_{\mathrm{p},r}\psi(q|\theta_{\mathrm{p},r}) - \sum_{l=1}^{C_\mathrm{n}} w_{\mathrm{n},l}\psi(q|\theta_{\mathrm{n},l}) \quad (4)$$

under the obvious restrictions on the weights $\mathbf{w} = [w_{\mathrm{p},\cdot}, w_{\mathrm{n},\cdot}]$: all the weights are non-negative and

$$\sum_{r=1}^{C_\mathrm{p}} w_{\mathrm{p},r} - \sum_{l=1}^{C_\mathrm{n}} w_{\mathrm{n},l} = 1 \quad (5)$$

To identify the LCDG-model including the numbers of its positive and negative components, we modify the EM algorithm to deal with the LCDG.

---

[1] The proof is provided on our web site: http://uofl.edu/speed/bioengineering/faculty/bioengineering-full/dr-ayman-el-baz/elbazlab.html.

First, the numbers $C_p - K$, C_n and parameters $\mathbf{w}$, Θ (weights, means, and variances) of the positive and negative DG components are estimated with a sequential EM-based initializing algorithm. The goal is to produce a close initial LCDG-approximation of the empirical distribution. Then under the fixed C_p and C_n, all other model parameters are refined with an EM algorithm that modifies the conventional one in [6] to account for the components with alternating signs.

Sequential EM-based initialization: Sequential EM-based initialization forms an LCDG-approximation of a given empirical marginal gray level distribution using the conventional EM-algorithm [6] adapted to the DGs. At the first stage, the empirical distribution is represented with a mixture of K positive DGs, each dominant mode being roughly approximated with a single DG. At the second stage, deviations of the empirical distribution from the dominant K-component mixture are modeled with other, "subordinate" components of the LCDG. The resulting initial LCDG has K dominant weights, say, $w_{p,1}, \ldots, w_{p,K}$ such that $\sum_{r=1}^{K} w_{p,r} = 1$, and a number of subordinate weights of smaller values such that $\sum_{r=K+1}^{C_p} w_{p,r} - \sum_{l=1}^{C_n} w_{n,l} = 0$.

The subordinate components are determined as follows. The positive and negative deviations of the empirical distribution from the dominant mixture are separated and scaled up to form two new "empirical distributions". The same conventional EM algorithm is iteratively exploited to find the subordinate mixtures of positive or negative DGs that approximate best the scaled-up positive or negative deviations, respectively. The sizes $C_p - K$ and C_n of these mixtures are found by sequential minimization of the total absolute error between each scaled-up deviation and its mixture model by the number of the components. Then the obtained positive and negative subordinate models are scaled down and then added to the dominant mixture yielding the initial LCDG model.

Modified EM algorithm for LCDG: Modified EM algorithm for LCDG maximizes the log-likelihood of the empirical data by the model parameters assuming statistically independent signals:

$$L(\mathbf{w}, \Theta) = \sum_{q \in \mathbf{Q}} f(q) \log p_{\mathbf{w},\Theta}(q) \qquad (6)$$

A local maximum of the log-likelihood in Eq. (6) is given with the EM process extending the one in [6] onto alternating signs of the components. Let $p_{\mathbf{w},\Theta}^{[m]}(q) = \sum_{r=1}^{C_p} w_{p,r}^{[m]} \psi(q|\theta_{p,r}^{[m]}) - \sum_{l=1}^{C_n} w_{n,l}^{[m]} \psi(q|\theta_{n,l}^{[m]})$ denote the current LCDG at iteration m. Relative contributions of each signal $q \in \mathbf{Q}$ to each positive and negative DG at iteration m are specified by the respective conditional weights

$$\pi_p^{[m]}(r|q) = \frac{w_{p,r}^{[m]} \psi(q|\theta_{p,r}^{[m]})}{p_{\mathbf{w},\Theta}^{[m]}(q)}; \qquad \pi_n^{[m]}(l|q) = \frac{w_{n,l}^{[m]} \psi(q|\theta_{n,l}^{[m]})}{p_{\mathbf{w},\Theta}^{[m]}(q)} \qquad (7)$$

such that the following constraints hold:

$$\sum_{r=1}^{C_p} \pi_p^{[m]}(r|q) - \sum_{l=1}^{C_n} \pi_n^{[m]}(l|q) = 1; \quad q = 0, \ldots, Q-1 \qquad (8)$$

The following two steps iterate until the log-likelihood changes become small:

E– step[m+1]: Find the weights of Eq. (7) under the fixed parameters $\mathbf{w}^{[m]}$, $\Theta^{[m]}$ from the previous iteration m, and

M– step[m+1]: Find conditional MLEs $\mathbf{w}^{[m+1]}$, $\Theta^{[m+1]}$ by maximizing $L(\mathbf{w}, \Theta)$ under the fixed weights of Eq. (7).

Considerations closely similar to those in [6] show this process converges to a local log-likelihood maximum. Let the log-likelihood of Eq. (6) be rewritten in the equivalent form with the constraints of Eq. (8) as unit factors:

$$L(\mathbf{w}^{[m]}, \Theta^{[m]}) = \sum_{q=0}^{Q} f(q) \left[\sum_{r=1}^{C_p} \pi_p^{[m]}(r|q) \log p^{[m]}(q) - \sum_{l=1}^{C_n} \pi_n^{[m]}(l|q) \log p^{[m]}(q) \right] \quad (9)$$

Let the terms $\log p^{[m]}(q)$ in the first and second brackets be replaced with the equal terms $\log w_{p,r}^{[m]} + \log \psi(q|\theta_{p,r}^{[m]}) - \log \pi_p^{[m]}(r|q)$ and $\log w_{n,l}^{[m]} + \log \psi(q|\theta_{n,l}^{[m]}) - \log \pi_n^{[m]}(l|q)$, respectively, which follow from Eq. (7). At the E-step, the conditional Lagrange maximization of the log-likelihood of Eq. (9) under the Q restrictions of Eq. (8) results just in the weights $\pi_p^{[m+1]}(r|q)$ and $\pi_n^{[m+1]}(l|q)$ of Eq. (7) for all $r = 1, \ldots, C_p$; $l = 1, \ldots, C_n$ and $q \in \mathbf{Q}$. At the M-step, the DG weights $w_{p,r}^{[m+1]} = \sum_{q \in \mathbf{Q}} f(q) \pi_p^{[m+1]}(r|q)$ and $w_{n,l}^{[m+1]} = \sum_{q \in \mathbf{Q}} f(q) \pi_n^{[m+1]}(l|q)$ follow from the conditional Lagrange maximization of the log-likelihood in Eq. (9) under the restriction of Eq. (5) and the fixed conditional weights of Eq. (7). Under these latter, the conventional MLEs of the parameters of each DG stem from maximizing the log-likelihood after each difference of the cumulative Gaussians is replaced with its close approximation with the Gaussian density (below "c" stands for "p" or "n", respectively):

$$\mu_{c,r}^{[m+1]} = \frac{1}{w_{c,r}^{[m+1]}} \sum_{q \in \mathbf{Q}} q \cdot f(q) \pi_c^{[m+1]}(r|q)$$

$$(\sigma_{c,r}^{[m+1]})^2 = \frac{1}{w_{c,r}^{[m+1]}} \sum_{q \in \mathbf{Q}} \left(q - \mu_{c,i}^{[m+1]}\right)^2 \cdot f(q) \pi_c^{[m+1]}(r|q)$$

This modified EM-algorithm is valid until the weights $\mathbf{w}$ are strictly positive. The iterations should be terminated when the log-likelihood of Eq. (6) does not change or begins to decrease due to accumulation of rounding errors.

The final mixed LCDG-model $p_C(q)$ is partitioned into the K LCDG-submodels $P_{[k]} = [p(q|k) : q \in \mathbf{Q}]$, one per class $k = 1, \ldots, K$, by associating the subordinate DGs with the dominant terms so that the misclassification rate is minimal.

The whole iterative segmentation process is as follows:

- **Initialization:** Find an initial map by the voxelwise Bayesian MAP classification of a given LDCT image after initial estimation of X LCDG-models of signals of each object class represented by one of the dominant modes.
- **Iterative refinement:** Refine the initial map by iterating these two steps:
  1. Estimate the potential values for region map model using Eq. (3).
  2. Re-collect the empirical gray level densities for the current regions, re-approximate these densities, and update the map.

3 Experimental Results and Conclusions

Experiments were conducted with the Low Dose Computed Tomography (LDCT) images acquired with a multidetector GE Light Speed Plus scanner (General Electric, Milwuakee, USA) with the following scanning parameters: slice thickness of 2.5 mm reconstructed every 1.5 mm, scanning pitch 1.5, 140 KV, 100 MA, and F.O.V 36 cm. The size of each 3D data set is $512 \times 512 \times 182$. The LDCT images contain two classes ($K = 2$), namely, darker lung tissues and brighter chest region. A typical LDCT slice, its empirical marginal gray level distribution $f(q)$, and the initial 2-component Gaussian dominant mixture $p_2(q)$ are shown in Fig. 2. Figure 3 presents the final estimated LCDG-model using the proposed modified EM-algorithm. The final LCDG of each class are obtained with the best separation threshold $t = 109$ as shown in Fig 3(c).

Table 1. Accuracy of our segmentation in comparison to five algorithms (IT, MRS [7], ICM [8], the gradient-based deformable model DMG [9], and the deformable model based on the gradient vector flow GVF [10])

Error, %	Segmentation algorithm					
	Our	IT	MRS	ICM	DMG	GVF
Minimum	**0.1**	2.81	1.90	2.03	10.1	4.10
Maximum	**2.15**	21.9	9.80	17.1	29.1	18.2
Mean	**0.32**	10.9	5.10	9.80	15.1	13.2
St.dev.	**0.71**	6.04	3.31	5.11	7.77	4.81
Significance less than		10^{-4}	10^{-3}	10^{-4}	10^{-4}	10^{-4}

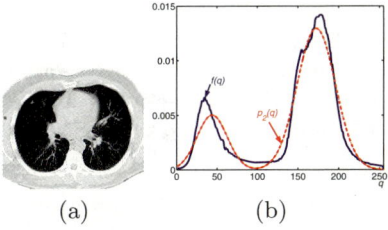

Fig. 2. Typical LDCT scan slice (a) and the empirical distribution $f(q)$ and the estimated dominant 2-component mixture $p_2(q)$ (b)

The region map obtained first with only the class LCDG-models is further refined using the iterative segmentation algorithm. Changes in the likelihood $L(\mathbf{g}, \mathbf{m})$ become very small after 12 iterations. For this map the initial estimated parameters are $V_{a,eq} = -V_{a,ne} = 1.02$, and the final estimated parameters are $V_{a,eq} = -V_{a,ne} = 1.67$. The final region map produced with these parameters using the Metropolis voxelwise relaxation is shown in Fig. 4. For comparison, Fig. 4 presents also the initial region map, the map refined with the randomly

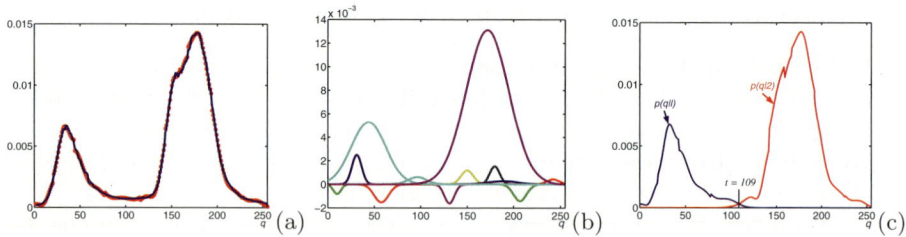

Fig. 3. Final 2-class LCDG-model overlaying the empirical density (a), the LCDG model components (b), and the estimated density for each class using LCDG-models (c)

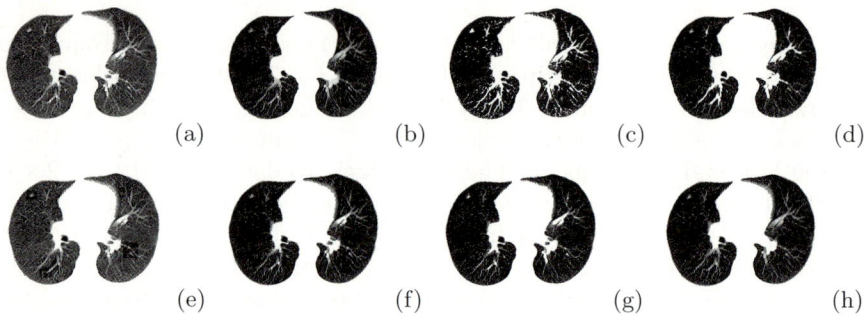

Fig. 4. Initial (a) and final (b) segmentation by the proposed approach (the final error 1.1% comparing to the ground truth); initial (c) and final (d) segmentation using the conventional normal mixture obtained by the EM algorithm (the final error 5.1%); refined lung regions (e) obtained from (a) using the randomly chosen Gibbs potentials of the map model (the final error 1.8%); (f) best segmentation obtained by the MRS algorithm with the potential values 0.3 and three level of resolution (error 2.3%); (g) best segmentation obtained by the ICM algorithm with the potential values 0.3 (error 2.9%), and the ground truth (h) produced by a radiologist

selected potentials, segmentation obtained by MRS algorithm [7], segmentation obtained by ICM algorithm [8], and the "ground truth" segmentation done by a radiologist. More 3D segmentation results are shown in Fig. 5.

The above experiments, as well as additional experiments with 1820 different bi-modal LDCT slices, have shown that our segmentation yields much better results than several more conventional algorithms. As indicated in Table 1, the most accurate algorithm among these latter algorithms, namely, the MRS [7], has the larger error range of 1.9 – 9.8% the mean error of 5.1% with respect to the ground truth. Our segmentation has the notably smaller error range of 0.1 – 2.15% and its mean error of 0.32% is more than fifteen times less.

Our experiments show that the proposed accurate identification of the Markov–Gibbs random field model demonstrates promising results in segmenting the lung region from LDCT images. Our present implementation on C++ programming language on the Intel quad processor (3.2GHz each) with 16 GB

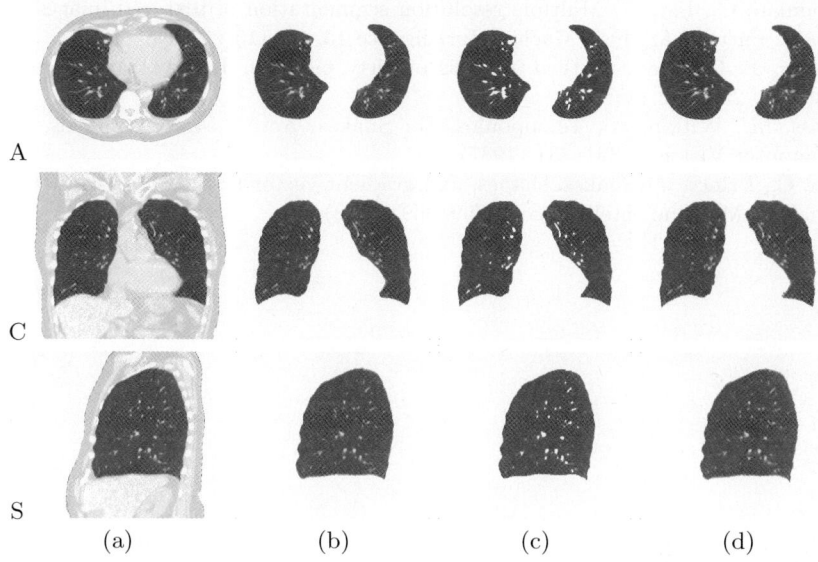

Fig. 5. Results of 3D Lung segmentation projected onto 2D axial (A), coronal (C), and saggital (S) planes for visualization: 2D profiles of the original LDCT images (a), our segmentation (b), IT segmentation, and (d) the radiologist's segmentation. Note that our segmentation errors are only around the outer edge (Error 0.79%. and the IT-based segmentation error is 4.57%. The errors are highlighted by yellow color.

memory and 2 TB hard drive with RAID technology takes about 296 sec for processing 182 LDCT slices of size 512×512 pixels each, i.e about 1.65 sec per slice.

Acknowledgement. This research work has been supported by Wallace H. Coulter Foundation.

References

1. American Cancer Society: Cancer Facts and Figures (2006)
2. Sluimer, I., Schilham, A., Prokop, M., van Ginneken, B.: Computer analysis of computed tomography scans of the lung: a survey. IEEE TMI 25(4), 385–405 (2006)
3. Hu, S., Hoffman, E., Reinhardt, J.: Automatic lung segmentation for accurate quantitation of volumetric X-ray CT images. IEEE TMI 20, 490–498 (2001)
4. Sluimer, I., Prokop, M., van Ginneken, B.: Toward automated segmentation of the pathological lung in CT. IEEE TMI 24(8), 1025–1038 (2005)
5. Gimel'farb, G.: Image textures and Gibbs random fields. Kluwer Academic, Dordrecht (1999)
6. Schlesinger, M., Hlavac, V.: Ten Lectures on Statistical and Structural Pattern Recognition. Kluwer Academic, Dordrecht (2002)

7. Bouman, C., Liu, B.: Multiple resolution segmentation of textured images. IEEE Trans. Pattern Analysis Machine Intelligence 13, 99–113 (1991)
8. Besag, J.: On the statistical analysis of dirty pictures. J. Royal Statistical Society B48, 259–302 (1986)
9. Kass, M., Witkin, A., Terzopoulos, D.: Snakes: Active contour models. Int. J. Computer Vision 1, 321–331 (1987)
10. Xu, C., Prince, J.: Snakes, shapes, and gradient vector flow. IEEE Trans. Pattern Analysis Machine Intelligence 7, 359–369 (1998)

Active Volume Models with Probabilistic Object Boundary Prediction Module

Tian Shen[1], Yaoyao Zhu[1], Xiaolei Huang[1],
Junzhou Huang[2], Dimitris Metaxas[2], and Leon Axel[3]

[1] Department of Computer Science and Engineering, Lehigh University,
Bethlehem, PA 18015
[2] Computational Biomedicine Imaging and Modeling Center, Rutgers University,
NJ 08854
[3] Department of Radiology, New York University School of Medicine,
New York, NY 10016

Abstract. We propose a novel Active Volume Model (AVM) which deforms in a free-form manner to minimize energy. Unlike Snakes and level-set active contours which only consider curves or surfaces, the AVM is a deforming object model that has both boundary and an interior area. When applied to object segmentation and tracking, the model alternates between two basic operations: deform according to current object prediction, and predict according to current appearance statistics of the model. The probabilistic object prediction module relies on the Bayesian Decision Rule to separate foreground (i.e. object represented by the model) and background. Optimization of the model is a natural extension of the Snakes model so that region information becomes part of the external forces. The AVM thus has the efficiency of Snakes while having adaptive region-based constraints. Segmentation results, validation, and comparison with GVF Snakes and level set methods are presented for experiments on noisy 2D/3D medical images.

1 Introduction

Boundary extraction is an important task in medical image analysis. The main challenge is to retrieve high-level information from low-level image signals while minimizing the effect of noise, intensity inhomogeneity, and other factors. Model-based methods have been widely used with considerable success. Most noticeable are two types of models: deformable models [1,2], and statistical shape and appearance model [3,4].

Kass et al. proposed Snakes [1], which are energy-minimizing splines with smoothness constraints and influenced by image forces. Other parametric models were proposed to incorporate overall shape model constraints [5] and to increase the attraction range of the original Snakes by *Gradient Vector Flow* (GVF) [6]. Depending solely on image gradient information, however, these methods may be trapped by noise and spurious edges. Region analysis strategies [7,8] have been incorporated in Snake-like models to improve their robustness to noise.

Another class of deformable models commonly used in medical image analysis is level set based geometric models [2]. This approach represents curves and surfaces implicitly as the level set of a higher-dimensional scalar function and the evolution of these implicit models is based on the theory of curve evolution, with speed function specifically designed to incorporate image gradient information. The integration of region information in geometric models has been mostly based on solving the frame partition problem as in *Geodesic Active Region* [9] and *Active contours without edges* [10].

In noisy medical images, statistical modeling approaches are adopted by adding some constrains from prior offline learning. Cootes et al. proposed methods for building *active shape models* [4] and *active appearance models* [3], by learning patterns of variability from a training set of annotated images. Integrating high-level knowledge, these models deform in ways constrained by the training data. Thus they are often more robust in image interpretation. Image interpretation by shape-appearance joint prior models can be based on image search [4], or by maximizing posterior likelihood of the model given image information, in a Bayesian framework [11]. Shape priors particularly have been introduced to level-set based cardiac segmentation [12], and to deformable models for constrained segmentation of bladder and prostate [13].

In this paper, we propose an Active Volume Model (AVM) which deforms with constraints from both Region Of Interest (ROI) and image gradient information. The ROI, which represents the predicted object, is obtained from a classification of image features based on model-interior statistics. An approximation of the object appearance statistics, the model-interior statistics are learned adaptively during model evolution. An advantage of the AVM model is that its formulation allows the ROI information to naturally become part of the Snakes external forces; in this way, rapid model deformations can be derived by finding the solution of the Euler equations in a variational framework [1]. In our experimental evaluation on various noisy medical images in 2D/3D, we found that AVM achieved comparable speed with the original Snakes and GVF [6] but with much better robustness and accuracy. The probabilistic ROI boundary-prediction module provides a meaningful classification, in comparison with the thresholding technique in [8]. With similar model initialization, AVM converges much faster (typically within $30 \sim 40$ iterations) than *Active contours without edges* (ACWE) [10]. While AVM produces a single smooth object boundary surface, the segmentation by ACWE often contains small holes and islands.

2 Methodology

An active volume model is a deforming solid that minimizes internal and external energy. The internal constraint ensures the model has smooth boundary. The external constraints come from image data, priors, and/or user-defined features.

Representing the model boundary parametrically, $\mathbf{v}(s) = (x(s), y(s))$, the internal energy term of AVM is defined similar to Active Contour Models.

$$E_{int} = \int_0^1 (\alpha(s)|\mathbf{v}_s(s)|^2 + \beta(s)|\mathbf{v}_{ss}(s)|^2)ds \qquad (1)$$

The external energy function consists of two terms: the gradient term E_g and the region term E_R. So the overall energy function is:

$$E = E_{int} + E_{ext} = E_{int} + k \cdot (E_g + k_{ext} \cdot E_R) \qquad (2)$$

where k is a constant that balances the internal and external forces. k_{ext} is a constant that balances the contributions of the gradient term and the region term.

Gradient Data Term. The gradient data term can be defined using the gradient map, edge distance map, or a combination of both. Denote a gradient magnitude map or the distance transform of an edge map as F_g, the gradient data term is defined as:

$$E_g = \int_0^1 F_g(\mathbf{v}(s))ds \qquad (3)$$

$$F_g = \begin{cases} D_{edge}^2, & \text{edge distance map; or} \\ -|\nabla I|^2, & \text{gradient magnitude map} \end{cases} \qquad (4)$$

where D_{edge} refers to the unsigned distance transform of the edge map, and ∇I represents the image gradient.

Region Data Term. A novel aspect of the active volume model is that it learns the appearance statistics of the object of interest dynamically and the model's deformation is driven by the predicted object-region boundary. External constraints from various sources can be accounted in the Region Data Term by probabilistic integration. Let us consider that each constraint corresponds to a probabilistic boundary prediction module, and it generates a confidence-rated probability map to indicate the likelihood of a pixel being: +1 (*object* class), or -1 (*non_object* class). Suppose we have n independent external constraints, the feature used in the kth constraint is f_k, and $L(\mathbf{v})$ denotes the label of a pixel $\mathbf{v}$, our approach to combining the multiple independent modules is applying the Bayes rule in order to evaluate the final confidence rate:

$$Pr(L(\mathbf{v})|f_1, f_2, ..., f_n) = \frac{Pr(f_1, f_2, ..., f_n|L(\mathbf{v}))Pr(L(\mathbf{v}))}{Pr(f_1, f_2, ..., f_n)}$$
$$\propto Pr(f_1|L(\mathbf{v}))Pr(f_2|L(\mathbf{v}))...Pr(f_n|L(\mathbf{v}))Pr(L(\mathbf{v})) \qquad (5)$$

For each independent module, the probability $Pr(f_k|L(\mathbf{v}))$ is estimated based on the active volume model's interior statistics. Considering a module using intensity statistics, the object region can be predicted according to the current model-interior intensity distribution. For instance, for a pixel $\mathbf{v}$ with intensity feature value $I(\mathbf{v}) = i$ where i ranges from 0 to 255, we have:

$$Pr(i|I) = Pr(i, object|I) + Pr(i, non\_object|I)$$
$$= Pr(i|object, I)Pr(object|I) + Pr(i|non\_object, I)Pr(non\_object|I) \quad (6)$$

In the equation, the intensity distribution over the entire image I, $Pr(i|I)$ is known, and we estimate the object-interior distribution $Pr(i|object, I)$ by the current model-interior intensity distribution. Therefore, the background distribution can be derived:

$$Pr(i|non\_object, I) = \frac{Pr(i|I) - Pr(i|object, I)Pr(object|I)}{Pr(non\_object|I)} \quad (7)$$

Assuming a uniform prior, $Pr(object|I) = Pr(L(\mathbf{v}) = object) = 0.5$ and $Pr(non\_object|I) = Pr(L(\mathbf{v}) = non\_object) = 0.5$, in Eqn. 7, we are able to compute the background probability $Pr(i|non\_object, I)$. Applying the Bayesian Decision rule, we can obtain a binary map P_B that represents the predicted object region; that is, $P_B(\mathbf{v}) = 1$ if $Pr(i|object, I) \geq Pr(i|non\_object, I)$, and $P_B(\mathbf{v}) = 0$ otherwise. We then apply a connected component analysis algorithm on P_B to retrieve the connected component that overlaps the current model. This connected region is considered as the current ROI. Due to noise, there might be small holes that need to be filled before extracting the shape of the ROI, R. (We will discuss how to detect and handle actual holes in the object in Section 2.3). Let us denote the signed distance transform of the current model's shape as Φ_M, and the signed distance transform of the ROI shape as Φ_R, the region-based external energy term is defined as:

$$E_R = \int_0^1 \Phi_M(\mathbf{v}(s))\Phi_R(\mathbf{v}(s))ds \quad (8)$$

The multiplicative term provides two-way balloon forces that deform the model toward the predicted ROI boundary. This allows flexible model initializations either overlapping the object or inside the object. Some example results are demonstrated in Fig. 3.

As one can see in Figure 1(C), the ROI evolves according to the changing object appearance statistics (estimated by model-interior statistics). And the image forces generated by the region term deform the model to converge to the object boundary. The Bayesian-Decision based ROI boundary prediction method outperforms other simple thresholding-on-the-probability-map techniques. For instance, we show the binary map P_B generated by applying a threshold of the mean of the model-interior probability in Figure 1(5) for comparison purposes; the ROIs and the converged model result significantly under-estimate the true object volume.

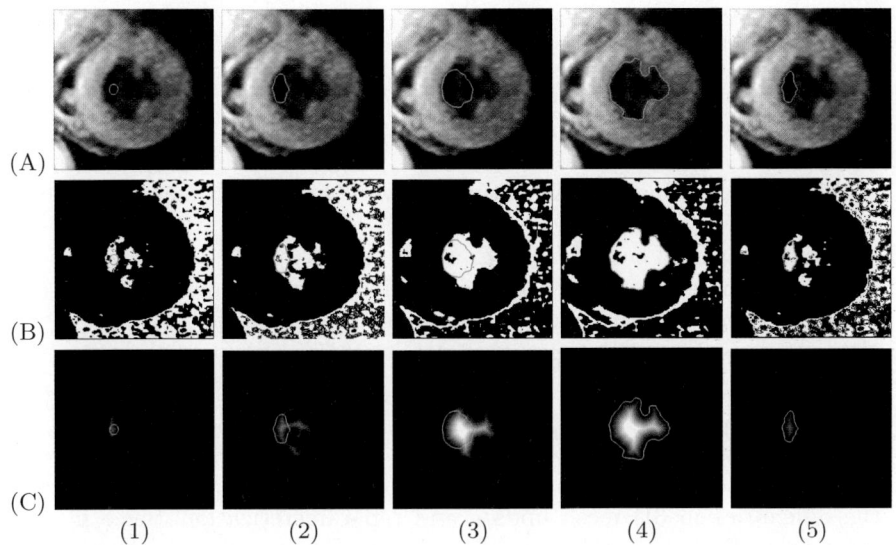

Fig. 1. Left Ventricle segmentation using AVM. (A) The model on the original image. (B) The binary map P_B estimated by intensity-based likelihood maps and applying the Bayesian Decision rule. (C) Distance transform of the ROI boundary. (1) Initial model. (2)-(3) The model after 8 and 18 iterations respectively. (4) Final result after 26 iterations. (5) Converged result using the mean model-interior probability as the threshold.

2.1 Model Dynamic Deformation

Summarizing all terms, the overall energy function is:

$$E = \int_0^1 \left(E_{int}(\mathbf{v}(s)) + k \cdot \left(F_g(\mathbf{v}(s)) + k_{ext} \cdot (\Phi_M(\mathbf{v}(s))\Phi_R(\mathbf{v}(s))) \right) \right) ds \quad (9)$$

The minimization of E can be achieved by finding the solution of the Euler Equations:

$$Ax + \partial E_{ext}(x,y)/\partial x = 0 \quad (10)$$

$$Ay + \partial E_{ext}(x,y)/\partial y = 0 \quad (11)$$

where A is the pentadiagonal banded matrix that specifies the internal smoothness constraints of the model [1]. And the model points at iteration t are calculated from model points at iteration $t-1$ as follows:

$$x_t = (A + \gamma I)^{-1}(\gamma x_{t-1} - \partial E_{ext}(x_{t-1}, y_{t-1})/\partial x) \quad (12)$$

$$y_t = (A + \gamma I)^{-1}(\gamma y_{t-1} - \partial E_{ext}(x_{t-1}, y_{t-1})/\partial y) \quad (13)$$

where matrix I is the identity matrix and γ is the step size.

Using the above optimization method, we adopt the following steps to deform the active volume model toward desired object boundary.

1. Initialize the active volume model, smoothness matrix A, step size γ, and calculate the gradient magnitude or edge map.
2. Compute Φ_M based on the current model; predict R by applying the Bayesian Decision rule to binarizing the estimated *object* probability map, and compute Φ_R.
3. Deform the model according to Eqns. 12 and 13.
4. Reparameterize the model by resampling along model-boundary curve length, and update the smoothness matrix A.
5. Repeat steps 2-4 until convergence.

2.2 Pseudo-3D Reconstruction

Parametric models often encounter efficiency and modeling issues in 3D because of the difficulties in 3D mesh update and reparameterization. Since most 3D volumetric medical images consist of stacks of 2D slices, we adopt an efficient and practical pseudo-3D reconstruction method, which is applicable in a variety of 3D segmentation problems. The basic idea is to perform 2D segmentation in one slice, and then propagate the contour to initialize models in neighboring slices (e.g. above and below). A previous slice's converged result is used to initialize a new AVM on the current slice and the model then deforms till convergence. To construct a 3D mesh model from the stack of 2D contours, we apply a shape registration algorithm using the implicit distance-transform representation [14] on pair-wise contours. Fifty sample points are taken from the first contour model, and correspondences for these points are computed sequentially on all other contours by shape registration. Once the segmentation is complete in 3D and correspondences between the stack of 2D contours are established, the 3D result is rendered as a triangle mesh in OpenGL. Interactive editing of the segmentation

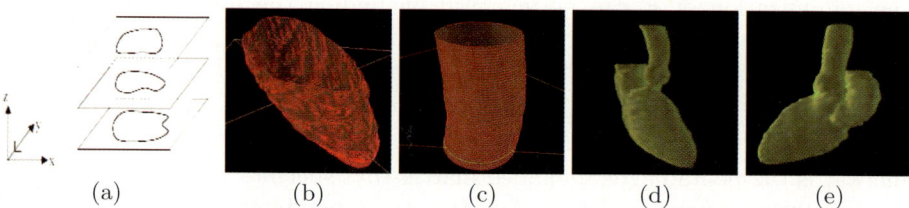

(a)   (b)   (c)   (d)   (e)

Fig. 2. Pseudo-3D segmentation and reconstruction. (a) Illustrating the "stack of contours" concept. (b)-(c) left ventricle (LV) and aorta showing segmentation on individual slices; LV is based on 82 slices and aorta 50 slices. (d)-(e) Complete reconstruction result with aorta, left atrium (LA) and LV. The aorta consists of 136 slices, LA consists of 101 and LV of 146 slices.

can be performed on individual 2D slices, and after editing, correspondences need to be recomputed only for the slices immediately adjacent to the edited slice. Figure 2 shows an example pseudo-3D reconstruction result of the left ventricle using a heart CT volume.

2.3 Detecting Change of Topology

We explicitly model topology changes by detecting holes in the volumetric model. Different from level set methods, our explicit hole-detection step has stricter requirement so that the only pixels considered belonging to a hole inside the AVM are those that are consistently classified to the background class for a number of iterations and connect to cover a relatively large fraction ($\geq 10\%$) of the model volume. It should be noted that we always exclude pixels that are classified to background inside the AVM when updating object statistics. If a hole is detected, a new model spawns off to represent the hole structure. The original model is now a compound object with geometry defined by Constructive Solid Geometry (CSG). Interior of the hole is excluded from computing the compound model statistics and the new hole model evolves and deforms on its own without affecting the compound model.

3 Experimental Results

We have experimented with the active volume model for extracting boundaries in various medical images. For images with no clear edges, such as ultrasound images, a smaller step size γ is required. For MRI or CT images, we use a larger step size.

We first test the model by using a set of cardiac CT images. Considering that the CT images give relatively reliable edges and gradients, we select a large step size. On a CT image with a stack of 303 2D slices, the model converges within 15 iterations for every slice (see Figure 3). Figure 3(A) also shows that model

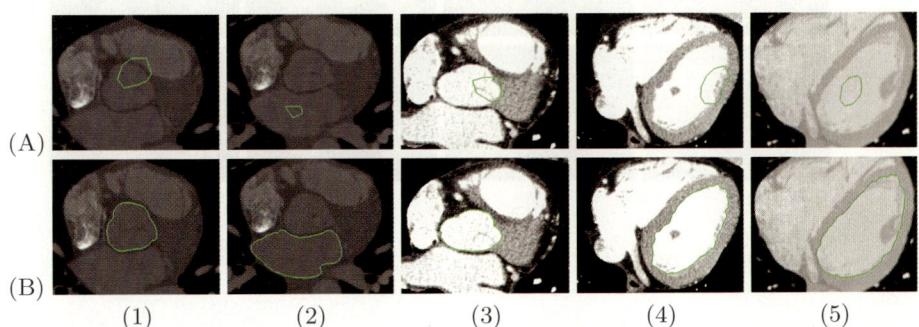

Fig. 3. Cardiac CT images. (A) Initial model. (B) Final converged result after (1)7 (2)8 (3)5 (4)6 (5)14 iterations.

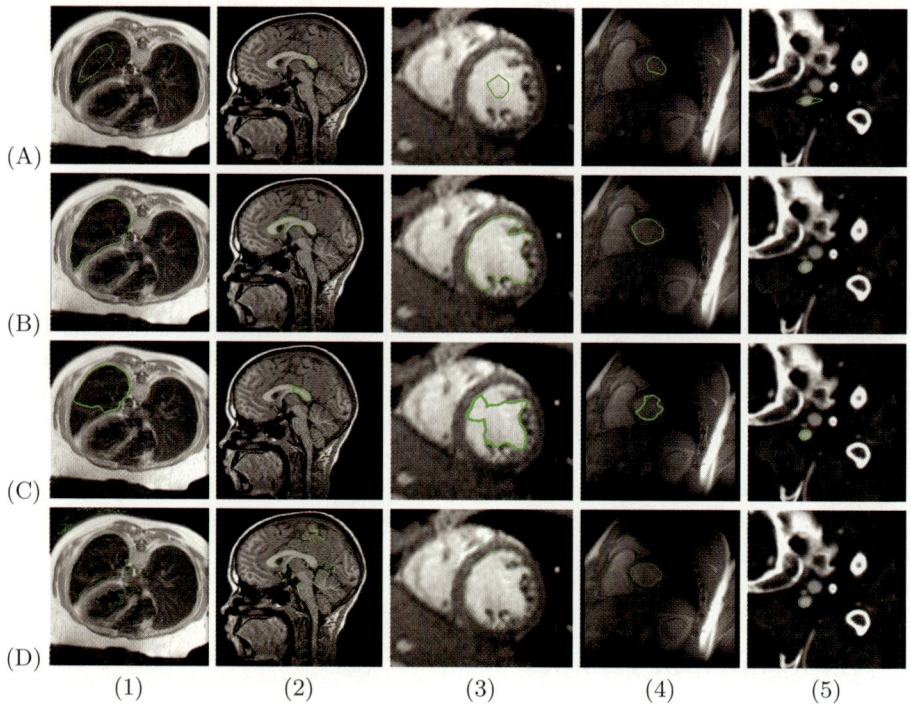

Fig. 4. Segmentation result for MRI and CTA images. (A) Initial model. (B) Final coverged result after (1)10 (2)26 (3)31 (4)8 (5)9 iterations. (C) Results from GVF after (1)80 (2)40 (3)30 (4)70 (5)15 iterations. (D) Results from Active contours without edges after (1)1600 (2)800 (3)200 (4)100 (5)100 iterations.

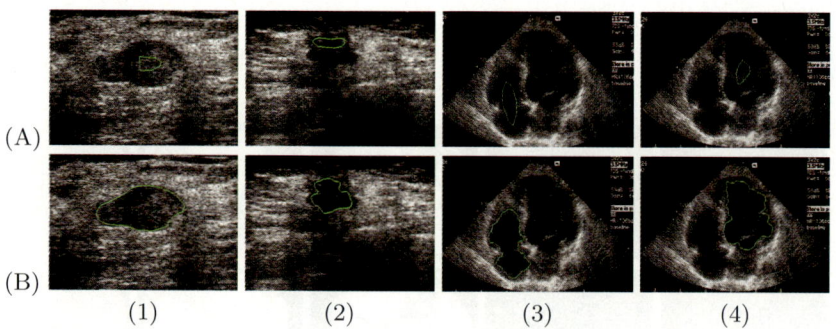

Fig. 5. Segmentation result for ultrasound images. (A) Initial model. (B) Final converged result after (1)21 (2)27 (3)35 (4)23 iterations.

initialization can either partially overlap the object or be completely inside the object. The model is able to expand or shrink to converge to the boundary of the object that dominates the model appearance.

Table 1. Parameters used in implementations when comparing AVM, GVF, and ACWE methods in Figure 4

Active volume model	k			k_{ext}		
	30.0			30.0		
Gradient vector flow	α	β	γ	κ	μ	σ
	0.05	0.0	1.0	0.6	0.1	5.0
Active contours without edges	λ_1	λ_2	ϵ	μ	ν	
	1.0	1.0	1.0	506.25	0.0	

Table 2. Running time and number of iterations for Figure 4

Model	Case	1	2	3	4	5
Active volume model	Iteration number	10	26	31	8	9
Gradient vector flow	Iteration number	80	40	30	70	15
Active contours without edges	Running time(seconds)	253.5	185.8	15.1	16.5	12.9
	Iteration number	1600	800	200	100	100

We also test the model on a variety of CTA and MRI medical images. Figure 4 shows example segmentation results. When segmenting vessel boundaries in CTA images (Figure 4(4) & (5)), we chose a greater coefficient k in Eqn. 9 to avoid the model shrinking to a dot, since the object covers a very small region in the image.

For all the images shown in Figure 4, we present comparison between the proposed active volume model (AVM), the *Gradient Vector Flow* (GVF) model [6], and the level-set based *Active Contours without Edges* (ACWE) [10]. The GVF implementation is from the original authors (http://iacl.ece.jhu.edu/projects/gvf/snakedemo/) and the ACWE implementation is by Michael Wasilewski (http://www.postulate.org/segmentation.php); we kept the default parameter settings in their original code. The parameters in AVM and the two compared methods are listed in Table 1. The efficiency of AVM is comparable to the original Snakes and to GVF, while the AVM's accuracy is better. AVM runs much faster than ACWE. AVM produces a smooth boundary directly while the ACWE result contains small holes and islands. Table 3 summarizes the comparison in efficiency, and Figure 4(C)&(D) demonstrate the GVF and ACWE results, in comparison with the AVM result in Figure 4(B).

We use a set of ultrasound images to test the robustness of the model to noise. Since there is no clear contrast edges in ultrasound images to certify the object boundary, the region-based properties of AVM become very important. Figure 5 shows segmentation results for ultrasound images, in which there are noisy gradients and spurious edges inside the ROI. In this case, the object prediction represented by the ROI is the only reliable information that enabled the finding of object boundary.

Finally, we test the running time and perform validation of the pseudo-3D reconstruction. On a workstation with Intel processor Xeon 5160, the processing time for segmentation and reconstruction shown in Figure 2(a) is 62 seconds, and the time for Figure 2(b) is 26 seconds. Therefore the active volume model is fast enough to be used in near real-time 3D reconstruction. Segmentation accuracy is also validated by comparing to gold standard generated by an expert using methods described in [15]. We performed validation on the 3D left ventricle reconstruction based on 82 slices (Figure 2(a)). The mean values of sensitivity and specificity are 95.7% and 99.7%, respectively. The mean value of the Dice similarity coefficient (DSC) is 97.6%.

4 Discussion

In this paper, we proposed a novel active volume model, which is a natural extension of parametric deformable models to integrate object appearance and region information. The main contributions include: (1) a clean formulation to integrate online learning and adaptive region statistics into active contours, (2) an efficient optimization framework that enables very fast gradient- and appearance-statistics based model deformations, and (3) the combination of multiple sources of information in a unified framework for object region and boundary prediction. Using various experiments on medical images, we demonstrated that our model can perform segmentation efficiently and reliably on CT, CTA, MRI and ultrasound images. In the future, we plan to experiment with true 3D active volume models so that data in the 3D evolving model can be incorporated into the ROI estimation. We will also integrate texture statistics and offline-learned prior models in the framework.

Acknowledgments. We would like to thank Dr. Yong Zhang and Dr. Stephen Wong for providing the CTA images, Dr. Chenyang Xu for the heart and brain MRI images, and Dr. Kaisar S. Alam for the ultrasound images. This work is supported by a research award to Dr. Xiaolei Huang from the Christian R. and Mary F. Lindback Foundation.

References

1. Kass, M., Witkin, A., Terzopoulos, D.: Snakes: Active contour models. Int'l. Journal on Computer Vision 1, 321–331 (1987)
2. Malladi, R., Sethian, J., Vemuri, B.: Shape modeling with front propagation: A level set approach. IEEE Trans. on Pattern Analysis and Machine Intelligence 17(2), 158–175 (1995)
3. Cootes, T., Edwards, G., Taylar, C.: Active appearance models. In: Proc. Of European Conf. on Computer Vision, vol. 2, pp. 484–498 (1998)
4. Cootes, T., Taylor, C., Cooper, D., Graham, J.: Active shape model - their training and application. Computer Vision and Image Understanding 61, 38–59 (1995)
5. Staib, L., Duncan, J.: Boundary finding with parametrically deformable models. IEEE Trans. on Pattern Analysis and Machine Intelligence 14(11), 1061–1075 (1992)

6. Xu, C., Prince, J.: Snakes, shapes and gradient vector flow. IEEE Trans. on Image Processing 7, 359–369 (1998)
7. Zhu, S., Yuille, A.: Region Competition: Unifying snakes, region growing, and Bayes/MDL for multi-band image segmentation. IEEE Trans. on Pattern Analysis and Machine Intelligence 18(9), 884–900 (1996)
8. Huang, X., Metaxas, D., Chen, T.: Metamorphs: Deformable shape and texture models. In: Proc. of IEEE Computer Society Conf. on Computer Vision and Pattern Recognition, pp. 496–503
9. Paragios, N., Deriche, R.: Geodesic active regions and level set methods for supervised texture segmentation. The International Journal of Computer Vision 46(3), 223–247 (2002)
10. Chan, T., Vese, L.: Active contours without edges. IEEE Trans. on Image Processing 10, 266–277 (2001)
11. Yang, J., Duncan, J.: 3D image segmentation of deformable objects with joint shape-intensity prior models using level sets. Medical Image Analysis 8(3), 285–294 (2004)
12. Kohlberger, T., Cremers, D., Rousson, M., Ramaraj, R., Funka-Lea, G.: 4D shape priors for a level set segmentation of the left myocardium in spect sequences. In: Larsen, R., Nielsen, M., Sporring, J. (eds.) MICCAI 2006. LNCS, vol. 4190, pp. 92–100. Springer, Heidelberg (2006)
13. Costa, M., Delingette, H., Novellas, S., Ayache, N.: Automatic segmentation of bladder and prostate using coupled 3D deformable models. In: Ayache, N., Ourselin, S., Maeder, A. (eds.) MICCAI 2007, Part I. LNCS, vol. 4791, pp. 252–260. Springer, Heidelberg (2007)
14. Huang, X., Paragios, N., Metaxas, D.: Shape registration in implicit spaces using information theory and free form deformations. IEEE Trans. on Patt. Anal. & Mach. Intell. 28(8), 1303–1318 (2006)
15. Popovic, A., de la Fuente, M., Engelhardt, M., Radermacher, K.: Statistical validation metric for accuracy assessment in medical image segmentation. International Journal of Computer Assisted Radiology and Surgery, 169–181 (2007)

Improving Parenchyma Segmentation by Simultaneous Estimation of Tissue Property T_1 Map and Group-Wise Registration of Inversion Recovery MR Breast Images

Ye Xing[1], Zhong Xue[2], Sarah Englander[2], Mitchell Schnall[2], and Dinggang Shen[2,3]

[1] Dept of Bioengineering
[2] Dept of Radiology, University of Pennsylvania, PA 19104
{Ye.Xing,Sarah.Englander,Mitchell.Schnall}@uphs.upenn.edu,
zxue@tmhs.org
[3] Dept of Radiology and Biomedical Research Imaging Center, University of North Carolina,
Chapel Hill, NC 27599
dgshen@med.unc.edu

Abstract. The parenchyma tissue in the breast has a strong relation with predictive biomarkers of breast cancer. To better segment parenchyma, we perform segmentation on estimated tissue property T_1 map. To improve the estimation of tissue property (T_1) which is the basis for parenchyma segmentation, we present an integrated algorithm for simultaneous T_1 map estimation, T_1 map based parenchyma segmentation and group-wise registration on series of inversion recovery magnetic resonance (MR) breast images. The advantage of using this integrated algorithm is that the simultaneous T_1 map estimation (E-step) and group-wise registration (R-step) could benefit each other and jointly improve parenchyma segmentation. In particular, in E-step, T_1 map based segmentation could help perform an edge-preserving smoothing on the tentatively estimated noisy T_1 map, and could also help provide tissue probability maps to be robustly registered in R-step. Meanwhile, the improved estimation of T_1 map could help segment parenchyma in a more accurate way. In R-step, for robust registration, the group-wise registration is performed on the tissue probability maps produced in E-step, rather than the original inversion recovery MR images, since tissue probability maps are the intrinsic tissue property which is invariant to the use of different imaging parameters. The better alignment of images achieved in R-step can help improve T_1 map estimation and indirectly the T_1 map based parenchyma segmentation. By iteratively performing E-step and R-step, we can simultaneously obtain better results for T_1 map estimation, T_1 map based segmentation, group-wise registration, and finally parenchyma segmentation.

1 Introduction

Breast cancer is the most common cancer in women. Breast cancer surveillance is improved through accurate assessment of the risk to develop cancer, which can be carried out by studying certain predictive biomarkers. Mammogram breast density has been demonstrated to be a biomarker of breast cancer risk [1]. The proposed MRI based predictive biomarkers are parenchyma volume and parenchyma enhancement pattern. Parenchyma volume should represent a more precise anatomic measure than mammogram density, while parenchyma enhancement intensity should correlate with an active proliferation and thus a risk of cancer [2]. Therefore, to diagnose breast cancer early and prevent morbidity and mortality, the quantitative analysis of these predictive biomarkers in parenchyma is desired. As a basis to analyze the proposed MRI based biomarkers, it is essential to accurately segment parenchyma, one of the two main breast tissues, from breast.

So far, there are mainly two types of methods proposed for segmenting parenchyma tissue from breast MR images, i.e., intensity-based segmentation and tissue property based segmentation. Intensity-based segmentation differentiates tissues from their intensities and has its own drawbacks in images with intensity inhomogeneity. Tissue property based segmentation uses MR physics to characterize the intrinsic properties of tissue, which is believed to be more robust to intensity inhomogeneity. T_1 value based parenchyma segmentation belongs to this category, which utilizes the intrinsic physical fact that parenchyma and fat have different T_1 values [3]. To develop T_1 value based parenchyma segmentation, the accurate estimation of T_1 value for each pixel in the image is an extremely important step. Our paper focuses on how to improve T_1 map estimation for achieving a better segmentation of parenchyma.

To estimate T_1 value, our group uses a 3D inversion recovery spoiled gradient echo sequence to collect series of inversion recovery images with T_i varying from 0.2 second to 1.6 seconds, and T_1 value is estimated by fitting the intensities of these inversion recovery images to the solution of Bloch equation. There are two main problems in T_1 estimation, and both of them decrease the accuracy of T_1 estimation:

1) The estimated T_1 is rather noisy due to the complexity of the non-linear equations to be fitted;
2) The estimated T_1 is inaccurate due to body motions during the imaging acquisition.

Accordingly, we here present a novel framework of joint T_1 map *estimation*, T_1 map based parenchyma *segmentation* and group-wise *registration* of inversion recovery images. It has its merit in solving T_1 map estimation, tissue segmentation, and image registration simultaneously, thus eventually improving parenchyma segmentation. In particular, parenchyma segmentation based on the estimated T_1 map could reduce the noise in T_1 map estimation by using an edge-preserving smoothing, and could produce tissue probability maps to guide the group-wise registration for more robust registration. Meanwhile, group-wise registration based on the previously produced probability maps could compensate the effect of body motions and thus improve T_1 estimation and parenchyma segmentation. By iteratively repeating these steps, we could improve T_1 estimation and finally parenchyma segmentation, which is important for quantitative analysis of predictive biomarkers of breast cancer.

2 Method

In the following, T_1 map estimation and T_1 map based parenchyma segmentation, as well as group-wise registration of probability maps, are described in Subsections 2.1 and 2.2, respectively.

2.1 T_1 Map Estimation and T_1 Map Based Parenchyma Segmentation

Our novel parenchyma segmentation is based on intrinsic tissue parameter T_1, which is more robust to intensity inhomogeneity. To get better segmentation results, the accuracy of T_1 estimation is important. In this step of T_1 map estimation and T_1 map based parenchyma segmentation: T_1 map *estimation* provides a basis for segmentation. Meanwhile, *segmentation* based on T_1 map not only provide the parenchyma segmentation results to guide group-wise registration (with details in Subsection 2.2), but also help perform a same-tissue-type-smoothing on previous estimated noisy T_1 map, which would eventually improves parenchyma segmentation.

2.1.1 T_1 Map Estimation

The image data were acquired using a 3D inversion recovery spoiled gradient echo sequence [4]. For each breast, five series of 3D images, $\{I^m, m=1,\ldots,5\}$, were acquired by using five different sets of inversion time T_i and repetition time T_R, i.e., $\{(T_i^m, T_R^m), m=1,\ldots,5\}=\{(1600, 280), (800, 280), (400, 280), (200, 280), (140, 280)\}$ in a unit of *ms*. The observation flip angle is fixed to $\alpha=20^0$ during all data acquisition. It takes 10-15 minutes to acquire 5 series of 56*256*256 inversion recovery (IR) images.

The intensities in each acquired image I^m can be theoretically represented by a solution of Bloch equation as defined next. Given T_i^m, T_R^m, and α for each image I^m, the theoretical intensity at each voxel v is $\hat{I}^m(v)$, which is a function of three position-dependent parameters, i.e., T_1 value $T_1(v)$, equilibrium magnetization $S_0(v)$, and inversion pulse flip angle $\beta(v)$. Notice that $T_1(v)$ is tissue-dependent, while two parameters $S_0(v)$ and $\beta(v)$ are generally tissue-independent. The relationship among these parameters is mathematically defined as follows:

$$\hat{I}^m(v)\Big|_{T_1(v),S_0(v),\beta(v)} = S_0(v)\left(1-\exp\left(-\frac{T_i^m}{T_1(v)}\right)\right) + \frac{S_0(v)\left(1-\exp\left(-\frac{T_R^m}{T_1(v)}\right)\right)\exp\left(-\frac{T_i^m}{T_1(v)}\right)\cos(\beta(v))}{1-\exp\left(-\frac{T_R^m}{T_1(v)}\right)\cos(\alpha)}. \quad (1)$$

This equation indicates that three parameters $T_1(v)$, $S_0(v)$, and $\beta(v)$ on each voxel v can be estimated from five acquired intensities, $\{I^m(v), m=1,\ldots,5\}$, by minimizing the fitting errors as defined in equation (2) below. This equation requires that the theoretically estimated intensities $\hat{I}^m(v)$ should best fit with the practically acquired intensities $I^m(v)$ on each voxel v, e.g.,

$$E_{estimation} = \sum_v \sum_{m=1}^{M} \left(I^m(v) - \hat{I}^m(v)\Big|_{T_1(v),S_0(v),\beta(v)}\right)^2, \quad (2)$$

where $M=5$ in our study. A gradient-based optimization algorithm can be used to search for suboptimal solutions, based on the initializations provided for $T_1(v)$, $S_0(v)$, and $\beta(v)$. As indicated above, random values will be provided in the first iteration of T_1 map estimation, while in other iterations the previously estimated T_1 map after edge-preserving smoothing will be used as an initialization for new T_1 map estimation.

2.1.2 T_1 Map Based Parenchyma Segmentation

Improving parenchyma segmentation based on T_1 map is our final goal, which could result in a potentially important breast cancer risk biomarker. Besides, the tentative segmentation results produced during the T_1 map estimation procedure can also help to perform an edge-preserving smoothing for the iteratively estimated noisy T_1 map. In particular, Fuzzy C-means is used for parenchyma segmentation [5].

In T_1 map estimation, the energy function $E_{estimation}$ in Eq. (2) can be very complex, thus the estimated T_1 map can be noisy due to the lack of spatial smoothness constraints on estimated T_1 map. To avoid this, we perform a T_1 map based parenchyma segmentation to determine tissue class by which an edge-preserving smoothing filter is built to smooth T_1 values only for the voxels with the same tissue class. Meanwhile, the improved T_1 map estimation helps produce more accurate and less noisy parenchyma segmentation. By iteratively repeating these steps, we can achieve both better estimation and segmentation of T_1 map. Also, with the segmentation results, tissue probability maps would be built for group-wise registration, as detailed in Section 2.2.1 below.

2.2 Group-Wise Registration

As mentioned above, registration among different time images is necessary to compensate for the patient's motion during image acquisition, and can benefit for the T_1 map estimation, T_1 map based parenchyma segmentation, and eventually parenchyma segmentation. We will use group-wise registration method to align all different time images simultaneously, rather than using pair-wise registration methods which can potentially produce bias due to the selection of template [6].

Generally, group-wise image registration is based on the similarity of image intensities, e.g., using correlation coefficient and mutual information. For our application, we first calculate the tissue probability map in each time point image, and the registration of different time point images is based on the respective tissue probability maps. This is because, based on physiological fact, the tissue probability is a consistent factor and the same tissue should have similar probability in different time point images.

Before giving the details of our proposed group-wise registration method, we first define $I^{virtual}$ as a virtual image where all collected images $\{I^m, m=1,\ldots,5\}$ will be registered. The transformation from the m-th inversion recovery image to the virtual image $I^{virtual}$ is defined as $h^m(v)$, where $v=1,\ldots,N$ is a voxel in the image space. $H^m=\{h^m(v), v=1,\ldots,N, m=1,\ldots,5\}$ represents all estimated transformations for all inversion recovery images. The segmentation result in $I^{virtual}$ is defined as $S=\{S(v), v=1,\ldots,N\}$, where $S(v)$ denotes the segmentation result for a pixel v in $I^{virtual}$.

2.2.1 Tissue Probability Map

The tissue probability map in each time image $I^m(v)$ can be estimated with the help of T_1 map segmentation result $S(v)$ in the space of virtual image $I^{virtual}$. Assume for each image $I^m(v)$, all pixels with the same tissue label c, i.e., $S(v)=c$, form a Gaussian distribution. This way, we can obtain a probability map for each image in $I=\{I^m(v), m=1,\ldots,5\}$, e.g., $P=\{P^m(v,c), m=1,\ldots,5, c$ is a tissue label$\}$. Here, $P^m(v,c)$ is the tissue probability of $I^m(v)$ belonging to a tissue class c, which can be defined as:

$$P^m(v,c) = P^m(I^m(v)|S(v)=c) = \frac{1}{\sqrt{2\pi}\sigma_{m,c}} \exp^{-\frac{(I^m(v)-\mu_{m,c})^2}{2\sigma_{m,c}^2}}, \quad (3)$$

where $\sigma_{m,c}$, $\mu_{m,c}$ are the standard deviation and mean of image intensities, belonging to the tissue class c, in the image I^m (v). The average of all tissue probability maps $\boldsymbol{P}=\{P^m(v,c)\}$ is the virtual probability map $P^{virtual}$, where all individual probability maps should be registered during the group-wise registration.

2.2.2 Group-Wise Deformable Registration Using Tissue Probability Maps

Our group-wise registration on tissue probability maps is implemented using B-spline based image registration [7]. As mentioned, $\boldsymbol{H}^m = \{h^m(v), v=1,\ldots,N, m=1,\ldots,5\}$ is a transformation from individual tissue probability map P^m to the common virtual tissue map space $P^{virtual}$. The energy function that our group-wise registration will minimize is:

$$E_{reg} = \sum_{m=1}^{M}\sum_{i=1}^{N}\left(P^m(h^m(v),c) - P^{virtual}(v,c)\right)^2. \quad (4)$$

Based on the estimated transformation $\boldsymbol{H}^m$, we can align each inversion recovery image I^m to the common space as I'^m, $(m=1,\ldots,5)$, where I'^m is the aligned image of I^m.

2.3 Summary of Algorithm

Fig. 1 summarizes the overall framework of our proposed joint T_1 map estimation, T_1 map based parenchyma segmentation, and group-wise registration technique. It takes approximately 15-20 minutes to process 5 series of 56*256*256 IR images, by a Linux machine with 1.6GHz CPU and 8GB RAM.

Step (1): T_1 map estimation of inversion recovery images $\boldsymbol{I}=\{I^m\}$. Use random values as initialization for $T_1(v)$, $S_0(v)$ and $\beta(v)$, and then independently estimate their true values by minimizing the errors between the practically acquired intensities $I^m(v)$ and theoretically estimated intensities $\hat{I}^m(v)$ as detailed in Subsection 2.1.1.

Step (2): Segment the currently estimated T_1 map into two classes, i.e., parenchyma and fat, by using a tissue segmentation algorithm such as fuzzy segmentation algorithm [5].

Step (3): Perform an edge-preserving smoothing on the currently estimated T_1 map, therefore achieving a smoothed version of T_1 map. By repeating Step (2), we can obtain better tissue segmentation, and the corresponding voxels in $\boldsymbol{I}=\{I^m(v)\}$ has the same tissue label c.

Step (4): Calculate tissue probability maps $\boldsymbol{P}=\{P^m(v,c)\}$ of $\boldsymbol{I}=\{I^m\}$. Assume the intensities of a same tissue class c is distributed at a Gaussian way, and then the tissue probability for pixel v in the image I^m can be calculated as $P^m(I^m(v)|S(v)=c)$. (Details are in Subsection 2.2.1.)

Step (5): Compute an average probability map $P^{virtual}$ from $\boldsymbol{P}=\{P^m(v,c)\}$, where all individual probability maps $P^m(v,c)$ will be registered during the group-wise registration in Step (6).

Step (6): Group-wise registration of $P=\{P^m(v,c)\}$ to the virtual average probability map $P^{virtual}$. The registration is implemented by B-spline based registration to minimize the differences between $P^m(v,c)$ and $P^{virtual}(v,c)$ as defined in Eq.(4).

Step (7): Generate the registered images $\{I'^m\}$, and check their differences with the corresponding results in the previous iteration. If total difference is smaller than a certain threshold, update $I=I'$, perform Steps (1)-(3) to obtain the final segmentation result and stop; otherwise, repeat Steps (1)-(7).

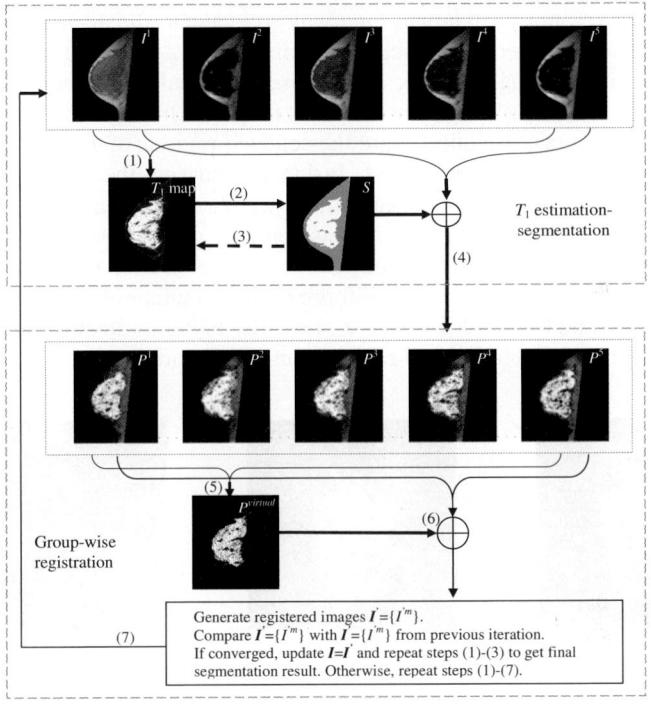

Fig. 1. The overall framework of joint T_1 map estimation, T_1 map based parenchyma segmentation and group-wise registration for MR breast inversion recovery images

3 Results

Experimental results are provided for demonstrating the performance of the proposed algorithm in joint T_1 map estimation, segmentation, and registration. *First*, the T_1 map estimation results are visually compared between the methods with and without using our joint framework of parenchyma segmentation and group-wise registration; validation of T_1 estimation on phantoms would also be presented. *Second*, quantitative comparisons on parenchyma segmentation are performed to show whether group-wise registration, rather than pair-wise registration, can improve the parenchyma segmentation.

3.1 Improvement of T_1 Map Estimation

We evaluated whether the use of joint T_1 map estimation, T_1 map based parenchyma segmentation and registration framework can effectively improve T_1 map estimation. Thus, in Fig. 2, we provide T_1 map estimation results, obtained by using or without using our joint framework. The maps in (b) and (a) represent, respectively, the T_1 maps estimated using our joint framework and without using our joint framework. For T_1 map in Fig. 2, the brighter pixels mean higher T_1 values, and they are more likely to be segmented as parenchyma in the breast tissue segmentation.

The difficulty of evaluating the improvement of T_1 map estimation is that the actual T_1 value of breast is not pre-known. One way to evaluate the accuracy of T_1 estimation is to evaluate the parenchyma segmentation results, as detailed in Subsection 3.2. The other way is to visually check the estimated T_1 values at the breast boundary where T_1 values should be lower, since there is no parenchyma at that region.

The red curves in (a), (b), and (c) are the selected regions of T_1 map for comparing the differences of T_1 values estimated. Inside red curves, the brighter pixels (with higher T_1 values) in (a) become darker in (b), which means that T_1 values in (b) are more accurately estimated since there is less parenchyma around the breast boundary. It can be better observed in the subtraction map (c). Also, the T_1 map in (b) is smoother than that in (a), which would improve the accuracy of parenchyma segmentation as demonstrated next. All of these show the better estimation of T_1 map with the proposed joint segmentation and registration framework.

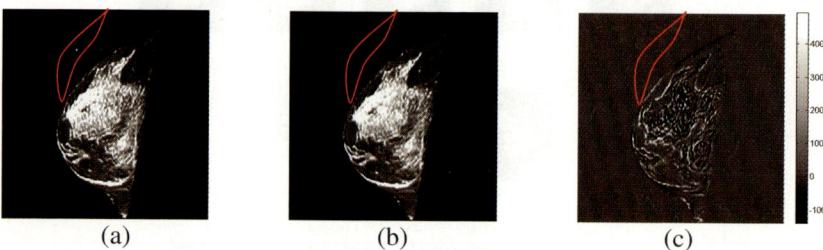

Fig. 2. T_1 map estimation results. (a) Estimated T_1 map without using joint parenchyma segmentation and group-wise registration. (b) Estimated T_1 map using joint parenchyma segmentation and group-wise registration. (c) Subtraction of (a) and (b).

We also performed a phantom test to validate the T_1 estimation. Phantoms containing six gadolinium-DTPA-BMA (Gd) saline solutions with different concentrations were studied. In practice, the relation of T_1 values between different Gd concentration solutions is modeled with a simple relationship as in Eq.(5):

$$\frac{1}{T_1(\rho_i)} - \frac{1}{T_1(\rho_0)} = \gamma \times (\rho_i - \rho_0), \tag{5}$$

where ρ_i ($i=1,\ldots,5$) is Gd concentration and ρ_0 is the baseline of Gd concentration; γ is the relaxation rate of Gd; $T_1(\rho_i)$ is the mean estimated T_1 values for Gd concentration ρ_i and $T_1(\rho_0)$ is the mean estimated T_1 for baseline Gd concentration ρ_0.

The ground truth of relaxation rate for Gd is 4.04. The estimated relaxation rate by Eq.(5) using the estimated T_1 of each Gd concentration is 4.10, so the error rate is 1.5%. This test means that our method has the potential to provide accurate T_1 values between different tissues.

3.2 Validation of Parenchyma Segmentation Results

Parenchyma segmentation is validated by comparing automated segmentation results with manual segmentation results by radiologists. Note, by performing this comparison, we could indirectly evaluate the improvement of T_1 map estimation by the proposed method, since the parenchyma segmentation is based on T_1 map and thus its accuracy can reflect the accuracy of estimated T_1 map indirectly.

Table 1. Overlay percentage and volume error between automated segmentation (P) and manual segmentation (R). P1, P2, P3 are the automated segmentation results on three patients.

		P1 vs. R	P2 vs. R	P3 vs. R
Overlay percentage	w/o reg	85.5%	88.7%	89.9%
	w/ reg	**87.4%**	**90.2%**	**91.9%**
Volume error	w/o reg	16.0%	12.0%	10.6%
	w/ reg	**13.5%**	**10.3%**	**8.4%**

From Table 1, we could observe: *first*, our automated segmentation using estimated T_1 map has a great potential of segmenting parenchyma tissue as good as human raters, with the overlay percentage ($\frac{V_A \cap V_B}{(V_A+V_B)/2}$) around 87%-92% and volume error ($\frac{|V_A - V_B|}{(V_A+V_B)/2}$) around 10%, where V_A and V_B denote the segmentation results by automated or manual methods respectively; *second,* the algorithm with group-wise registration has a better segmentation results, compared to the algorithm without using group-wise registration, which shows the importance of using group-wise registration to align the inversion recovery images and to improve parenchyma segmentation and T_1 map estimation.

4 Conclusion

We have presented a joint T_1 map estimation, T_1 map based parenchyma segmentation, and group-wise registration framework for improving parenchyma segmentation from MR inversion recovery images. By using this joint framework, we can jointly solve the two main problems in T_1 map estimation which is essential for parenchyma segmentation, e.g., noises in the estimated T_1 map and body motions among inversion recovery images. Experimental results show the improved accuracy in parenchyma segmentation using our proposed joint framework. In the future, we will test the performance of our joint framework by more breast image data. Also, we will apply this developed method to several large breast cancer studies performed in our institute.

References

1. Brisson, J., Merletti, F., Sadowsky, N.L., Twaddle, J.A., Morrison, A.S., Cole, P.: Mammographic features of the breast and breast cancer risk. American Journal of Epidemiology 115, 428–437 (1982)
2. Hayton, P., Brady, M., Tarassenko, L., Moore, N.: Analysis of dynamic MR breast images using a model of contrast enhancement. Medical Image Analysis 1(3), 207–224 (1996)
3. Boston, R.C., Schnall, M.D., Englander, S.A., Landis, J.R., Moate, P.J.: Estimation of the content of fat and parenchyma in breast tissue using MRI T1 histograms and phantoms. Magnetic Resonance Imaging 23(4), 591–599 (2005)
4. Foo, T.K.F., Sawyer, A.M., Faulkner, W.H., Mills, D.G.: Inversion in the Steady State: Contrast Optimization and Reduced Imaging Time with Fast Three-dimensional Inversion-Recovery-prepared GRE Pulse Sequences. Radiology 191, 85–90 (1994)
5. Bezdek, J., Ehrlich, R., Full, W.: FCM: Fuzzy C-Means Clustering Algorithm. Computers & Geosciences 10(2-3), 191–203 (1984)
6. Bhatia, K.K., Hajnal, J.V., Puri, B.K., Edwards, A.D., Rueckert, D.: Consistent groupwise non-rigid registration for atlas construction. In: IEEE International Symposium on Biomedical Imaging: Nano to Macro, 2004, April 15-18 (2004)
7. Rueckert, D., Sonoda, L.I., Hayes, C., Hill, D.L.G., Leach, M.O., Hawkes, D.J.: Non-rigid registration using free-form deformations: Application to breast MR images. IEEE Transactions on Medical Imaging 18(8), 712–721 (1999)

Atlas-Based Segmentation of the Germinal Matrix from in Utero Clinical MRI of the Fetal Brain

Piotr A. Habas[1,2], Kio Kim[1,2], Francois Rousseau[3],
Orit A. Glenn[2], A. James Barkovich[2], and Colin Studholme[1,2]

[1] Biomedical Image Computing Group
{piotr.habas,colin.studholme}@ucsf.edu
http://radiology.ucsf.edu/bicg
[2] Department of Radiology & Biomedical Imaging,
University of California San Francisco, San Francisco, CA 94143, USA
[3] LSIIT, UMR CNRS/ULP 7005, 67412 Illkirch, France

Abstract. Recently developed techniques for reconstruction of high-resolution 3D images from fetal MR scans allows us to study the morphometry of developing brain tissues in utero. However, existing adult brain analysis methods cannot be directly applied as the anatomy of the fetal brain is significantly different in terms of geometry and tissue morphology. We describe an approach to atlas-based segmentation of the fetal brain with particular focus on the delineation of the germinal matrix, a transient structure related to brain growth. We segment 3D images reconstructed from in utero clinical MR scans and measure volumes of different brain tissue classes for a group of fetal subjects at gestational age 20.5–22.5 weeks. We also include a partial validation of the approach using manual tracing of the germinal matrix at different gestational ages.

1 Introduction

Imaging of the human fetus using magnetic resonance (MR) imaging is emerging as an important clinical tool in the early detection of brain abnormalities [1,2]. The ability to evaluate morphometric measures of brain development that can be reliably derived from clinical imaging promises a range of new quantitative biomarkers that can be used in clinical evaluation of pregnancy and to form a better understanding of brain development [3,4]. Typical clinical MR image (MRI) acquired in utero is severely corrupted by motion of the fetus. Recently developed methods of image reconstruction using registration to correct for fetal motion [5,6,7] have permitted the formation of true 3D MR images of the fetal brain and have opened up the possibility of using methodology developed for adult brain image analysis to study the developing brain in utero. However, the underlying anatomy of the developing fetal brain is significantly different both in terms of geometry as well as underlying tissue morphology [8].

The fetal brain consists of a mixture of developed white matter and grey matter regions and other transient structures related to brain growth. One of the

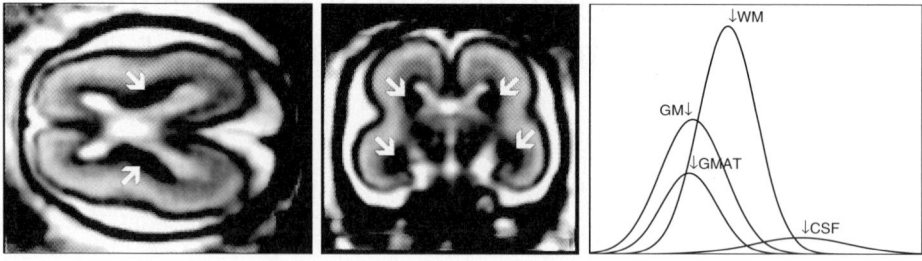

Fig. 1. Axial and coronal views of an MR T2w image with clearly visible hypointense regions of the germinal matrix. Distribution of voxel intensities for grey matter (GM), the germinal matrix (GMAT), white matter (WM), and cerebrospinal fluid (CSF).

most important of these is the germinal matrix, a deep brain region of developing cells adjacent to ventricules that is present in the fetal brain between 8 and 28 weeks gestational age (GA) [9,10]. During embryology and early fetal life, the germinal matrix is the site of production of both neurons and glial cells which then migrate out to their final location. Due to its high cell-packing density, the germinal matrix appears hypointense on T2-weighted (T2w) MR images as shown in Fig. 1. The volume of the germinal matrix increases exponentially reaching its peak at about 23–26 weeks GA and decreases subsequently [9,10]. There is little published material about the volume or the shape of the germinal matrix in normal fetuses and most of the work is derived from pathology [10]. The recent development of 3D MRI reconstruction techniques allows us to study the morphology and morphometry of developing tissues in utero. In this work we describe an approach to atlas-based tissue segmentation which is aimed at extracting key tissue regions from reconstructed 3D fetal MRI data, with particular focus on the delineation of the germinal matrix from developed white and grey matter regions.

2 Method

2.1 Problem Overview

Current clinical practice at our institution makes use of fast T2-weighted MR imaging to provide contrast for main tissue types in the fetal brain. Figure 1 illustrates the structures visible in this type of data. Segmentation of developing anatomy, even in neonates [11] and young children [12], is challenging due to evolving states of tissue and how this is reflected in MR images. In fetal imaging, there is a number of basic tissue states that are of interest including developed grey matter (GM) and white matter (WM), the germinal matrix (GMAT) and the coritcal plate (CP). As the germinal matrix generally appears with a similar intensity to the grey matter as shown in Fig. 1, its interpretation is dependent on the location around the ventricles. There are key areas where ventricles, GMAT and GM cortex are adjacent, particularly in regions of the parietal and occipital lobes. As some form of spatial context will be required to achieve meaningful segmentation, we approach the problem using an atlas-based tissue segmentation methodology.

2.2 MR Imaging Procedure

MR imaging was performed on a 1.5T scanner according to an IRB-approved protocol without sedation or contrast agent administration. A quick low-resolution localizer sequence was obtained during maternal free breathing to determine the location of the fetal head. Then, single-shot fast spin-echo (SSFSE) T2-weighted images were acquired using an eight channel torso phased array coil during normal maternal breathing. Based on the initial localizer, sets of contiguous slices were obtained in the approximately axial, coronal and sagittal planes with respect to the fetal brain. All images were acquired in an interleaved manner to reduce saturation of spins in adjacent slices. The following MR parameters were used: relaxation time TR ranging from 4000 ms to 8000 ms, effective echo time TE = 91 ms, flip angle 130°, in plane resolution 0.469mm × 0.469mm, slice thickness ≈ 3mm. These MR parameters were originally designed for clinical scans and have not been adjusted for tissue segmentation in this study or any other type of image analysis.

The following study was performed using clinical MR scans of 5 women at 20.5–22.5 weeks of pregnancy. The patients were referred for fetal MRI due to questionable abnormalities on prenatal ultrasound or a prior abnormal pregnancy. All women had normal fetal MRI and all newborns have had normal postnatal neurodevelopment.

2.3 Atlas Construction

To create a reference anatomy, a set of 3D high-resolution isotropic volumes (0.469mm × 0.469mm × 0.469mm) was formed from subject MR scans using the registration-based reconstruction technique [5]. An average shape and intensity image was constructed from these subject images by spatial normalization of the scans using a sequence of global linear registrations driven by normalized mutual information [13], followed by multiple elastic deformations driven by mutual information [14,15]. These were used to iteratively form an averagely shaped anatomy in an approach similar to [16]. The intensity of each scan was normalized and the spatially normalized images were averaged to form a high quality reference image. The reference average image was manually segmented into regions of white matter, grey matter, CSF, ventricular CSF and germinal matrix by expert observers. For this preliminary work, we have not delineated other subregions of white matter such as the cortical plate. Tissue label maps were extracted from the manual segmentation, convolved with a Gaussian kernel ($\sigma = 3.0 \times$ voxelsize) and normalized to simulate a probabilistic atlas shown in Fig. 2.

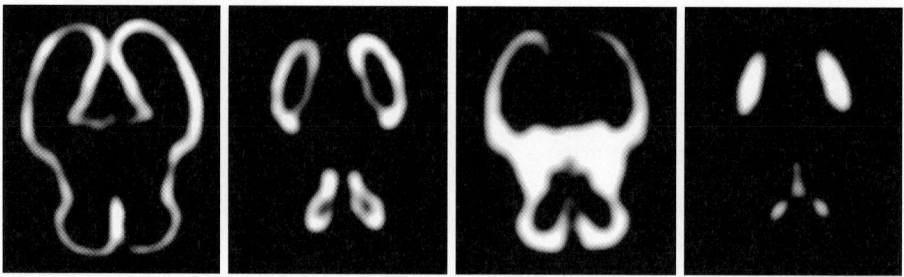

Fig. 2. Probabilistic atlas for grey matter, germinal matrix, white matter and cerebrospinal fluid (left to right, respectively) derived from the segmentation of the average MRI anatomy model

2.4 Volume Segmentation

General EM framework. Expectation-Maximization (EM) is a general technique for finding maximum likelihood estimates of model parameters in problems with missing data. The EM algorithm maximizes the likelihood of the observed data by interleaving the expectation step (E-step) which performs statistical classification of the observed data into K classes and the maximization step (M-step) which updates the current parameter estimation. In the context of brain MRI segmentation [17,18], the observed data are the voxel intensities $y = \{y_1, y_2, ..., y_N\}$, the missing data are the voxel labels $c = \{c_1, c_2, ..., c_N\}$ (image segmentation), and the model parameters are the class-conditional intensity distribution parameters $\theta = \{\theta_1, \theta_2, ..., \theta_K\}$.

Assuming that each voxel value is selected at random from one of the K classes and each class k is modeled by a Gaussian distribution $G_{\sigma_k}(y_i - \mu_k)$ [17] with mean μ_k and variance σ_k^2 ($\theta_k = \{\mu_k, \sigma_k\}$), the probability density that class k generated the voxel value y_i at position x_i is $p(y_i|k) = G_{\sigma_k}(y_i - \mu_k)$ and the corresponding class posterior probability $p(k|y_i)$ computed in the E-step is

$$p(k|y_i) = \frac{p(y_i|k)P(k)}{\sum_k p(y_i|k)P(k)} \quad (1)$$

where $P(k)$ is the prior probability for tissue class k. The estimation of current class distribution parameters in the M-step is performed according to

$$\mu_k = \frac{\sum_i p(k|y_i)y_i}{\sum_i p(k|y_i)} \qquad \sigma_k^2 = \frac{\sum_i p(k|y_i)(y_i - \mu_k)^2}{\sum_i p(k|y_i)} \quad (2)$$

and the intermediate segmentation of the MR image is given by voxel labels $c(x_i)$ assigned using the maximum posterior probability rule.

$$c(x_i) = \arg\max_k p(k|y_i) \quad (3)$$

Bias estimation. Intensity inhomogeneity or bias field can be major problems for automated MR image segmentation. Although it may not be visible for a human reader, such a bias may cause tissue mislabeling in intensity-based segmentation. This is particularly an issue for our fetal MR scans where we have an eight channel torso phased array coil.

Assuming a standard multiplicative bias model, intensity inhomogeneity is approximated by a linear combination of spatially smooth basis functions (low order polynomials). The bias field parameters are calculated in each iteration of the EM algorithm as the weighted least-squares fit to the difference between measured intensities y_i and predicted intensities $\tilde{y}_i$ calculated from intermediate estimates of class distribution parameters [19].

Prior probabilities. The independent segmentation model from Eqns. 1 and 2 performs labeling of MRI voxels based solely on their intensities y_i and assumes that different classes are well separated in the intensity space. This, however, is not the case for fetal brain segmentation where the overlap of intensities between tissue classes is substantial, especially for grey matter and germinal matrix, as shown in Fig. 1. Moreover, the resulting brain segmentation may be noisy or not anatomically feasible. To address these issues, we use the probabilistic atlas described in Section 2.3 to provide spatially varying class prior probabilities $P_a(k|x_i)$ at every voxel x_i.

The voxel labeling process is be further constrained by introduction of neighborhood dependencies where the probability that a voxel belongs to tissue k depends on the tissue types of its neighbors. We use an additional neighborhood-based prior $P_n(k|x_i)$ calculated from voxels x_j located not farther than d_k from x_i ($|x_i - x_j| \leq d_k$) and currently assigned to class k ($c(x_j) = k$).

$$P_n(k|x_i) = \sum_j \frac{P[c(x_j) = k]}{|x_i - x_j|^2} \quad \forall x_j : |x_i - x_j| \leq d_k \quad (4)$$

As a result, the prior probabilities $P(k)$ in Eqn. 1 become spatially varying as they are calculated from both the atlas and the neighborhood of the voxel.

$$P(k) = P(k|x_i) = P_a(k|x_i)P_n(k|x_i) \quad (5)$$

3 Results

High-resolution 3D volumes reconstructed from the subject scans were non-rigidly registered to the average anatomy model described in Section 2.3. The number of classes, $K = 6$, was selected to cover four types of brain tissue (GM, GMAT, WM, CSF) and two types of non-brain voxels (the fluid around the brain and the skull). Class probabilities $p(k|y_i)$ for brain tissues were initialized with values from the atlas and used to calculate initial estimates of intensity distribution parameters $\{\mu_k, \sigma_k\}$ according to Eqn. 2. The values of μ_k and σ_k for the two non-brain classes were copied from estimates for GM and CSF, respectively.

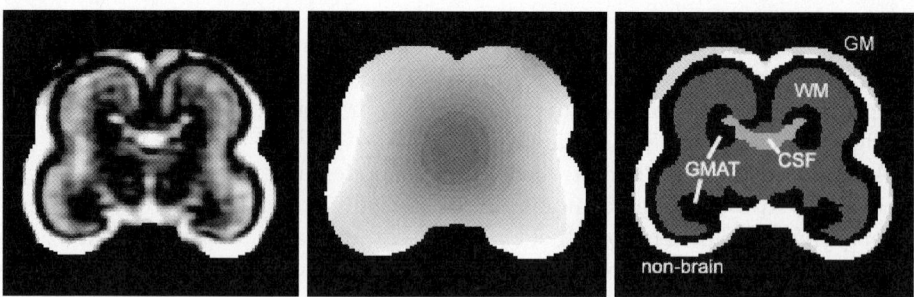

Fig. 3. A coronal view of the original MRI (left), bias field estimation (center) and final segmentation (right) for subject C

Table 1. Volumes of brain tissues (in mm^3) for fetal subjects of different gestational age (GA, in weeks) obtained from automatic and manual segmentation

Fetus	GA	automatic segmentation				man. seg.	rel. diff.
		CSF	GM	WM	GMAT	GMAT	GMAT
A	20.57	3155	13436	19287	4497	4920	8.6%
B	21.57	2831	13985	19555	4892	5229	6.4%
C	21.57	3588	18543	26549	6186	5872	5.3%
D	21.86	3223	20523	26215	6685	6495	2.9%
E	22.57	3894	18834	25339	6561	6146	6.7%

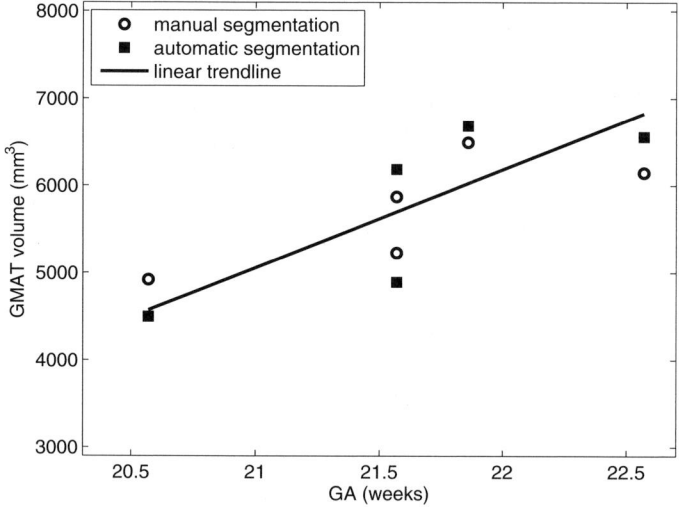

Fig. 4. The volume of germinal matrix (GMAT) for different gestational age (GA)

The segmentation was confined to regions where the atlas indicated the probability of any brain tissue to be larger than 0.01 as shown in Fig. 3. For each volume, 20 steps of the EM-based segmentation algorithm were performed as no significant changes were observed afterwards. Volumes of brain tissue were originally measured in the reference/atlas space and then corrected for the non-rigid transformation to achieve actual volumes in the original space of each subject. Additionally, the germinal matrix was manually traced for all fetal subjects by a field expert. The resulting tissue volumes and the relative difference between GMAT volumes obtained from automatic and manual segmentation are reported in Table 1.

4 Conclusions

In this paper we have described the development of the first in utero 3D MRI atlas of the human fetus which incorporates both developing and developed tissue classes. The approach builds on earlier work on 3D fetal image reconstruction techniques from clinical MRI data, making use of standard clinical protocols. This initial work has focussed on a narrow age range capturing the early brain development visible using MRI, with particular focus on extracting the germinal matrix, which is a key area of cell formation in the developing brain.

We have created an unbiased intensity and shape average template from a set of example MRI studies and formed an ideal segmentation of tissue classes in this reference anatomy. This is then used as a target for spatial normalization of individual scans to provide spatial priors for an EM-based segmentation scheme. We have automatically delineated 3D structures in the developing brain from clinically acquired MR images and have calculated volumes for both developed and transient tissue types.

The presented study will be further extended by analysis of other WM classes such as the cortical plate, incorporating manual tracing of multiple subjects in the probabilistic atlas and forming multiple atlases for different developmental stages.

References

1. Coakley, F.V., Glenn, O.A., Qayyum, A., Barkovich, A.J., Goldstein, R., Filly, R.A.: Fetal MRI: a developing technique for the developing patient. Am. J. Roentgenol. 182(1), 243–252 (2004)
2. Prayer, D., Kasprian, G., Krampl, E., Ulm, B., Witzani, L., Prayer, L., Brugger, P.C.: MRI of normal fetal brain development. Eur. J. Radiol. 57(2), 199–216 (2006)
3. Huppi, P.S., Warfield, S.K., Kikinis, R., Barnes, P.D., Zientara, G.P., Jolesz, F.A., Tsuji, M.K., Volpe, J.J.: Quantitative magnetic resonance imaging of brain development in premature and mature newborns. Ann. Neurol. 43(2), 224–235 (1998)
4. Grossman, R., Hoffman, C., Mardor, Y., Biegon, A.: Quantitative MRI measurements of human fetal brain development in utero. Neuroimage 33(2), 463–470 (2006)

5. Rousseau, F., Glenn, O.A., Iordanova, B., Rodriguez-Carranza, C., Vigneron, D.B., Barkovich, A.J., Studholme, C.: Registration-based approach for reconstruction of high-resolution in utero fetal MR brain images. Acad. Radiol. 13(9), 1072–1081 (2006)
6. Jiang, S., Xue, H., Glover, A., Rutherford, M., Rueckert, D., Hajnal, J.V.: MRI of moving subjects using multislice snapshot images with volume reconstruction (SVR): application to fetal, neonatal, and adult brain studies. IEEE Trans. Med. Imaging 26(7), 967–980 (2007)
7. Kim, K., Hansen, M.F., Habas, P.A., Rousseau, F., Glenn, O.A., Barkovich, A.J., Studholme, C.: Intersection-based registration of slice stacks to form 3d images of the human fetal brain. In: Proc. IEEE International Symposium on Biomedical Imaging: From Nano to Macro, Paris, France, pp. 1167–1170 (2008)
8. Kostovic, I., Judas, M., Rados, M., Hrabac, P.: Laminar organization of the human fetal cerebrum revealed by histochemical markers and magnetic resonance imaging. Cereb. Cortex 12(5), 536–544 (2002)
9. Battin, M.R., Maalouf, E.F., Counsell, S.J., Herlihy, A.H., Rutherford, M.A., Azzopardi, D., Edwards, A.D.: Magnetic resonance imaging of the brain in very preterm infants: visualization of the germinal matrix, early myelination, and cortical folding. Pediatrics 101(6), 957–962 (1998)
10. Kinoshita, Y., Okudera, T., Tsuru, E., Yokota, A.: Volumetric analysis of the germinal matrix and lateral ventricles performed using MR images of postmortem fetuses. Am. J. Neuroradiol. 22(2), 382–388 (2001)
11. Prastawa, M., Gilmore, J.H., Lin, W., Gerig, G.: Automatic segmentation of MR images of the developing newborn brain. Med. Image Anal. 9(5), 457–466 (2005)
12. Murgasova, M., Dyet, L., Edwards, D., Rutherford, M., Hajnal, J., Rueckert, D.: Segmentation of brain MRI in young children. Acad. Radiol. 14(11), 1350–1366 (2007)
13. Studholme, C., Hill, D.L.G., Hawkes, D.J.: An overlap invariant entropy measure of 3D medical image alignment. Pattern Recognit. 32(1), 71–86 (1999)
14. Collignon, A., Maes, F., Delaere, D., Vandermeulen, D., Suetens, P., Marchal, G.: Automated multi-modality image registration based on information theory. In: Proc. Information Processing in Medical Imaging, Brest, France, pp. 263–274 (1995)
15. Viola, P., Wells, W.M.: Alignment by maximization of mutual information. Int. J. Comput. Vis. 24(2), 137–154 (1997)
16. Guimond, A., Meunier, J., Thirion, J.P.: Average brain models: a convergence study. Comput. Vis. Image Underst. 77(2), 192–210 (2000)
17. Wells, W.M., Grimson, W.E.L., Kikinis, R., Jolesz, F.A.: Adaptive segmentation of MRI data. IEEE Trans. Med. Imaging 15(4), 429–442 (1996)
18. Van Leemput, K., Maes, F., Vandermeulen, D., Suetens, P.: Automated model-based tissue classification of MR images of the brain. IEEE Trans. Med. Imaging 18(10), 897–908 (1999)
19. Van Leemput, K., Maes, F., Vandermeulen, D., Suetens, P.: Automated model-based bias field correction of MR images of the brain. IEEE Trans. Med. Imaging 18(10), 885–896 (1999)

Segmenting Brain Tumors Using Pseudo–Conditional Random Fields

Chi-Hoon Lee[1,4], Shaojun Wang[2], Albert Murtha[3], Matthew R.G. Brown[1], and Russell Greiner[1]

[1] Department of Computing Science, University of Alberta, Canada
{chihoon,mbrown,greiner}@cs.ualberta.ca
[2] Department of Computing Science, Wright State University, USA
shaojun.wang@wright.edu
[3] Cross Cancer Institute, University of Alberta, Canada
albertmu@cancerboard.ab.ca
[4] Yahoo! Inc, USA
chihoon@yahoo-inc.com

Abstract. Locating Brain tumor segmentation within MR (magnetic resonance) images is integral to the treatment of brain cancer. This segmentation task requires classifying each voxel as either tumor or non-tumor, based on a description of that voxel. Unfortunately, standard classifiers, such as Logistic Regression (LR) and Support Vector Machines (SVM), typically have limited accuracy as they treat voxels as *independent* and *identically distributed* (*iid*). Approaches based on random fields, which are able to incorporate spatial constraints, have recently been applied to brain tumor segmentation with notable performance improvement over iid classifiers. However, previous random field systems involved computationally intractable formulations, which are typically solved using some approximation. Here, we present *pseudo-conditional random fields* (PCRFs), which achieve accuracy similar to other random fields variants, but are significantly more efficient. We formulate a PCRF as a regularized discriminative classifier that relaxes the classification decision for each voxel by considering the labels and features of neighboring voxels.

1 Introduction

Segmenting brain tumors in magnetic resonance (MR) images involves classifying each voxel as tumor or non-tumor [1,2,3]. This task, a prerequisite for treating brain cancer using radiation therapy, is typically done by hand by expert medical doctors, who find this process laborious and time-consuming. Replacing this manual effort with a good automated classifier would save doctors time; the resulting labels may also be more accurate, or at least more consistent.

We treat this as a binary classification task, using a classifier to map each MR image voxel described as a vector of values $\mathbf{x} \in \Re^d$ to a bit $y \in \{+1, -1\}$, corresponding to either tumor or non-tumor. We first *learn* this classifier from a set of data instances $\{\langle \mathbf{x}_i, y_i \rangle\}_i$ [4]. Here, we focus on *probabilistic classifiers* that actually return a class likelihood value $P(y = +1 \mid \mathbf{x}) \in [0,1]$ for each voxel; our classifier can then return $+1$ (tumor) if $P(y = +1 \mid \mathbf{x}) \geq 0.5$. In general, given an entire $n \times m$ image, our classifier will seek the most likely labeling over $\{-1, +1\}^{n \times m}$: $\mathbf{Y}^{(*)} = \operatorname{argmax}_{\mathbf{Y}} P(\mathbf{Y} \mid \mathbf{X})$. (This use of probabilities distinguishes these approaches from many other segmentation approaches, such as those based on variational and level set techniques [5,6].)

Standard machine learners, such as Naïve Bayes, logistic regression (LR), and support vector machines (SVMs), produce effective classifiers in many domains [7,8]. However, these algorithms assume that the individual instances are iid. This is appropriate if the instances correspond to, say, a patients in a study, as finding that one patient responds well to some treatment does not mean that the next patient will also respond well. However, this assumption is problematic in our current situation, where each instance corresponds to a voxel: Here, finding that one voxel is labeled a tumor strongly suggests that its neighbors will have a similar label; similarly non-tumor voxels tends to be next to other non-tumor voxels. Algorithms that assume the data is iid typically perform poorly when the data is not, which is why these algorithms do relatively poorly at segmentation tasks.

This has motivated researchers to apply Markov Random Fields (MRFs; [9]) and Conditional Random Fields (CRFs; [10]) to various segmentation tasks. These techniques are able to represent complex dependencies among data instances, giving them higher accuracy on the segmentation task than iid classifiers [11,12]. However, these random field approaches are based on computationally intractable formulations. Although there are approximation techniques that can deal with these computational challenges, CRF variants such as Discriminative Random Fields (DRFs) and Support Vector Random Fields (SVRFs) still require computationally expensive learning procedures [11,13].

In this paper, we present a novel supervised learning system, PCRF, that can efficiently produce high-quality segmenters, incorporating spatial constraints among MR image voxels. PCRF can be viewed as a regularized iid discriminative classifier that is first trained assuming the data is iid; this makes the training computationally efficient. It then relaxes the iid assumption during inference, by including a regularizing term that uses the class labels and feature vectors of neighboring voxels of a given voxel. We demonstrate that PCRF is robust and efficient by illustrating its performance at segmenting MR images of the brains of tumor patients. We show that PCRF is significantly more accurate than the corresponding base iid classifiers, and is significantly more efficient that other random field methods during training, while producing similar accuracy.

Section 2 reviews related work, including random field models. Section 3 introducing our framework and novel PCRF system. Section 4 presents experiments that empirically demonstrate the efficiency and effectiveness of our model.

2 Background

We view brain tumor segmentation on a 2D MR image as classifying each image voxel as either tumor or non-tumor. The challenge is finding the most likely configuration of (tumor vs. non-tumor) labels $\mathbf{Y} = (y_1, y_2, \ldots, y_r) \in \{-1, +1\}^r$ for the voxels of a 2D MR image $\mathbf{X} = (\mathbf{x}_1, \mathbf{x}_2, \ldots, \mathbf{x}_r)$, where each set ranges over the set of indices S of all voxels in the $r = m \times n$ image, each $y_i \in \{-1, +1\}$ is the label for voxel i, and $\mathbf{x}_i$ is the feature vector for voxel i.

A pair-wise MRF is formulated as

$$P(\mathbf{Y} \mid \mathbf{X}) \propto P(\mathbf{Y}, \mathbf{X}) = \frac{1}{Z(\mathbf{X})} \exp\left(\sum_{i \in S} D(\mathbf{x}_i, y_i) + \sum_{i \in S} \sum_{j \in N_i} V(y_i, y_j)\right) \quad (1)$$

where $D(\mathbf{x}_i, y_i)$ corresponds to the local log likelihood $\log(P(\mathbf{x}_i \mid y_i))$ of $\mathbf{x}_i$ given a class label y_i; $V(y_i, y_j)$ is a potential function that explicitly encodes the dependencies between labels at i and its neighbor j, based on N_i, which is the set of voxels neighboring $\mathbf{x}_i$. $Z(\mathbf{X})$ is a normalizing factor to make the formulation a probability distribution. We can read-off the MRF assumptions from Equation 1: that the voxels are conditionally independent given their class labels, and that spatial correlations are modelled based only on the labels of neighboring voxels (y_i and y_j) but not on the observations ($\mathbf{x}_i$ and $\mathbf{x}_j$). These factors limit the advantages of using MRFs to model spatial dependencies in MR images [11,12,13].

CRFs attempt to overcome these disadvantages by relaxing the conditional independence assumption and incorporating observations into the formulation of spatial dependencies.

$$P(\mathbf{Y} \mid \mathbf{X}) = \frac{1}{Z(\mathbf{X})} \exp\left(\sum_{i \in S} A(y_i, \mathbf{X}) + \sum_{i \in S} \sum_{j \in N_i} I(y_i, y_j, \mathbf{X})\right) \quad (2)$$

where $A(y_i, \mathbf{X})$ corresponds to the *conditional* probability distribution (while the MRF's $D(\mathbf{x}_i, y_i)$ corresponds to the log conditional probability), and the $I(y_i, y_j, \mathbf{X})$ term incorporates observations of data instances (unlike MRF's $V(y_i, y_j)$ which does not). The Discriminative Random Field (DRF) is a variant of the CRF that performs robustly in 2D image region classification problems [13]. The Support Vector Random Field (SVRF) is a modification of DRFs that address high dimensional feature vectors and imbalanced datasets effectively [11].

Unfortunately, DRFs and SVRFs are computationally expensive, especially during learning, as their computations are exponential in the number of data points. This is basically due to their need to compute the partition function, corresponding to the $Z(\mathbf{X})$ in Equation 2. (Note that Gaussian assumption of MRF makes $Z(\mathbf{X})$ in Equation 1 simpler.) This has led to many approximation methods, such as pseudo-likelihood, contrastive divergence, and pseudo-marginal approximation [10,13,14,12]. Unfortunately these approximations reduce the accuracy of the learned segementor. This motivated *Decoupled Conditional Random Fields* (DCRFs [15]), which speed up the CRF-based computation by approximating a CRF as the combination of two classifiers that are each trained separately. As the DCRF framework searches for the parameter values that optimize each model separately, the combined parameter values are not necessarily globally optimal.

3 Pseudo Conditional Random Fields – PCRFs

The PCRF framework attempts to obtain the advantage of both the MRF and CRF approaches by relaxing the iid assumption of a simple discriminative classifier by adding a regularization term. We want to find the most-likely labelling $P_\theta(\mathbf{Y}\,|\,\mathbf{X}) = \prod_{i\in S} P_\theta(y_i\,|\,\mathbf{X}, \mathbf{Y}-y_i)$. Given feature vectors (observations) $\mathbf{x}_i$ for each voxel i as well as the class labels y_{N_i} over neighboring voxels $j \in N_i$, the PCRF formulation defines

$$P_\theta(y_i\,|\,\mathbf{x}_i, \mathbf{x}_{N_i}, y_{N_i}) = \psi_\theta(\mathbf{x}_i, y_i) \times \prod_{j\in N_i} \phi^o(\mathbf{x}_i, \mathbf{x}_j) \times \phi^c(y_i, y_j), \quad (3)$$

where the potential functions $\phi^o(\mathbf{x}_i, \mathbf{x}_j)$ quantifies the similarity of the feature vectors for voxels i and j, and $\phi^c(y_i, y_j)$ models the interactions between the two class labels y_i and y_j. We can adjust $\phi^c(.)$ to alter the degree of continuity with respect to class labels expected by the model; e.g., if we set ϕ^c to give high weight when neighboring voxels share the same class label, then the resulting PCRF will prefer having the same class labels among neighboring voxels. Alternatively, setting $\phi^o \equiv 1$ and $\phi^c \equiv 1$ would remove all spatial dependencies, leading to an iid classifier. Note we use a fixed pair of potential functions: here we set $\phi^o(\mathbf{x}_i, \mathbf{x}_j) = \mathbf{x}_i^T \mathbf{x}_j$, as the similarity measure between neighboring voxels; note this measure is maximum value when the two vectors are co-linear. We also set $\phi^c(y_i, y_j) = \alpha$ if $y_i \equiv y_j$, and $1 - \alpha$ otherwise, where α weighs the continuity of identical class labels. Here we used $\alpha = 0.6$.

For now, we define $\psi_\theta(\mathbf{x}_i, y_i) = \sigma(\theta^T \mathbf{x}_i) = \frac{1}{1+exp(-\theta^T \mathbf{x}_i)}$ as a simple logistic regression classifier. We chose a discriminative approach rather than a generative one because the former empirically shows better performance than the latter [8].

Learning. Learning the PCRF parameters is more efficient than for other CRF variants as a PCRF needs to fit only the parameter vector θ for a local potential function $\psi_\theta(.)$, which does not involve any spatial interactions. Here, we use the standard way to maximize the conditional log-likelihood $\theta^{(*)} = \arg\max_\theta \sum_{i\in S} \left[y_i \log \sigma(\theta^T \mathbf{x}_i) + (1 - y_i) \log(1 - \sigma(\theta^T \mathbf{x}_i)) \right]$.

Inference. The PCRF inference process incorporates regularization based on neighbor relationships. In general, the objective of inference is to maximize the log likelihood:

$$\mathbf{Y}^* = \arg\max_{\mathbf{Y}} \log P(\mathbf{Y}\,|\,\mathbf{X})$$

$$= \arg\max_{\mathbf{Y}} \sum_{i\in S} \log \psi_\theta(\mathbf{x}_i, y_i) + \sum_{i\in S}\sum_{j\in N_i} \log \phi^c(\mathbf{x}_i, \mathbf{x}_j) + \log \phi^o(y_i, y_j) \quad (4)$$

The graph cuts algorithm solves image pixel classification tasks by minimizing an energy function when spatial correlations among pixels are independent of the observations; this involves using linear programming to find the max-flow/min-cut on a graph whose nodes correspond to voxels and edges correspond to connections between neighboring voxels [16]. We reformulate this graph cuts approach to apply to our PCRF framework (Equation 4), where neighbor relationships are dependent on both the labels and the observations (feature vectors).

4 Brain Tumor Segmentation

We applied our PCRF model to the challenging real world problem of segmenting brain tumors in MR images. Since a PCRF can be viewed as a regularized discriminative iid classifier, we first show the differences between PCRF and its degenerate iid classifier – LR.

To quantify the performance of each model, we used the percentage Jaccard score $J = 100 \times \frac{TP}{(TP+FP+FN)}$, where TP denotes the number of true positives, FP false positives, and FN false negatives, taken over the entire image. We used this score for brain tumor segmentation task as this data is very imbalanced in that only a small percentage of voxels are in the "tumor" class; hence scores like "accuracy" would be high as the "true negative" class is typically huge.

We applied several different models – LR, PCRF, SVRF – to the task of classifying MR image slices, where each slice is defined with 258 by 258 pixels, each of which is described using 33 features [17]. We considered data from 11 patients with brain tumors; for each patient, we annotated each voxel with values based on three different MR imaging modalities: *T1*, *T2*, and *T1 with gadolinium contrast*("T1c"). We focus on 2D images; this is sufficient to illustrate the challenges as the neighborhood structure here involves cycles, which makes both inference and learning procedures computationally challenging[1]. Testing and training were done in a patient-specific manner: for each patient, each algorithm was trained on a subset of the patient's data, then tested on another (disjoint) subset. This is similar to the approach taken in many other studies of automatic brain tumor segmentation such as [18,19,20,21].

Our systems attempted to segment the "enhancing" tumor area — the region that appears bright on T1c images. Note that it is not sufficient to simply threshold T1c images by "brightness" because other tissues can have the same range of intensities. In the case of glioblastomas with necrotic cores, which appear dark on T1 images, we defined the enhancing rim of the tumor as well as the dark necrotic core as the target tumor region.

Fig. 1 shows one example of segmentation results. One test and its correct label ("ground truth") slice are shown in first two columns respectively. The result from LR, shown in third from Fig. 1, indicates that LR correctly classifies the tumor region but that it also misclassifies several small non-tumor regions as "tumor". PCRF's result, which appears on the far right, is more accurate. (See [22] for the complete set of larger images.)

Fig. 2(a) presents the Jaccard percentage scores from the 11 studies, where points above the diagonal line denote instances in which the PCRF performed better than its degenerative model, LR. Overall, the PCRF's accuracy was statistically significantly higher than LR's at $p < 0.005$ on a paired sample t-test.

---

[1] We are beginning to explore extending this approach to 3D, which involves simply redefining the neighborhood structure.

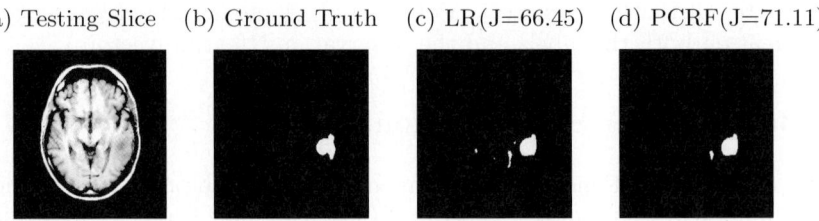

(a) Testing Slice (b) Ground Truth (c) LR(J=66.45) (d) PCRF(J=71.11)

Fig. 1. Classification results. The PCRF shows almost 4% improvement of Jaccard score over LR.

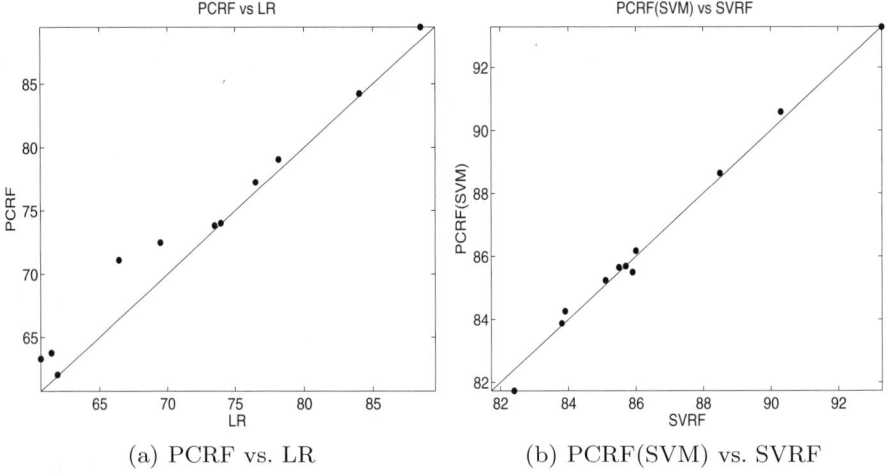

(a) PCRF vs. LR   (b) PCRF(SVM) vs. SVRF

Fig. 2. Jaccard Scores (percentage)

We also compared our PCRF system with the state-of-the-art CRF variant, the Support Vector Random Field (SVRF [11]), whose potential functions are based on Support Vector Machines (SVMs). Here, we implemented PCRF(SVM), which differed from the PCRF system only by using an SVM to compute the $\psi(\mathbf{x}, y)$ (from Equation 4) which models the relationship between a voxel's feature vector and its label. An SVM produces the distance between a hyperplane and a data instance as its decision value $f_{SVM}(\mathbf{x}_i) \in (-\infty, +\infty)$. To normalize this unbounded range, we fit this value to a sigmoid function: $g_{\beta_0,\beta_1}(\mathbf{x}) = P(y = +1 \mid \mathbf{x}) = \frac{1}{1+\exp(\beta_0+\beta_1(\mathbf{x}))}$, estimating the parameters β_0 and β_1 from the training data $\{(f_{SVM}(\mathbf{x}_i), y_i)\}_i$ [11]. Figure 2(b) compares the percentage Jaccard scores of PCRF(SVM)[2] vs SVRF. It is clear that PCRF(SVM) is comparable with SVRF.

We next considered the timing. As our PCRF did not need to learn parameters for its spatial correlation model, we anticipated it would be significantly faster

---

[2] PCRF(SVM) outperformed the SVM, which is a robust i.i.d. classifier ($p < 0.001$); see [22] for details.

during the learning stage. The learning times (average across 11 patients, in seconds) confirm this:

	DRF	SVRF	DCRF	PCRF
Tumor segmentation	1697	1276	63	**38**

Our PCRF was over 40 times faster than the DRF and over 30 times faster than the SVRF ($p < 10^{-37}$ and $p < 10^{-29}$, paired-samples t-tests for DRFs and SVRFs, respectively). Even DCRF, known as the fastest CRF variant, is significantly slower than our PCRF ($p < 10^{-26}$).

5 Conclusion

We found that the PCRF(SVM) system, which uses a linear SVM to map from voxel to label, worked effectively. We might be able to obtain further performance improvements by using a non-linear kernel function. In addition, we might be able to produce a more robust model by incorporating a prior $P(\theta)$ over θ to further reduce the possibility of overfitting. We are extending this work to develop effective systems to overcome the limitations of patient-specific training, by taking advantage of semi-supervised learning principles.

Contributions. This paper has presented the Pseudo Conditional Random Field (PCRF) model, a CRF-inspired formulation that incorporates a specified potential function to model the relationships between neighboring voxels. Our PCRF is fast to train as it does not need to fit parameters that model the neighbor relationships. It can be viewed as a regularized iid classifier, whose classification decisions for each pixel involve the labels and features of neighboring voxels. Thus, during inference, PCRF avoids the iid assumption, which is inappropriate for image segmentation tasks. We demonstrate that PCRF is effective by showing it can effectively segment brain tumors from MR images, achieving state-of-the-art segmentation results, but at a small fraction of the training time.

Acknowledgments. R. Greiner is supported by NSERC and the Alberta Ingenuity Centre for Machine Learning (AICML). C-H Lee is supported by the AICML. M. Brown is supported by Alberta Cancer Board. Our thanks to Dale Schuurmans for helpful discussions on problem formulation and to BTAP members for help in data processing.

References

1. Corso, J.J., Sharon, E., Yuille, A.L.: Multilevel segmentation and integrated bayesian model classification with an application to brain tumor segmentation. In: Larsen, R., Nielsen, M., Sporring, J. (eds.) MICCAI 2006. LNCS, vol. 4191, pp. 790–798. Springer, Heidelberg (2006)

2. Gering, D.T.: Diagonalized nearest neighbor pattern matching for brain tumor segmentation. In: Ellis, R.E., Peters, T.M. (eds.) MICCAI 2003. LNCS, vol. 2879, pp. 670–677. Springer, Heidelberg (2003)
3. Corso, J.J., Sharon, E., Dube, S., El-Saden, S., Sinha, U., Yuille, A.: Efficient Multilevel Brain Tumor Segmentation with Integrated Bayesian Model Classification. IEEE Transactions on Medical Imaging 27(5), 629–640 (2008)
4. Mitchell, T.: Machine Learning. McGraw-Hill, New York (1997)
5. Liu, J., Udupa, J.K., Odhner, D., Hackney, D., Moonis, G.: A system for brain tumor volume estimation via mr imaging and fuzzy connectedness. Computational Medical Imaging and Graphics 29(1), 21–34 (2005)
6. Cobzas, D., Birkbeck, N., Schmidt, M., Jagersand, M., Murtha, A.: A 3D variational brain tumor segmentation using a high dimensional feature set. In: MMBIA (2007)
7. Joachims, T.: Making large-scale svm learning practical. In: Scholkopf, B., Burges, C., Smola, A. (eds.) Advances in Kernel Methods - Support Vector Learning. MIT Press, Cambridge (1999)
8. Ng, A., Jordan, M.: On discriminative vs. generative classifiers: A comparison of logistic regression and naive bayes. In: NIPS, vol. 14 (2002)
9. Li, S.Z.: Markov Random Field Modeling in Image Analysis. Springer, Tokyo (2001)
10. Lafferty, J., Pereira, F., McCallum, A.: Conditional random fields: Probabilistic models for segmenting and labeling sequence data. In: ICML (2001)
11. Lee, C.H., Greiner, R., Schmidt, M.: Support vector random fields for spatial classification. In: Jorge, A.M., Torgo, L., Brazdil, P.B., Camacho, R., Gama, J. (eds.) PKDD 2005. LNCS (LNAI), vol. 3721, pp. 121–132. Springer, Heidelberg (2005)
12. Lee, C.H., Wang, S., Jiao, F., Schuurmans, D., Greiner, R.: Learning to model spatial dependency: Semi-supervised discriminative random fields. In: NIPS, vol. 19 (2007)
13. Kumar, S., Hebert, M.: Discriminative fields for modeling spatial dependencies in natural images. In: NIPS (2003)
14. Kumar, S., August, J., Hebert, M.: Exploiting inference for approximate parameter learning in discriminative fields: An empirical study. In: Rangarajan, A., Vemuri, B.C., Yuille, A.L. (eds.) EMMCVPR 2005. LNCS, vol. 3757, pp. 153–168. Springer, Heidelberg (2005)
15. Lee, C.H., Greiner, R., Zaiane, O.R.: Efficient spatial classification using decoupled conditional random fields. In: Fürnkranz, J., Scheffer, T., Spiliopoulou, M. (eds.) PKDD 2006. LNCS (LNAI), vol. 4213, pp. 272–283. Springer, Heidelberg (2006)
16. Boykov, Y., Veksler, O., Zabih, R.: Fast approximate energy minimization via graph cuts. In: ICCV, pp. 377–384 (1999)
17. Schmidt, M.: Automatic brain tumor segmentation. Master's thesis, University of Alberta (2005)
18. Garcia, C., Moreno, J.: Kernel based method for segmentation and modeling of magnetic resonance images. In: Lemaître, C., Reyes, C.A., González, J.A. (eds.) IBERAMIA 2004. LNCS (LNAI), vol. 3315, pp. 636–645. Springer, Heidelberg (2004)
19. Zhang, J., Ma, K., Er, M., Chong, V.: Tumor segmentation from magnetic resonance imaging by learning via one-class support vector machine. In: Int. Workshop on Advanced Image Technology, pp. 207–211 (2004)
20. Chen, T., Metaxas, D.N.: Gibbs prior models, marching cubes, and deformable models: A hybrid framework for 3d medical image segmentation. In: Ellis, R.E., Peters, T.M. (eds.) MICCAI 2003. LNCS, vol. 2879, pp. 703–710. Springer, Heidelberg (2003)
21. Kaus, M., Warfield, S., Nabavi, A., Black, P., Jolesz, F., Kikinis, R.: Automated segmentation of MR images of brain tumors. Radiology 218, 586–591 (2001)
22. http://www.cs.ualberta.ca/~btap/research/pcrf/ (2008)

Localized Priors for the Precise Segmentation of Individual Vertebras from CT Volume Data

Hong Shen[1], Andrew Litvin[2], and Christopher Alvino[1]

[1] Siemens Corporate Research, Inc., 755 College Road East, Princeton, NJ 08540
{shen.hong,christopher.alvinvo}@siemens.com
[2] Analogic Corporation, 8 Centennial Drive, Peabody, MA 01960
alitvin@analogic.com

Abstract. We present algorithms for the automatic and precise segmentation of individual vertebras in CT Volume data. When a local surface evolution method such as the level set is applied to such a complex structure, global shape priors will not be sufficient to avoid the leakage and local minima problems, particularly if precise object boundary is desired. We propose a prior knowledge base that contains localized priors—a group of high-level features whose detection will augment the surface model and be the key to success. Base on this a set of context blockers are applied to prevent the leakages. Carefully designed initial surface when registered with the data helps avoid the local minimum problem. The results of segmentation well approximate the human delineated object boundaries. We also present the validation result of the segmentation of 150 vertebras.

1 Introduction

The vertebra in high-contrast CT images as shown in Fig.1(a)-(i) represents a type of 3D structure that is complex yet prominent. The images differ from many other medical images, such as organs in MR or Ultrasound data, in which the shape is relatively simple, but with obscure boundaries even for a human observer. The vertebra in CT data has well-defined boundaries from a human observer's point of view, in that an educated observer can perform consistent and relatively precise delineation of the object boundaries on 2D slice images. On the other hand, the boundaries when viewed in detail are full of challenges for any segmentation algorithm. The vertebra of interest is usually adjacent or even connected to neighboring structures that have similar intensities. The internal regions are highly inhomogeneous, and the weak and diffused boundaries contain many gaps. Segmentation of the vertebra is also a typical 3D problem not to be solved on a slice-by-slice basis, due to the large variation of 2D cross-sectional shape from the 3D structural complexity, as shown in Fig.1(e)-(i). To appreciate the complexity, our timing for a human observer to delineate the 2D boundaries of a single vertebra slice-by-slice using a digital tablet is typically around 45 minutes.

The segmentation of the vertebra is of high importance to orthopedic applications. Interactive [1] and automatic methods were reported [2-5]. For an overview please see

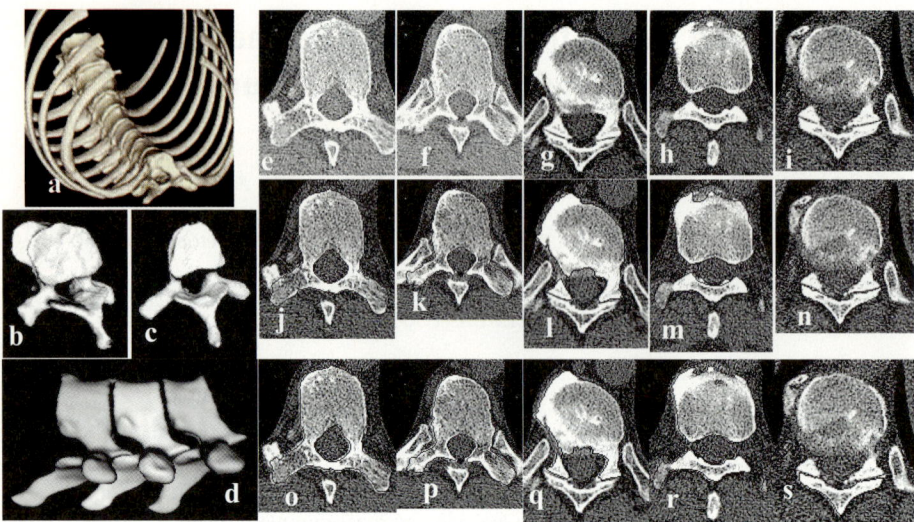

Fig. 1. 3D views of (a) the vertebras and rib structures form the thoracic cage. (b)(c) two segmented vertebras (d) three individually segmented and adjacent vertebras. (e)-(i): Cross-sections of one vertebra on sample axial slices, together with its neighboring vertebra and rib structures. (j)-(n): Corresponding 2D boundaries of the vertebra of interest delineated by a human observer on axial slices. The regions not enclosed by the boundaries belong to a neighboring vertebra or rib structure.(o)-(s) 2D boundaries of the vertebra segmented by the automatic algorithm.

Naegel [3]. None of the works however were able to automatically and precisely segment the complete individual vertebras from the complex neighboring structures.

In our previous work [6], we presented a preliminary solution for such a problem. We also discussed the problems of such typical method as described in [7], in which the level set is constrained by a global PCA model. The summary of discussion is as follows. First, the high consistency of human manual segmentation (Fig. 1(j)-(n)) requires precise matching of the auto-segmentation (Fig. 1(o)-(s)) to the actual object boundary, including any pathological deformation (e.g. Fig. 1(g); We recently measured the typical consistency between two independent human observers on the manual segmentation of a vertebra as over 94%). Second, a representative PCA model space covering the high variation and complex structure as well as unpredictable pathologies is theoretically and practically unachievable. Third, therefore we cannot solve the leakage and local minimum problem of level set using tight constraints from a global PCA model. Fourth, adding the model force and local image force together--and using a global multiplier to adjust relative strength [7] --creates competition between global model and local data forces. The dilemma lies in whether the model should be made stronger to prevent leakage or weaker to allow the surface convergence to the local data that is not covered in the incomplete model space. From the above, we believe the global model should serve as the optimal initialization for the level set rather than as a soft constraint applied during surface evolution. In this paper, we further propose the concept of *localized priors* that will guide the level set to avoid leakage and local minima at the places where most necessary.

2 Methods

2.1 The Mean Shape Model and the Vertebra Coordinate System

As shown in Fig. 2(a), the centerline of the spinal canal formed by the central cavity of all the vertebras was automatically extracted. Our system also fitted a set of planes to the inter-vertebral disc spaces at every interface of the adjacent vertebra bodies. The automated extraction of the spinal cord and inter-vertebra planes from a CT volume are yet to be detailed in a future publication. On any vertebra, a vertebra coordinate system (O, u_x, u_y, u_z) can be defined from the extracted local centerline section and the top and bottom inter-vertebra planes, as shown in Fig. 2(b). The spinal canal centerline makes two intersections T and B at the top and bottom inter-vertebra planes, and we define the origin O as the middle point of T and B. We define the z-axis unit vector u_z as the average of the two plane normals. On the plane orthogonal to u_z and passing through O, u_y is defined as the symmetrical axis of the 2D image on the plane. This comes from the 2D axial symmetric property of the vertebra and the rib structures. u_x is obtained by applying the right-hand rule. The scales on the three directions can be computed from the original axial, coronal, and sagittal resolutions.

We manually segmented a small number of vertebras and registered the surfaces of the vertebras such that u_x, u_y, u_z and O of all the vertebras coincided. In this common coordinate system, we constructed from the transformed surfaces a set of signed distance functions $S = \{\phi_1, \phi_2, ..., \phi_n\}$ such that the vertebra surfaces were represented as $\Gamma = \{\vec{x} \mid \vec{x} \in R^3, \phi(\vec{x}) = 0\}$. The mean shape shown in Fig. 2(b) was constructed as

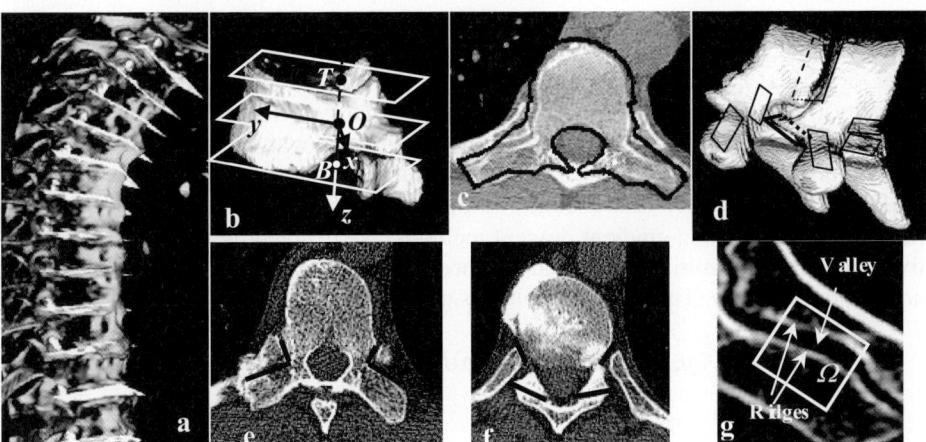

Fig. 2. (a) Spinal canal centerline and inter-vertebra planes overlaid on the spine. (b) The vertebra coordinate system based on the mean shape model. (c) The mean shape registered to data being used as the initial front. (d) Plane models at object interfaces representing high-level context features registered with the shape model. (e)(f) The axial projections of the plane models (g) Sandwich structure of the interface and the search ROI for the plane fitting.

$$\bar{\phi} = \frac{1}{n}\sum_{i=1}^{n}\phi_i \qquad (1)$$

The mean shape model was not intended to cover the shape variation among the vertebras, but it can be used to construct the initial front for level set evolution. Prior to the level set evolution, the whole data volume is automatically divided into volume of interests (VOI) centered at the vertebras, using the inter-vertebra planes (Fig. 2(a)) as references. The mean shape model was transformed into each of the VOI's. The registered surface was augmented such that its surface is close to and outside of the vertebra boundaries. [6] The augmented shape as shown in Fig. 2c was used as the initial front, thus to avoid the energy minimums inside the vertebra from the start.

2.2 Localized Priors

At the interfaces between two bright bone regions, where level set leakage usually occurred due to close contact of the surfaces, we defined plane models as illustrated in Fig. 2(d)-(f). These plane models were approximations of the curved surfaces at these interfaces, and we record them as high-level context features in the vertebra coordinate system associated with the mean shape model. In contrast to a global shape model, they represent prior knowledge at key locations and therefore are *localized priors*. The plane model was a simple and hence more robust representation, even though the interface may actually be a curved surface.

Given a VOI, the localized priors were transformed together with the mean shape model. In the local neighborhood of each mapped prior, we applied 3D steer-able filter [8] to detect the local primitives. We tuned the steer-able filter such that it only detected the primitives with orientations in the neighborhood of the prior orientation, thus reducing the noise and irrelevant primitives. We also switched the parameters of the steer-able filter to detect edges, ridges, and valleys, respectively. [8] As can be seen on Fig.2(g), the typical interface was a sandwich structure, with two layers of intensity ridges and one intensity valley between the two ridges. Instead of only fitting the plane model to the valley, three parallel planes with a fixed distance s apart were jointly fitted to the sandwich structure to improve robustness.

The search for the optimal location of the planes was conducted in a limited local neighborhood Ω, using gradient descent method. We denoted the set of valley primitives as V, ridge primitives as R, and the three sandwich planes to be detected as L, L^s and L^{-s}, respectively. The cost function was given by

$$E = \sum_{p \in V \cap \Omega} S_V(p)D(p,L) + 0.5 \sum_{p \in R \cap \Omega} S_R(p)D(p,L^s) + 0.5 \sum_{p \in R \cap \Omega} S_R(p)D(p,L^{-s}) \qquad (2)$$

where $S_V(p)$ and $S_R(p)$ were the filter responses of the valley and ridge primitives, respectively. $D(p, L)$ was the robust distance computed from the Euclidean point-to-plane distance $d(p, L)$ through differentiable p-norm with cut-off re-descending:

$$D(p,L) = \begin{cases} \left(d(p,L)^2 + \alpha\right)^{m/2} & d(p,L) < T \\ 0 & else \end{cases} \qquad (3)$$

where m was the p-norm parameter, and T was the distance threshold.

Most of the optimal planes fitted using gradient decent method closely approximated the actually interfaces. However, the interface between the rib and the transverse process of the vertebra was a rather curved surface. We therefore performed refinement in the neighborhood of the fitted plane. As shown in Fig. 3(a), we represented the initial surface with a mesh computed by uniform sampling of the plane. The element (i, j) was allowed only to move in the direction orthogonal to the plane, i.e., within the parallelepiped C_{ij}. The final mesh was estimated by solving the optimization problem

$$\{\hat{d}_{ij}\} = \arg\min_{d_{ij} \in [-R,R]} [\sum_{i,j} \sum_{k \in V \cap C_{ij}} S_V(k) \mid d(k,L) - d_{ij} \mid + \sum_{ij} d_{ij}^2] \quad (4)$$

where d_{ij} was the displacement of the mesh element with respect to the starting plane L, $S_v(k)$ was the strength of the valley primitive set V, and R was the maximum allowable displacement. The first term measures the weighted distance sum of the valley points in the parallelepiped to the mesh element, and becomes minimal when the mesh element is close to or on the valley primitives. The second term restricts the mesh element from being too far away from the original plane. The energy is the sum over all mesh elements. The estimated optimal displacements of all mesh elements define the final surface mesh. Shown in Fig. 3(b)(c) are the two final surfaces at the interface of the transverse process and the ribs.

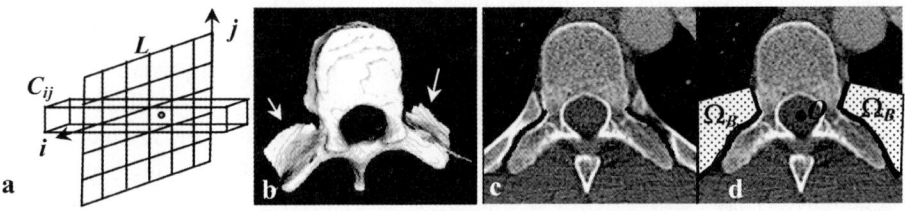

Fig. 3. Surface refinement based on fitted planes. (a) Mesh refinement scheme. (b) 3D rendering of the final surface (c) Axial projection of the surface. (d) The blocker regions formed based on the high-level features.

As shown in Fig. 3(d), the fitted planes and surfaces as detected high-level features are used to form blocker regions. To decide if a point is inside or outside of the blocker region, the origin O of the vertebra coordinate system is used as the reference. [6] Given the block region Ω_B, we define the "blocker speed" as

$$V_B(\vec{x}) = \begin{cases} 1, & \vec{x} \in \Omega_B \\ 0, & \text{else} \end{cases} \quad (5)$$

2.3 Level Set Formulation

The image speeds included both region-based terms and the primitive-bases terms. [6]

$$F_{image}(\vec{x}) = \alpha[(I(\vec{x}) - c_1)^2 - (I(\vec{x}) - c_2)^2] + \beta \nabla g(\vec{x}) \cdot \nabla \phi(\vec{x}, t), \quad (6)$$

where c_1 and c_2 were the intensity constants for soft tissues and cortical bones, respectively, and

$$g(\vec{x}) = \frac{1}{1 + D_E(\vec{x}) + D_R(\vec{x})}, \qquad (7)$$

D_E and D_R represented the edge and ridge responses from the 3D steerable filter [8],

$$F_{final}(\vec{x}) = [1 - v_B(\vec{x})]F_{image}(\vec{x}) - v_B(\vec{x}) + \varepsilon\kappa \qquad (8)$$

where κ was the mean curvature of the level set. The evolution of the surface was embedded in the evolution of a level set function $\phi(t)$:

$$\frac{\partial\phi}{\partial t} = F_{final}(\vec{x})\,|\nabla\phi| \qquad (9)$$

3 Results

We tested our algorithm on 21 thoracic CT volumes with axial resolution of 0.6~1 mm, each containing 6-8 thoracic vertebras. The total number of vertebras came up to 150. To provide quantitative validation for the automatic segmentations, we compared to human delineated results. The complete manual delineation of the vertebra by a human observer was very tedious and time consuming (e.g., 45 minutes for a single vertebra traversing 78 axial slices), which was the very reason that we needed an automatic algorithm. It was even more prohibitive to have a physician to perform such a task. As an alternative, we used the automatic segmentation result as the starting point of human delineation and the edited result were used as the ground truth for evaluation. To justify this, we tested the consistency between the edited results and the completely manual results on a couple of vertebras. Two human observers independently delineated these vertebras, and the results were examined by an orthopedic surgeon as acceptable. A third observer edited the automatic results of these same vertebras. The consistency between two result point sets S_1 and S_2 using S_2 as the reference was measured by the under-segment rate

$$u(S_1|S_2) = |U|/|S_2| \times 100\%, \quad \text{where} \quad U = \{p | p \in S_2 \text{ and } p \notin S_1\}, \qquad (10)$$

and the over-segment rate

$$o(S_1|S_2) = |O|/|S_2| \times 100\%, \quad \text{where} \quad O = \{p | p \in S_1 \text{ and } p \notin S_2\}, \qquad (11)$$

and |.| was the size of the point set. Shown in Table 1 are the under-segment and over-segment rates using the completely manual results as the references. From these we concluded that the inter-personal consistency was high enough that any educated human observer would be able to perform a consistent manual segmentation that was acceptable to an orthopedic surgeon. Further, the edited result based on the auto segmentation result was as good as a completely manual segmentation. Therefore to use the edited result as the reference for validation was reasonable and sound.

The 150 vertebras were segmented using our algorithm. The result of each vertebra was manually edited by a human observer and recorded as the reference. Shown in Fig. 4 are the histograms of the under-segment and over-segment rates of the automatic results using the edited results as the references. From the histogram we observed that the general segmentation results were satisfactory, but under-segmentation happened more frequently than over-segmentation.

Shown in Fig. 5 is a typical segmentation result. The 2D boundaries of the results were overlaid on the original data, which matched reasonably to the vertebra boundaries despite the adjacent and connected neighboring structures. Strictly speaking, the level set surface does appear to be a bit over-smoothed to preserve every details of the vertebra surface. Minor under-segmentation also existed at a few places. The blocker regions and initial level set front shown in Fig. 5(k)-(o) helps us understand the reason for success: The initial front was close to and outside of the vertebra boundaries, which avoided the internal local minimums; the blocker region forced the level-set to evolve outside of the neighboring structures so that leakage was prevented.

The un-optimized automatic algorithm took about 7 minutes in average for each vertebra, and the manual editing based on the automatic result took about 5 minutes in average.

Table 1. Consistency measures of manual and edited results

S_1	Manual result 1		Manual result 2	
	$u(S_1 \mid S_2)$	$o(S_1 \mid S_2)$	$u(S_1 \mid S_2)$	$o(S_1 \mid S_2)$
Manual result 1	n/a	n/a	5.3%	5.1%
Manual result 2	5.7%	5.5%	n/a	n/a
Edited result	6.2%	5.9%	5.8%	6.4%

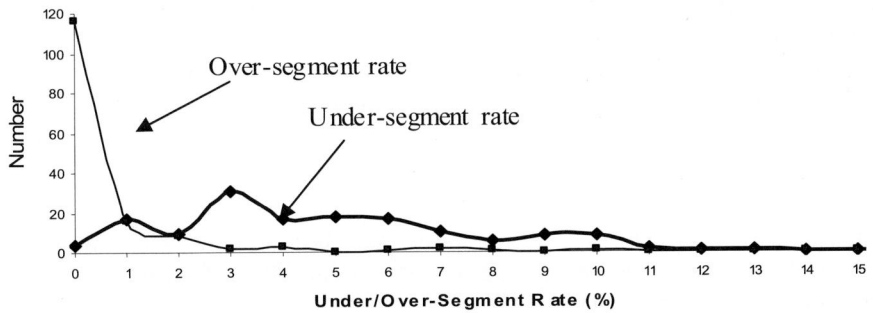

Fig. 4. Histogram of the under and over-segment rates

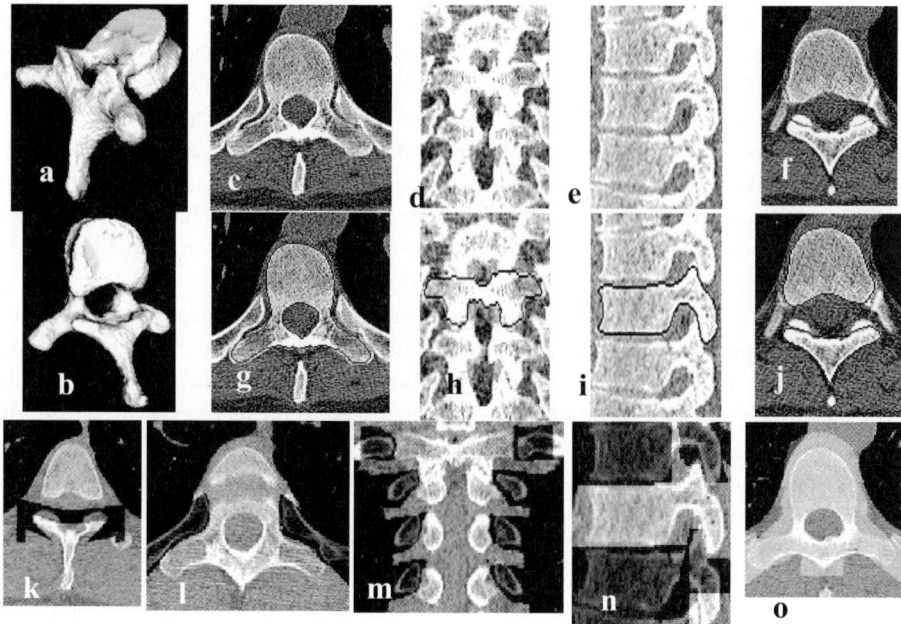

Fig. 5. A sample automatic segmentation result before human editing. (a)(b) 3D surface rendering of the segmented vertebra. (c)-(f) Sample axial, coronal and sagittal views of the original data (g)-(j) 2D boundaries of the segmentations. (k)-(n) Blocker regions (dark) as an intermediate result of the algorithm. (o) The initial front of the level set (white).

4 Conclusions

We reported in this paper an automatic method and the validated results for the precise segmentation of individual vertebras from a CT volume. The algorithm can be further improved; we should also investigate the effect of the key components such as the blocker extraction and the initial front in more detail. The current result, however, is useful with minor user edits. The concept of localized priors should be further explored to provide a more general framework, e.g. a statistical description to cover the variations. It is imaginable that such a set of localized statistical models should form a much smaller model space compared to a global model.

References

1. Kaminsky, J., Klinge, P., Rodt, T., Bokemeyer, M., Luedemann, W., Samii, M.: Specially adapted interactive tools for an improved 3D-segmentation of the spine. Computerized Medical Imaging and Graphics 28, 119–127 (2004)
2. Tan, S., Yao, J., Ward, M.M., Yao, L., Summers, R.M.: Computer aided evaluation of ankylosing spondylitis. In: 3rd IEEE International Symposium on Biomedical Imaging: Nano to Macro, pp. 339–342 (2006)

3. Naegel, B.: Using mathematical morphology for the anatomical labeling of vertebrae from 3D CT-scan images. Computerized Medical Imaging and Graphics 31(3), 141–156
4. Smyth, P.P., Taylor, C.J., Adams, J.E.: Automatic measurement of vertebral shape using active shape models. Image Vis. Computing 15, 575–581 (1997)
5. Lorenz, C., Krahnstover, N.: 3D Statistical Shape Models for Medical Image Segmentation. In: Second International Conference on 3-D Imaging and Modeling, p. 0414 (1999)
6. Shen, H., Shi, Y., Peng, Z.: Applying Prior Knowledge in the Segmentation of 3D Complex Anatomic Structures. In: The 1st International Workshop on Computer Vision for Biomedical Image Applications, Beijing, China (October 2005)
7. Leventon, M.E., Grimson, W.E., Faugeras, O.: Statistical shape influence in geodesic active contours. In: Proceedings IEEE Conference on Computer Vision and Pattern Recognition, vol. 1(1), pp. 316–323 (2000)
8. Freeman, W.T., Adelson, E.H.: The design and use of steerable filters. IEEE Transactions on Pattern Analysis and Machine Intelligence 13(9), 891–906 (1991)

Cell Spreading Analysis with Directed Edge Profile-Guided Level Set Active Contours

I. Ersoy[1], F. Bunyak[1], K. Palaniappan[1], M. Sun[2], and G. Forgacs[2]

[1] Department of Computer Science
[2] Department of Physics and Astronomy
University of Missouri-Columbia, Columbia MO 65211, USA*

Abstract. Cell adhesion and spreading within the extracellular matrix (ECM) plays an important role in cell motility, cell growth and tissue organization. Measuring cell spreading dynamics enables the investigation of cell mechanosensitivity to external mechanical stimuli, such as substrate rigidity. A common approach to measure cell spreading dynamics is to take time lapse images and quantify cell size and perimeter as a function of time. In our experiments, differences in cell characteristics between different treatments are subtle and require accurate measurements of cell parameters across a large population of cells to ensure an adequate sample size for statistical hypothesis testing. This paper presents a new approach to estimate accurate cell boundaries with complex shapes by applying a modified geodesic active contour level set method that directly utilizes the halo effect typically seen in phase contrast microscopy. Contour evolution is guided by edge profiles in a perpendicular direction to ensure convergence to the correct cell boundary. The proposed approach is tested on bovine aortic endothelial cell images under different treatments, and demonstrates accurate segmentation for a wide range of cell sizes and shapes compared to manual ground truth.

1 Introduction

Endothelial cells (ECs) reside in the innermost layer of blood vessels, and constantly experience mechanical stimulation such as shear stress and cyclic stretching. Increasing evidence shows the direct effects of these mechanical signals on endothelial structure and functions [1]. One particular example is that atherosclerotic lesions usually locate at the bifurcations and curvatures in the arterial tree, areas that are characterized by disturbed flow with low shear stress magnitudes [2]. This indicates that EC mechanosensitivity plays a critical role in atherosclerosis development. Atherosclerosis development is a complex, multiple stage process with various causing factors, among which high level of cholesterol is one of the most important. The corresponding biological study is to investigate cholesterol effects on EC mechanosensitivity by studying cell spreading

---

* Research partially supported by NIH NIBIB award R33-EB00573 (KP), NIH-HL64388 (GF), American Heart Association (MS).

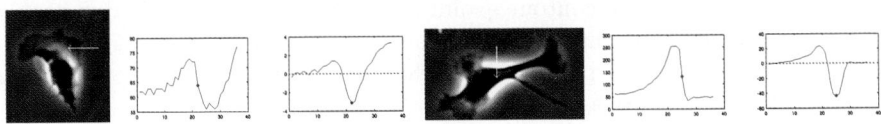

Fig. 1. Phase contrast cell images. Left to right: sample cell, intensity profile at the marked direction, derivative of the directed profile. The actual cell boundary point is marked on the graphs.

dynamics (e.g. cell spreading area as a function time) on substrates of different rigidity. This is of particular importance for ECs because mechanics of the endothelium changes during the development of atherosclerosis. Cell cholesterol level may be either elevated or decreased using chemical drugs (e.g. methyl-beta-cyclodextran) [3] and cell spreading is recorded for further cell area analysis. Under some conditions, cells show subtle difference between different cholesterol modulations (e.g. cholesterol enrichment and cholesterol depletion). To get good statistics, accurate cell area measurement and large sample size are needed. This requires automatic and accurate methods, especially when large volume of data are collected to obtain better statistics. In recent years, active contours have become increasingly popular for cell segmentation [4]. Geometric model of active contours [5] provides advantages such as eliminating the need to reparameterize the curve and automatic handling of topology changes via level set implementation [6]. The major drawbacks of the classical edge-based active contours are the leakage due to weak edges and stopping at local maximums in noisy images. While the region-based active contours [7, 8, 9] overcome these drawbacks, they require a bimodal image model to discern background and foreground which is not applicable in some high resolution cell images. Figure 1 shows typical phase contrast images of cells. The white regions surrounding the cells are the typical phase halo. A straight-forward implementation of [7] converges to the boundaries between phase halo and the rest of the image. Using various features in Chan and Vese formulation such as variance to discern cells from background gives satisfactory results [10] but the sharp phase halos contribute to the variance and cause early stopping of curve evolution. Similarly, edge stopping functions used in regular geodesic active contours, if initialized outside of the cells, respond to the outer edges of phase halos and cause early stopping which produces an inaccurate segmentation. When the curve is initialized inside the cells, the texture inside the cell also causes premature stopping. Often phase halo is compensated by normalizing the image but this weakens the cell boundaries further, especially in the areas where cells are flattened, and leads to leakage of the curve. One remedy is to enforce a shape model, but it fails for cells with highly irregular shapes. Nucleus-based initialization and segmentation [11] is also not applicable to images such as in figure 1. To obtain an accurate segmentation, we propose an approach that exploits the phase halo effect instead of compensating it. The intensity profile perpendicular to the local cell boundary is similar along the whole boundary of a cell; it passes from the brighter phase halo to the darker cell boundary. We propose to initialize the curve outside the cell and phase halo, and guide the active contour evolution based on the desired edge profiles which effectively lets the curve evolve through the halos and stop at the actual boundaries. We also use a spatially adaptive force to slow the curve evolution at boundaries to prevent leakage.

2 Methods

2.1 Ridge-Based Cell Detection

An initial curve close to the actual cell boundary needs to be detected to capture the desired characteristic of the local directional derivative as shown in figure 1. Shape-based properties of the intensity surface are utilized to produce the initial coarse cell detection. These properties are chosen because of their robustness to image contrast and intensity variations. In phase contrast microscopy images, the cell membrane boundaries and phase halos around the cells produce crest lines (ridges and valleys), and subcellular structures produce blob- or ridge-like patterns so the use of ridge detection methods are ideal for the initial detection. In curvature based detection, ridges can be defined as local extrema of principal curvatures [12]. Principal curvatures and directions of a hypersurface L correspond to the eigenvalues $\kappa_1 \geq ... \geq \kappa_{n-1}$ and eigenvectors $\xi_1 \geq ... \geq \xi_{n-1}$ of the shape operator matrix on the tangent space W. In 2D case, W is given by:

$$W = \mathbf{I}^{-1}\mathbf{II} = \begin{bmatrix} L_x \cdot L_x & L_x \cdot L_y \\ L_x \cdot L_y & L_y \cdot L_y \end{bmatrix}^{-1} \begin{bmatrix} L_{xx} \cdot c & L_{xy} \cdot c \\ L_{xy} \cdot c & L_{yy} \cdot c \end{bmatrix} \quad (1)$$

where $\mathbf{I}$ and $\mathbf{II}$ are the first and second fundamental forms and $c = \frac{L_x \times L_y}{|L_x \times L_y|}$ [12]. Since computation of principal curvatures is expensive, mean curvature $H = \frac{1}{2}(\kappa_1 + \kappa_2) = \frac{1}{2}trace(W)$ is often used [13,14] to classify surface patches ($H < 0$: peak, ridge, or saddle ridge; $H = 0$: flat or minimal surface; $H > 0$: pit, valley, or saddle valley). In generalization of local extrema for real-valued functions of a vector variable [12], a point x_0 is classified as maximum if $\nabla L(x_0) = 0$ (critical point) and $\mathcal{H}(L(x_0))$ is negative definite (all eigenvalues $\lambda_i < 0$) where $\mathcal{H}$ is the Hessian matrix:

$$\mathcal{H} = \begin{bmatrix} L_{xx} & L_{xy} \\ L_{xy} & L_{yy} \end{bmatrix} \quad (2)$$

For critical points ($\nabla L(x_0) = 0$), according to the Taylor series expansion and curvature definitions eigenvalues λ_i and eigenvectors v_i of the Hessian matrix correspond to principal curvatures κ_i and principal directions ξ_i respectively [15]. Eigenvalues and eigenvectors of the Hessian matrix have been used in many medical image processing applications as a ridgeness measure [16,17]. Since we want to detect membrane boundaries, phase halos, and subcellular structures associated with cells (dark ridges, bright ridges and dark blobs respectively), we use $|\lambda_1(\mathcal{H})|$. Initial cell detection is done by thresholding $|\lambda_1(\mathcal{H})|$. Threshold value T_r is selected based on mean and standard deviation (σ) of $\lambda_1(\mathcal{H})$. Regions where $|\lambda_1(\mathcal{H})| > T_r$ are classified as cells. The obtained mask is further refined using morphological closing to make cell masks more compact, and morphological opening and area opening to remove spurious detections and to refine cell contours.

2.2 Directed Edge Profile-Guided Level Set Active Contours

Initial detection of cells produce cell masks that have discontinuities and spurious results and they are larger than the actual cells, particularly where the phase halos are thick. To refine the initial cell detection, we propose a novel geodesic active contour evolution with spatially adaptive force and guided by edge profiles. In level set based active contour methods, a curve $\mathcal{C}$ is represented implicitly via a Lipschitz function ϕ by $\mathcal{C} = \{(x,y)|\phi(x,y) = 0\}$, and the evolution of the curve is given by the zero-level curve of the function $\phi(t,x,y)$ [7]. We propose use of a modified version of the geodesic active contours [5]. In regular geodesic active contours [5] the level set function ϕ is evolved using the speed function,

$$\frac{\partial \phi}{\partial t} = g(\nabla \mathbf{I})(F_c + \mathcal{K}(\phi))|\nabla \phi| + \nabla \phi \cdot \nabla g(\nabla \mathbf{I}) \quad (3)$$

where F_c is a constant, $\mathcal{K}$ is the curvature term (Eq.4) and $g(\nabla \mathbf{I})$ is the edge stopping function, a decreasing function of the image gradient which can be defined as in Eq.5.

$$\mathcal{K} = div\left(\frac{\nabla \phi}{|\nabla \phi|}\right) = \frac{\phi_{xx}\phi_y^2 - 2\phi_x\phi_y\phi_{xy} + \phi_{yy}\phi_x^2}{(\phi_x^2 + \phi_y^2)^{\frac{3}{2}}} \quad (4)$$

$$g(\nabla \mathbf{I}) = exp(-|\nabla G_\sigma(x,y) * \mathbf{I}(x,y)|) \quad (5)$$

The constant balloon force F_c pushes the curve inwards or outwards depending on its sign. The regularization term $\mathcal{K}$ ensures boundary smoothness and $g(\mathbf{I})$ is used to stop the curve evolution at cell boundaries. The term $\nabla g \cdot \nabla \phi$ is used to increase the basin of attraction for evolving the curve to the boundaries of the objects. The geodesic active contours are more suitable for our application where intensity inside the cell boundaries is highly heterogeneous, and there is no clear difference between inside and outside intensity profiles so intensity thresholding or Chan-Vese type minimal variance models are not applicable. However, since they are designed to stop at edges, they suffer from: (1) early stopping on background or foreground edges, (2) contour leaking across weak boundaries, and (3) for our particular application, early stopping at outer edges of phase halos. To overcome the first problem, we use the ridge-based initialization to start the contour from outside, close to the actual boundary. To reduce the effects of the second problem, we propose replacing the constant balloon force F_c in Eq. 3 with an intensity adaptive force F_A :

$$F_A(x,y) = c\mathbf{I}(x,y) \quad (6)$$

This intensity adaptive force increases the speed of contraction on bright phase halos and reduces it on thin dark extensions and prevents leaking across weak edges. To handle the third problem, we propose a modified edge stopping function. The existence of phase halo increases the edge strength at cell boundaries. We propose the edge stopping function g_d (Eq. 9) guided by the directed edge profile, that lets the curve evolve through the outer halo edge and stop at the actual boundary edge. As shown in figure 1, if initialized close to the actual boundary, the first light-to-dark edge encountered in the local perpendicular direction corresponds to the actual boundary. By choosing this profile as the stopping criterion we avoid the outer edge of phase halo. This stopping function is obtained as follows. Normal vector $\boldsymbol{N}$ to the evolving contour/surface can be determined directly from the level set function:

$$\boldsymbol{N} = -\frac{\nabla \phi}{|\nabla \phi|} \qquad (7)$$

Edge profile is obtained as the intensity derivative in opposite direction to the normal:

$$\mathbf{I}_{-\boldsymbol{N}} = \frac{\nabla \phi}{|\nabla \phi|} \cdot \nabla \mathbf{I} \qquad (8)$$

Dark-to-light transitions produce positive response in $\mathbf{I}_{-\boldsymbol{N}}$. We define the edge profile-guided edge stopping function g_d as:

$$g_d(\nabla \mathbf{I}) = 1 - \mathrm{H}(-\mathbf{I}_{-\boldsymbol{N}})(1 - g(\nabla \mathbf{I})) \qquad (9)$$

where H is the heaviside step function:

$$\mathrm{H}(x) = \begin{cases} 1 \text{ if } x > 0 \\ 0 \text{ elsewhere} \end{cases}$$

This sets g_d to 1 at regions where there is a dark-to-light (background-to-halo) transition perpendicular to boundary, and keeps regular edge stopping function everywhere else. Thus it lets the active contour evolve through the edges with a dark-to-light profile and stop at edges with light-to-dark profile. Eq.10 shows the speed function of the proposed curve evolution.

$$\frac{\partial \phi}{\partial t} = (1-\mathrm{H}(-\mathbf{I}_{-\boldsymbol{N}})(1-g(\nabla \mathbf{I})))(c\mathbf{I}+\mathcal{K}(\phi))|\nabla \phi|+\nabla \phi \cdot \nabla (1-\mathrm{H}(-\mathbf{I}_{-\boldsymbol{N}})(1-g(\nabla \mathbf{I}))) \qquad (10)$$

3 Experiments and Results

Bovine aortic endothelial cells (BAECs; Cambrex East Rutherford, NJ) between passages 12 and 16 were grown in DMEM (Invitrogen, Carlsbad, CA) containing 10% fetal bovine serum (FBS; Sigma-Aldrich, St. Louis, MO), 10 g/ml penicillin, streptomycin and kanamycin sulfate (Invitrogen, Carlsbad, CA). Cell cultures were maintained in a humidified incubator at 37C, with 5% CO_2. Cells were split every 3-4 days. Rat-tail collage I (BD Biosciences, Bedford, MA) at 0.3 mg/ml in acidic acid was absorbed onto the glass coverslip for 24 hours. Then the coverslip was rinsed in PBS to remove unbound collagen. A glass coverslip in a 35 mm

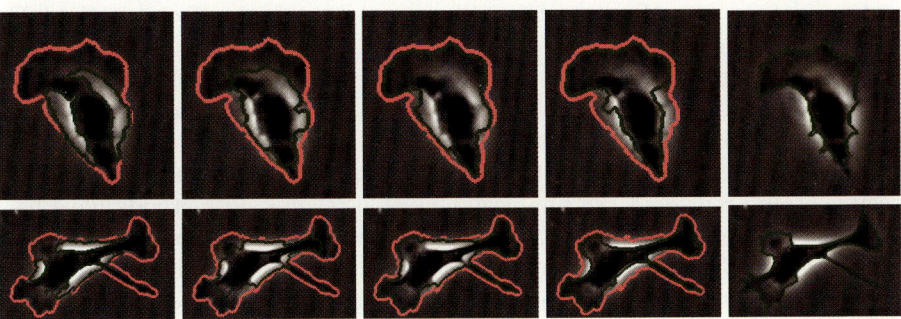

Fig. 2. Magnified results on sample cells from BAEC data set. light red: ridge-based initialization, dark green: final segmentation. From left to right: Chan and Vese, GAC, GAC with adaptive force, proposed method, manual ground truth.

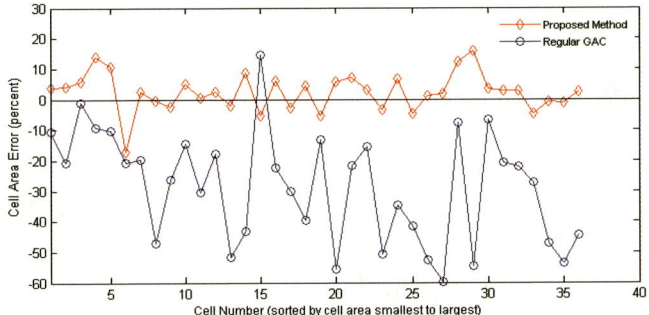

Fig. 3. Percentage error of cell area with respect to ground truth: proposed method vs. regular GAC

Table 1. Error analysis with respect to manual ground truth

Image	Cells	Method	Avg. Area (pixels)	Avg. Error (%)	RMS
1	9	Regular GAC	1872	-51.9%	2038
		Proposed	3947	1.4%	243
2	6	Regular GAC	2259	-21.1%	838
		Proposed	3137	7.2%	213
3	12	Regular GAC	2797	-14.9%	692
		Proposed	3327	0.4%	130
4	9	Regular GAC	2367	-28.7%	1216
		Proposed	3476	2.5%	262
Total	36	Regular GAC	2368	-28.6%	1298
		Proposed	3488	2.3%	212

Petri dish with 1 ml cell culture medium is placed on an Olympus IX70 inverted microscope. 2×10^4 cells from cell suspension were added to the Petri dish. Images of spreading cells were recorded in phase contrast mode with a CoolSNAPfx digital video camera (Photometrics, Tucson, AZ), using a 10× objective. The proposed method was tested on a data set of BAECs obtained as described above. Each image in the data set is 1300×1030 pixels in size and contains about 30–50 BAECs. Figure 2 shows segmentation results of four methods and the manually drawn ground truth on magnified sample cells. Light red contours represent the ridge-based initialization as described in previous section. Dark green contours represent the final segmentation results, all methods have been initialized with the red contours. Chan and Vese method, as expected, converges to phase halos. Geodesic active contour with fixed force and regular edge stopping function (regular GAC) leaks through weak edges and is stopped by the strong phase halo edges. If the spatially adaptive force is applied, the contour tends to stop at weak edges most of the time as well as on strong halo edges. The proposed edge profile-guided stopping function with spatially adaptive force assures the desired result, it is stopped by weak halo-to-boundary edges, but evolves through the strong outer halo edges and converges to the desired boundary, producing a very tight cell segmentation. To obtain a quantitative validation of the proposed method, a small set of images have been selected and cells not in direct contact have been manually segmented by an expert in the art. Majority of cells have been successfully segmented by the proposed method except a few cells that were merged or separated. Table 1 shows error analysis with respect to this ground truth. The same parameters are used for all images, 0.5σ is chosen as the threshold at the ridge-based initial detection phase. Fourth and fifth columns of the table show the average cell area and average percentage error for each image respectively, regular GAC has a big error due to leakage through the actual boundaries whereas the proposed method gives good results. In total (36 cells) the average error of regular GAC is -28.6%, that of proposed method is 2.3%. Sixth column shows the RMS error, again the proposed method results in better performance as opposed to regular GAC. Figure 3 compares regular GAC and proposed method with respect to the manual ground truth in terms of percentage deviation from the actual cell area for each of the 36 cells.

4 Discussion and Conclusion

A new approach to obtain accurate cell boundaries in phase contrast microscopy is presented in this paper. The use of ridge and blob measures provides a robust initial detection. The active contour is implemented with level set and its evolution is guided by edge profiles to stop it at the desired boundaries. This enables the active contour to pass through phase halo edges and stop at the actual cell boundary. Also, the use of spatially adaptive force prevents leakage at the boundaries. The proposed method is tested on time lapse images of bovine aortic endothelial cells with highly complex structure, it provides very robust performance compared to other methods and ground truth. Methods that cannot successfully exclude phase halos skew the statistics because at different times and substrates, the amount of halo around a cell is variable. The proposed method provides an automatic estimate of cell area that is of sufficient accuracy to test various biological hypotheses.

References

1. Aplin, A., Hogan, B., Tomeu, J., Juliano, R.: Cell adhesion differentially regulates the nucleocytoplasmic distribution of active map kinases. J. Cell Sci. 115, 2781–2790 (2002)
2. Parker, K., Brock, A., Brangwynne, C., Mannix, R., Wang, N., Ostuni, E., Geisse, N., Adams, J., Whitesides, G., Ingber, D.: Directional control of lamellipodia extension by constraining cell shape and orienting cell tractional forces. FASEB J. 16, 1195–1204 (2002)
3. Sun, M., Northup, N., Marga, F., Huber, T., Byfield, F., Levitan, I., Forgacs, G.: The effect of cellular cholesterol on membrane-cytoskeleton adhesion. J. Cell Sci. 120, 2223–2231 (2007)
4. Wang, X., He, W., Metaxas, D., Matthew, R., White, E.: Cell segmentation and tracking using texture-adaptive snakes. In: Proc. 4th IEEE Int. Symp. Biomed. Imaging (ISBI), pp. 101–104. IEEE Comp. Soc., Los Alamitos (2007)
5. Caselles, V., Kimmel, R., Sapiro, G.: Geodesic active contours. Int. J. of Comp. Vision 22, 61–79 (1997)
6. Sethian, J.: Level Set Methods and Fast Marching Methods, 2nd edn. Cambridge Univ. Press, Cambridge (1999)
7. Chan, T., Vese, L.: Active contours without edges. IEEE Trans. Image Process 10, 266–277 (2001)
8. Nath, S., Palaniappan, K., Bunyak, F.: Cell segmentation using coupled level sets and graph-vertex coloring. In: Larsen, R., Nielsen, M., Sporring, J. (eds.) MICCAI 2006. LNCS, vol. 4190, pp. 101–108. Springer, Heidelberg (2006)
9. Bunyak, F., Palaniappan, K., Nath, S.K., Baskin, T.I., Dong, G.: Quantitative cell motility for in vitro wound healing using level set-based active contour tracking. In: Proc. 3rd IEEE Int. Symp. Biomed. Imaging (ISBI), pp. 1040–1043. IEEE Comp. Soc., Los Alamitos (2006)
10. Palaniappan, K., Ersoy, I., Nath, S.: Moving object segmentation using the flux tensor for biological video microscopy. In: Ip, H.H.-S., Au, O.C., Leung, H., Sun, M.-T., Ma, W.-Y., Hu, S.-M. (eds.) PCM 2007. LNCS, vol. 4810, pp. 483–493. Springer, Heidelberg (2007)
11. Yan, P., Zhou, X., Shah, M., Wong, S.: Automatic segmentation of high throughput RNAi fluorescent cellular images. IEEE Trans. Inf. Tech. Biom. 12, 109–117 (2008)
12. Eberly, D.: Ridges in Image and Data Analysis. Kluwer Academic Publishers, Dordrecht (1996)
13. Lopez, A., Lumbreras, F., Serrat, J., Villanueva, J.: Evaluation of methods for ridge and valley detection. IEEE Trans. PAMI 21, 327–335 (1999)
14. Besl, P.J., Jain, R.C.: Segmentation through variable-order surface fitting. IEEE Trans. PAMI 10, 167–192 (1988)
15. Bronshtein, I., Semendyayev, K.: 4.3 Differential Geometry. In: Handbook of mathematics, 3rd edn. Springer, London (1997)
16. Staal, J., Abràmoff, M., Niemeijer, M., Viergever, M., van Ginneken, B.: Ridge-based vessel segmentation in color images of the retina. IEEE Trans. Med. Imag. 23, 501–509 (2004)
17. Zhou, J., Chang, S., Metaxas, D., Axel, L.: Vessel boundary extraction using ridge scan-conversion deformable model. In: Proc. 3rd IEEE Int. Symp. Biomed. Imaging (ISBI), pp. 189–192. IEEE Comp. Soc., Los Alamitos (2006)

Brain MR Image Segmentation Using Local and Global Intensity Fitting Active Contours/Surfaces

Li Wang[1], Chunming Li[2,*], Quansen Sun[1], Deshen Xia[1], and Chiu-Yen Kao[3]

[1] School of Computer Science & Technology,
Nanjing University of Science and Technology, China
[2] Institute of Imaging Science, Vanderbilt University, USA
chunming.li@vanderbilt.edu
[3] Department of Mathematics, The Ohio State University, USA

Abstract. In this paper, we present an improved region-based active contour/surface model for 2D/3D brain MR image segmentation. Our model combines the advantages of both local and global intensity information, which enable the model to cope with intensity inhomogeneity. We define an energy functional with a local intensity fitting term and an auxiliary global intensity fitting term. In the associated curve evolution, the motion of the contour is driven by a local intensity fitting force and a global intensity fitting force, induced by the local and global terms in the proposed energy functional, respectively. The influence of these two forces on the curve evolution is complementary. When the contour is close to object boundaries, the local intensity fitting force became dominant, which attracts the contour toward object boundaries and finally stops the contour there. The global intensity fitting force is dominant when the contour is far away from object boundaries, and it allows more flexible initialization of contours by using global image information. The proposed model has been applied to both 2D and 3D brain MR image segmentation with promising results.

1 Introduction

The segmentation of the brain magnetic resonance (MR) images into white matter (WM), gray matter (GM), and cerebral spinal fluid (CSF) has been an important and fundamental step in research and clinical applications, including diagnosis of pathology, presurgical planning and computer integrated surgery. A major difficulty in segmentation of MR images is the intensity inhomogeneities due to the radio-frequency coils or acquisition sequences.

Active contour models have been widely used in medical image segmentation [1,2,3,4,5,6,7,8,9,10,11]. The existing active contour models can be categorized into two classes: edge-based models [1,2,3,4] and region-based models [5,6,7,8,9,10,11]. Edge-based models may suffer from boundary leakage problem

---
* Corresponding author.

for brain MR images, in which some parts of WM and GM boundaries are quite fuzzy due to low contrast there. Region-based models have better performance than edge-based models in the presence of weak boundaries. However, most of region-based models [5,6,7,8] tend to rely on intensity homogeneity. For example, the well-known piecewise constant (PC) models [7,10,8] are based on the assumption that image intensities are statistically homogeneous (roughly a constant) in each region, therefore they fail to segment MR images with intensity inhomogeneity. In [10] and [11], two similar active contour models were proposed to minimize the Mumford-Shah functional [12]. These models, widely known as piecewise smooth (PS) models, have exhibited certain capability of handling intensity inhomogeneity. However, the computational cost of the PS model is rather expensive due to the complicated procedures [13]. Moreover, to the best of our knowledge, the PS models have not been used to segment brain MR images.

Recently, Li et al. proposed a local binary fitting (LBF) model [14,15] to overcome intensity inhomogeneity. The LBF model draws upon local intensity information, which enables the model to cope with intensity inhomogeneity. With accurate local intensity information, the LBF model is able to recover object boundaries precisely. Some related methods were recently proposed in [13,16], which have similar capability of handling intensity inhomogeneity as the LBF model. However, these methods [14,15,13,16] are to some extent sensitive to initialization, which limit their practical applications.

In this paper, we propose an improved active contour/surface model, which combines the advantages of both local and global intensity information. We define an energy functional with two terms: one is a local intensity fitting term and the other is an auxiliary global intensity fitting term. The local intensity fitting term induces a local force to attract the contours and stop it at object boundaries, which enables the model to cope with intensity inhomogeneity. The global intensity fitting term drives the motion of the contour far away from object boundaries, and therefore allows for flexible initialization of the contours.

2 Background

2.1 Chan-Vese Model

Chan and Vese [7] proposed an active contour approach to the Mumford-Shah problem [12] for a special case where the original image is a piecewise constant function. The global data fitting term in the Chan-Vese (CV) model is defined as follows

$$\mathcal{F}^{\text{CV}}(c_1, c_2, C) = \int_{outside(C)} (I - c_1)^2 d\mathbf{x} d\mathbf{y} + \int_{inside(C)} (I - c_2)^2 d\mathbf{x} d\mathbf{y} \quad (1)$$

where *outside(C)* and *inside(C)* represent the regions outside and inside the contour C, respectively, and c_1 and c_2 are two constants that fit the image intensities in the entire regions *outside(C)* and *inside(C)*. Obviously, the constants c_1 and

c_2 that best fit the intensity are not accurate, if the intensities in each region separated by C are inhomogeneous. Without taking local image information into account, the CV model generally fails to segment images with intensity inhomogeneity. Likewise, more general piecewise constant models in a multiphase level set framework [10,8] are not applicable for such images either.

2.2 Local Binary Fitting Model

To overcome the difficulty caused by intensity inhomogeneities, Li *et al.* proposed the local binary fitting (LBF) model, which utilizes the local intensity information [14,15]. Two spatially varying fitting functions $f_1(\mathbf{x})$ and $f_2(\mathbf{x})$ are introduced to approximate the local intensities on the two sides of the contour. In the LBF model, the local data fitting term was defined as follows

$$\mathcal{F}^{\text{LBF}}(\phi, f_1, f_2) = \lambda_1 \int [\int K_\sigma(\mathbf{x}-\mathbf{y})|I(\mathbf{y})-f_1(\mathbf{x})|^2 H(\phi(\mathbf{y}))d\mathbf{y}]d\mathbf{x}$$
$$+ \lambda_2 \int [\int K_\sigma(\mathbf{x}-\mathbf{y})|I(\mathbf{y})-f_2(\mathbf{x})|^2(1-H(\phi(\mathbf{y})))d\mathbf{y}]d\mathbf{x} \quad (2)$$

where H is Heaviside function, and K_σ is a Gaussian kernel with standard deviation σ. Due to the localization property of the kernel function, the local data fitting energy is dominated by the intensities $I(\mathbf{y})$ in a neighborhood of $\mathbf{x}$. This localization property enables the LBF model to deal with intensity inhomogeneity. Moreover, the LBF model can recover object boundaries more precisely than other region-based models without using local intensity information. However, at the cost of introducing the localization property, the LBF model becomes more sensitive to initialization than the PC models.

3 Local and Global Intensity Fitting Energy

Our method combines the advantages of the CV model and the LBF model by taking the local and global intensity information into account. In this section, we will detail our active contour model based on local and global intensity fitting (LGIF) to handle intensity inhomogeneity.

The local intensity fitting energy [14] is defined as follows, which is similar with Eq. (2):

$$\mathcal{E}^{\text{LIF}}(\phi, f_1, f_2) = \int [\int K_\sigma(\mathbf{x}-\mathbf{y})|I(\mathbf{y})-f_1(\mathbf{x})|^2 H(\phi(\mathbf{y}))d\mathbf{y}]d\mathbf{x}$$
$$+ \int [\int K_\sigma(\mathbf{x}-\mathbf{y})|I(\mathbf{y})-f_2(\mathbf{x})|^2(1-H(\phi(\mathbf{y})))d\mathbf{y}]d\mathbf{x} \quad (3)$$

We use the CV model's global intensity fitting energy

$$\mathcal{E}^{\text{GIF}}(\phi, c_1, c_2) = \int |I(\mathbf{x})-c_1|^2 H(\phi(\mathbf{x}))d\mathbf{x} + \int |I(\mathbf{x})-c_2|^2(1-H(\phi(\mathbf{x})))d\mathbf{x} \quad (4)$$

Now, we define the following energy functional

$$\mathcal{E}^{\text{LGIF}}(\phi, c_1, c_2, f_1, f_2) = (1-\omega)\mathcal{E}^{\text{LIF}}(\phi, f_1, f_2) + \omega\mathcal{E}^{\text{GIF}}(\phi, c_1, c_2) \quad (5)$$

where ω is a positive constant ($0 \leq \omega \leq 1$). When the intensity inhomogeneity in the image is severe, the parameter value ω should be chosen small enough. For more accurate computation involving the level set function, we need to regularize the level set function by penalizing its deviation from a signed distance function [17], which can be characterized by the following energy functional

$$\mathcal{P}(\phi) = \int \frac{1}{2}(|\nabla\phi(\mathbf{x})| - 1)^2 d\mathbf{x} \quad (6)$$

In addition, it is necessary to smooth the zero level set contour by penalizing its length, which is computed by

$$\mathcal{L}(\phi) = \int |\nabla H(\phi(\mathbf{x}))| d\mathbf{x} \quad (7)$$

Now, we define the entire energy functional

$$\mathcal{F}(\phi, f_1, f_2, c_1, c_2) = \mathcal{E}^{\text{LGIF}}(\phi, c_1, c_2, f_1, f_2) + \nu\mathcal{L}(\phi) + \mu\mathcal{P}(\phi) \quad (8)$$

It can be shown that the optimal fitting functions f_1 and f_2 and constants c_1 and c_2 that minimize the energy (8) are given by

$$f_1(\mathbf{x}) = \frac{K_\sigma(\mathbf{x}) * [H(\phi(\mathbf{x}))I(\mathbf{x})]}{K_\sigma(\mathbf{x}) * H(\phi(\mathbf{x}))}, \quad f_2(\mathbf{x}) = \frac{K_\sigma(\mathbf{x}) * [(1-H(\phi(\mathbf{x})))I(\mathbf{x})]}{K_\sigma(\mathbf{x}) * [1-H(\phi(\mathbf{x}))]} \quad (9)$$

$$c_1 = \frac{\int I(\mathbf{x})H(\phi(\mathbf{x}))d\mathbf{x}}{\int H(\phi(\mathbf{x}))d\mathbf{x}}, \quad c_2 = \frac{\int I(\mathbf{x})(1-H(\phi(\mathbf{x})))d\mathbf{x}}{\int (1-H(\phi(\mathbf{x})))d\mathbf{x}} \quad (10)$$

Minimization of the energy functional $\mathcal{F}$ in Eq. (8) with respect to ϕ is achieved by solving the gradient descent flow equation

$$\frac{\partial\phi}{\partial t} = -\delta(\phi)(F_1 + F_2) + \nu\delta(\phi)\text{div}\left(\frac{\nabla\phi}{|\nabla\phi|}\right) + \mu\left(\nabla^2\phi - \text{div}\left(\frac{\nabla\phi}{|\nabla\phi|}\right)\right) \quad (11)$$

where $\delta(\cdot)$ is the Dirac delta function, and $F_1 = (1-\omega)[\int K_\sigma(\mathbf{y}-\mathbf{x})|I(\mathbf{x}) - f_1(\mathbf{y})|^2 d\mathbf{y} - \int K_\sigma(\mathbf{y}-\mathbf{x})|I(\mathbf{x}) - f_2(\mathbf{y})|^2 d\mathbf{y}]$, $F_2 = \omega[(I-c_1)^2 - (I-c_2)^2]$. We call F_1 and F_2 the local intensity fitting (LIF) force and global intensity fitting (GIF) force, respectively.

3.1 Influence of the LIF and GIF Forces

The influence of the LIF force and GIF force on the curve evolution is complementary. When the contour is near object boundaries, the LIF force is dominant, which attracts the contour toward object boundaries and finally stops the contour there. Therefore, the location of the final contour is determined by the LIF

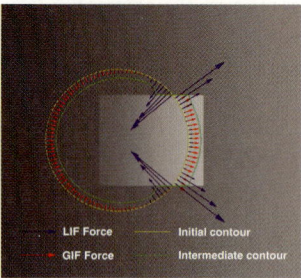

Fig. 1. Influence of LIF and GIF forces

force. When the contour is far away from object boundaries, the GIF force is dominant, while the LIF force is close to zero. This can be illustrated by an example shown in Fig. 1. The initial contour and the contour after 10 iterations are plotted in yellow and green respectively. The blue and red arrows represent the LIF and GIF force, respectively. The magnitude of the force is represented by the length of the arrow. It can be seen that the LIF force is dominant near the object boundaries, while the GIF force is dominant at locations far away from object boundaries.

3.2 Extension to Multi-phase Formulation

In this subsection, we extend the LGIF model to a multi-phase level set formulation, so that WM, GM, and CSF can be segmented simultaneously. By using n level set functions, at most 2^n regions can be segmented [10]. In a four-phase level set representation, two level set functions ϕ_1, ϕ_2 are used to define the following four regions: $\{\phi_1 > 0, \phi_2 > 0\}$, $\{\phi_1 > 0, \phi_2 < 0\}$, $\{\phi_1 < 0, \phi_2 > 0\}$, $\{\phi_1 < 0, \phi_2 < 0\}$. We define the following energy functional

$$\mathcal{F} = (1-\omega)\sum_{i=1}^{4}\int\int K_\sigma(\mathbf{x}-\mathbf{y})|I(\mathbf{y})-f_i(\mathbf{x})|^2 m_i(\mathbf{y})d\mathbf{y}d\mathbf{x}$$
$$+ \omega\sum_{i=1}^{4}\int |I(\mathbf{x})-c_i|^2 m_i(\mathbf{x})d\mathbf{x}$$
$$+ \nu(\mathcal{L}(\phi_1)+\mathcal{L}(\phi_2)) + \mu(\mathcal{P}(\phi_1)+\mathcal{P}(\phi_2)) \qquad (12)$$

where $m_1 = H(\phi_1)H(\phi_2)$, $m_2 = H(\phi_1)(1-H(\phi_2))$, $m_3 = (1-H(\phi_1))H(\phi_2)$, $m_4 = (1-H(\phi_1))(1-H(\phi_2))$.

It can be shown that the optimal fitting functions $f_1, \cdots, f_4$ and constants $c_1, \cdots, c_4$ that minimize the energy (12) are given by

$$f_i(\mathbf{x}) = \frac{K_\sigma(\mathbf{x}) * [m_i I(\mathbf{x})]}{K_\sigma(\mathbf{x}) * m_i}, \quad c_i = \frac{\int_\Omega I(\mathbf{x})m_i d\mathbf{x}}{\int_\Omega m_i d\mathbf{x}}, \quad i = 1, \cdots, 4 \qquad (13)$$

Minimization of the energy functional $\mathcal{F}$ in Eq. (12) with respect to ϕ_1 and ϕ_2 is achieved by solving the gradient descent flow equations

$$\frac{\partial \phi_1}{\partial t} = -\delta(\phi_1)\Big(H(\phi_2)(e_1 - e_3) + (1 - H(\phi_2))(e_2 - e_4)\Big) + \nu\delta(\phi_1)\mathrm{div}\left(\frac{\nabla \phi_1}{|\nabla \phi_1|}\right)$$
$$+ \mu\left(\nabla^2 \phi_1 - \mathrm{div}\left(\frac{\nabla \phi_1}{|\nabla \phi_1|}\right)\right) \qquad (14)$$

$$\frac{\partial \phi_2}{\partial t} = -\delta(\phi_2)\Big(H(\phi_1)(e_1 - e_2) + (1 - H(\phi_1))(e_3 - e_4)\Big) + \nu\delta(\phi_2)\mathrm{div}\left(\frac{\nabla \phi_2}{|\nabla \phi_2|}\right)$$
$$+ \mu\left(\nabla^2 \phi_2 - \mathrm{div}\left(\frac{\nabla \phi_2}{|\nabla \phi_2|}\right)\right) \qquad (15)$$

where $e_i(\mathbf{x}) = (1 - \omega)\int K_\sigma(\mathbf{y} - \mathbf{x})|I(\mathbf{x}) - f_i(\mathbf{y})|^2 d\mathbf{y} + \omega|I(\mathbf{x}) - c_i|^2$.

4   Experimental Results

In this paper, we use the following default setting of the parameters $\sigma = 3.0$, $\mu = 1.0$, $\nu = 0.001 \times 255 \times 255$, time step $\Delta t = 0.1$, and $\omega = 0.01$. When the intensity inhomogeneity in the image is more severe, the parameter value ω should be chosen smaller. We first apply our multi-phase model to segment a MR image from McGill Brain Web [18] with noise level 3%, and intensity non-uniformity (INU) 40%, as shown in the first row of Fig. 2. We have increased INU to test the validity of our method to handle intensity inhomogeneity. The second row shows a real brain MR image with obvious intensity inhomogeneity. For this image, we set $\omega = 0.005$. In fact, some intensities of the white matter in the upper part are even lower than those of the gray matter in the lower part. Nevertheless, our method achieves satisfactory segmentation results for these two images, as shown in the second column of Fig. 2. To demonstrate the advantage of our model in terms of accuracy, we compare it with the PC model [10]. We used Wells *et al.*'s algorithm [19] to correct intensity inhomogeneity before we applied the PC models. The third column shows the results of the PC model. We use the Jaccard similarity [20] as a metric to evaluate the performance of image segmentation algorithms. For this McGill Brain Web image, the JS for WM, GM and CSF obtained by the PC model are 0.87, 0.79, and 0.77 respectively. The corresponding JS coefficients of the segmentation result obtained by our method are 0.91, 0.81, and 0.82 respectively. Compared with the results obtained by the PC model, the results of our method are more accurate.

Fig. 3 shows the surfaces of the GM and WM segmentation of real 3D brain MR images with obvious intensity inhomogeneity. The upper and lower row show the results obtained by PC model and our model, respectively. It can be seen that GM obtained by the PC model is a little bit thinner at the top of the

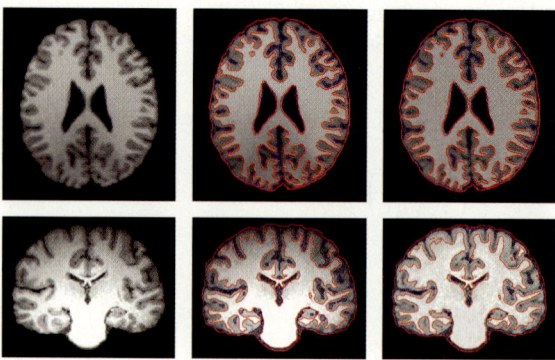

Fig. 2. Results for brain MR images. The red and blue curves are zero level set of ϕ_1 and ϕ_2. Column 1: Original images; Column 2: Results of our model; Column 3: Results of PC model applying to corrected images.

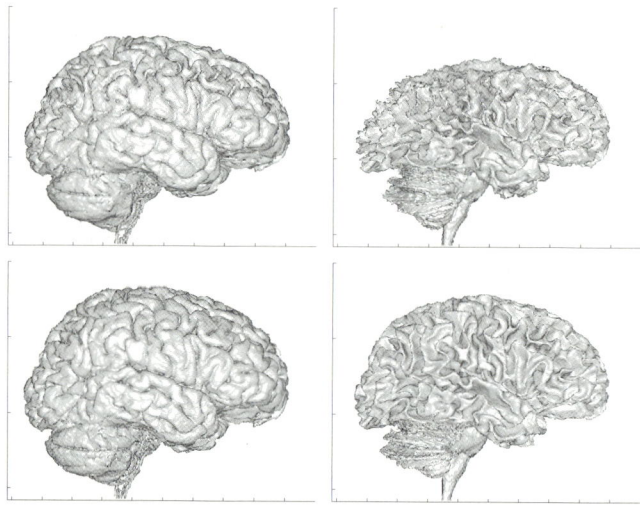

Fig. 3. Results for 3D brain MR images. Row 1: GM and WM surfaces obtained by the PC model; Row 2: GM and WM surfaces obtained by our model.

brain and WM is seriously misclassified as GM. While the surfaces obtained by our method are more accurate. To demonstrate the advantage of our method clearly, we show two sagittal slices and the corresponding contours obtained by the PC model and our method in Fig. 4. It can be clearly seen that the PC model does not correctly segment images: part of the WM is incorrectly identified as the GM, while part of the GM is labeled as the WM. By contrast, our method recovers the boundaries of WM, GM, and CSF accurately.

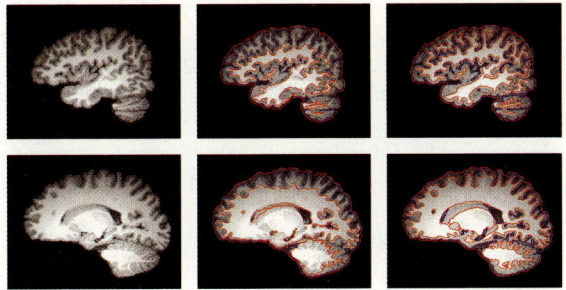

Fig. 4. Sagittal view of 3D segmentation of Fig. 3. Column 1: Original images; Column 2: Results of the PC model; Column 3: Results of our method.

5 Conclusion

In this paper, we provide an improved region-based active contour/surface model for 2D and 3D brain MR image segmentation by drawing upon both local and global intensity information, which is better adapted to the intensity inhomogeneity problem. Experimental results demonstrate desirable performance of our method for brain MR images with intensity inhomogeneity.

References

1. Kass, M., Witkin, A., Terzopoulos, D.: Snakes: active contour models. Int'l J. Comp. Vis. 1, 321–331 (1987)
2. Caselles, V., Catte, F., Coll, T., Dibos, F.: A geometric model for active contours in image processing. Numer. Math. 66, 1–31 (1993)
3. Kimmel, R., Amir, A., Bruckstein, A.: Finding shortest paths on surfaces using level set propagation. IEEE Trans. Patt. Anal. Mach. Intell. 17, 635–640 (1995)
4. Xu, C., Prince, J.: Snakes, shapes, and gradient vector flow. IEEE Trans. Imag. Proc. 7(3), 359–369 (1998)
5. Ronfard, R.: Region-based strategies for active contour models. Int'l. J. Comp. Vis. 13, 229–251 (1994)
6. Samson, C., Blanc-Feraud, L., Aubert, G., Zerubia, J.: A variational model for image classification and restoration. IEEE Trans. Patt. Anal. Mach. Intell. 22(5), 460–472 (2000)
7. Chan, T., Vese, L.: Active contours without edges. IEEE Trans. Imag. Proc. 10, 266–277 (2001)
8. Paragios, N., Deriche, R.: Geodesic active regions and level set methods for supervised texture segmentation. Int'l. J. Comp. Vis. 46, 223–247 (2002)
9. Rousson, M., Cremers, D.: Implicit active shape models for 3D segmentation in MR imaging. In: Barillot, C., Haynor, D.R., Hellier, P. (eds.) MICCAI 2004. LNCS, vol. 3216, pp. 209–216. Springer, Heidelberg (2004)
10. Vese, L., Chan, T.: A multiphase level set framework for image segmentation using the Mumford and Shah model. Int'l. J. Comp. Vis. 50, 271–293 (2002)

11. Tsai, A., Yezzi, A., Willsky, A.S.: Curve evolution implementation of the Mumford-Shah functional for image segmentation, denoising, interpolation, and magnification. IEEE Trans. Imag. Proc. 10, 1169–1186 (2001)
12. Mumford, D., Shah, J.: Optimal approximations by piecewise smooth functions and associated variational problems. Commun. Pure Appl. Math. 42, 577–685 (1989)
13. Piovano, J., Rousson, M., Papadopoulo, T.: Efficient segmentation of piecewise smooth images. In: Scale Space and Variational Methods in Computer Vision, pp. 709–720 (2007)
14. Li, C., Kao, C., Gore, J., Ding, Z.: Implicit active contours driven by local binary fitting energy. In: IEEE Conference on Computer Vision and Pattern Recognition(CVPR) (2007)
15. Li, C., Kao, C., Gore, J., Ding, Z.: Minimization of region-scalable fitting energy for image segmentation. IEEE Trans. Imag. Proc. (to appear)
16. Brox, T., Cremers, D.: On the statistical interpretation of the piecewise smooth Mumford-Shah functional. In: Sgallari, F., Murli, A., Paragios, N. (eds.) SSVM 2007. LNCS, vol. 4485, pp. 203–213. Springer, Heidelberg (2007)
17. Li, C., Xu, C., Gui, C., Fox, M.D.: Level set evolution without re-initialization: A new variational formulation. In: IEEE Conference on Computer Vision and Pattern Recognition(CVPR), vol. 1, pp. 430–436 (2005)
18. http://www.bic.mni.mcgill.ca/brainweb/
19. Wells, W., Grimson, E., Kikinis, R., Jolesz, F.: Adaptive segmentation of MRI data. IEEE Trans. Med. Imag. 15(4), 429–442 (1996)
20. Jaccard, P.: The distribution of flora in the alpine zone. New Phytol. 11(2), 37–50 (1912)

Model-Based Segmentation Using Graph Representations

D. Seghers, J. Hermans, D. Loeckx, F. Maes, D. Vandermeulen, and P. Suetens

Katholieke Universiteit Leuven, Faculties of Medicine and Engineering, Medical Image Computing (Radiology - ESAT/PSI), University Hospital Gasthuisberg, Herestraat 49, B-3000 Leuven, Belgium
dieter.seghers@uz.kuleuven.ac.be

Abstract. A generic supervised segmentation approach is presented. The object is described as a graph where the vertices correspond to landmarks points and the edges define the landmark relations. Instead of building one single global shape model, a priori shape information is represented as a concatenation of local shape models that consider only local dependencies between connected landmarks. The objective function is obtained from a maximum a posteriori criterion and is build up of localized energies of both shape and landmark intensity information. The optimization problem is discretized by searching candidates for each landmark using individual landmark intensity descriptors. The discrete optimization problem is then solved using mean field annealing or dynamic programming techniques. The algorithm is validated for hand bone segmentation from RX datasets and for 3D liver segmentation from contrast enhanced CT images.

1 Introduction

Supervised segmentation has become very popular in the medical image processing domain due to its generic nature, robustness and high accuracy. In general these methods extract shape and gray-value appearance information from a set of training images and corresponding segmentations. A very popular approach is to build a global model of the shape as for example proposed by [1]. Unfortunately, these global models do not fit accurately to unseen images, especially in the case of a low number of training shapes. A way to cope with this is the use of more flexible models, either by superimposing local degrees of freedom onto a global shape description as for example the work of Heimann *et al.* [2], or by limiting the shape model to local descriptors as for example [3, 4]. In a previous contribution [5] the segmentation problem was formulated as a minimal cost path problem (MCP) where intensity costs are assigned to the nodes (landmarks) and shape costs are assigned to node-to-node transitions. A drawback of this method is that the shapes are limited to contours. The objective of this work is to generalize the MCP method to a more generic graph-based object representation.

2 Method

2.1 Training Set

The training set consists of a set of images and a set of corresponding segmentations. The segmented object is mathematically represented as an undirected graph $\mathcal{G} = (\mathcal{V}, \mathcal{E})$: the vertices $\mathcal{V} = \{1, \ldots, n\}$ correspond to the landmark points $\mathbf{l}_1, \ldots, \mathbf{l}_n$ and the edges $\mathcal{E}$ contain unordered pairs of distinct vertices $\{i, j\}$. The number of edges will be denoted with t. An alternative way to formulate the interrelationship between the landmarks is by defining the neighborhood system $\mathcal{N} = \{\mathcal{N}_i | \forall i \in \mathcal{V}\}$ where $\mathcal{N}_i$ is the set of vertices neighboring i. The presented approach assumes that the images in the training set are aligned affinely, either by acquisition or by registration.

The behavior of the object will be described statistically by building a model of the gray-level appearance in the image around each landmark and by modeling the shape.

2.2 Intensity Model

The intensity model is constructed by estimating the probability distribution functions (PDF) of the intensity patterns $\mathbf{f}_i$ in the image around each landmark i individually. First, an intensity descriptor $\mathbf{f}_i = F(I, \mathbf{l}_i)$ is defined that extracts the pattern $\mathbf{f}_i$ around the location $\mathbf{l}_i$ in the image I.

In the learning phase, the pattern $\mathbf{f}_i$ is extracted from each training image and at each landmark $\mathbf{l}_i$. From these samples, the PDF $p(\mathbf{f}_i)$ is estimated for each landmark individually. Writing the PDF as a Gibbs function

$$p(\mathbf{f}_i) = \frac{1}{z_i} \exp\left(-\frac{1}{2} d_i(\mathbf{f}_i)\right) \quad (1)$$

allows to work with energies $d_i(\mathbf{f}_i)$ instead of probabilities $p(\mathbf{f}_i)$. A location in a test image with a low intensity energy has an intensity pattern which is similar to what is found in the training images and is likely to coincide with the true landmark location from an intensity point of view.

When the PDF is modeled as a Gaussian distribution, the energy $d_i(\mathbf{f}_i)$ becomes the mahalanobis distance between $\mathbf{f}_i$ and its mean:

$$d_i(\mathbf{f}_i) = (\mathbf{f}_i - \boldsymbol{\mu}_i)^\mathrm{T} \boldsymbol{\Sigma}_i^{-1} (\mathbf{f}_i - \boldsymbol{\mu}_i) \quad (2)$$

with $\boldsymbol{\mu}_i$ and $\boldsymbol{\Sigma}_i$, respectively the mean and covariance of $\mathbf{f}_i$.

The intensity features of different landmarks are modeled independently, hence the joint PDF of $\mathbf{f} = (\mathbf{f}_1, \ldots, \mathbf{f}_n)$ becomes

$$p(\mathbf{f}) = \frac{1}{Z_\mathbf{f}} \exp\left(-\frac{1}{2} E_\mathrm{f}(\mathbf{f})\right) \quad (3)$$

with $E_\mathrm{f}(\mathbf{f}) = \sum_{i=1}^n d_i(\mathbf{f}_i)$ the global intensity energy and Z_f a normalizing constant.

The same approach as in [5] is adopted to define the intensity descriptor $F(I, \mathbf{l}_i)$. First, a set of N feature images is computed from the original image I. Secondly, intensity profiles $\mathbf{f}_i^{(k)}$ are extracted from the feature images $I^{(k)}$ by taking samples on a sphere centered at $\mathbf{l}_i$. Alternatively, linear instead of spherical profiles can be used by taking samples along the image gradient in $\mathbf{l}_i$. The intensity pattern $\mathbf{f}_i = F(I, \mathbf{l}_i)$ is then constructed by concatenating the N feature profiles $\mathbf{f}_i^{(k)}$ resulting in one large intensity pattern $\mathbf{f}_i$. The PDF $p(\mathbf{f}_i)$ (Eq. 1) is estimated by modeling each feature vector $\mathbf{f}_i^{(k)}$ individually. In the case of a Gaussian, the covariance Σ_i in the energy (Eq. 2) becomes a block diagonal matrix as the dependencies between different features are ignored. Consequently, the computed energy is an overestimation of the true value.

2.3 Shape Model

The shape is described by the positions of the landmarks $\mathbf{l} = \mathbf{l}_\mathcal{V} = (\mathbf{l}_1, \ldots, \mathbf{l}_n)$. Similar as for the intensity patterns, a model of the shape is built by estimating the joint shape PDF $p(\mathbf{l})$ from a set of training shapes. The model relies on two assumptions. First, the probability function of an edge vector does not depend on its location in space: $p(\mathbf{l}_j - \mathbf{l}_i | \mathbf{l}_i) = p(\mathbf{l}_j - \mathbf{l}_i)$ with $j \in \mathcal{N}_i$, implying $p(\mathbf{l}_j | \mathbf{l}_i) = p(\mathbf{l}_j - \mathbf{l}_i)$. This assumption also implies that the shape PDF is invariant for translations: $p(\mathbf{l}_i) = c^{\text{te}}$. A second model supposition (*markovianity*) is that a landmark i only interacts with its neighbors : $p(\mathbf{l}_i | \mathbf{l}_{\mathcal{V}-\{i\}}) = p(\mathbf{l}_i | \mathbf{l}_{\mathcal{N}_i})$. Hence, the shape obeys the definition of a markov random field (MRF). According to the Hammersley-Clifford theorem [6] the joint PDF of an MRF can be written as

$$p(\mathbf{l}) = \frac{1}{Z_\mathbf{l}} \exp\left(-\frac{1}{2} E_\mathbf{l}(\mathbf{l})\right) \quad (4)$$

The energy $E_\mathbf{l}(\mathbf{l})$ is a sum of local energy functions over all possible cliques[1] of the graph and $Z_\mathbf{l}$ is a normalizing constant. First, the shape energy is computed for a trivial graph consisting of only one triangle: $\mathcal{V} = \{1, 2, 3\}$ and $\mathcal{E} = \{\{1, 2\}, \{1, 3\}, \{2, 3\}\}$. The joint PDF written in the energy space becomes

$$\log p(\mathbf{l}_1, \mathbf{l}_2, \mathbf{l}_3) = \log p(\mathbf{l}_1) + \log p(\mathbf{l}_2 | \mathbf{l}_1) + \log p(\mathbf{l}_3 | \mathbf{l}_1, \mathbf{l}_2) \quad (5)$$

If only the influence of the edges $\{1, 2\}$ and $\{1, 3\}$ is considered, the log equation (Eq. 5) can be approximated as

$$\log p(\mathbf{l}_1, \mathbf{l}_2, \mathbf{l}_3) \approx \log p(\mathbf{l}_1) + \log p(\mathbf{l}_2 | \mathbf{l}_1) + \log p(\mathbf{l}_3 | \mathbf{l}_1) \quad (6)$$

In order to obtain an approximation that takes all edges into account, Eq. 6 is considered for all three possible combinations. Averaging them leads to

$$\log p(\mathbf{l}_1, \mathbf{l}_2, \mathbf{l}_3) \approx c^{\text{te}} + \frac{2}{3} \left(\log p(\mathbf{l}_2 - \mathbf{l}_1) + \log p(\mathbf{l}_3 - \mathbf{l}_1) + \log p(\mathbf{l}_3 - \mathbf{l}_2)\right) \quad (7)$$

---

[1] A clique is a subset of a graph such that every two vertices in the clique are neighbors.

Similar as in Eq. 1, the PDF of an edge $\mathbf{l}_j - \mathbf{l}_i$ can be written using the *edge energy* $d_{ij}(\mathbf{l}_i, \mathbf{l}_j)$ expressing the likelihood of the edge $\mathbf{l}_j - \mathbf{l}_i$. When the edge distribution is modeled as a Gaussian, the energy $d_{ij}(\mathbf{l}_i, \mathbf{l}_j)$ is the mahalanobis distance between $\mathbf{l}_j - \mathbf{l}_i$ and its expected value. Remark that the edge energy is symmetrical, i.e. $d_{ij}(\mathbf{l}_i, \mathbf{l}_j) = d_{ji}(\mathbf{l}_j, \mathbf{l}_i)$. From Eq. 4 and Eq. 7, the triangle shape energy becomes

$$E_\mathrm{l}(\mathbf{l}_1, \mathbf{l}_2, \mathbf{l}_3) = \frac{2}{3}\left(d_{12}(\mathbf{l}_1, \mathbf{l}_2) + d_{13}(\mathbf{l}_1, \mathbf{l}_3) + d_{23}(\mathbf{l}_2, \mathbf{l}_3)\right) \qquad (8)$$

For a general graph with n vertices and t edges, a similar expression as Eq. 8 can be derived

$$E_\mathrm{l}(\mathbf{l}) = \frac{n-1}{t} \sum_{\{i,j\}\in\mathcal{E}} d_{ij}(\mathbf{l}_i, \mathbf{l}_j) \qquad (9)$$

2.4 Objective Function

Criterion. The segmentation problem is formulated using a maximum a posteriori (MAP) probability criterion:

$$\mathbf{l}^* = \arg\max_{\mathbf{l}} p(\mathbf{l}|I) = \arg\max_{\mathbf{l}} \frac{p(I|\mathbf{l})p(\mathbf{l})}{p(I)} \qquad (10)$$

The shape prior $p(\mathbf{l})$ is given by Eq. 4 and Eq. 9. The probability $p(I|\mathbf{l})$ is proportional to $p(\mathbf{f})$ as given by Eq. 3 with $\mathbf{f} = F(I, \mathbf{l})$. Hence, the criterion (Eq. 10) becomes

$$\mathbf{l}^* = \arg\min_{\mathbf{l}} \left(E_\mathrm{f}(F(I,\mathbf{l})) + E_\mathrm{l}(\mathbf{l})\right) \qquad (11)$$

$$= \arg\min_{\mathbf{l}} \left(\sum_{i=1}^{n} d_i(F(I,\mathbf{l}_i)) + \gamma \sum_{\{i,j\}\in\mathcal{E}} d_{ij}(\mathbf{l}_i, \mathbf{l}_j)\right) \qquad (12)$$

with $\gamma = (n-1)/t$.

Discretization. As the objective function (Eq. 12) has many local optima it is difficult to optimize in the continuous domain. Therefore, the segmentation task is converted to a discrete labeling problem. For each landmark i, a set of candidate locations is obtained by evaluating the intensity energy $d_i(F(I,\mathbf{l}))$ at each point $\mathbf{l}$ of a search grid and selecting the m lowest-energy locations. The result is a set of candidates $\mathcal{C} = \{\{\mathbf{l}_{ik}, \mathbf{f}_{ik}\}_{k=1}^{m}\}_{i=1}^{n}$. At this point, the segmentation problem becomes a labeling problem $\mathbf{x} = (\mathbf{x}_1, \ldots, \mathbf{x}_n)$ where one candidate per landmark needs to be selected. $\mathbf{x}_i$ represents the choice for landmark i: $\sum_{k=1}^{m} x_{ik} = 1$ and $x_{ik} = 1$ if candidate k is selected. The PDF $p(\mathbf{l}|I)$ is now converted into a discrete probability distribution $P(\mathbf{x}|\mathcal{C})$ with energy

$$E(\mathbf{x}) = \sum_{i=1}^{n}\sum_{a=1}^{m} (x_{ia} d_i(\mathbf{f}_{ia})) + \frac{\gamma}{2}\sum_{i=1}^{n}\sum_{a=1}^{m}\left(x_{ia}\sum_{j\in\mathcal{N}_i}\sum_{b=1}^{m} x_{jb} d_{ij}(\mathbf{l}_{ia}, \mathbf{l}_{jb})\right) \qquad (13)$$

Hence, an intensity energy is assigned to each selected candidate landmark (first term in Eq 13), and a local shape energy is assigned to each selected edge. The theoretical value for γ is $(n-1)/t$. In the implementation of this method, the value for γ is also used to compensate for the overestimated intensity energy (Eq. 2). The optimal γ-value is obtained from a leave-one-out strategy during the training phase yielding a value always larger than $(n-1)/t$.

2.5 Optimization

Dynamic Programming (DP). In the case when the graph is an open contour with n landmarks and $n-1$ edges, the problem is reduced to a minimal cost path problem which can be solved using dynamic programming [6, 5] with computational complexity $O(nm^2)$. Also more complex graphs can be handled using DP, but with increasing complexity. The computational complexity can be found out by eliminating the graph landmark by landmark. The computational complexity is $O(nm^{a+1})$ with a the number of edges that disappear each time a landmark is eliminated.

Iterative DP. From a computational point of view, DP is not acceptable for complex graphs. An approximating iterative procedure is proposed instead. Prior to optimization, the graph is divided into a number of (overlapping) subgraphs (paths). The paths are generated randomly, starting from a specific edge and iteratively adding concatenating edges as long as the path is not self-intersecting. From every edge in $\mathcal{E}$ a random path is started resulting into a total of t subgraphs $\mathcal{V}^{(i)}$. Once all the paths are generated, an iterative optimization procedure is started as follows. Each subgraph $\mathcal{V}^{(i)}$ is optimized globally using DP and the result yields votes for the selected landmark candidates. After optimizing every random path, the least voted candidates are removed. This procedure is repeated till only one candidate is left for every landmark.

Mean field annealing. The discrete labeling $\mathbf{x}$ satisfies the condition of an MRF and listens to the Gibbs distribution

$$P(\mathbf{x}|\mathcal{C}) = \frac{1}{Z_\mathbf{x}} \exp\left(-\frac{1}{T}E(\mathbf{x})\right) \qquad (14)$$

with $T=2$ and with $E(\mathbf{x})$ computed as in Eq. 13. According to Eq. 14, the temperature T can be altered without influencing the optimum $\mathbf{x}^*$. At the other hand, the mean $\overline{\mathbf{x}}$ changes with T as follows:

$$\lim_{T\to 0+} \overline{\mathbf{x}}_T = \lim_{T\to 0+} \sum_\mathbf{x} \mathbf{x} P(\mathbf{x}) = \mathbf{x}^* \qquad (15)$$

The rationale behind mean field annealing [6] is that instead of minimizing the energy $E(\mathbf{x})$ directly, one can try to estimate the mean field $\overline{\mathbf{x}}_T$ at a sufficiently high temperature and then track it down as the temperature is lowered towards zero. The estimated mean field β is computed from the following set of nonlinear equations:

$$\alpha_{ik} = \exp\left(-\frac{1}{T}\left(d_i(\mathbf{f}_{ik}) + \gamma \sum_{j \in \mathcal{N}_i} \sum_{b=1}^{m} \beta_{jb} d_{ij}(\mathbf{l}_{ik}, \mathbf{l}_{jb})\right)\right) \quad (16)$$

$$\beta_{ik} = \frac{\alpha_{ik}}{\sum_{a=1}^{m} \alpha_{ia}} \quad (17)$$

$\forall i = 1, \ldots, n$ and $\forall k = 1, \ldots, m$. The set is solved using iterative resubstitution: The values for $\beta_{ik}^{(i)}$ are computed from $\alpha_{ik}^{(i)}$ using Eq. 17. The updated values $\alpha_{ik}^{(i+1)}$ are computed with Eq. 16. This procedure is started from an initial point $\alpha_{ik}^{(0)}$ and iterated till the values for α_{ik} and β_{ik} are sufficiently stable. The mean field equations are solved several times, starting at a sufficiently high T, and gradually decreasing the temperature towards zero resulting in a mean β that converges to a binary assignment.

3 Experiments and Results

The algorithm is validated for two applications: segmentation of hand bones from RX and liver segmentation from contrast enhanced CT scans.

3.1 Hand Bones

The segmentation task consists of the delineation of 11 bones in the hand (bones of the thumb, the small and middle finger) from RX datasets. A hierarchical segmentation strategy is illustrated in Fig. 1. In a first step, the algorithm of Sect. 2 is applied with a model trained from graphs consisting of 11 vertices positioned at the centers of the hand bones as shown in Fig. 1(a). Applying a segmentation with this model enables the localization of each bone individually. Fig. 1(b) shows an unseen hand radiograph to be segmented. The intensity PDF's (Eq. 1) of landmarks 1, 4 and 11 are superimposed on the image in the corresponding search regions. The search region of $\mathbf{l}_i$ is chosen such that each $\mathbf{l}_i$ of the training shapes is covered. In a second step, eleven individual contour models consisting of 20 to 40 landmarks (Fig. 1(c)) are used to delineate each bone individually. The segmentation is performed on sub-images centered around the detected centers from the first step. Fig. 1(d) shows such an extracted image together with the intensity PDF's of landmarks 8 and 18. The delineation of bone 11 is shown in Fig. 1(e).

This hierarchical segmentation setup is validated on a set of 50 training images (width of 256 pixels) of both adults and children using a leave-one-out approach. The intensity model was built using spherical profiles with a radius of 8 pixels for the first model and profiles with a radius of 1 pixel to delineate the individual bones. Optimizing with iterative DP resulted in a mean overlap and mean distance error of 87.5% and 1.36 pixels respectively. Using mean field annealing scored slightly worse with an overlap of 86.2% and 1.46 pixels distance error.

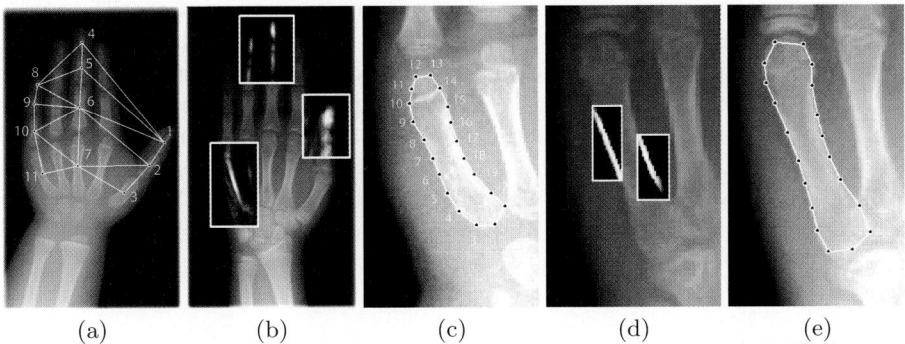

Fig. 1. Hand segmentation strategy: (a) model for bone localization; (b) intensity PDF of landmark 1, 4 and 11; (c) model for bone delineation; (d) intensity PDF of landmark 8 and 18; (e) automated bone delineation

3.2 Liver

A set of 20 contrast enhanced CT datasets and corresponding segmentations of the liver were obtained from [7]. Prior to segmentation, an affine registration step was applied to align the images. The liver was described as a surface mesh consisting of $n = 3277$ landmarks and $t = 9825$ edges. Segmentation is carried out with a multi-resolution-approach starting from large profiles (large radius) and large search regions and ending with smaller and more accurate profiles in smaller search regions. Three resolution stages were carried out with linear profiles sampled along the image gradient with sizes ranging between 30 and 6 millimeters. In between consecutive resolution stages, a postprocessing step was needed to counter the following problem. Prior to optimization, candidate locations are searched for every landmark. If no proper locations were generated for a particular landmark due to a failing intensity descriptor, the segmented object contained outliers. To overcome this, the outlier locations with excessive shape energies were relaxed to lower shape energy locations.

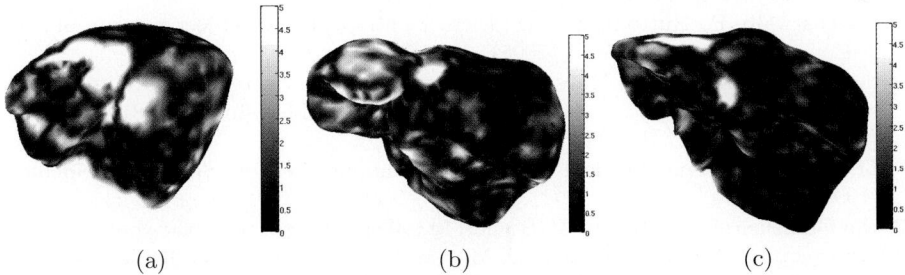

Fig. 2. Surface distance errors for (a) the worst (3.5mm), (b) an average (1.4mm) and (c) the best (0.9mm) segmentation. Black and white correspond to 0 and 5mm respectively.

The segmentation scheme was validated using leave-one-out on the training set and applying the scoring system as in [7] which is based on five metrics (volumetric overlap, volume difference, surface distance, root mean square surface distance and maximum surface distance). For comparison, a score of 75% implies a performance as good as human. The best results were obtained with iterative DP with an mean score of 67% compared to 57% for mean field annealing. The mean overlap and closest distance error was 91.7% and 1.47mm respectively. Fig. 2 displays the distance errors of the worst, middle and best case with scores of 33%, 72% and 83% respectively.

4 Discussion

A supervised image segmentation method based on graph representations is proposed. The model is built from local statistical models of both shape and gray-level appearance resulting in an approach that accurately fits to unseen data. The discretization of the objective function obtained from a MAP criterion, allows to formulate the segmentation task as a labeling problem and thus enables robust optimization techniques as dynamic programming and mean field annealing. The generic nature of the method is illustrated for hand bone delineation from RX datasets and for liver segmentation from contrast enhanced CT scans. Despite the heuristic nature of the iterative DP method, better results were obtained than optimizing with mean field annealing.

References

[1] Cootes, T., Taylor, C., Cooper, D., Graham, J.: Active shape models - their training and applications. Computer Vision and Image Understanding 61(1), 38–59 (1995)

[2] Heimann, T., Wolf, I., Meinzer, H.: Active shape models for a fully automated 3D segmentation of the liver – an evaluation on clinical data. In: Larsen, R., Nielsen, M., Sporring, J. (eds.) MICCAI 2006. LNCS, vol. 4191, pp. 41–48. Springer, Heidelberg (2006)

[3] Amit, Y., Kong, A.: Graphical templates for model registration. IEEE Trans. Pattern Anal. Machine Intell. 18(3), 225–236 (1996)

[4] Felzenszwalb, P., Huttonlocker, D.: Pictorial structures for object recognition. Int. J. Comput. Vis. 61(1), 55–79 (2005)

[5] Seghers, D., Loeckx, D., Maes, F., Vandermeulen, D., Suetens, P.: Minimal intensity and shape cost path segmentation. IEEE Trans. Med. Imag. 26(8), 1115–1129 (2007)

[6] Li, S.: Markov Random Field Modeling in Computer Vision. Springer, Heidelberg (1995)

[7] van Ginneken, B., Heimann, T., Styner, M.: 3D segmentation in the clinic: A grand challenge. In: Heimann, T., Styner, M., van Ginneken, B. (eds.) 3D Segmentation in the Clinic: A Grand Challenge, pp. 7–15 (2007)

3D Brain Segmentation Using Active Appearance Models and Local Regressors

K.O. Babalola, T.F. Cootes, C.J. Twining, V. Petrovic, and C.J. Taylor

Division of Imaging Science and Biomedical Engineering,
The University of Manchester, Manchester, UK
kola.babalola@manchester.ac.uk
http://www.isbe.man.ac.uk/~kob

Abstract. We describe an efficient and accurate method for segmenting sets of subcortical structures in 3D MR images of the brain. We first find the approximate position of all the structures using a global Active Appearance Model (AAM). We then refine the shape and position of each structure using a set of individual AAMs trained for each. Finally we produce a detailed segmentation by computing the probability that each voxel belongs to the structure, using regression functions trained for each individual voxel. The models are trained using a large set of labelled images, using a novel variant of 'groupwise' registration to obtain the necessary image correspondences. We evaluate the method on a large dataset, and demonstrate that it achieves results comparable with some of the best published.

1 Introduction

Accurately segmenting structures from 3D medical images is an important step in a wide range of applications, particularly when diagnosing disease, monitoring patients or evaluating the effects of pharmaceutical compounds.

Many approaches to automatic and semi-automatic segmentation are being developed. In this paper we describe a system which uses volumetric Active Appearance Models (AAMs) [4] to locate the shape and positions of each structure, then refines the segmentation with a set of local regressors which estimate the probability that voxels near the boundary belong to the structure.

One of the most effective methods of segmentation of subcortical structures in the brain is that of Aljabar et al.[11]. Given a set of labelled training images, a new image can be segmented by registering each of a subset of the training images to the new image, transfering the labels and using these to vote for the most likely label for each voxel. By selecting the subset to be those training images with similar properties to the target image, state of the art performance can be achieved.

This approach is effective, but relatively time-consuming, due to the number of full 3D registrations required. The method described below is inspired by this classifier fusion approach, but is much more efficient. Rather than perform many individual registrations, we use a combination of AAMs to locate the structures rapidly. Rather than retaining all the training set to use to perform label voting, we summarise the information by training local regressors, one per voxel in a model reference image. These are able to correct small boundary errors, leading to a good final result.

The contributions of the paper include

- An improved method of finding correspondences by applying groupwise registration to multi-plane images containing both intensity and label data
- A two layer system for locating deep brain structures using a global AAM followed by the use of individual AAMs for each part.
- A method of refining the solution using simple linear regressors trained in the reference frame
- An evaluation of the performance on multiple structures on a large dataset

In the following we describe the key components of the system in more detail, and present quantitative results on a large dataset.

2 Background

There are many approaches to segmenting structures from 3D volumetric images, including deformable surface meshes, medial representations, segmentation by registration, and shape constrained level set approaches, amongst others e.g. see [12]. However, here we concentrate on methods using statistical shape models, based on the original work of Cootes et al.[5]. In particular, the Active Appearance Model, a fast method of matching appearance models to new images, has been found to be effective for analysing medical images [3]. It was extended to volumetric images (2D+time) by Mitchell et al.[10]. To construct such models each image in a training set must be annotated with corresponding points. Frangi et al.[8] obtained correspondences by using volumetric deformation of binary images. Klemencic et al.[9] extended this to build 3D (volumetric) AAMs of the hippocampus. In related work, Duchesne and Collins [7] used an AAM trained on deformation fields to estimate the deformation of a new image. The target image was then segmented by transferring labels from the reference volume.

3 Methodology

To train the system we have access to a set of 3D MR images, for each of which we have voxel label images (i.e. an image of label values indicating which structure each voxel belongs to).

In order to construct statistical models of shape and appearance, it is necessary to find a set of points in each image which define the correspondences.

3.1 Computing Correspondence

The label images allow us to construct binary images for each structure. To find correspondences for a given structure we could use the approach of Frangi et al.[8] and apply non-rigid registration to such binary images. However, we use a variant of the "groupwise" registration approach of Cootes et al.[2]. This seeks to find the deformations of space which allow us to construct the most compact model of a set of images. A key novelty in this work is that rather than registering a set of binary label images, we generate a set of two plane images in which the first plane is the binary label, and the second is a locally normalised intensity image. Groupwise registration involves estimating the volumetric deformations which best match each two-plane image to the group mean. The inclusion of both intensity and labels in the process means that the correspondences are estimated to both match the label boundaries, as well as nearby structures in the grey-level image. This extra information leads to better final shape and appearance models. Yeo et al.[13] also register intensity and label images to build probabistic atlases.

The deformations are represented by the movements of a tetrahedral mesh, covering the region of interest. The nodes of the mesh are control points. The positions of the control points on two images define a sparse set of corresponding points across the images, and a dense correspondence can be found efficiently using affine interpolation within each tetrahedra of the mesh.

3.2 Model Construction

By aligning the sets of control points on each image and applying Principal Component Analysis we can generate a statistical shape model [5].

By warping each grey-level image into the mean reference image (using the tetrahedral mesh) we can apply PCA to the resulting textures to generate a statistical texture model. We can combine the shape and texture models to build a combined statistical model of appearance [4], with the form

$$\begin{aligned} \mathbf{x} &= \bar{\mathbf{x}} + \mathbf{Q}_s \mathbf{c} \\ \mathbf{g} &= \bar{\mathbf{g}} + \mathbf{Q}_g \mathbf{c} \end{aligned} \quad (1)$$

where $\bar{\mathbf{x}}$, $\bar{\mathbf{g}}$ are vectors of the mean shape and mean texture, $\mathbf{x}$, $\mathbf{g}$ are the shape and texture vectors in the reference frame, $\mathbf{Q}_s$, $\mathbf{Q}_g$ are matrices describing the modes of variation derived from the training set, and $\mathbf{c}$ is a vector of parameters controlling both shape and texture. For a given $\mathbf{c}$ we can generate a texture, then warp this using the generated shape to create a synthetic image of the modelled object. For instance, Figure 1 shows a slice through the 3D image generated by the model of the region around the left ventricle.

Such a model can be matched to a new image rapidly using the Active Appearance Model algorithm [4]. This seeks to minimise a sum-of-squares problem of the form

$$F(\mathbf{p}) = |\mathbf{r}(\mathbf{p})|^2 = \mathbf{r}^T \mathbf{r} \quad (2)$$

where $\mathbf{p}$ contains the t model parameters (the appearance parameters $\mathbf{c}$, together with global pose parameters - see [4]), and $\mathbf{r} = \mathbf{r}(\mathbf{p})$ is a function returning the n_g residual differences between model and data for parameters $\mathbf{p}$. By making assumptions about the Jacobian, a fast updating algorithm can be derived which can match the model to a new image in a few iterations.

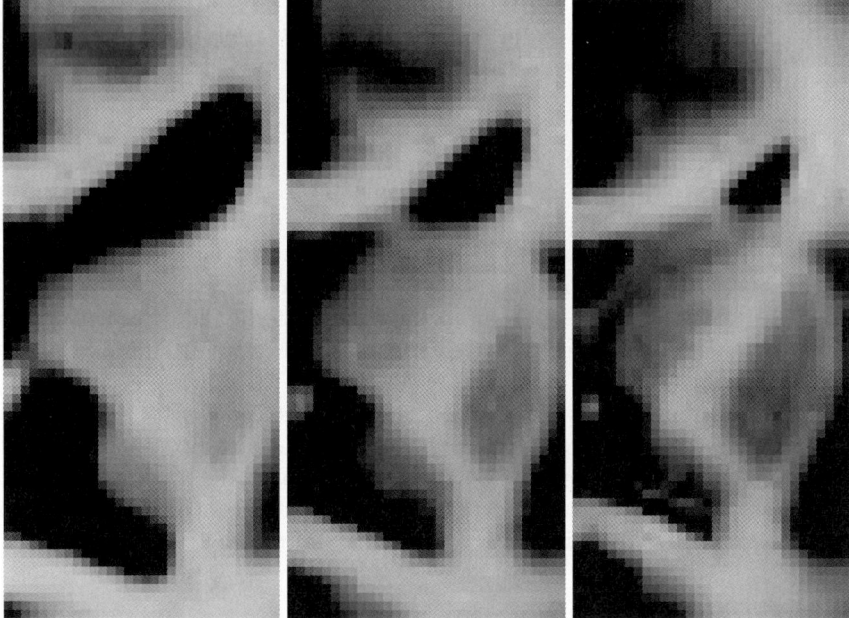

Fig. 1. Slice through images synthesized by varying the first mode of the appearance model of the left ventricle between -2.5 and +2.5 standard deviations

3.3 Segmenting Voxels

Given the correspondences estimated by the groupwise registration, we can warp each binary label image into the reference frame. If we compute the mean of these warped images, across the training set, we derive a mean probability image. Each voxel of this gives the probability that it belongs to the object of interest in the reference frame. For instance, Figure 2a shows a slice through the mean probability image for the left ventricle.

One approach to segmenting a new image is to first match the appearance model using the AAM, then to project the mean probability image into the target image using the resulting model points. The resulting warped probability image can be thresholded at 0.5 to obtain a hard estimate of voxels inside and outside of the object of interest.

However, in some cases the result of the AAM search may not be accurate enough to give a good segmentation. Mis-matches can occur because of poor initialisation, unmodelled image structures or because the model does not contain enough degrees of freedom to accurately deform to a particular image.

Such sub-optimal matching may mean that the object boundaries are incorrectly delineated. However, where such mis-matches are relatively small, we can correct for them by analysing the local image structure.

Rather than use the mean probability image, we generate a new probability image based on pixel intensities warped into the model frame.

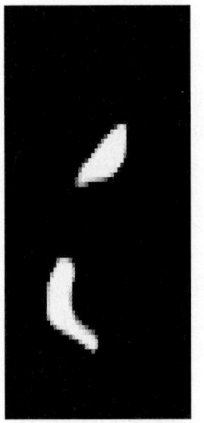 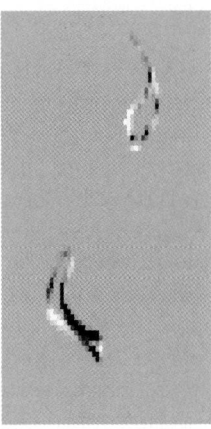

a) Mean Probability Image b) Difference in probability due to regression

Fig. 2. Probability images in reference frame for the left ventricle. The image on the left is the mean probability image. That on the right is a difference image of the probabilities computed from the mean for one subject before and after application of regression.

During a training phase we warp each normalised intensity image into the model reference frame using the known correspondences. For any given voxel in this frame we then have a set of probabilities, p_i, $i = 1..n_{images}$, that it is inside the object (by warping the binary label images)[1] together with corresponding vectors of intensity values $\mathbf{g}_i$ sampled in the region around the voxel.

We then perform linear regression to learn a function to estimate the probability given the intensity pattern

$$p = f(\mathbf{g}) = \mathbf{a}^T \mathbf{g} + d \qquad (3)$$

This is repeated for every voxel near the boundary. Voxels away from the boundary are assumed to have either p=0 (outside) or p=1 (inside).

Given a new image, we can then segment it using the following steps

- Match a volumetric AAM to estimate correspondence with the model frame
- Use the resulting correspondences to warp the normalised intensities into the model frame
- Use the voxel probability estimators (Eq.3) to compute the probability image in the reference frame
- Use the correspondences to warp this into the image frame
- Obtain a labelled image by selecting the structure with maximum probability ≥ 0.5 at each voxel

Figure 2b shows the difference in the resulting probability image before and after regression.

---

[1] We use trilinear interpolation during warping, leading to values of p in the range $(0, 1)$ for voxels near boundaries.

4 Experiments

We were provided with 270 T1 MR images and corresponding manually labelled images which included the labels of 18 subcortical structures – the brain stem, fourth ventricle and the left and right pairs of the accumbens, amygdala, caudate, hippocampus, lateral ventricles, thalamus, pallidum and putamen (see figure 3). There was a wide variation in the subject pool age (4.5 years – 83 years), and disease (controls, Alzheimer's disease, Schizophrenia, Attention Deficit Hyperactivity Disorder and prenatal drug exposure).

We established correspondence using the groupwise registration method described in section 3.1. We then constructed both a global AAM (containing all structures) and a set of individual AAMs, one for each structure. The voxel regressors were constructed as described above.

To evaluate the performance of the method a set of 27 leave-10-out experiments were performed, in which the models are trained on 260 images, then tested on the remaining 10. The search is fully automatic, involving three stages:

i) a global search with the AAM of all structures,
ii) local search with each individual structure AAM to refine the matches
iii) segmentation by combining the generated probability images into a single label image

The quality of the resulting segmentations were quantitatively evaluated using the corresponding manually labelled image as a gold standard and the Dice overlap coefficient [6] as the evaluation metric.

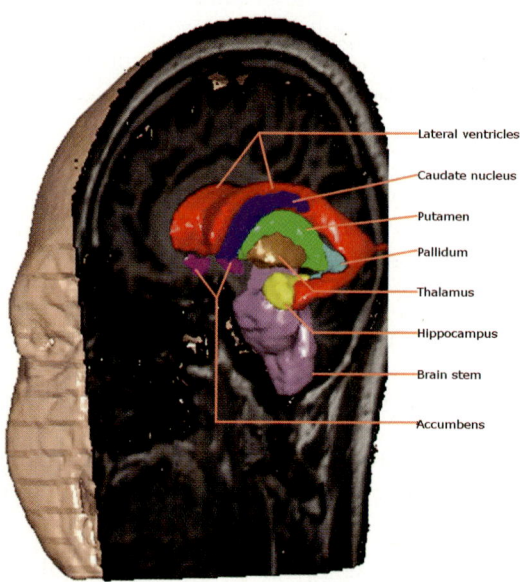

Fig. 3. Surface rendering of an MR image showing subcortical structures used in model building

5 Results

Columns 2 and 3 of Table 1 shows the Dice coefficients for the results of the leave 10 out segmentations using the AAM, both with and without the final regressor estimate of the probability image. It demonstrates the the regressors are able to significantly improve the Dice overlap results for almost every structure.

Table 1. Mean Dice overlap coefficients for segmentation results. Standard errors are shown in parenthesis ($n = 270$ for fourth ventricle and brain stem, $n = 540$ for other structures). The last column shows results for the method of Aljabar et al.[11] on the same dataset (figures obtained from [1]).

Structure	AAM + mean prob	AAM + regressor	Classifier Fusion
Accumbens	73.1% (0.4)	73.7% (0.4)	75.8%
Amygdala	75.0% (0.4)	76.1% (0.4)	77.7%
Brain Stem	91.3% (0.4)	92.5% (0.4)	94.2%
Caudate	85.9% (0.2)	88.7% (0.2)	88.1%
Fourth ventricle	78.7% (0.4)	82.9% (0.3)	83.2%
Hippocampus	80.9% (0.2)	83.7% (0.2)	83.5%
Pallidum	81.7% (0.2)	83.1% (0.2)	81.9%
Putamen	88.6% (0.1)	90.8% (0.1)	89.8%
Thalamus	89.9% (0.1)	90.8% (0.1)	90.8%
Lateral ventricles	83.2% (0.4)	90.2% (0.3)	91.3%

6 Discussion and Conclusions

We have described a system for segmenting sub-cortical structures from 3D MR images of the brain. The method first finds the approximate positions of all structures using a global AAM. It refines the positions using individual AAMs of each structure, then produces a final segmentation by computing a labelled image from probability images of each structure. These probability images can be derived from the mean of the training set. However, we have demonstrated that better results can be obtained by using simple regressors at each voxel to estimate the probability of object occupancy based on the pattern of grey level intensities nearby. Because this is able to correct for some mis-matching of the shape models, it generally leads to better overall results.

The results for most structures are comparable to the best published results for these structures, though most other results are on much smaller datasets. Direct comparison with four different algorithms from four different groups [1] shows that the method is achieving results similar to the best known method on this dataset (the fusion of predictions from registering many atlases [11]).

The proposed method is relatively swift, taking less than 20 minutes to segment all structures in a single image using a standard single processor PC.

The tool and models will be made freely available for research purposes.

We anticipate it will be possible to improve the results still further by tuning the model building and search parameters for each structure individually, and by exploring more sophisticated regression models for predicting the probability images.

Acknowledgements

This work was funded by the EPSRC. David Kennedy of the Center for Morphometric Analysis, Boston, provided the MR images used.

References

1. Babalola, K., Patenaude, B., Aljabar, P., Schnabel, J., Kennedy, D., Crum, W., Smith, S., Cootes, T.F., Jenkinson, M., Rueckert, D.: Comparison and evaluation of segmentation techniques for subcortical structures in brain MRI. In: Proc. MICCAI. LNCS, vol. 5241 (2008)
2. Cootes, T., Twining, C., Petrović, V., Schestowitz, R., Taylor, C.: Groupwise construction of appearance models using piece-wise affine deformations. In: 16th British Machine Vision Conference, vol. 2, pp. 879–888 (2005)
3. Cootes, T.F., Beeston, C., Edwards, G.J., Taylor, C.J.: A unified framework for atlas matching using Active Appearance Models. In: Proc. Information Processing in Medical Imaging, pp. 322–333 (1999)
4. Cootes, T.F., Edwards, G.J., Taylor, C.J.: Active Appearance Models. IEEE Transactions on Pattern Analysis and Machine Intelligence 23(6), 681–685 (2001)
5. Cootes, T.F., Taylor, C.J., Cooper, D., Graham, J.: Active Shape Models - their training and application. Computer Vision and Image Understanding 61(1), 38–59 (1995)
6. Dice, L.R.: Measures of the amount of ecologic association between species. Ecology 26, 297–302 (1945)
7. Duchesne, S., Pruessner, J.C., Collins, D.L.: Appearance-based modelling and segmentation of the hippocampus from MR images. In: Proceedings of the 23rd Annual International Conference of the IEEE on Engineering in Medicine and Biology Society, vol. 3, pp. 2677–2680 (2001)
8. Frangi, A.F., Rueckert, D., Schnabel, J.A., Niessen, W.J.: Automatic 3D ASM construction via atlas-based landmarking and volumetric elastic registration. In: Insana, M.F., Leahy, R.M. (eds.) IPMI 2001. LNCS, vol. 2082, pp. 78–91. Springer, Heidelberg (2001)
9. Klemencic, J., Pluim, J., Viergever, M., Schnack, H., Valencic, V.: Non-rigid registration based Active Appearance Models for 3D medical image segmentation. Journal of Imaging Science and Technology 48(2), 166–171 (2004)
10. Mitchell, S., Boudewijn, P., Lelievedt, P.F., van der Geest, R., Bosch, H., Reiber, J., Sonka, M.: Time continuous segmentation of cardiac MR image sequences using active appearance motion models. In: SPIE Medical Imaging (February 2001)
11. Aljabar, P., Heckemann, R., Hammers, A., Hajnal, J., Rueckert, D.: Classifier selection strategies for label fusion using large atlas databases. In: Ayache, N., Ourselin, S., Maeder, A. (eds.) MICCAI 2007, Part I. LNCS, vol. 4791, pp. 523–531. Springer, Heidelberg (2007)
12. Pizer, S.M., Fletcher, P., Joshi, S., et al.: Deformable M-Reps for 3D medical image segmentation. International Journal of Computer Vision 2-3(55), 85–106 (2003)
13. Yeo, B., Sabuncu, M., Desikan, R., Fischl, B., Golland, P.: Effects of registration regularization and atlas sharpness on segmentation accuracy. In: Ayache, N., Ourselin, S., Maeder, A. (eds.) MICCAI 2007, Part I. LNCS, vol. 4791, pp. 683–691. Springer, Heidelberg (2007)

Comparison and Evaluation of Segmentation Techniques for Subcortical Structures in Brain MRI

K.O. Babalola[1], B. Patenaude[2], P. Aljabar[3], J. Schnabel[4], D. Kennedy[5], W. Crum[6], S. Smith[2], T.F. Cootes[1], M. Jenkinson[2], and D. Rueckert[3]

[1] Division of Imaging Science and Biomedical Engineering (ISBE), University of Manchester, UK
{kola.babalola,tim.cootes}@manchester.ac.uk
[2] FMRIB Centre, John Radcliffe Hospital, University of Oxford, OX3 9DU, UK
{mark,brian}@fmrib.ox.ac.uk
[3] Department of Computing, Imperial College London, SW7 2BZ, UK
{dr,pa}@doc.ic.ac.uk
[4] Department of Engineering Science, University of Oxford, Oxford, OX1 3PJ, UK
julia.schnabel@eng.ox.ac.uk
[5] MGH/MIT/HMS Athinoula A. Martinos Center for Biomedical Imaging, Building 149, 13th Street, Radiology/CNY149-Room 2301, Charlestown, MA 02129, USA
dave@cma.mgh.harvard.edu
[6] Institute of Psychiatry, Box P089, De Crespigny Park, London, UK, SE5 8AF
bill.crum@iop.kcl.ac.uk

Abstract. The automation of segmentation of medical images is an active research area. However, there has been criticism of the standard of evaluation of methods. We have comprehensively evaluated four novel methods of automatically segmenting subcortical structures using volumetric, spatial overlap and distance-based measures. Two of the methods are atlas-based – classifier fusion and labelling (CFL) and expectation-maximisation segmentation using a dynamic brain atlas (EMS), and two model-based – profile active appearance models (PAM) and Bayesian appearance models (BAM). Each method was applied to the segmentation of 18 subcortical structures in 270 subjects from a diverse pool varying in age, disease, sex and image acquisition parameters. Our results showed that all four methods perform on par with recently published methods. CFL performed significantly better than the other three methods according to all three classes of metrics.

1 Introduction

Functional and structural brain imaging are playing an expanding role in neuroscience and experimental medicine. The amount of data produced by imaging increasingly exceeds the capacity for expert visual analysis, resulting in a growing need for automated image analysis. In particular, accurate and reliable methods for segmentation (classifying image regions) are a key requirement for the extraction of qualitative or quantitative information from images.

Image segmentation aims to separate an image into anatomically meaningful regions. The objective evaluation of image segmentation methods is crucially important in order to get automated image segmentation methods accepted in clinical practice. One of the key challenges for the evaluation of automated image segmentation methods is the lack of a gold standard against which to compare segmentation methods. In most cases expert manual segmentations are regarded as a gold standard. Given any gold standard segmentation there exist a large number of different methodologies that can be used to evaluate the quality of a given segmentation. These can be broadly divided into three groups. The first group, spatial overlap measures e.g. the Dice [1] coefficient and generalised overlap indicies [2], quantify the overlap between regions. Secondly, distance measures, e.g. signed surface distances, the mean absolute distance and the Hausdorff distance [3], quantify the distance between manually and automatically segmented surfaces. Thirdly, there are volumetric measures based solely on the volumes of the segmented regions e.g. the difference between volumes [4]. The selection of a class of metric depends on the clinical application of interest.

In this paper we compare four different state-of-the-art algorithms for automatic segmentation of subcortical structures in MR brain images. Two of these are model-based, and the other two are based on image registration. For objective comparisons and to address the limitations mentioned above, they have been evaluated using the same data and criteria. The dataset was large (270 subjects) and varied in age, disease and sex (see section 2). 18 subcortical structures were segmented from each subject and evaluated using a mixture of spatial overlap, distance and volumetric measures. We present qualitative and quantitative results of the evaluation of each method with respect to manually annotated data, and with respect to the other methods.

2 Materials and Method

The dataset consisted of 270 T1-weighted MR brain images which had been extensively labelled manually using methods similar to those described in [5]. For the purposes of this study, we used the a subset of the labels of 18 structures – the brain stem, the fourth ventricle and the left and right pairs of the accumbens, amygdala, caudate nucleus, hippocampus, lateral ventricles, pallidum, putamen and thalamus. The imaged cohorts included control subjects as well as subjects with Alzheimer's Disease, Schizophrenia, Attention Deficit Hyperactivity Disorder (ADHD), and prenatal drug exposure. Their ages ranged from 4.5yrs to 83yrs.

Four different methods have been used for segmentation. In each case the automatic segmentation, A has been compared to the manually labelled image which has been regarded as gold standard, G, by computing the metrics described below.

2.1 Segmentation Methods

Classifier Fusion and Labelling (CFL). [6] obtains segmentations by propagating labels from multiple atlases to the query subject and fusing them using a voting rule. When presented with a large repository of atlases it addresses problems of scale by ranking the atlases based on similarity with the query subject and choosing the best 20.

Profile Active Appearance Models (PAM). [7] are a variation of active appearance models which model the intensities along profiles normal to the boundary of a structure. A composite model of all structures and local models for each structure are coupled to perform a global search followed by more refined structure specific searches.

Bayesian Appearance Models (BAM). [8] Similar to the profile AAM, the BAM models texture along profiles normal to a surface. The BAM differs from the PAM mainly in that it models the relationship between shape and intensity via the conditional distribution of intensity given shape. Rather than synthesising intensities, BAM predicts intensity distributions and maximises the probability of the shape given the observed intensities.

Expectation-Maximisation-based segmentation using a dynamic brain atlas (EMS). [9] is a probabilistic approach combining a standard EM-based segmentation [10] with a dynamic brain atlas construction [11].

2.2 Evaluation Metrics

Dice coefficient. The Dice coefficient D [1] is one of a number of measures of the extent of spatial overlap between two binary images. It is commonly used in reporting performance of segmentation and gives more weighting to instances where the two images agree. Its values range between 0 (no overlap) and 1 (perfect agreement). In this paper the Dice values are expressed as percentages and obtained using Equation 1.

$$D = \frac{2(A \bigcap G)}{(A \bigcap G + A \bigcup G)} \times 100 \qquad (1)$$

Hausdorff distance. The directed Hausdorff distance H_{ag}, between two sets of points A and G can be obtained in a two stage manner. First, for each point in A the minimum distance to all points in G is obtained. H_{ag} is the maximum of this set of minimum distances. In the present case, the minimum distance for the ith surface voxel in A to the set of surface voxels in G is d_i^{ag}, therefore H_{ag} is the maximum value of the surface distance of all surface voxels in A (Equation 2). The Hausdorff distance, H, is the maximum of the directed form for $A \rightarrow G$ and $G \rightarrow A$ (Equation 3).

$$H_{ag} = max\{d_i^{ag}\}, i = \{1 \ldots n_a\} \qquad (2)$$

$$H = max(H_{ag}, H_{ga}) \qquad (3)$$

Volumes. For each individual segmentation result we find the volume, V, as the number of labelled voxels multiplied by the voxel dimensions. We then calculate the percentage absolute volumetric difference (AVD) as the ratio of the absolute difference between the original volume and the segmented volume, to the original volume (Equation 4). The absolute value is used to account for some segmentation results having a lower volume than the gold standard, and others having a higher volume.

$$AVD = \frac{|V_a - V_g|}{V_g} \times 100 \qquad (4)$$

2.3 Experiments

The 270 subjects were randomly assigned into 27 groups of 10. Each of the methods described in section 2.1 was applied to segment each image in one of the groups of 10 using data from the other 26 groups. The results from each method were converted into binary voxel images with the same resolution as the input images. One binary file was obtained for each structure for each subject, and the measures described in section 2.2 applied to obtain quantitative results. Qualitative results were obtained by superimposing contours derived from the binary images onto the respective T1 images.

3 Results

Table 1 shows the results of applying the metrics of section 2.1 to the segmentation results of each structure using the manual labels as gold standards. The results are averages for each structure (left and right pairs combined) over the 27 sets of leave ten out experiments ($n = 540$ for all structures except brain stem and fourth ventricle where $n = 270$). summary box and whisker plots of the values of the Dice coefficient, Hausdorff distance and percentage absolute volumetric difference are given in Figure 1. The *p-values* of two-sample *t-tests* on the differences between the means were obtained at a structure by structure level and also over all structures pooled together. Differences were taken to be significant for *p-values* less than 0.05.

4 Discussion

Summary of results relative to gold standard
Table 1 contains results for each method relative to the gold standard as measured by spatial overlap, volumetric and distance-based metrics. The results are shown by structure, and a summary over all structures is given in Figure 1. Using the summary over all structures and the significance levels, the methods can be ranked in order of decreasing performance by a spatial overlap, a distance-based, and a volumetric metric as follows:

Table 1. Summary table for results of all methods applied on all structures over all measures with respect to manual annotations

Structure	Method	Dice Coefficient	Hausdorff Distance (mm)	Percent mean abs vol diff
accumbens	CFL	75.8 (7.2)	3.1 (1.0)	17.6 (16.9)
	PAM	67.7 (9.9)	3.8 (1.2)	18.2 (13.5)
	BAM	68.7 (7.9)	3.5 (1.0)	31.7 (29.1)
	EMS	67.9 (7.9)	4.3 (1.5)	28.6 (33.1)
amygdala	CFL	77.7 (5.8)	4.4 (1.6)	17.0 (15.8)
	PAM	66.9 (12.3)	5.3 (2.2)	20.9 (17.6)
	BAM	73.1 (6.9)	4.8 (2.2)	24.7 (22.8)
	EMS	70.8 (7.4)	5.4 (1.6)	22.1 (22.7)
brain stem	CFL	94.2 (1.4)	4.8 (1.5)	4.0 (3.0)
	PAM	87.8 (3.0)	6.0 (1.8)	6.8 (5.7)
	BAM	88.5 (2.0)	6.4 (2.1)	7.8 (5.8)
	EMS	82.9 (3.6)	7.7 (2.1)	21.1 (8.4)
caudate	CFL	88.1 (2.8)	4.1 (1.9)	7.7 (6.2)
	PAM	83.4 (5.1)	4.1 (2.0)	5.0 (5.5)
	BAM	85.6 (3.5)	4.6 (2.1)	13.2 (11.5)
	EMS	82.6 (5.7)	6.4 (3.2)	14.0 (12.9)
fourth ventricle	CFL	83.3 (4.7)	6.6 (2.9)	15.0 (11.5)
	PAM	70.6 (9.9)	7.7 (3.1)	15.4 (13.9)
	EMS	77.4 (8.6)	9.0 (4.2)	39.1 (34.2)
hippo-campus	CFL	83.5 (3.7)	4.5 (1.5)	9.2 (8.7)
	PAM	76.8 (6.2)	5.2 (1.6)	12.0 (7.4)
	BAM	79.12 (4.3)	5.0 (1.7)	22.1 (16.5)
	EMS	76.4 (5.9)	6.4 (2.0)	14.5 (13.3)
lateral ventricle	CFL	91.3 (3.7)	9.8 (7.3)	6.5 (6.3)
	PAM	80.9 (6.8)	14.0 (8.4)	7.3 (9.9)
	BAM	79.5 (9.6)	16.2 (9.5)	39.0 (34.7)
	EMS	82.9 (12.0)	10.5 (6.8)	39.4 (53.3)
pallidum	CFL	81.9 (4.8)	3.6 (1.1)	9.9 (7.1)
	PAM	79.3 (5.1)	3.8 (1.0)	9.4 (9.9)
	BAM	79.5 (4.3)	3.8 (1.0)	22.8 (15.7)
	EMS	80.5 (4.5)	3.9 (1.1)	13.8 (10.5)
putamen	CFL	89.8 (2.4)	3.6 (1.1)	6.9 (6.2)
	PAM	86.3 (2.8)	3.8 (1.1)	4.0 (4.2)
	BAM	86.4 (2.6)	4.4 (1.5)	14.6 (8.9)
	EMS	86.6 (2.5)	4.5 (1.2)	8.2 (6.6)
thalamus	CFL	90.8 (1.6)	4.0 (1.0)	4.8 (4.1)
	PAM	87.7 (2.8)	4.1 (1.0)	4.0 (3.3)
	BAM	87.6 (2.5)	4.3 (1.0)	13.7 (9.3)
	EMS	85.2 (2.1)	5.5 (1.4)	10.6 (6.5)

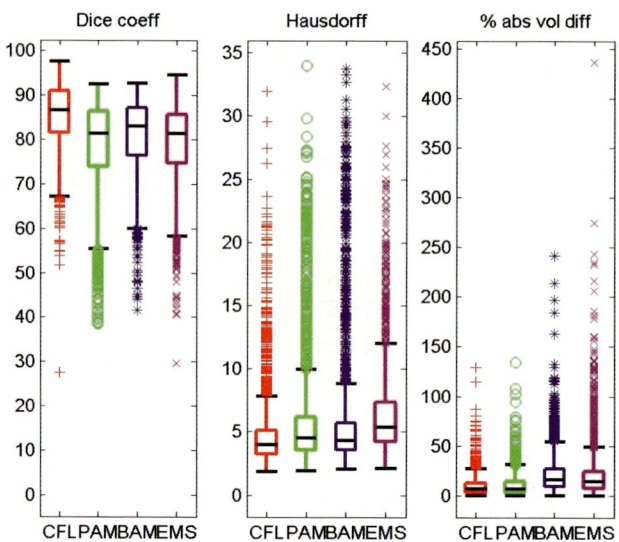

Fig. 1. Box and whisker plots of Dice coefficients, Hausdorff distance, and percentage absolute volumetric difference over all structures for each method. The whiskers are 1.5 × the inter-quartile range, and values outside these are plotted individually.

Spatial overlap (Dice): CFL → BAM → EMS → PAM
Distance-based (Hausdorff): CFL → BAM and PAM → EMS
Volumetric (AVD): CFL and PAM → EMS and BAM

The CFL method clearly gives the best overall performance with respect to the gold standard. When considering performance on a structure by structure basis the Dice coefficients of CFL are significantly better than those of the other three methods for all structures. The Dice values of BAM are either the same or better than those of PAM and EMS for all structures except the lateral ventricles (and pallidum for EMS). The Dice values of EMS were better than those for PAM for the amygdala, fourth ventricle, lateral ventricle and pallidum.

The Hausdorff distances of CFL at the structure level are better than those of all other methods for all structures except the caudate, pallidum and thalamus where it performs at least as well or better than the other methods. BAM and PAM have a mixture of better and same results relative to each other for this metric. EMS only performed better than BAM and PAM for the lateral ventricle.

CFL performed better than BAM and EMS for all structures, according to AVD. However, it didn't performed as well as PAM on the caudate, putamen and thalamus. PAM was better than EMS and BAM for all structures except the amygdala where it performed the same as EMS, and the brain stem where it was the same with BAM. EMS performed better than PAM on the hippocampus, pallidum, putamen and thalamus.

When comparing how well a method performed on the different structures, the order of best performance depends on the metric used to judge the performance.

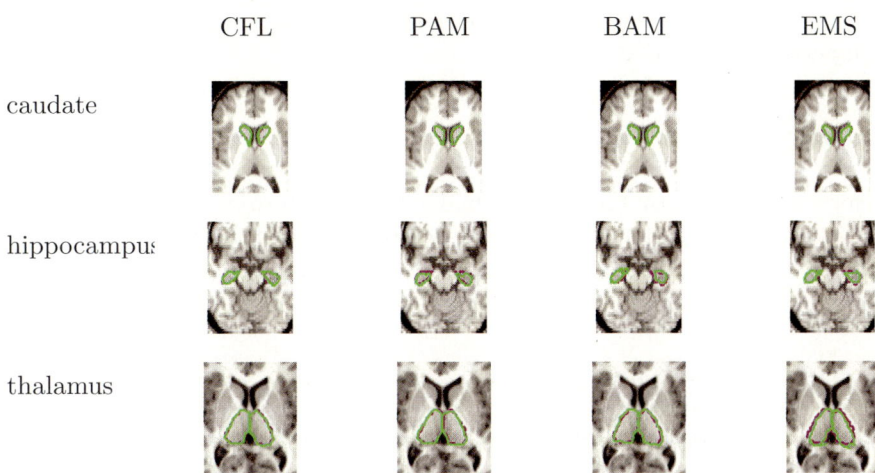

Fig. 2. Overlays of the segmentation results of all four methods for the subjects that gave the best Dice value for some structures for the CFL method. Pink is gold standard, green is result of method.

According to the spatial overlap metrics, the accumbens gives the worst overlap results for all methods, and the brain stem gives the best results. However the accumbens gives the best (lowest) Hausdorff distance and the lateral ventricles the worst for all methods. These differences are a combination of the fact that the accumbens are the smallest structures (hence small errors in overlap give high changes in the spatial overlap measures), and the shape of the lateral ventricles (in particular the length of the occipital horns coupled with partial volume effects along them) means that they are difficult to segment especially for methods relying on prior shape topology (BAM and PAM).

In terms of computing time and resources required, the CFL method is most expensive taking the order of a few hours to segment a 3D volumetric image. The model based methods perform faster in the order of tens of minutes and the EMS method falls in between these two.

5 Conclusion

We have presented a comprehensive comparison of four methods for fully automatic segmentation of 18 subcortical structures in the brain. These methods perform at least on par with currently available methods. The results will be of use to those needing to make a decision about a tool to use for applied research in brain imaging. The BAM method has been implemented as FIRST in the widely used FSL software suite[1], and the PAM method will be available for download over the internet from the University of Manchester[2] UK. The binaries and code

---

[1] www.fmrib.ox.ac.uk/fsl/first
[2] www.isbe.man.ac.uk/~kob/ibim

to implement the CFL method on a database of images is also freely available from Imperial College, UK [3].

Acknowledgements

This work was funded by the EPSRC under the IBIM project. David Kennedy of the Center for Morphometric Analysis, Boston, provided the MR images used.

References

1. Dice, L.R.: Measures of the amount of ecologic association between species. Ecology 26, 297–302 (1945)
2. Crum, W.R., Camara, O., Hill, D.L.G.: Generalised overlap measures for evaluation and validation in medical image analysis. IEEE Transanctions on Medical Imaging 25(11), 1451–1461 (2006)
3. Gerig, G., Jomier, M., Chakos, M.: Valmet: A new validation tool for assessing and improving 3D object segmentation. In: Niessen, W.J., Viergever, M.A. (eds.) MICCAI 2001. LNCS, vol. 2208, pp. 516–523. Springer, Heidelberg (2001)
4. Collins, D.L., Holmes, C.J., Peters, T.M., Evans, A.C.: Automatic 3-D model-based neuroanatomical segmentation. Human Brain Mapping 3(3), 190–208 (1995)
5. Filipek, P., Richelme, C., Kennedy, D., Caviness, V.: The young adult human brain: An MRI-based morphometric analysis. Cereb. Cort. 4, 344–360 (1994)
6. Aljabar, P., Heckemann, R., Hammers, A., Hajnal, J., Rueckert, D.: Classifier selection strategies for label fusion using large atlas databases. In: Ayache, N., Ourselin, S., Maeder, A. (eds.) MICCAI 2007, Part I. LNCS, vol. 4791, pp. 523–531. Springer, Heidelberg (2007)
7. Babalola, K.O., Petrovic, V., Cootes, T.F., Taylor, C.J., Twining, C.J., Williams, T.G., Mills, A.: Automated segmentation of the caudate nuclei using active appearance models. In: 3D Segmentation in the clinic: A grand challenge. Workshop Proceedings, MICCAI 2007, Brisbane, pp. 57–64 (2007)
8. Patenaude, B., Smith, S., Kennedy, D., Jenkinson, M.: Bayesian shape and appearance models, Technical report TR07BP1, FMRIB Centre - University of Oxford
9. Murgasova, M., Dyet, L., Edwards, A.D., Rutherford, M., Hajnal, J., Rueckert, D.: Segmentation of brain MRI in young children. Acad. Rad (in press, 2007)
10. Leemput, K.V., Maes, F., Vandermeulen, D., Suetens, P.: Automated model-based tissue classification of MR images of the brain. IEEE TMI 18(10), 897–908 (1999)
11. Hill, D.L.G., Hajnal, J.V., Rueckert, D., Smith, S.M., Hartkens, T., McLeish, K.: A dynamic brain atlas. In: Dohi, T., Kikinis, R. (eds.) MICCAI 2002. LNCS, vol. 2488, pp. 532–539. Springer, Heidelberg (2002)

---

[3] www.doc.ic.ac.uk/~dr/software

Hierarchical Shape Statistical Model for Segmentation of Lung Fields in Chest Radiographs

Yonghong Shi[1] and Dinggang Shen[2,*]

[1] Digital Medical Research Center, Fudan University, Shanghai, 200032, China
Yonghong.Shi@fudan.edu.cn
[2] Department of Radiology and Biomedical Research Imaging Center
University of North Carolina, Chapel Hill, NC 27599
dgshen@med.unc.edu

Abstract. The standard Active Shape Model (ASM) generally uses a whole population to train a single PCA-based shape model for segmentation of all testing samples. Since some testing samples can be similar to only sub-population of training samples, it will be more effective if particular shape statistics extracted from the respective sub-population can be used for guiding image segmentation. Accordingly, we design a set of hierarchical shape statistical models, including a whole-population shape model and a series of sub-population models. The whole-population shape model is used to guide the initial segmentation of the testing sample, and the initial segmentation result is then used to select a suitable sub-population shape model according to the shape similarity between the testing sample and each sub-population. By using the selected sub-population shape model, the segmentation result can be further refined. To achieve this segmentation process, several particular steps are designed next. *First*, all linearly aligned samples in the whole population are used to generate a whole-population shape model. *Second*, an affinity propagation method is used to cluster all linearly aligned samples into several clusters, to determine the samples belonging to the same sub-populations. *Third*, the original samples of each sub-population are linearly aligned to their own mean shape, and the respective sub-population shape model is built using the newly aligned samples in this sub-population. By using all these three steps, we can generate hierarchical shape statistical models to guide image segmentation. Experimental results show that the proposed method can significantly improve the segmentation performance, compared to conventional ASM.

Keywords: Active shape model, Hierarchical shape statistics; Chest radiograph.

1 Introduction

The utility of image processing technique in diagnostic chest radiology has increased with the growing acceptance of digital radiography. Many methods, such as automatic

---

* Corresponding author. This work was partially supported by Shanghai Leading Academic Discipline Project (Project No. B112) and Science and Technology Commission of Shanghai Municipality (Project No. 06dz22103).

detection of lung nodules, characterization of interstitial disease, and delineation of ribs, have been developed. In all these applications, the information inside the lung region is most interesting. Thus, the segmentation of lung regions becomes an important image processing procedure that has to be performed in most practical applications [1-3].

Various methods have been applied to segment the lung fields from posterior-anterior chest radiographs [1-5], and they roughly fall into four categories: 1) rule-based segmentation methods have been used to detect the outline of ribcage or the diaphragm; 2) pixel-based methods were proposed to classify each pixel of an image into either lung field or background based on a multi-scale filter bank of Gaussian derivatives and a K-NN classifier; 3) hybrid methods were formulated by combining rule-based methods and pixel-based classification for lung field segmentation; and 4) deformable model-based methods, such as active shape model and active appearance model have been successfully applied in lung field segmentation.

Among these four categories of segmentation algorithms, the active shape model (ASM) developed by Cootes *et al.* [4] was a prosperous starting point because of its ability to incorporate *a priori* information extracted from a training set and its flexibility to represent object shapes. In ASM, the use of PCA-based shape statistics trained on population samples ensures that the segmentation can produce plausible shapes. However, current shape-based segmentation methods generally use the whole population samples to train a single PCA-based shape model and use it for segmentation of all testing samples. Since some testing samples can be similar to only sub-population of training samples, it will be more effective if particular shape statistics extracted from the respective sub-population can be used for guiding the segmentation [10-14]. However, it is not pre-known which sub-population shape information should be used for a new test image before segmenting it.

We accordingly design a set of hierarchical shape statistical models, including a whole-population shape model and a series of sub-population shape models, to hierarchically guide image segmentation. In particular, the whole-population shape model is used to guide the initial segmentation of the testing sample, and the resulted segmentation is used to select a suitable sub-population shape model according to the shape similarity between the testing sample and each sub-population. Thus, by using the selected sub-population shape model, the segmentation result can be further refined.

To achieve this designed segmentation process, we will produce a set of hierarchical shape statistical models in the training stage as follows. *First*, all linearly aligned samples in the whole population are used to generate a whole-population shape model. *Second*, an affinity propagation method [9] is used to cluster all linearly aligned samples into several clusters, to determine samples belonging to the same sub-populations. *Third*, the original samples of each sub-population are linearly aligned to their own mean shape, and the respective sub-population shape model is built using the newly aligned samples in the sub-population. By using all these three steps, we can generate hierarchical shape statistical models to guide image segmentation.

This paper is organized as follows. Section 2 introduces a strategy of our hierarchical shape statistical models for segmenting lung fields from chest radiographs. Section 3 describes the experiments, and Section 4 concludes the paper.

2 Method

2.1 Summary of ASM Algorithm

For better describing our proposed method, we first summarize the main idea of ASM algorithm, and point out its potential limitation [2, 4]. The ASM scheme consists of two main elements: a global shape model and a local appearance model.

A global shape model is built from a set of training samples, e.g., segmented lung fields [2, 6]. Each training image is described by n correspondence points, using a shape vector $x = (x_1, y_1, ..., x_n, y_n)^T$. All shape vectors are linearly aligned by minimizing the sum of squared distances among all aligned shape vectors. By calculating the mean shape $\bar{x}$ and the covariance matrix, the principal modes can be estimated. Thus, a new shape x can now be represented as $x = \bar{x} + \Phi b_x$, where Φ contains the principal modes of variation of the shape model and b_x contains shape parameters. It has been proved that, if the specific shape statistics can be used for guiding the segmentation, the accuracy of segmentation can be highly improved [5]. This motivates us to build hierarchical shape statistical models for hierarchically guiding the image segmentation in this study.

In ASM, a local appearance model is constructed for each landmark by using the normalized first derivative profile. For enhancing the performance of ASM, several improvements for the local appearance model have been proposed. For example, the moments of local histograms extracted from the filtered versions of the images using a filter bank of Gaussian derivatives are considered to enhance the accuracy of ASM [7]. Also, scale invariant feature transform (SIFT) [8] is used to significantly improve the performance of ASM [5]. In this study, we will use SIFT to construct local appearance model.

2.2 Hierarchical Shape Statistical Models

In Introduction, we mentioned that we will build a set of hierarchical shape statistical models to guide image segmentation. A whole-population shape statistical model will be first built from all linearly aligned samples (c.f. Fig. 1(F)) as described in Section 2.1 above. Then, a series of sub-population shape statistical models will be built to better represent the shape variations within each sub-population. Sub-populations will be generated from all aligned samples using an affinity propagation method [9], which can adaptively cluster the samples into a number of clusters (or sub-populations). The number of clusters (or sub-populations) will be automatically determined, based on the given shape similarity measure. Once we know the samples belonging to a particular sub-population, we can obtain their original shapes and then linearly normalize them into their own mean shape (c.f. Fig. 1(A)~(E)), which can be very different from the mean shape of whole population (c.f. Fig. 1(F)). Accordingly, we can use those particularly aligned samples to build a sub-population shape statistical model for each sub-population, using PCA technique. Details of this process are described next.

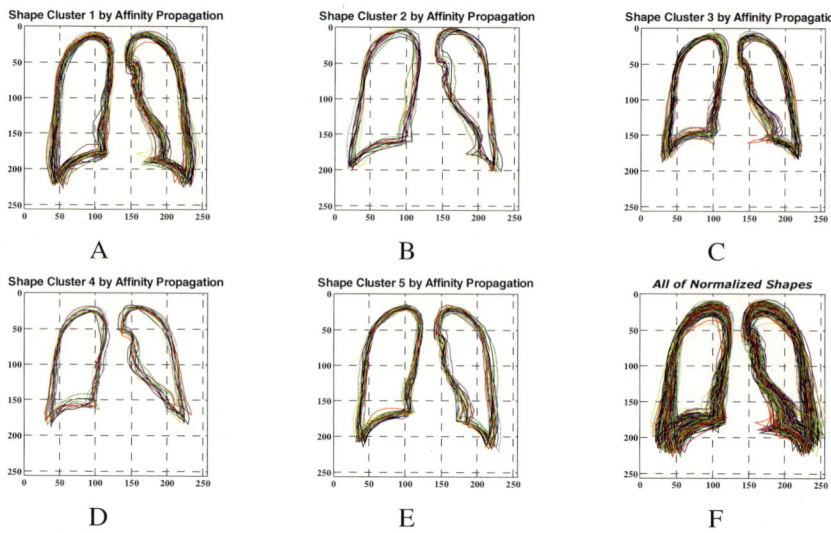

Fig. 1. Normalized samples in whole population (F), or in sub-populations (A~E). Sub-populations are clustered by affinity propagation. There are totally five sub-populations from our normalized training samples. Note, the original samples belonging to the same sub-population are re-normalized to their own mean shape (A~E), to represent their own variations.

Clustering of sub-populations

Clustering data by identifying a subset of representative examples (or exemplars) is important in many applications including ours. The k-means algorithm can be used to find such "exemplars", by first randomly choosing an initial subset of data points and then iteratively refining it. However, this works well only when initial choice is close to a good solution. Contrary to the k-means algorithm, affinity propagation method [9] simultaneously considers all data points as potential exemplars, and then recursively exchanges real-valued messages between data points until a high-quality set of exemplars and corresponding clusters emerges. Affinity propagation method can find clusters with much lower error than other methods, and it can complete in less time.

Thus, we select this method to cluster our training samples into a number of sub-populations. For example, for those spatially normalized samples (c.f. Fig. 1(F)), we obtained five sub-populations using affinity propagation (c.f. Fig. 1(A)~(E)). Original samples in each of these five sub-populations are re-normalized to their own mean shape. By overlapping all re-normalized shapes in each sub-population, we can obtain five figures in Fig. 1(A~E), which is different from the overlay of all normalized shapes in the whole population Fig. 1(F).

These five figures clearly indicate that five sub-populations have very different emphases. For example, a sub-population in Fig. 1(A) has shapes of larger size, compared to other sub-populations. For the sub-populations in Fig. 1(B) and Fig. 1(D), the size of right lung (left in the figure) is both larger than that of left lung, while the shapes of left lung in these two sub-populations are very different. On the other hand, sub-populations in Fig. 1(C) and Fig. 1 (E) have different sizes of lung, although their

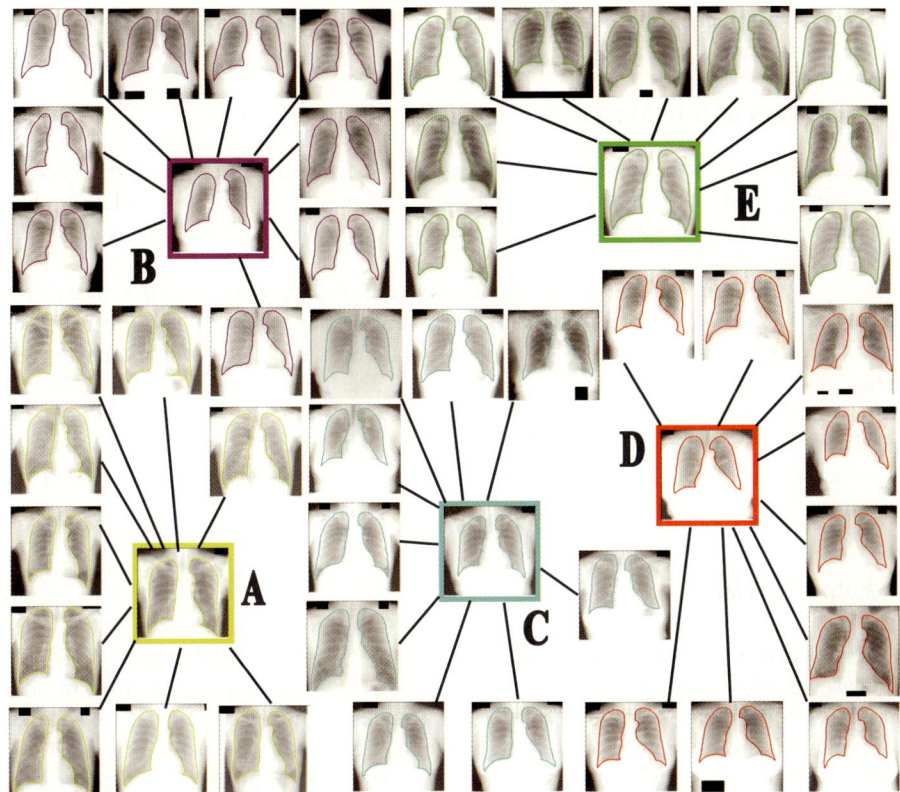

Fig. 2. Original shape samples in five sub-populations of chest radiographs. Exemplars are highlighted by colored boxes. Shapes in the same sub-population are drawn by same color.

overall global shapes are similar. This example intuitively indicates the importance of using sub-population shape statistics for better guiding image segmentation.

Fig. 2 shows the selected original samples in each subpopulation. It can be observed that different sub-populations have very different original shapes.

Construction of hierarchical shape statistical models

Both whole population shape statistical model and a series of sub-population shape statistical models are built using their own samples, as detailed below:

- The whole population shape statistical model is built from all samples. All samples will be first normalized to the common shape space, to remove the difference of scale, size, shape and position among samples. The normalized samples are shown in Fig. 1(F) for visual inspection. Then, using PCA, these normalized samples can be used to build a whole-population shape statistical model, as used in ASM.
- These normalized samples are clustered into sub-populations, such as five sub-populations in our study (c.f. Fig. 1(A~E) and Fig. 2), by the affinity propagation method. Then, all original samples belonging to the same sub-population are re-normalized to their own mean shape (c.f. Fig. 1(A~E)). Thus, using PCA, a

sub-population shape statistical model can be built for each sub-population using its own normalized shape samples.

2.3 Summary of Our Algorithm

Our algorithm has two components, i.e., *training* and *testing*. In the *training stage*, we build hierarchical shape statistical models, which include a whole-population shape statistical model and a series of sub-population shape statistical models, as detailed in the subsection above.

In the *testing stage*, for a given new testing sample, we first use SIFT-based local appearance model to deform our whole-population shape model. The obtained segmentation will be constrained by the whole-population shape statistics. After the segmentation is converged, we use the segmented shape to compute its similarity to each of sub-populations. The most similar one is selected as the particular sub-population that the testing sample belongs to. Thus, we can use the corresponding sub-population shape statistical model to refine the segmentation of the testing sample until the segmentation procedure converges.

3 Experiments

The performance of our algorithm is evaluated by a JSRT/SCR database [2, 6]. The 247 cases in this database are subdivided in two folds. Each fold contains an equal amount of normal cases and abnormal cases. Images in one fold were segmented with the images in the other fold as training set, and vice versa. All of the original radiographs were down-sampled to the 256 by 256 resolution images. Two quantitative measures are used to evaluate the performance of the algorithms, i.e., the average overlay percentage and the average contour distance between automated segmentation result and manual segmentation result.

To evaluate the performance of our hierarchical shape statistical model (*SIFT-H*), we compare the following four methods. *SIFT-H* denotes our algorithm which uses SIFT features for lung field matching and hierarchical shape statistical models for shape constraining. *Intensity-H* denotes the method that is similar to *SIFT-H*, except we use image intensity and gradient features to replace the SIFT features for lung field matching. The last two methods, *SIFT-W* and *Intensity-W*, are, respectively, similar to *SIFT-H* and *Intensity-H*, except that *SIFT-W* and *Intensity-W* use only whole-population shape statistics for shape constraining.

Some qualitative segmentation results by *SIFT-H* are provided in Fig. 3. The top row shows the manual segmentations, and the bottom row shows the results by *SIFT-H*. It can be seen that the results by *SIFT-H* are similar to the manual segmentations.

For quantitative comparison, the average overlay percentage and the average contour distance between the segmentation results and the ground truth of all 247 images are reported in Table 1 and Table 2, respectively. It can be seen that, when hierarchical shape statistical models are used, the average overlay percentages of *SIFT-H* (93.6%) and *Intensity-H* (89.1%) are much higher than those of *SIFT-W* (92.0%) and *Intensity-W* (87.0%). Similar conclusion can be drawn for the average contour distances in Table 2. It can be observed that the average contour distance is decreased

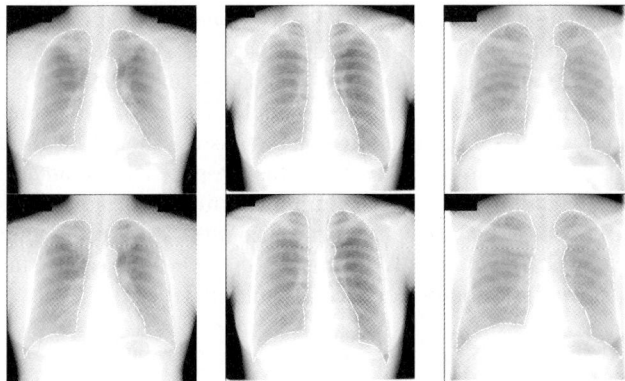

Fig. 3. Three chest radiographs with (top) manual and (bottom) automated segmentation of lung fields by *SIFT-H*

Table 1. Average overlay percentage between manual segmentation and automated segmentation of all 247 images in the JSRT/SCR database (%)

Algorithm	Mean±std	Minimum	Median	Maximum
SIFT-H	93.6±2.88	80.0	93.9	96.3
Intensity-H	89.1±4.42	70.6	90.8	95.8
SIFT-W	92.0±3.1	78.3	92.8	96.1
Intensity-W	87.0±7.4	60.8	89.2	95.4

Table 2. Average contour distance between manual segmentation and automated segmentation of all 247 images in the JSRT/SCR database (unit in pixel)

Algorithm	Mean±std	Minimum	Median	Maximum
SIFT-H	1.56±0.62	0.85	1.53	4.62
Intensity-H	2.82±0.77	0.94	2.76	5.63
SIFT-W	1.78±0.78	0.96	1.64	6.79
Intensity-W	3.10±1.95	1.03	2.36	9.69

from *SIFT-W* (1.78 pixels) and *Intensity-W* (3.10 pixels) to *SIFT-H* (1.56 pixels) and *Intensity-H* (2.82 pixels), respectively, because of using hierarchical shape statistics. All of these results indicate that, no matter which kind of image features are used, the methods using hierarchical shape statistical models outperform those using only a whole-population shape statistical model.

4 Conclusion

We have presented a hierarchical shape statistical model to hierarchically guide the segmentation of lung fields from chest radiographs. This hierarchical shape statistical model includes both whole-population shape statistics and sub-population shape statistics. The clustering of sub-populations from the whole training samples is completed by an affinity propagation technique. Then, samples belonging to the same sub-population are used to train the sub-population shape statistical model using PCA technique. In the applications, the whole-population shape statistical model is first used to guide the initial segmentation of a new test sample. The resulted segmentation is then used to determine which sub-population shape statistics should be used to refine the segmentation of the test sample. By using this proposed hierarchical segmentation strategy, the segmentation performance is highly improved, compared to the ASM using only whole-population shape statistics and the ASM using intensity/gradient features, rather than SIFT features. In this paper, the two-level shape statistical models are used, which can be potentially extended to multiple levels.

References

1. van Ginneken, B., ter Haar Romeny, B.M., Viergever, M.A.: Computer-Aided Diagnosis in Chest Radiography: a Survey. IEEE Trans. on Medical Imaging 20(12), 1228–1241 (2001)
2. van Ginneken, B., Stegmann, M.B., Loog, M.: Segmentation of Anatomical Structures in Chest Radiographs using Supervised methods: a Comparative Study on a Public Database. Medical Image Analysis 10, 19–40 (2006)
3. Luo, H., Gaborski, R., Acharya, R.: Automatic segmentation of lung regions in chest radiographs: a model guided approach. In: ICIP 2000, vol. 2, pp. 483–486 (2000)
4. Cootes, T.F., Taylor, C.J.: Statistical Models of appearance for Computer Vision. Technical Report, Wolfson Image Analysis Unit, University of Manchester (2001)
5. Shi, Y., Qi, F., Xue, Z., Chen, L., Ito, K., Matsuo, H., Shen, D.: Segmenting Lung Fields in Serial Chest Radiographs Using Both Population-based and Patient-specific Shape Statistics. IEEE Trans. on Medical Imaging 27(4), 481–494 (2008)
6. Shiraishi, J., et al.: Development of a Digital Image Database for Chest Radiographs with and without a Lung Nodule: Receiver Operation Characteristic Analysis of Radiologists' Detection of Pulmonary Nodules. American Journal of Roentgenology 174(1), 71–74 (2000)
7. van Ginneken, B., Frangi, A.F., Staal, J.J., ter Haar Romeny, B.M., Viergever, M.A.: Active shape model segmentation with optimal features. IEEE Trans. on Medical Imaging 21(8), 924–933 (2002)
8. Lowe, D.G.: Distinctive Image Features from Scale-Invariant Keypoints. International Journal of Computer Vision 60(2), 91–110 (2004)
9. Brendan, J.: Frey and Delbert Dueck. Clustering by Passing Messages between Data Points. Science 315, 972–976 (2007)
10. Heap, A.J., Hogg, D.C.: Improving specificity in PDMs using a hierarchical approach. In: British Machine Vision Conference 1997, Colchester, Essex (1997)
11. Bregler, C., Omohundro, S.: Surface learning with applications to lipreading. In: Advances in neural information processing systems, vol. 6 (1994)
12. Stegmann, M.B., Larsson, H.B.W.: Motion-compensation of cardiac perfusion MRI using a statistical texture ensemble. In: Magnin, I.E., Montagnat, J., Clarysse, P., Nenonen, J., Katila, T. (eds.) FIMH 2003. LNCS, vol. 2674, pp. 151–161. Springer, Heidelberg (2003)
13. Stegmann, M.B., Larsson, H.B.W.: Fast registration of cardiac perfusion MRI. In: Proceeding of International Society of Magnetic Resonance in Medicine, Toronto, Canada (2003)
14. Cootes, T.F., Taylor, C.J.: A mixture model for representing shape variation. Image and Vision Computing 17(8), 567–573 (1999)

Sample Sufficiency and Number of Modes to Retain in Statistical Shape Modelling

Lin Mei*, Michael Figl, Daniel Rueckert, Ara Darzi, and Philip Edwards*

Dept. of Biosurgery and Surgical Technology Imperial College London, UK
l.mei,eddie.edwards@imperial.ac.uk*

Abstract. Statistical shape modelling is a popular technique in medical imaging, but the issue of sample size sufficiency is not generally considered. Also the number of principal modes retained is often chosen simply to cover a percentage of the total variance. We show that these simple rules are unreliable. We propose a new method that uses bootstrap replication and a t-test comparison with noise to decide whether each mode direction has stabilised. We establish mode correspondence by minimising the distance between the space spanned by the replicates and their mean. By retaining only stable modes, our method distinguishes real anatomical variation from modes dominated by random noise. This provides a lower stopping rule when the sample is small and converges as the sample size increases. We use this convergence to determine sample sufficiency. For validation we use synthetic datasets of the left ventricle generated with a known number of structural modes and added noise. Our stopping rule detected the correct number of modes to retain where other methods failed. The methods were also tested on real 2D (22 points) and 3D (500 points) face data, retaining 24 and 70 modes with sample sufficiency being reached at approximately 50 and 150 samples respectively. For a 3D database of the left ventricle (527 points), 319 samples are not sufficient, but at this level we can retain around 55 stable modes. Our method provides a principled foundation for appropriate selection of the number of modes to retain and determination of sample size sufficiency for statistical shape modelling.

1 Introduction

Statistical shape modelling (SSM) is a technique for characterising variation of shape and fitting to unseen shapes. A set of sample shapes is collected and principal component analysis (PCA) is performed to determine the principal modes of shape variation. Since the surfaces are usually extracted from 3D image data the dimensionality of the shape vector will typically be high, perhaps several thousand. The number of samples used in constructing the model varies, but is generally in the range 10-50 [1,2,3,4]. While these training sets are sufficient

---

* We would like to thank Tyco Healthcare for funding Lin Mei's PhD studentship. We are also grateful to many other members of the Department of Computing and the Department of Biosurgery and Surgical Technology at Imperial College.

to prove the principle of a technique, the sample may not be large enough to ensure that the resulting model reflects the true background anatomical variation. Limited literature can be found discussing PCA sample size sufficiency. In the related field of common factor analysis (CFA), early guidelines for a minimum sample size requirement involved either a universal size regardless of the data dimension or a ratio to the number of dimensions. However, there is inconsistency between the suggestions, implying that the minimum size depends on some intrinsic characteristics of the data other than its dimension. MacCallum et al. proposed that for CFA they are communality and overdeterminaton level [5].

Methods which identify the number of modes to retain for a PCA model are called *stopping rules*. A number of methods have been proposed for PCA [6,7,8,9]. The most commonly used rule in SSM is to use a threshold, e.g. 95%, on the cumulative percentage of principal modes' variance [8,10]. However, the choice of threshold is somewhat arbitrary, and we will show in section 5 that the number of modes retained varies with sample size.

Stability measurements for SSM have been proposed to determine the number of modes. Given two shape models trained from different sample sets, Daudin et al [11] used a sum of correlation coefficients between pairs of principal components; Besse et al [12] used a loss function derived from an Euclidean distance between orthogonal projectors; Babalola et al [13] used the Bhattacharya Metric to measure the similarity of PCA models from different sample sets. Resampling techniques such as bootstrapping [11] and jackknifing [12] are used. The distribution of PCA modes across the replicates reflects their distribution in the population, allowing stability analysis to be performed. The selected principal modes span a subspace. Besse et al. proposed a framework for choosing the number of modes based on their spanned-space stability [14]. This method differentiates structural modes and noise-dominated modes when the sample set is large. However, as will be shown in the section 5, this method can only provide a estimation of the number of modes when the sample size is large enough.

In this paper, we establish mode correspondence by minimising the distance between principal spanned spaces. We then apply bootstrapping to estimate the distribution of each eigenmode direction and perform a t-test against pure Gaussian noise to determine the number of modes that should be retained for SSM. This leads to a procedure to test for the sufficiency of the current sample size by convergence of the number of modes retained. These methods are validated on synthetic data generated with a known number of modes, and applied to a real dataset of the left ventricle from MRI and datasets of 2D and 3D faces.

2 Stopping Rule by Stability of Mode Direction

Our stopping rule is based on bootstrap stability analysis on mode directions. This requires correspondence of the PCA modes trained from different replicates.

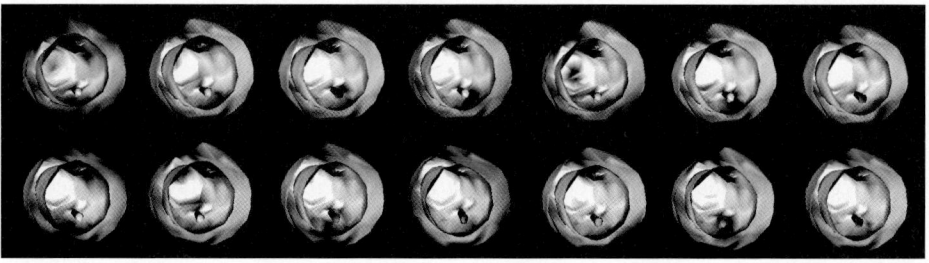

Fig. 1. Comparison of Leading 7 Eigenmodes from two mutually exclusive sets of 50 samples from our 3D heart mesh database. Darker texture implies larger variation.

2.1 Establishing Mode Correspondence

Examining individual modes requires mode correspondence. Normally, this is done by matching those with the same eigenvalue ranks. This method may fail if the variances along two modes are quite similar. As can be seen in figure 1, there can be significant variation of individual mode directions between sample sets. However, the combined modes from different sample sets may still span similar subspaces. Mode alignment can be achieved by minimising the distance between these subspaces.

For the leading PCA modes $\{(a_i, \lambda_i) | a_i| = 1\}$ of an n-dimensional distribution, we define the principal spanned space (PSS) as the subspace $\mathbb{S}^k$ spanned by $\{a_i\}$, where distance measurement used by Besse et al.[12] can be applied:

$$d(\mathbb{A}^k, \mathbb{B}^k) = k - trace(AA^T BB^T) \qquad (1)$$

where the columns of A and B are the modes spanning PSS $\mathbb{A}^k$ and $\mathbb{B}^k$.

For two sets of PCA modes, a_i and b_i, trained from different sample sets of a common distribution, the following rule can be used to establish correspondence. The first mode in a_i corresponds to the mode of a replicate that minimises $d(\mathbb{S}_a^1, \mathbb{S}_b^1)$, and we proceed iteratively. Assume we have already aligned $\mathbb{S}_a^k$, the PSS from the first k modes in a_i, to the spanned space $\mathbb{S}_b^k$ from k modes in the replicate b_i. The mode in b_i that corresponds to the k+1th mode in a_i will be the one that minimises $d(\mathbb{S}_a^{k+1}, \mathbb{S}_b^{k+1})$.

2.2 t-Test on Mode Stability

There is a risk with tests using the magnitude of the variance that stopping rules will be dominated by the first few modes and fail to identify the correct cut-off point. Also, it is the mode directions that define the basis of a shape model for fitting or synthetic shape generation. Therefore we propose a stopping rule based on the stability of the mode direction only.

Averaged dot-product between corresponding modes and their mean was used as the stability of mode direction [9]. We apply the same principle to the modes from different bootstrap replicates, but for clarity we use the angles between mode directions. The instability, ξ, of mode $\boldsymbol{a}_i$ is given by:

$$\xi(\boldsymbol{a}_i) = \frac{\sum_{j=1}^{m} arccos(\boldsymbol{a}'_{ij} \cdot \widehat{\boldsymbol{\alpha}_i})}{m\pi} \qquad (2)$$

where $\widehat{\boldsymbol{\alpha}_i}$ is the mean mode vector and m is the number of bootstrap replicates.

Since noise-dominated modes should have higher instability, a threshold on ξ can be used to differentiate them from structural modes. However, the choice for the threshold is arbitrary and is found to be sensitive to the size of replicates. Instead, assuming the distribution of angles between corresponding modes is Gaussian, an one-tailed t-test can be used to establish whether a mode is dominated by noise to a given significance level.

We generate a pure Gaussian noise dataset to compare with the test dataset. All conditions must be the same – the dimensionality, the number of samples in the dataset, the number of replicates, and the number of samples in each replicate. Since we are only interested in mode directions, the level of noise is not important. Let the angle for the first pure noise mode to be $\boldsymbol{\alpha}_1$ and the angle for the i-th mode of the test samples to be $\boldsymbol{a}_i$, The null hypothesis of the t-test is $H_0 : \xi(\boldsymbol{\alpha}_1) > \xi(\boldsymbol{a}_i)$. By rejecting H_0 at a given confidence level, one can safely conclude that the i-th mode is not dominated by noise.

3 Sample Size Sufficiency

Studies on CFA showed that the sample size requirement for a statistical model really depends on certain characteristics of the data that are modelled. For CFA these are communality and overdetermination level [5]. For SSM, such factors could be the compactness and the number of genuine anatomical modes not hidden by noise. With increasing sample size, more PCA modes of the background variance are well covered. Once the training set becomes sufficient, no further modes will be revealed. We propose the following procedure to determine the sample size sufficiency. For a sample set, X, of n samples:

1) Apply PCA on X, to get a set of modes B.
2) Starting with a reasonably small number, n^*, Construct a set of resampled sets $\{X_j^*\}$, in which each set, X_j^* contains n^* samples randomly drawn from X allowing repeats.
3) Apply PCA to $\{X_j^*\}$ to get each set of modes $\{B_j^*\}$ and align them to B using the algorithm described in section 2.1.
4) With modes in $\{B_j^*\}$ aligned, calculate the number of structural modes, k can be tested using our t-Test based stopping rule.
5) Repeat 2-4 with an increased n^*. If k converges before n^* reaches n, we have sufficient samples. Otherwise, further samples are required.

An effective stopping rule for part 4 in this procedure should converge.

4 Real Datasets

As sample data we use a set of 319 surface models of the left ventricle, each with 527 corresponding points. These are derived from 4D CT scans of 29 subjects. Eleven shapes for each subject are chosen at different points in the cardiac cycle. Two other real shape datasets are also used to verify our sample size sufficiency test – 135 samples from the landmarks of the 2D AR face database (22 points) [15] and 150 samples of 3D faces (decimated to 500 points) from University of Notre Dame [16], preprocessed using Papatheodorou's method [17].

5 Validation on Synthetic Data

We have validated previous stopping rules and our method using synthetic data generated using the leading 40 modes of the model built from all the 319 cardiac samples. Gaussian noise with 1mm standard deviation is added to each element of the shape vector. The average noise vector length is 41.3mm, which is significantly larger than variance along the 40th genuine mode which is 9.9mm, stopping rules applied to this dataset should not retain more than 40 modes.

5.1 Validation of Previous Methods

We validated the rule of 95% cumulative variance using synthetic datasets sized from 50 to 200. Compactness plots are shown in the figure 2. With increasing sample size, the number of modes retained by this rule increases beyond 40, where the noise dominates the variance. These noise modes contribute to an increasing proportion of the total variance with increasing sample size, and the number of modes covering 95% of total variance increases accordingly. A similar trend was also found for the real data, strongly suggesting that this rule is unreliable and should not be used.

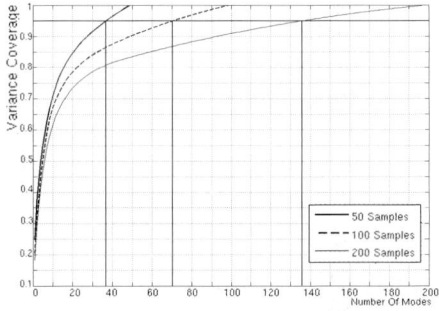

Fig. 2. 95% thresholded compactness plots for synthetic datasets

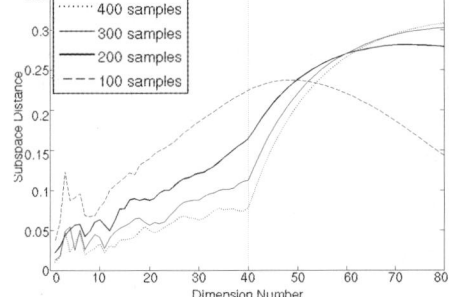

Fig. 3. Instability of PSS for synthetic datasets

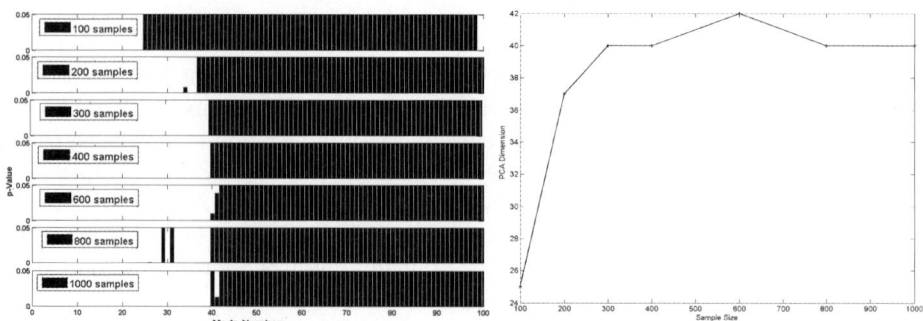

Fig. 4. *t*-Test Based stopping rule on synthetic cardiac datasets of different size

The method of Besse et al [14] was validated with synthetic datasets sized from 100 to 400. A plot of instability, measured as the distance between subspaces spanned by different replicates, is shown in figure 3. Although this method provides a visible indication of the correct number of modes to retain when the sample size is sufficiently large, it cannot identify the lower number of modes that should be retained when the sample size is insufficient.

5.2 Validation of *t*-Test Comparison with Noise

Our method was validated with synthetic datasets sized from 100 to 1000. Figure 4 shows the bar graphs of the p-Value (up to our 0.05 confidence level) from *t*-Tests for each mode trained from different sample sizes. The number of modes to retain versus the sample size is also shown. Our stopping rule does not have the tendency of going beyond 40 under large sample sizes. It also identifies a lower number of stable modes to retain for smaller sample sizes. It appears a sample size of around 300 is sufficient.

6 Results on Real Datasets

Figure 5 shows the results of sample sufficiency tests applied to the real cardiac dataset. The plot on the left side is the p-value for different replicate sizes. It shows that the number of modes determined by our stopping rule with 0.05 confidence level does not converge before the replicate size reaches the total sample size. This suggests that 319 samples are not enough. However, if an SSM is built from these samples, the number of modes to retain should be around 55.

Figure 6 shows sample size sufficiency tests on the real face datasets. For the 2D dataset, the plot obviously converges at 24 modes with 50 samples. With the 3D faces, the graph appears close to convergence at around 70 modes for the 150 samples. These results suggest both face datasets are sufficient.

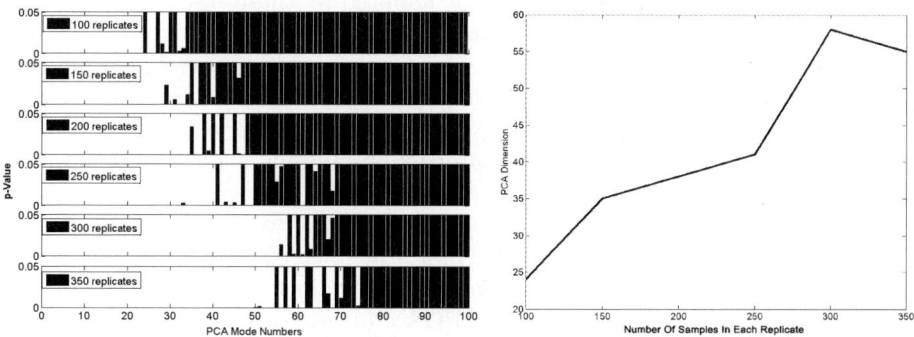

Fig. 5. Real heart dataset sufficiency test

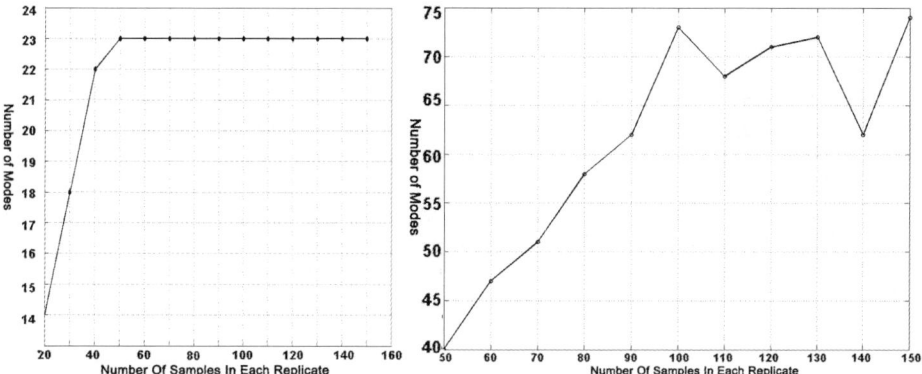

Fig. 6. Result of real face datasets sufficiency test. Left: 2D faces; Right: 3D faces.

7 Discussion

We propose a stopping rule for determining the number of modes to include for SSM based on mode direction stability. For a synthetic cardiac dataset generated with 40 real structural modes plus added noise our method converges correctly where conventional methods did not. We provide mode correspondence by minimising the distance between the principal spanned spaces rather than by the rank of their variances. We apply our stopping rule in a procedure we introduce to determine PCA sample size sufficiency. Results on real data suggest 319 samples are not sufficient for SSM of left ventricle (527 points) where both cardiac deformation and population variance are combined, but around 55 modes can be retained. However, 150 samples is sufficient for the 3D face meshes (500 points), where around 70 modes are retained. There is no trivial relationship between dimension of the shape vector, number of true anatomical modes and the required sample size. A more sophisticated method such as ours should be used instead.

It is hoped that our techniques will be adopted by those researchers working in SSM. Currently the number of samples used in most published studies is unlikely to be sufficient in the sense described in this paper. We hope that medical imaging researchers will gather more data and combine their sample sets in the aim of sufficient sample size for producing a standard, validated SSM for each organ. We aim to begin this process by building a significant database for two anatomical regions, the thorax and the lower abdomen. In time we intend to make the data and resulting models freely available to other research groups.

We provide what we believe to be the first principled test for sample sufficiency and determination of the number of modes to retain for SSM. Our method is also applicable to other applications of PCA and related fields.

References

1. Lee, S.L., Horkaew, P., Caspersz, W., Darzi, A., Yang, G.Z.: Assessment of shape variation of the levator ani with optimal scan planning and statistical shape modeling. Journal Of Computer Assisted Tomography 29, 154–162 (2005)
2. Rueckert, D., Frangi, A.F., Schnabel, J.A.: Automatic construction of 3-D statistical deformation models of the brain using nonrigid registration. IEEE Transactions On Medical Imaging 22, 1014–1025 (2003)
3. Lotjonen, J., Kivisto, S., Koikkalainen, J., Smutek, D., Lauerma, K.: Statistical shape model of atria, ventricles and epicardium from shortand long-axis MR images. Medical Image Analysis 8, 371–386 (2004)
4. Heimann, T., Wolf, I., Meinzer, H.P.: Active shape models for a fully automated 3d segmentation of the liver - an evaluation on clinical data. In: Larsen, R., Nielsen, M., Sporring, J. (eds.) MICCAI 2006. LNCS, vol. 4191, pp. 41–48. Springer, Heidelberg (2006)
5. MacCallum, R., Widaman, K., Zhang, S., Hong, S.: Sample size in factor analysis. Psychological Methods 4, 84–99 (1999)
6. Osborne, J., Costello, A.: Sample size and subject to item ratio in principal components analysis. Practical Assessment, Research and Evaluation 9(11) (2004)
7. Jackson, D.: Stopping rules in principal components analysis: a comparison of heuristical and statistical approaches. Ecology 74(8), 2204–2214 (1993)
8. Jolliffe, I.: Principal Component Analysis, 2nd edn. Springer, Heidelberg (2002)
9. Sinha, A., Buchanan, B.: Assessing the stability of principal components using regression. Psychometrika 60(3), 355–369 (2006)
10. Cootes, T., Taylor, C., Cooper, D., Graham, J.: Training models of shape from sets of examples. In: Proc. British Machine Vision Conference, pp. 266–275. Springer, Berlin (1992)
11. Daudin, J., Duby, C., Trecourt, P.: Stability of principal component analysis studied by the bootstrap method. Statistics 19, 341–358 (1988)
12. Besse, P.: PCA stability and choice of dimensionality. Statistics& Probability 13, 405–410 (1992)
13. Babalola, K., Cootes, T., Patenaude, B., Rao, A., Jenkinson, M.: Comparing the similarity of statistical shape models using the bhattacharya metric. In: Larsen, R., Nielsen, M., Sporring, J. (eds.) MICCAI 2006. LNCS, vol. 4190, pp. 142–150. Springer, Heidelberg (2006)

14. Besse, P., de Falguerolles, A.: Application of resampling methods to the choice of dimension in PCA. Computer Intensive Methods in Statistics. In: Hardle, W., Simar, L. (eds.), pp. 167–176. Physica-Verlag, Heidelberg (1993)
15. Cootes, T.: The AR face database 22 point markup,
    http://www.isbe.man.ac.uk/~bim/data/tarfd_markup/tarfd_markup.html
16. University of Notre Dame Computer Vision Research Laboratory: Biometrics database distribution, http://www.nd.edu/~cvrl/UNDBiometricsDatabase.html
17. Papatheodorou, T.: 3D Face Recognition Using Rigid and Non-Rigid Surface Registration. PhD thesis, VIP Group, Department of Computing, Imperial College, London University (2006)

Optimal Feature Point Selection and Automatic Initialization in Active Shape Model Search

Karim Lekadir and Guang-Zhong Yang

Visual Information Processing, Department of Computing
Imperial College London, United Kingdom
{lekadir,gzy}@doc.ic.ac.uk

Abstract. This paper presents a novel approach for robust and fully automatic segmentation with active shape model search. The proposed method incorporates global geometric constraints during feature point search by using inter-landmark conditional probabilities. The A* graph search algorithm is adapted to identify in the image the optimal set of valid feature points. The technique is extended to enable reliable and fast automatic initialization of the ASM search. Validation with 2-D and 3-D MR segmentation of the left ventricular epicardial border demonstrates significant improvement in robustness and overall accuracy, while eliminating the need for manual initialization.

1 Introduction

Active Shape Models (ASM) [1] are well recognized for their ability to capture significant and complex variability within a family of anatomical shapes. They can also act as a deformable template for medical image segmentation, where the search procedure involves in an iterative manner the identification of target feature points followed by the ASM model fitting. The method, however, is also known to have a number of difficulties in practice. First, the ASM search requires a suitable initialization to achieve satisfactory convergence. Generally, this is carried out by subjective manual interaction through which the user places the mean shape close to the anatomical structure under investigation. For shapes with complex geometry or shape variability, this may not be a satisfactory initialization and the search may be trapped in a local minimum. Some global search methods have been investigated for automatic initialization [2,3] but they are time consuming especially in 3-D. Another common problem with the ASM search is the presence of outliers, *i.e.*, when some of the detected feature points lie on incorrect boundary positions, a situation that is inevitable in practice due to confusing or missing image structures. These misplaced points significantly affect the segmentation outcome due to the least squares minimization nature of the subsequent pose and shape parameters estimation. Some robust ASM extensions have been suggested [4,5] but their performance is limited depending on the level of noise, as well as the dimensionality and complexity of the problem. Finally, the feature point detection is traditionally carried out using normal search profiles, which are not guaranteed to cover the features of interest on the boundary, as these types of search regions lack tangential coverage. Consequently, some target structures may not be reached at any iteration of the search procedure and some additional manual interaction may be necessary to define key landmarks, such as the valve and apex points in long axis left ventricular segmentation.

These three challenges are addressed in this paper within a single framework. The fundamental theoretical basis behind this work is the optimal feature point selection algorithm, based on inter-landmark conditional probabilities and the A* graph search algorithm. Instead of selecting the feature candidates with the best grey-level properties within each search region independently, the proposed algorithm finds in one step the least grey-level cost and geometrically consistent combination of feature candidates from all search regions, ensuring the elimination of erroneous feature points. The optimality of the algorithm enables the use of large search regions instead of the normal search profiles, resulting in extended coverage of the target features and improved adaptation to complex structures. With some modifications, the proposed algorithm allows reliable and fast automatic initialization of the ASM search without user interaction. The validation is carried out on the challenging MR segmentation of the left-ventricular epi-cardial border both in 2-D and 3-D.

2 Methods

2.1 Optimal Feature Point Selection

In ASM search, the feature point selection is achieved by estimating for the candidate points p_{ij} within each search region H_i the degree of match between the underlying grey-level profile and its corresponding model built during the training stage. The grey-level cost function $d_g(p_{ij})$ used for this purpose can be derived for example by calculating the Mahalanobis distance to the mean grey-level profile [6].

In addition to the grey-level based cost function, the proposed framework introduces for optimal feature point selection the notion of inter-landmark conditional probability, which describes the statistical distribution of a landmark point p_i given the known positions of a set of m points (out of n landmark points in the shape), i.e.,

$$P(p_i \mid p_{s(1)}, \ldots, p_{s(m)}) = P(\mathbf{x}_i \mid \mathbf{x}_{s(1)}, \ldots, \mathbf{x}_{s(m)}) \tag{1}$$

where s is an indexing function and $\mathbf{x}_i$ denotes the coordinates of the point p_i. The estimation of the conditional p.d.f. requires a suitable regression model that relates the points p_i and $p_{s(1)}, \ldots, p_{s(m)}$. Based on a generalization of the barycentric coordinates [7], the introduced formulation describes $\mathbf{x}_i$ as an affine combination of $\mathbf{x}_{s(1)}, \ldots, \mathbf{x}_{s(m)}$ which is invariant to the position of the points, as follows:

$$\mathbf{x}_i = \sum_{k=1}^{m} c_k \mathbf{x}_{s(k)} + \mathbf{t} + \mathbf{e} \quad \text{with} \quad \sum_{k=1}^{m} c_k = 1 \tag{2}$$

The weights c_k and translation vector $\mathbf{t}$ are calculated at the training stage by differentiation such that the model residuals $\mathbf{e}$ are minimized. With the proposed landmark-based regression model, the probability density function of $\mathbf{x}_i$ conditioned on the known values of $\mathbf{x}_{s(1)},...,\mathbf{x}_{s(m)}$ can be described using a multivariate Gaussian distribution with mean $\mathbf{x}_i^*$ and covariance $\mathbf{S}_i^*$:

$$\mathbf{x}_i^* = \sum_{k=1}^{m} c_k \mathbf{x}_{s(k)} + \mathbf{t} \qquad \mathbf{S}_i^* = \mathrm{Cov}(\mathbf{e}_i) \qquad (3)$$

The inter-landmark conditional probabilities incorporate geometric constraints to the feature point selection in order to ensure that erroneous feature points are not considered during the procedure. A domain $A(p_i \mid p_{s(1)},...,p_{s(m)})$ of geometrically allowable candidates for the point p_i can be derived at each stage of the algorithm given the points $p_{s(1)},...,p_{s(m)}$:

$$A(p_i \mid p_{s(1)},...,p_{s(m)}) = \left\{ \mathbf{x}_{ij} \mid (\mathbf{x}_{ij} - \mathbf{x}_i^*)^T \mathbf{S}_i^{*-1} (\mathbf{x}_{ij} - \mathbf{x}_i^*) < U \right\} \qquad (4)$$

where U is a threshold that controls the size of the landmark allowable domain and which can be calculated from the chi-squared distribution [8].

The aim of the proposed algorithm is to select the least grey-level cost set of candidate points amongst all geometrically consistent combinations. For this purpose, a tree search algorithm based on the A* algorithm [9] is introduced for optimal feature point selection. Let s be the sequence function describing the order in which search regions are explored and starting from the initial region $H_{s(1)}$, a number of paths can be explored. All the paths are stored in a priority queue Q and at each stage of the algorithm, the choice of the path to be further expanded is based on the calculation of a cost function of the actual path g and a heuristic estimation h of the remaining cost to reach the final landmark point. The cost function is calculated by summing all individual grey-level costs in the actual path:

$$g(L_k) = \sum_{i=1}^{|L_k|} d_g \left(p_{s(i) L_k(i)} \right) \qquad (5)$$

where $|L_k|$ denotes the size of the path L_k and $L_k(i)$ the index of the feature candidate selected within the corresponding search region.

The heuristic function estimates the most optimistic remaining cost to reach the final landmark point, by summing the minimum grey-level cost amongst the geometrically consistent candidates within each remaining search region, i.e.,

$$h(L_k) = \sum_{i=|L_k|+1}^{n} \min_j \left[d_g \left(p_{s(i)j} \right) \right] \qquad (6)$$

with $p_{s(i)j} \in A\left(p_{s(i)} \mid p_{s(1)},...,p_{s(i-1)} \right) \cap H_{s(i)}$

The cost function g favors paths with the best grey-level characteristics, whilst the heuristic function h is used to penalize paths that lead to poor intensity characteristics within the remaining landmark allowable domains. At each stage of the algorithm, the path L_k with the minimal sum of the cost and heuristic functions is selected from the priority queue, *i.e.*,

$$L_k = \arg\min_{L_k \in Q}\left[g(L_k) + h(L_k) \right] \qquad (7)$$

The expansion of each path is only allowed using feature candidates that are geometrically consistent with the points in the current path based on the allowable conditional domain in Eq. (4). The tree search is carried out until a path reaches one of the candidates of the last search region $H_{s(n)}$. Because the heuristic in Eq. (6) is admissible, *i.e.*, it never overestimates the remaining cost to the final feature point, it can be shown [9] that the selection achieved using the A* algorithm is optimal and therefore is guaranteed to be the best valid set of feature points within the search regions.

The order in which the search regions are visited in the tree can be defined at the training stage as follows. The first point $p_{s(1)}$ is preferably chosen as a key landmark (corner or high curvature point). Then the ith index in the sequence s corresponds to the point that correlates most with the points already in the sequence, *i.e.*, the point with the smallest allowable domain calculated from the inter-landmark conditional probability $P(\mathbf{x}_{s(i)} | \mathbf{x}_{s(1)},...,\mathbf{x}_{s(i-1)})$. This is equivalent to choosing the point with the minimal determinant of the covariance matrix calculated from Eq. (3). The procedure continues until all n landmark points indices are within the sequence.

It is worth noting that the conditional probability $P(\mathbf{x}_{s(i)} | \mathbf{x}_{s(1)},...,\mathbf{x}_{s(i-1)})$ can be approximated by using only a subset of the points $p_{s(1)},...,p_{s(i-1)}$ that most correlates with the point $p_{s(i)}$. Furthermore, the effect of rotation and scaling is eliminated by using the values from the initialization.

2.2 Automatic Initialization

As a result of the optimality of the introduced algorithm, the method is guaranteed to output the geometrically valid set of feature points with the best intensity profiles independently of the size of the input search regions. This enables the use of considerably large search regions instead of the traditional normal search profiles. By using the entire image for each feature search region, it is evident that the ASM initialization becomes unnecessary. Such a method, however, would require a lot of computations to reach the final solution and is therefore not desirable. The automatic initialization can be significantly speeded up by finding one or a few potential candidates for the initial points $p_{s(1)}$ and then deriving search regions for all other landmark points by estimating the inter-landmark conditional probabilities $P(p_{s(i)} | p_{s(1)})$ and the corresponding allowable domains. To this end, the entire image or a region of interest is scanned and the positions with high heuristic values as calculated from Eq. (7) are eliminated, as this indicates that the induced landmark allowable domains are unlikely to intersect with the target features. The remaining candidates in the image with low heuristic values, on the other hand, are very likely to lie close to the true position of $p_{s(1)}$. To achieve faster elimination of incorrect initial points, the heuristic is replaced by an average minimal grey-level cost calculated over the m_k first search regions:

$$h_0\left(p_{s(1)k}\right) = \frac{1}{m_k}\left[d_g\left(p_{s(1)k}\right) + \sum_{i=2}^{m_k}\min_j\left[d_g\left(p_{s(m_k)j}\right)\right]\right] \quad (8)$$

$$\text{with } p_{s(m_k)j} \in A\left(p_{s(m_k)} \mid p_{s(1)k}\right)$$

At the start of automatic initialization, all candidates for the initial point are stored in a priority queue with m_k set to 1. At each subsequent iteration, the candidate with the lowest heuristic value calculated from Eq. (8) is further considered by incriminating its m_k and updating the heuristic accordingly. With this method, candidates inducing landmark allowable domains that intersect the target boundary are brought forward in the priority queue and the algorithm stops when the first few candidates in the priority queue reaches a value of m_k equal to n. The optimal feature point selection algorithm from previous section is then applied to the identified initial points and to the corresponding landmark allowable domains and the result followed by model fitting is used as the ASM initialization.

It must be noted that if the initial orientation and scaling are not known, these can be also efficiently estimated by using the exact same approach presented in this section, by copying the candidate points for different rotations and scale factors and calculating the inter-landmark allowable domains and the heuristic in Eq. (8) accordingly. In left ventricular segmentation with MR, the intersection between the horizontal and vertical long axis views provides initial estimates of these parameters and allows the definition of a region of interest. Typically, the automatic initialization procedure and one iteration of the proposed ASM technique are sufficient to obtain satisfactory convergence. The automatic initialization step is carried out within a few seconds in both 2-D and 3-D.

2.3 Validation

The proposed fully automatic ASM framework is validated with 2-D and 3-D segmentation of the epi-cardial border of the left ventricle from long and short axis MR images. In cardiac MR, reliable segmentation of the epi-cardial boundary without user interaction is challenging because of its intensity appearance that displays faint/weak edges often surrounded by fat and confusing structures. Additionally, the automatic definition of the valve and apex points is difficult.

The LV datasets were collected by scanning 20 subject (13 normal, 5 locally abnormal, 2 severely abnormal) using a 1.5T MR scanner (Sonata, Siemens, Erlangen Germany) and a TrueFISP sequence (TE = 1.5 ms, TR = 3 ms, slice thickness = 10 mm, pixel size of 1.5 to 2 mm) within a single breath-hold. The long and short axis images were annotated by an expert clinician using a manual contouring tool. The estimation of the inter-landmark conditional probabilities and their evaluation using the proposed ASM framework were carried out on a leave-one-out basis. For automatic initialization, the initial point $P_{s(1)}$ was chosen as the apex for the 2-D segmentation and as the lower RV/LV junction point of the mid-ventricular slice for the 3-D case. For comparison, the datasets were also segmented using the original ASM [1] and a robust ASM extension [4] based on robust estimators. These methods were initialized by placing the mean shapes for each long and short axis image at the centre of the corresponding manual segmentations. The same local intensity models and grey-level cost function was used for all methods, based on the standard ASM search formulation [6].

3 Results

Table 1 summarizes the segmentation error statistics (mean, standard deviation, min and max) for both the 2-D and 3-D epi-cardial datasets, as obtained using the existing ASM methods, the automatic initialization alone and the entire proposed ASM framework. To aid visualization, the segmentation errors for the 20 datasets are also displayed for the 3-D case in Fig. 1. It can be seen from the results that the original ASM lacks robustness for epi-cardial segmentation, as the target structures, unlike the endo-cardial borders, are often poorly defined and coupled with considerable artifacts. The robust ASM improves upon the original ASM results (14 % average improvement in 2-D and 22 % in 3-D), but its performance is not consistent for all datasets. It is evident from the obtained results that the proposed fully automatic framework outperforms the existing techniques used for comparison. In particular, it can be seen that on average the automatic initialization alone performs better in shape localization, which demonstrates its robustness. The entire framework using automatic initialization and the optimal feature selection performs well for all datasets, with a maximal segmentation error less than 2 mm and an average improvement with respect to ASM of 46 % and with respect the robust ASM of 33 %. This performance can be explained by the nature of the proposed method, which ensures outlier-free image search due to the geometrically constrained selection of feature points, while existing ASM methods become more instable as the imaging conditions or the boundary appearance characteristics deteriorate.

Fig. 2 shows 2-D/3-D illustrations of the strength of the proposed algorithm when applied to challenging segmentation tasks. The 2-D long axis view displays a dilated left ventricle with poor signal definition of the boundaries, especially at the apex and lateral apical regions. As a result, the original ASM fails to recover the boundary of

Table 1. Detailed error analysis of the ASM methods (in *mm*)

	2-D				3-D			
	Mean error	Std.	Min error	Max error	Mean error	Std.	Min error	Max error
Original ASM [1]	2.01	1.12	0.87	4.98	2.13	1.01	0.98	4.94
Robust ASM [4]	1.71	0.92	0.86	4.38	1.65	1.00	0.92	4.66
Auto. initialization	1.23	0.32	0.82	1.88	1.60	0.41	0.96	2.67
Proposed method	1.13	0.32	0.64	1.82	1.11	0.25	0.79	1.84

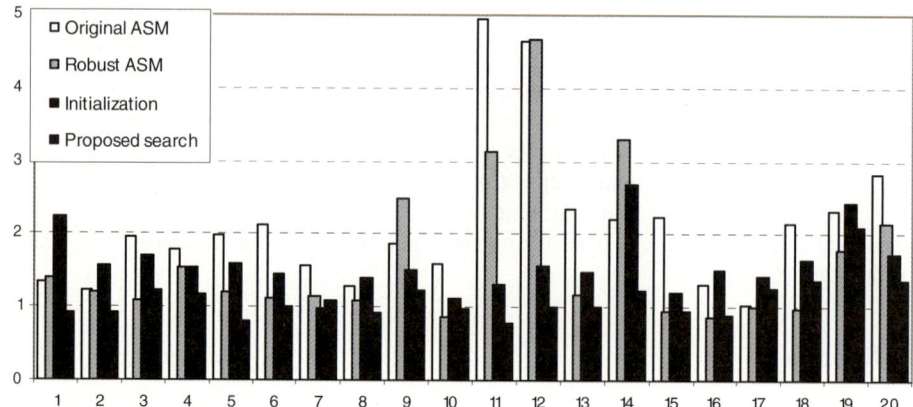

Fig. 1. 3-D segmentation errors (in *mm*) as obtained with the proposed technique and initialization, with comparison to the existing ASM methods

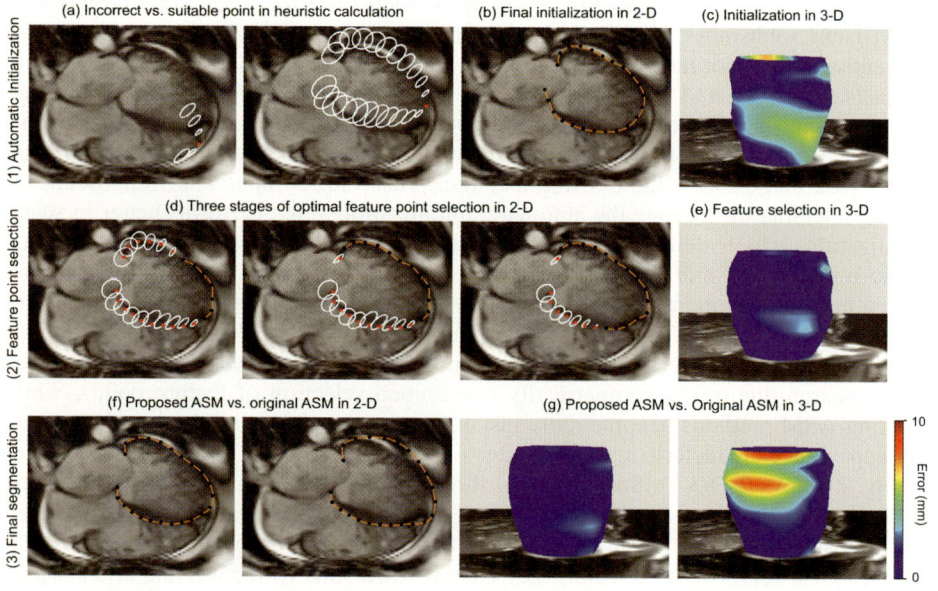

Fig. 2. Illustration of each stage of the proposed technique in 2-D and 3-D

interest (see (f), average segmentation error equal to 4.58 mm). The automatic initialization is illustrated in (a)-(b). The apex of the right ventricle is investigated as a possible initial point due to resemblance with the left ventricular apex. This point is, however, rejected after only a few conditional search regions considered in the heuristic calculation (Eq. (8)), as these landmark allowable domains do not intersect with the target image features, and therefore return high minimal grey-level cost values. In contrast, although the left ventricular apex is poorly displayed in the image, the corresponding allowable domains are located on the boundary of interest and the candidate point under investigation is therefore successfully selected as an initial point (a). The subsequent final 2-D initialization is shown in (b) after feature point selection. The automatic initialization achieves a reasonably good localization of the boundary, with only minor errors at the apex and valve points. The optimal feature point selection algorithm in subsequent iterations is illustrated in (d), where three intermediate stages of the procedure are shown. It can be noticed that the landmark allowable domains, calculated using the inter-landmark conditional probabilities, become smaller as the path approaches the corresponding landmark points, therefore restricting the selection algorithm to valid candidate positions on the boundary. The final 2-D segmentation is shown in (f), demonstrating high accuracy along the entire boundary, as well as for the key landmark points (valve and apex points). Similarly, the proposed method achieves significant improvement in 3-D (see (g)), due to more suitable initialization (c) and robust identification of the feature points (e).

4 Conclusion

This paper presents a novel technique for robust feature point detection and automatic initialization in ASM-based segmentation. Due to the use of the A* algorithm and inter-landmark conditional probabilities, the introduced method ensures optimal selection of the feature points according to both geometric and appearance criteria. With some modifications in the heuristic calculation, the algorithm enables fast and reliable automatic initialization of the ASM search. The validation on 2-D and 3-D MR segmentation of the left-ventricular epi-cardial border shows significant increase in overall accuracy and robustness, while eliminating the need for manual initialization.

References

1. Cootes, T.F., Cooper, D., Taylor, C.J., Graham, J.: Active shape models - Their training and application. Computer Vision and Image Understanding (CVIU) 61, 38–59 (1995)
2. Brejl, M., Sonka, M.: Object localization and border detection criteria design in edge-based image segmentation: automated learning from examples. IEEE Transactions on Medical Imaging 19, 973–985 (2000)
3. de Bruijne, M., Nielsen, M.: Shape particle filtering for image segmentation. In: Barillot, C., Haynor, D.R., Hellier, P. (eds.) MICCAI 2004. LNCS, vol. 3216, pp. 168–175. Springer, Heidelberg (2004)
4. Rogers, M., Graham, J.: Robust active shape model search. In: Heyden, A., Sparr, G., Nielsen, M., Johansen, P. (eds.) ECCV 2002. LNCS, vol. 2353, pp. 517–530. Springer, Heidelberg (2002)
5. Lekadir, K., Merrifield, R., Yang, G.-Z.: Outlier detection and handling for robust 3-D active shape models search. IEEE Transactions on Medical Imaging 26, 212–222 (2007)
6. Cootes, T.F., Taylor, C.J.: Active shape model search using local grey-level models: a quantitative evaluation. In: Proc. British Machine Vision Conf (BMVC) (1993)
7. Coxeter, H.S.M.: Barycentric coordinates. In: Introduction to geometry, 2nd edn., pp. 216–221. Wiley, New York (1969)
8. Becker, C., Gather, U.: The masking breakdown point of multivariate outlier identification rules. Journal of the American Statistical Association 94, 947–955 (1999)
9. Russell, S.J., Norvig, P.: Artificial intelligence: a modern approach. Prentice-Hall, Englewood Cliffs (2003)

MR-Less High Dimensional Spatial Normalization of ^{11}C PiB PET Images on a Population of Elderly, Mild Cognitive Impaired and Alzheimer Disease Patients

Jurgen Fripp[1], Pierrick Bourgeat[1], Parnesh Raniga[1,3], Oscar Acosta[1], Victor Villemagne[2], Gareth Jones[2], Graeme O'keefe[2], Christopher Rowe[2], Sébastien Ourselin[1,4], and Olivier Salvado[1]

[1] Australian e-Health Research Centre, CSIRO ICT Centre, Brisbane, Australia
[2] Department of Nuclear Medicine and Centre for PET, Austin Hospital, Melbourne, Australia
[3] School of Electrical and Information Engineering, The University of Sydney, Sydney, Australia
[4] (Current Affiliation) Centre for Medical Image Computing, University College London, London, United Kingdom

Abstract. $\beta - amyloid$ (Aβ) plaques are one of the neuropathological hallmarks of Alzheimer's disease (AD) and can be quantified using the marker ^{11}C PiB. As ^{11}C PiB PET images have limited anatomical information, an Magnetic Resonance Image (MRI) is usually acquired to perform the spatial normalization needed for population analysis. We designed and evaluated a high dimensional spatial normalization approach that only uses the ^{11}C PiB PET image. The non-rigid registration (NRR) is based on free form deformation (FFD) modelled using B-splines. To compensate for the limited anatomical information, the FFD is constrained to an allowable transform space using a model trained from MR registrations. Aβ deposition is dependent on disease staging, so a spatially normalized ^{11}C PiB PET appearance model selects and refines the atlas. The approach was compared with MR NRR using data from healthy elderly, mild cognitive impaired and Alzheimer disease participants. Using segmentation propagation, an average Dice similarity coefficient of 0.64 and 0.73 was obtained for white and gray matter. The R-squared correlation between the uptake obtained in the frontal, parietal, occipital and temporal was 0.789, 0.843, 0.871 and 0.964. These are very promising results, considering the low resolution of ^{11}C PiB PET images.

1 Introduction

$\beta - amyloid$ (Aβ) plaques are one of the neuropathological hallmarks of Alzheimer's disease (AD) and appear many years before cognitive symptoms become apparent. ^{11}C PiB PET [1] is one of the most promising imaging agents

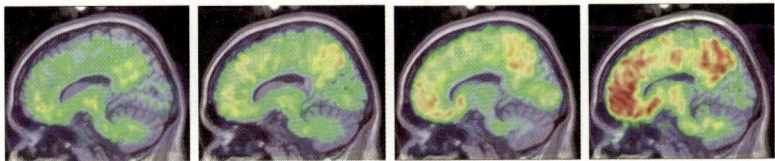

Fig. 1. Four example spatially normalized ¹¹C PiB PET cases overlaid on the Colin atlas *left* Healthy elderly *middle left* mild cognitive impaired *middle and far right* Alzheimer's

for assessing Aβ deposition. PiB has been shown to be more specific than other markers at binding to amyloid. In previous studies, it has been observed that the pattern of uptake found in ¹¹C PiB PET images can vary significantly and in some cases overlap between AD, mild cognitive impaired (MCI) and healthy elderly (NC). Example ¹¹C PiB PET images are presented in Fig. 1, which highlight this variability and indicate why high dimensional non-rigid registration is problematic.

Variation in brain structure and Aβ deposition between individuals, as well as differences in image resolution and field of view can make direct comparisons of ¹¹C PiB PET images difficult. To perform statistical analysis some form of spatial normalization is necessary. The standard approach is through linear scaling and non-linear warping, which is often performed using Statistical Parametric Mapping (SPM) [2]. This involves the patients ¹¹C PiB PET and MR being co-registered, the patients MR being affinely and non-rigidly warped to an atlas, then the warping is applied to the co-registered PET to obtain spatially normalized PET images [3,4]. The main disadvantages of this approach are the accumulation of registration errors and requiring an MR for each patient.

For future clinical use into the early detection of Alzheimers disease it is desirable to be able to analyse and compare ¹¹C PiB PET images accurately without requiring a MR image. There are several reasons why this is important: minimise the cost required for neurological assessment, reduce the burden on the patient and allow its implementation when MRs cannot be acquired (e.g. claustrophobic patients and/or metalic implants).

In some Fluorodeoxyglucose (FDG) and PiB PET studies, an average PET atlas has been used with linear and low dimensional warping [5,6,7]. However, ¹¹C PiB PET images exhibit highly variable and even non-corresponding regions of $\beta - amyloid$ deposition (often related to disease staging). Hence, the use of a single average atlas for ¹¹C PiB PET registration is not ideal and may adversely affect the registration results for some patients [7]. The use of a specifically selected atlas or a generated atlas that in some way best matches the participant's scan has been pursued in MR [8,9], and in many applications can allow more accurate non-rigid registration results [10]. In this paper we utilize a generative appearance model of spatially normalized ¹¹C PiB PET images to allow us to select and refine the atlas for each participant.

A popular approach for non-rigid registration is to use spline-based transformations [11]. In this paper the deformation is represented by a free form deformation (FFD) based on B-splines. Statistical control point model (SCPM) constraints can then be used to restrict these deformations to an allowable deformation space [12]. In general it has been found to improve robustness, although it can reduce precision. This is less of a concern for ^{11}C PiB PET images which have much lower resolution, higher noise and limited structural information compared to the MRs used to train the SCPM. We use SCPM in the non-rigid registration to provide constraints on the transformation model, and hence implicitly embed anatomical information.

We present an approach to perform MR-less ^{11}C PiB PET-PET spatial normalization. This is validated in a leave-one-out fashion on a large sample of real clinical participants from an Alzheimer study by comparing the spatial normalization obtained with that obtained using MR.

2 Method

2.1 Subjects

PiB PET scans from 98 participants enrolled in a longitudinal study assessing ^{11}C PiB PET for early diagnosis of AD were used in this study [13]. Participants were excluded if they were not fluent in English, mini-mental state examination (MMSE) was less than 12, or there was a history of brain injury or alcoholism. The 24 AD participants met NINCDS/ADRDA criteria for probable AD. The 20 MCI participants met Petersen's recently published consensus criteria. The remaining 54 participants were healthy elderly participants. Objective impairment was established as at least one neuropsychological test score falling 1.5 SD or more below relevant normative data.

2.2 Image Acquisition Protocols

The ^{11}C PiB PET scans were acquired using a Philips ADAC Allegro full-ring tomograph with PIZELAR germanium oxyorthosilicate crystal detectors. Each participant was injected with 370 MBq of ^{11}C-PiB and were scanned for 20 minutes starting 40 minutes post-injection. Summed images for the 40 to 60 minutes time frame were used (2x2x2mm). Sagittal MR images were acquired using a T_1 weighted 3D SPGR sequence 1.5T (1.1x1.1x1.5mm) and 3T scanners (0.5x0.5x2mm).

2.3 Registration for Training

The rigid PET to MR co-registration and MR to Atlas affine image registration was performed using the automated method of Ourselin et al [14]. This approach uses a block matching strategy to estimate the global transformation with a matching criteria of normalized cross correlation. The MR to atlas non-rigid registration was performed using an inhouse implementation of B-splines based FFD [11]. The B-spline transformation model describing the deformation is written by the tensor product of the 1D cubic B-splines:

$$T_{local}(x,y,z) = \sum_{l=0}^{3}\sum_{m=0}^{3}\sum_{n=0}^{3} B_l(u) B_m(v) B_n(w) \phi_{i+l,j+m,k+n} \quad (1)$$

Where u, v and w are the relative positions of the index point along each axis and ϕ are the parameters of the B-splines. The matching criteria used in the FFD was normalized mutual information (NMI) [15], with the cost function $C_{total} = (1-\omega)C_{similarity} - \omega C_{constraint}$ where $C_{constraint}$ is the smoothness constraint from [16] with $\omega = 0.01$. This was optimised in a three level multi-resolution scheme, with the image sub-sampled by a factor of 4, 2 and 1, and the control point spacing changed from 20, 10 to 5 mm respectively.

Using the aforementioned affine registration [14] and B-Spline based FFD [11] all participant's co-registered MR scans were spatially normalized to the Colin atlas [17]. The obtained transformations were then used to warp the participants ^{11}C PiB PET image to the Colin atlas and hence obtain spatially normalized ^{11}C PiB PET images. We will refer to this process as PET-MR spatial normalization, while the MR-less ^{11}C PiB PET spatial normalization approach will be referred to as PET-PET spatial normalization.

2.4 Principal Component Analysis

Given N images with M voxels we can construct a $X = M \times N$ matrix (each column i is the voxel data from the i th image x_i). Then the mean image is simply $\mu = \frac{1}{N}\sum_{i=1:N} x_i$. The principal component model was calculated using a singular value decomposition with the covariance matrix $\frac{1}{N}DD^T$ decomposed as $U\sum U^T = \frac{1}{N}DD^T$ where D is the mean-offset map (column i given by $D_i = x_i - \mu$), and U has column vectors that represent the orthogonal modes of variation and $\sum$ is a diagonal matrix of corresponding eigenvalues. An image x_{unseen} can be decomposed into a N dimensional vector of weights $w = U^T(x_{unseen} - \mu)$, which we will refer to as eigen-weights. Given eigen-weights w, an image x_{new} can be reconstructed by $x_{new} = Uw + \mu$. The principal component scores were constrained to be within 3 standard deviations.

Generative ^{11}C PiB PET Appearance Model: The ^{11}C PiB PET images was intensity normalized using a zero mean unit variance filter. Performing PCA on the intensity and spatially normalized ^{11}C PiB PET images allowed a generative appearance model to be created that could be used to generate intensity and spatially normalized ^{11}C PiB PET atlases. The number of modes used was 61 and accounted for 95% of the variation in the training data.

Statistical Control Point Model (SCPM): Performing PCA on the parameters ϕ of the B-spline obtained in the PET-MR spatial normalization allowed a SCPM to be computed for each level that was used to provide an allowable deformation space. This was used to constrain deformations to be close to those previously seen in training. The number of modes used in each level was (84, 82, 79) and accounted for 95% of the variation in the training data.

2.5 PET-PET Spatial Normalization

The PET-PET spatial normalization approach extends SCPM constrained non-rigid registration to include the generative ^{11}C PiB PET appearance model. To initialize this approach, the original ^{11}C PiB PET image is affinely propagated to the Colin atlas. In this paper we want to directly compare the PET-MR and PET-PET spatial normalization, so the affine transformation obtained in training is used for both approaches, in practice a PET-PET affine registration would be used [7]. The initial atlas is generated using the affinely registered ^{11}C PiB PET image.

The PET-PET spatial normalization is then performed using the same FFD based non-rigid registration between the affinely registered ^{11}C PiB PET image and the generated atlas. This was performed in the same three level multi-resolution scheme with the same parameters used in the training. However, unlike the MR-PET spatial normalization, no smoothness constraints were used, instead every third iteration the current ϕ parameters were reconstructed (and constrained) using the SCPM. As well as this, the current atlas was refined every fifth iteration using the current spatially normalized ^{11}C PiB PET image with the generative appearance model. This approach tends to result in the appearance of the generated ^{11}C PiB PET atlas and the transformed ^{11}C PiB PET image becoming similar.

2.6 Validation

For validation we assume that the results obtained by the PET-MR spatial normalization is correct and treat it as ground truth. All experiments were performed in a leave one out fashion. The MRs were segmented into gray (GM), white matter (WM) and cerebral spinal fluid (CSF) [18]. The Dice similarity coefficient (DSC = $2T_P/(2T_P + F_P + F_N)$, where T_P is true positive, T_N is true negative, F_P is false positive and F_N is false negative) was calculated between the propagated segmentations obtained using PET-MR and PET-PET spatial normalization. The mean uptake in various regions was also calculated for all images with the R-squared correlation calculated between the PET-PET (or affine) and MR-PET spatial normalization.

3 Results

Figure 2 qualitatively illustrates the typical spatial normalization. Qualitative assessment indicated that the PET-PET spatial normalization was very good, which was most evident in the ventricles, skull and outer cortex where more anatomical information is present. It was found that a realistic spatial normalization could **not** be obtained if only the generative atlas (using smoothness constraints) or SCPM (using mean spatially normalized ^{11}C PiB PET image as atlas) was used (results not shown).

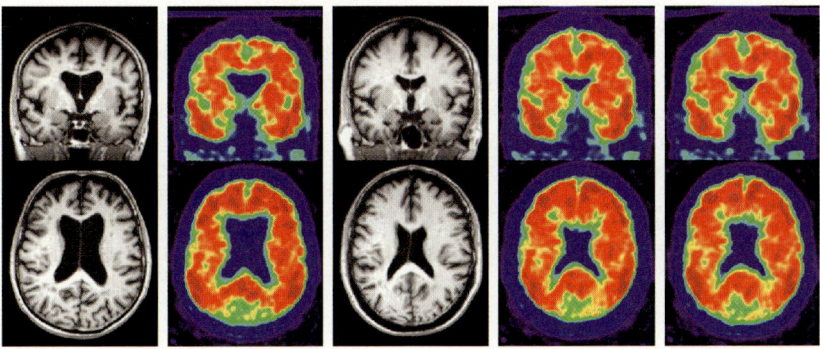

Fig. 2. Example registration results for one case *left to right* Affinely registered MR, Propagated Affinely Co-registered PiB, Non-rigidly registered MR, PET-MR spatial normalization and PET-PET spatial normalization

By propagating the GM, WM and CSF segmentation of each participant into the spatially normalized space, it can be seen (Figure 3) that the PET-PET approach is slightly inferior to MR-PET. By propagating the segmentations using the PET-MR and PET-PET spatial normalizations, an average DSC of 0.64 and 0.73 was obtained for the GM and WM. This is quite good, considering the average DSC for GM and WM obtained by comparing direct MR and ^{11}C PiB PET segmentation is 0.59 and 0.69 [19]. There was no obvious bias in the algorithm due to the disease staging, with all results similar in quality (Table 1). The minimum (and maximum) DSC for the GM, WM and CSF was 0.56 (0.69), 0.67 (0.78) and 0.40 (0.56).

In clinical studies, the primary interest is to extract statistics from various regions in the brain and to see whether changes in these regions are related to disease staging. So to further validate this approach we also consider the quantitative statistics obtained automatically from various regions (using composite regions defined with the AAL mask). An example of the average uptake (image

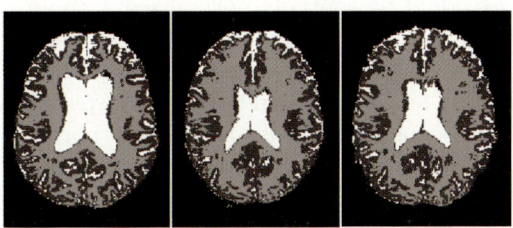

Fig. 3. Example GM, WM and CSF segmentation propagation using *left* Affine *middle* PET-MR and *right* PET-PET spatially normalization. This image illustrates the quality of the approach, with only minor errors in finer details, brain shape and ventricle size. **Note:** This is the same case and slice used in Figure 2.

Table 1. Mean (standard deviation) DSC results of the propagated segmentations on the spatially normalized atlas. The segmentation propogations were obtained using PET-MR and PET-PET transforms.

Class	GM	WM	CSF
AD	0.64 (0.02)	0.73 (0.02)	0.49 (0.04)
MCI	0.64 (0.02)	0.73 (0.02)	0.49 (0.04)
NC	0.65 (0.02)	0.74 (0.02)	0.49 (0.03)

Table 2. R-squared correlation between the uptake obtained in a region using PET-MR spatial normalization and the results of affine and our PET-PET spatial normalization

	Affine	PET-PET NRR
Frontal	0.726	0.789
Occipital	0.769	0.871
Parietal	0.779	0.843
Hippocampus	0.935	0.949
Precuneus	0.939	0.965
Temporal	0.952	0.964

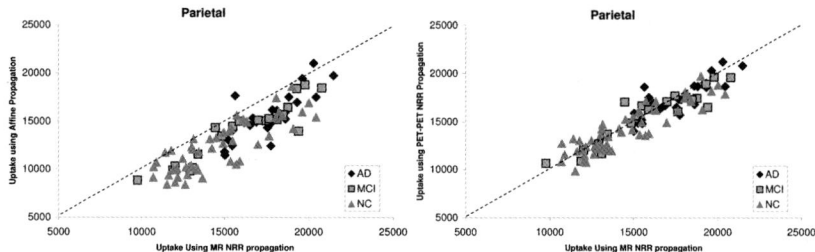

Fig. 4. Uptake found in the parietal region using MR spatial normalization compared to that found using *left* Affine and *right* PET-PET spatial normalization

intensity) in the parietal cortex is illustrated in Figure 4 by comparing affine and PET-PET to PET-MR. The R-squared correlation for several regions is also presented in Table 2, which show the close match between PET-PET and PET-MR spatial normalization, especially compared to the affine spatial normalization.

4 Conclusion

^{11}C PiB PET images could be spatially normalized with an accuracy almost as high as when using an MR scan, despite the limited anatomical resolution of the PET image. This was achieved by 1) constraining the approach to only use brain deformations that had been learn't from MR spatial normalization on a large database of MR scans, and 2) use a spatially normalized ^{11}C PiB PET atlas that was continually updated using a generative appearance model. This approach was validated using segmentation propagation and regional analysis and was shown to obtain results which are comparable to the traditional MR based spatial normalization, especially in regions where anatomical information is present (e.g. ventricles). The primary limitations of this approach are the computational cost ($\frac{1}{4}$, 1 and 5 hours for each respective level), requirement for significant training data and use of the same levels and control point spacing as the training data.

In conclusion, in the absence of MRs, it is possible to perform high dimensional spatial normalization of ^{11}C PiB PET image. This approach is relevant for widespread clinical use of amyloid imaging. Future work will involve refining this approach to include partial volume correction of the PiB PET images and to impose diffeomorphic constraints.

References

1. Klunk, W.E., et al.: Imaging brain amyloid in Alzheimer's disease with Pittsburgh Compound-B. Ann. Neurol. 55(3), 306–319 (2004)
2. Ashburner, J., et al.: Nonlinear Spatial Normalization Using Basis Functions. Human Brain Mapping 7, 254–266 (1999)
3. Ziolko, S., et al.: Evaluation of voxel-based methods for the statistical analysis of PIB PET amyloid imaging studies in Alzheimer's disease. NeuroImage 33(1), 94–102 (2006)
4. Lopresti, B., et al.: Simplified quantification of Pittsburgh Compound B amyloid imaging PET studies: a comparative analysis. J. Nucl. Med. 46(12), 1959–1972 (2005)
5. Lee, S., et al.: FDG-PET images quantified by probabilistic atlas of brain and surgical prognosis of temporal lobe epilepsy. Epilepsia (9), 1032–1038 (2002)
6. Kemppainen, N.M., et al.: PET amyloid ligand [11C] PIB uptake is increased in mild cognitive impairment. Neurology 68(19), 1603–1606 (2007)
7. Fripp, J., et al.: Generative atlases and atlas selection for C11-PIB PET-PET registration of Elderly. In: Mild cognitive impaired and Alzheimer disease patients IEEE Symp. on Biom. Imag., pp. 1155–1158 (2008)
8. Rohlfing, T., et al.: Evaluation of atlas selection strategies for atlas-based image segmentation with application to confocal microscopy images of bee brains. NeuroImage 21, 1428–1442 (2004)
9. Blezek, D., et al.: Atlas stratification. Med. Imag. Anal. 11(5), 443–457 (2007)
10. Wu, M., et al.: Optimum template selection for atlas-based segmentation. NeuroImage 34(4), 1612–1618 (2007)
11. Rueckert, D., et al.: Nonrigid registration using free-form deformations: Application to breast MR images. IEEE Trans. Med. Imag. 18, 712–721 (1999)
12. Rueckert, D., et al.: Automatic construction of 3-D statistical deformation models of the brain using nonrigid registration. IEEE Trans. Med. Imag. 8, 1014–1025 (2003)
13. Rowe, C.C., et al.: Imaging beta-amyloid burden in aging and dementia. Neurology 68(20), 1718–1725 (2007)
14. Ourselin, S., et al.: Reconstructing a 3D structure from serial histological sections. IVC 19, 25–31 (2001)
15. Studholme, C., et al.: An Overlap Invariant Entropy Measure of 3D Medical Image Alignment. Pattern Recognition 32(1), 71–86 (1999)
16. Rohlfing, T., et al.: Volume-preserving nonrigid registration of MR breast images using free-form deformation with an incompressibility constraint. IEEE Trans. Med. Imag. 22, 730–741 (2003)
17. Collins, D., et al.: Design and construction of a realistic digital brain phantom. IEEE Trans. Med. Imag. 17(3), 463–468 (1998)
18. Bourgeat, P., et al.: Improved cortical thickness measurement from MR images using partial volume estimation. In: IEEE Symp. on Biom. Imag., pp. 205–208 (2008)
19. Raniga, P., et al.: PIB-PET Segmentation for Automatic SUVR Normalization Without MR Information. In: IEEE Symp. on Biom. Imag., pp. 348–351 (2007)

Computational Atlases of Severity of White Matter Lesions in Elderly Subjects with MRI

Stathis Hadjidemetriou[1], Peter Lorenzen[1], Norbert Schuff[2], Susanne Mueller[2], and Michael Weiner[2]

[1] NCIRE/VA UCSF, 4150 Clement St., San Francisco, CA 94121, USA
[2] UCSF, 4150 Clement St., San Francisco, CA 94121, USA

Abstract. MRI of cerebral white matter may show regions of signal abnormalities. These changes may be associated with hypertension, inflammation, or ischemia, as well as altered brain function. The goal of this work has been to construct computational atlases of white matter lesions that represent both their severity as well as the frequency of their occurrence in a population to achieve a better classification of white matter disease. An atlas is computed with a pipeline that uses 4T FLAIR and 4T T1-weighted (T1w) brain images of a group of subjects. The processing steps include intensity correction, lesion extraction, intra-subject FLAIR to T1w rigid registration, and seamless replacement of lesions in T1w images with synthetic white matter texture. Subsequently, the T1w images and lesion images of different subjects are registered nonrigidly to the same space. The decrease in T1w intensities is used to obtain severity information. Atlases were constructed for two groups of subjects, elderly normal controls or with mild cognitive impairment, and subjects with cerebrovascular disease. The lesion severities of the two groups have a significant statistical difference with the severity in the atlas of cerebrovascular disease being higher.

Keywords: Intensity correction, brain lesion segmentation, lesion severity, computational atlas construction.

1 Introduction

In the aging brain, MRI of cerebral white matter can exhibit increased intensity on T2-weighted (T2w) images and decreased intensity on T1-weighted (T1w) images, these effects are attributed to white matter lesions and MRI is the method of choice for their detection. They have been associated with hypertension, inflammation, or ischemia. They can also decrease cognitive performance, and have been associated with a variety of pathological conditions that include Alzheimer's disease [1], multiple sclerosis, and stroke. However, knowledge of their pathological underpinnings is limited [1].

Several protocols exist, mostly based on a T2w MR image, for the qualitative visual rating of age related lesions [2]. However, the visual protocols are not all mutually consistent and can saturate. The qualitative evaluations can also be time consuming, biased, and rarely use the radiometric information of the lesions.

In automatic lesion analysis the use of T2w imaging has been limited due to the overlap between the lesion intensity range and that of the cerebrospinal fluid [3,4]. Atlases have been constructed directly from T2w images in the form of FLAIR with affine co-registration [4] or from binary lesion maps extracted from FLAIR images followed by non-rigid registration [5]. These atlases are being increasingly investigated as means for improved diagnosis. In multiple sclerosis T2w and FLAIR MRI have been found very sensitive to the presence of lesions, but often not very specific to lesion severity [6]. Physical disability in multiple sclerosis has been found to correlate with the T1w intensity of lesions [6].

The segmentation of white matter lesions often involves coregistration of images of multiple contrasts followed by vectorization of their radiometric information [7]. Spatial information has also been used with techniques that include normalized cuts [8] and active contours [9]. Lesion segmentation often requires a threshold for their intensities [3] or its determination through manual seeding [8]. The latter is time consuming and may be biased. In general, lesion intensities depend on the subject as well as the instrumentation [5] and can vary throughout the image. Lesions can also be diffuse and they can have irregular shapes, which further complicates their extraction [3,4].

The aim of this work has been to construct computational atlases of white matter lesion information. A FLAIR and a T1w image are co-analyzed, which is expected to provide a better assessment of white matter lesions than either one alone. The intensity values of lesions in FLAIR and T1w images do not correspond uniquely. Thus, the two images are examined serially starting with the FLAIR image whose processing provides the lesion template. The binary classification of the lesions is extended into a gradual one. The atlases represent both the severity of lesions as well as the frequency of their occurrence in a population. The analysis in this study is used to assess lesion severity of elderly subjects with normal or mildly impaired cognition and due to cerebrovascular disease. The two atlases are shown to have a significant statistical difference.

2 Methods

The atlases are constructed with a pipeline which uses a $4T$ FLAIR image I_{FLAIR} and a $4T$ T1w image I_{T1w} of N elderly subjects, $i = 0, \ldots, N-1$. The FLAIR image is processed first. Its processing starts with a robust correction for the $4T$ intensity non-uniformities [10]. The correction does not make use of anatomic priors and hence it can accommodate variations in anatomy of elderly subjects such as ventricle enlargement.

2.1 Segmentation of White Matter Lesions from the FLAIR Image

The brain region from $I_{FLAIR,i}$ is extracted using BET [11] and is denoised with median filtering. Many focal intensity distortions occur at the peripheral brain region such as those due to magnetic susceptibilities from the nose and ears, blood flow, as well as chemical shift artifacts from extracranial lipids. Hence, the brain template is eroded for $6mm$. The self-co-occurrence statistics of the remaining region are analyzed with expectation maximization into a mixture of two Gaussians. The distribution in the low intensity range corresponds to CSF and is backprojected to the image to cancel the ventricle region. The largest connected component of the valid FLAIR region gives the inner region of the parenchyma, $I_{F,P}(\mathbf{x})$, where $\mathbf{x}$ are the voxel coordinates.

The diffuse nature of lesions causes an extensive partial volume between normal and abnormal parenchyma. This results in an overlap between the intensity distribution of the normal appearing parenchyma and that of the lesions, particularly at the intermediate intensity range [3,4]. The intensities corresponding exclusively to normal appearing white matter and abnormal parenchyma are located at the extremes of the dynamic range. The extremes are extracted using reference measures from FLAIR intensity statistics. The first is the intensity of maximum density, which is the mean intensity of the normal appearing white matter, $\mu_{F,P}$. The second is the full width half maximum ($fwhm$), which gives the standard deviation of the distribution of the normal appearing white matter, $\sigma_{F,P} = 2\sqrt{2\pi} fwhm$.

In a FLAIR image the lesion intensity is not directly proportional to severity [12]. The maximum intensity is reached at the early stages of lesion development and an advanced lesion evolves to a scar which contains a dark water cyst. This makes the maximum lesion intensity a common feature in FLAIR images. It is computed as the maximum image intensity, $I_{F,P,max} = max_{\mathbf{x}} I_{F,P}(\mathbf{x})$, in the inner parenchyma. The intensity range considered to correspond exclusively to normal appearing white matter in the inner parenchyma is $[0, \mu_{F,P} + 0.25(I_{F,P,max} - \mu_{F,P})]$. The intensity range considered to correspond exclusively to abnormal white matter is $[(\mu_{F,P} + 0.51(I_{F,P,max} - \mu_{F,P}), I_{F,P,max}]$. To avoid false positives in images that do not contain lesions, the intensitity ranges are readjusted considering z-scores based on $\mu_{F,P}$ and $\sigma_{F,P}$ of the distribution of the normal appearing white matter. The lower threshold for lesion intensity is set to $\mu_{F,P} + 4\sigma_{F,P}$.

The intensity ranges provide seed regions in a FLAIR image both for the normal appearing and the abnormal parenchyma. These regions initialize the graph cut segmentation algorithm [13], which resolves ambiguous regions with the path of maximum simulated flow to provide the lesion template $L_i(\mathbf{x})$. An example of white matter lesion detection is shown in figure 1 (a). The first row shows the FLAIR image of a subject with a high lesion load, the second row shows the extracted white matter lesion template, and in the third row the outer contours of the lesions are superimposed upon the FLAIR image.

2.2 Assessment of the Severity of White Matter Lesions

The severity of the lesions is extracted from the T1w image. Its intensity restoration can be confounded by the presence of white matter lesions whose statistics have been shown to have a variance larger than those of the normal appearing white matter [14]. Thus, prior to the intensity restoration of a T1w image, $I_{T1w,i}$, the intensity corrected FLAIR image is co-registered rigidly to $I_{T1w,i}$ with

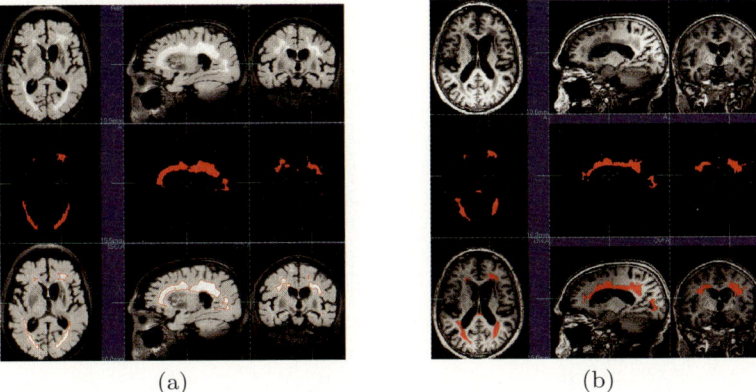

Fig. 1. Segmentation of white matter lesions from the FLAIR image in (a). The lesions are nulled in the T1 image in (b), prior to its intensity correction.

transformation f_i. The same transformation is applied to the lesion mask $L_i(\mathbf{x})$ to project it to the $T1w$-image $I_{T1w,i}$ and the regions corresponding to the projection are nulled. An example of the lesion template of a subject in the space of the T1w image is shown in figure 1 (b). The remaining region corresponds to normal appearing parenchyma and is corrected for intensity uniformity [10]. The estimated non-uniformity over the healthy region is kept fixed, and is extrapolated to the region occupied by the abnormal tissue numerically with the Laplacian $\nabla B_{T1w,i} = 0$, where $B_{T1w,i}$ is the intensity non-uniformity of the $T1w$ image.

The darkening of the white matter in a T1w image is used to assess lesion severity. The region of the normal parenchyma in the T1w image is segmented into white matter, gray matter, and cerebrospinal fluid. The segmentation is performed by analyzing the self-co-occurrence statistics into a Gaussian mixture using expectation maximization. The mean intensity of the white matter, $\mu_{wm,i}$, and the mean intensity of the cerebrospinal fluid, $\mu_{csf,i}$, are used as references for voxel-wise severity evaluation. The mean intensity of the white matter, $\mu_{wm,i}$ corresponds to zero severity. As the lesion intensity in a T1w image, $I_{T1w,i}(\mathbf{x})$, decreases towards the mean intensity of the cerebrospinal fluid, in cysts, the severity index increases linearly. The lesion severity index $S_i(\mathbf{x})$ at voxel $\mathbf{x}$ is postulated as:

$$S_i(\mathbf{x}) = \frac{(\mu_{wm,i} - I_{T1w,i}(\mathbf{x}))}{(\mu_{wm,i} - \mu_{csf,i})}. \tag{1}$$

Voxels with intensity higher than $\mu_{wm,i}$ are also considered as normal. An example of severity assessment for white matter lesions is shown in figure 2 (a) and in the third row it is superimposed upon the T1w image.

2.3 Seamless Lesion Replacement in T1w Images

The intensity corrected T1w images are further processed to replace white matter lesions with synthetic texture representing healthy white matter. To this end

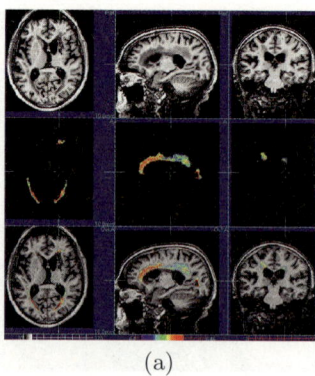 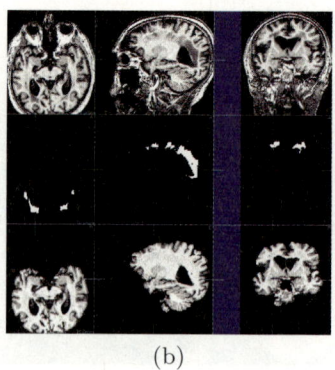

(a)   (b)

Fig. 2. An intensity corrected T1 image together with its severity map in (a). Replacement of white matter lesion regions in the third row in (b).

the image is smoothed with median filtering and the brain region is eroded to eliminate bright artifacts in the outer brain. Then, the voxel of maximum intensity is selected, which corresponds to normal appearing white matter. Starting from the selected voxel a region growing algorithm is used to extract a part of the normal appearing white matter. This region is used to provide a sample of the histogram and intensity co-occurrences of the normal appearing white matter.

A texture is randomly generated with approximately the same zero order histogram as that of the normal appearing white matter [14,15]. The generated texture is altered iteratively to also enforce the local co-occurrence statistics of the normal appearing white matter $C_{NAWM,i}$ into the synthetic white matter $C^t_{synth,i}$, where t is the iteration. The match criterion between the co-occurrences is the L_2 norm. A pair of neighboring voxels in the synthetic texture is randomly selected. Their intensities are interchanged and the co-occurrence matrix is updated efficiently by considering only the co-occurrences of the two voxels. The interchanges that improve the match of the co-occurrences,

$$\|C^{t+1}_{synth,i} - C_{NAWM,i}\|_2 < \|C^t_{synth,i} - C_{NAWM,i}\|_2, \qquad (2)$$

are retained [14]. The iterations continue until the rate of retained changes is very low. A possible discontinuity at the boundary is eliminated by randomly interchanging the intensities of the local cross-border co-occurrences [15]. In the first row of figure 2 (b) is an example of an image with a considerable white matter lesion load. In the second row is the extracted lesion image in T1w space, and in the last row the lesions are replaced with synthetic white matter texture.

2.4 Spatial Normalization to a Common T1w Anatomic Space

The atlases are created with an unbiased method based on Frechet means in metric spaces [16]. It uses an iterative algorithm for the simultaneous deformation of the subject images into an evolving average image. The images are transformed with the large deformation fluid based algorithm performed in multiresolution [16]. A common T1w atlas space is constructed from the T1w images of several healthy subjects in their sixties. The common space is used as a reference for the coregistration of the lesion replaced T1w images with 9-parameter affine transformations $h_{a,i}^{-1}$. The co-registered images are further transformed non-rigidly, $h_{nr,i}^{-1}$, to form an unbiased atlas [16]. The concatenation of the intra-subject and inter-subject registrations are applied to every lesion template, $S_i^R(\mathbf{x}) = S_i(f_i h_{a,i}^{-1} h_{nr,i}^{-1} \mathbf{x})$, to transform them to the common T1w space. The co-registered severity maps in a group are averaged to give the atlas:

$$S^G(\mathbf{x}) = \frac{1}{N} \sum_{i=0}^{N-1} S_i^R(\mathbf{x}), \qquad (3)$$

which represents lesions severity as well as population frequency.

3 Experimental Results

Two groups of subjects were drawn each from a different study. A group of 15 subjects that were normal or with mild cognitive impairment, but not demented (mean age of 72 +/- st.dev. of 9, 10 men/5 women). The second was a group of 7 subjects diagnosed with cerebrovascular disease with varying degrees of cognitive impairment (mean age of 66 +/- st.dev. of 8, 2 men/5 women). All subjects or their legal guardian provided written informed consent before participating in the respective studies. The protocol was approved by the Committees of Human Research at UCSF and VA. The brain images of the subjects were acquired with a $4Tesla$ whole-body Siemens/Bruker MRI scanner. The T1w images $I_{T1w,i}$ were volumetric based on MPRAGE acquisitions. Their nominal resolution was $1.0 \times 1.0 \times 1.0\, mm^3$ at a matrix of $176 \times 256 \times 256$ voxels. The FLAIR acquisitions

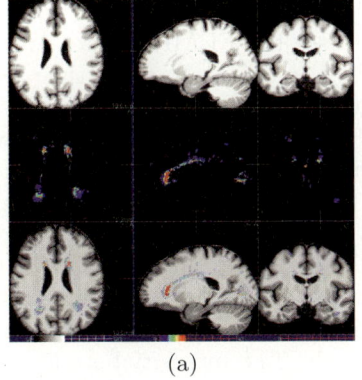
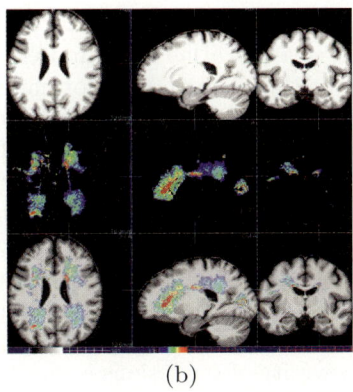

(a)   (b)

Fig. 3. The lesion severity atlas of the elderly subjects in (a) and of the subjects with cerebrovascular disease in (b) in the common anatomic space

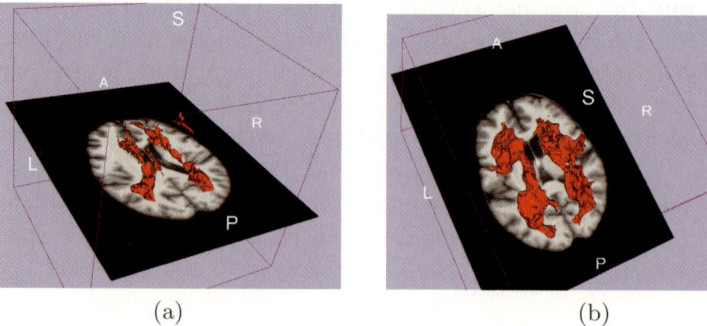

Fig. 4. Visualizations of the severity atlases shown in figure 3 (a) and figure 3 (b), in (a) and (b), respectively, at the 0.8 iso-severity-frequency level

$I_{FLAIR,i}$ were also volumetric. Their nominal resolution was $1.0 \times 1.0 \times 1.0\ mm^3$ at a matrix size of $176 \times 224 \times 256$ voxels.

The atlas of the elderly subjects that were normal or with mild cognitive impairment is shown with cross-sections in figure 3 (a). The first row shows the reference T1w atlas. The second row shows the combined atlas of lesion severity and frequency in the population. In the third row is the combined lesion atlas superimposed over the reference T1w atlas. The atlas in figure 3 (a) is also shown with a simulation of a viewpoint in 3D at the 0.8 iso-severity-frequency contour in figure 4 (a). Similarly, figure 3 (b) shows cross-sections of the atlas of the subjects with cerebrovascular disease and in figure 4 (b) is a viewpoint of the atlas in 3D at the 0.8 iso-severity-frequency contour. The lesion severity of the elderly subjects diagnosed with cerebrovascular disease is significantly higher. The two atlases have been compared with a voxelwise Wilcoxon signed rank test. They have a significant statistical difference with $p \approx 0$.

4 Discussion

A lesion severity atlas is computed, which uses the FLAIR images to localize lesions and the radiometric information of the T1w images to assess their severity. The method used provides an unbiased atlas that represents both lesion severity as well as frequency in a population. The atlases computed in this work show that lesion severity of elderly subjects with cerebrovascular disease is significantly higher than that of elderly subjects that were normal or with mild cognitive impairment. The non-rigid registration of images with enlarged ventricles or small brains to a reference atlas of normal subjects can increase the volume of the lesions in the atlas. An atlas can be further processed to classify the lesion templates into categories such as periventricular versus deep white matter.

The severity of the lesions is assessed from the T1w intensity because it varies monotonically with lesion development, in contrast to the T2-weighted intensity of FLAIR, which is designed to suppresses the signal from the cerebrospinal fluid that advanced lesions may contain [12]. Hence, the severity of advanced lesions may be underestimated if the FLAIR image intensities are used alone. Moreover, the T1w intensity has been found more specific than the T2w information in terms of lesion severity, primarily in multiple sclerosis [6]. The severity scale can be improved by considering the non-linearity between the intensities in a T1-MPRAGE image and relaxation as well as by using an inter-subject reference for the healthy white matter intensity.

References

1. Erkinjuntti, T., Gao, F., Lee, D.: Lack of difference in brain hyperintensities between patients with early Alzheimer's disease and control subjects. Arch. Neurol. 51, 260–268 (1994)
2. Pantoni, L., Simoni, M., Pracucci, G.: European task on age-related white matter changes. Visual rating scales for age-related white matter changes (leukoaraiosis). Can the heterogeneity be reduced? Stroke 33, 2827–2833 (2002)
3. Jack, C., O'Brien, P., Rettman, D., Shiung, M., Xu, Y., Muthupillai, R., Manduca, A., Avula, R., Erickson, B.: FLAIR histogram segmentation for measurement of leukoaraiosis volume. Journal of Magnetic Resonance Imaging 14, 668–676 (2001)
4. Wen, W., Sachdev, P.: The topography of white matter hyperintensities on brain MRI in healthy 60-to 64-year-old individuals. Neuroimage 22, 144–154 (2004)
5. Yoshita, M., Fletcher, E., DeCarli, C.: Current concepts of analysis of cerebral white matter hyperintensities on magnetic resonance imaging. Topics in Magnetic Resonance Imaging 16(6), 399–407 (2005)
6. Walderveen, M., Kamphorst, W., Scheltens, P.: Histopathologic correlate of hypointense lesions on T1-weighted spin-echo MRI in multiple sclerosis. Neurology 50, 1282–1288 (1998)
7. Pham, S., Shen, D., Herskovits, E., Resnick, S., Davatzikos, C.: Automatic segmentation of white matter lesions in T1-weighted brain MR images. In: Proc. of ISBI, pp. 253–256 (2002)
8. Ballin, A., Galun, M., Gomori, M., Filippi, M., Valsasina, P., Basri, R., Brandt, A.: An integrated segmentation and classification approach applied to multiple sclerosis analysis. In: Proc. of CVPR, pp. 1122–1129 (2006)
9. Warfield, S., Dengler, J., Zaers, J., Guttmann, C., Wells, W., Ettinger, G., Hiller, J., Kikinis, R.: Automatic identification of grey matter structures from MRI to improve the segmentation of white matter lesions. Journal of Image Guided Surgery 1(6), 326–338 (1995)
10. Hadjidemetriou, S., Studholme, C., Mueller, S., Weiner, M., Schuff, N.: Restoration of MRI data for field nonuniformities using high order neighborhood statistics. In: Proc. of SPIE Medical Image Processing, vol. 6512 (2007)
11. Smith, S.: Fast robust automated brain extraction. Proc. of Human Brain Mapping 17, 143–155 (2002)
12. Rovaris, M., Comi, G., Rocca, M., Cercignani, M., Colombo, B., Santuccio, G., Filippi, M.: Relevance of hypointense lesions on fast fluid-attenuated inversion recovery MR images as a marker of disease severity in cases of multiple sclerosis. American Journal of Neuroradiology 20, 813–820 (1999)

13. Boykov, Y., Veksler, O., Zabih, R.: Fast approximate energy minimization via graph cuts. IEEE Trans. on PAMI 23(11), 1222–1239 (2001)
14. Kovalev, V., Kruggel, F., Gertz, H., Cramon, D.: Three-dimensional texture analysis of MRI brain datasets. IEEE Trans. on Medical Imaging 20(5), 424–433 (2001)
15. Zalesny, A., Ferrari, V., Caenen, G., Gool, L.: Composite texture synthesis. International Journal of Computer Vision 62(1/2), 161–176 (2005)
16. Joshi, S., Davis, B., Jomier, M., Gerig, G.: Unbiased diffeomorphic atlas construction for computational anatomy. Neuroimage 23, S151–S160 (2004)

Simulation of Ground-Truth Validation Data Via Physically- and Statistically-Based Warps

Ghassan Hamarneh, Preet Jassi, and Lisa Tang

Medical Image Analysis Lab., Simon Fraser University, Burnaby, BC, V5A 1S6, Canada
{hamarneh,preetj,lisat}@cs.sfu.ca

Abstract. The problem of scarcity of ground-truth expert delineations of medical image data is a serious one that impedes the training and validation of medical image analysis techniques. We develop an algorithm for the automatic generation of large databases of annotated images from a single reference dataset. We provide a web-based interface through which the users can upload a reference data set (an image and its corresponding segmentation and landmark points), provide custom setting of parameters, and, following server-side computations, generate and download an arbitrary number of novel ground-truth data, including segmentations, displacement vector fields, intensity non-uniformity maps, and point correspondences. To produce realistic simulated data, we use variational (statistically-based) and vibrational (physically-based) spatial deformations, nonlinear radiometric warps mimicking imaging non-homogeneity, and additive random noise with different underlying distributions. We outline the algorithmic details, present sample results, and provide the web address to readers for immediate evaluation and usage.

Keywords: validation, segmentation, deformation, simulation, vibration, variation, non-uniformity.

1 Introduction

Medical images provide a wealth of data about internal anatomy and physiology essential for computer-aided modeling, diagnosis, treatment, and tracking of diseases. This, in turn, imposes high demands for automated, accurate, fast, and robust medical image analysis methods. This need has resulted in a plethora of alternative medical image segmentation, registration, and shape correspondence algorithms. Ironically, the wealth of data, from the ever growing high-dimensional images of millions of pixels and meshes with thousands of vertices, is also the cause of scarcity of ground-truth data sets of labeling, spatial transformation, and point correspondences, on which the medical image analysis algorithms must be evaluated and validated.

Aside from a few exceptions [26][34][35], assessing the performance of image analysis algorithms requires ground-truth data, such as expert-labeled images, physical or computational phantoms with known segments, deformations, or corresponding intrinsic landmarks or external markers [36][33][20]. Some of the notable efforts for providing simulated and ground-truth data include BrainWeb simulated brain MR images [4], the internet brain segmentation repository [15], PET-SORTEO for simulated PET data [24], and STAPLE for image segmentation validation [31]. Frameworks for evaluating and validating medical image registration techniques include the retrospective image registration evaluation projects [32][12][21][14], the non-rigid image registration evaluation project (NIREP) [3], and others [23][2]. Gerig et al. were the first to assess and visualize differences between multiple segmentations through their publicly available VALMET software [13]. Standard approaches for evaluating segmentation results given ground-truth segmentation include the Hausdorff distance, Dice coefficient [9], and the Jaccard index [16]. More recently, alternative approaches were proposed [25][10][11][30]. Evaluating point correspondence between pairs or within a group of shapes is also of interest in the computational anatomy community, which is primarily based on either geodesic distances between corresponding points found by the algorithm and known ground-truth, or via assessing the statistical shape model's generality, specificity, or description length [17][28][29][8].

In addition to validating medical image analysis algorithms, large amounts of ground-truth data is important for machine learning and statistical modeling techniques, such as learning relationships (e.g. regression) between shape and appearance [5]. In medical imaging, learning techniques suffer from the problem of high-dimensional, small sample size datasets ("the curse of dimensionality"), in which even the smallest of typical 2D scalar medical images (few hundred pixels, squared) can be seen as samples in tens-of-thousands dimensional space. Clearly, the situation is much more severe for 3D, or 4D (3D+time) data sets with vector (e.g. color or displacements) or matrix (e.g. diffusion tensor) entries.

To the best of our knowledge, none of the existing ground-truth databases or validation methods allows the user to simulate novel data from a single reference dataset (an image, its segmentation, and its landmark points) capturing the exact anatomy on which the developed algorithms need to be trained or validated. In this work, we contribute to addressing the problem of scarcity of ground-truth data through the simulation of an arbitrarily large number of novel ground-truth datasets from a single reference data set and the creation of a web interface to this simulation tool. Although it is difficult to evaluate the validity and realism of the simulated data, we employ a physically- and statistically-based generative model to ensure data realism to a large degree by adopting the formulation proposed in [7]. We also extend [7] to operate on images rather than landmarks along contours of shapes, and extend it from 2D to 3D. While we focus on data simulation for validating or training generic, modality-independent segmentation algorithms, the simulated images will possess appearance characteristics according to the modality of the reference data set.

2 Methods

Combinations of statistically- and physically-based spatial deformations, smoothly varying intensity non-uniformity warps, and random noise are applied to a reference data set which is uploaded by the user through our web-interface, in order to generate new ground-truth data. The reference set consists of a reference image I_i, its corresponding binary or multi-label segmentation S_i, and a set of landmark coordinates L_i. A few user-selected parameters, including the number of desired ground-truth data, are also supplied as input to the algorithm. The user is then notified via email of the URL from which to download the generated novel ground-truth data.

2.1 Spatial Transformations

Spatial deformations of the image are generated as follows[1]. An M×N uniform grid of control points $\mathbf{x}=\{(cx_{ij},cy_{ij}); i=1$ to M; $j=1$ to N$\}$ is initialized in the image plane. The control points are displaced as described below and the displacements are interpolated over the image plane. Displacements can be either random, where each component of the displacement vector field is sampled from a uniform random distribution ($[-a,a]\times[-a,a]$); from a statistically-driven point distribution model (PDM) [6]; through a physically-based, vibrational model; or a combined model [7] as described below.

2.1.1 Generative Statistically-Based Model

Given a training set of deformed grids of control points, each represented as a 2MN-vector, their linear variational modes can be obtained via principal component analysis of their covariance matrix $\mathbf{S}$ [6]. A PDM approximates control point grids as the sum of a mean grid and $t<2MN$ main modes of variation: $\mathbf{x} = \overline{\mathbf{x}} + \mathbf{Pb}$, where $\overline{\mathbf{x}}$ is a 2MN-vector of average locations of the control points and $\mathbf{P}$ is a 2MN×t matrix of principal components. By choosing different weights (within ±3std) for the t-vector $\mathbf{b}$, new control point locations are obtained and used to synthesize new images.

2.1.2 Generative Physically-Based Model

We follow Cootes and Taylor's approach to calculating the vibrational modes of shapes [7]. However, in this work, the coordinates of the grid of control points are treated as the shape's landmarks. Physically-based vibrational modes of the grid are generated through modal analysis of a finite element model (FEM). This gives rise to control points' displacements, which are then used to synthesize new deformed images. The grid of control points are considered nodes with masses interconnected by springs with constant stiffness and with rest lengths equal to the distance between the locations of the control points in the original, undeformed grid. New control point locations are then generated using $\mathbf{x} = \hat{\mathbf{x}} + \mathbf{\Phi u}$, where $\hat{\mathbf{x}}$ is a 2NM-vector of the original locations of the coordinates in the grid, $\mathbf{\Phi}$ is a 2MN square matrix of eigenvectors representing the vibrational modes, and $\mathbf{u}$ is a 2MN-vector of weights. The matrix $\mathbf{\Phi}$ is the solution of the generalized eigen-system $\mathbf{K\Phi} = \mathbf{M\Phi\Omega}^2$, where $\mathbf{K}$ is a 2MN square stiffness matrix calculated as in [7], $\mathbf{M} = \mathbf{I}$ is a 2MN square mass matrix, $\Omega^2 = diag\left(\omega_1^2, \omega_2^2, ..., \omega_{2MN}^2\right)$ is a matrix of eigenvalues associated with the eigenvectors in $\mathbf{\Phi}$, and ω_i is the frequency of ith vibrational mode.

2.1.3 Combined Vibrational-Variational Model

FEM generates new control point locations through vibrations of a single grid. PDM generates new grids by sampling the allowable space constructed from a training set.

---

[1] Our simulation can generate 2D or 3D data. We only write the 2D equations for clarity.

We generate new grids with displaced control points similar to the PDM approach but relying on a combined covariance matrix $\mathbf{S}_c = \mathbf{S} + \alpha \left(1/m \sum_{i=1}^{m} \mathbf{\Phi}_i \mathbf{\Lambda} \mathbf{\Phi}_i^T \right)$, where $\mathbf{\Lambda} = diag\left(\omega_i^{-2} \right)$ is used to generate more low frequency vibrations and less high frequency, m is the current number of available grid samples, and α balances variational vs. vibrational deformations. Starting with a single uniform grid (m=1), $\mathbf{S} = \mathbf{0}$ and hence only vibrational modes generate new shapes. As more grids are available, we gradually reduce the effect of vibrational modes by setting $\alpha = \alpha_1/m$, where α_1 is a constant.

2.2 Intensity Non-uniformity Via Radiometric Warps

Intensity non-homogeneity is modeled via a smoothly varying, additive intensity field, parameterized by the number U of modes (minima or maxima) in the field. U spatial locations {$(ux_i,uy_i); i=1,2,...,U$} are sampled from a bivariate uniform distribution extending throughout the image domain, or selected on a uniform grid. At each location, a random, uniformly-distributed bias in $[-b:b] \times I_{max}$ is generated, where I_{max} is the maximum intensity bias.

2.3 Spatial and Radiometric Interpolation

Different types of interpolation are involved in the simulation of novel ground-truth data. We interpolate the spatial displacements of the gray-level and segmentation image domains, and of landmark coordinates using bi-cubic interpolation. There are several possible interpolation methods for interpolating the pixel intensities from the original spatially un-warped intensity image [19]. To generate the results in this paper, we used bi-linear intensity interpolation in 2D and thin plate splines in 3D. We used nearest-neighbor interpolation for warping the ground-truth labels to avoid erroneous interpolated labels. We interpolate the intensity non-uniformity fields from the intensity biases at the non-uniformity mode centers using bi-cubic interpolation. To resemble ground-truth segmentation, the warped segmentation images are not affected by intensity non-uniformity or by noise.

2.4 Additive Noise

The warped intensity images are deteriorated by additive Gaussian noise [18] or other distributions (e.g. uniform or impulse noise) by specifying the appropriate parameters (e.g. the mean and variance of Gaussian noise).

2.5 Web Simulation Tool and Implementation Details

The simulation code is written in MATLAB (Mathworks, Natwick, MA). MATLAB Compiler for Linux is used to compile M files into stand-alone executables. The web-server interface and MATLAB Component Runtime (MCR) alleviate the need for

MATLAB during run-time. The web interface is created using XHTML, CSS and DHTML. PHP handles the form submissions, uploading the reference images, invoking the simulation code, creating and compressing the appropriate folders and ground-truth files, sending email notifications, and updating an XML file queue to handle the different user submissions. To access the web-based tool, visit http://mialweb.cs.sfu.ca/. There, the user selects 2D or 3D simulation, uploads an image (I) and corresponding segmentation (S) and landmark coordinates (L), and specifies simulation parameters. The parameters are: density of the control grid (M×N); extent of random spatial displacement (a); number of variational modes (t), or alternatively, fraction of explained variance; parameter balancing variational vs. vibrational modes (α_1); number of modes for the intensity non-uniformity (U), and whether the mode locations are at uniform grid points; extent of non-uniformity (b); noise parameters (e.g. mean and variance of Gaussian); and number of simulated samples to generate (G). The user is then notified by email of the URL from which the generated files can be downloaded. This data includes G samples of each of the following: spatially warped intensity images; spatially warped segmentation labels; warped intensity + non-uniformity; warped intensity + noise; warped intensity + non-uniformity + noise; the noise field; the non-uniform intensity bias field; and the displacement vector field.

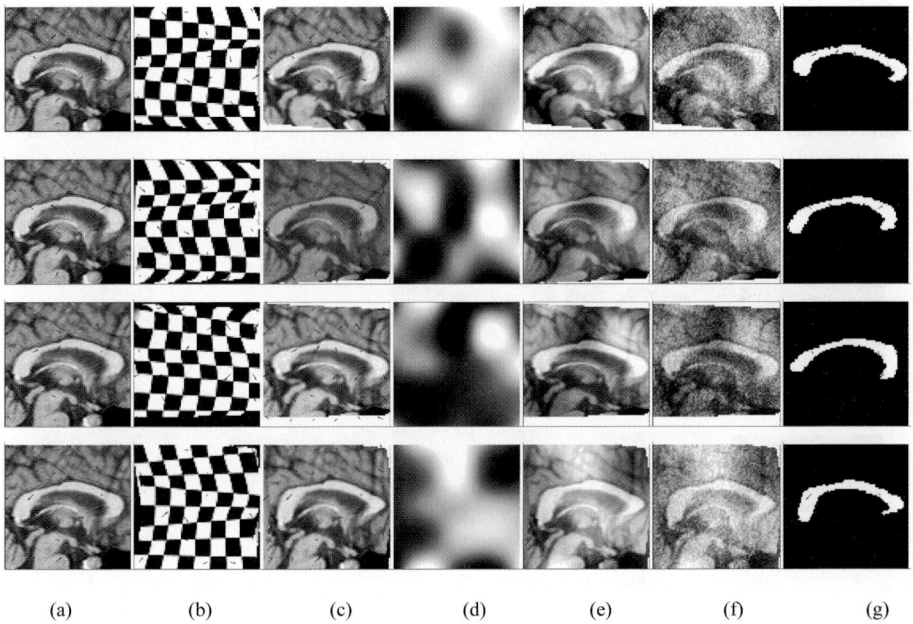

Fig. 1. 2D Simulation: (a) Reference image with different grid displacements (small arrows), (b) deformed checkerboard, (c) deformed image, (d) non-uniformity field, (e) 'c+d', (f) 'e+noise', (g) simulated segmentation (reference segmentation not shown)

3 Results

Figure 1 shows sample simulations of novel 2D MR brain images, deformations and displacement vector fields, segmentations, non-uniformity maps, and noisy images. Figure 2 shows sample simulations of 3D pelvic CT data. Figure 3 shows sample simulations of 2D and 3D ground-truth point correspondences. Figure 4 shows snapshots of the progress of using the simulation web-interface.

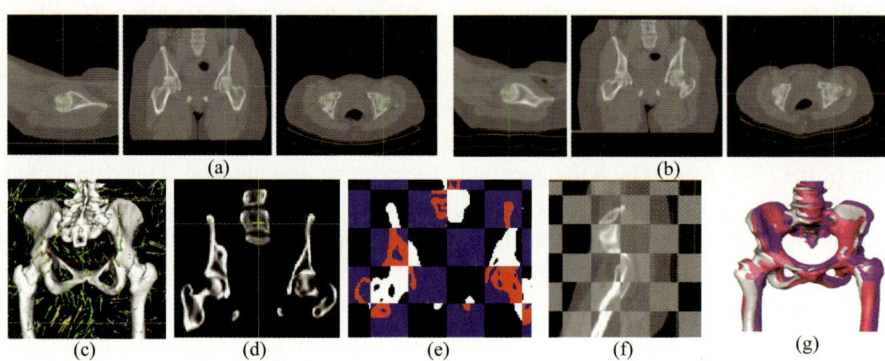

Fig. 2. 3D Simulation: Three orthogonal views of (a) reference CT pelvic volume, (b) one of the simulated volumes, (c) displacement vector field and surface rendering of simulated pelvic and neighboring bone, (d) close-up on simulation result, (e) simulated segmentation (checkerboard overlay with reference segmentation), (f) checkerboard overlay of reference and simulated data, (g) several other simulated datasets shown with different colors

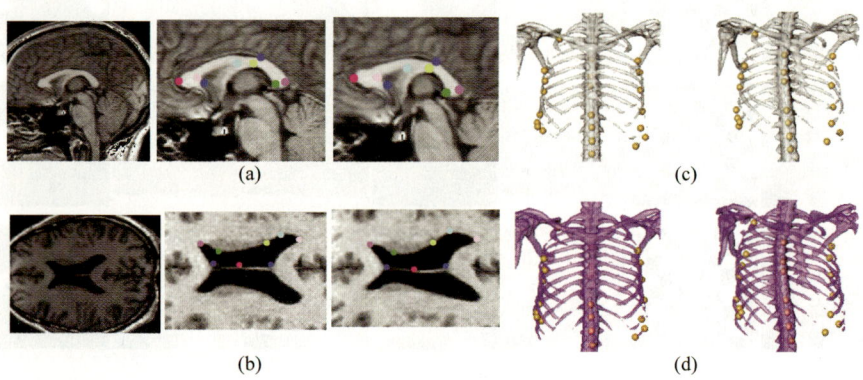

Fig. 3. Simulating 2D and 3D ground-truth point correspondence. (a,b) 2D reference image (left), close up on reference landmarks (middle), and simulated corresponding landmarks (right). (c,d) Two examples of reference thoracic segmentation and landmarks (left) and simulated segmentation and corresponding landmarks (right).

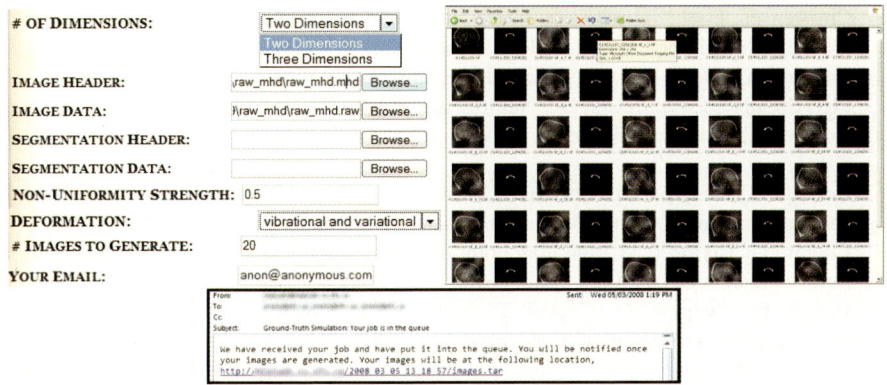

Fig. 4. Simulation progress. The user fills a web-form (sample fields are shown top-left) and receives an email notification (bottom) to download the simulated images (top-right).

4 Conclusions

Lack of sufficient ground-truth data in medical imaging is evident, despite the pressing need to validate a large number of medical image analysis algorithms and to address the high dimension, small sample size problem plaguing machine learning. We present a preliminary proof-of-concept system for simulating ground-truth data, which requires a single reference dataset, generates physically and statistically plausible deformations, applies radiometric warps and noise, and is easily accessed through a web-interface. Although the resulting simulated data may not represent "real" changes, they still appear realistic and are useful for validation, benchmarking, and machine learning (e.g. capturing relationships between spatial warps and intensity variations). Further, the so-called "unrealistic" simulations may stand in lieu of unpredictable, pathological cases, which unfortunately have not been properly addressed by almost all existing algorithms, let alone validated. The work presented here is only a first step towards a more elaborate ground-truth simulator under development. Future work includes adopting advanced models of intensity non-uniformity (e.g. [27][22]), modal analysis reflecting real tissue properties (from the literature or via MR elastography measurements), modality-specific customization of the simulated data (e.g. to simulate diffusion tensor images, one must ensure that the diffusion tensor in each voxel is transformed correctly [1]).

Acknowledgements

We thank Parisa Shooshtari and Omer Ishaq for assistance in code development, James Peltier for assistance in setting up the web server, and NSERC for funding.

References

[1] Alexander, D., Pierpaoli, C., Basser, P., Gee, J.: Spatial transformations of diffusion tensor magnetic resonance images. IEEE TMI 20(11), 1131–1139 (2001)

[2] Chou, Y., Skrinjar, O.: Ground truth data for validation of nonrigid image registration Algorithms. In: ISBI, pp. 716–719 (2004)

[3] Christensen, et al.: Introduction to the Non-Rigid Image Registration Evaluation Project (NIREP). In: Biomedical Image Registration Workshop, pp. 128–135 (2006)
[4] Cocosco, C., Kollokian, V., Kwan, R., Evans, A.: BrainWeb: Online Interface to a 3D MRI Simulated Brain Database. NeuroImage 5(4), part 2/4, S425 (1997)
[5] Cootes, T., Edwards, Taylor, C.: Active Appearance Models. PAMI 23(6), 681–685 (2001)
[6] Cootes, T., Taylor, C., Cooper, D., Grahamet, J.: Active Shape Models - Their Training and Application. Computer Vision and Image Understanding 61(1), 38–59 (1995)
[7] Cootes, T., Taylor, C.: Combining point distribution models with shape models based on finite element analysis. Image and Vision Computing 13(5), 403–409 (1995)
[8] Davies, R., Twining, C., Cootes, T., Waterton, J., Taylor, C.: A minimum description length approach to statistical shape Modeling. IEEE TMI 21(5), 525–537 (2002)
[9] Dice, L.: Measures of the Amount of Ecologic Association Between Species. Ecology 26(3), 297–302 (1945)
[10] Everingham, M., Muller, H., Thomas, B.: Evaluating image segmentation algorithms using monotonic hulls in fitness/cost space. BMVC, 363–372 (2001)
[11] Everingham, M., Muller, H., Thomas, B.: Evaluating image segmentation algorithms using the Pareto front. ECCV (IV), 34–48 (2002)
[12] Fitzpatrick, et al.: Visual assessment of the accuracy of retrospective registration of MR and CT images of the brain. IEEE TMI 17, 571–585 (1998)
[13] Gerig, G., Jomier, M., Chakos, M.: VALMET: A new validation tool for assessing and improving 3D object segmentation. In: Niessen, W.J., Viergever, M.A. (eds.) MICCAI 2001. LNCS, vol. 2208, pp. 516–523. Springer, Heidelberg (2001)
[14] Hellier, et al.: Retrospective Evaluation of Inter-subject Brain Registration. IEEE TMI 22(9), 1120–1130 (2003)
[15] Internet Brain Segmentation Repository, http://www.cma.mgh.harvard.edu/ibsr/
[16] Jaccard, P.: Étude comparative de la distribution florale dans une portion des Alpes et des Jura. Bulletin de la Société Vaudoise des Sciences Naturelles 37, 547–579 (1901)
[17] Karlsson, J., Ericsson, A.: A ground truth correspondence measure for benchmarking. In: ICPR, pp. 568–573 (2006)
[18] Kwan, R., Evans, A., Pike, B.: MRI Simulation-Based Evaluation of Image-Processing and Classification Methods. IEEE TMI 18(11), 1085–1097 (1999)
[19] Lehman, T., Gonner, C., Spitzer, K.: Survey: Interpolation Methods in Medical Image Processing. IEEE TMI 18(11), 1049–1075 (1999)
[20] Maintz, J., Viergever, M.: A survey of medical image registration. MIA 2(1), 1–36 (1998)
[21] Maurer, C., Fitzpatrick, J., Wang, M., Galloway, R., Maciunas, R., Allen, G.: Registration of head volume images using implantable fiducial markers. IEEE TMI 16(4), 447–462 (1997)
[22] Pawluczyk, O., Yaffe, M.: Field nonuniformity correction for quantitative analysis of digitized mammograms. Medical Physics 28(4), 438–444 (2001)
[23] Pennec, X., Thirion, J.: A Framework for Uncertainty and Validation of 3-D Registration Methods based on Points and Frames. IJCV 25(3), 203–229 (1997)
[24] Reilhac, et al.: PET-SORTEO: validation and development of database of Simulated PET volumes. IEEE Transactions on Nuclear Science 52(5), part 1, 1321–1328 (2005)
[25] Rosenberger, C.: Adaptive evaluation of image segmentation results. In: ICPR, pp. 399–402 (2006)
[26] Schestowitz, R., Twining, C., Petrovic, V., Cootes, T., Crum, B., Taylor, C.: Non-Rigid Registration Assessment Without Ground Truth. In: MIUA, vol. 2, pp. 151–155 (2006)

[27] Sled, J., Pike, B.: Understanding Intensity Non-uniformity in MRI. In: Wells, W.M., Colchester, A.C.F., Delp, S.L. (eds.) MICCAI 1998. LNCS, vol. 1496, pp. 614–622. Springer, Heidelberg (1998)
[28] Styner, M., Rajamani, K., Nolte, L., Zsemlye, G., Székely, G., Taylor, C., Davies, R.: Evaluation of 3D Correspondence Methods for Model Building. In: Taylor, C.J., Noble, J.A. (eds.) IPMI 2003. LNCS, vol. 2732, pp. 63–75. Springer, Heidelberg (2003)
[29] Twining, C., Cootes, T., Marsland, S., Petrovic, V., Schestowitz, R., Taylor, C.: Information-Theoretic Unification of Groupwise Non-Rigid Registration and Model Building. In: MIUA, pp. 226–230 (2006)
[30] Unnikrishnan, R., Pantofaru, C., Hebert, M.: A Measure for Objective Evaluation of Image Segmentation Algorithms. In: CVPR Workshop on Empirical Methods in Computer Vision, p. 34 (2005)
[31] Warfield, S., Zho, K., Wells, W.: Simultaneous Truth and Performance Level Estimation (STAPLE): An Algorithm for the Validation of Image Segmentation. IEEE TMI 23(7), 903–921 (2004)
[32] West, et al.: Comparison and evaluation of retrospective inter-modality brain image registration techniques. J. Computer Assisted Tomography 21(4), 554–566 (1997)
[33] Zhang, Y.: A review of recent evaluation methods for image segmentation. In: ISSPA, pp. 148–151 (2001)
[34] Zhang, H., Fritts, J., Goldman, S.: An entropy-based objective evaluation methods for image segmentation. In: SPIE, vol. 5307, pp. 38–49 (2003)
[35] Zhang, H., Cholleti, S., Goldman, S.: Meta-Evaluation of Image Segmentation Using Machine Learning. In: CVPR, pp. 1138–1145 (2006)
[36] Zhang, Y.: A survey on Evaluation Methods for Image Segmentation. Pattern Recognition 29(8), 1335–1346 (1996)

Shape Analysis with Overcomplete Spherical Wavelets

B.T. Thomas Yeo[1,4,*], Peng Yu[2], P. Ellen Grant[3,4],
Bruce Fischl[1,3], and Polina Golland[1]

[1] Computer Science and Artificial Intelligence Laboratory, MIT, USA
[2] Division of Health Sciences and Technology, MIT, USA
[3] Athinoula A. Martinos Center for Biomedical Imaging, MGH/HMS, USA
[4] Division of Pediatric Radiology, MGH, USA

Abstract. In this paper, we explore the use of over-complete spherical wavelets in shape analysis of closed 2D surfaces. Previous work has demonstrated, theoretically and practically, the advantages of over-complete over bi-orthogonal spherical wavelets. Here we present a detailed formulation of over-complete wavelets, as well as shape analysis experiments of cortical folding development using them. Our experiments verify in a *quantitative* fashion existing *qualitative* theories of neuro-anatomical development. Furthermore, the experiments reveal *novel* insights into neuro-anatomical development not previously documented.

1 Introduction

In this paper, we explore the use of overcomplete spherical wavelets [1,16] for shape analysis of closed 2D surfaces. Wavelets offer a tradeoff between entirely local and global features more commonly used in shape analysis.

In the Euclidean space, a pixel representation of an image provides precise pointwise features, but suffers from noise and can benefit from a multiscale representation using global contextual information. At the other extreme, the Fourier transform creates a global summary of an image at the expense of localization ability. The orthogonal/bi-orthogonal wavelet transform [5] provides a tradeoff between pixel-wise and Fourier representation by projecting an image onto basis functions with compact support, at different spatial scales and locations.

Unfortunately, each level of the multi-scale orthogonal/bi-orthogonal wavelet transform suffers from sampling aliasing. Practically, this results in a loss of translational invariance: translation of an image by even one pixel causes dramatic changes in the wavelet coefficients [13]. A related problem is unidentifiability [13,18]. Suppose a tumor of a certain size exists at a certain spatial location. Ideally, one would want a large wavelet coefficient at that particular scale and spatial location. But due to undersampling, the tumor's location might not be sampled at that scale, resulting in two moderate wavelet coefficients on either

---

[*] Corresponding author: ythomas@csail.mit.edu

side of the actual tumor. Considering coefficients from that scale leads to a false hypothesis of the existence of two moderate-sized tumors.

Over-complete wavelets resolve these problems by ensuring each wavelet scale is sufficiently sampled [13]. Overcomplete transforms result in more coefficients than pixels, hence the name "overcomplete". This inefficiency is compensated for by their increased accuracy and robustness.

Pioneering work using landmarks for shape analysis include the Procrustes method [8] and active shape models (ASM) [4]. The individual landmarks provide precise local information about the shape, but lack global contextual information. ASM performs principal component analysis on the landmarks of training images, thus avoiding some limitations of landmark-based methods. However, this requires training data, while we are interested in generic shape representations.

The desire for a global shape representation motivates the introduction of global basis functions. Since closed 2D shapes can be spherically parameterized, one can treat each coordinate function $\{x, y, z\}$ of a closed 2D surface as a spherical image and project it onto spherical bases, such as spherical harmonics [2] and polynomials [14].

Schroder and Sweldens [12] proposed the bi-orthogonal spherical wavelet transform for scalar spherical images. The application of these wavelets to closed 2D surfaces demonstrated great utility in both segmentation and shape analysis [11,17]. Unfortunately, the bi-orthogonal wavelet transform on the sphere suffers from the same aliasing problems observed in Euclidean images. Overcomplete spherical wavelets [1,16] overcome these problems by ensuring sufficient sampling at each scale and have been shown to be both more robust and more sensitive to group differences than bi-orthogonal spherical wavelets in shape analysis [18].

In this paper, we present a detailed formulation of overcomplete spherical wavelets and incorporate them into the growth model of neonatal cortical folding, extending the experiments in the workshop paper [18]. Our analysis yields quantitative characterizations of cortical folding development consistent with previous studies, which were based on visual inspection of post-mortem brains [3]. The results also provide novel insights into neuro-anatomical development, suggesting directions for future experimental verification, and potentially providing a basis for early detection of neurodevelopmental disorders.

2 Overcomplete Spherical Wavelets for Shape Analysis

In this section, we outline the theory and implementation details of overcomplete spherical wavelets for shape analysis. While several related formulations of wavelet transforms on the sphere exist, we follow the continuous spherical filter bank and sampling framework of [16].

Continuous Spherical Filter Bank Theory. In the Euclidean domain, convolution is defined as the inner product of two functions translated relative to each other. In the spherical domain, we define spherical convolution as the inner product between spherical functions rotated relative to each other.

Let $I(\theta, \phi)$ be a spherical scalar image (function) and $\{\widetilde{h}_n(\theta, \phi)\}_{n=1}^N$ be a set of N spherical scalar filters (functions) parameterized by the spherical coordinates (θ, ϕ). We apply each filter $\widetilde{h}_n$ to the image via spherical convolution, resulting in the continuous outputs $w_n = I \circledast \widetilde{h}_n$. In wavelet theory, $\{\widetilde{h}_n\}$ are called the analysis filters. We can then convolve $\{w_n\}$ with another set of spherical filters $\{h_n\}$, called the synthesis filters, producing reconstructed image components $\widehat{I}_n = w_n \circledast h_n$. We define $\widehat{I} = \sum_n \widehat{I}_n$ to be the reconstructed image.

If $\{\widetilde{h}_n, h_n\}_{n=1}^N$ are such that $\widehat{I} = I$ for all input images I, the analysis-synthesis filter bank is invertible and $\{w_n\}$ is a lossless representation of the original image I. In particular, if the filters $\{\widetilde{h}_n\}$ are dilated versions of a template filter, then $\{w_n\}$ is a continuous wavelet transformation (CWT) that captures the original image properties at multiple scales. While conceptually similar to the Euclidean case, there are significant differences between planar and spherical convolutions. For example, unless $\widetilde{h}_n$ is axisymmetric (i.e., radially symmetric about the north pole), w_n is a function on $SO(3)$ rather than a spherical function.

For a general non-axisymmetric analysis-synthesis filter bank, the relationship between the input and reconstructed image is as follows [16]:

$$\widehat{I}^{l,m} = I^{l,m} \frac{8\pi^2}{2l+1} \sum_{n=1}^{N} \sum_{m'=-l}^{l} \left[h_n^{l,m'}\right] \left[\widetilde{h}_n^{l,m'}\right]^* \qquad (1)$$

where $I^{l,m}$ is the degree l and order m spherical harmonic coefficient of function $I(\theta, \phi)$ and $*$ denotes complex conjugation. We define the frequency response of a filter bank to be

$$H_{\widetilde{h},h}(l) = \frac{8\pi^2}{2l+1} \sum_{n=1}^{N} \sum_{m=-l}^{l} [h_n^{l,m}][\widetilde{h}_n^{l,m}]^*. \qquad (2)$$

It is easy to see that a filter bank is invertible if and only if its frequency response $H_{\widetilde{h},h}(l)$ is equal to 1 for all l such that $I^{l,m} \neq 0$.

We now construct a spherical continuous wavelet transform (SCWT). We define the analysis filters $\widetilde{h}_n = D_n \psi$ to be dilations of a template wavelet ψ and

$$h_n^{l,m} = \begin{cases} \frac{1}{H_{\widetilde{h},\widetilde{h}}(l)} \widetilde{h}_n^{l,m} & \text{for } H_{\widetilde{h},\widetilde{h}}(l) > 0 \\ 0 & \text{otherwise} \end{cases} \qquad (3)$$

One can verify that this analysis-synthesis filter bank is invertible for frequencies (l, m) for which $H_{\widetilde{h},\widetilde{h}}(l) \neq 0$.

Sampling Theory for SCWT. In the above formulation, the spherical images, filters and SCWT are defined continuously. While fast algorithms exist for computing and representing these continuous functions via coefficients of basis functions (e.g., spherical harmonics, and wigner-D functions), in practice, effective analysis requires sampling the SCWT. The sampling scheme and the discrete convolution between the wavelet samples and the continuous synthesis filter bank must be defined in a way that ensures invertibility.

It turns out that for axisymmetric analysis-synthesis filter banks of a finite spherical harmonic degree, latitude-longitude (lat-lon) sampling – at a sufficient rate dependent on the maximum spherical harmonic degree – guarantees that the filter bank has the same frequency response under the continuous and discrete convolution [16]. Thus an invertible continuous filter bank remains invertible under sampling and discrete convolution. The sampling guarantee implies that we can sample the SCWT defined in Eq. (3) while maintaining invertibility.

Implementation. In practice, we first establish a minimal metric-distortion spherical coordinate system [6] for an input shape consisting of mesh vertices $\{x_i, y_i, z_i\}$, resulting in the coordinate samples $\{x(\theta_i, \phi_i), y(\theta_i, \phi_i), z(\theta_i, \phi_i)\}$. Fast spherical convolution requires representing the coordinate functions in the spherical harmonic domain. We interpolate the coordinate samples onto the lat-lon grid and use the fast spherical harmonic transform [9] to obtain the spherical harmonic coefficients $\{x^{l,m}, y^{l,m}, z^{l,m}\}$. We verify by visual inspection and by computing percentage errors that interpolation errors are small.

For multi-scale shape analysis, we choose the template wavelet ψ to be the Laplacian-of-Gaussian [18]. We compute the SCWT of each coordinate function via convolutions with the analysis-synthesis filter bank in the spherical harmonic domain. As required by the sampling theories, the wavelet coefficients are sampled onto the lat-lon grid. For computational convenience, we interpolate the sampled wavelet coefficients onto a subdivided icosahedron grid (160k vertices). Theoretically, the coarser wavelet scales require smaller number of samples to prevent aliasing. In this work, we over-sample the wavelets coefficients on the same dense grid at all scales to increase the precision of our analysis. By re-interpolating the wavelet coefficient samples from the subdivided icosahedron back to the lat-lon grid, we again verify that interpolation errors are small.

Since metric distortion is invariant under rotations of the coordinate system, the resulting shape analysis is also rotation invariant, unlike bi-orthogonal wavelets. Rotational invariance of the overcomplete wavelet transform was theoretically and experimentally demonstrated in [18].

To summarize, given an input shape as a set of mesh vertices $\{x_i, y_i, z_i\}$, the spherical wavelet transforms output a set of wavelet coefficients samples $\{w_n^j(x), w_n^j(y), w_n^j(z)\}$ on the subdivided icosahedron grid, where j denotes the vertex index on the grid and n denotes the index of the filter, which corresponds directly to the resolution level of the wavelet transform.

3 Experiments and Discussion

Cortical folds in humans start developing at about 9 weeks in gestation and change dramatically until birth. The mechanism involved remains unclear. Cortical folds are known to correlate with function and cytoarchitecture [7]. The study of the folding formation process can therefore deepen our understanding of structure-function relationship and neurological diseases originating from abnormal structural and functional connectivity in neuro-development. A previous postmortem study reports regional and hemispheric differences in folding patterns in gestation [3]. Recent advances in MR imaging allow us to study the cortical folding pattern of premature newborns in-vivo.

We consider 11 MRI scans of eight normal neonates at gestational ages of 30.57, 31.1, 34, 37.71, 38.1, 38.4, 39.72, and 40.43 weeks, and three children (2, 3 and 7 years old). The cortical surfaces corresponding to the gray-white matter boundary were manually segmented, automatically registered [6] and manually checked for correspondence. We then apply the overcomplete spherical wavelets and employ the Gompertz function [15] to characterize the folding development:

$$F(t) = me^{-e^{-r(t-p)}} + \epsilon(t) \quad (4)$$

where $F(t)$ is some feature derived from the wavelet coefficients $w_t(x), w_t(y), w_t(z)$ at age t [17]. m is the maximum value of F at maturity, r is the maximum growth rate, p is the age of fastest growth and $\epsilon(t)$ is i.i.d. zero mean Gaussian noise. We assume a zero mean Gaussian prior on m, p, and r and estimate them using the maximum-a-posteriori framework. The variance of the Gaussian noise and priors on m, p and r are tuned via cross-validation. We estimate the confidence intervals of the estimated parameters using the Laplace approximation [10] and measure the goodness-of-fit with an R^2 statistic. An R^2 of 0.6 implies the model explains 60% of the variation in the data, and is considered a good fit.

Global Analysis of Folding Development. At each frequency level $n \in \{0, \ldots, 4\}$, for each cortical surface, we compute $F_n(t) = \sum_{j=1}^{J} w_{n,t}^j(x)^2 + w_{n,t}^j(y)^2 + w_{n,t}^j(z)^2$, where t is the age of the subject and J is the number of sampled wavelet coefficients per level. $F_n(t)$ summarizes the amount of cortical folding at the n-th scale: coefficients on the coarser level add details to the primary folds while coefficients on the finer level contribute to the smaller folds. For each wavelet level n, we then regress $F_n(t)$ against time t using Eq. (4). A good fit indicates that folding development at that scale obeys the characteristic of the Gompertz curve: fast exponential growth followed by slowing down and tapering off.

The estimated model parameters provide intuitive notions of growth. Fig. 1 shows that the speed of folding development r increases from level 0 to level 2 in both hemispheres and the age of fastest folding development p increases monotonically with frequency levels from approximately 29 to 33 weeks. The maximum development ages and speeds are significantly different across frequency levels. This temporal developmental order from the larger scale folds to smaller scale folds is consistent with the postmortem study [3] and more salient than in the previous imaging study based on bi-orthogonal spherical wavelets [17].

Furthermore, we find that in the left hemisphere, the fastest folding development occurs at a younger age than in the right at all levels (Fig. 1b), suggesting that cortical folds in the left hemisphere develop earlier, but slower than the right (Fig. 1a). In the postmortem study [3], structures in the temporal lobe, including the superior frontal, superior temporal and transverse temporal gyri were found to appear at an earlier gestational age on the right hemisphere. In

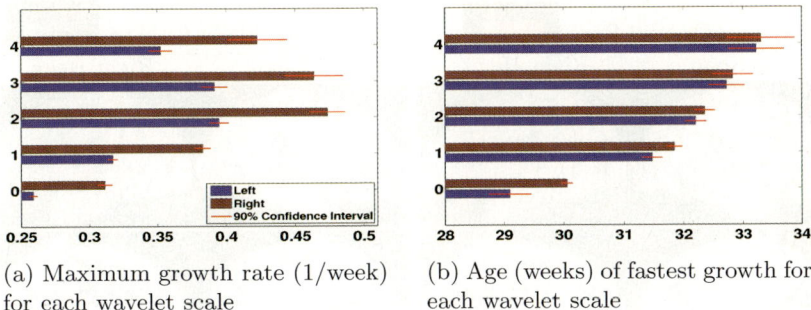

(a) Maximum growth rate (1/week) for each wavelet scale

(b) Age (weeks) of fastest growth for each wavelet scale

Fig. 1. Summary of Gompertz model fit to the global wavelet energies for wavelet scales $\{0,\ldots,4\}$. Parameters of the Gompertz model provide intuitive notion of growth. Red bars indicate 90% confidence intervals.

contrast, our result predicts an earlier folding development age, but a slower development speed on the left. The inconsistency between the two studies is probably due to a difference in definitions. For example, the definition of age of appearance in [3] is different from the age of fastest development in our model.

Regional Analysis of Folding Development. At each frequency level $n \in \{0,\ldots,4\}$, for each cortical surface, and for each spatial location j, we compute $F_{n,j}(t) = w_{n,t}^j(x)^2 + w_{n,t}^j(y)^2 + w_{n,t}^j(z)^2$. Once again, we regress $F_{n,j}(t)$ against t using Eq. (4) and study both when and where folding of the cortical surface occurs at different spatial scales.

Fig. 2 shows the results of the regional analysis. At each frequency scale, spatial locations with $R^2 > 0.6$ are color-coded with the corresponding development speed and age, and superimposed on the youngest newborn surface. To visualize the different spatial scales, the support of the corresponding wavelet basis function at that scale is shown in dark gray around each color-coded vertex.

Consistent with the global development results, regions that develop earlier (darker blue) also grow more slowly (more red). For example, the lateral side of the parietal lobe on the left hemisphere develops earlier than the right, but at a slower speed. In particular, the post-central sulcus and inter-parietal sulcus develop two weeks earlier in the left hemisphere than in the right.

Also consistent with the global analysis, we find that larger folds develop earlier but slower. On the lateral side, the pre- and post-central gyri develop the fastest during 30-31 weeks in both hemispheres while smaller structures such as supramarginal and angular gyri develop the fastest at much later time, as can be seen on level 3. Another example is the superior temporal gyrus developing much earlier than the smaller middle and inferior temporal gyri.

Discussion. Modeling cortical folding in the wavelet domain allows us to localize and study its regional development. Consistent with previous studies, we find that larger cortical folds develop at younger gestational ages with slower speeds. We also find that the left hemisphere develops earlier but slower than

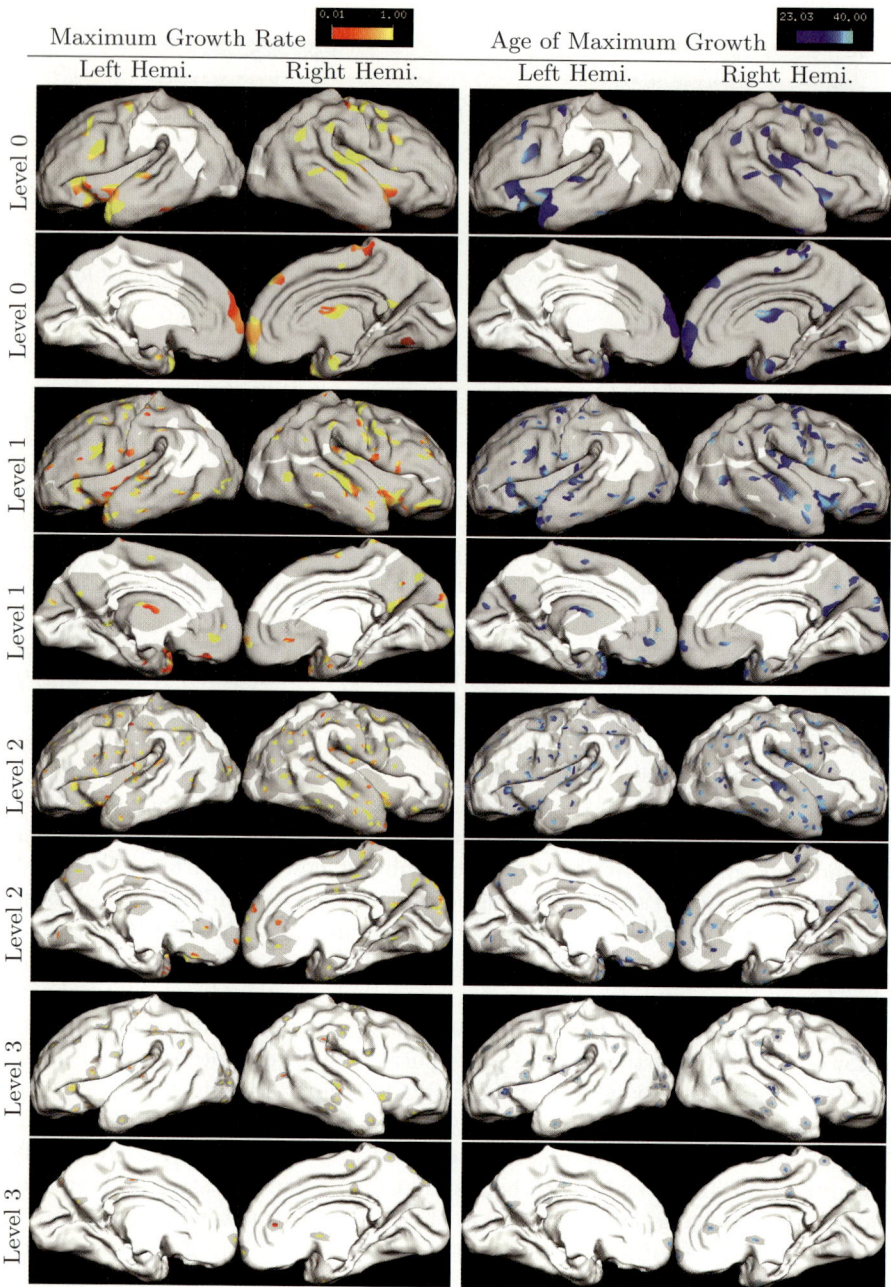

Fig. 2. Regional Growth Pattern. Colored regions indicated areas whose wavelet coefficients fit well to the Gompertz model. Each region has an accompanying support region shown in dark gray. The size of the supports correspond to the support of the wavelet basis at that scale, which decreases with increasing level.

the right. The study of individual wavelet coefficients detects and quantifies the regional differences in folding development at different spatial scales.

Because the overcomplete wavelet bases are not orthogonal, the correlation between wavelet coefficients at different levels should be taken into account, requiring further development of computational methods that model such dependencies. We note that for orthogonal representations, this problem is avoided at the price of losing rotational invariance and sensitivity.

While more analysis is needed to characterize the probability of false positives in the local analyses, our general agreement with the postmortem study [3] is encouraging. Furthermore, the improvement over biorthogonal wavelets is grounded in rigorous wavelet theory that cannot be attributed to multiple comparisons.

4 Conclusion

In this work, we explore the use of over-complete spherical wavelets in cortical shape analysis. We present a theoretic formulation of over-complete spherical wavelet filter banks and demonstrate their application on a study of cortical folding in newborns. Our experiments quantitatively verify previous experiments based on visual examination of postmortem brains and offer new insights into neuro-anatomical development.

Acknowledgments. Support for this research is provided in part by the NAMIC (NIH NIBIB NAMIC U54-EB005149), the NAC (NIT CRR NAC P41-RR13218), the mBIRN (NIH NCRR mBIRN U24-RR021382), the NIH NINDS R01-NS051826 grant, the NSF CAREER 0642971 grant, NCRR (P41-RR14075, R01 RR16594-01A1), the NIBIB (R01 EB001550, R01EB006758), the NINDS (R01 NS052585-01) and the MIND Institute. Additional support was provided by The Autism & Dyslexia Project funded by the Ellison Medical Foundation. B.T. Thomas Yeo is funded by A*STAR, Singapore.

References

1. Bogdanova, I., et al.: Stereographic Wavelet Frames on the Sphere. Applied and Computational Harmonic Analysis 19, 223–252 (2005)
2. Brechbüler, C., et al.: Parametrization of closed surfaces for 3-D shape description. Computer Vision and Image Understanding 61, 154–179 (1995)
3. Chi, J., et al.: Gyral development of the human brain. Ann. Neurol. 1 (1997)
4. Cootes, T., et al.: Active Shape Models-Their Training and Application. Computer Vision and Image Understanding 61(1), 38–59 (1995)
5. Daubechies, I.: Ten Lectures on Wavelets. SIAM, Philadelphia (1992)
6. Fischl, B., et al.: Cortical Surface-Based Analysis II: Inflation, Flattening, and a Surface-Based Coordinate System. NeuroImage 9(2), 195–207 (1999)
7. Fischl, B., et al.: Cortical Folding Patterns and Predicting Cytoarchictecture. Cerebral Cortex (2007)

8. Goodall, C.: Procrustes Method in the Statistical Analysis of Shape. Journal of the Royal Statistical Society B 53(2), 285–339 (1991)
9. Driscoll, J., Healy, D.: Computing Fourier Transforms & Convolutions on the 2-Sphere. Adv. in Appl. Math. 15, 202–250 (1994)
10. Minka, T.: Using Lower Bounds to Approximate Integrals, Technical Report (2001)
11. Nain, D., et al.: Multiscale 3-D shape representation and segmentation using spherical wavelets. IEEE Transactions on Medical Imaging 26, 598–618 (2007)
12. Schroder, P., Sweldens, W.: Spherical Wavelets: Efficiently Representing Functions on the Sphere. In: Computer Graphics Proceedings (SIGGRAPH), pp. 161–172 (1995)
13. Simoncelli, E., et al.: Shiftable Multi-scale Transforms. IEEE Transaction Information Theory 38(2), 587–607 (1992)
14. Staib, L., Duncan, J.: Model-based deformable surface finding for medical images. IEEE Transactions on Medical Imaging 15, 720–731 (1996)
15. Virene, E.: Reliability Growth and its Upper Limit. In: Proc. 1968 Annu. Symp. Reliability, pp. 265–270 (1968)
16. Yeo, B.T.T., et al.: On the Construction of Invertible Filter Banks on the 2-Sphere. IEEE Transactions on Image Processing 17(3), 283–300 (2008)
17. Yu, P., et al.: Cortical Surface Shape Analysis Based on Spherical Wavelets. IEEE Transactions on Medical Imaging 26(4), 582–598 (2007)
18. Yu, P., et al.: Cortical Folding Development Study based on Over-complete Spherical Wavelets. In: MMBIA (2007)

Particle-Based Shape Analysis of Multi-object Complexes

Joshua Cates[1], P. Thomas Fletcher[1], Martin Styner[2], Heather Cody Hazlett[2], and Ross Whitaker[1]

[1] Scientific Computing and Imaging Institute, Univ. Utah, Salt Lake City, UT, USA
[2] Depts. Psychiatry & Computer Science, Univ. North Carolina, Chapel Hill, NC, USA

Abstract. This paper presents a new method for optimizing surface point correspondences for shape modeling of multiobject anatomy, or shape *complexes*. The proposed method is novel in that it optimizes correspondence positions in the full, joint shape space of the object complex. Researchers have previously only considered the correspondence problem separately for each structure, thus ignoring the interstructural shape correlations that are increasingly of interest in many clinical contexts, such as the study of the effects of disease on groups of neuroanatomical structures. The proposed method uses a nonparametric, dynamic particle system to simultaneously sample object surfaces and optimize correspondence point positions. This paper also suggests a principled approach to hypothesis testing using the Hotelling T^2 test in the PCA space of the correspondence model, with a simulation-based choice of the number of PCA modes. We also consider statistical analysis of object poses. The modeling and analysis methods are illustrated on brain structure complexes from an ongoing clinical study of pediatric autism.

1 Introduction

Statistical shape modeling is an increasingly important tool for the analysis of anatomical objects derived from 3D medical images. In many areas of clinical psychiatric and neurological research, the joint analysis of *complexes* of multiple anatomical structures is of increasing interest because certain spectrum disorders, such as autism, are thought to represent a confluence of several underlying abnormalities, impacting the *relationships* between brain regions [1]. Shape models of anatomical complexes are also important tools for geneticists and developmental biologists, who rely on quantifications of phenotype in gene targeting studies (e.g., [2]).

We define a *multiobject complex* as a set of solid shapes, each representing a single, connected biological structure, assembled into a scene within a common coordinate frame. A multiobject complex contains shape, pose, scale, and positional information for each structure. Some examples include the segmentations of multiple brain structures from a single MRI of a patient and sets of bones segmented from a CT scan. Point-based models, which we consider in this work, represent shape by sampling each shape surface in a consistently ordered fashion in order to define homologous object surface points called *correspondences*. The set of correspondences for a population is then used for statistical analysis, including hypothesis testing for group differences[3,4].

The choice of correspondence positions is a critical step for point-based modeling. State-of-the-art methods typically rely on parameterized surface models that assume a spherical or toroidal topology, and are thus not suitable for multiobject complexes, which are nonmanifold, and consist of disconnected sets of discrete surfaces. Some parametric methods have been applied to shape complexes by finding correspondences for each structure independently, and then treating those correspondences as the *marginal* distributions of the multiobject complex [5]. This particular approach, however, is not consistent with standard methods in statistics, which generally seek to use the simplest model that explains the observed data. For point-based modeling, this means that ideally one should seek a compact distribution for the correspondences in the full, joint shape space. Several methods for optimizing correspondence positions for collections of single objects have been proposed (e.g.,[6,4]), but a *joint optimization* for a multiobject model has yet to be demonstrated and analyzed.

Optimization in the full, joint shape space of complexes is important for several reasons. If variabilities between individual shapes in a complex are correlated, for example, the marginal variabilities can appear small, and might not otherwise be preserved. By modeling these correlations among variabilities, optimization in the joint space may also produce more compact distributions for correspondences. The specific choice of optimization methods is also an important factor. Parametric approaches, for example, are potentially limited for multiobject modeling because they typically rely on individual *anchor shapes* to regularize the optimization process, and thus would restrict the degree to which parameterizations of different objects in the ensemble could interact.

In this paper we propose a novel, nonparametric approach to multiobject shape modeling that is an extension of the entropy-based particle system method given for single objects in [4]. The proposed method optimizes correspondence positions in the full, joint shape space of the object complex. Because statistical analysis of shape models is in itself a difficult problem due to the very high dimensionality of the shape space and the relatively low numbers of samples, we also present a systematic approach to shape analysis using Hotelling T^2 tests in the PCA space of the correspondences, with a simulation-based approach to the dimensionality reduction. Additionally, we show how point-based models can be used to analyze group differences in object position, pose, and scale. The proposed modeling framework is applied to a proof-of-concept analysis of brain structure complexes from a study of pediatric autism. Our analysis shows group differences in shape between normal and patient populations that have not been seen previously in this data, and show how an optimized joint model yields results with a higher statistical power than a model constructed by simply optimizing the marginal distributions.

This paper builds on previous work on statistical shape parameterization and analysis that has mostly focused on single objects. For instance, Styner et al. [3] use geometric considerations on individual shapes, without ensemble statistics. Finding correspondence positions that minimize information content (log-determinant of the covariance matrix) across an ensemble of simple, closed, 2D objects was first proposed by Kotcheff and Taylor[7], and extended by Davies et al. [6] using a minimum description length (MDL) minimization to compute 3D surface parameterizations. In previous work, Cates et al. [4] propose a nonparametric, particle-based method, which minimizes the entropy of the resulting description. This strategy includes an explicit penalty for geometric regularity, and thus does not require a regularization based on a-priori anchor shapes, as is typically done with MDL. Previous results on statistical analysis of multiobject complexes have been shown using sampled medial mesh (m-rep) representations [8,5], but do not include an ensemble-based parameterization. The contributions of this paper are, therefore, the generalization of an ensemble-based, statistical correspondence algorithm to shape complexes, and a systematic statistical analyses of multiobject shape, size, and pose, as well as a demonstration of hypothesis testing with this framework in a compelling clinical application.

2 Methodology

This section gives a brief overview of the particle-system correspondence optimization method for single object surfaces given in [4], and then describes its extension to multiobject complexes of surfaces. We also present our approach to the statistical analysis of the shape, scale, and pose in the resulting models.

Correspondence Optimization for Single Objects. We define a surface as a smooth, closed manifold of codimension one, which is a subset of $\Re^d$ (e.g., $d = 3$ for volumes). We sample a surface $S \subset \Re^d$ using a discrete set of N points that are considered random variables $Z = (X_1, X_2, \ldots, X_N)$ drawn from a probability density function (PDF), $p(X)$. We denote a realization of this PDF with lower case, and thus we have $z = (x_1, x_2, \ldots, x_N)$, where $z \in S^N$. The probability of a realization x is $p(X = x)$, which we denote simply as $p(x)$.

The amount of information contained in such a random sampling is, in the limit, the differential entropy of the PDF, which is

$$H[X] = -\int_S p(x) \log p(x) dx = -E\{\log p(X)\}, \tag{1}$$

where $E\{\cdot\}$ is the expectation. Approximating the expectation by the sample mean, we have $H[X] \approx -\frac{1}{N-1} \sum_i \log p(x_i)$. To estimate $p(x_i)$, we use a nonparametric Parzen windowing estimation from the particle positions, modified to adaptively oversample in regions of higher curvature by the inclusion of a scaling term that is proportional to local curvature magnitude. This results in a set of points on the surface that repel each other with Gaussian-weighted forces.

Now consider an ensemble $\mathcal{E}$, which is a collection of M surfaces, each with their own set of particles, i.e., $\mathcal{E} = z^1, \ldots, z^M$. The ordering of the particles on each shape implies a correspondence among shapes, and thus we have a matrix of particle positions $P = x_j^k$, with particle positions along the rows and shapes across the columns. We model $z^k \in \Re^{Nd}$ as an instance of a random variable Z, and minimize a combined ensemble and shape cost function

$$Q = H(Z) - \sum_k H(P^k), \qquad (2)$$

which favors a compact ensemble representation balanced against a uniform distribution of particles on each surface. Given the low number of samples relative to the dimensionality of the space, we use a parametric approach for density estimation in the space of shapes, modeling $p(Z)$ parametrically as a Gaussian with covariance Σ. The entropy is then given by

$$H(Z) \approx \frac{1}{2}\log|\Sigma| = \frac{1}{2}\sum_{j=1}^{Nd} \log \lambda_j, \qquad (3)$$

where $\lambda_1, ..., \lambda_{Nd}$ are the eigenvalues of Σ.

The cost function Q is minimized using a gradient descent strategy to manipulate particle positions. The negative gradient $-\partial H(Z)/\partial P$ gives a vector of updates for the entire system, which is recomputed once per iteration of the entire particle system. This gradient term is added to the individual shape-based updates $\partial H(P^k)/\partial P^k$ to give the update for each particle. The surface constraint is specified by the zero set of a scalar function $F(x)$, and maintained by projecting the gradient of the cost function onto the tangent plane of the surface, followed by iterative reprojection of the particle onto the nearest root of F by the method of Newton-Raphson. The optimization function balances entropy of individual surface samplings with the entropy of the shape model, maximizing the former for geometric accuracy (a good sampling) and minimizing the latter to produce a compact model.

Correspondences Across MultiObject Complexes. The particle-based correspond method outlined above *can* be directly applied to multiobject complexes by treating all of the objects in the complex as one. However, if the objects themselves have distinct identities (i.e., object-level correspondence is known a priori), we can assign each particle to a specific object, decouple the spatial interactions between particles on different shapes, and constrain each particle to its associated object, thereby ensuring that each correspondence stays on a particular anatomical structure. The shape-space statistics remain coupled, however, and the covariance Σ (Eqn. 3) includes all particle positions across the entire complex, so that optimization takes place on the joint, multiobject model.

Any set of implicitly defined surfaces is appropriate as input to this framework. In the case of binary segmentations, the input is a set of M segmentations of N-object complexes, which contains $N \times M$ distinct, volumetric label masks. A binary mask contains an implicit shape surface at the interface of the labeled pixels and the background, but contains aliasing artifacts that must first be removed. We have found that the r-tightening algorithm given by Williams et al. [9] is effective in removing these artifacts without compromising the precision of the segmentation. Typically we follow the antialiasing step with a very slight Gaussian blurring to remove the high-frequency artifacts that can occur as a result of numerical approximations. We initialize the optimization using the splitting strategy described in [4], starting with a single particle on each object. For the hypothesis testing that will follow, it is important that correspondences be computed without knowledge of the group classification of the shapes. We therefore compute shape models for the shape complexes that include both the control and study data, which we will refer to as *combined* models.

Statistical Analysis for Correspondence-Based Shape Models. The goal of statistical analysis in the context of this paper is to quantify shape differences of the targeted anatomy between control and study populations, and to perform hypothesis testing for statistical significance of those differences. An important consideration is to quantify differences in a way that accounts for desirable invariances, which is typically done by explicitly normalizing for size and pose variation. In a multiobject setting, we must decide the level of granularity at which to align shapes in order to analyze pose and scale. Previous work [5,10] employs a hierarchical strategy, with a *global* coordinate frame for the entire complex, followed by a set of *local* coordinate frames for each object. The global frame is established by alignment of the entire complex, resulting in M sets of global pose parameters. Remaining pose discrepancies among the individual objects constitute the local coordinate frames, and are determined by alignment of each ensemble of individual shapes, to give a set of N local pose parameters for each of the M complexes.

For the analysis of object pose and scale, we first align shapes with respect to their centers of mass and the orientation of their first principal eigenvectors. We then align shapes with respect to rotation, translation, and scaling using a Procrustes algorithm, which is run at regular intervals between the correspondence optimization updates (see [4]). Hypothesis testing on object scale can now be done using standard, two-tailed parametric t-test, and group differences in relative position analyzed with a parametric Hotelling T^2 test. For relative pose, we use a general nonparametric hypothesis test for metric spaces [11], which relies only on pairwise distances between the data, and we use geodesic distances in the rotation group.

We refer to the differences in correspondences that remain in the population after pose and scale alignment as *shape*. The high dimensionality of the shape space, coupled with the relatively low sample size of our data, precludes the use of traditional low-dimensional statistical metrics directly in the full shape space. Instead, we use a standard, data-driven approach to dimensionality reduction and project the correspondences into a lower dimensional space determined by choosing a number of basis vectors from principal component analysis (PCA). Ideally, we would like to choose only PCA modes that account for variance that cannot be explained by random noise. *Parallel analysis* is commonly recommended for this purpose [12]. Parallel analysis works by comparing the percent variances of each of the PCA modes with the average percent variances obtained

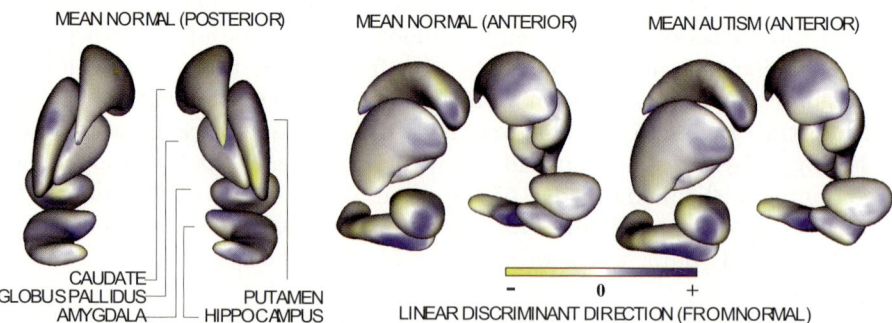

Fig. 1. Mean brain structure complexes with average pose. Colormap indicates the magnitude and direction of the linear discriminant.

via PCA of Monte Carlo simulations of samplings from isotropic, multivariate, unit Gaussian distributions. We choose only modes with greater variance than the simulated modes for the dimensionality reduction, and use use a standard, parametric Hotelling T^2 test to test for group differences, with the null hypothesis that the two groups are drawn from the same distribution.

To visualize group differences that are driving the statistical result, we compute the linear discriminant vector implicit in the Hotelling T^2 statistic, which is the is the line along which the between-class variance is maximized with respect to the within-class variance. This line is also known as Fisher's linear discriminant, and is given by

$$\mathbf{w} = (\mathbf{\Sigma_a} + \mathbf{\Sigma_b})^{-1}(\mu_\mathbf{a} - \mu_\mathbf{b}), \quad (4)$$

where μ are the group means for groups a and b, and $\mathbf{\Sigma}$ are their covariance matrices. Vector $\mathbf{w}$ can be rotated back from PCA space into the full dimensional shape space, and then mapped onto the mean group shape visualizations to give an indication of the significant morphological differences between groups.

3 Results and Discussion

For the experimental analysis, we used multiobject segmentation data taken from an ongoing longitudinal pediatric autism study[13], which includes MRI brain scans of autistic subjects and typically-developing controls at time points of 2 and 4 years of age. The data consists of binary segmentations of 10 subcortical brain structures (see Fig 1), which were done by trained experts using semi-automated procedures[5]. For this analysis, we had 10, 2-year old male controls available, and chose 15 matched autism subjects for comparison. Multiobject correspondences were computed from the segmentations as described in Section 2 to produce a combined model of the groups. We sampled each complex of segmentations with 10,240 correspondence points, using 1024 particles per structure. For comparison, we also computed point-correspondence models for each of the 10 structures separately and concatenated their correspondences together to form a *marginally optimized* joint model.

Scale and pose were calculated for structures in the complex as described in Sect. 2. Hypothesis testing indicates significant group differences in scale only for the right and left amygdala, with p-values of 0.0017 and 0.018, respectively. Hotelling T^2 tests on mean structure positions do not suggest any differences between the groups, with $p > 0.05$ for all structures. Similarly, group difference in pose are not indicated by the statistical pose analysis, and we obtained $p > 0.05$ for all structures. This result for pose is also consistent with results given in [5] on this data.

The hypothesis test method outlined in Sect. 2 gives a highly significant p-value of 0.0087, with 8 PCA modes chosen by parallel analysis. This result is the first evidence shown for this data for group differences in shape alone. Gorczowski [5] reports group differences when scale is included with shape, but reports insignificant shape discrimination between groups when the shapes are normalized to the same size. Parallel analysis of the marginally-optimized model indicates that the first 6 modes should be used, which gives a p-value of 0.0480. While the test still suggests group differences at the 5% significance level, we note that the result is an order of magnitude lower in statistical power.

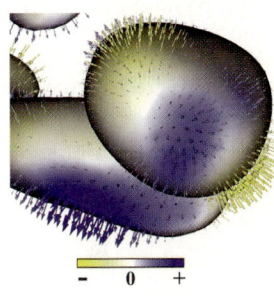

Fig. 2. Detail from Fig. 1

Previous work in shape analysis has suggested hypothesis testing on individual correspondence point positions instead of working in the full dimensional shape space [14]. For comparison, we ran statistical tests at every correspondence point location, using an open-source implementation of the nonparametric Hotelling T^2 method described in [14], with 20,000 permutations among groups and an FDR bound set to 5%. Uncorrected p-values show widespread differences, but no significance remains after FDR correction. This result is in contrast to the global shape result, and illustrates one of the difficulties with point-based shape analysis at a local feature scale: the unavoidable reduction in statistical power due to the necessary correction for multiple comparisons.

Figure 1 shows the mean shape surfaces for the normal and autistic groups, as reconstructed from the Euclidean averages of the correspondence points. Each structure is displayed in its mean orientation, position, and scale in the global coordinate frame. We computed the average orientation for each structure using methods for averaging in curved spaces [15]. We used the arithmetic mean of position and the geometric mean of scale. Mean pose differences between the two groups appear small, as might be expected from their statistical analyses.

To illustrate the morphological differences that are driving the global shape result, we visualize the linear discriminant vector **w** (Equation 4) in Fig. 1, as described in the previous section. The length in the surface normal direction of each of the point-wise discriminant vector components for the autism data is given by the colormap. Yellow indicates a negative (inward) direction, and blue indicates a positive (outward) direction. The right amygdala for the normals is shown in Fig. 2 as a more detailed example, with the vectors depicted as arrows. Note the clear trend towards a shortening of the anterior end of the amygdala in the autistic versus the normal population.

In summary, our results suggest that the proposed modeling and analysis framework can effectively model group differences in the autism data that have not been seen with other methods, and more powerful statistical results are obtained by optimization in the joint space than by optimization in the marginal space. This analysis, however, is only a proof-of-concept example of how the particle method may be applied to multiobject data. A more rigorous study, which remains for future work, is required in order draw clinical conclusions.

Acknowledgments

This work is supported by the Center for Integrative Biomedical Computing, (NIH 2-P41-RR12553-07), the National Alliance for Medical Image Computing (NIH U54-EB005149), NIH grant HD03110, and the Autism Speaks Foundation.

References

1. Chultz, R., Robins, D.: Functional neuroimaging studies of autism spectrum disorders. In: Handbook of autism and pervasive developmental disorders, 3rd edn., pp. 515–533. J. Wiley and Sons, Chichester (2005)
2. Davis, A., Capecchi, M.: Axial homeosis and appendicular skeleton defects in mice with targeted disruption of hoxd-11. Development 120, 2187–2198 (1995)
3. Styner, M., Lieberman, J.A., Pantazis, D., Gerig, G.: Boundary and medial shape analysis of the hippocampus in schizophrenia. Medical Image Analysis (2004)
4. Cates, J., Fletcher, P.T., Styner, M., Shenton, M., Whitaker, R.: Shape modeling and analysis with entropy-based particle systems. In: Karssemeijer, N., Lelieveldt, B. (eds.) IPMI 2007. LNCS, vol. 4584, pp. 333–345. Springer, Heidelberg (2007)
5. Gorczowski, K., Styner, M., Jeong, J., Marron, J., Piven, J., Hazlett, H., Pizer, S., Gerig, G.: Statistical shape analysis of multi-object complexes. In: Proceedings of IEEE Conference on Computer Vision and Pattern Recognition, pp. 1–8. IEEE, Los Alamitos (2007)
6. Davies, R.H., Twining, C.J., Cootes, T.F., Waterton, J.C., Taylor, C.J.: 3D statistical shape models using direct optimisation of description length. In: Heyden, A., Sparr, G., Nielsen, M., Johansen, P. (eds.) ECCV 2002. LNCS, vol. 2352, pp. 3–20. Springer, Heidelberg (2002)
7. Kotcheff, A., Taylor, C.: Automatic Construction of Eigenshape Models by Direct Optimization. Medical Image Analysis 2, 303–314 (1998)
8. Pizer, S.M., Jeong, J.Y., Lu, C., Muller, K.E., Joshi, S.C.: Estimating the statistics of multi-object anatomic geometry using inter-object relationships. In: Fogh Olsen, O., Florack, L.M.J., Kuijper, A. (eds.) DSSCV 2005. LNCS, vol. 3753, pp. 60–71. Springer, Heidelberg (2005)
9. Williams, J., Rossignac, J.: Tightening: curvature-limiting morphological simplification. In: Proc. 9th ACM Symp. on Solid and Physical Modeling, pp. 107–112 (2005)

10. Gerig, G., Joshi, S., Fletcher, T., Gorczowski, K., Xu, S., Pizer, S., Styner, M.: Statistics of populations of images and its embedded objects: Driving applications in neuroimaging. In: IEEE Symp. on Biomed. Imaging ISBI, pp. 1120–1123 (2006)
11. Hall, P., Tajvidi, N.: Permutation tests for equality of distributions in high-dimensional settings. Biometrika 89(2), 359–374 (2002)
12. Glorfeld, L.W.: An improvement on horn's parallel analysis methodology for selecting the correct number of factors to retain. Educational and Psychological Measurement 55, 377–393 (1995)
13. Hazlett, H., Poe, M., Gerig, G., Smith, R., Provenzale, J., Ross, A., Gilmore, J., Piven, J.: Magnetic resonance imaging and head circumference study of brain size in autism: Birth through age 2 years. Arch. Gen. Psych. 62, 1366–1376 (2005)
14. Styner, M., Oguz, I., Xu, S., Brechbühler, C., Pantazis, D., Levitt, J., Shenton, M., Gerig, G.: Framework for the statistical shape analysis of brain structures using SPHARM-PDM. The Insight Journal (2006)
15. Fletcher, P., Lu, C., Pizer, S., Joshi, S.: Principal geodesic analysis for the study of nonlinear statistics of shape. IEEE Trans. Med. Imaging 23(8), 995–1005 (2004)

Multivariate Statistical Analysis of Whole Brain Structural Networks Obtained Using Probabilistic Tractography

Emma C. Robinson[1], Michel Valstar[1], Alexander Hammers[2], Anders Ericsson[1], A. David Edwards[3], and Daniel Rueckert[1]

[1] Department of Computing, Imperial College, London. SW7 2BZ, UK
[2] MRC Clinical Sciences Centre and Division of Neuroscience, Faculty of Medicine, Imperial College, London. W12 ONN, UK
[3] Department of Paediatrics, Imperial College, London. W12 ONN, UK

Abstract. This paper presents a new framework for the analysis of anatomical connectivity derived from diffusion tensor MRI. The framework has been applied to estimate whole brain structural networks using diffusion data from 174 adult subjects. In the proposed approach, each brain is first segmented into 83 anatomical regions via label propagation of multiple atlases and subsequent decision fusion. For each pair of anatomical regions the probability of connection and its strength is then estimated using a modified version of probabilistic tractography. The resulting brain networks have been classified according to age and gender using non-linear support vector machines with GentleBoost feature extraction. Classification performance was tested using a leave-one-out approach and the mean accuracy obtained was 85.4%.

1 Introduction

Key to better understanding of brain function is a mapping of its underlying anatomical connectivity. Diffusion tensor MRI offers the possibility for approximation of this underlying neural microstructure through estimation of the diffusive profile of water molecules within brain tissue; known to be anisotropic or directed along white matter bundles. Connections between brain regions can then be estimated using tractography. In their simplest form tractography algorithms break down in areas of low diffusion anisotropy making them unsuited to studies of whole brain connectivity. In contrast, probabilistic tractography methods such as [1] have been shown to accurately represent thalamo-cortical grey matter connectivity in a wide variety of subject groups [2][3]. In a natural progression of this approach we therefore seek to extend use of this technique to generate an approximation of the coordinated network of these connections in the whole brain.

Previous attempts at modelling functional and structural brain connections exist in [4][5][6][15]. All of these studies have used graph theory and in particular the properties of small world graphs to characterise brain networks. Unfortunately, while this is useful for making generalised statements about the nature and development of brain networks, it offers no quantifiable means of comparing the brain networks of different subjects. In this study we explore the potential for characterising brain networks of different subject groups using state-of-the-art classification techniques from pattern recognition; performing classification through a combination of non linear support vector machines (SVM) [7] with Gentle Boosting[8].

This paper makes two contributions: first, we present a model for the estimation of structural brain networks in adults which includes the calculation of parameters determining the probability as well as the strength of connections. Secondly we show how this model can be applied to a group of adult subjects on which classification is performed. Our results show that the brains of different subject groups can be distinguished by nature of their patterns of neural connectivity alone.

2 Methods

2.1 Probabilistic Tractography and Connection Probability Estimation

Traditional streamline tractography algorithms work by following the direction of maximum diffusion at each voxel, estimated from the principal eigenvector of the diffusion tensor. Unfortunately, this maximum likelihood approach offers no measurement of the confidence in the trajectory of the fibre tract. Thus, these approaches have problems tracking into areas of low diffusion anisotropy. Probabilistic schemes on the other hand, allow for tracking into areas of low certainty by directly estimating confidence in the model using, for example, Bayesian inference [1]. This results in a range of possible principal diffusion directions that can be sampled from during repeated streamlining resulting in a series of possible end points for each tract. Thus, given two regions of interest (ROIs) A and B, the probability of B being connected to the seed region A (given the data, Y) can be calculated as the proportion of the total number of streamlines which reach region B:

$$P(\exists\, A \to B | Y) = \frac{n_{A \to B}}{n_A}\ . \tag{1}$$

Here $n_{A \to B}$ denotes the number of streamlines seeded in region A which reach region B and n_A denotes the number of streamlines seeded in region A.

In most cases the manually defined seed and target regions will however be very large in comparison to the tract volumes and thus division by entire seed volumes leads to an under-representation of the true likelihood of connection. Probability is therefore better defined in terms of the sub-region $s \in A$, whose voxels have a non-zero probability of seeding streamlines to B:

$$P(\exists\, s \to B | Y) = \frac{n_{A \to B}}{n_s}\ . \tag{2}$$

Here n_s denotes the number of streamlines seeded in sub-region s.

2.2 Connectivity Strength Estimation

Whilst the probabilistic measures defined above give us some idea of the strength of belief that a connection exists, it does not measure the strength of the connection, i.e. the tract size. Influenced by confounding factors such as measurement noise and model inaccuracies, variations of the connection probability between subjects become difficult to interpret. Therefore we define another measure for the estimation of connection strength based on the concept of information flow and adapted from [6]. In this approach, local connection weights between voxels are determined by estimation of the diffusive transfer between them using integration of the orientation distribution function (ODF) over the solid angle β ($= \frac{4\pi}{26}$) where the ODF radially projects a Gaussian probability density estimation ($P(\boldsymbol{R})$) of the diffusion displacement (R) along each of the 26 unit vectors ($\hat{u}$) joining each voxel ($\boldsymbol{r_i}$) with its neighbours:

$$\text{ODF} = \psi(\hat{u}) = \int_0^{+\inf} R^2 P(\boldsymbol{R}) dR \qquad (3)$$

$$P(\boldsymbol{R}) = (4\pi t)^{-\frac{3}{2}} (|D|)^{-\frac{1}{2}} exp^{\frac{-\boldsymbol{R}^T D^{-1} \boldsymbol{R}}{4t}} \; . \qquad (4)$$

Here D represent the diffusion tensor and $\boldsymbol{R} = \hat{u}R$ is the projection of relative spin displacement of the water molecules along the unit vector $\hat{u}$.

By integrating over the solid angle β (which describes the volume proportion over the unit sphere) it is possible to approximate the diffusion proportion ($P_{\text{diff}}(\hat{u})$, proportionality constant C) calculated along each of the 26 projected directions in turn:

$$P_{\text{diff}}(\hat{u}) = \frac{1}{C} \int_\beta \psi(\hat{u}) dS \; . \qquad (5)$$

Local weights between voxels sampled during probabilistic tractography are determined by averaging this diffusion proportion in both directions along the unit arc joining voxels. Path or connection weights (ζ) between regions are determined by the mean of all $P_{\text{diff}}(\hat{u})$ obtained at each step of the probabilistic tracking. Finally, (anatomical) connection strengths (ACS) are determined by multiplication of ζ by an approximation of tract cross section taken from the mean number of voxels ($\boldsymbol{r_i}$) in the seed and target volumes ($V_{\text{seed}}, V_{\text{target}}$):

$$\text{ACS} = \frac{\zeta}{2} \Big(\sum_{\forall \boldsymbol{r_i} \in V_{\text{seed}}} \boldsymbol{r_i} + \sum_{\forall \boldsymbol{r_i} \in V_{\text{target}}} \boldsymbol{r_i} \Big) \qquad (6)$$

2.3 Experiment: Extraction of Structural Brain Networks

ROIs for seeding tractography were obtained by segmentation of the brain into 83 regions by label propagation [9] from multiple, manually-generated brain atlases. The resulting segmentations were then estimated using decision fusion as described in [10]. As neurological connections typically start and end in the grey matter, cortical white matter was removed by multiplication of the anatomical

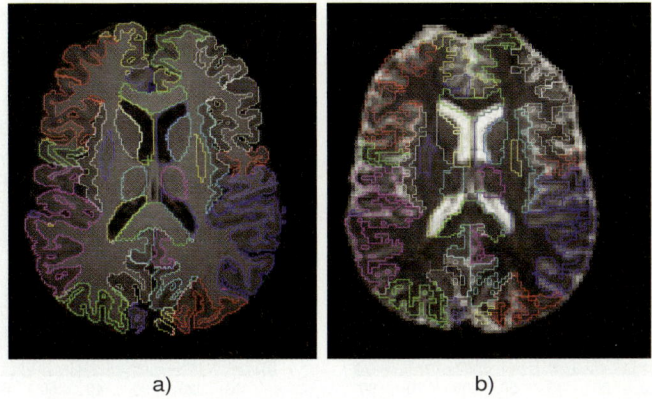

Fig. 1. a) Structural (T1) segmentation and b) diffusion space segmentation after multiplication of anatomical segmentations with tissue segmentations to remove cortical white matter. Registration to diffusion space was performed by affine registration in two stages via T2 space.

segmentation with a tissue segmentation obtained using SPM5 [11]. Segmentations were transformed to the diffusion space (where tractography is traditionally performed) using affine registrations via intermediary T2 space (Fig. 1).

Next tractography was performed between pairs of regions in turn with only direct connections between regions being retained and connectivity being determined both probabilistically (2) and in terms of the connection strength (ACS) previously defined (6).

Results were represented as indices in 83x83 connection matrices (Fig. 2). Self-connections along the diagonal were removed and symmetry was enforced (since DTI is incapable of distinguishing between afferent and efferent biological connections). Connection vectors were formed by concatenating rows of each connectivity matrix. Finally, due to symmetry reasons, connections below the diagonal were removed as was the quadrant representing left-to-right connectivity which should be empty (assuming that all connections between brain lobes pass through and thus terminate at the corpus callosum).

2.4 Statistical Analysis of Structural Brain Networks

Gentle Boosting for Feature Extraction. Boosting is a technique which greatly improves the performance of classifiers by sequentially re-training weak classifiers on weighted data. It is used here solely for the purpose of feature extraction [8] choosing essentially orthogonal features on which to perform training using SVM. Over several boosting rounds weighted-least-squares regression was performed for every parameter. The best performing parameters were then selected as features and training samples were re-weighed according to their performance at each stage.

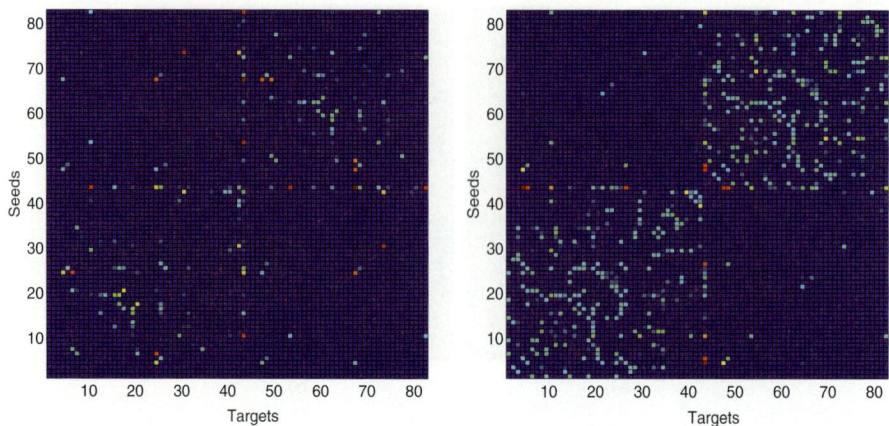

Fig. 2. Figure 1 Matrices representing mean ACS (left) and connection probability (right) for the network of connections between the 83 regions defined during anatomical segmentation

Classification using Support Vector Machines. Classification was performed using binary non-linear support vector machines [7].

In this technique, n-dimensional data $\mathbf{x_i}$, $i = 1, 2...n$; where n, in this case, is the number of GentleBoost features; is mapped through ϕ to a higher dimensional space H ($\phi : \mathbf{R}^n \mapsto H$), in the hope that the data is linearly separable in that space. Separation is achieved by maximising the distance between the two parallel hyperplanes which form the boundaries between each class $y_i \in \{+1, -1\}$. Training points which define these hyperplanes are called the support vectors $\mathbf{s}$ (total number N_s).

Optimal separation is found by formulating the problem as a Lagrangian with multipliers α_i. This has the added benefit of representing the problem in inner product form allowing for the higher dimensional problem to be solved in a lower dimensional space using a Mercer kernel [8] : $K(\mathbf{x_i}, \mathbf{x_j}) = \langle \phi(\mathbf{x_i}), \phi(\mathbf{x_j}) \rangle$. After training the decision function on a test point $\mathbf{x}$ is then given by:

$$f(x) = \sum_{i=1}^{N_s} \alpha_i y_i K(\mathbf{s_i}, \mathbf{x}) = b \qquad (7)$$

Where, b refers to the bias of the hyperplanes from the origin. A Gaussian radial basis function kernel was used: $K(\mathbf{x_i}, \mathbf{x_j}) = e^{-\|\mathbf{X} - \mathbf{Y}\|^2 / 2\sigma_2}$

Leave one out tests. Classification was performed N times each with N-1 image vectors in the training set. The remaining image vector was then used for testing.

Performance was calculated using the F_{measure}, the harmonic mean of classification precision and recall, where precision (P) is a measure of the number of true positives (those correctly labelled as belonging to a class) over the total (true positives plus false positives) and, recall (R) is a measure of true positives divided by the number of objects that should have been labelled in that class (true positives plus false negatives): $F_{\text{measure}} = \frac{2 \cdot P \cdot R}{P+R}$

3 Results

Connectivity analysis was performed on 174 adult brains (89 female); median age 45 years (range: 20-86 years). Scanning was performed on a Philips 3 Tesla system. T1 and T2 images were acquired prior to diffusion weighted imaging using 3D MRPRAGE and dual echo weighted imaging. Single shot echo planar DTI was acquired in 15 non collinear directions using the following parameters: TR 12000ms, TE 51ms, slice thickness 2mm, voxel size = 1.75 x 1.75 x 2mm^3, b value 1000s/mm^2.

Connectivity results are shown in Fig. 2. Rows and columns have been permuted such that left and right brain regions are separated and corpus callosum runs through the middle. Left-right quadrants are predominantly empty (as expected) except for connections across the mid-line caused by registration error (Fig. 1). In addition results for connection strength and probability show significantly different intensity patterns reflecting the differences in interpretation between a high probability that a connection exists and inference of a strong connection.

Leave one out results for classification according to age (group 1 = 20-49 years; group 2 = 50-86 years) or gender are shown in Table 1. In both cases the classifier performed better on the results for connectivity strength. Discriminating features (connections) identified by the classifiers are shown in Tables 2 and 3. For men and women these predominantly include connections to and from the corpus callosum, temporal gyri and areas of the limbic system known to differ between

Table 1. F_{measure} results of the classification

	Age	Gender
Strength	87.9%	86.8%
Probability	85.1%	81.6%

Table 2. Discriminating features defining classification for connection strength: P = posterior; A=anterior; S=superior; I=inferior; L=left; R=right. Derivation described in 2.4.

Age	Gender
Postcentral to A Temporal (L)	Presubgenual Frontal to Cingulate (A) (L)
Subgenual Frontal to I. Frontal (L & R)	Corpus to Cingulate (P) (L)
Straight Gyrus to Medial Temporal (R)	Corpus to S. Temporal (A) (L)
Nucleus Accumbens to I. Frontal (R)	Putamen to Pallidum (L)

Table 3. Discriminating features defining classification for connection probability: P = posterior; A=anterior; S=superior; I=inferior; L=left; R=right. See 2.4.

Age	Gender
Putamen to Cingulate (P) (L and R)	Presubgenual Frontal to Cingulate (P) (L)
Brainstem to Cingulate (P) (L)	Insula to Lingual (L)
Brainstem to S. Frontal (L)	Thalamus to P. Orbital (L)
S.Temporal (P) to Cingulate (P) (R)	Thalamus to Putamen (L)

genders. For age, differences predominantly include features of the frontal lobe and its associated connections.

4 Discussion

Fundamental to understanding differences in brain function between the sexes or over time is identification of differences in the underlying connectivity which monitors behaviour. Studies into structural brain connectivity across subject groups thus far have been limited mostly to major white matter structures. These have pointed to an overall degeneration in fractional anisotropy (FA) and therefore connection strength with age [12] and regional differences in FA in the corpus callosum between men and women[13]. However this is the first study that has pointed to global changes in connectivity across subject groups.

Whilst it is possible that ACS; calculated from seed and target volumes; may be sensitive to changes in brain size and therefore interpretation of any features should be approached with caution, there are similarities here with reports from functional studies which suggest that female brains exhibit higher bilateral connectivity [14] (reflected by the significance of connections to the corpus callosum) as well as a prominence of age-discriminating features connecting the pre-frontal lobes, whose white matter integrity is known to correlate with changes in behavioural performance over time[12].

It is true that more sophisticated diffusion models such as diffusion spectrum imaging have produced more detailed connected networks [15] and therefore we acknowledge that steps do need to be taken to improve accuracy of the model through better registration (so that ROIs can be assumed correct with a high degree of accuracy) and extension to multiple-fibre tractography models (such that all connections are well approximated). Nevertheless, notwithstanding any limitations, this group study has shown great potential for the discrimination of subject groups by nature of their whole brain connectivity. Studies of this kind have the potential to highlight the key connective features which best describe anatomical segregation across subject groups. And, though care must be taken to verify the results with histology and current clinical opinion, if studied in line with functional research such features may help to vastly improve understanding of the origins of behavioural change. Furthermore, extensions to multiple class or unsupervised learning approaches may allow us to model healthy ageing.

References

1. Behrens, T., Woolrich, M., Jenkinson, M., Johansen-Burg, H., Nunes, R., Clare, S., Matthews, P., Brady, J., Smith, S.: Characterization and propagation of uncertainty in diffusion-weighted mr imaging. Magn. Res. Med. Anal. 50, 1077–1088 (2003)
2. Behrens, T., Johansen-Burg, H.: Relating connectional architecture to grey matter function using diffusion imaging. Phil. Trans. R. Soc. B 360, 903–911 (2005)
3. Counsell, S., Dyet, L., Larkman, D., Nunes, R., Boardman, J., Allsop, J., Fitzpatrick, J., Srinivasan, L., Cowan, F., Hajnal, J., Rutherford, M.: Edwards: Thalamo-cortical connectivity in children born preterm mapped using probabilistic magnetic resonance tractography. Neuroimage 34, 896–904 (2006)
4. Honey, C., Kötter, R., Breakspear, M., Sporns, O.: Network structure of cerebral cortex shapes functional connectivity on multiple time scales. PNAS 24, 10240–10245 (2007)
5. Achard, S., Salvador, R., Whitcher, B., Suckling, J., Bullmore, E.: A resilient low frequency small-world human brain functional network with highly connected association cortical hubs. J. Neuroscience 26, 63–72 (2006)
6. Iturria-Medina, Y., Canales-Rodrígues, E., Melie-García, L., Valdés-Hernández, P., Martínez-Montes, E., Alemán-Gómez, Y., Sánchez-Bornot, J.: Characterizing brain anatomical connections using diffusion weighted MRI and graph theory. Neuroimage 36, 645–660 (2007)
7. Burges, C.: A tutorial on support vector machines for pattern recognition. Data mining and knowledge discovery 2, 121–167 (1998)
8. Valstar, M.F., Pantic, M.: Fully automatic facial action unit detection and temporal analysis. In: CVPR, pp. 149–126 (2006)
9. Heckemann, R., Hajnal, J., Aljabar, P., Rueckert, D., Hammers, A.: Automatic anatomical brain MRI segmentation combining label propagation and decision fusion. Neuroimage 33, 115–126 (2006)
10. Aljabar, P., Heckemann, R., Hammers, A., Hajnal, J.V., Rueckert, D.: Classifier selection strategies for label fusion using large scale atlas databases. In: Medical Image Computing and Computer-Assisted Intervention, pp. 523–531 (2006)
11. Ashburner, J., Friston, K.: Unified segmentation. Neuroimage 26, 839–851 (2005)
12. Madden, D., Whiting, W., Huettel, S., White, L., MacFall, J., Provenzale, J.: Diffusion tensor imaging of adult age differences in cerebral white matter:relation to response time. NeuroImage 21, 1174–1181 (2004)
13. Oh, J., Song, I., Lee, J., Kang, H., Park, K., Kang, E., Loo, D.: Tractography guided statistics in diffusion tensor imaging for the detection of gender difference in fiber integrity of the corpora callosa. NeuroImage 36, 606–616 (2007)
14. Davatzikos, C., Resnick, S.: Sex differences in anatomic measures of interhemispheric connectivity; correlations with cognition in women but not men. Cerebral Cortex 8, 635–640 (1998)
15. Hagmann, P., Kurant, M., Gigandet, X., Thiran, P., Wedeen, V., Meuli, R., Thiran, J.: Mapping human whole-brain structural networks with diffusion MRI. PLoSONE 7, 597 (2007)

Optimized Conformal Parameterization of Cortical Surfaces Using Shape Based Matching of Landmark Curves

Lok Ming Lui[1], Sheshadri Thiruvenkadam[1], Yalin Wang[1,2], Tony Chan[1], and Paul Thompson[2]

[1] Department of Mathematics, UCLA, Los Angeles, CA 90095-1555
[2] Laboratory of Neuro Imaging and Brain Research Institute, UCLA School of Medicine, CA 90095-1555

Abstract. In this work, we find *meaningful* parameterizations of cortical surfaces utilizing prior anatomical information in the form of anatomical landmarks (sulci curves) on the surfaces. Specifically we generate close to conformal parametrizations that also give a *shape-based* correspondence between the landmark curves. We propose a variational energy that measures the harmonic energy of the parameterization *maps*, and the shape dissimilarity between mapped points on the landmark curves. The novelty is that the computed maps are guaranteed to give a *shape-based* diffeomorphism between the landmark curves. We achieve this by intrinsically modelling our search space of maps as flows of smooth vector fields that do not flow across the landmark curves, and by using the local surface geometry on the curves to define a shape measure. Such parameterizations ensure consistent correspondence between anatomical features, ensuring correct averaging and comparison of data across subjects. The utility of our model is demonstrated in experiments on cortical surfaces with landmarks delineated, which show that our computed maps give a shape-based alignment of the sulcal curves without significantly impairing conformality.

1 Introduction

Parametrization of the cortical surface is a key problem in brain mapping research. Applications include the registration of functional activation data across subjects, statistical shape analysis, morphometry, and processing of signals on brain surfaces (e.g., denoising or filtering). Applications that compare surface data often make use of surface *diffeomorphisms* that result from parameterization. For the above diffeomorphisms to map data consistently across surfaces, parametrizations are required that preserves the original surface geometry as much as possible. Parameterizations should also be chosen so that the resulting diffeomorphisms between surfaces align key anatomical features consistently.

Conformal mapping [1,2] is particularly convenient for genus-zero cortical surface models since it gives a parameterization without angular distortions, and comes with computational advantages when solving PDEs on surfaces using grid-based and metric-based computations [3]. However, the above parameterization is not guaranteed to map anatomical features, such as sulcal landmarks, consistently from subject to subject [2,4].

Landmark-based *diffeomorphisms* [4,5,6,7,8,9] are often used to compute, or adjust, cortical surface parameterizations. Similarly to the above works, given two cortical surfaces with anatomical landmarks (sulci curves), we want to find close to conformal parameterizations for the surfaces driven by shape based correspondences (*registration*) between the curves. Our work has three main contributions; first, the surface diffeomorphism resulting from our parameterization maps the sulcal curves *exactly*; second, the correspondence is shape based, i.e., maps similarly-shaped segments of sulcal curves to each other; finally, the conformality of the surface parameterizations is preserved to the greatest possible extent.

Optimization of surface diffeomorphisms by landmark matching has been studied intensively. Gu et al. [2] optimized the conformal parametrization by composing an optimal Möbius transformation so that it minimizes a landmark mismatch energy. The resulting parameterization remains conformal. Glaunes et al.[6] proposed to generate large deformation diffeomorphisms of the sphere onto itself, given the displacements of a finite set of template landmarks. The diffeomorphism obtained can match landmark features well, but it is, in general, not a conformal mapping, which can be advantageous for solving PDEs on the resulting grids. Leow et al.[7] proposed a level-set based approach for matching different types of features, including points and 2D or 3D curves represented as implicit functions.

Tosun et al. [8] proposed a more automated mapping technique that results in good sulcal alignment across subjects, by combining parametric relaxation, iterative closest point registration and inverse stereographic projection. Wang et al. [4] proposed an energy that computes maps that are close to conformal and also driven by a landmark matching term that measures the Euclidean distance between the specified landmarks.

Many of the above methods e.g. [4,6] require corresponding landmark points on the surfaces to be labeled in advance. Secondly, the landmark match measures used above are based on Euclidean distance, or overlap of level set functions representing the landmarks, and do not use shape information to guide correspondences of features within curves. So, the resulting correspondences would be unreliable in the case of landmark curves that differ by non-rigid deformations. Finally, constraining the surface diffeomorphism to exactly align the landmark curves during minimization is difficult, e.g. [4,8].

To resolve the above issues, we propose a method to optimize the conformal parameterization of the surfaces while non-rigidly registering the landmark curves. Specifically, we formulate our problem as a variational energy defined on a search space of diffeomorphisms generated as flows of smooth vector fields. The vector fields are restricted only to those that *do not flow* across the landmark curves (to enforce exact landmark correspondence). Our energy has 2 terms: (1) a shape term to map similar shaped segments of the landmark curves to each other, and (2) a harmonic energy term to optimize the conformality of the parametrization maps.

2 Model

Given two cortical surfaces M_1 and M_2, with sulcal landmark curves $\hat{C}_1$ and $\hat{C}_2$ labeled on them. The curves $\hat{C}_i$ have the same topology relative to M_i. These landmarks curves can be detected automatically by the automatic landmark tracking technique introduced by Lui et al. [10]. Here, we want to find diffeomorphisms $\hat{f}_1 : \Omega \subset \Re^2 \to M_1$, $\hat{f}_2 : \Omega \to M_2$ such that $\hat{f}_2 \circ \hat{f}_1^{-1}|_{\hat{C}_1}$ is a shape based diffeomorphism onto $\hat{C}_2$, i.e $\hat{f}_2 \circ \hat{f}_1^{-1}$ maps *similarly shaped* segments of $\hat{C}_1$ and $\hat{C}_2$ to each other. Also we want $\hat{f}_i$ to be as conformal as possible.

To simplify our computations, M_i are firstly conformally parameterized onto the conformal parameter domain D_i. Assume that $\hat{C}_i$ are mapped to C_i on the parameter domain D_i. Thus, our problem is reduced to the 2D problem of finding diffeomorphism $\tilde{f}_i : \Omega \to D_i$ such that $\tilde{f}_2 \circ \tilde{f}_1^{-1}|_{C_1} = C_2$ is a shape-based diffeomorphism onto C_2. We propose our problem as the minimization of a variational energy with respect to diffeomorphisms $\tilde{f}_i : \Omega \to D_i$, subject to the correspondence constraint $\tilde{f}_2 \circ \tilde{f}_1^{-1}(C_1) = C_2$. The energy consists of two terms. The first term measures the harmonic energy of the maps $\tilde{f}_i$, and the second term measures the shape dissimilarity between C_1 and $\tilde{f}_2 \circ \tilde{f}_1^{-1}(C_1)$.

To handle the above correspondence constraint, we move all our computations to the parameter domain Ω using initial diffeomorphisms $f_{0,i} : \Omega \to D_i$. Let $C \subset \Omega$ be a topological representative of C_i, with $f_{0,i}(C) = C_i$. With the above framework, the energy is formulated over Ω, and the search space of diffeomorphisms $\tilde{f}_i : \Omega \to D_i$, subject to $\tilde{f}_2 \circ \tilde{f}_1^{-1}(C_1) = C_2$, can be constructed as time-1 flows of smooth vector fields on Ω that do not flow across C. For the shape term, we measure the shape dissimilarity between the corresponding landmarks which minimizes the difference in *geodesic curvatures* on the corresponding pairs of points on C_1 and C_2. We discuss the details in the following sections.

2.1 Formulation

The initial diffeomorphisms $f_{0,i}$ give us a convenient way to perform our computations on the domain Ω. Diffeomorphisms $\tilde{f}_i : \Omega \to D_i$ with $\tilde{f}_2 \circ \tilde{f}_1^{-1}(C_1) = C_2$ can be realized through unique diffeomorphisms $f_i : \Omega \to \Omega$ with $f_i(C) = C$, satisfying $\tilde{f}_i = f_{0,i} \circ f_i$ (Fig. 1(left)). Thus we formulate our problem as the minimization of the following energy over diffeomorphisms $f_i : \Omega \to \Omega$ with $f_i(C) = C$. Denote $\tilde{f}_i = f_{0,i} \circ f_i$, $F = [\tilde{f}_1, \tilde{f}_2]$,

$$E[f_1, f_2] = \int_\Omega |\nabla \tilde{f}_1|^2 + |\nabla \tilde{f}_2|^2 \, dx + \lambda \int_C \left(\kappa_1(\tilde{f}_1) - \kappa_2(\tilde{f}_2)\right)^2 |F_x \wedge F_y| \, ds \quad (1)$$

The first term is the harmonic energy of $\tilde{f}_i$. The second term is a *symmetric* shape term defined as an arc length integral over $F(C)$, similar to Thiruvenkadam et al. [11]. Here, the shape measure $\kappa_i(p_i)$ is determined by the geodesic curvature of M_i corresponding to the point p_i. Defining the symmetric shape measure over $F(C)$ makes the term independent of the choice of the initial maps $f_{0,i}$, and also avoids local minima problems that occur while matching flat curve segments.

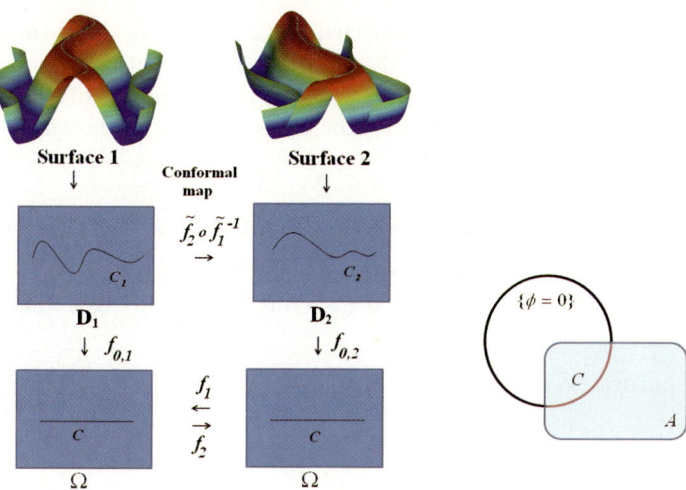

Fig. 1. The left panels show the framework of our algorithm. The right panel shows the level set representation for C (Brown open curve), $C = \{\phi = 0\} \cap A$. A is the shaded region, $\{\phi = 0\}$ is the circle.

In the above energy, using a search space of diffeomorphisms $f_i : \Omega \to \Omega$, and then imposing $f_i(C) = C$ as a constraint during minimization is difficult. Hence we propose a method to directly consider a *reduced search space* of diffeomorphisms $f_i : \Omega \to \Omega$ that satisfy $f_i(C) = C$.

2.2 Level Set Representation for C

Since we are dealing with the sulcal curves as our landmarks, we assume that $C = \cup_{k=1}^{N} \Gamma_k$, a union of open curves $\Gamma_k \subset \Omega$. We represent C implicitly in level set form to be able to write the second integral in energy (1) with respect to x. Being the union of open curves, C can be represented as the intersection of the 0-level set of a signed distance function ϕ, and a region A (Fig. 1(right)). Then the arc length integral of C becomes

$$\int_C ds = \int_\Omega \chi_A \, |\nabla H(\phi)| \, dx,$$

where $H(t)$ is a regularized version of the Heaviside function.

2.3 Modelling the Search Space for f_i

To construct an appropriate search space for f_i, we consider smooth vector fields, $\boldsymbol{X_i} = a_i \frac{\partial}{\partial x} + b_i \frac{\partial}{\partial y}$, where $a_i, b_i : \Omega \to \Re$ are C^1 functions with compact support. Then the flow of $\boldsymbol{X_i}$, $\Phi^{\boldsymbol{X_i}}(\mathbf{x}, t)$ is given by the differential equation,

$$\frac{\partial \Phi^{\boldsymbol{X_i}}}{\partial t}(\mathbf{x}, t) = \boldsymbol{X_i}(\Phi^{\boldsymbol{X_i}}(\mathbf{x}, t)),$$

$$\Phi^{\boldsymbol{X_i}}(\mathbf{x}, 0) = \mathbf{x}.$$

Then the time-1 flow $\Phi^{\boldsymbol{X_i}}(\mathbf{x}, 1) : \Omega \to \Omega$ is a diffeomorphism.

Now let $\boldsymbol{n} := \tilde{\delta}(\phi) \, \tilde{\chi}_A \nabla \phi$, for regularized versions $\tilde{\delta}, \tilde{\chi}_A$ of the Dirac-δ function, and χ_A. We see that $\boldsymbol{n}$ coincides with the unit-normal vector field on C. Let η_{ep} be a smooth function on Ω such that $\eta_{ep} = 0$ at the endpoints of the open curves $\Gamma_k \subset C$, $k = 1, 2, ..N$. Consider the vector fields $\boldsymbol{Y}_i$ that do not *flow across* C,

$$\boldsymbol{Y}_i = P_C \boldsymbol{X}_i := \eta_{ep} \left(\boldsymbol{X}_i - (\boldsymbol{X}_i \cdot \boldsymbol{n})\boldsymbol{n}_i \right).$$

We notice the following properties for the time-1 flow, $\Phi^{\boldsymbol{Y}_i}(.,1)$,

- $\Phi^{\boldsymbol{Y}_i}(.,1) : \Omega \to \Omega$ is a diffeomorphism since $\boldsymbol{Y}_i$ is C^1.
- Also $\boldsymbol{Y}_i|_C$ is a C^1 vector field *on* C. Thus $\Phi^{\boldsymbol{Y}_i}(.,1)|_C$ is a diffeomorphism onto C.

Hence it is natural to set $f_i = \Phi^{\boldsymbol{Y}_i}(.,1)$.

2.4 Energy

We formulate the energy (1) over the space of C^1 smooth vector fields on Ω, $\boldsymbol{X}_i = a_i \frac{\partial}{\partial x} + b_i \frac{\partial}{\partial y}$,
$J[a_i, b_i] =$

$$\int_\Omega |\nabla \tilde{f}_1|^2 + |\nabla \tilde{f}_2|^2 \, dx + \lambda \int_\Omega \chi_A \left(\kappa_1(\tilde{f}_1) - \kappa_2(\tilde{f}_2) \right)^2 |\nabla H(\phi)| \, |F_x \wedge F_y| \, dx$$
$$+ \beta \int_\Omega |D\boldsymbol{X}_1|^2 + |D\boldsymbol{X}_2|^2 \, dx \quad (2)$$

Here, as before $\tilde{f}_i = f_{0,i} \circ f_i$, and $f_i = \Phi^{\boldsymbol{Y}_i}(.,1)$, the time-1 flow of the vector field $\boldsymbol{Y}_i = P_C \boldsymbol{X}_i$. The last integral in the energy is the smoothness term for the vector fields $\boldsymbol{X}_i$. To minimize the above energy, we can iteratively modify the vector field $\boldsymbol{X}_i$ by the following Euler-Lagrange equation:

$$\frac{da_i}{dt} = \int_0^1 B_i(\phi_s^{\boldsymbol{Y}_i}) \, \Psi_i(\phi_s^{\boldsymbol{Y}_i}, 1) \, \Psi_i^{-1}(\phi_s^{\boldsymbol{Y}_i}, s) \, P_C e_1 \, |D\phi_s^{\boldsymbol{Y}_i}| \, ds - \beta \Delta a_i$$

$$\frac{db_i}{dt} = \int_0^1 B_i(\phi_s^{\boldsymbol{Y}_i}) \, \Psi_i(\phi_s^{\boldsymbol{Y}_i}, 1) \, \Psi_i^{-1}(\phi_s^{\boldsymbol{Y}_i}, s) \, P_C e_2 \, |D\phi_s^{\boldsymbol{Y}_i}| \, ds - \beta \Delta b_i,$$

where: $B_i := -\Delta \tilde{f}_i \, Df_{0,i} + \lambda \chi_A \left((-1)^{i-1} (\kappa_1(\tilde{f}_1) - \kappa_2(\tilde{f}_2)) \nabla \kappa_i - \nabla \cdot C_i \right) Df_{0,i} \, |\nabla H(\phi)|$;
Ψ_i is the orthogonal fundamental matrix for the homogeneous system of

$$\frac{\partial}{\partial t} P_i(x,t) = \eta P_C e_1 \left(\Phi^{\boldsymbol{Y}_i}(x,t) \right) + D\boldsymbol{Y}_i(\Phi^{\boldsymbol{Y}_i}(x,t)) \, P_i(x,t), \quad P_i(x,0) = \boldsymbol{0}.$$

3 Experimental Results

We have tested our automatic landmark tracking algorithm on cortical hemispheric surfaces extracted from brain MRI scans, acquired from normal subjects at 1.5 T (on a GE Signa scanner). Experimental results show that our algorithm can effectively compute cortical surface parameterizations that align the landmark features in a way that also enforces shape correspondence, while preserving

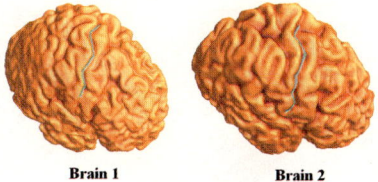

Fig. 2. The figure shows two different cortical surfaces with sulcal landmarks

the conformality of the surface-to-surface mapping to the greatest extent possible. The computed map is guaranteed to be a diffeomorphism because the map is formulated as the integral flow of a smooth vector field.

Figure 2 shows two different cortical surfaces with sulcal landmarks labeled on them. We seek parameterizations of these surfaces that align the landmark features consistently while optimally preserving conformality. A diffeomorphism between the two surfaces is then obtained by computing the composition of the two parameterizations. Figure 3 shows the result of matching the cortical surfaces with one landmark labeled (for purposes of illustration) on each brain. Figure 3(A) shows the cortical surface of Brain 1. It is mapped to the cortical surface of Brain 2 under the conformal parameterization as shown in Figure 3(B). Note that the sulcal landmark on Brain 1 is only mapped approximately to the sulcal region on Brain 2. It is not mapped exactly to the corresponding sulcal landmark on Brain 2. Figure 3(C) shows the matching result under the parameterization we propose in this paper. Note that the corresponding landmarks are mapped exactly. Also, the correspondence between the landmark curves follows the shape information.

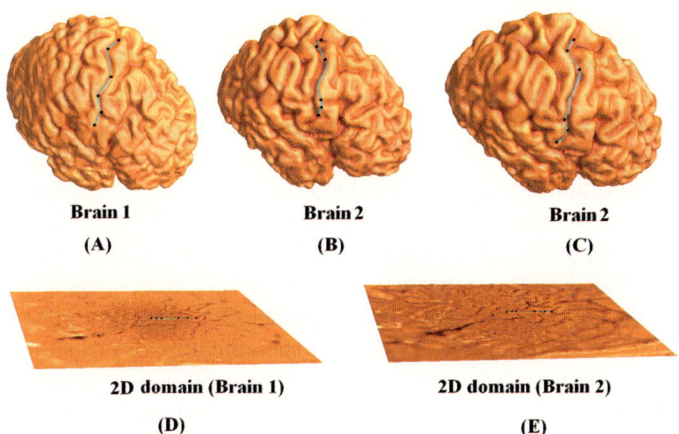

Fig. 3. This figure shows the result of matching the cortical surfaces with one landmark labeled. (A) shows the surface of Brain 1. It is mapped to Brain 2 under conformal parameterization, as shown in (B). (C) shows the result of matching using our proposed algorithm. (D) and (E) show the standard 2D parameter domains for Brain 1 and Brain 2 respectively.

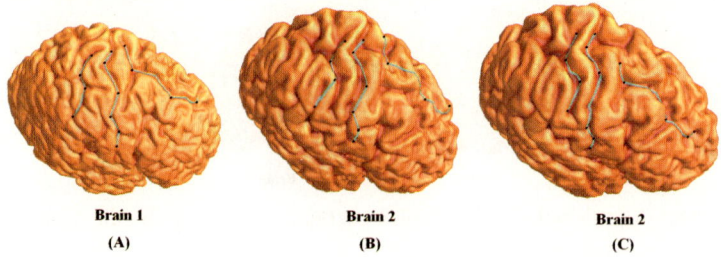

Fig. 4. Illustration of the result of matching the cortical surfaces with several sulcal landmarks. (A) shows the brain surface 1. It is mapped to brain surface 2 under the conformal parameterization as shown in (B). (C) shows the result of matching under our proposed parameterization.

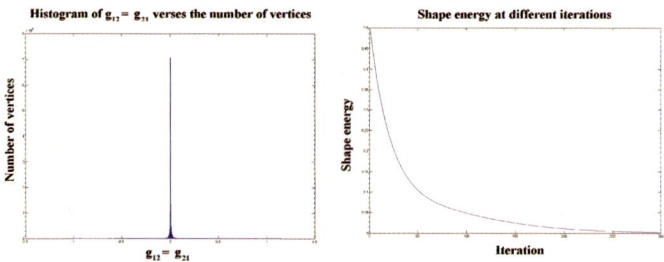

Fig. 5. The left shows the histogram of $g_{12} = g_{21}$ of the brain surface under the parameterization computed with our algorithm. The right shows the shape energy at different iterations.

It maps the secondary features of one landmark curve to the secondary features of the other landmark curve (See the black dots). Figure 3(D) and (E) show the standard 2D parameter domain of Brain 1 and Brain 2 respectively. The landmark curve is mapped to same horizontal line and the shape feature are mapped to the same positions (see the black dots). This is advantageous as the surface average of many subjects would retain features that consistently occur on sulci, while uniform speed parameterizations may cause these features to cancel out. Figure 4 gives an illustration of the matching results for cortical surfaces with several sulcal landmarks labeled on them. Figure 4(A) shows the brain surface 1 with several landmarks labeled. It is mapped to brain surface 2 under the conformal parameterization as shown in Figure 4(B). Again, the sulcal landmarks on Brain 1 are only mapped approximately to the sulcal regions on Brain 2. Figure 4(C) shows the matching result under the parameterization we proposed. The corresponding landmarks are mapped exactly. Also, the correspondence between the landmark curves follows the shape information (corners to corners [See the black dot]). To examine the conformality of the parameterization, we show in Figure 5($Left$) the histogram of $g_{12} = g_{21}$ of the Riemannian metric under the parameterization computed with our proposed algorithm. Observe that $g_{12} = g_{21}$ are very close to zero at most vertices. This means that the Riemannian metric is a diagonal matrix, thus the parameterization computed is very close to conformal. It also shows that conformal map being intrinsic to global surface geometry, is not significantly affected by small changes in the local geometry induced by the shape term. Figure 5(*Right*) shows that the shape energy is decreasing with iterations, implying an improving shape based correspondence between the landmark curves.

4 Conclusion and Future Work

In this paper, we developed an algorithm to find parametrizations of the cortical surfaces that are close to conformal and also give a *shape based* correspondence between embedded landmark curves. We propose a variational approach by minimizing an energy that measures the harmonic energy of the parameterization *maps*, and the shape dissimilarity between mapped points on the landmark curves. The parameterizations computed are guaranteed to give a *shape-based* diffeomorphism between the landmark curves. Experimental results show that our algorithm can effectively compute parameterizations of cortical surfaces that align landmark features consistently with shape correspondence, while preserving the conformality as much as possible. As future work, we plan to apply this algorithm to cortical models from healthy and diseased subjects to build population shape averages. The enforcement of higher-order shape correspondences may allow subtle but systematic differences in cortical patterning to be detected, for instance in neurodevelopmental disorders such as Williams syndrome, where the scope of cortical folding anomalies is of great interest but currently unknown. Another area of interest is to work on better numerical schemes to improve computational efficiency and accuracy.

References

1. Haker, S., Angenent, S., Tannenbaum, A., Kikinis, R., Sapiro, G., Halle, M.: IEEE TVCG 6(2), 181–189 (2000)
2. Gu, X., Wang, Y., Chan, T.F., Thompson, P.M., Yau, S.T.: IEEE TMI 23(8), 949–958 (2004)
3. Lui, L., Wang, Y., Chan, T.F.: VLSM. In: ICCV (2005)
4. Wang, Y., Lui, L., Chan, T.F., Thompson, P.: In: Duncan, J.S., Gerig, G. (eds.) MICCAI 2005, Part I. LNCS, vol. 3750, pp. 675–683. Springer, Heidelberg (2005)
5. Gu, X., Yau, S.: ACM Symp. on Geom. Processing 2003 (2003)
6. Glaunés, J., Vaillant, M., Miller, M.: J. Maths. Imaging and Vision 20, 179–200 (2004)
7. Leow, A., Yu, C., Lee, S., Huang, S., Protas, H., Nicolson, R., Hayashi, K., Toga, A., Thompson, P.: NeuroImage 24(3), 910–927 (2005)
8. Tosun, D., Rettmann, M., Prince, J.: Med. Image Anal. 8(3), 295–309 (2004)
9. Thompson, P., Hayashi, K., Sowell, E., Gogtay, N., Giedd, J., Rapoport, J., de Zubicaray, G., Janke, A., Rose, S., Semple, J., Doddrell, D., Wang, Y., van Erp, T., Cannon, T., Toga, A.: NeuroImage 23, S2–S18 (2004)
10. Lui, L.M., Wang, Y., Chan, T.F., Thompson, P.: IEEE (CVPR), New York 2, 1784–1792 (2006)
11. Thiruvenkadam, S., Groisser, D., Chen, Y.: VLSM (2005)

Construction of Hierarchical Multi-Organ Statistical Atlases and Their Application to Multi-Organ Segmentation from CT Images

Toshiyuki Okada[1,2], Keita Yokota[1,2], Masatoshi Hori[3], Masahiko Nakamoto[2,1], Hironobu Nakamura[3], and Yoshinobu Sato[2,1]

[1] Graduate School of Information Science and Technology, Osaka University,
[2] Division of Image Analysis,
[3] Department of Radiology,
Graduate School of Medicine, Osaka University, Suita, Osaka 565-0871, Japan

Abstract. Hierarchical multi-organ statistical atlases are constructed with the aim of achieving fully automated segmentation of the liver and related organs from computed tomography images. Constraints on inter-relations among organs are embedded in hierarchical organization of probabilistic atlases (PAs) and statistical shape models (SSMs). Hierarchical PAs are constructed based on the hierarchical nature of inter-organ relationships. Multi-organ SSMs (MO-SSMs) are combined with previously proposed single-organ multi-level SSMs (ML-SSMs). A hierarchical segmentation procedure is then formulated using the constructed hierarchical atlases. The basic approach consists of hierarchical recursive processes of initial region extraction using PAs and subsequent refinement using ML/MO-SSMs. The experimental results show that segmentation accuracy of the liver was improved by incorporating constraints on inter-organ relationships.

1 Introduction

Statistical atlases, which represent anatomical variations among individuals, have been shown to be useful for segmentation and quantification of medical images [1]. In previous work, statistical atlases have typically been constructed for a single organ in a uniform manner [1]. However, multiple organs are interrelated in the human body. Furthermore, the hierarchical nature is involved in the shape of a single organ, as well as multi-organ inter-relationships. Our previous study developed hierarchically decomposed statistical shape models (SSMs) [2]. Although the developed models were shown to be useful for accurate segmentation due to the hierarchical nature, the results in [2] clarified that explicit incorporation of the constraints of adjacent organs is essential to further improve accuracy. Statistical modeling of multi-organ structures will thus provide useful information for robust segmentation and shape recovery from medical images. Recent work [3] has tried to incorporate inter-organ relationships into SSMs. The basic limitation, however, is that quite large variations need to be statistically modeled for inter-organ relationships compared with a single organ. A quite large number of learning datasets are needed to model complex structures. Due to this limitation, previous works limited applications to 2D or simple 3D shapes [3].

In this paper, we embed the constraints for multi-organ inter-relationships into hierarchically organized statistical atlases to deal with the large variations involved. Hierarchical organization schemes have been developed for two atlas representations: probabilistic atlases (PAs) [4] and SSMs [1]. Spatial normalization for constructing and utilizing PAs is progressively performed based on the predefined hierarchy of organ structures. SSMs are also hierarchically constructed within single organ shape, as well as across multiple organs. Sub-shapes within a single organ shape or sub-shapes across multiple organ shapes are hierarchically organized. By restricting SSM construction to local sub-shapes in inter-related organs rather than to whole shapes, variations in multi-organ inter-relationships are effectively modeled using a moderate number of training datasets. Further, multi-organ SSMs of whole shapes are realized by hierarchical organization of SSMs constructed for decomposed sub-shapes. Hierarchy in constructed PAs and SSMs is directly linked to a hierarchical automated segmentation procedure, where hierarchically normalized PAs are utilized to provide good initial conditions for subsequent multi-organ SSM fitting. We experimentally evaluated the effects of integrating multi-organ inter-relationships on performance improvements in segmentation results of the liver from computed tomography (CT).

2 Methods

2.1 Hierarchical Probabilistic Atlas

Given hierarchical relationships of inter-related organ structures, spatial normalization is performed according to the given hierarchy. Here, we considered the hierarchy of the abdominal cavity, liver, vena cava and gallbladder (Fig. 1). Shape and position of the anatomical structures of lower hierarchy levels, e.g., the gallbladder and vena cava, are strongly constrained by those of higher hierarchy levels, e.g., the liver. Spatial normalization for an organ of interest is performed by mapping the dataset for an individual patient into the normalized space through nonrigid registration [5] using the organ shape of the next highest hierarchy level to remove unwanted shape and positional variations as well as represent datasets in the canonical frame (left side of Fig. 2).

Before the PA is constructed, we assume that the regions of each anatomical structure have already been segmented from the CT datasets. In the case of normalization for the gallbladder and vena cava, a dense three-dimensional (3D) deformation field is obtained by nonrigid registration of individual liver shapes to the average liver shape. Gallbladder and vena cava regions are normalized based on the average liver shape by warping individual CT datasets using the obtained deformation fields. The PA is constructed by averaging the warped segmented binary images of each structure. The right side of Fig. 2 shows constructed PAs of the gallbladder and vena cava normalized using the liver in comparison with those using the abdominal cavity and those without normalization. The high-probability area (colored red) was increased in the liver-normalized PA, showing high predictive performance.

We refer to the hierarchy described in this subsection as "inter-organ hierarchy", to differentiate from "intra-organ hierarchy" described in the next section.

2.2 Hierarchical Organization of Multi-Organ Statistical Shape Models

We considered two inter-related organ shapes. Let S (e.g., the liver) and T (e.g., the vena cava or gallbladder) be the sets of vertices comprised in the surface models of the two shapes. All training datasets of S and T are nonrigidly registered to the surface model of the standard shape of S and T, respectively [5], so that they have the same topology of the vertices as the standard shape. That is, correspondences of all vertices are known among the datasets. Let S' and T' be the sets of vertices of the sub-shapes (hereafter called "patches") of S and T, respectively. Let U be the union of S' and T'. We defined multi-organ SSM (MO-SSM) as the SSM of U.

A multi-level SSM (ML-SSM) [2] of S is defined as the set of SSMs of hierarchically decomposed patches S_i and S_{ij}, which denote all patches and the j-th patch of "intra-organ hierarchy" level i, respectively, where $i = 0, 1, \cdots m$. As correspondences of all vertices among datasets are known, these decompositions can be determined for all datasets automatically if the decomposition is defined only for the standard shape dataset. T_i and $T_{ij} (i = 0, 1, \cdots, n)$ are defined similarly. Principal component analysis is performed for each patch.

In constructing MO-SSM, we assume that the set of the patches of U ($= S' \cup T'$) satisfy the conditions, $S' \subseteq S_n$ and $T' \subseteq T_m$, that is, $U \subseteq (S_n \cup T_m)$. Figure 3 shows an example of MO-SSM, where S and T are the liver and gallbladder (or vena cava), respectively, $m = 2$, and $n = 0$. The patches on S (the liver), which are closely inter-related to T are selected as S', while the whole shape of the gallbladder (or vena cava), that is T_0, is selected as T'. In this case, two patches on S at intra-organ hierarchy level 2 are selected for S', at least one vertex of which is located within the pre-determined distance to the surface of T through all datasets.

To connect two ML-SSMs for different organs with MO-SSM, the adhesiveness constraints [2] are combined. Adhesiveness constraint was originally introduced to remove inconsistencies in adjacent patches at the same hierarchy level in ML-SSM. The decomposition of patches is performed so that adjacent patches overlap each other along the boundaries. The adhesive constraint ensures that two adjacent patches adhere to each other in the overlapped area to recover the consistent whole single shape. MO-SSM of U overlaps with S and T only on patches S' and T', respectively. The adhesive constraint is applied to the overlap areas S' and T' so that the sum of the distances between vertices of MO-SSM for U and the corresponding vertices for S' or T' in ML-SSM of S or T, respectively, is sufficiently small. As the MO-SSM is limited to local region S' rather than the whole shape of S (the liver in this case), the involved variations can be efficiently encoded even without a large number of training datasets.

2.3 Hierarchical Approach to Multi-Organ Segmentation from CT

Based on the constructed hierarchical PAs and ML/MO-SSMs, a hierarchical automated segmentation procedure is derived by assuming that anatomical structure at inter-organ hierarchy level 0 has already been extracted. In this paper, we assumed that the anatomical structure at level 0 is the approximated abdominal cavity region (as shown in Fig. 1 and Fig. 2), which is extracted based on the lung and bone regions. We confirmed that the approximated abdominal cavity region can be reliably extracted using more than 100 CT datasets.

The basic approach is as follows:

Step 0: Inter-organ hierarchy level $k \leftarrow 0$.
Step 1: Region extraction of anatomical structures at inter-organ hierarchy level $k+1$ and refinement of those extracted at level k, in which datasets are spatially normalized using anatomical structures obtained at level k or higher (a smaller number means higher level).
  Step 1-1: Initial region extraction using PAs [2][6].
  Step 1-2: Refinement of extracted regions of structures at level $k+1$ using ML-SSMs [2], wherein intra-organ hierarchy is embedded (only when $k = 0$ in the experiments).
  Step 1-3: Refinement of extracted regions of structures at levels k and $k+1$ using MO-SSMs (only when $k = 1$ in the experiments).
Step 2: $k \leftarrow k + 1$. Go to Step 1.

In Step 1-1, likelihood based on position and intensity is estimated at each voxel position from PA and CT data, then voxel-based segmentation is performed [6]. In Step 1-2, ML-SSM is successively fitted to refine the segmentation. The details of these methods are described in [2][6]. In this paper, we have added new Step 1-3 for refinement of segmentation results of anatomical structures at levels $k+1$ and k using the inter-organ constraints.

Let $\mathbf{s}'$ and $\mathbf{t}'$ be the shape parameter (coefficient) vector of S' and T' in single organ ML-SSMs of S and T, respectively, and $\mathbf{u}'$ be that of the MO-SSM of U (S' and T'). Let P_S and P_T be the sets of detected edge points for S and T from CT data, respectively. The detection method for edge points is described in [1]. Given P_S and P_T, we estimate the shape parameter vector $\mathbf{s}'$, $\mathbf{t}'$, and $\mathbf{u}'$ by minimizing

$$C_1\left(\mathbf{s}', \mathbf{t}', \mathbf{u}'; P_S, P_T\right) = C_D\left(\mathbf{s}'; P_S\right) + C_D\left(\mathbf{t}'; P_T\right) + \lambda_1 C_N\left(\mathbf{s}', \mathbf{t}', \mathbf{u}'\right), \quad (1)$$

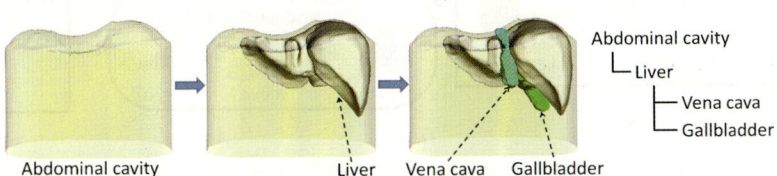

Fig. 1. Hierarchy in inter-organ relationships of the abdominal cavity, liver, vena cava and gallbladder

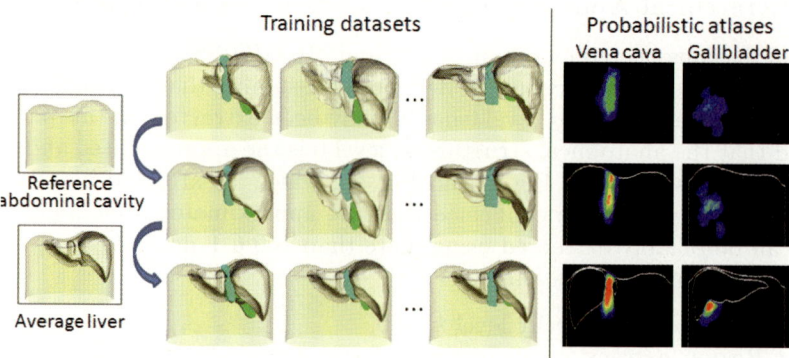

Fig. 2. Hierarchical spatial normalization (left) and resulting probabilistic atlases (right). Upper row: Original datasets. Middle row: Normalized datasets by the abdominal cavity. Lower row: Normalized datasets by the liver. In the liver-normalized space, probabilistic atlases have high probability area (colored red) compared with other probabilistic atlases having relatively wide low probability areas (colored blue).

where $C_D(\mathbf{s}'; P)$ is the sum of distances between model surface S' and edge points P, and $C_N(\mathbf{s}', \mathbf{t}', \mathbf{u}')$ is the inter-organ constraint. λ_1 is a weight parameter balancing these constraints. The edge detection process and minimization process of Eq. (1) are repeatedly performed. After this, final refinement is performed. Let $\mathbf{s}''$ be a shape parameter vector of $\mathbf{s}$ but not included in $\mathbf{s}'$ and R be the estimated shape by minimization Eq. (1). As a final process of segmentation, by fixating $\mathbf{s}'$ obtained by minimizing Eq. (1), we estimate the remaining shape parameters $\mathbf{s}''$ by minimizing

$$C_2(\mathbf{s}''; R) = C_D(\mathbf{s}''; R) + \lambda_2 C_A(\mathbf{s}''), \tag{2}$$

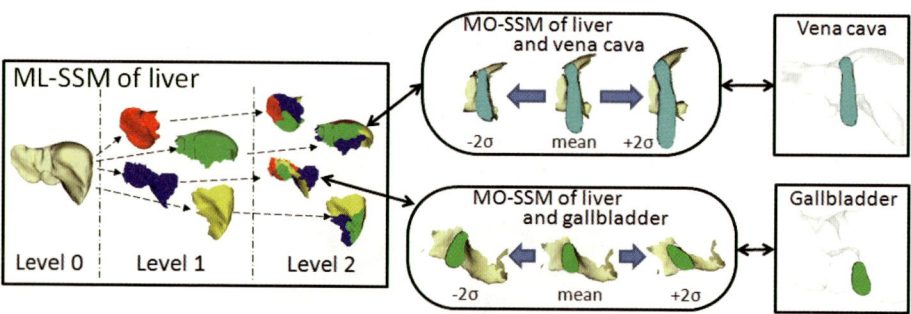

Fig. 3. Hierarchical multi-organ statistical shape models (MO-SSMs). In this case, an MO-SSM (middle) is constructed for the union of small local patches of the liver and the whole shape of the vena cava or gallbladder.

where $C_D(\mathbf{s}''; R)$ is the sum of distances between the current model surface and R, and $C_A(\mathbf{s}'')$ is the adhesiveness constraint for overlap regions to eliminate inconsistency among adjacent patches [2]. λ_2 is a weight parameter balancing the two constraints.

3 Results

Twenty-eight abdominal CT datasets (slice thickness, 2.5 mm; pitch, 1.25 mm; Field of view (FOV) 350×350 mm^2, 512×512 matrix, 159 slices) were used. Contrast agent was used for CT. We randomly selected 8 datasets for evaluation, and others for training. The hierarchical PA and ML-SSMs for the liver, vena cava and gallbladder, and MO-SSMs of liver-vena cava and liver-gallbladder were constructed from the 20 training datasets. In ML-SSMs for the vena cava and gallbladder, the number of intra-organ hierarchy levels was 1, thus representing just conventional SSMs. ML-SSM for the liver used in the experiments was the same as described in [2]. We used $\lambda_1 = 2.0$ and $\lambda_2 = 0.4$ for the MO-SSMs of liver-vena cava and liver-gallbladder, respectively, which were experimentally determined. Segmentation of the liver was performed first, then the vena cava and gallbladder were segmented. Finally, segmentation results for these three organs were refined using MO-SSMs. Given the CT datasets input for evaluation, all procedures were performed in a fully automated manner according to the basic approach described in the previous subsection.

Figures 4 (a) and (b) show the results of segmentation accuracy of the liver around the vena cava and gallbladder, respectively. Absolute surface distance (ASD) [7] was used as a measure of segmentation accuracy. Manually traced regions were used for reference. By combining MO-SSMs of liver-vena cava and liver-gallbladder, accuracy was improved in all cases compared with using the ML-SSM of the liver alone (on average from 2.69 mm to 2.04 mm around the vena cava and from 2.51 mm to 1.87 mm around the gallbladder). Figure 5 shows segmentation results for two illustrative cases. In Fig. 5 (a), MO-SSM of the liver

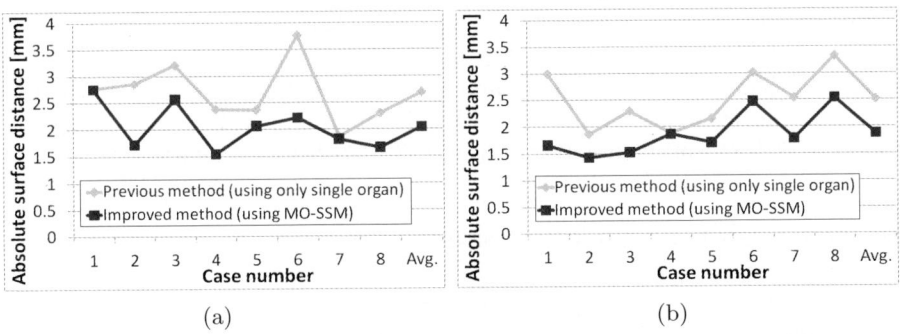

Fig. 4. Evaluation results of segmentation accuracy of the liver around (a) the vena cava and (b) gallbladder

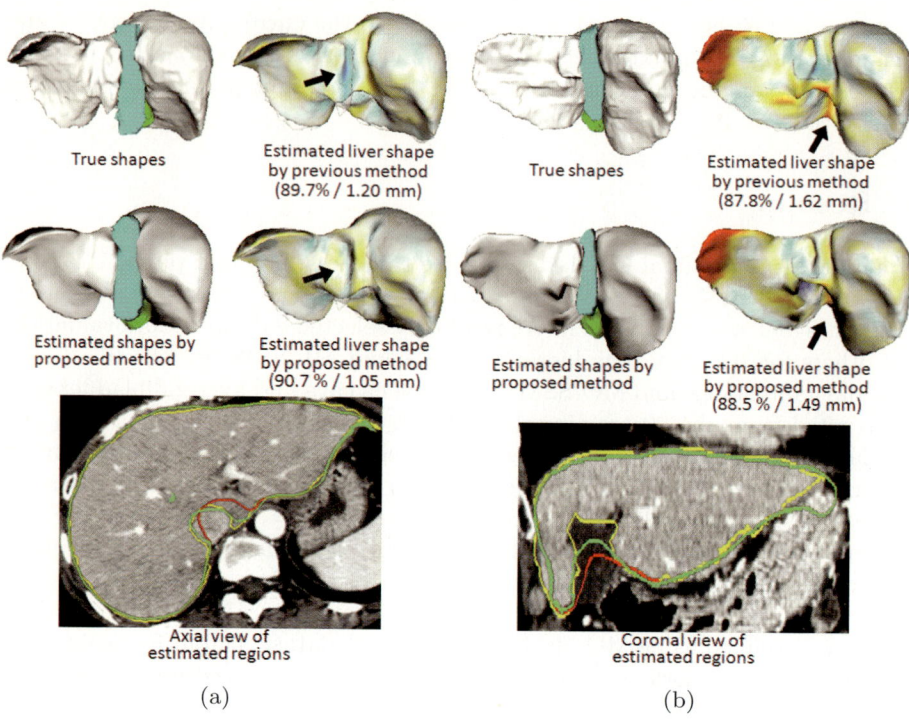

Fig. 5. Results of illustrative cases. (a) Case 2. MO-SSM of the vena cava was effective in this case (shown by arrow). (b) Case 8. MO-SSM of the gallbladder was effective in this case (shown by arrow). Estimated liver shapes are shown as color codes representing signed surface distance errors (red, convex error; white, no error; blue, concave error). Typical CT cross-sections are also shown (red contour, estimated by previous method; green, proposed method; yellow, ground truth). Note that unshown parts of the red contours overlap with the green contours.

and vena cava was effective and the segmentation result was improved around the vena cava. In Fig. 5 (b), similar improvements were observed around the gallbladder. The proposed method improves the segmentation accuracy only for local regions around the vena cava and gallbladder. By averaging over the whole liver, the improvements become superficially small and ASD was improved from 1.59 to 1.46 mm and volumetric overlap (VO) [7] from 87.9 to 88.8 %.

4 Discussion and Conclusions

We have described construction of hierarchical multi-organ statistical atlases and application of this method to segmentation of the liver and other peripheral organs (vena cava and gallbladder) from CT. Using multi-organ statistical atlases, segmentation accuracy of the liver was improved. In particular, segmentation accuracy around the caudate lobe located near the vena cava was significantly improved. The caudate lobe is a small but clinically important liver lobe, and semi-automated segmentation is considered difficult [8]. Improved segmentation accuracy around the caudate lobe is thus worthy of note.

The methods described in this paper were performed in a fully automated manner. Hierarchically organized PAs were particularly useful for automation. The initial regions of the vena cava and gallbladder were effectively extracted using PAs normalized by the average liver. Without hierarchical normalization, automation would often fail. Hierarchical organization of PAs and MO/ML-SSMs is directly linked to the hierarchical segmentation procedure.

In this work, we constructed multi-organ statistical atlases for the vena cava and gallbladder for modeling inter-relationships with the liver. However, other organs, such as the stomach, heart, and kidney, are inter-related with the liver in addition to the vena cava and gallbladder. As shown in Fig. 5 (a), large segmentation error was observed in the left lobe in two out of eight cases. This error was caused by ambiguity in boundaries of the liver and stomach. Similar error was observed at boundaries of the liver and heart in one case. Since we used contrast CT images, the boundaries of the liver and kidney were clear, and segmentation error was not observed at the boundaries. We considered that the vena cava and gallbladder are strongly constrained by the liver rather than the stomach and heart, and were incorporated into MO-SSMs first. More organs can be incorporated using the proposed method to improve segmentation accuracy of the liver. As future work, we plan to incorporate other organs, such as the stomach and heart.

References

1. Lamecker, H., et al.: Segmentation of the liver using a 3D statistical shape model. Technical report, Zuse Institue, Berlin (2004)
2. Okada, T., et al.: Automated segmentation of the liver from 3D ct images using probabilistic atlas and multi-level statistical shape model. In: Proc. Medical Image Computing and Computer-Assisted Intervention, pp. 86–93 (2007)
3. Yang, J., et al.: Neighbor-constrained segmentation with level set based 3-D deformable models. IEEE Transactions on Medical Imaging 34(8), 940–948 (2004)
4. Park, H., et al.: Construction of an abdominal probabilistic atlas and its application in segmentation. IEEE Transactions on Medical Imaging 22(4), 483–492 (2003)
5. Chui, H., et al.: A new point matching algorithm for non-rigid registration. Computer Vision and Image Understanding 89, 114–141 (2003)
6. Zhou, X., et al.: Constructing a probabilistic model for automated liver region segmentation using non-contrast X-ray torso CT images. In: Proc. Medical Image Computing and Computer-Assisted Intervention, pp. 856–863 (2006)
7. Heimann, T., et al.: MICCAI workshop on 3D segmentation in the clinic (2007), http://mbi.dkfz-heidelberg.de/grand-challenge2007/
8. Hermoye, L., et al.: Liver segmentation in living liver transplant donors: Comparison of semiautomatic and manual methods. Radiology 234(1), 171–178 (2005)

Shape-Based Alignment of Hippocampal Subfields: Evaluation in Postmortem MRI

Paul A. Yushkevich[1], Brian B. Avants[1], John Pluta[1,2], David Minkoff[1,2], John A. Detre[1,2], Murray Grossman[2], and James C. Gee[1]

[1] Department of Radiology, University of Pennsylvania
[2] Department of Neurology, University of Pennsylvania

Abstract. This paper estimates the accuracy of hippocampal subfield alignment via shape-based normalization. Evaluation takes place in postmortem MRI dataset acquired at 9.4 Tesla with many averages and approximately 0.01 mm^3 voxel resolution. Continuous medial representations (cm-reps) are used to establish geometrical correspondences between hippocampal formations in different images; the extent to which these correspondences match up subfields is evaluated and compared to normalization driven by image forces. Shape-based normalization is shown to perform only slightly worse than image-based normalization; this is encouraging because the former is more applicable to *in vivo* MRI, which typically lacks features that distinguish hippocampal subfields.

1 Introduction

The hippocampus is arguably one of the most fascinating structures in the brain, and much remains unknown about its precise role in the memory system [13]. Neurons in the hippocampus are uniquely susceptible to neurodegenerative disorders, and, in particular, Alzheimer's disease (AD) [5]; imaging-based hippocampal volumetry is a reliable early predictor of AD onset [9, 15]. The hippocampus is not a uniform structure: it is formed by two interlocking folded layers of neurons, the *cornu Ammonis (CA)* and the *dentate gyrus (DG)*, which are further divided into subfields and subserve different functional roles. Non-uniform neuron loss across the hippocampal subfields has been reported in neurodegenerative disorders [3, 4, 18], as has a non-uniform rate of neuroplasticity [8, 10, 14].

Recently, these has been much interest in measuring subfield-level changes associated with neurodegenerative diseases using MRI. However, it is very difficult to identify the boundaries of hippocampal layers in clinical MRI modalities, since the dark band separating these layers, formed by the vestigial hippocampal sulcus (VHS) and strata radiata (SR), is thinner than the typical voxel resolution. In the absence of MRI acquisitions that specifically target the hippocampus (e.g., [22]), the labeling of subfields relies primarily on shape cues, i.e., on the position of the subfields relative to the overall hippocampus shape. The primary instance of this approach is the Washington University hippocampus atlas [6, 16], in which the hippocampus template was manually labeled with the help of an anatomical reference [7].

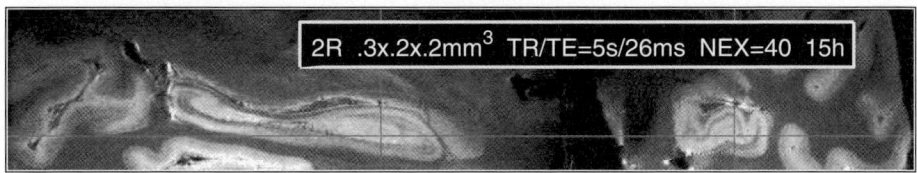

Fig. 1. Sagittal and coronal views of one of the postmortem hippocampus MRIs

Our group is developing an atlas of the human hippocampus using high-field postmortem MRI [19]. Imaging at 0.01 mm^3 voxel resolution, we are able to separate hippocampal layers and label the major subfields of the hippocampus. However, one of the main challenges associated with this atlas is how to effectively apply it to *in vivo* studies in which there are few reliable intensity features within the hippocampus. A natural approach is to use shape cues to map subfields from the atlas to manually or automatically generated segmentations of the hippocampus from *in vivo* data; as is typically done for the Washington University atlas [12, 16]. The goal of this paper is to evaluate how accurately shape-based normalization aligns hippocampal subfields between subjects.

A full evaluation of this kind would require a dataset where *in vivo* and *postmortem* images for the same subjects would be available. In absence of such data, we restrict our attention to the postmortem dataset, making a somewhat strong assumption that the segmentation of the overall hippocampus in the postmortem dataset would be sufficiently similar to the segmentation in *in vivo* data. Clearly, both manual and automatic hippocampus segmentation in *in vivo* MRI are quite challenging problems in themselves, and whatever subfield alignment errors we report in this paper would be exacerbated by errors in the segmentation of the overall hippocampus shape. Nevertheless, given the recent interest in subfield-level inference in *in vivo* MRI, we believe that the results reported in the postmortem dataset will be valuable to the field.

The evaluation experiment compares how well shape-based normalization, which does not use intensity cues, performs vis-à-vis diffeomorphic image registration driven by intensity. The latter is treated as a "gold standard", since it is using all the cues that are available in the *postmortem* dataset, and which would not be available in typical *in vivo* data.

2 Materials and Methods

2.1 Specimens and Imaging

Formalin-fixed brain specimens ($\geq$21 days) from three autopsy cases with no abnormal neuropathological findings were studied. Hemispheres were separated from the cerebellum and brain stem, and samples containing the intact hippocampus and not larger than 70mm in diameter were extracted from each hemisphere by making two incisions: the first, orthogonal to the midsagittal plane and parallel to the main axis of the hippocampus, passing through the

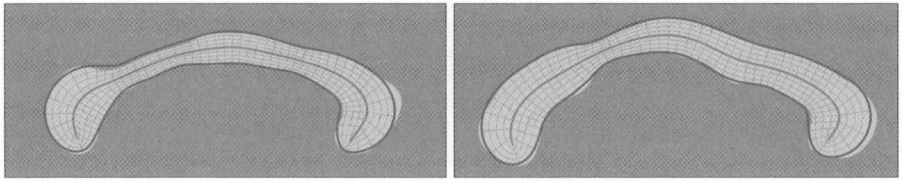

Fig. 2. A conceptual 2D illustration of shape-based normalization via the cm-rep coordinate system. The central curve is the skeleton **m**; the radial lines from the skeleton to the boundary are the spokes; the shape-based mapping between the two models is given by the locations of corresponding grid vertices.

corpus callosum; the second, parallel to the midsagittal plane, removing the lateral-most third of the sample. In our observation, the deformation caused to the hippocampus while cutting the brain was minimal, as the cuts were made a good distance away from the hippocampus.

Images of five hippocampus samples (3 right, 2 left) were acquired on a 9.4 Tesla Varian 31cm horizontal bore scanner (Varian Inc, Palo Alto, CA) using a 70mm ID TEM transmit/receive volume coil (Insight Neuroimaging Systems, Worchester, MA) and a stock multi-slice spin echo sequence. MRI parameters varied slightly across the samples; typical values are TR/TE=5000/26ms; voxel size: 0.2mm × 0.3mm × 0.2mm; matrix: 300 × 280; 130 slices; 45 averages; acquisition time around 15 hours.

2.2 Manual Segmentation

The layered structure of the hippocampus is clearly visible in our images (Fig. 1). One of the authors ([omitted for blind review]) performed the segmentation manually in ITK-SNAP (itksnap.org), using the Duvernoy atlas [7] as the main reference, and taking as much as 80 hours to label each hippocampus. The segmentation included the following labels: CA1, CA2+CA3, DG and VHS+SR. The CA4 subfield was also segmented but, following [1], we treat is a as component of the DG.

2.3 Shape-Based Normalization

Shape-based normalization uses the continuous medial representation (cm-rep) method [20, 21]. A deformable cm-rep model is fitted to each binary segmentation of the hippocampus, so as to maximize the overlap between the model and the binary image, while minimizing distortion across models. As the cm-rep model deforms, the method preserves the branching topology of the its skeleton, making it possible to leverage medial geometry for normalization and shape analysis.

A cm-rep model is defined as follows. A triangle mesh is used to represent the skeleton of the model. Each mesh node consists of a point $\mathbf{m} \in \mathbb{R}^3$ and a positive *radius* value R. The mesh is constructed by recursive subdivision of a coarse mesh using Loop subdivision rules [11]. The boundary of the model consists of two surface patches $\mathbf{b}^+$ and $\mathbf{b}^-$, one on each side of the skeleton. These boundary patches are derived from the skeleton mesh using the *inverse skeletonization* formula:

$$\mathbf{b}^\pm = \mathbf{m} + R\left(-\nabla_\mathbf{m} R \pm \sqrt{1 - \|\nabla_\mathbf{m} R\|^2}\,\mathcal{N}_\mathbf{m}\right), \tag{1}$$

where $\nabla_\mathbf{m} R$ denotes the Riemannian (surface) gradient of R on $\mathbf{m}$ and $\mathcal{N}_\mathbf{m}$ denotes the unit normal to $\mathbf{m}$. These first-order properties are computed using finite difference approximations. Constraints are in place to ensure that the two boundary patches share a common edge and do not self-intersect, thus forming a boundary of a simple region in $\mathbb{R}^3$ [21].

The interior of the cm-rep model is spanned by line segments, called *spokes*, which extend from points $\mathbf{m}_i$ on the skeleton to the corresponding points $\mathbf{b}_i^+$ and $\mathbf{b}_i^-$ on the model's boundary and which are orthogonal to the boundary. As argued in [20] and illustrated in Fig. 2, the spokes form a shape-based coordinate system on the interior of the cm-rep model.

In order to establish correspondences between cm-rep models fitted to different hippocampi, we minimize the variance in Euclidean distance between corresponding pairs of points in the shape-based coordinate system. This is done in an iterative process, to allow each model to be fitted in parallel. The correspondence energy function for model s at iteration t has the form

$$E_{\text{corr}}^{s,t} = \sum_i \sum_{j \in N(i)} \left(d_{ij}^{s,t} - \bar{d}_{ij}^{t-1}\right)^2, \tag{2}$$

where $N(i)$ denotes the grid points adjacent to grid point i, $d_{ij}^{s,t}$ is the Euclidean distance between grid points i and j in model s at iteration t, and $\bar{d}_{ij}^{t-1}$ is the average of this distance across all models at the previous iteration.

2.4 Deformable Registration

We use a diffeomorphic fluid warping method known as *Symmetric Normalization (SyN)* [2] to perform pairwise registration between hippocampus images. Given an image match metric Π (in our case, normalized cross-correlation), registration of images I and J seeks a pair of diffeomorphic maps ϕ_1, ϕ_2 that minimize

$$E(I, J, \phi_1, \phi_2) = \Pi[I(\phi_1(\mathbf{x}, \tfrac{1}{2})), J(\phi_2(\mathbf{x}, \tfrac{1}{2}))] +$$
$$+ \int_0^{\frac{1}{2}} \|\mathbf{v}_1(\mathbf{x}, t)\|_L \, dt + \int_0^{\frac{1}{2}} \|\mathbf{v}_2(\mathbf{x}, t)\|_L \, dt \;,$$
$$\text{subj. to } \frac{\partial \phi_i(\mathbf{x}, t)}{\partial t} = \mathbf{v}_i(\phi_i(\mathbf{x}, t), t)\,, \quad i = 1, 2\,. \tag{3}$$

Symmetric diffeomorphic maps from I to J and from J to I are given, respectively, by $\phi_2^{-1} \circ \phi_1$ and $\phi_1^{-1} \circ \phi_2$. Binary masks of the hippocampus are incorporated into the registration because the goal of registration in this experiment is to establish an upper bound on the performance of shape-based normalization.

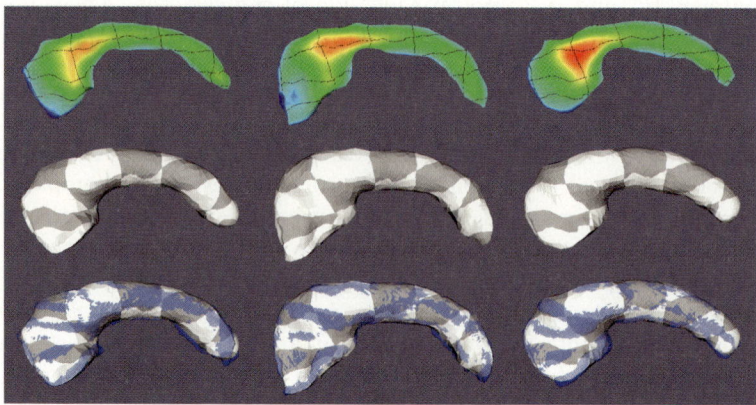

Fig. 3. Examples of cm-rep model fitting. The models' skeletons are shown in the top row, with color representing the radius field R (red: thicker, blue: thinner). The boundary is plotted in the middle row, with the checkerboard pattern showing the correspondence between models. The last row superimposes in semi-transparent blue the boundaries binary segmentations to which these models were fitted.

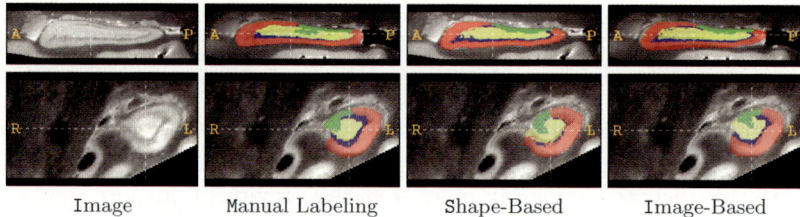

      Image   Manual Labeling   Shape-Based   Image-Based

Fig. 4. Comparison of subfield labeling in two leave-one-out experiments (top row shows sample 3L in sagittal plane; second row shows sample 2R in coronal plane). Shown are the manual segmentation of the subfields, the labeling using shape-based normalization (via cm-reps) and the labeling using image registration.

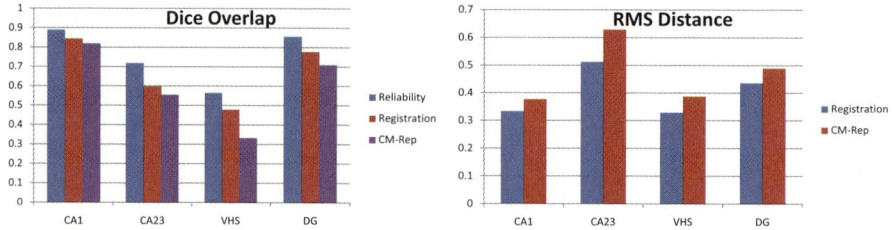

Fig. 5. Average Dice overlap (left) and average root mean square boundary distance (right) between cm-rep based subfield labeling and the manual segmentation, compared to registration-based labeling. The overlap plot also includes overlap between repeated manual segmentations by the same rater as a reference.

2.5 Evaluation of Subfield Alignment

Quantitative evaluation of the alignment of hippocampal subfields via shape-based and image-based normalization is performed in the leave-one-out framework. For a given hippocampus image I_s, a deformation field from each other hippocampus image to I_s is constructed. In the case of image registration, this field is produced by the registration algorithm; in the case of cm-rep normalization, the field is interpolated from the correspondences assigned by the coordinate system. The manually generated subfields labels for every image except I_s are deformed into the space of I_s using these warp fields, and a consensus labeling of I_s is produced by applying the STAPLE algorithm [17] to the warped labels. This consensus segmentation of I_s is compared to the manual segmentation of I_s in terms of Dice overlap and root mean square boundary distance.

3 Results

Fig. 3 illustrates cm-rep models fitted to binary hippocampus segmentations. A checkerboard map is used to illustrate the correspondence between different models. The cm-rep models do not fit the binary segmentations with complete accuracy. This is caused by the fact that the cm-rep model is constrained to have a skeleton of predefined branching topology, as well as by the contribution of the correspondence term. The average Dice overlap between the fitted models and the segmentations is 0.93. The greatest mismatch occurs in the head of the hippocampus, which has complex folding features. These features are not typically seen in hippocampus segmentations in *in vivo* data, for which the accuracy of cm-rep fitting is somewhat higher (0.95) [20].

Fig. 4 compares the labeling of hippocampal subfields in some of the cross-validation experiments. For each experiment, the labeling achieved by image-based registration, cm-rep normalization and the target manual segmentation are shown. The average over all five samples of the overlap between the manual segmentation of the subfields in each hippocampus and the segmentation generated by cm-rep normalization is plotted in Fig. 5 for each subfield, compared to the same overlap computed for image-based normalization. These overlaps are also compared to the average overlap between repeated manual segmentations by the same rater (these reliability measurements were computed only on a subset of slices). A similar comparison of root mean square distance is also shown in Fig. 5.

4 Discussion and Conclusions

The results of our evaluation experiment are encouraging but also open to interpretation. The fact that shape-based normalization, which does not use any intensity information, performs only slightly worse than image registration for subfield labeling is significant. It suggests that it may be possible to use subfield maps in the analysis of low resolution *in vivo* datasets where intensity information inside of the hippocampus is not informative for subfield differentiation. On the other hand, it has to be recognized that the overall error associated with subfield labeling, whether manual, image-based or shape-based, is substantial, even in this high-resolution postmortem dataset. It is likely that additional improvements to the segmentation protocol and the computational techniques used in this paper would result in greater consistency. Nevertheless, subfield mapping in *in vivo* datasets, which is exacerbated by the difficulty of segmenting the hippocampus itself, will likely be of limited accuracy for years to come.

Limitations of this paper include the fact that evaluation was performed on postmortem data, thus the results we report may not be representative of performance in *in vivo* datasets. There may be nonuniform shape changes introduced across the hippocampus by the preparation of brain samples after autopsy. Also, the current postmortem dataset is small and does not include pathology. We are working to address these limitations, by acquiring additional data, as well as by incorporating more advanced hippocampus-specific *in vivo* imaging techniques (e.g. [22]) into our analysis. Despite the limitations, we believe that the proposed technique, as well as the postmortem hippocampus atlas on which is is based, will be of value to morphometric studies of aging and dementia. Perhaps the 'safest' way to apply the technique is in a longitudinal study, where fluid registration can be used to derive a subject-specific atlas image, and shape-based subfield labeling would be applied to the atlas.

Acknowledgement

This project is supported by NIH grants AG027785, NS061111, MH068066 and NS045839, and the Pilot Project Award from the Penn Comprehensive Neuroscience Center.

References

1. Amaral, D.G., Scharfman, H.E., Lavenex, P.: The dentate gyrus: fundamental neuroanatomical organization (dentate gyrus for dummies). Prog. Brain. Res. 163, 3–22 (2007)
2. Avants, B.B., Epstein, C.L., Grossman, M., Gee, J.C.: Symmetric diffeomorphic image registration with cross-correlation: Evaluating automated labeling of elderly and neurodegenerative brain. Med. Image Anal. (June 2007) (in press)
3. Bobinski, M., Wegiel, J., Tarnawski, M., Bobinski, M., Reisberg, B., de Leon, M.J., Miller, D.C., Wisniewski, H.M.: Relationships between regional neuronal loss and neurofibrillary changes in the hippocampal formation and duration and severity of alzheimer disease. J. Neuropathol. Exp. Neurol. 56(4), 414–420 (1997)
4. Braak, H., Braak, E.: Neuropathological stageing of alzheimer-related changes. Acta Neuropathol. 82(4), 239–259 (1991)
5. Braak, H., Braak, E.: Staging of alzheimer's disease-related neurofibrillary changes. Neurobiol Aging 16(3), 271–278 (1995) (discussion 278–284)

6. Csernansky, J.G., Wang, L., Swank, J., Miller, J.P., Gado, M., McKeel, D., Miller, M.I., Morris, J.C.: Preclinical detection of alzheimer's disease: hippocampal shape and volume predict dementia onset in the elderly. Neuroimage 25(3), 783–792 (2005)
7. Duvernoy, H.M.: The human hippocampus, functional anatomy, vascularization and serial sections with MRI, 3rd edn. Springer, Heidelberg (2005)
8. Eriksson, P.S., Perfilieva, E., Björk-Eriksson, T., Alborn, A.M., Nordborg, C., Peterson, D.A., Gage, F.H.: Neurogenesis in the adult human hippocampus. Nat. Med. 4(11), 1313–1317 (1998)
9. Jack, C.R., Petersen, R.C., Xu, Y., O'Brien, P.C., Smith, G.E., Ivnik, R.J., Tangalos, E.G., Kokmen, E.: Rate of medial temporal lobe atrophy in typical aging and Alzheimer's disease. Neurology 51(4), 993–999 (1998)
10. Kuhn, H.G., Dickinson-Anson, H., Gage, F.H.: Neurogenesis in the dentate gyrus of the adult rat: age-related decrease of neuronal progenitor proliferation. J. Neurosci. 16(6), 2027–2033 (1996)
11. Loop, C., DeRose, T.: Generalized b-spline surfaces of arbitrary topology. In: Computer Graphics (ACM SIGGRAPH Proceedings), pp. 347–356 (1990)
12. Miller, M.I., Trouvé, A., Younes, L.: Geodesic shooting for computational anatomy. J. Math. Imaging Vis. 24(2), 209–228 (2006)
13. Squire, L.R., Stark, C.L., Clarkx, R.E.: The medial temporal lobe. Annu. Rev. Neurosci. 27, 279–306 (2004)
14. van Praag, H., Schinder, A.F., Christie, B.R., Toni, N., Palmer, T.D., Gage, F.H.: Functional neurogenesis in the adult hippocampus. Nature 415(6875), 1030–1034 (2002)
15. Visser, P.J., Verhey, F.R.J., Hofman, P.A.M., Scheltens, P., Jolles, J.: Medial temporal lobe atrophy predicts Alzheimer's disease in patients with minor cognitive impairment. J. Neurol Neurosurg Psychiatry 72(4), 491–497 (2002)
16. Wang, L., Miller, J.P., Gado, M.H., McKeel, D.W., Rothermich, M., Miller, M.I., Morris, J.C., Csernansky, J.G.: Abnormalities of hippocampal surface structure in very mild dementia of the Alzheimer type. Neuroimage 30(1), 52–60 (2006)
17. Warfield, S.K., Zou, K.H., Wells, W.M.: Simultaneous truth and performance level estimation (STAPLE): an algorithm for the validation of image segmentation. IEEE Trans. Med. Imaging 23(7), 903–921 (2004)
18. West, M.J., Kawas, C.H., Stewart, W.F., Rudow, G.L., Troncoso, J.C.: Hippocampal neurons in pre-clinical alzheimer's disease. Neurobiol. Aging 25(9), 1205–1212 (2004)
19. Yushkevich, P., Avants, B., Pluta, J., Minkoff, D., Pickup, S., Liu, W., Detre, J., Grossman, M., Gee, J.: Building an atlas of hippocampal subfields using postmortem MRI. In: IEEE International Symposium on Biomedical Imaging: Macro to Nano (to appear, 2008)
20. Yushkevich, P.A., Zhang, H., Gee, J.: Continuous medial representation for anatomical structures. IEEE Trans. Med. Imaging 25(2), 1547–1564 (2006)
21. Yushkevich, P.A., Zhang, H., Simon, T.J., Gee, J.C.: Structure-specific statistical mapping of white matter tracts. Neuroimage 41(2), 448–461 (2008)
22. Zeineh, M.M., Engel, S.A., Thompson, P.M., Bookheimer, S.Y.: Dynamics of the hippocampus during encoding and retrieval of face-name pairs. Science 299(5606), 577–580 (2003)

Customized Design of Hearing Aids Using Statistical Shape Learning

Gozde Unal[1], Delphine Nain[2], Greg Slabaugh[3], and Tong Fang[3]

[1] Faculty of Engineering and Natural Sciences, Sabanci University, Turkey
gozdeunal@sabanciuniv.edu
[2] McKinsey& Company, USA
[3] Siemens Corporate Research, Princeton NJ, USA*

Abstract. 3D shape modeling is a crucial component of rapid prototyping systems that customize shapes of implants and prosthetic devices to a patient's anatomy. In this paper, we present a solution to the problem of customized 3D shape modeling using a statistical shape analysis framework. We design a novel method to learn the relationship between two classes of shapes, which are related by certain operations or transformation. The two associated shape classes are represented in a lower dimensional manifold, and the reduced set of parameters obtained in this subspace is utilized in an estimation, which is exemplified by a multivariate regression in this paper. We demonstrate our method with a felicitous application to estimation of customized hearing aid devices.

1 Introduction

3D shape modeling and estimation is a crucial task in custom design of anatomical shapes. A sample shape estimation problem in systems for rapid prototyping of hearing aid devices is depicted in Figure 1. For a comfortable fit, it is important that the shape of the hearing aid match the patient's ear geometry. The two classes of shapes, here patients' 3D raw ear impressions and the output hearing aid shapes, are normally related by certain operations or a transformation R. Current practice involves mainly a manual design (even in an electronic environment), and the goal is to automate this process for increasing efficiency, patient comfort, repeatability, and throughput in audiologist offices.

Our work is similar in spirit to the image analogy problem [1], where a new painting D is produced by the input photograph C, by copying matching patches from a prior painting/photo pair A/B. The explicit relation between the pairs is not learned however, which is our aim in this work. The celebrated active shape models work [2] developed a compact description of the variation of shapes in a class using statistical methods. In [3], a statistical shape model is built for the human ear canal (as point clouds), where the correspondences are obtained by warping a template onto shapes, which are annotated with 18 landmarks by a specialist. In [4] a smoother dense mesh is obtained by a Markov field regularization of the correspondence field. In these works, the ear canal model is used for analysis of gender differences in its shape, and for its deformation

---

* This work is supported by Siemens Corporate Research, Princeton NJ, USA.

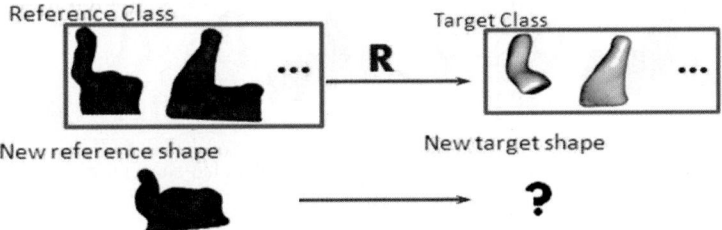

Fig. 1. Shape Estimation Problem

by mandibular movement [5]. Manual marking of landmarks is not suitable for rapid prototyping systems, moreover, finding stable feature points in all shapes is difficult due to individual variations. The correspondence problem was alleviated in an Eulerian shape representation framework in [6], which used PCA to build a shape prior to guide the segmentation of objects in images. Variations on PCA such as kernel PCA [7] and principal factor analysis [8] were employed for statistical shape analysis, although PCA is preferred here for its optimality in dimensionality reduction. In a recent work [9], regression techniques are utilized to investigate degrees of correlation and dependence variation between shapes of different structures within the brain. Our method is different in mathematical details and includes deformation of predicted shapes via predicted difference masks and fitted planes, with a focus on shape generation for prosthetic devices. [10] took a machine learning approach for image segmentation, and [11] used Frèchet expectation to generalize univariate regression to manifold-valued data to study the effect of aging on brain shape in patient populations.

Our main contribution is the development of an automatic shape transformation method to be used in various applications like customized design of anatomical parts. Our system learns the relationship between two classes of shapes and generates a shape from one class when given as an example a shape from another class. We design an asymmetric registration for shapes that significantly differ in geometry in Sec 2.1. We then propose a novel shape generation technique based on multivariate regression in Sec 2.2 and 2.3.

2 Method

There are various styles of hearing aids such as canal, and in-the-ear [12], and the design process starts with a rough mold of the patient's ear, so called undetailed shell (or shape), that is then detailed by a specialist. The detailing process includes cutting unused parts based on the desired shell style and the geometry of the patient's mold (Fig 2), rounding edges and other operations needed to fit the electronics in the shell. This is a time-consuming process that is based on the skills and experience of the specialist. Alternatively, the specialist now can carry out the detailing on digitized ear shells using CAD software systems, which are still not-fully automatic. Our work aims at removing this bottleneck in rapid prototyping systems for hearing aid devices.

We obtained 90 digitized undetailed molds and their corresponding detailed molds from a specialist. We define a "Ground truth" (GT) shape as the shape, which is detailed

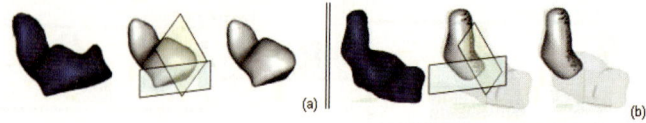

Fig. 2. Ear impressions;(a) Half shell, (b) Canal shell; undetailed shapes (left); detailed shapes with (middle) and without cutting planes (right)

by the audiologist, and is later digitized. Ear shells were digitized by a 3D laser scanner, a 3D point cloud is obtained and triangulated to build a polygonal mesh surface, which is then converted to a voxel and signed distance function (SDF) representation [6]. The dataset consisted of 41 molds of Half-Shell type (Figure 2-a), and 49 molds of Canal Shell type (2-b). The undetailed shell is made of two main parts: the long and thin structure on the top is the ear canal and the round bowl-like structure is the concha which funnels sound to the ear canal [13]. We see that the detailed half shells occupy most of the ear canal and a large part of the concha, and the detailed canal shells occupy mostly the ear canal.

2.1 Asymmetric Shape Registration

The reference (undetailed) shapes must be registered with their corresponding target (detailed) shapes in the training set. In a variational registration setting, we propose an asymmetric distance restricted to a band around both the detailed shape Φ^d and undetailed shape Φ^u, but constrained mainly by the smaller of the two shapes. This provides a new asymmetric rigid registration differential equation, which is derived from sum of squared distances energy functional between Φ^u and Φ^d:

$$\frac{\partial g_i}{\partial t} = \int_\Omega \mathcal{X}_\beta \left(\Phi^u(\boldsymbol{X}), \Phi^d(g(\boldsymbol{X})) \right) \left[\Phi^u(\boldsymbol{X}) - \Phi^d(g(\boldsymbol{X})) \right] \left\langle \nabla \Phi^d(g\boldsymbol{X}), \frac{\partial g(\boldsymbol{X})}{\partial g_i} \right\rangle d\boldsymbol{X} \quad (1)$$

where g is a rigid transformation $g(\boldsymbol{X}) = R\boldsymbol{X} + \boldsymbol{T}$, $\boldsymbol{X} \in \mathbb{R}^3$, with parameters g_i of 3D rotation matrix R, and 3D translation $\boldsymbol{T}$. Φ^u and Φ^d are the undetailed and detailed shell SDFs defined over the domain Ω. The new characteristic function takes the form

$$\mathcal{X}_\beta(\Phi_u, \Phi_d) = \begin{cases} 0, \max(|\Phi_u|, |\Phi_d|) > \beta \\ 1, \max(|\Phi_u|, |\Phi_d|) < \beta \end{cases} \quad (2)$$

Figure 3 depicts an application to ear shell registration, where the symmetric one [14] in (b) fails because the detailed shape Φ_d is significantly smaller than the undetailed shape Φ_u and parts of the undetailed shape that do not exist in the detailed shell still influence the registration. In the asymmetric version, the alignment was successful as shown in (c).

Note that in addition, all undetailed shapes in the training are aligned with the symmetric registration so that the variation in the data is due to the geometry and not the pose.

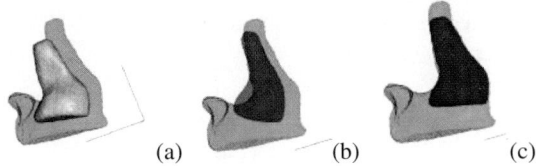

Fig. 3. Registration of detailed ear impressions to undetailed: (a) shapes before registration; (b) shape (red) after symmetric registration; (c) shape (red) after registration by Eq.(1)

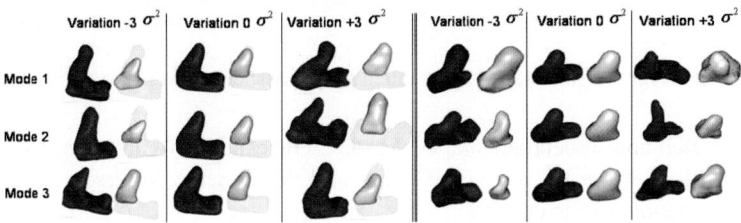

Fig. 4. The first 3 modes for both the undetailed (dark) and detailed (light) shapes. The weights are varied from $-3\sigma^2 \leq w_i \leq 3\sigma^2$. Left: Canal shell, Right: Half shell.

2.2 Shape Estimation

After alignment of the shapes, we will represent them in a lower dimensional manifold and relate the undetailed shapes with the detailed shapes on this manifold as explained next.

We conduct a standard statistical analysis on a training set of N undetailed shapes to obtain a shape variability matrix $\boldsymbol{S}^u = [\tilde{\boldsymbol{\Phi}}_1^u \; \tilde{\boldsymbol{\Phi}}_2^u \; \cdots \; \tilde{\boldsymbol{\Phi}}_N^u]$ on which a PCA is carried out: $\frac{1}{N}\boldsymbol{S}^u \boldsymbol{S}^{u\,T} = \boldsymbol{U}^u \boldsymbol{\Sigma}^u \boldsymbol{U}^{u\,T}$. Here the columns e_i^u of the matrix $\boldsymbol{U}^u$ represent the orthogonal modes of variation in the undetailed shapes, called eigenshapes, and the diagonal matrix $\boldsymbol{\Sigma}^u$ contains the corresponding eigenvalues, σ_i^u. A similar analysis is carried out for the detailed shapes. Each shape $\boldsymbol{\Phi}_i^u$ and $\boldsymbol{\Phi}_i^d$ in the undetailed and detailed classes then can be represented by a vector of weights as:

$$w_i^u = \boldsymbol{U}^{u\,T}(\boldsymbol{\Phi}_i^u - \boldsymbol{m}^u), \text{ and } w_i^d = \boldsymbol{U}^{d\,T}(\boldsymbol{\Phi}_i^d - \boldsymbol{m}^d), \quad (3)$$

where $\boldsymbol{m}^*$'s are the mean shapes. A small number of principal modes, k, which is selected as the same for both the undetailed and detailed shape classes, explains a significant portion of the variability in the ear impression shape space (see Sec 3).

Figure 4 depicts the first 3 modes of variations for both the undetailed and detailed shape datasets. In the Canal Shell dataset, we see similar variations as observed in [3]. The mode 1 deformation corresponds to a bending of the canal and a flattening of the concha for the undetailed shape, and a widening at the base of the canal and a height shift for the detailed shape. Mode 2 corresponds to a thickening of the concha and a bending of the canal for the undetailed shape and a general size change for the detailed shape. Mode 3 corresponds to a flattening of the ear canal for both shapes. For the Half Shell variations, we see that mode 1 corresponds to a general size change of the concha

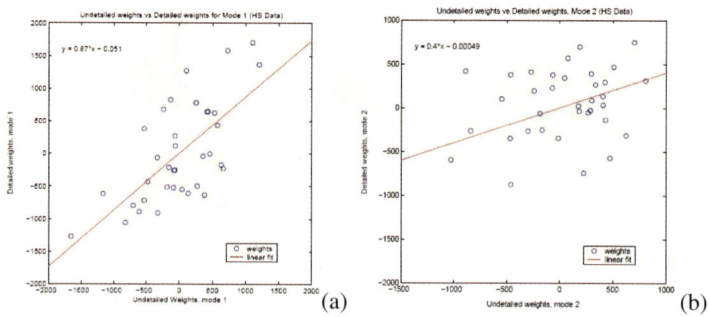

Fig. 5. The weights of undetailed vs. detailed shapes associated to 1st (a), 2nd mode (b)

for both detailed and undetailed shapes. Mode 2 corresponds to an overall size change with a flattening of the tip of the ear canal and the concha. Mode 3 corresponds to narrowing/widening of the concha and the ear canal.

For the undetailed set, we form the Nxk weight matrix $\boldsymbol{W^u}$ where row i is the vector $\boldsymbol{w_i^u}$ representing the ith undetailed shape. Similarly, $\boldsymbol{W^d}$ represents the weight matrix for the detailed shapes. We would like to find a model that best describes the relation between the two shape classes in this highly reduced dimensional space, i.e., a mapping $\boldsymbol{R}$ between the two shape representations as:

$$\boldsymbol{R} \circ \boldsymbol{W^u} = \boldsymbol{W^d}. \tag{4}$$

We discuss the nature of this mapping we would like to find next. Figure 5 shows the first mode of variation plotted for each detailed (y-axis) and undetailed (x-axis) pair of shapes in the Half Shell Data. It can be observed that there exists a correlation that is close to linear between both sets of weights. As expected, the y-intercept is close to 0 since an undetailed weight of 0 on the major axis of variation means that the undetailed shape is very close to the mean and therefore the detailed shape should also be expected to be close to the mean. Similarly a linear relationship is observed for the second mode as shown in Fig. 5(b). We also examined other mode combinations such as first mode vs. second mode and third mode, and found close to linear correlations. Intuition gained from these experiments lead us to assume a linear relationship between the two classes of shapes. In order to find a general multivariate regression between all the weights, we construct a linear least squares optimization problem:

$$\boldsymbol{W^u} \boldsymbol{X^d} = \boldsymbol{W^d} \tag{5}$$

where $\boldsymbol{X^d}$ is a transformation matrix that encodes the detailing process: it transforms the undetailed shape class into the detailed shape class. To find $\boldsymbol{X^d}$, $\boldsymbol{W^u}$, which is of size Nxk, where $N > k$ (hence overdetermined problem), is inverted by an SVD decomposition [15]:

$$\boldsymbol{W^u} = \boldsymbol{U^w} \boldsymbol{D^w} \boldsymbol{V^w}^T, \tag{6}$$

then the least squares solution $\boldsymbol{X^d}$ is given by:

$$\boldsymbol{X^d} = \boldsymbol{V^w} (\boldsymbol{D^w})^{-1} \boldsymbol{U^w}^T \boldsymbol{W^d} \tag{7}$$

where $(\boldsymbol{D^w})^{-1}$ is the simple inverse of a diagonal matrix with singular values.

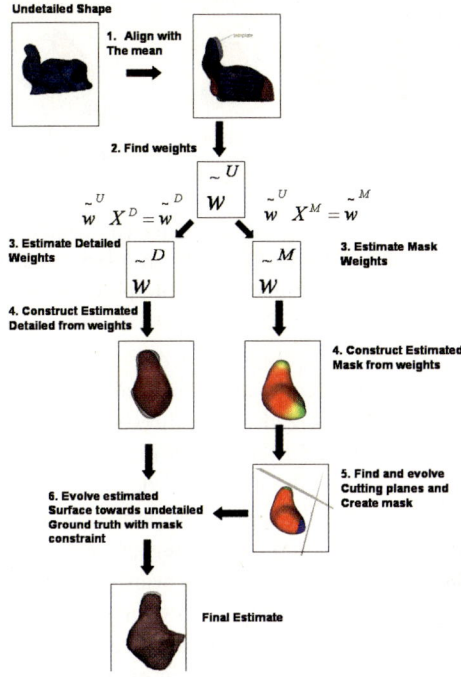

Fig. 6. Flowchart describing the proposed automatic shape generation method

We build a statistical model for a class of auxiliary shapes, called mask shapes, to help deform the estimated model towards the patient ear canal anatomy for an exact fit. 3D mask shapes M_i are formed from the difference of shapes in the two training sets, i.e. $\Phi_i^u - \Phi_i^d$. This mask will be used to indicate regions in the estimated detailed shape that are allowed to propagate towards the undetailed shell, except at the parts that we detected as "cuts" by our algorithm during the final deformation phase. Hence along with the estimated matrix for the detailed shapes X^d, a second regression matrix X^m is estimated and stored during the training phase.

2.3 Automatic Shape Generation

After the training phase, a new undetailed shape is given as input to the system, and the expected output is a corresponding detailed shell similar to one that would have been produced by a specialist. We note that since different types of detailed shells exist, the training phase must be done on the type that is expected as an output of the estimation.

Flowchart in Figure 6 summarizes our automatic shape generation method: The new undetailed shape is registered to the mean shape from the training data as explained in Section 2.1. The weight vector for the new undetailed shape is computed and the weight vector for the detailed shape is estimated through the stored regression matrix (7)

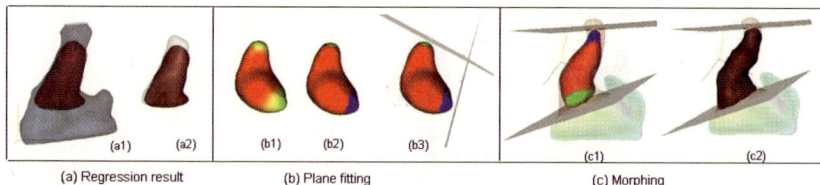

Fig. 7. (a) Detailed shape found through regression is depicted (in red/dark) on (a1) the undetailed shape; (a2) the GT detailed shape (in grey/light). **(b)** (b1) estimated mask; (b2) the resulting clustering with 2 clusters; (b3) the fitted planes. **(c)** Morph of an initial detailed surface (c1) towards the undetailed surface constrained by planes, final result in (c2).

(Fig 7-a). Next, difference mask weights are estimated via the regression matrix X^m to form the mask M, which is binarized with a threshold of 1. The regions of M that are 0 correspond to "cuts" that would have been made by the technician. Those cuts usually produce flat surfaces. Since the estimated detailed shapes do not always have flat surfaces where the mask is 0, first we cluster points on the mask surface by using the k-means algorithm, then we fit planes to these regions as shown in Figure 7-b. Finally, we morph the initially estimated detailed shape towards the undetailed shape where the evolution mask field is nonzero. It is allowed to evolve until it reaches the plane and flattens out as depicted in Figure 7-c. As for the surface deformation step, we utilized a simple morphing PDE as in [16] modified with our estimated mask and the planes.

3 Results

For both datasets (half-shell and canal shell), we randomly split the data so that 90% of the data was used for training and 10% used for testing. This operation is repeated three times for more robust validation. The number of modes needed to explain 95%, 97% and 99% variability in the data, were 12, 15, and 22, respectively. For a 95% variation, only 12 modes are retained, which is a significant decrease from 22 modes needed to explain 99% of the variability in the data. This also shows the huge dimensionality reduction given that the shapes in our training dataset were represented on a voxel grid of 80^3.

The sum of squared difference (SSD) in millimeters between the estimated shape $\tilde{\Phi}_d$ and the ground truth shape Φ_d is used as a validation measure. Table 1 shows the average SSD values obtained for both datasets. The overall SSD value between the estimated shape and the ground truth was smaller than $1.5mm$ in all cases.

Table 1. Average SSD (in mm) between the estimated shapes and the ground truth shapes in the Half-Shell (HS) and Canal (C) dataset for all three test sets and three variation values

SSD (HS)	95% variation	97% variation	99% variation	SSD (C)	95% variation	97% variation	99% variation
test 1	1.16	1.19	1.17	test 1	1.51	1.47	1.40
test 2	1.07	1.17	0.97	test 2	1.41	1.40	1.35
test 3	1.37	1.35	1.32	test 3	1.32	1.32	1.31

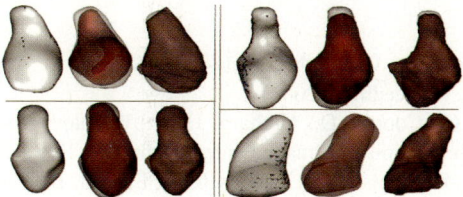

Fig. 8. (Each Quadrant)Left: GT detailed shape; Middle: Estimated detailed shape before evolution; Right: Estimated Detailed Shape after evolution (all are superimposed on the GT shape)

We show qualitative results for the Half-Shell dataset in Figure 8, where the estimated shapes are observed to be in good agreement with the GT shapes, particularly in the canal region. The errors as expected are distributed around the cut points since the shape evolution is restricted to the cutting planes which are estimated through our shape learning process on a mask field. Our preliminary but extensive experiments have shown that our algorithm is robust to different shell types, and a low SSD value is obtained for all tests. As part of our future studies, further validation will be performed on our system.

4 Conclusions and Discussions

We presented a general framework to automatically generate a target shape from a reference shape via learning the relation of these two shape classes on a much lower dimensional manifold than the original shape space. As a specific application, our system learns how to detail a hearing aid shape by estimating a mapping from a patient's digitized ear mold to the detailed shell. Further refinement of the shape is achieved by deforming the estimated shell towards the undetailed shell in regions where the shapes should fit using an estimated auxiliary shape class. We learned the relation between two shape classes through a linear multivariate regression due to the underlying assumption that the two shape classes have a linear relation, which is demonstrated to be a reasonable assumption by our results.

Our proposed framework is quite general in that a mapping between the two classes of shapes can be estimated in a proper setting. This framework contains several known components such as variational registration, PCA in the distance transform space for shape analysis, and linear regression used in an interesting and novel system for automatic shape transformation. Some of these components can be replaced with other ones: for instance, using non-linear regression instead of linear regression (to account for more complex relations between associated classes of shapes), kernel PCA or manifold learning instead of PCA, Eulerian vs. Lagrangian shape representation, and others. While such changes may improve the results, they would not change the overall concept. However, we plan to apply our technique with different components to other applications in custom design of various anatomical parts such as dental implants and prosthetic hips.

References

1. Hertzmann, A., Jacobs, C., Oliver, N., Curless, B., Salesin, D.: Image analogies. In: SIGGRAPH Conference Proceedings (2001)
2. Cootes, T., Taylor, C., Cooper, D., Graham, J.: Active shape models - their training and application. Computer Vision and Image Understanding 61(1), 38–59 (1995)
3. Paulsen, R., Larsen, R., Nielsen, C., Laugesen, S., Ersboll, B.: Building and testing a statistical shape model of the human ear canal. In: Dohi, T., Kikinis, R. (eds.) MICCAI 2002. LNCS, vol. 2489, pp. 373–380. Springer, Heidelberg (2002)
4. Paulsen, R.R., Hilger, K.B.: Shape modelling using markov random field restoration of point correspondences. In: Taylor, C.J., Noble, J.A. (eds.) IPMI 2003. LNCS, vol. 2732, pp. 1–12. Springer, Heidelberg (2003)
5. Darkner, S., Larsen, R., Paulsen, R.: Analysis of deformation of the human ear and canal caused by mandibular movement. In: Ayache, N., Ourselin, S., Maeder, A. (eds.) MICCAI 2007, Part II. LNCS, vol. 4792, pp. 801–808. Springer, Heidelberg (2007)
6. Leventon, M., Grimson, W., Faugeras, O.: Statistical shape influence in geodesic active contours. In: IEEE CVPR, Hilton Head, vol. 1 (2000)
7. Rathi, Y., Dambreville, S., Tannenbaum, A.: Statistical shape analysis using kernel pca. In: IS&T, SPIE Symposium on Electronic Imaging (2006)
8. Aguirre, M., Linguraru, M., Marias, K., Ayache, N., Nolte, L.P., Ballester, M.: Statistical shape analysis via principal factor analysis. In: IEEE Int. Symp. Biomedical Imaging (2007)
9. Rao, A., Aljabar, P., Rueckert, D.: Hierarchical statistical shape analysis and prediction of sub-cortical brain structures. Medical Image Analysis 12 (2008)
10. Zhou, K., Comaniciu, D.: Shape regression machine. In: Karssemeijer, N., Lelieveldt, B. (eds.) IPMI 2007. LNCS, vol. 4584, pp. 13–25. Springer, Heidelberg (2007)
11. Davis, B., Fletcher, P., Bullitt, E., Joshi, S.: Populations shape regression from random design data. In: IEEE Int. Conf. Computer Vision (2007)
12. NIH-NICD: National institute on deafness and other commnunication disorders: Hearing aids information,
    http://www.nidcd.nih.gov/health/hearing/hearingaid.asp
13. Gray, H.: Gray's anatomy of the human body (1918),
    http://www.bartleby.com/107/229.html
14. Paragios, N., Rousson, M., Ramesh, V.: Distance tranforms for non-rigid registration. Computer Vision and Image Understanding (CVIU) 89(2-3), 142–165 (2003)
15. Press, W.H., Teukolsky, S.A., Vetterling, W., Flannery, B.P.: Numerical Recipes in C. Cambridge University Press, Cambridge (1992)
16. Whitaker, R.T., Breen, D.E.: Level-set models for the deformation of solid objects. In: Eurographics/Siggraph, Proceedings of Implicit Surfaces, pp. 19–35 (1998)

A Novel Explicit 2D+t Cyclic Shape Model Applied to Echocardiography

Ramón Casero and J. Alison Noble

Institute of Biomedical Engineering, Department of Engineering Science,
University of Oxford, UK
{rcasero,noble}@robots.ox.ac.uk*

Abstract. In this paper, we propose a novel explicit 2D+t cyclic shape model that extends the Point Distribution Model (PDM) to shapes like myocardial contours with cyclic dynamics. We also propose an extension to Procrustes alignment that removes pose and subject size variability while maintaining dynamic effects. Our model draws on ideas from Principal Component Analysis (PCA), Multidimensional Scaling (MDS) and Kernel PCA (KPCA) and solves 3 shortcomings of previous implicit models: 1) cardiac cycles in the data set do not each need to have the same number of frames, 2) the required number of subjects for statistically significant results is substantially reduced and 3) the displacement of contour points incorporates time as an explicit variable. We illustrate our method by computing models of the myocardium in the 4 principal planes of 2D+t echocardiography data.

1 Background

Principal Component Analysis (PCA) [1], also known as the Karhunen-Loève transform, is one of the most popular methods in Statistics for modeling, dimensionality reduction and denoising, and widely employed in biomedical image analysis. It was introduced into the computer vision literature as a dimensionality reduction method for face images [2]. PCA finds a basis of orthonormal vectors that span the data set. The first vector is in the direction of maximum variance of the data. The next component has the direction of maximum variance amongst those orthogonal to the first, and so on. Cootes et al. [3] proposed computing a shape space by applying PCA to Procrustes aligned point configurations, and called it the Point Distribution Model (PDM)

$$x = \bar{x} + V \cdot b \tag{1}$$

---

* We are thankful to Prof A. Zisserman, whose unwavering enthusiasm for scientific discussion gave us the motivation and tools to write this paper; to Dr H. Becher and Dr J. Timperley, John Radcliffe Hospital, Oxford, for the data acquisition and tracing of the contours; and to Prof J.M. Brady, for his comments and suggestions. Part of this research has been funded by the EPSRC, Mirada Solutions Ltd., Oriel College and the Department of Engineering Science, University of Oxford.

where $\bar{x}$ is the mean shape, V is the shape space matrix, and b is the *coefficient or Principal Components (PC)* vector. In this model, x is a vector with the Euclidean uv-coordinates of $n/2$ points or landmarks

$$x_{2D} = [u(1), \ldots, u(n/2), v(1), \ldots, v(n/2)]^\top \quad (2)$$

One of the main applications of the PDM in medical imaging is to provide a shape space on which segmentation boundaries can be constrained to physiologically viable organs. In terms of statistical analysis, x is a vector with n random variables. The model is learned from a training set of M examples $X = [x_1, \ldots, x_M]$. The mean shape is $\bar{x} = 1/M \sum_{i=1}^{M} x_i$. The eigenvectors or *loading vectors* $V = [v_1, \ldots, v_M]$ are computed using PCA; that is, as solutions to the eigenproblem $Sv = \lambda v$, where λ is an eigenvalue, and S is the covariance matrix $S = \frac{1}{M}\tilde{X}\tilde{X}^\top$ of the centered training set $\tilde{X}$ with elements $\tilde{x}_i = x_i - \bar{x}$.

This formulation is not restricted to 2D, and can be generalized to 3D or higher dimensions. PCA has been used in computer vision to build 2D or 3D deformable models with uncorrelated modes of variation, e.g. in Active Shape Models (ASMs) [4] or Active Appearance Models (AAMs) [5,6]. Some medical imaging modalities, especially echocardiography, depend strongly on temporal information, and implicit time extensions have been proposed to 2D and 3D PCA models [7,8]. Such models are implicit because instead of adding a time variable, they are built from the concatenation of shape vectors

$$x_{\text{implicit 2D+t}} = [x_{2D}^{1\top}, x_{2D}^{2\top}, \ldots, x_{2D}^{F\top}]^\top \quad (3)$$

where x_{2D}^i is the shape at time $t(i)$. Then PCA is computed in the usual way. This approach, which we call the implicit 2D+t model, has 3 important shortcomings. First, all cardiac cycles in the data set need to have the same number of frames; considering the variability of heart rates in subjects and sampling rates between studies, this is never going to be the case in practice. Thus, it becomes necessary to interpolate the image data to a fixed number of frames, a hard and computationally expensive problem that requires 2D+t volume registration and can introduce new artifacts, e.g. double edges.

Second, even though linear models are relatively immune to the curse of dimensionality problem, in order to start obtaining significant results with PCA, the number of training samples M needs in principle to increase linearly with the number of variables n [9]. When F frames are stacked together, the size of the data set is reduced by a factor F, and the number of variables increases by the same amount. That is, implicit 2D+t models require $\mathcal{O}(F^2)$ times more subjects than simple 2D to approximate the data. With $F \approx 16$ in typical studies, this becomes effectively infeasible. A computational issue also arises, even if there is enough data, as the matrices of the eigenproblem are very large.

Third, implicit 2D+t models assume that consecutively occurring positions of the same landmark are separate independent variables, while it is more realistic and informative to model the variability of each point as a 2-dimensional random variable that changes with time.

The main contribution of this paper is to propose a novel explicit 2D+t cyclic shape model that addresses the above shortcomings. We also propose an extension to Procrustes alignment that removes pose and subject size variability while maintaining dynamic effects. We illustrate our new method by computing 2D+t models from expert traced contours of the myocardium in the 4 principal planes of 2D+t echocardiography data.

2 Method

It may seem that a 3D model [6] could be used for 2D+t, just by replacing the third spatial coordinate by time. But because all the contour points in the same frame share the same value of t, this is equivalent to concatenating the same variable n times to the shape vector. It follows that the determinant $|S| = 0$, and it is not so straightforward to solve the eigenproblem. To avoid this, we propose an extended shape vector with a single time variable $t \in [0, 1]$

$$x_{\text{explicit 2D+t}} = [x_{\text{2D}}^\top, rt]^\top \tag{4}$$

where r is a scaling factor that will be discussed below. The vector in Eq. (4) has important shortcomings of its own for cyclic dynamics. Fig. 1a illustrates the typical horizontal displacement of a 2D contour point in the middle of the left wall of a 2-chamber view. First, the horseshoe-like curve means that any linear model such as PCA will poorly approximate the relationship between spatial coordinates and time. Second, PCA is dual to linear Multidimensional Scaling (MDS) [10], where the distance matrix is defined by the scalar products between the training vectors, i.e. PCA tries to preserve Euclidean distances between training vectors. In Fig. 1a, points near $t = 0$ and $t = 1$ are far apart according to the Euclidean distance for the model; in reality, we know that they are close in the cardiac cycle.

We contend that both the lack of linearity and the distance problem can be tackled with Kernel PCA (KPCA) [11], a non-linear generalization of PCA. The main idea that we borrow from KPCA is that shape+time vectors can be mapped to a higher dimensional space in which the relations between variables are linear, and then we can compute PCA in that space. We propose the transformation

$$x_{\text{explicit 2D+t}} = [x_{\text{2D}}^\top, rt_1, rt_2]^\top \tag{5a}$$
$$t_1 = \cos(2\pi t) \tag{5b}$$
$$t_2 = \sin(2\pi t) \tag{5c}$$

To define r, it should be noted 1) that PCA searches not only for those directions in which relationships between variables are more linear, but also for those with larger variance; and 2) that because there are many more shape than time variables, the model tends to underestimate the temporal effect. We propose

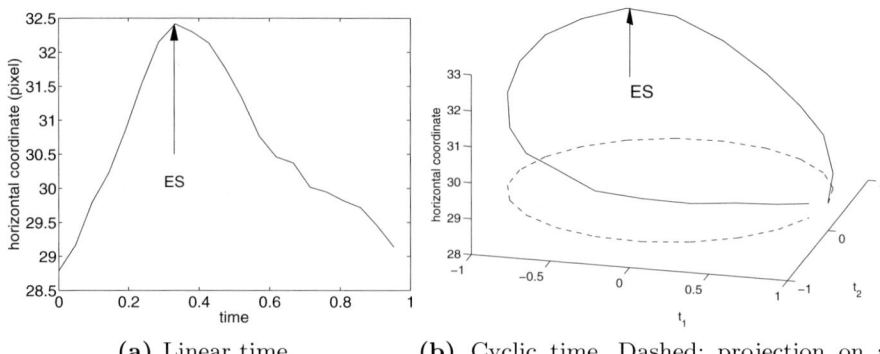

(a) Linear time.   **(b)** Cyclic time. Dashed: projection on a horizontal plane.

Fig. 1. Mean horizontal coordinate of a 2D contour point in the middle of the left wall of a 2-chamber view (see point marked with a 'o' in Fig. 3a). Curve computed as the mean of 21 subjects. Time for the cardiac cycle has been normalized to $t \in [0, 1]$, with $t = 0$ end diastole. The arrow points to end systole (ES). Coordinate units are pixels.

$$r = \sqrt{\frac{\sum_{i=1}^{n/2} \mathrm{Var}(u(i)) + \sum_{i=1}^{n/2} \mathrm{Var}(v(i))}{\mathrm{Var}(t_1) + \mathrm{Var}(t_2)}} \quad (6)$$

so that the total variance contributed to the model by shape variables is the same as that contributed by time variables, where the variance estimate Var is computed over the sample of size M.

While KPCA usually maps the data to a much higher dimensional space and uses MDS and the kernel trick to make computations tractable, Eq. (5) only increases the dimensionality by 2, so it is possible to work directly in feature space. Fig. 1b illustrates the advantages of the map in Eq. (5). First, the curve and the manifold that contains it can be reasonably approximated by an ellipse and a plane, respectively, which suggests a good linear approximation $u \approx \alpha_1 t_1 + \alpha_2 t_2$ for some scalars α_1, α_2. And second, the points near $t = 0$ and $t = 1$ are now close in Euclidean distance.

The PDM of Eq. (1) can now be expanded using Eq. (5). In centered block matrix form we have

$$\begin{bmatrix} \tilde{x} \\ r\tilde{t}' \end{bmatrix} = \begin{bmatrix} V_{1,1} & V_{1,2} \\ V_{2,1} & V_{2,2} \end{bmatrix} \begin{bmatrix} b' \\ b_r \end{bmatrix} \quad (7)$$

where $t' = [t_1, t_2]^\top$, $b' = [b_1, b_2]^\top$. An explicit relationship between shape and time can be obtained noticing that

$$\tilde{x} = V_{1,1} b' + V_{1,2} b_r \quad (8a)$$
$$r\tilde{t}' = V_{2,1} b' + V_{2,2} b_r \quad (8b)$$

Substituting $[b_1, b_2]^\top$ from Eq. (8b) in Eq. (8a), and uncentering $\tilde{x}$, the shape model can be formulated as

$$x = c + A_b b_r + A_t t' \tag{9a}$$
$$c = \bar{x} - A_t \bar{t'} \tag{9b}$$
$$A_t = rV_{1,1}V_{2,1}^{-1} \tag{9c}$$
$$A_b = -\frac{1}{r}A_t V_{2,2} + V_{1,2} \tag{9d}$$

Finally, we propose an extension to Procrustes alignment for 2D+t data. Procrustes alignment is used to remove pose and subject size variability from the training set. But if it is applied to a stack of our 2D+t contours, then temporal variability is removed too. Procrustes alignment could be applied to $x_{\text{implicit 2D+t}}$ vectors, as in AAMM, but then it would be necessary to interpolate each volume to the same number of frames. Instead, we propose applying standard Procrustes alignment (e.g. Least-Squares Fit Generalized Orthogonal Procrustes Analysis [12]) to the mean shape $\bar{x}$ of each cardiac cycle. Procrustes alignment computes a similarity transformation for each mean shape (translation, scaling and rotation) that can be applied to each frame of the corresponding volume. This method is illustrated by Fig. 2.

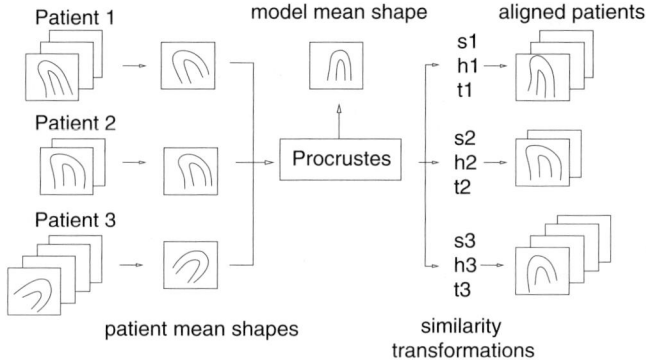

Fig. 2. Procrustes alignment for 2D+t data. Similarity transformations are composed of a scaling s, a rotation h and a translation t.

3 Results

To illustrate our method, we computed 2D+t models using Eq. (9) on 21 contrast echocardiography studies at rest in the 4 standard planes: 2-, 3- and 4-chamber (2C, 3C, 4C) and short axis (SAX). Contours for the endocardium and epicardium were traced by 2 experts, who placed anatomical landmarks (6 in apical, 2 in SAX). Pseudolandmarks were interpolated at equal arclengths (to a total of 50 in apical, 30 in SAX), and aligned using the method in Fig. 2.

The time effect was studied making $b_r = 0$ and sampling $t \in [0, 1]$ uniformly at 11 instants. For the 2C plane all resulting contours were plotted together in Fig. 3a. A point on the endocardium was selected and marked with a 'o' to help

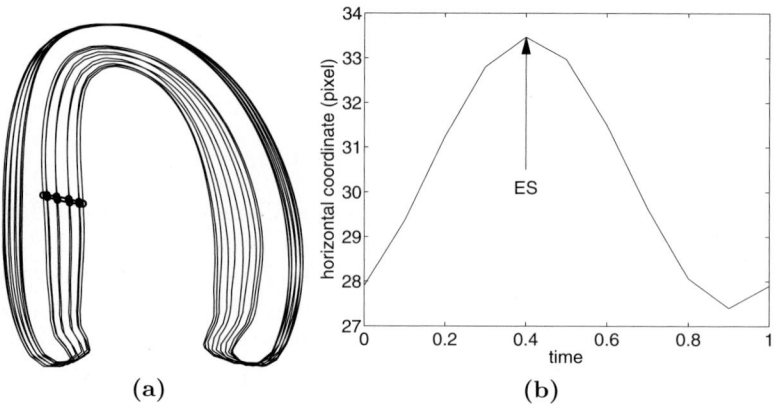

Fig. 3. Endocardium and epicardium in 2C plane cyclic time linear PCA model using Eq. (9). Time variation with $b_r = 0$. The model was trained on the same data as Fig. 1. (a) One cardiac cycle sampled at 11 instants in $t \in [0, 1]$. The 'o' marks the point selected to plot the horizontal displacement in (b).

visualize its displacement. The modelled horizontal displacement of the 2C point in Fig. 3b is a good approximation of the empirical one in Fig. 1a, and seems to reflect the temporal effect sensibly, although with a limitation: the model does not reflect the asymmetry of the data, so all points in the model show a small phase shift $\Delta t = .07$, with the end systole (ES) peak moving from $t_{ES} = 0.33$ to $t_{ES} = 0.40$. Different regions of the endocardium display different degrees of excursion and larger than for the epicardium, as would be expected. Fig. 4 shows results for the other planes. Quite interestingly, the SAX plane model has counterclockwise rotation in the endocardium and clockwise in the epicardium, an indication of torsion.

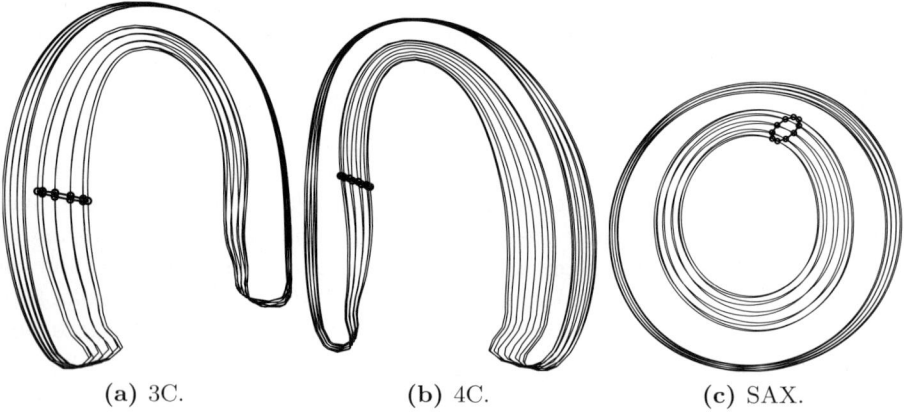

Fig. 4. Similar to Fig. 3a, for the other 3 principal echocardiography planes

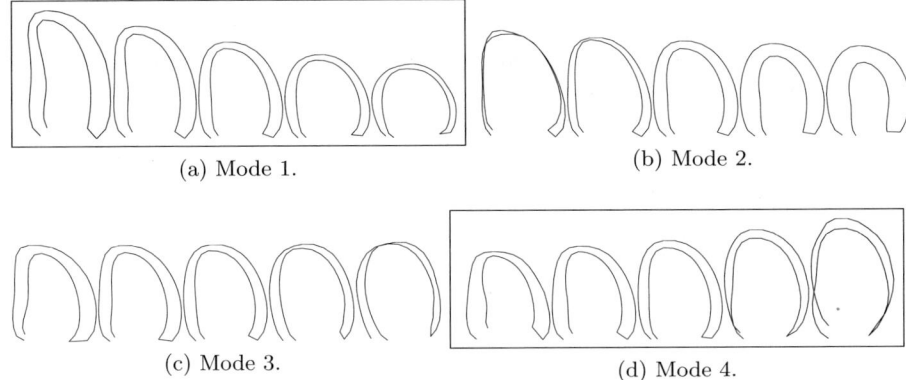

Fig. 5. 2C plane cyclic time linear PCA model using Eq. (9). Shape coefficient variation $\pm 3\sigma$ in first frame ($t = 0$).

The shape coefficients effect was studied by setting $t = 0$. Fig. 5 displays the first 4 modes of variation for the 2C plane. For the i-th mode we plotted curves for coefficient values in $-3\sigma_i \leq b_r(i) \leq 3\sigma_i$, to point out that extreme coefficient values can generate spurious shapes. The results suggest that contractility dynamics have been largely removed from the shape coefficients, and are modelled by the time variable.

The first coefficients appear to have a physiological interpretation: Mode 1 controls the elongation of the ventricle, while mode 2 controls the thickness of the myocardium.

4 Discussion

In this paper we have presented a novel explicit 2D+t cyclic shape model that we contend is better suited to cyclic dynamics than previous implicit models. Our model is built on observations drawn from PCA, MDS and KPCA theory to offer a linear approximation of cyclic data. A limitation of the model is that it can not express asymmetries in the displacement of contour points well, and thus suffers from a small phase shift. Future work will be finding a reparameterization of the displacement curve to take into account said asymmetries. Otherwise, it provides a sensible approximation to the expected dynamics of human hearts adding just 2 time variable to shape vectors. We have also presented an extension to Procrustes Analysis that maintains temporal effects in heart dynamics while removing pose and subject size variability. Finally, while our presentation and experiments have been limited to echocardiography 2D+t data, the model itself is not limited in dimensionality or imaging modality, and could be easily extended to 3D+t studies using 3D Procrustes Alignment [6], or applied to data extracted from other modalities, e.g. MRI. It could also accommodate other cyclic effects, e.g. respiration in liver imaging.

References

1. Hotelling, H.: Analysis of a complex of statistical variables into principal components. Journal of Educational Psychology 24(6), 417–441 (1933)
2. Sirovich, L., Kirby, M.: Low-dimensional procedure for the characterization of human faces. Journal of the Optical Society of America 4(3), 519–524 (1987)
3. Cootes, T., Taylor, C., Cooper, D., Graham, J.: Training models of shape from sets of examples. In: Procs. of the BMVC, pp. 266–275. Springer, Berlin (1992)
4. Cootes, T., Taylor, C.: Active shape models - 'Smart snakes'. In: Procs. of the BMVC, pp. 266–275. Springer, Heidelberg (1992)
5. Edwards, G., Taylor, C., Cootes, T.: Learning to identify and track faces in image sequences. In: Procs. of the BMVC (1997)
6. Mitchell, S., Bosch, J., Lelieveldt, B., van der Geest, R., Reiber, J., Sonka, M.: 3-D active appearance models: segmentation of cardiac MR and ultrasound images. IEEE Transactions on Medical Imaging 21(9), 1167–1178 (2002)
7. Bosch, J., Mitchell, S., Lelieveldt, B., Nijland, F., Kamp, O., Sonka, M.: Automatic segmentation of echocardiographic sequences by active appearance motion models. IEEE Transactions on Medical Imaging 21(11), 1374–1383 (2002)
8. Stegmann, M., Pedersen, D.: Bi-temporal 3D active appearance models with applications to unsupervised ejection fraction estimation. In: Proc. of SPIE, International Symposium on Medical Imaging 2005, vol. 5747, pp. 336–350 (2005)
9. Henry, R., Lewis, C., Hopke, P., Williamson, H.: Review of receptor model fundamentals. Atmospheric Environment 18, 1507–1515 (1984)
10. Gower, J.: Some distance properties of latent root and vector methods used in multivariate analysis. Biometrika 53(3,4), 325–338 (1966)
11. Schölkopf, B., Smola, A., Müller, K.R.: Nonlinear component analysis as a kernel eigenvalue problem. Neural Computation 10(5), 1299–1319 (1998)
12. Rohlf, F., Slice, D.: Extensions of the Procrustes method for the optimal superimposition of landmarks. Systematic Zoology 39(1), 40–59 (1990)

Spatial Consistency in 3D Tract-Based Clustering Statistics

Matthan Caan[1,2], Lucas van Vliet[2], Charles Majoie[1], Eline Aukema[1], Kees Grimbergen[1], and Frans Vos[1,2]

[1] Department of Radiology, Academic Medical Center, University of Amsterdam, NL
[2] Quantitative Imaging Group, Delft University of Technology, NL
m.w.a.caan@tudelft.nl

Abstract. We propose a novel technique for tract-based comparison of DTI-indices between groups, based on a representation that is estimated while matching fiber tracts. The method involves a non-rigid registration based on a joint clustering and matching approach, after which a 3D-atlas of cluster center points is used as a frame of reference for statistics. Patient and control FA-distributions are compared per cluster. Spatial consistency is taken to reflect a significant difference between groups. Accordingly, a non-parametric classification is performed to assess the continuity of pathology over larger tract regions. In a study to infant survivors treated for medulloblastoma with intravenous methotrexate and cranial radiotherapy, significant decreases in FA in major parts of the corpus callosum were found.

1 Introduction

Over the past decade Magnetic Resonance Diffusion Tensor Imaging (MR-DTI) has been used to characterize the local white matter structure in the human brain. Typically, properties derived from the tensor, such as the Fractional Anisotropy (FA) [1], are involved to study differences between diseased subjects and normals.

It may be observed that not all the tensor information (represented by orientation and shape) is used in the latter analysis. For instance, connectivity information is neglected as tensor shape properties are studied on a voxel- or region-of-interest-basis. Alternatively, fiber tracts are used as a subspace in which properties are averaged. However, high variation in white matter anatomy exists along white matter tracts [2]. Not surprisingly, analysis is currently focusing on profiles along tracts. For instance, in a study to Amyotrophic Lateral Sclerosis (ALS), it was recently found that only parts of the corticospinal tract were affected by the disease [3]. Here, a Mann-Whitney U-test was performed to assess local spatial consistency.

Prior to such inter-subject comparison of tract-based features, correspondence between the tracts is to be achieved. Anatomical variability across subjects needs to be accounted for in a non-rigid manner. Preferably, correspondence is not only obtained along, but also in the plane normal to the local tract orientation.

In case of small patient and control groups, diffusion properties need to be spatially combined to ensure sufficient sensitivity for discrimination. This may be achieved by a statistical description, e.g. some mean property such as FA over the tract and the corresponding standard deviation in case of a unimodal distribution. Clearly, such averaging goes at the cost of losing spatial information. A more specific approach is to employ the correlation in the data, after which it is found which voxels do or do not contribute to an observable difference between patients and controls [4].

Relevant related work includes affine matching of fibers [5], such that diffusion properties are represented along tracts. Inter-subject comparison is not facilitated by either approach, though. Joint probabilistic clustering and point-by-point mapping achieves arc-length tract representations [6]. Tract-based morphometry also uses such an arc-length representation, based on matched tract regions to a chosen prototype. Subsequently, it is used for detecting white matter differences between groups of subjects [7]. Neither do these methods achieve non-rigid tract correspondence, nor is an unsupervised partitioning of tracts facilitated. Tract based spatial statistics projects non-rigidly registered volumes onto a skeletonization of the FA [8], but tensor orientation information is not used in the alignment, nor in the analysis.

We propose a framework for tract-based analysis that partitions tracts in an unsupervised manner. The method involves a non-rigid registration based on a joint clustering and matching approach, after which a 3D-atlas of cluster center points is used as a frame of reference for statistics. Underlying shape coherence of trajectories is captured in anisotropic cluster shapes. Patient and control FA-distributions are compared per cluster. Spatial consistency is taken to reflect a significant difference between groups. Accordingly, a non-parametric classification is performed to assess the continuity of pathology over larger tract regions.

2 Method

2.1 Feature Selection

The analysis starts with selecting fiber tracts of interest both in patients and controls. We perform a full brain tractography using the FACT algorithm in DTIStudio software [9], after which ROIs are placed that, combined by logical operators, define a sub-selection of fibers, here the corpus callosum.

2.2 Registration

Initially, the fibers need to be brought into spatial correspondence. The concept of point set matching is applied to points along the fiber tracts in order to do so [10].

Suppose that in total, P datasets are to be aligned. Each dataset $p \in \{1, \ldots, P\}$, is represented by sampling the selected fiber tracts, yielding point-set consisting of N^p points $X^p = \{x_i^p, i = 1 \ldots N^p\}$. For each point set, a set of K cluster center points is defined, denoted by $C^p = \{c_a^p | a = 1 \ldots K\}$. An atlas cluster point set $\mathcal{Z} = \{z_a | a = 1 \ldots K\}$ is defined that is to explain the cluster centers over all point sets. By means of a deterministic annealing approach, the registration process gradually refines from global to local matching. The initial temperature T_{init} and final temperature T_{final} are a priori defined. T is lowered after each iteration: $T_{ind+1} = \alpha T_{ind}$, with $0 < \alpha < 1$.

A mixture of Gaussians models the density of the point set, in which the membership variable m_{ai}^p indicates the degree to which a point "feature" x_i^p belongs to cluster center point c_a^p. The membership m_{ai}^p is now defined as

$$m_{ai}^p = \frac{q_{ai}^p}{\sum_{a=1}^K q_{ai}^p}, \forall a, i, \quad (1)$$

with

$$q_{ai}^p = \exp\left(-\frac{1}{2\sigma^2}|x_i^p - c_a^p|^2\right). \quad (2)$$

assuming isotropic covariance matrices ($\Sigma_a^p = \sigma^2 I$), and, and, after normalization, $\sum_{a=1}^K m_{ai}^p = 1$. The temperature is defined to be the variance in equation 2, $T = \sigma^2$.

The algorithm proceeds in an iterative manner. The cluster center points are initiated at randomly chosen points in the dataset. They are recomputed after the membership has been updated (eq. 1), using

$$c_a^p = \frac{\sum_{i=1}^{N_p} m_{ai}^p x_i^p}{\sum_{i=1}^{N_p} m_{ai}^p}, \forall a \in \{1, \ldots, K\}, \forall p \in \{1, \ldots, P\}. \quad (3)$$

Then, the atlas points are formed by averaging the cluster center points, $z_a = 1/P \sum_{p=1}^P c_a^p$. The atlas points can be seen as a "common frame of reference", representing the mean shape of the point sets. An affine and non-rigid thin plate spline transform is now computed to warp the atlas points to the cluster center points and vice versa. The next iteration is started by lowering the temperature and transforming the atlas points to the subsequent datasets. In the latter step, information from other datasets is implicitly included in clustering a single dataset.

2.3 Statistics

DTI is sensitive to detecting pathology that manifests itself along white matter pathways. The challenge is to be precise in describing which local regions specifically characterize a disease. We assume for our analysis that the voxels through which a fiber tract passes are somehow connected. By jointly analyzing such samples, statistical power is to be gained compared to per-voxel comparison. What is more, a multi-modal analysis of the data may actually be necessary: simply averaging data over the connected voxels delivers a physiologically feasible mean only if there is a unimodal distribution.

We propose to use the clustering outcome of the registration as the statistical frame of reference; i.e. correspondence is implicitly defined via the atlas cluster points z_a. The membership function (equation 1) defines the extend to which points x_i^p are assigned to cluster centers point c_a^p. It may be observed that in such a way fiber tract statistics are modeled in 3D since the data points emanate from several fibers that constitute a tract. To the best of our knowledge, previously proposed arc-length representations have not yet been generalized to higher dimensions. A cumulative distribution of FA-values per patient per cluster is build, in which the membership values act as relative weights. Consequently, distant voxels will get a low weight.

The clinical study described in this paper (see below) involves paired data of patients and controls. For each such pair, the distributions of FA data in the neighbourhood of a cluster center point is compared. In other words, a pair-wise comparison of FA-distributions is needed. As no prior information on the distribution is available, a non-parametric test is required. We use the Kolmogorov-Smirnov (KS)-test to do so in a two-tailed fashion: for each patient/control pair and for each cluster center point, it is determined if either the FA-distribution of the one is significantly above or below the other or if the difference is insignificant. The latter comparison is performed over all patient/control pairs from which the majority vote is retained. Effectively, this score boils down to either a higher or lower FA, ties are discarded.

Subsequently, the consistency of the outcome along the tract is checked. Here, the underlying hypothesis is that if the voting score is similar over a larger number of nearby clusters, it is an indication of a significant difference between the groups. In order to check the 'consistency' two classes are asserted, corresponding to dominance of either the patient or control distributions. Class assignment is obtained by unsupervised classification by means of a k-nearest neighbour classifier. A leave-one(-cluster)-out cross validation scheme is involved to train and test the classifier, resulting in the relative classification error over all clusters. It is taken that a small classification error indicates that the dominating distribution can be predicted from neighbouring data. This is considered to reflect a systematic difference between the groups.

For comparison purposes a paired t-test is performed on averaged FA-values over the clusters, using the membership values as relative weights. Notice that such a comparison does not include any spatial connectivity.

To assess the validity of both approaches, statistics are computed on ten randomly permuted data sets (i.e. by randomly assigning the class labels 'patient' or 'control' to the data).

3 Results

Six infant survivors treated for medulloblastoma with intravenous methotrexate and cranial radiotherapy were included in the study as well as age-, education- and sex-matched healthy controls. The aim of this study was to confirm the hypothesis that the treatment affects a major white matter tract, the corpus callosum. The number of subjects emanated from a power analysis performed a priori, expecting a major effect. All subjects were scanned on a 3.0T Philips Intera (Best, The Netherlands) MRI-scanner. After data inspection, it was found

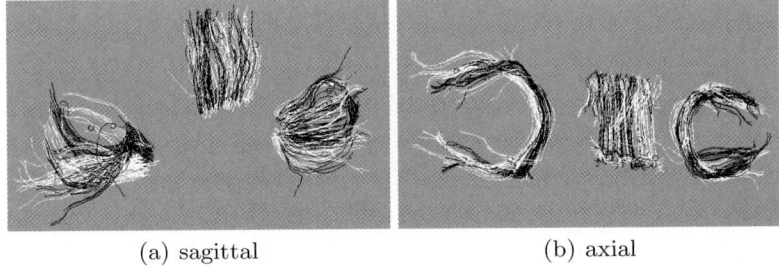

(a) sagittal (b) axial

Fig. 1. Transformed fibers of the corpus callosum (that could be reproducibly tracked in all subjects) after matching. Fibers of one patient and one control are shown in black and white.

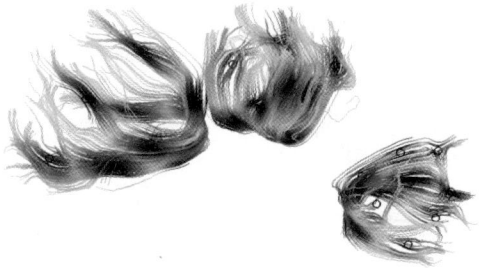

Fig. 2. The maximum membership per fiber-point $\max_i m_{ai}^p$ and cluster center points after one matching instance, in one dataset

that unfortunately one patient had incomplete data and had to be excluded (and simultaneously the matched control).

Fiber tracking was performed in the genu, center and splenium of the corpus callosum. Because of white matter degeneration, other corpus callosum parts could not be successfully tracked in all subjects. Fiber coordinates (in mm) were scaled by a factor of 0.01, such that increased numerical stability between translation and rotation parameters was obtained. The resulting tracts from the 10 datasets were jointly matched. The optimal cluster size is determined experimentally below (see figure 4). The temperature was step-wise lowered by a factor of 0.9, starting at $T_{init} = 10^{-2}$, until the final temperature of $T_{final} = 10^{-3}$ was reached. As an illustration, registered tracts of one randomly chosen patient/control pair are displayed in figure 1. To account for the inherent stochastic nature of the clustering, ten realizations of atlas points were combined.

Next, the membership m_{ai}^p was computed for all voxels included in the tracking. Here, $T = 5 \cdot 10^{-3}$ was chosen, yielding a uniform coverage of the clusters over the data. The result is depicted in figure 2. Subsequently, the cumulative FA-distributions were calculated using the membership function as weighting. In the Kolmogorov-Smirnov test to assess the difference per patient/control pair, the number degrees of freedom equaled the cluster size in voxels. The distributions in one cluster for all patients and corresponding KS-significances are given in figure 3.

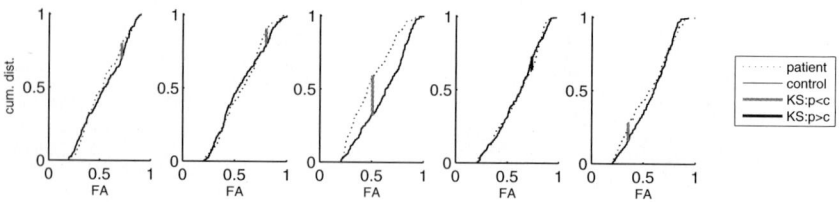

Fig. 3. Cumulative FA-distributions for five patient/control pairs in one arbitrarily chosen cluster, with Kolmogorov-Smirnov test results. Voting yields a lower FA for patients for this cluster.

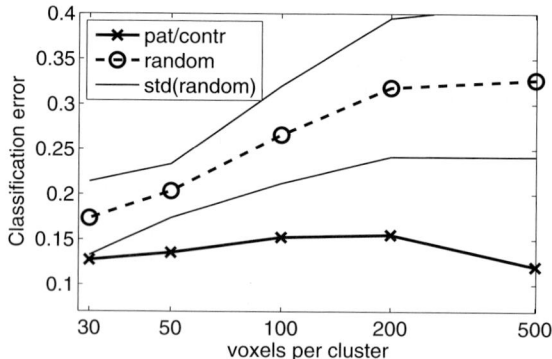

Fig. 4. Classification error as function of the cluster size for both patients/controls and randomly composed classes. The latter is a mean over ten different class compositions, for which the corresponding standard deviation is plotted in gray.

In a leave-one-out cross-validation, a $(3 \cdot 10)$-nearest neighbour classifier was trained on the voting outcome over all pairs of the 10 matching instances, and the classification error was determined. Registration and classification were executed ten times with a range of voxels per cluster. The results are shown in figure 4. The error for randomly composed classes is proportional to the cluster size. Due to the local continuity of the FA, neighbouring values can be predicted, regardless of the class composition. The difference with randomly assigned class labels was significant ($p<0.05$) for cluster sizes larger and 50 voxels [11]. The outcome of the voting and classification process for a cluster size of 200 voxels is displayed in figure 5. A globally decreased FA can be observed.

For comparison, a paired t-test per cluster center point was done (we did not include a correction for the number of comparisons at this stage). 22% of the total number of cluster center points yielded a significant difference ($p < 0.05$). These are annotated in figure 5. In comparison to the results of the 2-nn classifier, less consistent and more evenly distributed differing points can be observed, which we consider not trustworthy. Randomly permuting the class labels 500 times yielded that only in 4% of the permutations a significant difference was found

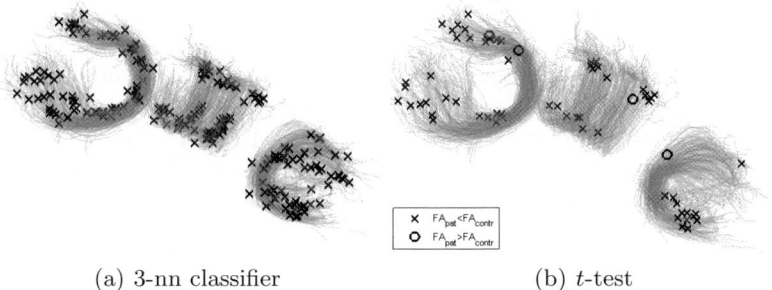

Fig. 5. Result of the voting and classification procedure, depicting correctly classified clusters with decreased (×) and increased FA (○) for patients. Also, the results of t-test statistics (without multiple comparison correction) are shown.

in 22% or more cluster center points. From this we conclude that the differences might be conceived as mathematically significant (since the percentage is lower than 5%), despite clinical reserves.

4 Discussion

We presented a novel approach to 3D, tract-based statistical analysis of FA data. Inter-subject correspondence was achieved by non-rigid registration based on a joint clustering and matching. The clustering delivered atlas points that served as a frame of reference for performing the analysis. A distribution of FA-values per cluster and per subject was calculated. Subsequently, the Kolmogorov-Smirnov test for inequality of distributions was used to pair-wise compare patients and controls. The latter comparison was performed over available patient/control pairs from which the majority vote was retained.

In a study into infant medulloblastoma survivors, corpus callosum tracts from patients and controls were pair-wise studied. A decreased FA in larger parts of the corpus callosum was observed. The decrease could be predicted by a 3-NN classifier with an error of 14% when 200 voxels per cluster were used, which indicated a significant difference. In comparison to t-test statistics per cluster, the proposed method was able to detect larger regions in which patients differed from controls.

Voxel-based analysis is well-known to be relatively sensitive to small misregistration. In contrast, the proposed method is merely affected by the misregistration component that is parallel to the tract. Due to the continuity of the FA, this effect could be limited. Actually, in figure 1, we illustrated a good overlap between tracts of an arbitrarily chosen patient/control pair.

Although manual tracking was performed in this study, we believe that this work can easily be adapted to (un)supervised full brain tractography clustering methods. Additionally, analyzing larger cohorts that are partitioned in several subgroups, could be facilitated by a multi-sample Kolmogorov-Smirnov test.

Acknowledgments

Matthan Caan is involved in the Virtual Laboratory for e-Science project, supported by a BSIK grant from the Dutch Ministry of Education, Culture and Science, and the ICT innovation program of the Ministry of Economic Affairs. This study was financially supported by the Gratama Foundation and Research School Neurosciences Amsterdam, The Netherlands.

References

1. Basser, P., Pierpaoli, C.: Microstructural and physiological features of tissues elucidated by quantitative-diffusion-tensor MRI. J. Magn. Reson. B 111, 209–219 (1996)
2. Gerig, G., Gouttard, S., Corouge, I.: Analysis of brain white matter via fiber tract modeling. Engineering in Medicine and Biology Society 426, 4421–4424 (2004)
3. Sage, C., Peeters, R., Gorner, A., Robberecht, W., Sunaert, S.: Quantitative diffusion tensor imaging in amyotrophic lateral sclerosis. NeuroImage 34, 486–499 (2007)
4. Caan, M., Vermeer, K., van Vliet, L., Majoie, C., Peters, B., den Heeten, G., Vos, F.: Shaving diffusion tensor images in discriminant analysis: A study into schizophrenia. Medical Image Analysis 10, 841–849 (2006)
5. Corouge, I., Fletcher, P., Joshi, S., Gouttard, S., Gerig, G.: Fiber tract-oriented statistics for quantitative diffusion tensor MRI analysis. Med. Im.Anal. 10, 786–798 (2006)
6. Maddah, M., Wells III, W., Warfield, S., Westin, C.F., Grimson, W.: Probabilistic clustering and quantitative analysis of white matter fiber tracts. In: Karssemeijer, N., Lelieveldt, B. (eds.) IPMI 2007. LNCS, vol. 4584, pp. 372–383. Springer, Heidelberg (2007)
7. O'Donnell, L., Westin, C.F., Golby, A.: Tract-based morphometry. In: Ayache, N., Ourselin, S., Maeder, A. (eds.) MICCAI 2007, Part II. LNCS, vol. 4792, pp. 161–168. Springer, Heidelberg (2007)
8. Smith, S., Jenkinson, M., et al.: Tract-based spatial statistics: Voxelwise analysis of multi-subject diffusion data. NeuroImage 31, 1487–1505 (2006)
9. Jiang, H., van Zijl, P., et al.: DtiStudio: Resource program for diffusion tensor computation and fiber bundle tracking. Computer Methods and Programs in Biomedicine 81, 106–116 (2006)
10. Chui, H., Rangarajan, A., Zhang, J., Leonard, C.: Unsupervised learning of an atlas from unlabeled point-sets. IEEE Trans. on Pattern analysis and Machine Intelligence 26, 160–172 (2004)
11. Alippi, C., Braione, P.: Classification methods and inductive learning rules: What we learn from theory. IEEE Trans. Systems Man. Cybernatics 36, 649–655 (2006)

Dynamic Probabilistic Atlas of Functional Brain Regions for Transcranial Magnetic Stimulation

Juha Koikkalainen[1], Mervi Könönen[2,4], Jari Karhu[3], Jarmo Ruohonen[3], Eini Niskanen[2,5,6], and Jyrki Lötjönen[1]

[1] VTT, P.O.B. 1300, FIN-33101 Tampere, Finland
[2] NBS-laboratory, Department of Clinical Neurophysiology, Kuopio University Hospital, P.O.B. 1777, FIN-70211 Kuopio, Finland
[3] Nexstim Ltd., Elimäenkatu 9 B, FIN-00510 Helsinki, Finland
[4] Department of Clinical Radiology, Kuopio University Hospital, P.O.B. 1777, FIN-70211 Kuopio, Finland
[5] Department of Physics, University of Kuopio, P.O.B. 1627, FIN-70211 Kuopio, Finland
[6] Department of Neurology, Kuopio University Hospital, P.O.B. 1777, FIN-70211 Kuopio, Finland

Abstract. Transcranial Magnetic Stimulation (TMS) is a technique to stimulate the brain non-invasively. The applications range from accurate localization of the primary motor areas to potential treatment of disorders such as tinnitus, severe depression, and pain. Stereotactic guidance requires individual MR images of the subject's head, which is in some applications typically omitted due to financial motivations. In this paper, we introduce a method that offers improved TMS pulse targeting also to those subjects who do not have MR examinations. A probabilistic brain model was constructed by spatially normalizing the locations of the functional brain areas in a study population, and modeling the distributions and estimates of the locations of the functional brain regions using probabilistic methods. The application of the probabilistic brain model to the target subject was based on a point set determined from the scalp and facial skin of the target subject. The methods were evaluated using data from four functional brain areas from 56 healthy subjects. The accuracy of the estimates of the locations of the functional brain regions was about nine millimeters.

1 Introduction

Transcranial Magnetic Stimulation (TMS) is a technique to stimulate the brain non-invasively [1,2]. The applications range from accurate localization of the primary motor areas to potential treatment of disorders such as tinnitus, severe depression, and pain [3,4]. The clinical usefulness of TMS is greatly improved when it is combined with Magnetic Resonance (MR) imaging-guided navigation. Such combined use can tell exactly which locations of the brain are stimulated in TMS examinations [5]. Stereotactically guided TMS has been termed as Navigated Brain Stimulation (NBS).

Stereotactic guidance requires individual MR images of the target subject's (the subject for whom the NBS study is performed) head. In some of the applications of NBS, especially in psychiatric applications, the patients typically do not undergo an MR examination for diagnostic reasons. In these applications, the acquisition of the MR images is typically limited by financial motivations. In this paper, we introduce a method that offers improved TMS pulse targeting also to those groups of subjects who do not routinely have MR examinations. The objective is to provide accurate, fast, and low-cost methods to give *a priori* information on the locations and distributions of functional brain regions. This *a priori* information is useful also when MR images are available.

The main principle of the methods studied was to probabilistically model the distributions of the locations of functional brain regions by combining data from 56 subjects, for which the locations of the hand and leg motor areas were mapped with NBS. A probabilistic functional brain map was constructed by spatially normalizing the NBS localization data to the coordinate system of a mean brain template. When a target subject without MR images enters an NBS examination, the probabilistic atlas, including the mean grayscale brain template, its segmentation and functional brain map, is non-rigidly transformed to match his or her head's external shape. The non-rigid transformation is based on a set of points determined from the scalp and facial skin of the target subject. Therefore, expensive and time-consuming anatomical imaging of the target subject is not needed.

Our probabilistic atlas can be used during NBS examinations in two ways: 1) individualized head model is obtained for the target subject by deforming the head model of the mean brain template. This enables the visualization of the distributions of the locations of the functional brain regions and the current location of stimulus on a subject-specific head model, either using grayscale data of the model or surfaces made from its segmentation. 2) The probabilistic functional brain map indicates the most probable regions for stimulating desired cortical areas. When the first target location is searched, the map is based solely on the previously analyzed data from 56 subjects. However, when information about the locations of different functional brain regions becomes available during the stimulation procedure, the functional brain map is updated dynamically. In other words, the probability for a specific cortical area does not depend only on the data from the study population, but also on the already located areas of the current target subject. While this paper focuses on TMS, the methods are readily applicable also to other electromagnetic brain imaging methods such as magnetoencephalography (MEG).

2 Materials

The study population consisted of 56 healthy subjects (29 females, 27 males, mean age 48 ± 16 years, range 20 − 80 years). NBS studies were performed for each subject to locate the hand and leg motor areas.

The stimulation setup consisted of the navigation system (Nexstim Ltd, Helsinki, Finland) combined with a magnetic stimulator (Nexstim Ltd, Helsinki,

Finland) and a 50 mm figure-of-eight biphasic TMS coil. During stimulation, muscle activity was recorded and monitored continuously by electromyography (EMG) (ME 6000, Mega Electronics Ltd, Kuopio, Finland). EMG was measured from the thenar and hypothenar muscles (opponens pollicis) when examining hand motor area on the cortex, and from the tibialis muscle when examining leg motor area on the cortex. The NBS system delivered trigger pulses that synchronized the TMS and EMG systems.

Three anatomical landmarks and 22 marker points were defined on the scalp and facial skin. The anatomical landmarks were the nasion and the left and right peri-auricular points. The marker points were defined as follows: six points approximately equidistantly on the mid-sagittal slice starting from the tip of the nose and ending to the back of the head, six points on the horizontal slice at the level of the nasion, six points on the horizontal slice at the level of forehead, and four points on the horizontal slice at the level of the top of the brain. The difference between landmarks and marker points was that the landmarks could be defined from the same exact anatomical location from each subject, whereas the locations of the marker points could slightly vary between subjects. The points for one subject are visualized in Fig. 1. These points had two roles: 1) they allowed the reconstruction of the geometry of the head when anatomical images were not available and 2) they guided the registration processes needed to construct the probabilistic model of the locations of the functional brain regions and to match this model to the coordinate system of the target subject.

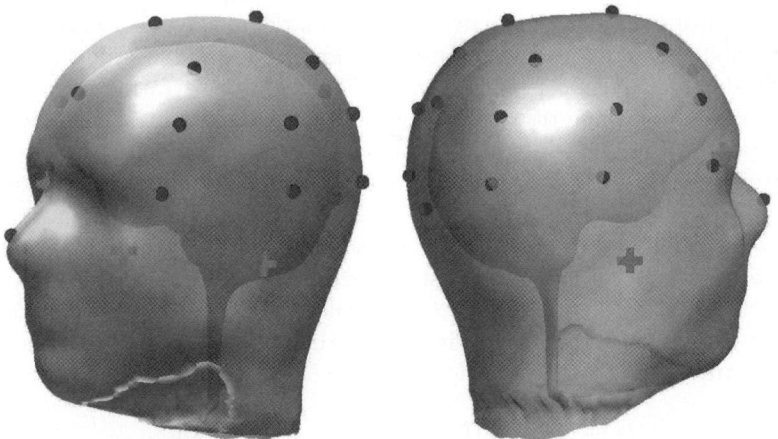

Fig. 1. The surfaces of the probabilistic atlas and the markers (spheres), and the anatomical landmarks (crosses)

3 Methods

The probabilistic brain model consists of a mean brain template representing the average brain anatomy and distributions and estimates of the locations of functional brain areas. In the NBS studies, the constructed probabilistic brain model is transformed into the target subject head providing the estimates of the locations of the functional brain areas for the target subject and enabling the visualization of the distributions of the functional brain areas on a subject-specific head model.

3.1 Construction of Probabilistic Brain Model

Mean Brain Template. A mean brain template representing the average anatomy of the healthy population was used as the reference in this study. The template had been constructed in the previous studies using the MR images of 31 healthy subjects (not included in the study population of this study) using methods presented in [6]. An MR volume representing the mean brain anatomy was generated from the MR images. This volume can be used in visualizing different spatial data related to NBS, such as the locations of functional regions, in subject specific anatomy. The surfaces representing the scalp, skull, and brain envelope, and the anatomical landmarks were also determined manually.

Registration of Training Set Data to Mean Brain Template. The study population has to be spatially normalized to study the distributions of the locations of functional brain areas. The normalization was performed by registering the study population subjects to the mean brain template.

The point-based registration method used in this work was originally presented in [6]. The method was composed of three steps: rigid, affine, and non-rigid registrations. First, the anatomical landmarks of the mean brain template were rigidly registered to the anatomical landmarks of the study population subject using the method proposed in [7]. Then, the registration was continued using 9-parameter affine transformation and all the anatomical landmarks and marker points. Finally, the scalp surface of the mean brain template was registered non-rigidly to the marker points of the study population subject using the free-form deformation (FFD) grid with linear basis functions and grid size $4 \times 4 \times 4$ [8]. The 9-affine and FFD transformations were optimized by minimizing a weighted sum of the mean distance from the markers of the subject, $\mathbf{p}_i$, to the scalp surface of the mean brain template, $\mathbf{M}$, and the distance between the corresponding anatomical landmarks of the subject, $\mathbf{l}_i$, and the mean brain template, $\mathbf{m}_i$:

$$E = \frac{1}{N_s} \sum_{i=1}^{N_s} d(\mathbf{M}, \mathbf{p}_i) + \alpha \frac{1}{N_l} \sum_{i=1}^{N_l} \|\mathbf{l}_i - \mathbf{m}_i\|. \tag{1}$$

The number of the anatomical landmarks and marker points were denoted by N_l and N_s, respectively. The distance $d()$ was defined from a distance map computed for the scalp surface. In this study, the optimal values for the weight α were searched by testing several values. The values used were $\alpha = 1$ in affine registration and $\alpha = 0.05$ in FFD registration.

Distributions and Estimates of Functional Brain Areas. After the NBS localization results of each study population subject had been transformed into the coordinate system of the mean brain template, the distributions of the functional brain areas were determined. These distributions give good first estimates for the locations of functional brain areas so that only small adjustments are needed to find the optimal locations during the stimulation.

The distributions of the functional brain areas were estimated using nonparametric probability density functions (Parzen windowing [9]). The probability that the jth functional brain area was located at location (x, y, z) was computed as

$$\hat{P}_j(x,y,z) = \sum_{i=1}^{N} \frac{1}{\sqrt{2\pi\sigma_1^2}} e^{-\frac{||(x,y,z)-X_{i,j}||^2}{2\sigma_1^2}}, \tag{2}$$

$$P_j(x,y,z) = \frac{\hat{P}_j(x,y,z)}{\sum_{x,y,z} \hat{P}_j(x,y,z)}, \tag{3}$$

where N was the number of subjects, $X_{i,j}$ the location of the jth functional brain area of the ith subject, and σ_1 was used to control the width of the Gaussian window. In this study, we used $\sigma_1 = 5$ mm. The normalization in Eq. 3 was done so that the probabilities would sum up to one. Similarly, the mean of the locations of a functional brain area in the study population was used as the estimate of the location of the jth functional brain area $\hat{Y}_j$:

$$\hat{Y}_j = \frac{1}{N} \sum_{i=1}^{N} X_{i,j}. \tag{4}$$

In the NBS studies, the hand motor area is usually located first, and after that the motor area of leg. In this study, a technique was proposed in which the optimal location of a functional brain area determined with NBS was utilized to improve the accuracy of the distribution and estimate of another functional brain area. It was hypothesized that if, for example, the motor area of hand of a study population subject is near to the corresponding area of the target subject the same is true also for the motor area of leg.

Based on this hypothesis, a Gaussian model was assumed for the dependency between the locations of different functional brain areas. Weights were determined for each study population subject based on the distance from the location of a functional brain area of the study population subject to the optimal location of the target subject obtained with NBS. A Gaussian function was used to determine the weights:

$$w_{i,j} = \frac{1}{\sqrt{2\pi\sigma_2^2}} e^{-\frac{||X_{i,j}-Y_j||^2}{2\sigma_2^2}}, \tag{5}$$

where Y_j was the real location of the jth functional brain area of the target subject obtained with NBS and σ_2 was used to control the width of the Gaussian function. With the small values of σ_2, those study population subjects for which $||X_{i,j} - Y_j||$ is small will get large weights. If σ_2 is large, also those subjects, for which $||X_{i,j} - Y_j||$ is large, will have moderate weights. The optimal value for σ_2 was searched and used in computing the results.

If the optimal localization results of several functional brain areas were used, the weights of all the areas were multiplied,

$$\hat{w}_i = \prod_j w_{i,j}, \qquad (6)$$

and, normalized so that they summed up to one:

$$\bar{w}_i = \frac{\hat{w}_i}{\sum_{j=1}^{N} \hat{w}_j}. \qquad (7)$$

Finally, the distribution of the functional brain area was approximated using the weighted version of Eq. 2:

$$P_j(x,y,z) = \sum_{i=1}^{N} \bar{w}_i \frac{1}{\sqrt{2\pi\sigma_1^2}} e^{-\frac{||(x,y,z) - X_{i,j}||^2}{2\sigma_1^2}}, \qquad (8)$$

and the estimate of the location of the functional brain area was computed as the weighted mean of the locations of the functional brain area in the study population:

$$\hat{Y}_j = \sum_{i=1}^{N} \bar{w}_i X_{i,j}. \qquad (9)$$

3.2 Evaluation

The accuracy of the estimates of the locations of functional brain areas was evaluated by measuring the Euclidean distances from the estimates $\hat{Y}_j$ to the real locations of the functional brain regions Y_j obtained using NBS. This was performed for all the subjects, and the mean of the estimation errors was computed for each functional brain region. Three techniques of determining the estimate were evaluated: Technique 1) The mean of the study population locations (Eq. 4). Technique 2) The weighted mean of the study population locations (Eq. 9) by utilizing *a priori* information on the optimal location of the corresponding functional brain area on the opposite hemisphere. Technique 3) The weighted mean of the study population locations (Eq. 9) by utilizing *a priori* information on the optimal locations of all the other functional brain areas.

The analysis was performed using full leave-one-out cross-validation: the subject representing the target subject was excluded from the study population, and the probabilistic model was generated using the remaining subjects. This was repeated for each one of the 56 study population subjects. As a result, the probabilistic brain models used in this paper were based only on 55 subjects and were slightly different for each target subject.

4 Results

The results for the estimation accuracy of the locations of the functional brain areas were 8.8 ± 4.3 mm, 9.2 ± 5.2 mm, 8.7 ± 5.2 mm and 8.8 ± 4.9 mm for opponens pollicis (right hemisphere), opponent pollicis (left hemisphere), tibialis (right hemisphere) and tibialis (left hemisphere), respectively. These numbers correspond to the Technique 1. The error was reduced by $0.5 - 1.5$ mm by utilizing the information on the optimal locations of the other functional brain areas located using NBS (Techniques 2 and 3). The best result was obtained by utilizing all the other functional brain areas (Technique 3) although the difference compared with the Technique 2 was small.

Examples of the distributions of the functional brain areas on a subject-specific head model using the navigation tool are shown in Fig. 2. In this example, the optimal locations of all the functional brain areas already obtained using NBS were utilized to provide *a priori* information.

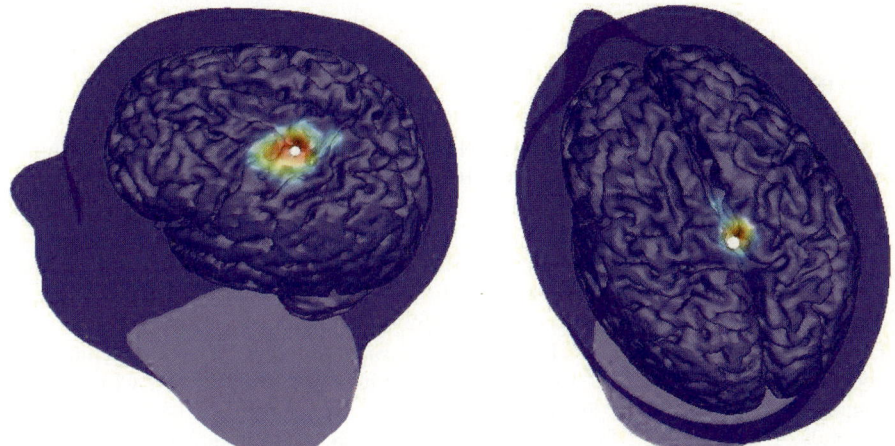

Fig. 2. Probability distributions for the two functional brain areas visualized on a subject-specific head model

5 Discussion

In the study described in this paper, a fast, accurate, and low-cost method was developed for NBS studies to provide an estimate of the locations of functional brain regions using a dynamic probabilistic atlas. In addition, methods for the visualization of the distributions of the functional brain areas on a subject-specific head model were developed. These methods enable reasonably accurate identification of the desired NBS target sites even without individual brain imaging results.

The accuracy of the estimates of the locations of the functional brain areas obtained using the probabilistic brain model was about nine millimeters. The estimation accuracy was better for the representation area of the tibialis than for the representation area of the opponens pollicis. Especially, the utilization of the localization information from the opposite hemisphere improved much more the localization accuracy of the representation area of the tibialis. This was because the representation area of the tibialis is located close to the mid-sagittal plane, and therefore, the distance to the opposite hemisphere is short. We have tested the utilization of the MR images in the registrations needed in the construction of the probabilistic brain model, but this has not improved the accuracy of the estimates.

The developed methods were fast. The non-rigid point-based registration of the mean brain template to the target subject head took approximately 3 − 4 seconds (implemented with C), the computation of the estimate of the location of a functional brain area less than one second (implemented with Matlab), and the computation of the distribution of the location of a functional brain area approximately eight seconds (implemented with Matlab) using a standard PC workstation. Especially the parts implemented with Matlab could be further hastened.

References

1. Barker, A., Jalinous, R., Freeston, I.: Non-invasive magnetic stimulation of human motor cortex. Lancet. 1(8437), 1106–1107 (1985)
2. Hallett, M.: Transcranial magnetic stimulation and the human brain. Nature 406, 147–150 (2000)
3. George, M., Nahas, Z., Molloy, M., Speer, A., Oliver, N., Li, X.B., Arana, G., Risch, S., Ballenger, J.: A controlled trial of daily left prefrontal cortex TMS for treating depression. Biological Psychiatry 48(10), 962–970 (2000)
4. Pridmore, S., Kleinjung, T., Langguth, B., Eichhammer, P.: Transcranial magnetic stimulation: Potential treatment for tinnitus? Psychiatry and Clinical Neurosciences 60(2), 133–138 (2006)
5. Hannula, H., Ylioja, S., Pertovaara, A., Korvenoja, A., Ruohonen, J., Ilmoniemi, R., Carlson, S.: Somatotopic Blocking of Sensation with Navigated Transcranial Magnetic Stimulation of the Primary Somatosensory Cortex. Human Brain Mapping 26(2), 100–109 (2005)
6. Koikkalainen, J., Lötjönen, J.: Reconstruction of 3-D Head Geometry from Digitized Point Sets: an Evaluation Study. IEEE Transactions on Information Technology in Biomedicine 8(3) (2004)
7. Arun, K., Huang, T., Blostein, S.: Least-squares fitting of two 3-D point sets. IEEE Transactions on Pattern Analysis and Machine Intelligence 9(5), 698–700 (1987)
8. Rueckert, D., Sonoda, L., Hayes, C., Hill, D., Leach, M., Hawkes, D.: Nonrigid Registration Using Free-Form Deformations: Application to Breast MR Images. IEEE Transactions on Medical Imaging 18(8), 712–721 (1999)
9. Duda, R., Hart, P.: Pattern Classification and Scene Analysis. John Wiley & Sons, New York (1973)

Unbiased Stratification of Left Ventricles

Rajagopalan Srinivasan, K.S. Shriram, and Srikanth Suryanarayanan

Imaging Technologies Lab, GE Global Research, India

Abstract. Image based quantitative stratification of the Left Ventricles (LV) across a population helps in unraveling the structure-function symbiosis of the heart. An unbiased, reference less grouping scheme that automatically determines the number of clusters and a physioanatomically relevant strategy that aligns the intra cluster LV shapes would enable the robust construction of pathology stratified cardiac atlas. This paper achieves this hitherto elusive stratification and alignment by adapting the conventional strategies routinely followed by clinicians. The individual LV shape models (N=127) are **independently** oriented to an "*attitudinally consistent orientation*" that captures the physioanatomic variations of the LV morphology. Affinity propagation technique based on the automatically identified inter-LV_landmark distances is used to group the LV shapes. The proposed algorithm is computationally efficient and, if the inter cluster variations are linked to pathology, could provide a clinically relevant cardiac atlas.

1 Introduction

The omnipresent manifestation of cardiovascular disease has necessitated the cross-disciplinary convergence towards creating computational tools that enable **P4** (**p**ersonalized, **p**redictive, **p**reemptive and **p**articipatory) medicine. Construction of pathology-specific cardiac atlases is a forerunner among these computational tools. By augmenting the epidemiological studies with the associated pathology stratified physioanatomic variations, cardiac atlases can benefit the practitioner, practice and the patient.

Image based quantitation of the pathology associated morphologic alterations and personalization of this knowledge to the patient specific multidimensional data helps in assessing the patient's cardiac wellness. While clinicians have acquired the skills to perform such stratification mentally, automatic stratification requires a machine-learning step that involves collating data across multiple subjects into a statistical atlas that captures the pathology-specific morphology variations.

The atlas construction is typically accomplished through an image alignment process that establishes pair wise correspondence between two datasets and subsequently stitches multiple such correspondences to establish a joint homology. Such approaches suffer from the biased choice of a reference dataset to which the rest are aligned. To overcome this discrepancy, a number of unbiased, simultaneous registration schemes have been proposed [1-3]. These schemes align the multiple subjects to a common coordinate system by determining the most consistent alignment of the joint data. Though technically elegant, these techniques do not adhere to the clinician friendly *"attitudinally consistent orientation"* [4] and require the simultaneous treatment of all the datasets under investigation.

In brain mapping, the Talairach space is often used as the unifying co-ordinate system that provides *"attitudinally consistent orientation"* to **independently** map inter and intra- subject brain datasets. Likewise, a unified space could be described to map LVs based on the following facts: (a) the LV pose serves as a unifying reference frame across different subjects [5]; (b) the motion of the LV through the cardiac cycle can be separated into global translation, longitudinal and circumferential shortening or elongation [6]; and (c) acquisition during the diastasic phase of the cardiac cycle provides a dataset with least motion artifacts [7].

By cascading the above-mentioned facts into an algorithmic pipeline, we propose an unbiased, referenceless approach that reorients the shape models of the individual LVs **independently** into a consistent physioanatomic space, and in the process maximizes the joint similarities between the datasets. The reoriented LV shapes can be subsequently aggregated into a crisp or statistical atlas. However, for a dynamic physioanatomically-varying organ such as the LV, a single crisp exemplar (atlas) cannot account for the complete family of shape space; blind statistical grouping of aligned shapes does not help in understanding the pathological influences. This necessitates the need for LV stratification into tighter subgroups. Though unsupervised, unbiased, and reference less shape clustering techniques exist, lack of methods to estimate the natural number of clusters in a population has probably hindered the construction of unbiased LV groupings. This paper explores the use of affinity propagation [8] to construct unbiased, natural clusters of LV shapes. In combination with the *"attitudinally consistent orientation"*, the proposed stratification strategy helps in constructing physioanatomically-stratified atlases. Linking the physioanatomic variations to the underlying pathology enables the construction of clinically relevant cardiac atlases.

2 Materials and Methods

2.1 Data Acquisition

The datasets for this study were selected from the cardiac CT scans acquired at Narayana Hrudhayalaya, Bangalore, India using a 64-slice Lightspeed VCT (GE Healthcare) MDCT scanner. Acquisitions from patients with atypical chest pain, those requiring corrective surgery and potentially normal subjects who participated in the mandatory executive screening were included in this study. In accordance with the clinical protocol, the heart rate of the subjects was, where required, ionotropically controlled using beta-blockers. Personalized BMI-adjusted tube current and retrospective ECG gating was used during the acquisition. High temporal resolution images were obtained by reconstructing the data with partial scan reconstruction at 75% interval (corresponding to the almost no-motion diastasic phase) in R-R ECG cycle.

2.2 Construction of LV Shape Model

The LV shape model was built using an interactive segmentation tool available in the GE Healthcare Advantage Windows (AW) workstation. Trained 3D technicians sparsely segmented the key LV sections using the border-tracing tool; the sparse segmentations were populated using a shape propagation technique. Out-of-plane edge incoherency was corrected using a topology preserving smoothing method based on curvature flow.

2.3 Generation of Attitudinally Consistent Orientation

As mentioned before, the motion of the LV through the cardiac cycle can be distinctly separated into global translation, longitudinal and circumferential shortening or elongation [6]. By **independently** translating the individual LV shape models to a common origin and reorienting them so that their orthogonal axes correspond to the directions of longitudinal and circumferential scaling, the respective models can be aligned to the clinically recognized "*attitudinally consistent orientation*". Grouping the LVs in this consistent position facilitates the quantification of the physioanatomic variations in the morphology.

The global translation is synchronized by computing the centroids of the individual LV and shifting them to a common origin. The longitudinal axis of the LV spans across the apex and the base; this axis corresponds to the pose of the LV shape model. The pose is captured from the shape's second order moment via the Principal Component Analysis (PCA). Aligning the dominant orientation of the individual models **independently** to a *"common axis"* (in this study x- axis was used as the common axis) establishes a consistent longitudinal framework across all the models. Figure 1 illustrates the longitudinal alignment.

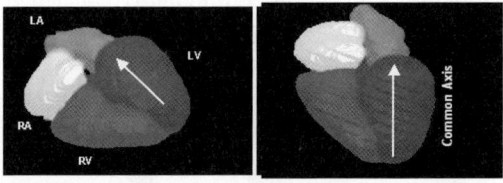

Fig. 1. Consistent inter-subject LV pose (right) is achieved by independently aligning the principal Eigen vectors of the individual LV shape models (left) to a common axis

While the PCA based alignment provides a referenceless, unbiased longitudinal orientation consistency across the LV shape models, it does not guarantee a consistent in-plane orientation. Correcting for this inconsistency in an independent, unbiased and referenceless manner is a challenge and requires exploiting the salient features of the cardiac architecture.

Within the LV, an organ in perpetual flux, the aortic vestibule and the immediate vicinity of the mitral valve are stationary across the cardiac cycle [5]. Identifying and suitably orienting key landmarks within this region provides a consistent in-plane orientation and hence better overall alignment. These landmarks were identified by traversing through the medial surface (MS) of the LV shape model.

A number of efficient algorithms exist for constructing the MS of a given shape. In this study, the Parameter controlled skeletonization proposed in [9] was used. Briefly, the method uses the fact that any point on the MS should be the local maxima in the

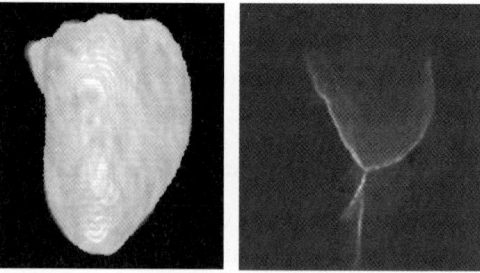

Fig. 2. Parameter-skeleton based MS (right) of a LV shape model (left)

distance transform space. The local maxima locations greater than the mean neighborhood distance is identified as a candidate location in MS. Figure 2 shows the MS generated by this method for a representative LV.

As clearly seen in Figure 2, the MS of LV originates at the apex and bifurcates towards the aortic and mitral valves. The landmarks of our choice lie at the terminal of the "Y". The landmark corresponding to the aortic valve is used to fix the in-plane rotation. Since the aortic valve is closed during the *diastasic* phase, the distance coding of the prong terminating on this valve will be stronger (this can be clearly seen in the left prong of Figure 2). The plane formed by the principal eigen vector of the LV and the aortic valve (terminal of the dominant prong of the MS) is rotated about the "*common axis*" until it aligns with the XZ plane as shown in Figure 3. This procedure ensures that all the datasets are in an *"attitudinally consistent orientation"* that captures the physioanatomic variations of the LV morphology.

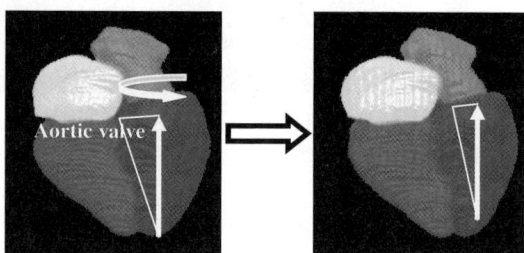

Fig. 3. In-plane alignment of using planed formed by LV principal axis and the aortic valve

2.4 Stratification of LV Shapes

As mentioned before, crisp or statistical aggregation of consistently oriented LV models does not provide a clinically relevant cardiac atlas. An unsupervised clustering technique that automatically finds the natural number of clusters is required to create an unbiased stratification of LVs. Affinity propagation [8] readily meets this stringent requirement. Briefly, affinity propagation iteratively finds clusters given pair wise similarities of a point cloud of n-dimensional data. Further to resolving the clusters in the point cloud, the algorithm identifies the exemplar that is most 'central' to each of the clusters.

In each iteration, every candidate i is considered as a potential exemplar of a cluster and its 'responsibility' to every potential member k of the cluster computed as:

$$r(i,k) = s(i,k) - \max_{k' \neq k}\{a(i,k') + s(i,k')\}$$

where, $s(i,k)$ is the similarity between candidates i and k and the 'availability' $a(i,k)$ of data point k to a cluster exemplified by i is defined as:

$$a(i,k) = \min\{0, r(k,k) + \sum_{i' \notin \{i,k\}} \max\{0, r(i',k)\}\}$$

Iteratively, competing exemplars claim data points at every turn and convergence is achieved when data points coalesce into distinct clusters.

For clustering the LV shapes, similarity metric based on the inter-distances between the apex(Ap), aortic valve (Av) and mitral valve (Mv) as deduced from the terminals of the dominant "Y" in the medial surface was used. Specifically, the similarity metric $s(i,k)$ between datasets i and k is defined as

$$s(i,k) = (((D(Ap_i, Av_i) + D(Ap_i, Mv_i) + D(Av_i, Mv_i)) - ((D(Ap_k, Av_k) + D(Ap_k, Mv_k) + D(Av_k, Mv_k)))^2$$

where $D(x,y)$ is the distance between points x and y.

3 Results

On a database of 127 LV shape models, the affinity propagation yielded six unique clusters based on the similarity measure described above. The glyphs in Figure 4 shows the pair wise similarities before and after stratification in the form of a 'confusion' matrix; the darker shade implies a low similarity between two datasets. Results for the LV landmark based stratification (right panel) qualitatively reveals the maximization and minimization respectively of intra (diagonal sub blocks) and inter (off-diagonal sub blocks) cluster similarities.

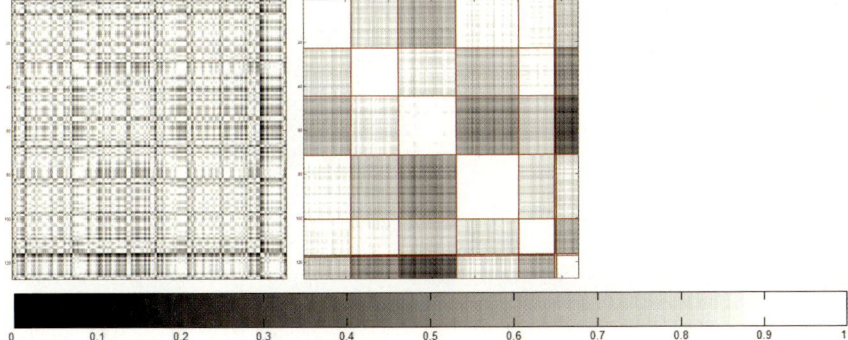

Fig. 4. Pair wise similarity between LV shape models before (left) and after (right) affinity propagation based clustering. Lighter the shade, higher the similarity.

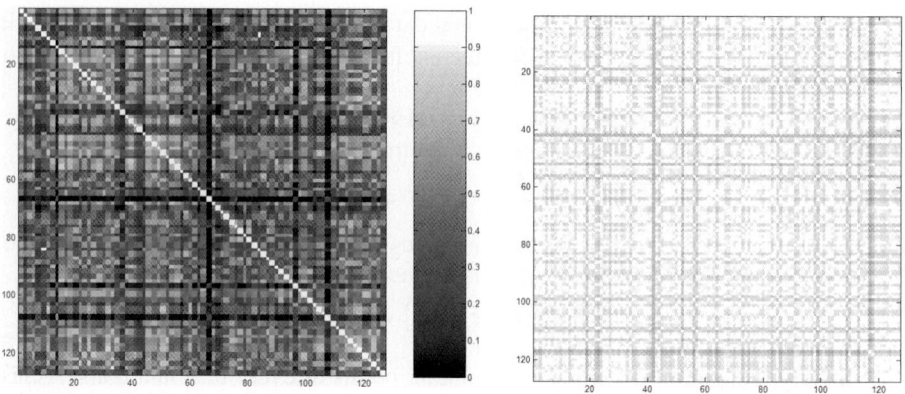

Fig. 5. Pair wise DSCs between the LV shapes before (left) and after (right) ***independent*** orientation of the individual LVs into the "*attitudinally consistent orientation*" space

Quantitative efficacy of the stratification was established by computing the Analysis of Similarity (ANOSIM) R that indicates the magnitude of difference among clusters. Value of 1 indicates that the communities completely differ among defined

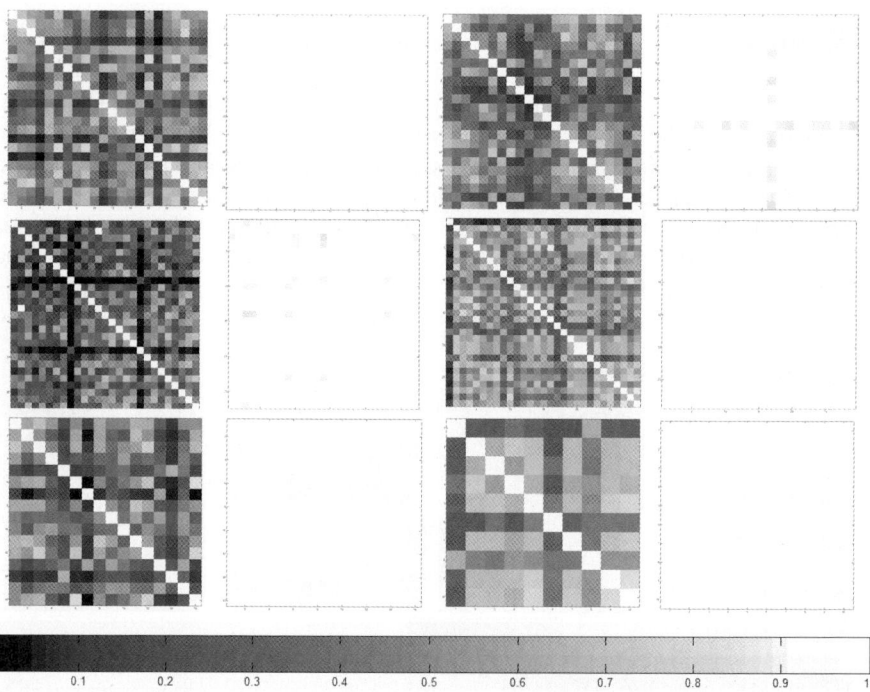

Fig. 6. Pair wise DSC between LV shapes within the six clusters. The DSCs shown in the left and right columns correspond respectively to those before and after the independent alignment to the *"attitudinally consistent orientation"* space.

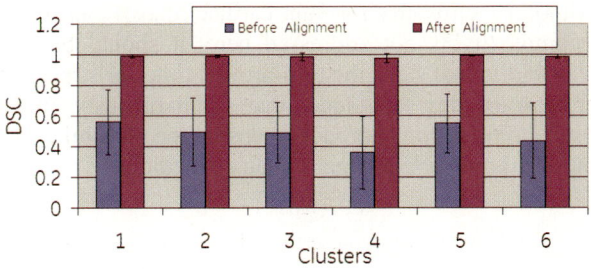

Fig. 7. Pair wise DSC of LV shape volumes in each of the six clusters before and after alignment. The mean DSC shows marked improvement after alignment; concomitantly, the standard deviation has also reduced in the aligned space.

groups, value of 0 indicates no difference among groups. The combined R for the six LV clusters was found to be 0.9213 ± 0.023 highlighting the greater agreement of candidates within each of the clusters.

To capture the efficacy of the *"attitudinally consistent orientation"* step, pairwise similarity between the models was computed both in the native and aligned space. Dice Similarity Coefficient (DSC) was used as the similarity metric. The glyphs in Figure 5 show the effect of the **independent** alignment of the individual LVs to the *"attitudinally consistent orientation"* space. It is clear that the DSC numbers show marked improvement after the unbiased, reference less, anatomically relevant alignment indicating closeness of match. The results also attest the fact that much of the mismatch across LVs can be accounted for by an affine transformation.

Figure 6 shows the pair wise DSC for the LVs within the six clusters. The graph in Figure 7 shows the mean DSCs before and after alignment of the LVs within the six clusters; the statistics agrees with the visual glyphs shown in Figure 7.

4 Discussion and Conclusions

The quintessential feature for grouping LV across multiple subjects should preferably be one that has a coeval existence across the life span of the humans. The ballooning of the secondary myocardium from the outer curvature of the "**Y**" shaped primary heart tube results in the formation of the atrial and ventricular chambers [10]. The apical portion of the left ventricle (LV) originates from the stem of the primary heart tube. Subsequently the mitral and aortic valves develop along the prongs of the heart tube. The signature of the Y tube about which the LV twirled around can be clearly seen even in adult hearts from its medial axis (Figure 2). This justifies the clinical relevance of the *mitral-aortic-LV_base* landmarks as key points for LV stratification.

Grouping data automatically into natural clusters has hitherto been a hard problem. The advent of affinity propagation has enabled the possibility of creating unbiased clusters. By combining the quintessential LV landmarks with a robust affinity propagation based LV stratification and unbiased, referenceless, **independent** orientation of the LVs into *"attitudinally consistent orientation"* space, this paper made the first attempt to represent multi subject Left Ventricles within a unified space to optimally characterize the physioanatomic variations. By linking the physioanatomic variations to the underlying pathology clinically relevant cardiac atlases can be created. While the computational complexity is not addressed here, it should be convincing that given the simplicity of individual steps the turn-around time for stratification is orders of magnitude faster than existing techniques that simultaneously operate on all the datasets. The proposed stratification approach opens up the possibility of image based personalized, preemptive, predictive and participatory medicine.

References

1. Bhatia, K.K., et al.: Consistent group-wise non-rigid registration for atlas construction. In: Proc. IEEE Symposium on Biomedical Imaging (ISBI), pp. 908–911 (2004)
2. De Craene, M., et al.: Multi-subject registration for unbiased Statistical Atlas Construction. In: Barillot, C., Haynor, D.R., Hellier, P. (eds.) MICCAI 2004, Part I. LNCS, vol. 3216, pp. 655–662. Springer, Heidelberg (2004)
3. Zollie, L., et al.: Efficient population registration of 3D data. In: Liu, Y., Jiang, T., Zhang, C. (eds.) CVBIA 2005. LNCS, vol. 3765, pp. 291–301. Springer, Heidelberg (2005)
4. McAlpine, W.A.: Heart and Coronary Arteries. An anatomical atlas for Clinical Diagnosis, Radiological Investigation, and Surgical Treatment. Springer, Berlin (1995)
5. Edwards, L.: The Vortex of Life. Floris Books (1993)
6. Gould, K.L., et al.: Analysis of wall dynamics and directional components of left ventricular contraction in man. Am. J. Cardiol. 38, 322 (1976)
7. Mahesh, M., Cody, D.D.: Physics of Cardiac imaging with multiple-row detector CT. Radiographics 27, 1495–1509 (2007)
8. Frey, B., Dueck, D.: Clustering by Passing Messages between Data Points. Science 315, 972 (2007)
9. Gagvani, N., Silver, D.: Parameter controlled skeletonization of three dimensional objects. Technical Report CAIP-TR-216, Rutgers State University of New Jersey (1997)
10. Moorman, A., et al.: Development of the heart: formation of the cardiac chambers and arterial trunks. Heart 89, 806–814 (2003)

3D Cerebral Cortical Morphometry in Autism: Increased Folding in Children and Adolescents in Frontal, Parietal, and Temporal Lobes

Suyash P. Awate[1,*], Lawrence Win[2], Paul Yushkevich[1],
Robert T. Schultz[2], and James C. Gee[1]

[1] Penn Image Computing and Science Lab (PICSL), University of Pennsylvania
awate@mail.med.upenn.edu
[2] Center for Autism Research (CAR), Children's Hospital of Philadelphia, USA

Abstract. This paper presents a systematic evaluation of cortical folding, or complexity, in autism. It introduces two *novel measures* to analyze folding in a specific region of interest, which, unlike traditional measures, produce an intuitive easily-interpretable description of folding and inform the nature of folding change by incorporating local surface-patch orientation. This study reports *new* findings of *increased* cortical folding in autistics in the frontal, parietal, and temporal lobes, as compared to controls. These differences are stronger in children than adolescents. The paper validates part of the findings using the new measures based on comparisons with traditional measures. Unlike studies in the literature, this paper reports new findings, via a *fully 3D* folding analysis on all brain lobes, based on the consensus of virtually *all* 6 folding measures used (2 new, 4 traditional) via rigorous statistical *permutation testing*. In these ways, this paper not only strengthens some previous clinical findings, but also extends the state of the art in autism research.

1 Introduction

Autism is a serious neurodevelopmental disorder that causes a variety of cognitive deficits impairing social interaction and communication. A good understanding of the underlying neurobiological causes is absent. Mostly, brain morphometry in autism [1,2,3,4,5,6], revealing abnormalities in both gray matter (GM) and white matter (WM), has been restricted to volumetry of tissues, lobes, brain, etc. For instance, Carper *et al.* [2] found volumetric abnormalities in the frontal, temporal, and parietal lobes, and attributed this finding to the role of these lobes in normal behavioral function. Levitt *et al.* [7] create maps of 22 major sulci and report anatomical shifts for some sulci in frontal and temporal lobes. Nordahl *et al.* [8] report increased sulcal depths for autistic subjects in the operculum and the intraparietal sulcus using surface-based morphometry

---

* The authors gratefully acknowledge the NIH support of this work through grants HD042974, HD046159, MH068066, NS045839, U19-HD35482, U54-MH066494-01.

(SBM). They found all abnormalities to be more pronounced in children than adolescents.

Studies on cortical folding, or complexity, in autism have received very little attention. The degree of cortical folding is actually closely tied to brain volume [9]. Qualitative, *visual scoring-based*, analyses by Piven et al. [10] and Bailey et al. [11] report irregularities in folding patterns in the form of polymicrogyria and hyperconvoluted temporal lobes. Polymicrogyria typically increases the irregularity of the GM-WM interface [12]. A recent *preliminary* study by Hardan et al. [13] reports increased gyrification on one 2D coronal slice anterior to the corpus callosum. They compute a gyrification index (GI) by *manually tracing* the outer and inner cortical 2D contours. They *hypothesize* that the increased cortical convolutions in autistics will be more pronounced in children than in adults, finding negative correlation between GI and the autistics' age.

Apart from GI, there are several other measures [14,15,16] to characterize different aspects of cortical folding. These include measures defined using the properties of individual cortical-surface patches (*local measures*) and measures designed to extract information from the entire cortical surface taken as a whole (*global measures*). While Batchelor et al. [15] use a subset of these measures to study folding in the developing human fetal brain (region-based folding computation), Tosun et al. [16] use another subset to quantify cortical folding in Parkinson-plus syndrome (voxel-based folding computation).

2 Materials and Methods

2.1 Clinical Cohort and MRI

The clinical cohort comprised 70 normal males and 90 autistic males, both divided into 3 age groups: (i) children: 7.5 to 12.5 years, (ii) adolescents: 12.5 to 19.5 years, and (iii) adults: 19.5 to 31 years. The age distributions in the corresponding normal and patient groups were well matched. The sample size, mean age (in years), and standard deviation of age (in years) for the *normal* groups were: (i) 20, 10.5, 1; (ii) 24, 15.9, 2.3; and (iii) 26, 25.6, 3.4; and for the *autistic* groups were: (i) 48, 10.3, 1.3; (ii) 32, 15.5, 1.9; and (iii) 10, 25.7, 3, respectively. MR images were acquired on a GE 1.5T scanner; sagittal SPGR; 2 NEX, 1.2mm^3; TR=24; flip angle=45; matrix=192x256; FOV=30cm; 124 slices.

2.2 Traditional Measures for Cortical Folding Analysis

This study employs the traditional cortical-folding measures to compare and validate the performance of the new measures introduced in the next section. Traditional measures, described as follows, can be difficult to interpret.

1. *Intrinsic curvature index* (ICI) [14]: counts hemispherical features by integrating across all surface patches with positive Gaussian curvature.

$$\text{ICI}(\mathcal{M}) = \frac{1}{4\pi} \int_{m \in \mathcal{M}} G^+(m) \, d\mathcal{M}, \qquad (1)$$

where $G^+(m) = \max(K_{\min}(m)K_{\max}(m), 0)$; $K_{\min}$, $K_{\max}$ are the principal curvatures. Any local bump/pit with a hemispherical shape, irrespective of its size, increases ICI by 0.5. However, ICI *ignores* cylindrical and saddle-like patches that have non-positive Gaussian curvature. This separation of curved patches, although mathematically sound, makes ICI *difficult to interpret*.

2. *Mean curvature L2 norm* (MCN) [15]: counts hemispherical and cylindrical features by integrating the mean curvature across all surface patches:

$$\text{MCN}(\mathcal{M}) = \left[\int_{m \in \mathcal{M}} H^2(m) d\mathcal{M} \right]^{0.5}, \tag{2}$$

where $H(m) = [K_{\min}(m) + K_{\max}(m)]/2$. However, similar to ICI, MCN *ignores* non-planar surface patches having saddle-like shapes ($H(m) = 0$), thereby complicating the semantics of its application to cortical folding.

3. *Convexity ratio* (CR): is a global measure of folding defined as the ratio of the areas of the surface and its convex hull. Increased convolution/gyrification will increase CR. CR generalizes GI to 3D.

4. *Isoperimetric ratio* (IPR): is a global measure of folding defined as the ratio of surface area to the enclosed volume to the power 2/3. Convoluted surfaces have increased IPRs. Both CR and IPR, being global measures, fail to probe deeply into the *local causes* for the changes in folding.

All aforementioned measures, furthermore, ignore the *orientation* of surface patches, e.g. they fail to distinguish a road surface with multiple bumps from another road where the bumps are replaced by potholes. The bumps and potholes on a surface might be compared to cortical gyri and sulci, respectively.

2.3 Novel Measures for Region-Based Cortical Folding Analysis

This section describes two novel measures to quantify the degree of cortical folding in a region of interest. These novel measures are based on Koenderink's seminal work in differential geometry [17], which completely characterizes local surface patches/neighborhoods in terms of their *shape index* and *curvedness*. While the shape index characterizes the orientation associated with a surface patch, i.e. concave, hyperbolic (saddle), or convex, curvedness quantifies the deviation of the surface patch from planarity. This systematic and intuitive *reparameterization* (shape index, curvedness) of the surface descriptors (principal curvatures) can lead to more meaningful studies of cortical folding.

The *shape index* $S(m)$, for a patch at point m on surface $\mathcal{M}$, is

$$S(m) = -\frac{2}{\pi} \arctan \frac{K_{\max}(m) + K_{\min}(m)}{K_{\max}(m) - K_{\min}(m)}. \tag{3}$$

For instance, (i) a patch on a sphere, which has the same curvature in all directions, has $S = 1$; (ii) a patch on a cylinder, which has no curvature along the axis of the cylinder, has $S = 0.5$; (iii) saddle-shaped patch, which is convex in one direction and concave in the orthogonal direction, has $S = 0$. The shape index changes sign based on the orientation (notion of inside versus outside) of the surface, e.g. a cap ($S = 1$) and a cup ($S = -1$). The shape index is independent of the scale associated with the surface patch. In this way, the shape index informs the *type* of the patch and its *orientation* (see Figure 1(e)).

The *curvedness* for the surface patch at point m, which perfectly complements the information captured by the shape index, is

$$C(m) = [0.5(K_{\max}^2(m) + K_{\min}^2(m))]^{0.5} \qquad (4)$$

and measures the deviation from flatness or planarity. Thus, more convoluted surface patches produce larger values of C. The curvedness is, however, sensitive to the scale associated with the surface patch. For instance, if lengths are scaled up by $\lambda > 1$, then the resulting surface patch now covers a smaller portion of the surface, thereby reducing $K_{\max}$ and $K_{\min}$ by a factor of λ. Extremely small patches have $C \to 0$; indeed, all sufficiently-small patches can be well approximated as being planar (corollary of the Taylor's theorem).

Based on this local parameterization of surface *patches* in terms of the shape index S and curvedness C, this paper proposes *two novel measures* to quantify folding characteristics of cortical-surface *regions*. These novel folding measures are, by design, *invariant to translation and rotation* (changes in the location or orientation of the slice planes during MRI) as well as the scale (changes in the resolution of the MR image) of the cortical surface representation (akin to measures in previous section).

1. **Average curvedness** (AC): We define AC by integrating the curvedness over the region of interest $\mathcal{M}$ on the cortical surface.

$$\mathrm{AC}(\mathcal{M}) = \left[\int_{m \in \mathcal{M}} C^2(m) d\mathcal{M} \right]^{0.5}, \qquad (5)$$

where $d\mathcal{M}$ is the area measure of a small surface patch. AC is *invariant to scale* because $C^2 d\mathcal{M}$ is invariant to scale. Planar surface patches do not contribute to AC. A *more-convoluted* cortex produces a *larger* value of AC.

2. **Average shape index** (AS): We define AS by integrating the shape index over the region of interest $\mathcal{M}$ on the cortical surface

$$\mathrm{AS}(\mathcal{M}) = \int_{m \in \mathcal{M}} \mathrm{S}(m) \frac{d\mathcal{M}}{\| d\mathcal{M} \|}. \qquad (6)$$

AS measures the average convexity/concavity of a surface. Planar components of a surface do *not* contribute to AS. For example, a surface having more number of (convex) *bumps/protrusions* or larger protrusions will produce a *larger* AS. On the other hand, a surface having more number of (concave) *pits* will produce a *smaller* AS. The protrusions and pits on a surface might be compared to gyri and sulci on the cerebral cortex, respectively.

2.4 Folding Analysis in a Level-Set Framework

The basic components of the pipeline, described as follows, are shown in Figure 1.

Brain Tissue Segmentation: The skull stripping and initial alignment of the images into AC-PC space were performed manually using Analyze (Figure 1(a)).

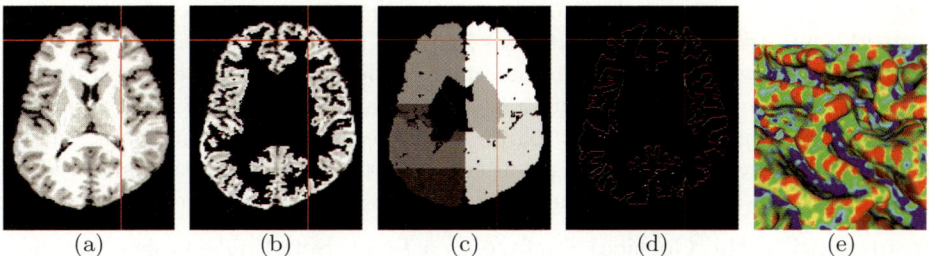

Fig. 1. (a) MR image, after skull stripping and CSF removal, showing GM and WM only. (b) Segmentation (only cortical GM shown) after labor-intensive manual editing of the WM-GM interface. (c) Parcellation of the GM+WM mask into lobes and subcortical region. (d) The cortical surface shown as a zero crossing of a level set (level-set embedding not shown). Note that the cortical surface is stored at a much higher resolution ($0.4mm^3$) as compared to (a)–(c) ($1.2mm^3$); so the view in (d) is an interpolated view at approximately the same slice as that in (a)–(c). (e) A visualization of the shape index computed at each point on a small part of the cortical surface. (red ≡ convex, blue ≡ concave, and yellow/green ≡ hyperbolic/saddle-like patch).

Cerebrospinal fluid (CSF) was removed by thresholding prior to the automatic *binary* GM segmentation by the method developed by Zeng *et al.* [18]. Although this segmentation method [18] has been shown in one comparison to be the most sensitive and accurate of more than half dozen such algorithms [19], it is imperfect. Thus, in a slice-by-slice manner (across 3 orthogonal views), an expert amongst us *manually* corrected the cortical GM-WM interface returned from the automated procedure. This allowed for extremely accurate measurements of the inner cortical surface (Figure 1(b)) (intraclass correlation coefficients for all component ROIs exceed 0.9). We use these binary segmentations, as initial segmentations to the method developed by Awate *et al.* [20,21], to produce accurate probabilistic/fuzzy tissue segmentations.

Brain Parcellation into Lobes: A standard procedure was employed to manually (expert) delineate the boundaries of the lobes in both hemispheres. The lobes are the regions of interest for the study in this paper (Figure 1(c)).

Cortical Surface Delineation: Typical clinical MR images, with limitations on resolution and the ensuing partial-volume effects, provide significantly better contrast at the GM-WM interface (inner cortical surface) than the GM-CSF interface (outer cortical surface). Consequently, some SBM studies [14] select the mid-cortical surface manually. Some SBM approaches estimate the outer cortical surface relying on the accuracy of the inner cortical surface and assuming that the outer cortical surface has a similar shape as the inner one. Subsequently, they select the mid-cortical surface [8] which is even more similar to the inner cortical surface than the outer surface.

The lobe-specific study in this paper treats the inner cortical-surface contour that corresponds to a GM membership of 0.5 as the fiducial surface (similar to the approach in [15]) in order to achieve reliable and clinically-relevant results.

Conducting this lobe-specific folding study on the outer- or mid-cortical surface, instead, *may not alter current findings* because: (i) clinical evidence shows that polymicrogyria specifically affects the inner cortical surface, increasing its irregularity [12], (ii) an estimated outer/mid cortical surface would have a similar shape as the inner one, (iii) all folding measures, being scale invariant, would be unaffected by isotropic changes in size, and (iv) the integration involved in computing lobe-based folding measures produces robust estimates.

Representing the Cortical Surface as a Level Set: Unlike typical methods that encode the cortical surface via an explicit mesh representation, we employ an implicit level-set representation [22]. To improve the accuracy of the distance map that embeds the cortical surface as the zero level set (Figure 1(d)), especially near adjacent sulci that can come quite close to each other, we first supersample the tissue segmentation maps/images to a high resolution (0.4mm^3) and then fit [22] a level set, to the cortical surface, to subvoxel accuracy.

Compute Folding Measures: For every lobe, we compute the novel and the traditional folding measures. The surface gradients and derivatives of the level set, used to compute the principal curvatures and area measures of the cortical-surface patches, are obtained via standard numerical schemes [22].

2.5 Statistical Analyses Via (Nonparametric) Permutation Testing

Typical statistical analyses use the (parametric) Student's t test [14,16], which assumes that the observations are *independent*. Permutation tests, on the other hand, are nonparametric and rely on the *less inclusive* assumption that the observations are *exchangeable*, thereby making the test more stringent. Under the permutation-test null hypothesis (both samples generated by one distribution), the independent and identically-distributed observations are exchangeable.

We performed one-tailed permutation testing (more stringent than the corresponding t tests) to test if the autistics exhibited higher values for novel and traditional cortical-folding measures, for every lobe. A larger AC implies a more convoluted surface, while a larger AS indicates a surface with more (convex) bumps/protrusions. The permutation-test *statistic* was the *difference of means* between the normal and autistic samples; $200,000$ permutations.

3 Results and Discussion

Significantly-Increased Folding in Children: P values and effect sizes (D) in Table 1 indicate that virtually all measures *consistently* inform significantly-increased folding in frontal, temporal, and parietal lobes in both hemispheres. Unlike traditional measures, increased AS informs that increased folding resulted from more *protrusions, not pits*, on the WM at the WM-GM interface. While the differences are most significant in frontal and parietal lobes, they are insignificant in the occipital lobe (not reported) at the $p = 0.05$ level. These results are consistent with the preliminary folding study (on one coronal slice) by Hardan *et al.* [13] and extend those findings to other brain regions.

Table 1. Children: Cohen's *effects sizes* (D) and permutation-test *p values* (P) for 6 folding measures. AC and AS are proposed novel measures; ICI, MCN, CR, IPR are traditional measures. D values indicate the separation of the distributions independent of sample size ($D < 0.2$ is low, $D > 0.8$ is large separation). * indicates $P \geq 0.10$.

	Lt. Parietal		Lt. Temporal		Lt. Frontal		Rt. Parietal		Rt. Temporal		Rt. Frontal	
	D	P	D	P	D	P	D	P	D	P	D	P
AC	0.72	0.002	0.44	0.04	0.65	0.009	1	0.0003	0.46	0.02	0.76	0.002
AS	0.61	0.001	0.34	0.02	0.60	0.002	0.64	0.0001	0.54	0.002	0.48	0.003
ICI	0.50	0.02	0.49	0.03	0.66	0.008	1	0.0001	0.71	0.0007	0.56	0.01
MCN	0.56	0.01	0.56	0.01	0.68	0.005	1	0.0001	0.72	0.0007	0.77	0.002
CR	0.84	0.0005	0.37	0.08	0.55	0.02	1.1	0.0001	1	0.0001	0.50	0.03
IPR	0.54	0.01	0.08	0.35*	0.92	0.0007	0.79	0.002	0.79	0.01	0.67	0.008

Table 2. Adolescents: Cohen's effects sizes (D) and permutation-test p values (P)

	Lt. Parietal		Lt. Temporal		Lt. Frontal		Rt. Parietal		Rt. Temporal		Rt. Frontal	
	D	P	D	P	D	P	D	P	D	P	D	P
AC	0.41	0.05	0.23	0.17*	0.70	0.005	0.56	0.02	0.44	0.05	0.59	0.01
AS	0.38	0.01	0.49	0.01	0.35	0.01	0.42	0.03	0.58	0.005	1	0.001
ICI	0.23	0.19*	0.22	0.18*	0.73	0.005	0.33	0.09	0.72	0.006	0.38	0.08
MCN	0.36	0.09	0.36	0.08	0.71	0.005	0.51	0.03	0.68	0.007	0.35	0.09
CR	0.58	0.01	0.33	0.10*	0.42	0.06	0.38	0.08	0.65	0.008	0.33	0.11*
IPR	0.44	0.05	0.29	0.13*	0.60	0.01	0.55	0.02	0.76	0.003	0.27	0.14*

Increased Folding in Adolescents: P values and effect sizes (D) in Table 2 indicate folding changes similar to those in children, but less significant overall. Most measures *consistently* inform significant, or close-to significant, increase in folding in all cases except the left temporal lobe. The differences were insignificant in the occipital lobe (not reported) at the $p = 0.05$ level. These findings are consistent with [13,8] where such differences were expected, but were found insignificant. Hardan et al. [13] also report that GI correlates negatively with autistics' age. In this way, these results extend previous research. Observe that many p values in this case are only slightly higher than 0.05 and the corresponding D values are not too low.

Adults: We found insignificant differences in adults, consistent with previous hypotheses/findings [13,8]. However, the autistic adult sample size (10) is small.

Age-Independent Comparison: Permutation tests comparing the entire normal sample to the entire autistic sample, irrespective of age, produced p values (not reported) for *all* measures in *all* lobes that were *consistently smaller* than the p values in tables 1 and 2, thus indicating most significant differences. This finding supports the claim that the close-to-significant findings ($0.05 < p < 0.1$) for adolescents may increase significance with larger sample sizes.

References

1. Courchesne, E., Press, G., Yeung-Courchesne, R.: Parietal lobe abnormalities deteced with MR in patients with infantile autism. Am. J. Rad. 160, 387–393 (1993)
2. Carper, R.A., Moses, P., Tigue, Z.D., Courchesne, E.: Cerebral lobes in autism: Early hyperplasia and abnormal age effects. NeuroImage 16(4), 1038–1051 (2002)
3. Aylward, E., Minshew, N., Field, K., Sparks, B., Singh, N.: Effects of age on brain volume and head circumference in autism. Neurology 59, 175–183 (2002)
4. Hardan, A., Muddasani, S., Vemulapalli, M., Keshavan, M., Minshew, N.: An MRI study of increased cortical thickness in autism. Am. J. Psych. 163(7), 1290–1292 (2006)
5. Neeley, E.S., Bigler, E.D., Krasny, L., Ozonoff, S., McMahon, W., Lainhart, J.E.: Quantitative temporal lobe differences: Autism distinguished from controls using classification and regression tree analysis. Brain and Develop. 29(7), 389–399 (2007)
6. Mostofsky, S., Burgess, M., Gidley-Larson, J.: Increased motor cortex white matter volume predicts motor impairment in autism. Brain 130, 2117–2122 (2007)
7. Levitt, J., Blanton, R., Smalley, S., Thompson, P., Guthrie, D., McCracken, J., Sadoun, T., Heinichen, L., Toga, A.: Cortical sulcal maps in autism. Cerebral Cortex 13(7), 728–735 (2003)
8. Nordahl, C., Dierker, D., Mostafavi, I., Schumann, C., Rivera, S., Amaral, D., Van-Essen, D.: Cortical folding abnormalities in autism revealed by surface-based morphometry. Journal of Neuroscience 27(43), 11725–11735 (2007)
9. Armstrong, E., Schleicher, A., Omran, H., Curtis, M., Zilles, K.: The ontogeny of human gyrification. Cerebral Cortex 5, 56–63 (1995)
10. Piven, J., Berthier, M., Starkstein, S., Nehme, E., Pearlson, G., Folstein, S.: Magnetic resonance imaging evidence for a defect of cerebral cortical development in autism. Am. J. Psych. 147, 734–739 (1990)
11. Bailey, A., Luthert, Dean, Harding, Janota, Montgomery, Rutter, Lantos: A clinicopathological study of autism. Brain 121(5), 889–905 (1998)
12. Sztriha, L., Guerrini, R., Harding, B., Stewart, F., Chelloug, N., Johansen, J.: Clinical, MRI, and pathological features of polymicrogyria in chromosome 22q11 deletion syndrome. Am. J. Med. Genetics 127(A), 313–317 (2004)
13. Hardan, A., Jou, R., Keshavan, Varma, Minshew, N.: Increased frontal cortical folding in autism: a preliminary MRI study. Psyc. Res. 131(3), 263–268 (2004)
14. Van-Essen, D., Drury, H.: Structural and functional analyses of human cerebral cortex using a surface-based ATLAS. J. Neuroscience 17(18), 7079–7102 (1997)
15. Batchelor, P.G., Castellano-Smith, A.D., Hill, D.L.G., Hawkes, D.J., Cox, T.C.S., Dean, A.F.: Measures of folding applied to the development of the human fetal brain. IEEE Trans. Medical Imaging 21(8), 953–965 (2002)
16. Tosun, D., Duchesne, S., Rolland, Y., Toga, A., Verin, M., Barillot, C.: 3D analysis of cortical morphometry in differential diagnosis of Parkinson's Plus Syndromes. In: Med. Imag. Comput. and Comp. Assist. Intervention, pp. 891–899 (2007)
17. Koenderink, J., van Doorn, A.: Surface shape and curvature scales. Image and Vision Computing 10(8), 557–565 (1992)
18. Zeng, X., Staib, L., Schultz, R., Duncan, J.: Segmentation and measurement of the cortex from 3D MR images using coupled surfaces propagation. IEEE Trans. Medical Imaging 18(10), 100–111 (1999)
19. Shattuck, D.W., Leahy, R.M.: Brainsuite: An automated cortical surface identification tool. Medical Image Analysis 6(2), 129–142 (2002)

20. Awate, S.P., Tasdizen, T., Foster, N.L., Whitaker, R.T.: Adaptive Markov modeling for mutual-information-based unsupervised MRI brain-tissue classification. Medical Image Analysis 10(5), 726–739 (2006)
21. Awate, S.P., Zhang, H., Gee, J.C.: A fuzzy, nonparametric segmentation framework for DTI and MRI analysis: With applications to DTI tract extraction. IEEE Trans. Med. Imag. 26(11), 1525–1536 (2007)
22. Osher, S., Paragios, N.: Geometric Level Set Methods in Imaging, Vision, and Graphics. Springer, Heidelberg (2003)

Prediction of Biomechanical Parameters of the Proximal Femur Using Statistical Appearance Models and Support Vector Regression

Karl Fritscher[1], Benedikt Schuler[1], Thomas Link[2], Felix Eckstein[3], Norbert Suhm[4], Markus Hänni[4], Clemens Hengg[5], and Rainer Schubert[1]

[1] Institute for Biomedical Image Analysis, UMIT, Austria
{Karl.Fritscher,Benedikt.Schuler,Rainer.Schubert}@umit.at
[2] Department of Radiology and Biomedical Imaging
University of California, San Francisco
Thomas.Link@radiology.ucsf.edu
[3] Institut für Anatomie und muskolosekelttale Forschung, Paracelsus University, Salzburg
Felix.Eckstein@pmu.ac.at
[4] AO Development Institute, Davos, Switzerland
{Norbert.Suhm, Markus.Haenni}@aofoundation.org
[5] Department of Trauma Surgery, Medical University Innsbruck, Austria
Clemens.Hengg@uki.at

Abstract. Fractures of the proximal femur are one of the principal causes of mortality among elderly persons. Traditional methods for the determination of femoral fracture risk use methods for measuring bone mineral density. However, BMD alone is not sufficient to predict bone failure load for an individual patient and additional parameters have to be determined for this purpose. In this work an approach that uses statistical models of appearance to identify relevant regions and parameters for the prediction of biomechanical properties of the proximal femur will be presented. By using Support Vector Regression the proposed model based approach is capable of predicting two different biomechanical parameters accurately and fully automatically in two different testing scenarios.

Keywords: Fracture load, bone strength, proximal femur, support vectors, appearance models.

1 Introduction

Fractures of the proximal femur are one of the principal causes of mortality among elderly persons. Hip fractures are primarily caused by an increased fragility of the proximal femur, due to osteoporosis or other conditions affecting bone strength. Techniques for the determination of fracture risk traditionally use methods for measuring bone mineral density (BMD) like e.g. DXA [1]. However, there is still a significant overlap in bone mineral density between osteoporotic and normal individuals and BMD alone is not sufficient to predict bone failure load for an individual patient [2].

As a consequence different other approaches were introduced using parameters based on bone geometry (e.g. [3]), trabecular (micro)-architecture (e.g. [4, 5]), and (micro)-finite element analysis (e.g. [6, 7]) to assess bone strength and estimate fracture risk.

Apart from improving the identification of patients with a high fracture risk another type of projects aims at improving the surgical treatment of femoral fractures, by predicting the risk of failure of an osteosynthesis, the so called "cut-out" risk. In [8] a tool has been developed which can be used during the surgical intervention by measuring the peak torque until complete breakaway of the cancellous bone in the femoral head. Moreover, several non invasive methods were introduced in order to predict the cut out risk using CT or x-ray images based on the calculation of Haralick texture features in CT images [9] or Minkowski functionals[10] in different regions of interest.

Beside of finding appropriate parameters most of approaches mentioned above are also dependent on defining a number of different regions of interest (ROIs) in which potentially relevant parameters are obtained. In many cases the placement of these ROIs for an individual patient needs user interaction and is therefore subjective.

Therefore in this work an approach that is based on the usage of statistical models will be presented. The key idea of this work is to use these models in order to identify relevant regions and parameters for the prediction of biomechanical properties of the proximal femur. By using these parameters as predictor variables for Support Vector Regression (=SVR) the proposed model based approach is capable of predicting two different biomechanical parameters accurately, objectively and fully automatically.

2 Methods

The workflow of the proposed algorithm can be summed up as follows:

Step 1: Create an accurate combined representation of shape and spatial intensity distribution of an object by applying an atlas based non-rigid registration on a training set of CT images (for more details refer to section 2.1)

Step 2: Apply Principal Component Analysis (=PCA) using the output of step 1 in order to reduce the dimensionality of the input space. By using a correlation-based feature selection method, a subset of n relevant Principal Components (=PCs) can be identified (for more details refer to 2.2).

Step 3: Regress the PC scores of the n relevant PCs obtained in step 2 against the biomechanical parameter of interest and find the best subset of the PCs as well as the optimal parameter values for Support Vector Regression using a stratified cross-validation scheme (for more details refer to 2.3).

Step 4: Select a subsample of the original set of input variables represented by the combined shape-intensity representations by using the eigenvector loadings of the n relevant PCs in order to reduce the number of non-relevant variables and identify relevant regions (for more details refer to 2.4).

Step 5: Repeat steps 2 and 3 with the subsample of the original set of input variables obtained in step 4.

2.1 Combined Shape-Intensity Representation

The method that is used to create a combined shape-intensity model is based on the approach presented in [11] and has been extended to generate combined representations of shape and spatial intensity-distribution [12]. The approach is based on the usage of rigid and non-rigid registration in order to align a number of subjects to an atlas subject. Performing this registration for n subjects results in n aligned intensity representations and *n* deformation fields $\{D_1, D_2, .., D_n\}$, which represent shape variations. The aligned intensity representations I_n and the shape representations D_n for each subject of the training set are placed in one vector *z*. The length of the vector z is 4 x number of pixels within the structure of interest (e.g. the proximal femur) for 3D images.

2.2 Combined Shape-Intensity Model

Using the representations described in section 2.1, PCA is applied to reduce the dimensionality of the input data: Given n, d-dimensional training vectors, $\{z_1,...,z_n\}$ a training matrix *M* can be defined. Using Singular Value Decomposition, the covariance matrix Σ of *M* can be decomposed [13]. In the case when $d >> n$, the system is underconstrained resulting in a large number of eigenvectors that will be zero. In these cases the Matrix *U*, containing the eigenvectors of Σ, can be calculated from the smaller Matrix *T*

$$T = \frac{1}{n}\sum_{i=1}^{n}(z_i - \mu)^T(z_i - \mu) \quad (1)$$

where μ is the mean of all training elements z [13].

The vector of PC scores α for a subject *x* of the training set can be calculated by using

$$\alpha = U_k^T(x - \mu) \quad (2)$$

U_k is a matrix consisting of the first k columns of *U* and represents the set of *k* orthogonal modes of shape-intensity variations. An approximation of a shape-intensity pair in 3D can then be represented by using *k* PCs and a *k* dimensional vector of PC scores α. In order to compensate the differences in scaling of the pixel intensities representing the spatial intensity distribution and the deformation field components, the pixel intensities are rescaled by a factor f in each combined shape-intensity distribution. This factor is calculated by dividing the average range between the minimum and maximum deformation of all subjects by the average range between the highest and lowest intensity value of all subject.

After performing PCA the PC scores of a subset of PCs will be used as predictor variables for SVR. This subset of PCs is determined in the next step.

2.3 Attribute Selection and Support Vector Regression

Using the PC scores and the biomechanical parameter of interest of all subjects in the training set a correlation-based feature selection method [14] with a greedy stepwise forward search method is used in order to identify a subset of k potentially relevant PCs. N-fold cross-validation (n=number of subjects in the training set) is applied for this purpose. The PC scores of the selected k PCs will then be used to train a Support Vector Regression [15] model. In this project an exponential kernel of the form $k(x,x') = \langle x,x' \rangle^p$ with $p \in \mathbb{N}$ was used for the Support Vector Regression. For details on Support Vector Regression please refer to [15]. The best subset of the k PCs as well as the optimal values for p and for the complexity parameter C (for details on the parameters of SVR please refer to [15]) are obtained by using a stratified cross-validation scheme: First, one of the n subjects is chosen as the test data set. The remaining n-1 subjects serve as training set. Using this leave-one out scheme a set of parameters for the SVR parameters $C(\{0.3,0.5,0.7,1,3,5,10,20,40,60,80,100\})$ and $p(\{1,2,3\})$ is defined. Starting with the subset of k PCs identified by the greedy stepwise forward search method, the best combination of p and C is determined by reducing the numbers of used PCs by one in each step from k PCs down to 1 PC. The order in which the PCs are excluded is determined by the ranking that results from the greedy stepwise search algorithm in the attribute selection step prior to SVR.

2.4 Reducing the Size of the Training Vectors Z_i

After the attribute selection the size of the training vectors z_i is reduced in order to remove non-relevant elements of the training vectors z_i and identify relevant properties. For this purpose the correlation coefficient r_k between the score values of the kth PC for each subject in the training set and the biomechanical parameter of interest are calculated for each of the PCs that have been determined in the attribute pre-selection step. Using r_k and L_k, which is the vector containing the eigenvector loadings of the kth PC, a vector U_w containing weights for each element of z_i can be calculated as follows:

$$U_w = \sum_{k=1}^{m} r_k |L_k| \qquad (3)$$

Using U_w the dimension of each original training vector z_i is reduced by removing the elements of z_i, whose weighting values in U_w are beneath a relative threshold T. This results in n reduced training vectors zs_i. Using the vectors zs_i, a second iteration of PCA, attribute selection and support vector regression is performed to obtain a final regression model. Analogously to the determination of the optimal numbers of PCs described in section 2.3 again a stepwise procedure is used to find the best values for T in this second iteration: Initially the calculations described in sections 2.2 and 2.3 are performed setting T=90%. Thereafter T is reduced by 10 % and the calculations are performed again. T is reduced stepwise by 10 % as long as the predictive quality of any of the regression models resulting from different parameter combinations for p and C does not decrease compared to the best working model in the previous step. In order to assess the predictive quality of a certain regression model the correlation between real and predicted parameter values, as well as the mean absolute error (MAE) and the relative absolute error (RAE) is measured.

2.5 Data Material

The pipeline described above was tested in two different test settings in which two biomechanical parameters should be predicted. In the first setting (=setting A) the parameter "peak torque until complete breakaway" (=PTB), which was obtained using the DensiProbe tool presented in [8], should be predicted for 14 proximal femora of men and women aged between 64 and 96 years. For this purpose CT images of cadaveric femora have been used. The values for PTB ranged from 3.9 to 12.41 Nm. The special challenge using these dataset was that the CT images were obtained using two different micro CT scanners and different image resolutions. Seven out of the 14 images had an original isotropic resolution of 0.082 x 0.082 x 0.082 mm and were acquired using a Scanco DensiScan 1000 microCT scanner. The remaining seven images were acquired using a Scanco XtremeCT scanner with an original image resolution of 0.246 x 0.246 x 0.246 mm. In order to simulate clinical conditions all images were resampled to images with an isotropic voxel spacing of 0.984 mm (using linear interpolation).

In test setting B, CT images of 26 femur specimen of men and women between 58 and 98 years with an original resolution of 0.2 x 0.2 x 0.5 mm were used. Again – in order to simulate the resolution of images that are acquired in clinical routine - the images were resampled to images with an isotropic pixel spacing 0.7x0.7x0.7 mm (using linear interpolation). The fracture load of the femora was obtained by simulating a fall on the greater trochanter (=side-impact configuration), which was leading to different types of fractures (cervical, intertrochanteric and shaft fractures) [16]. The values for the fracture load ranged from 2453 to 6359 N.

3 Results

The accuracy of the registration during the modeling process was evaluated by calculating the mean absolute error between the pixel intensities of the original CT images and the model instances that were created by using the appearance model with all PCs. Moreover, the original images and the created instance images were converted to 8-bit images (256 grey levels).

For test setting A, a statistical model of the femoral head and neck region was created. Analyzing the registration accuracy as described above a mean absolute error of 7.3 grey levels (σ=6.6), which corresponds to 2.8 % of the whole intensity range was measured. The results of the leave-one-out tests for testing scenario A are summed up in table 1. The table is showing the number of used PCs, the obtained correlation, the errors RAE and MAE, the used combination of parameters (kernel exponent and C) and the percentage of input variables that lead to the best results for 1 to k (in this case k=7) predictor variables (=PCs). Best results with R=0.975 (p<0.01) could be achieved using 100 % of the input variables (last line) and 7 PCs. Using the criterion defined above the maximum reduction of the variable input space was 30% (P=70%). Using only 3 predictor variables a correlation of R=0.862 (p<0.01) could be achieved.

Table 1. Evaluation of the predictive quality for the prediction of peak-torque to breakaway

PCs	R	RAE [%]	MAE[Nm]	exp	C	P [%]
1	0.630	74	1.66	1	0.5	70
2	0.800	49	1.1	2	3	90
3	0.862	42	0.94	3	1	100
4	0.850	44	1.34	2	0.3	70
5	0.905	40.2	1.26	1	0.3	80
6	0.952	30	0.67	1	0.5	80
7	0.975	22.4	0.503	1	0.5	100

For test setting B a model of the whole proximal femur including the small trochanter was created. Analyzing the registration accuracy a mean absolute error of 9.1 grey levels ($\sigma=7.1$), which corresponds to 3.6% of the whole intensity range, was measured. The results of the leave-one-out tests are summed up in table 2, which is having the same structure as table 1. Using 100 % of the input variables (last line), the highest correlation R=0.93 (p<0.01) could be obtained with 10 predictor variables. The variable input space could be reduced up to 50%, which also lead to the highest correlation (R=0.944, p<0.01). Using 3 predictor variables still a correlation of R=0.886 (p<0.01) could be achieved. Note, that for both testing scenarios all results have been obtained using n-fold cross-validation

Table 2. Evaluation of the predictive quality for the prediction of failure load

PCs	R	RAE [%]	MAE[N]	exponent	C	P [%]
1	0.755	59	602	2	0.5	50
2	0.763	55	552	1	5	60
3	0.886	36	368	3	1	50
4	0.830	45.6	459	3	0.7	50
5	0.880	41	412	2	0.3	50
6	0.944	29	301	2	10	50
7	0.891	39.8	401	1	0.7	60
8	0.910	34.3	344	1	3	100
9	0.930	30.6	308	1	5	100
10	0.930	27.6	278	1	10	100

For this study DXA measurements in 5 different regions in the head and neck region of the proximal femur were also obtained. The DXA values measured in the femoral neck showed the highest correlation to failure load with R=0.73. Figure 1 is illustrating what structures are described by the 3 PCs showing highest correlation to failure load on one coronal sample slice.

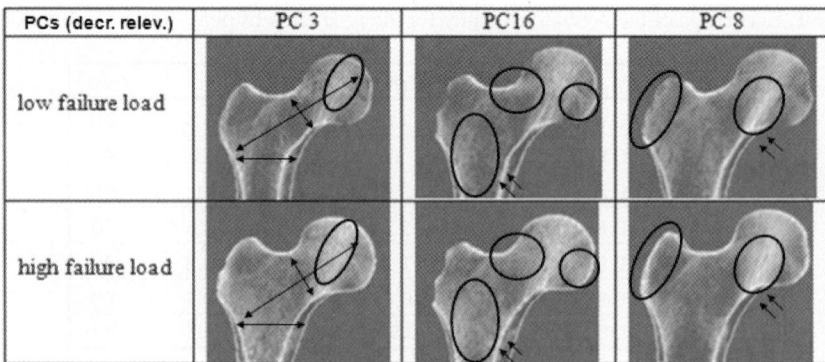

Fig. 1. Variations of the proximal femur described by the 3 Principal Components with highest correlation to failure load (Coronal cut through femoral head neck and shaft)

The images illustrate the major differences between femora with low (top) and high fracture load (bottom). PC 3 predominantly illustrates variations of the shape of the femur (neck thickness, shape of head, shape of greater trochanter) and the cancellous bone in the femoral head. The two other PCs mainly describe variations of the cancellous bone in the shaft, neck (PC 16) and head region (PCs 16 and 8). PC 8 also illustrates variations concerning the shape and length of the cortical region in the lower femoral neck. The regions around the greater and small trochanter, around the femoral head and neck as well as the cortical region in the shaft also remained in the model after 50 % reduction of the input variables.

4 Discussion

Using two different testing scenarios and an extensive cross-validation scheme it has been demonstrated that the model based approach presented in this work, can provide an excellent tool for estimating femoral fracture load and peak torque to breakaway with high accuracy using CT images with clinical resolution. By using this approach one has the possibility to depict a number of different geometric and structural properties that can be used to predict biomechanical bone parameters, accurately and reliably. Although the tests were performed using images with comparably low resolution, the quantitative results in terms of the amount of correlation between real and predicted parameter values are absolutely comparable to studies that partly use higher image resolutions [7-10].

Beside of the accuracy of the proposed method, another positive aspect of the algorithm is its ability to implicitly identify potential parameters as well as sub-regions that are useful for the prediction of biomechanical properties. The nature of the parameters that can be identified range from geometrical properties of the bone to variations of the spatial intensity distribution in medical images. In combination with the ease of use of the proposed algorithm this fact makes the approach useful for a wide field of applications. Having a valid (regression) model, the calculation of a shape-intensity representation and parameter prediction for a new unseen segmented dataset only takes ~5-15 minutes, depending on the resolution of the CT images. The next steps in this project will be the investigation of alternative methods for dimensionality reduction and the application of the proposed methods in a large clinical study, which has been started recently.

References

1. Adams, J.E.: Single and dual energy X-ray absorptiometry. Eur. Radiol. 7, 20–31 (1997)
2. Faulkner, K.G., Cummings, S.R., Black, D., Palermo, L., Gluer, C.C., Genant, H.K.: Simple measurement of femoral geometry predicts hip fracture: the study of osteoporotic fractures. J. Bone Miner. Res. 8, 1211–1217 (1993)
3. Bergot, C., Bousson, V., Meunier, A., Laval-Jeantet, M., Laredo, J.D.: Hip fracture risk and proximal femur geometry from DXA scans. Osteoporos Int. 13, 542–550 (2002)
4. Boehm, H.F., Link, T., Monetti, R., Mueller, D., Rummeny, E., Newitt, D., Majumdar, S., Raeth, C.W.: Application of the Minkowski Functionals in 3D to High Resolution MR Images of Trabecular Bone for the Prediction of the Biomechanical Strength. Microscopy and Microanalysi, 716–717 (2004)
5. Link, T.M., Majumdar, S., Lin, J.C., Augat, P., Gould, R.G., Newitt, D., Ouyang, X., Lang, T.F., Mathur, A., Genant, H.K.: Assessment of trabecular structure using high resolution CT images and texture analysis. J. Comput. Assist. Tomogr. 22, 15–24 (1998)
6. Bessho, M., Ohnishi, I., Matsuyama, J., Matsumoto, T., Imai, K., Nakamura, K.: Prediction of strength and strain of the proximal femur by a CT-based finite element method. J. Biomech. 40, 1745–1753 (2007)
7. Keyak, J.H.: Improved prediction of proximal femoral fracture load using nonlinear finite element models. Med. Eng. Phys. 23, 165–173 (2001)
8. Suhm, N., Hengg, C., Schwyn, R., Windolf, M., Quarz, V., Hänni, M.: Mechanical torque measurement predicts load to implant cut-out: a biomechanical study investigating DHS anchorage in femoral heads. Arch. Orthop. Trauma. Surg (2006) (online)
9. Fritscher, K.D., Schuler, B., Grünerbl, A., Hänni, M., Schwieger, K., Suhm, N., Schubert, R.: Assessment of femoral bone quality using co-occurrence matrices and adaptive regions of interest. In: Proceedings of SPIE Medical Imaging, vol. 6514, p. 65141K (2007)
10. Huber, M.B., Carballido-Gamio, J., Fritscher, K.D., Schubert, R., Haenni, M., Hengg, D., Majumdar, S., Link, T.M.: Morphological Texture Analysis of Radiographs of the Proximal Femur- in vitro study using biomechanical strength as a standard of reference. In: 29th ASBMR, Honolulu (2007)
11. Rueckert, D., Frangi, A.F., Schnabel, J.A.: Automatic Construction of 3-D Statistical Deformation Models of the Brain Using Nonrigid Registration. IEEE Trans. Med. Imaging 22, 1014–1025 (2001)
12. Fritscher, K.D., Gruenerbl, A., Schubert, R.: 3D image segmentation using combined shape-intensity prior models. International Journal of Radiology and Surgery 1(3), 123–135 (2007)
13. Leventon, M., Grimson, E., Faugeras, O.: Statistical Shape Influence in Geodesic Active Contours. Computer Vision and Pattern Recognition 1, 316–323 (2000)
14. Hall, M.: Correlation-based Feature Selection for Machine Learning. Department of Computer Science. PhD Thesis. Waikato University, New Zealand (1998)
15. Smola, A.J., Schoelkopf, B.: A tutorial on support vector regression. Statistics and Computing 14, 199–222 (2003)
16. Lochmüller, E.M., Eckstein, F.: Biomechanische Tests in der Evaluation osteodensitometrischer Verfahren - Hintergrund, Übersicht und aktuelle Befunde. Osteologie 11, 154–177 (2002)

Automatic Labeling of Anatomical Structures in MR FastView Images Using a Statistical Atlas

Matthias Fenchel[1,2], Stefan Thesen[1], and Andreas Schilling[2]

[1] Siemens Healthcare Sector, MR Division, Applications & Workflow,
Erlangen, Germany
matthias.fenchel.ext@siemens.com
[2] WSI-GRIS, Eberhard-Karls-Universität, Tübingen, Germany

Abstract. We present a method for fast and automatic labeling of anatomical structures in MR FastView localizer images, which can be useful for automatic MR examination planning. FastView is a modern MR protocol, that provides larger planning fields of view than previously available with isotropic 3D resolution by scanning during continuous movement of the patient table. Hence, full 3D information is obtained within short acquisition time. Anatomical labeling is done by registering the images to a statistical atlas created from training image data beforehand. The statistical atlas consists of a statistical model of deformation and a statistical model of grey value appearance. It is generated by non-rigid registration and principal component analysis of the resulting deformation fields and registered images. Labeling of an unseen FastView image is done by non-rigid registration of the image to the statistical atlas and propagating the labels from the atlas to the image. In our implementation, the statistical models of deformation and appearance are both implemented on the GPU (graphics processing unit), which permits computing the atlas based labeling using GPU hardware acceleration. The running times of about 10 to 30 seconds are of the same magnitude as the image acquisition itself, which allows for practical usage in clinical MR routine.

1 Introduction

In current clinical MR practice, it is desirable to have more automation and standardization of the examination workflows. Automation of manual tasks like slice positioning, coil selection, adaptations of sequence parameters, etc. would reduce the need for highly trained technical operators. It would also lead to more reproducibility, more comparability and shorter examination slots, which in turn increases the overall utilization of the scanner. Solutions based on image processing from fast pre-scan acquisitions for the automation of manual steps are highly appreciated. To name but a few of these methods, van der Kouwe et al. [1] presented a solution for reproducible MR head scan planning using a human brain atlas. Peschl [2] showed a method for the spine. In [3] a method for automatic liver scan planning from fast localizer scans was published.

This paper presents an algorithm for fast and automatic labeling of anatomical structures in fast MR whole-body pre-scans. We aim at a complete labeling or multi-organ segmentation of the patient's torso for an automation of the MR exam with respect to complex positioning, marking, reading and reporting features. The performance of the applications should be competitive with a human operator in terms of speed and precision. This requires a fast imaging protocol and a fast segmentation algorithm. The FastView protocol is a good basis for the anatomical labeling with the purpose of the desired applications as it provides full 3D information, large field of view, sufficient resolution (5 mm isotropic) and fast acquisition (about 20 seconds). It is a modern proton-density weighted 2D axial acquisition technique during continuous movement of the patient table similar to [4] and [5]. Keil et al. [6] already used this protocol for an estimation of the patient's position and orientation.

The labeling resp. segmentation algorithm uses a statistical atlas of deformation and appearance of the human torso, which captures the averages and main modes of variation in shape and intensity. The atlas is created from a set of representative training data instances. Registration of an unseen data set to the statistical atlas, which is accomplished by finding the deformation field and appearance that 'best' fits the data set, yields the anatomical labeling or multi-organ segmentation by label propagation.

Atlas based segmentation has been abundantly used throughout medical image segmentation literature. Most publications have been made in human brain image segmentation and diagnosis. Talairach presented an atlas with a complete reference coordinate system for the human brain [7]. Cootes introduced active shape models and active appearance models and published their application to atlas based matching in [8]. Rueckert proposed statistical analysis of the using non-rigid deformation fields for the creation of a statistical atlas [9] of the brain. Zhou and Bai [10] created an abdominal atlas from CT scans and used it in a fuzzy-connectedness approach for identification of abdominal organs. Park et al. [11] used a probabilistic abdominal atlas for supervised multi-organ segmentation from CT scans. To the best of our knowledge this paper is the first to create an atlas from whole-body MR images of the complete human torso, although with moderate resolution, and use it for multi-organ segmentation or anatomical labeling.

2 Building the Statistical Atlas

2.1 Training Data Acquisition and Preprocessing

For the statistical atlas, a representative group of 31 volunteers is scanned using the FastView protocol. The images are acquired with a resolution of 5 mm isotropic and an axial field of view of 1000 mm. The training group is selected in a way that ensures that a possibly large portion of natural variation is captured, which means that volunteers of different ages, sex and stature are scanned using different scanner devices with different hardware and B_0 field strengths. The images are first cropped and transformed to a common coordinate frame. As the arm positions of the volunteers during the acquisition are arbitrary, which can have harmful effects on the non-rigid registrations, the images are preprocessed with an automatic arm stripping algorithm. Further processing is done with pure torso images, as shown in figure 2. The image intensities are also normalized by piecewise linear scaling such that the peaks of the two-modal histograms coincide.

2.2 Non-rigid Inter-subject Registration

Modeling natural variation requires establishing spatial correspondence among the training image data sets from the volunteers. This is done implicitly by performing non-rigid registrations of all data sets to a reference data set.

The non-rigid transformation is set up by a global affine transformation and a local free-form transformation. For the free-form transformation, a regular 3D control grid is superimposed onto the image. The deformation of a single point is given by the deformations of the control grid with a cubic B-spline tensor product interpolation. This ensures both smoothness and local support of the deformation coefficients, which is similar to the deformation used by Rueckert et al. in [9]. The similarity measure of choice for inter-subject registration of MR images is mutual information [12], based upon minimizing histogram entropy and allowing for variations of contrast among different subjects.

The registration process is driven by a a cost function, which combines a normalized mutual information term NMI with an additional regularization term summing up the squared norm of differences of adjacent control point shifts v_i, which is similar to the well-known diffusion regularizer. This regularization term punishes 'unnatural' or rupturing deformations. A third term considers predefined correspondences, so called manual landmarks LM. The cost function reads as follows with the empirical constants λ and γ:

$$Cost(T) = NMI + \lambda \sum_{(i,j) \in NB} ||v_i - v_j||^2 + \gamma \sum_{x_i \in LM} ||x'_i - T(x_i)||^2 \quad (1)$$

where T is the non-rigid deformation, NB is the 27-neighborhood on the grid of control points, v_i is the movement of control point i, LM is the set of all manual landmarks, x'_i is a landmark in the reference image and x_i in the data image. λ and γ are empirical coefficients that weight the different terms.

The cost function is minimized using a gradient descent optimization with adaptive step length. This procedure increases the step length as long as the value decreases steadily, but decreases its step length if not. The registration is implemented using a multi-scale approach, starting with a coarse resolution of image data and control grid points and gradually refining the image data and the grid resolution. The maximum resolution of the control grid is 20 mm, i.e. one grid point for 4 voxels.

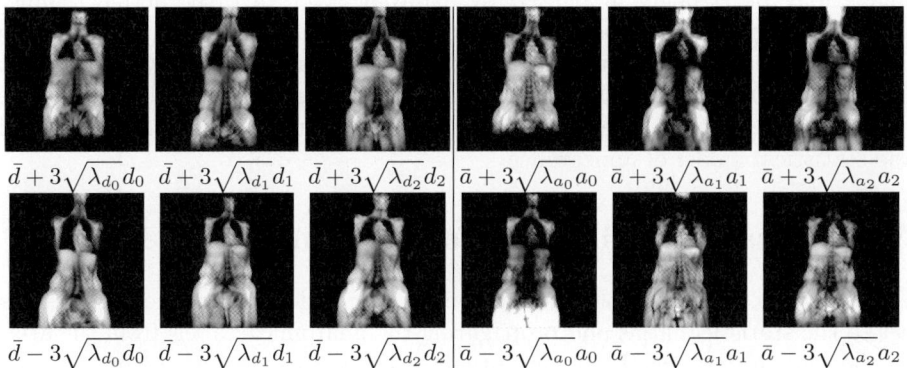

Fig. 1. This figure shows the major principal modes of deformation (first 3 columns) and appearance (second 3 columns) of the atlas. $\bar{d}$ is the average deformation, $\bar{a}$ the average intensity and λ_i the respective principal values i, with $\sqrt{\lambda_i}$ being the Gaussian standard deviation of mode i.

2.3 Statistical Model of Deformation

Registering all image data sets I_i to a reference data set I_{ref} produces n non-rigid transformations T_i and n registered data sets $I_i(T_i)$. Each of the transformations T_i contains an affine part M_i and a free-form part d_i, with the coefficients of the control grid point shifts. Since statistical analysis is to be performed exclusively on the free-form part, all affine content is removed from the d_i beforehand.

Statistical models of deformation [9] extend the concepts of active shape models. Instead of performing statistical analysis on point coordinates, principal component analysis is directly calculated on the deformation fields d_i. This yields the linear model:

$$d_{instance} = \bar{d} + \Phi_d \cdot d \qquad (2)$$

where $\bar{d}$ is the average deformation field, Φ_d a matrix whose columns contain the principal deformations and d the feature vector with the weights of the principal components. Setting the entries of the feature vector d to a range within $\pm 3\sqrt{\lambda_i}$ produces valid deformation fields within a $\pm 3\sigma_i$ interval of the implicit multivariate Gaussian distribution. Those deformation fields can be used to warp unseen image data for registration to the atlas. Figure 1 shows images of the final atlas and the statistical model of deformation.

2.4 Statistical Model of Appearance

The variety of the intensity appearances of identical organs in different subjects is handled by a statistical model of appearance, which is set up by performing principal component analysis on the pixelwise intensity values of the registered data sets $I_i(T_i)$. In contrast to active appearance models [13] or [14], however, the appearance statistics are kept independent of the deformation model without correlation. This is motivated by the fact that the intensity appearance of an image may be strongly influenced by external effects like the actual scanner hardware, e.g. coils, the basic magnetic field etc. and not only by the proton densities of the actual organs. As many of these effects are obviously independent of the deformation fields, they should be treated differently in order to keep the atlas free from biases. The last three columns of figure 1 show three modes of the statistical model of appearance.

3 Application of the Atlas for Fast Anatomical Labeling

Labeling resp. segmentation of an unseen data set is done by registering the data set to the statistical atlas and propagating the anatomical labels from the atlas to the unseen data set. First, an outline of the registration algorithm is given followed by a description of a fast implementation using programmable GPU hardware.

3.1 Atlas Based Registration

The labeling algorithm consists of 3 phases: First, a rough affine offset registration of the unseen image I_{uns} to the statistical atlas is computed by aligning the bounding boxes of binary images created from the data. Next, the affine transformation M, the instance of the deformation field d and the intensity appearance a of the atlas are calculated which best map I_{uns} to the atlas I_{atlas}. Finally, the labels of the anatomical structures are propagated to I_{uns} using the registration result.

The registration result is found by minimizing the following distance cost function:

$$(M_{opt}, d_{opt}, a_{opt}) = \arg \min_{M,d,a} \frac{\sum_{x_i \in \Omega} w_i \left(I_{atlas}(a, x_i) - I_{uns}(T(x_i))\right)^2}{\sum_{x_i \in \Omega} w_i} \quad (3)$$

where x_i are the world coordinates of pixel i and w_i a specific weight for the influence of pixel i to the registration. This is particularly important for certain structures of high variation, like head, legs or stomach, which should not affect organs with small variation like the lungs. If w_i is set to $\frac{1}{\sigma(x_i)^2}$, the squared standard deviation of each pixel in the training images, a Gaussian distance between the atlas and I_{uns} is obtained. Final division by the total sum of weights normalizes the distance measure with respect to the overlap size of I_{atlas} and I_{uns}.

The iterative registration algorithm repeats the following steps: First, an intensity instance I_{atlas} of the atlas is created using the appearance feature values a_i. An instance d of the deformation field is computed from the deformation feature values d_i. The unseen image I_{uns} is warped using the affine offset M and the free-form deformation d followed by the computation of the distance measure between I_{atlas} and I_{uns}. This is repeated until the optimum has been found.

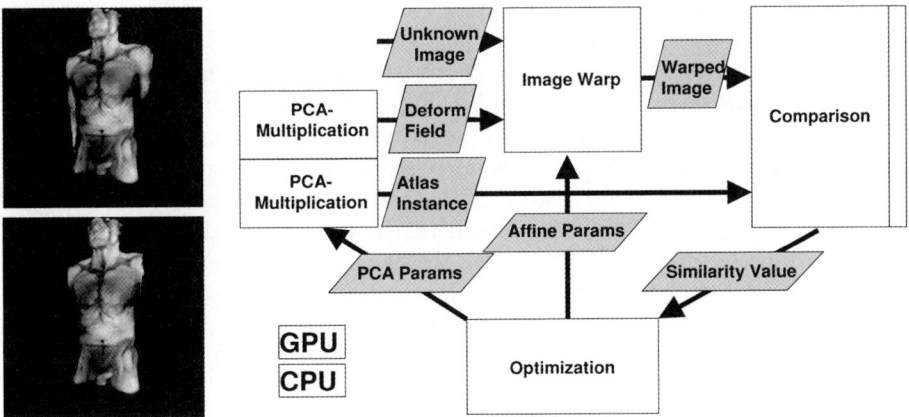

Fig. 2. Top shows FastView image in volume rendering, bottom the result after arm stripping

Fig. 3. Data flow and computation components of the registration algorithm. The white box indicates the CPU based computation component, while the boxes shaded in grey indicate GPU based computation components.

The registration runs in a hierarchical top-down way, starting with a coarse resolution and gradual refinement. A Gauss-Newton optimization scheme is chosen, with numerical derivatives being computed using symmetric differences. Gauss-Newton requires the image to be divided into blocks for which the distance measure values are calculated in parallel.

3.2 GPU Based Implementation

A basic implementation of the registration algorithm is slow, because each warping step requires B-spline tensor computations for each voxel. However, modern computer graphics hardware provides enormous floating-point, parallel computation and interpolation power off the shelf. This potential has proven to be powerful for general purpose computations like image registration [15]. Although warping the images by means of a fragment shader on the GPU results in an enormous performance boost, each warp requires the deformation field being transferred from memory to the graphics card and the warped volume being transferred back, which unnecessarily slows down the computation. Therefore, all image based computation steps are implemented as fragment shaders on the GPU, including the generation of a deformation field instance, (i.e. evaluating equation 2), generation of an intensity instance of the atlas, warping and evaluation of the distance function. This reduces data transfer between GPU and memory to the parameter values of the optimization and the values of the similarity measure resp. cost function. See figure 3 for an overview of the data flow and components of computation. All data needed for the registration, i.e. atlas data, image data, matrix data, etc. are stored using float textures in the GPU memory, which minimizes data traffic and boosts performance.

4 Results and Discussion

Validation of the atlas based segmentations is done by placing anatomical landmarks in all data sets. Between 2 and 4 landmark points per organ of interest are used. Reproducibility is studied by repeating the placements multiple times and with different operators. The mean positions of these landmarks are then considered to be the ground truth. The standard deviations were about 10.4 mm. The performance of the atlas based registrations and labelings is assessed by calculating the displacements of the propagated landmark positions to the ground truth. All tests are performed in leave-all-in and leave-one-out scenarios. Leave-all-in means that the atlas is built from all data sets and then compared to the result of the registration of one of those data sets. Table 1 gives an overview of the results.

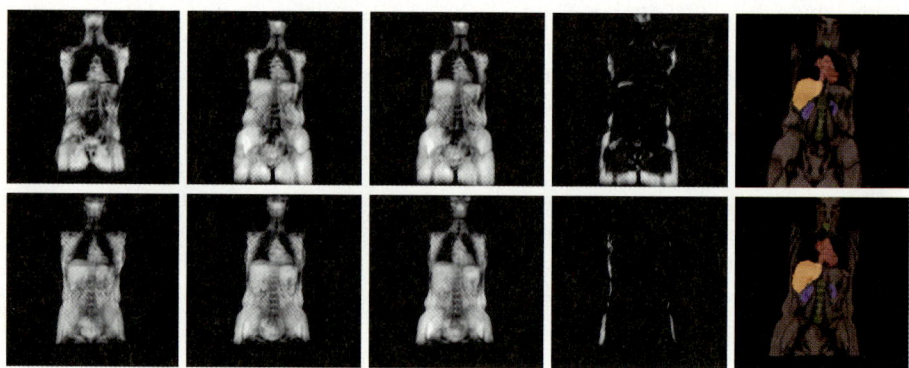

Fig. 4. This figure shows two registration results: from left to right, the original images, the warped images, the best fitting instances of the atlas, difference images and slice images of propagated labels for heart, kidneys, spine and liver

Table 1. The experimental results of the displacements between the manual landmarks and the landmarks determined by the atlas based registration

# Deformation modes	# Appearance modes	LM displacements (mm)	
		leave-all-in	leave one out
0	5	23.7	28.5
10	5	17.4	25.4
20	10	13.7	24.0
30	15	11.7	22.4

Average calculation times are about 10-30 seconds depending on the number of modes being used. Evidently, the results improve with an increasing number of modes. Overall, the deviations converge to a σ resp. 2σ interval of the ground truth for the leave-all-in resp. leave-one-out case.

5 Conclusion and Future Work

We presented a method for fast anatomical labeling in FastView MR localizer images. The results are promising and suitable for the desired applications. As for further applications, more exactness may be needed, future work will focus on improving the data basis of the atlas, which will lead to an atlas with more generalization ability. Considering its leave-one-out performance, the atlas would certainly benefit from additional training data. Another issue will be to further enhance performance by switching from numerical to analytical derivatives calculated on the GPU. Future work will also consider a final fine-tuning segmentation of the anatomical labels, using local histogram measures and shape priors. Currently, the search space of the registration is constrained to the space of valid deformation instances of the atlas. In the future this could be extended to a free non-rigid registration guided by a deformation prior imposed by the statistical model of deformation.

References

1. van der Kouwe, A., Benner, T., Fischl, B., Schmitt, F., Salat, D., Harder, M., Sorensen, A., Dale, A.: On-line automatic slice positioning for brain MR imaging. NeuroImage 27(1), 222–230 (2005)
2. Peschl, S., Ernst, T., Speck, O., Hennig, J.: Auto alignment of intervertebral disk. In: Proceedings of the 12th Annual Meeting of the ISMRM, vol. 2216 (May 2004)
3. Fenchel, M., Thesen, S., Schilling, A.: Fully automatic liver scan planning - slice and navigator positioning from stacked 2D localizer scans. In: Proceedings of the 14th Annual Meeting of ISMRM 2006, p. 467 (2006)
4. Barkhausen, J., Quick, H., Lauenstein, T., Goyen, M., Ruehm, S., Laub, G., Debatin, J., Ladd, M.: Whole-body MR imaging in 30 seconds with real-time TRUE-FISP and a continuously rolling table platform: feasibility study. Radiology 220, 252–256 (2001)
5. Kinner, S., Zielonka, A., Zenge, M.O., Ladd, S., Ladd, M.: Whole-body MR imaging with continuously moving table and multiplanar reformations: toward parameter optimization for SSFP imaging in patient examinations. In: Proceedings of the 14th Annual Meeting of ISMRM 2006, vol. 2421 (2006)
6. Keil, A., Wachinger, C., Brinker, G., Thesen, S., Navab, N.: Patient position detection for SAR optimization in magnetic resonance imaging. In: Larsen, R., Nielsen, M., Sporring, J. (eds.) MICCAI 2006. LNCS, vol. 4191, pp. 49–57. Springer, Heidelberg (2006)
7. Talairach, J., Tournoux, P.: Co-planar Stereotaxic Atlas of the Human Brain: 3-Dimensional Proportional System - an Approach to Cerebral Imaging. Thieme Medical Publishers, New York (1988)
8. Cootes, T.F., Beeston, C., Edwards, G.J., Taylor, C.J.: A unified framework for atlas matching using active appearance models. In: Kuba, A., Sámal, M., Todd-Pokropek, A. (eds.) IPMI 1999. LNCS, vol. 1613, pp. 322–330. Springer, Heidelberg (1999)
9. Rueckert, D., Frangi, A.F., Schnabel, J.A.: Automatic construction of 3D statistical deformation models of the brain using non-rigid registration. IEEE Trans. Med. Imaging 22(8), 1014–1025 (2003)

10. Zhou, Y., Bai, J.: Atlas based automatic identification of abdominal organs. Proceedings of the SPIE Medical Imaging 5747, 1804–1812 (2005)
11. Park, H., Bland, P.H., Meyer, C.R.: Construction of an abdominal probabilistic atlas and its application in segmentation. IEEE Trans. Med. Imaging 22(4), 483–492 (2003)
12. Wells, W., Viola, P., Atsumi, H., Nakajima, S., Kikinis, R.: Multi-modal volume registration by maximization of mutual information. In: Medical Image Analysis, pp. 35–51 (1996)
13. Cootes, T.F., Edwards, G.J., Taylor, C.J.: Active appearance models. In: European Conference on Computer Vision, vol. 2, pp. 484–498 (1998)
14. Stegmann, M.B., Ersbøll, B.K., Larsen, R.: Fame - a flexible appearance modelling environment. IEEE Trans. Med. Imaging 22(10), 1319–1331 (2003)
15. Harris, M.: GPGPU: General purpose computation on GPUs. In: Eurographics (2004)

Conformal Slit Mapping and Its Applications to Brain Surface Parameterization

Yalin Wang[1,2], Xianfeng Gu[3], Tony F. Chan[2], Paul M. Thompson[1], and Shing-Tung Yau[4]

[1] Lab. of Neuro Imaging, UCLA School of Medicine, Los Angeles, CA 90095, USA
ylwang@math.ucla.edu
[2] Mathematics Department, UCLA, Los Angeles, CA 90095, USA
[3] Comp. Sci. Department, SUNY at Stony Brook, Stony Brook, NY 11794, USA
[4] Department of Mathematics, Harvard University, Cambridge, MA 02138, USA

Abstract. We propose a method that computes a conformal mapping from a multiply connected mesh to the so-called *slit domain*, which consists of a canonical rectangle or disk in which 3D curved landmarks on the original surfaces are mapped to concentric or parallel lines in the slit domain. In this paper, we studied its application to brain surface parameterization. After cutting along some landmark curve features on surface models of the cerebral cortex, we obtain multiple connected domains. By computing exact harmonic one-forms, closed harmonic one-forms, and holomorphic one-forms, we are able to build a circular slit mapping that conformally maps the surface to an annulus with some concentric arcs and a rectangle with some slits. The whole algorithm is based on solving linear systems so it is very stable. In the slit domain parameterization results, the feature curves are either mapped to straight lines or concentric arcs. This representation is convenient for anatomical visualization, and may assist statistical comparisons of anatomy, surface-based registration and signal processing. Preliminary experimental results parameterizing various brain anatomical surfaces are presented.

1 Introduction

In this paper, we introduce a new method to conformally map a multiply connected domain to an annulus with multiple concentric arcs (called the *circular slit map*) or to a rectangle with multiple straight lines (the *parallel slit map*). It is a global conformal parameterization method without segmentation. First, it computes exact harmonic one-forms and closed harmonic one-forms. Secondly, it computes all bases of holomorphic one-forms. Given appropriate boundary conditions, it can compute a unique circular slit map up to a rotation around the center. The slit mapping computes the intrinsic structure of the given surface, which can be reflected in the shape of the target domain.

Most of brain conformal parameterization methods [1,2,3,4,5,6] can handle the complete brain cortex surface, but can not deal with cortex surfaces with boundaries. The holomorphic flow segmentation method [7] can match cortex surfaces with boundaries or landmarks, but the resulting mappings have singularities, which are very error-prone in practice. Only the Ricci flow method [8] and slit map method can handle surfaces with complicated topologies (boundaries and landmarks) without singularities. The Ricci flow method is a nonlinear optimization process, which is much more time consuming than slit map method. The Ricci flow method also has higher requirements for the quality for the tessellations of the surfaces. Because the Ricci flow method involves a lot of transcendental computations, it is not as stable as slit map method. Slit map method is a linear method, which is more efficient and robust.

1.1 Related Work

Brain surface parameterization has been studied intensively. Schwartz et al. [9], and Timsari and Leahy [10] computed quasi-isometric flat maps of the cerebral cortex. Drury et al. [11] presented a multiresolution method for flattening the cerebral cortex. Hurdal and Stephenson [1] reported a discrete mapping approach that uses circle packings to produce "flattened" images of cortical surfaces on the sphere, the Euclidean plane, and the hyperbolic plane. The maps obtained are quasi-conformal approximations of classical conformal maps. Haker et al. [2] implemented a finite element approximation for parameterizing brain surfaces via conformal mappings. They select a point on the cortex to map to the north pole of the Riemann sphere and conformally map the rest of the cortical surface to the complex plane by stereographic projection of the Riemann sphere to the complex plane. Gu et al. [3] proposed a method to find a unique conformal mapping between any two genus zero manifolds by minimizing the harmonic energy of the map. They demonstrate this method by conformally mapping a cortical surface to a sphere. Ju et al. [4] presented a least squares conformal mapping method for cortical surface flattening. Joshi et al. [5] proposed a scheme to parameterize the surface of the cerebral cortex by minimizing an energy functional in the pth norm. Ju et al. [6] reported the results of a quantitative comparison of FreeSurfer [12], CirclePack, and least squares conformal mapping (LSCM) with respect to geometric distortion and computational speed. Wang et al. [7] have used holomorphic 1-forms to parameterize anatomical surfaces with complex (possibly branching) topology. Wang et al. [8] introduced a brain surface conformal mapping algorithm based on algebraic functions. By solving the Yamabe equation with the Ricci flow method, it can conformally map a brain surface to a multi-hole disk.

2 Theoretical Background

Suppose S is a surface embedded in $\mathbb{R}^3$, with induced Euclidean metric $\mathbf{g}$. S is covered by an atlas $\{(U_\alpha, \phi_\alpha)\}$. Suppose (x_α, y_α) is the local parameter on the chart (U_α, ϕ_α). We say (x_α, y_α) is *isothermal*, if the metric has the representation $\mathbf{g} = e^{2\lambda(x_\alpha, y_\alpha)}(dx_\alpha^2 + dy_\alpha^2)$.

The *Laplace-Beltrami operator* is defined as

$$\Delta_\mathbf{g} = \frac{1}{e^{2\lambda(x_\alpha, y_\alpha)}}\left(\frac{\partial^2}{\partial x_\alpha^2} + \frac{\partial^2}{\partial y_\alpha^2}\right).$$

A function $f : S \to \mathbb{R}$ is *harmonic*, if $\Delta_\mathbf{g} f \equiv 0$.

Suppose ω is a differential one-form with the representation $f_\alpha dx_\alpha + g_\alpha dy_\alpha$ in the local parameters (x_α, y_α), and $f_\beta dx_\beta + g_\beta dy_\beta$ in the local parameters (x_β, y_β). Then

$$\begin{pmatrix} \frac{\partial x_\alpha}{\partial x_\beta} & \frac{\partial y_\alpha}{\partial x_\beta} \\ \frac{\partial x_\alpha}{\partial y_\beta} & \frac{\partial y_\alpha}{\partial y_\beta} \end{pmatrix} \begin{pmatrix} f_\alpha \\ g_\alpha \end{pmatrix} = \begin{pmatrix} f_\beta \\ g_\beta \end{pmatrix}.$$

ω is a *closed one-form*, if on each chart (x_α, y_α), $\frac{\partial f}{\partial y_\alpha} - \frac{\partial g}{\partial x_\alpha} = 0$. ω is an *exact one-form*, if it equals the gradient of some function. An exact one-form is also a closed one-form. If a closed one-form ω satisfies $\frac{\partial f}{\partial x_\alpha} + \frac{\partial g}{\partial y_\alpha} = 0$, then ω is a *harmonic one-form*. The gradient of a harmonic function is an exact harmonic one-form.

The so-called *Hodge star operator* turns a one-form ω to its *conjugate* $*\omega$, $*\omega = -g_\alpha dx_\alpha + f_\alpha dy_\alpha$.

A *holomorphic one-form* is a complex differential form $\omega + \sqrt{-1}*\omega$, where ω is a harmonic one-form.

Suppose S is an open surface with n boundaries $\gamma_1, \cdots, \gamma_n$. We can uniquely find a holomorphic one-form ω, such that

$$\int_{\gamma_k} \omega = \begin{cases} 2\pi & k = 1 \\ -2\pi & k = 2 \\ 0 & otherwise \end{cases} \quad (1)$$

Definition 1 (Circular Slit Mapping). *Fix a point p_0 on the surface, for any point $p \in S$, let γ be an arbitrary path connection p_0 and p, then the circular slit mapping is defined as $\phi(p) = e^{\int_\gamma \omega}$.*

Theorem 1. *The function ϕ effects a one-to-one conformal mapping of M onto the annulus $1 < |z| < e^{\lambda_0}$ minus $n - 2$ concentric arcs situated on the circles $|z| = e^{\lambda_i}, i = 1, 2, \cdots, n - 2$.*

The proof of the above theorem on slit mapping can be found in [13]. For a given choice of the inner and outer circle, the circular slit mapping is uniquely determined up to a rotation around the center. The parallel slit mapping can be defined in a similar way.

Definition 2 (Parallel Slit Mapping). *Let $\bar{S}$ be the universal covering space of the surface S, $\pi : \bar{S} \to S$ be the projection and $\bar{\omega} = \pi^*\omega$ be the pull back of ω. Fix a point $\bar{p}_0$ on $\bar{S}$, for any point $p \in \bar{S}$, let $\bar{\gamma}$ be an arbitrary path connection $\bar{p}_0$ and $\bar{p}$, then the parallel slit mapping is defined as $\bar{\phi}(\bar{p}) = \int_{\bar{\gamma}} \bar{\omega}$.*

3 Algorithm Pipeline

Suppose the input mesh has $n+1$ boundaries, $\partial M = \gamma_0 - \gamma_1 - \cdots - \gamma_n$. Without loss of generality, we map γ_0 to the outer circle of the circular slit domain, γ_1 to the inner circle, and all the others to the concentric slits.

The algorithm pipeline is as follows :
1 Compute the basis for all exact harmonic one-forms;
2. Compute the basis for all closed harmonic one-forms;

3. Compute the basis for all holomorphic one-forms;
4. Construct the slit mapping.

3.1 Basis for Exact Harmonic One-Forms

The first step of the algorithm is to compute the basis for exact harmonic one-forms. Let γ_k be an inner boundary, we compute a harmonic function $f_k : S \to \mathbb{R}$ by solving the following Dirichlet problem on the mesh M: $\begin{cases} \Delta f_k \equiv 0 \\ f_k|_{\gamma_j} = \delta_{kj} \end{cases}$, where δ_{kj} is the Kronecker function, Δ is the discrete Laplace-Beltrami operator using the co-tangent formula proposed in [14].

The exact harmonic one-form η_k can be computed as the gradient of the harmonic function f_k, $\eta_k = df_k$, and $\{\eta_1, \eta_2, \cdots, \eta_n\}$ form the basis for the exact harmonic one-forms.

3.2 Basis for Harmonic One-Forms

After getting the exact harmonic one-forms, we will compute the closed one-form basis. Let γ_k ($k > 0$) be an inner boundary. Compute a path from γ_k to γ_0, denote it as ζ_k. ζ_k cut the mesh open to M_k, while ζ_k itself is split into two boundary segments ζ_k^+ and ζ_k^- in M_k. Define a function $g_k : M_k \to \mathbb{R}$ by solving a Dirichlet problem,

$$\begin{cases} \Delta g_k \equiv 0 \\ g_k|_{\zeta_k^+} = 1 \\ g_k|_{\zeta_k^-} = 0. \end{cases}$$

Compute the gradient of g_k and let $\tau_k = dg_k$, then map τ_k back to M, where τ_k becomes a closed one-form. Then we need to find a function $h_k : M \to \mathbb{R}$, by solving the following linear system: $\Delta(\tau_k + dh_k) \equiv 0$.

Updating τ_k to $\tau_k + dh_k$, we now have $\{\tau_1, \tau_2, \ldots, \tau_n\}$ as a basis set for all the closed but non-exact harmonic one-forms.

With both the exact harmonic one-form basis and the closed non-exact harmonic one-form basis computed, we can construct the harmonic one-form basis by taking the union of them: $\{\eta_1, \eta_2, \cdots, \eta_n, \tau_1, \tau_2, \cdots, \tau_n\}$.

3.3 Basis for Holomorphic One-Forms

In Step 1 we computed the basis for exact harmonic one-forms $\{\eta_1, \cdots, \eta_n\}$. Now we compute their conjugate one-forms $\{*\eta_1, \cdots, *\eta_n\}$, so that we can combine all of them together into a holomorphic one-form basis set.

First of all, for η_k we compute an initial approximation η'_k by a brute-force method using the Hodge star. That is, rotating η_k by 90° about the surface normal to obtain η'_k. In practice such an initial approximation is usually not accurate enough. In order to improve the accuracy, we employ a technique utilizing the harmonic one-form basis we just computed. From the fact the η_k is harmonic, we can conclude that its conjugate $*\eta_k$ should also be harmonic.

Therefore, $^*\eta_k$ can be represented as a linear combination of the base harmonic one-forms: $^*\eta_k = \sum_{i=1}^n a_i\eta_i + \sum_{i=1}^n b_i\tau_i$.

Using the wedge product $\wedge$, we can construct the following linear system,

$$\int_M {}^*\eta_k \wedge \eta_i = \int_M \eta'_k \wedge \eta_i, \int_M {}^*\eta_k \wedge \tau_j = \int_M \eta'_k \wedge \tau_j.$$

We solve this linear system to obtain the coefficients a_i and b_i ($i = 1, 2, \cdots, n$) for the conjugate one-form $^*\eta_k$. Pairing each base exact harmonic one-form in the basis with its conjugate, we get a basis set for the holomorphic one-form group on M: $\{\eta_1 + \sqrt{-1}^*\eta_1, \cdots, \eta_n + \sqrt{-1}^*\eta_n\}$

3.4 Construct Slit Mapping

After computing the holomorphic one-form basis, we need to find a special holomorphic one-form $\omega = \sum_{i=1}^n \lambda_i(\eta_i + \sqrt{-1}^*\eta_i)$, such that the imaginary part of its integral satisfies

$$Im\left(\int_{\gamma_k} \omega\right) = \begin{cases} -2\pi & k = 1 \\ 0 & k > 1 \end{cases}$$

To get the coefficients λ_i, we solve the following linear system for λ_i, $i = 1, \cdots, n$:

$$\begin{pmatrix} \alpha_{11} & \alpha_{12} & \cdots & \alpha_{1n} \\ \alpha_{21} & \alpha_{22} & \cdots & \alpha_{2n} \\ \vdots & \vdots & \ddots & \vdots \\ \alpha_{n1} & \alpha_{n2} & \cdots & \alpha_{nn} \end{pmatrix} \begin{pmatrix} \lambda_1 \\ \lambda_2 \\ \vdots \\ \lambda_n \end{pmatrix} = \begin{pmatrix} -2\pi \\ 0 \\ \vdots \\ 0 \end{pmatrix}$$

where $\alpha_{kj} = \int_{\gamma_j} {}^*\eta_k$.

It can be proven that this linear system has a unique solution, which reflects the fact that γ_1 is mapped to the inner circle of the circular slit domain. Further, the system implies the following equation $\lambda_1\alpha_{01} + \lambda_2\alpha_{02} + \cdots + \lambda_n\alpha_{0n} = 2\pi$, which means that γ_0 is mapped to the outer circle in the circular slit domain.

After computing the desired holomorphic one-form ω, we are ready to generate the circular slit mapping. What we need to compute is a complex-valued function $\phi: M \to \mathbb{C}$ by integrating ω and taking the exponential map. Choosing a base vertex v_0 arbitrarily, and for each vertex $v \in M$ choosing the shortest path γ from v_0 to v, we can compute the map as the following: $\phi(v) = e^{\int_\gamma \omega}$.

Based on the circular slit map ϕ we just computed, we can compute a parallel slit map $\tau: M \to \mathbb{C}$: $\tau(v) = \ln \phi(v)$.

4 Experimental Results

We applied our algorithms to parameterize various anatomical surfaces extracted from 3D MRI scans of the brain. In this paper, the segmentations are regarded as given, and result from automated and manual segmentations detailed in our prior work. Figure 1 shows an example of our computation results. For the

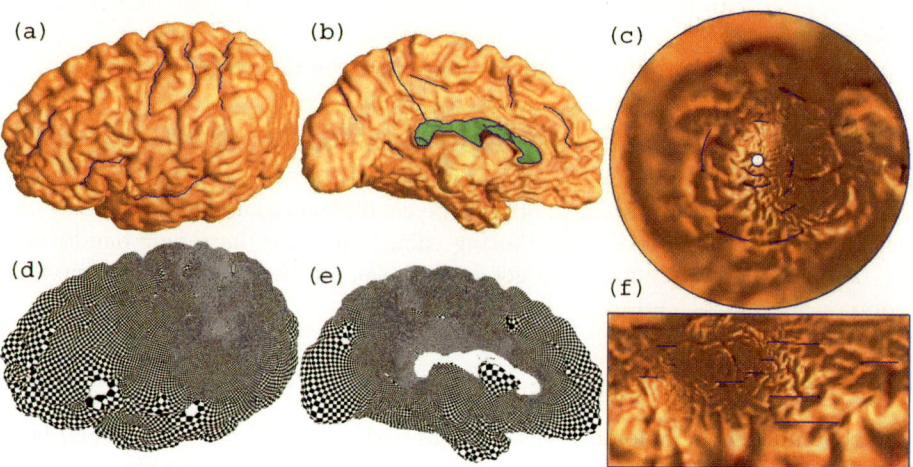

Fig. 1. (a) and (b) show the cortical surface with 12 landmarks cut open, including an open boundary at the corpus callosum (in green); (c) is the parallel slit map result; (f) is the circular slit map result; (d) and (e) show the conformal texture parameterized by the circular slit map (f)

cortical surface of the brain, we cut it open along twelve major landmarks. (a) and (b) show the brain surface from two different views. With our slit mapping algorithm, we can conformally map it to a rectangular domain with four slits (c) and an annulus with ten concentric arcs (d). (d) and (e) demonstrate the conformal texture mapping as the pull-back of the coordinates induced by the circular slit mapping of (f).

We also tested our algorithm on a left hippocampal surface, a key structure in the medial temporal lobe of the brain, for which parametric shape models are commonly developed for tracking shape differences and longitudinal atrophy in disease. The results are shown in the first row of Subfigure 1 in Figure 2. We leave two holes on the front and back of the hippocampal surface, representing its anterior junction with the amygdala and its posterior limit as it turns into the white matter of the *fornix*. We also randomly selected two curves lying in regions of high curvature, which are of interest for surface registration research (these could also be boundaries of the CA fields, or other architectonic boundaries, if high-field images are available). The parallel slit mapping result is shown with appropriate landmark curves labeled. We also applied our algorithm to lateral ventricular surface (second row in Subfigure 1 of Figure 2). We introduced three cuts. The motivation for these cuts are based on the topology of the lateral ventricles, in which several horns are joined together at the "atrium" or "trigone". In the parallel slit mapping result, two boundaries are mapped to left and right boundaries, respectively. The rectangle's lengthy aspect ratio reflects its intrinsically long horn-like shape. The third column shows the

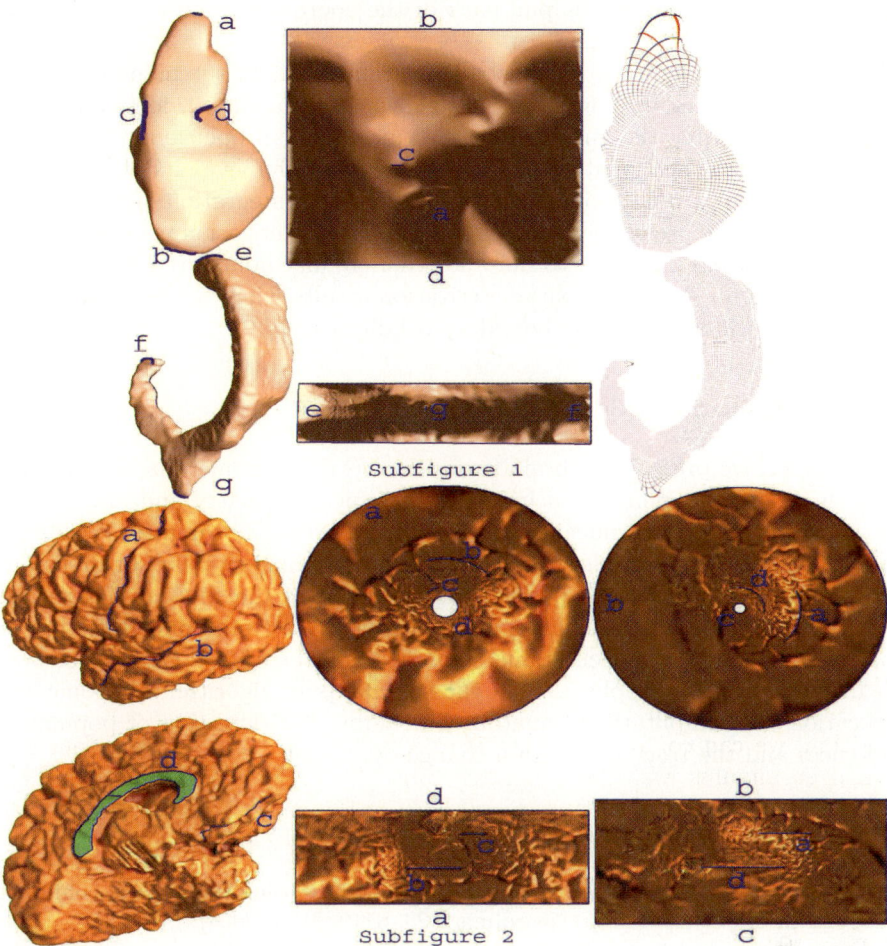

Fig. 2. Subfigure 1 illustrations the parallel slit mapping results for a hippocampal surface and a left lateral ventricle. Surfaces are cut open along various landmarks which are the blue curves on two pictures in the left column. Similar to previous other work, the landmarks are curves are either at the end of shape or follow significant curvatures. In the first row, four landmarks are cut open on a hippocampal surface. In the parallel slit map result, landmarks b and d are mapped to the upper and lower boundaries, respectively. On the second row, three landmarks are introduced on a lateral ventricle surface. In the parallel slit map, e and f are mapped to the left and right boundaries, respectively. Their conformal texture are also shown. In Subfigure 2,conformal parameterization results are shown with different boundary conditions. The first column shows a cerebral cortical surface is cut open along four major sulcal landmarks. The second column shows the circular slit map and parallel slit map results when a pair of landmarks are selected as boundaries landmark a as the exterior circular boundary and d as the inner circular boundary. The third column shows results the other pair of landmarks are selected as boundaries.

conformal texture mapping as pull-back of the coordinates induced by the slit mapping.

In Figure 2, Subfigure 2 demonstrates various parallel slit mapping results given different boundary conditions. As shown in Subfigure 2, four landmarks were cut open. After the cut, the surface turns into an open boundary genus three surface. For the Equation 1, we selected two different pairs of landmarks as the exterior and inner boundaries by putting the integration of different γ_k as 2π and -2π. The second column shows the parameterization results when we use landmark a and d as the exterior and inner circular boundaries, respectively. The third column shows the parameterization results when we select the other pair of landmark curves as the boundary conditions.

5 Conclusions and Future Work

In this paper, we presented a brain surface conformal parameterization method based on the slit mapping, which transfers cortical geometry and any embedded landmarks into a canonical domain, with conformal coordinates. With fixed boundary conditions, our algorithm can compute unique circular slit maps and parallel slit maps, where the positions and lengths of the slits are determined by the conformal equivalence class of the surface. We tested our algorithm on hippocampal, lateral ventricular and cerebral cortical surfaces. Our future work will include empirical application of the slit mapping algorithm to biomedical applications in computational anatomy, including the detection of population differences and the tracking of brain change over time.

References

1. Hurdal, M.K., Stephenson, K.: Cortical cartography using the discrete conformal approach of circle packings. NeuroImage 23, S119–S128 (2004)
2. Angenent, S., Haker, S., Tannenbaum, A., Kikinis, R.: Conformal geometry and brain flattening. Med. Image Comput. Comput.-Assist. Intervention, 271–278 (September 1999)
3. Gu, X., Wang, Y., Chan, T.F., Thompson, P.M., Yau, S.T.: Genus zero surface conformal mapping and its application to brain surface mapping. IEEE TMI 23(8), 949–958 (2004)
4. Ju, L., Stern, J., Rehm, K., Schaper, K., Hurdal, M.K., Rottenberg, D.: Cortical surface flattening using least squares conformal mapping with minimal metric distortion. In: IEEE ISBI, Arlington, VA, USA, pp. 77–80 (2004)
5. Joshi, A.A., Leahy, R.M., Thompson, P.M., Shattuck, D.W.: Cortical surface parameterization by p-harmonic energy minimization. In: IEEE ISBI, Arlington, VA, USA, pp. 428–431 (2004)
6. Ju, L., Hurdal, M.K., Stern, J., Rehm, K., Schaper, K., Rottenberg, D.: Quantitative evaluation of three surface flattening methods. NeuroImage 28(4), 869–880 (2005)
7. Wang, Y., Lui, L.M., Gu, X., Hayashi, K.M., Chan, T.F., Toga, A.W., Thompson, P.M., Yau, S.T.: Brain surface conformal parameterization using Riemann surface structure. IEEE TMI 26(6), 853–865 (2007)

8. Wang, Y., Gu, X., Chan, T.F., Thompson, P.M., Yau, S.T.: Brain surface conformal parameterization with algebraic functions. In: Larsen, R., Nielsen, M., Sporring, J. (eds.) MICCAI 2006, Part II. LNCS, vol. 4191, pp. 946–954. Springer, Heidelberg (2006)
9. Schwartz, E., Shaw, A., Wolfson, E.: A numerical solution to the generalized mapmaker's problem: Flattening nonconvex polyhedral surfaces. IEEE TPAMI 11(9), 1005–1008 (1989)
10. Timsari, B., Leahy, R.M.: An optimization method for creating semi-isometric flat maps of the cerebral cortex. In: Proceedings of SPIE, Medical Imaging, San Diego, CA (February 2000)
11. Drury, H.A., Van Essen, D.C., Anderson, C.H., Lee, C.W., Coogan, T.A., Lewis, J.W.: Computerized mappings of the cerebral cortex: A multiresolution flattening method and a surface-based coordinate system. J. Cognitive Neurosciences 8, 1–28 (1996)
12. Fischl, B., Sereno, M.I., Dale, A.M.: Cortical surface-based analysis II: Inflation, flatteningm and a surface-based coordinate system. NeuroImage 9, 179–194 (1999)
13. Ahlfors, L.V.: Complex Analysis. McGraw-hill, New York (1953)
14. Pinkall, U., Polthier, K.: Computing discrete minimal surfaces and their conjugate. Experimental Mathematics 2(1), 15–36 (1993)

Automatic Determination of Arterial Input Function for Dynamic Contrast Enhanced MRI in Tumor Assessment

Jeremy Chen, Jianhua Yao, and David Thomasson

Diagnostic Radiology Department, Clinical Center, National Institutes of Health, Bethesda, MD, 20892, USA

Abstract. Dynamic Contrast Enhanced MRI (DCE-MRI) is today one of the most popular methods for tumor assessment. Several pharmacokinetic models have been proposed to analyze DCE-MRI. Most of them depend on an accurate arterial input function (AIF). We propose an automatic and versatile method to determine the AIF. The method has two stages, detection and segmentation, incorporating knowledge about artery structure, fluid kinetics, and the dynamic temporal property of DCE-MRI. We have applied our method in DCE-MRIs of four different body parts: breast, brain, liver and prostate. The results show that we achieve average 89.5% success rate for 40 cases. The pharmacokinetic parameters computed from the automatic AIF are highly agreeable with those from a manually derived AIF (R^2=0.89, P(T<=t)=0.19) and a semiautomatic AIF (R^2=0.98, P(T<=t)=0.01).

Keywords: DCE-MRI, AIF, tumor imaging.

1 Introduction

In the U.S. for 2008 the American Cancer Society estimates 565,650 deaths due to cancer along with 437,180 new cases of cancer detected [1]. Excluding basal and squamous skin cancer, breast cancer has the highest incidence rate among women and is the second leading cause of cancer deaths in women after lung cancer [1]. In men prostate cancer has the highest incidence rate among men and is the leading cause of cancer death in men. Locating, identifying, and knowing the state of cancer tumors early is the best way to improve future prognosis.

Dynamic contrast enhanced MRI (DCE-MRI) is today one of the most popular methods for tumor assessment. Tumor growth beyond a certain size depends on the development of a vascular supply that meets the increased metabolic demand of neoplastic tissue. Studies show that tumor malignancy is highly correlated with increased vascularity. DCE-MRI allows the visualization of tumor vasculature.

The simplest pharmacokinetic model is the one-compartment model where it is assumed that all contrast agents are administered into a single blood vessel compartment [2]. Later a two-compartment model describing contrast agent exchange between the blood vessels and surrounding interstitium as a bi-directional process was proposed [3]. Most of these models such as the General Kinetic Model [4] are based on the indicator dilution theory and require the Arterial Input Function (AIF) to deconvolute with in order to find the concentration of blood (contrast agent) flowing into tissue. These models can [4] quantitatively characterize the permeability of tissue by calculating tracer dynamic parameters such as the extravasation rate (K_{trans}), reflux rate (k_{ep}), and the extravascular extracellular distribution volume (ve). Examining these parameters can be used to monitor the effects of therapy on tumor and normal tissue. These models are currently being used in trials to examine breast, liver, brain, and prostate tumors at our institute [4, 5, 6].

Automating the process of finding the AIF can save valuable human-operator time. It also removes the inherent inter-operator variability when choosing an AIF and reduces the variability when comparing changes in pharmacokinetic parameters in follow-up studies during treatment therapy.

There are several methods already developed that automatically extract an AIF from DCE-MRIs. Most of them pick an AIF by looking at various characteristics of image voxel's time-intensity curves, such as peak height, peak width, take-off time, and initial slope [7]. Parker et al. [8] proposed another method to automatically extract an AIF from various parts of the body in DCE-MRI; using a known characteristic of artery voxel time curves, high peak height, it chooses the top 5% of voxels that enhance the brightest and uses them to generate the AIF. However, this method may have some inaccuracy because voxels of an artery are not necessarily being used obtain an AIF. Also this method makes use of only 2d information and is not completely automatic because it requires an operator to pick one axial slice on which to find an AIF.

In this paper we propose a new method that automatically extracts an AIF in DCE-MRI by automatically segmenting the voxels of a major artery in 3d and using the averages of their time-intensity curves to define the AIF. The AIF can then be exported and used in pharmacokinetic models to calculate tumor permeability parameters. This method is versatile, able to extract an AIF from DCE-MRI of different body parts: brain, breast, liver, and prostate. We automatically detect the aorta near the breast and liver, the superior sagittal sinus in the brain and the iliac artery near the prostate and use them to computer AIF.

2 Materials and Methods

2.1 Imaging Protocol

There are currently four different IRB approved DCE-MRI imaging protocols in our institution used to examine different human body parts: breast, brain, liver and prostate, as in Fig 3.

In general the DCE-MRI image acquisition protocols were done using a 3D SPGRE sequence. The TR and TE are consistent with temporal and spatial resolution that varies between clinical studies (different body parts).

Axial Images were acquired 4-8 mm in slice thickness. The dynamic data sets were acquired during and after injection of 0.1mmol/Kg (typically between 12 and 20cc) of Gd-DTPA contrast at a rate of .2-3 cc/sec for a temporal resolution from 5-30 seconds; the values depend on imaging protocol used.

2.2 Flow Chart

The flow chart of our AIF determination method is summarized in Fig. 1. It has a detection stage and a segmentation stage. A height filter is applied on the DCE-MRI to keep voxels with signal intensity greater than a threshold. Then a slope filter keeps only the voxels with a fast enough wash-in. A 2d blob labeling process is used to form distinguishable 2d-connected regions. The 3D overlapping region that is most cylindrical in shape is detected as the vessel. A refined slope filter and region growing algorithm is then conducted to segment the vessel. The AIF is calculated from the vessel's intensity curves.

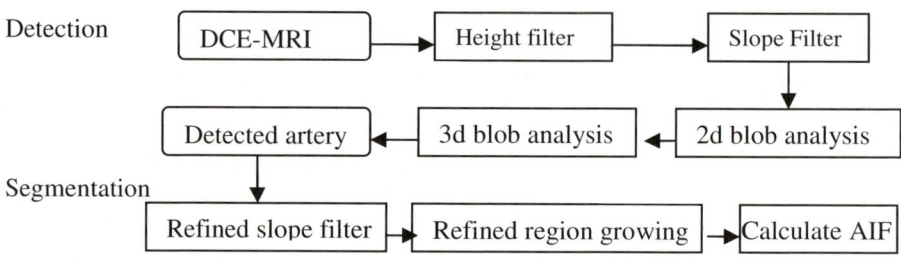

Fig. 1. Flow Chart of AIF Determination Method

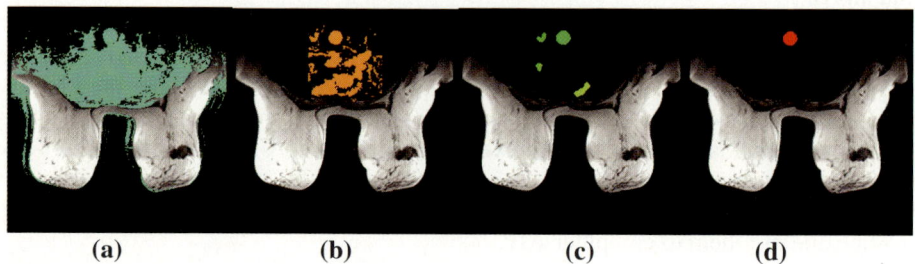

Fig. 2. Illustration of AIF determination (a) Height Filter, (b) Initial Uptake Slope Filter, (c) 2d Blob regions, (d) Segmented Image

2.3 Artery Detection

In the detection phase, each voxel's time intensity curve is examined. Major arteries have large amount of Gd-DTPA contrast agent flowing through them, causing the image voxels of the major arteries to brighten more than most other voxels. The peak height of an AIF is generally higher than the peak height of most others. Thus, a height filter is used to filter out voxels with small peak curves. The filter is written as,

$$S(t_p) > \mu \tag{1}$$

where t_p is the time to peak, and μ is the mean peak value of all voxels in the image. The voxels passing the height filter are shown in Fig 2a.

The second filter is based on the fact that the signal intensity of major artery voxels brightens quickly from a fast wash-in of gadolinium contrast agent. This is represented by a steep uptake slope, thus a slope filter is used to keep the voxels with a slope greater than a threshold. The signal enhancement ratio of every time point is defined as

$$R(t) = \frac{S(t)}{S_0} \qquad (2)$$

where $R(t)$ is the ratio of signal enhancement from baseline to time t, S_0 is the baseline signal which is computed as the average signal of the first three time points. The uptake slope is then computed as,

$$slope = \frac{R(t_p)-1}{t_p} \qquad (3)$$

where t_p is the signal peak time which is initially set to a time depending on the imaging protocol and body part. If the slope is greater than a preset threshold θ_1, then it is kept as major artery candidate. The voxels passing the slope filter are shown in Fig 2b.

After the two filters, a blob labeling process is run on the remaining voxels to form distinguishable 2d connected components (we call them blobs) from the candidate voxels in each axial slice. A size filter is used to keep only blobs that are big enough to possibly be part of the major artery (Fig. 2c). For each blob, the average peak time is calculated, and the earliest 20% time-to-peaks are averaged and set as the estimated major artery time-to-peak t_p'. The slope filter is repeated using the estimated t_p'. The next step is to calculate the compactness and circularity of each of the remaining blob as follows,

$$C_z = Circularity = \frac{1}{Compactness} = \frac{A}{P^2}. \qquad (4)$$

here P is the perimeter of the blob and A is the area.

The 2d blobs are then propagated in transverse direction to form 3d blobs. 2d blobs that overlap each other in axial slices above or below are considered to be part of the same object in 3d. The cylindricality of each 3d object is calculated by summing across the axial slices the circularity of each 2d blob belonging to the same 3d object.

$$Cylindricality = \sum_z C_z. \qquad (5)$$

C_z is the circularity of the object on the axial slice z. The most cylindrical object is selected as the artery to determine AIF. We recompute the new time-to-peak (t_p") using the detected artery and use it for the rest of the slope calculations. The center of the detected artery is used as the seed for the artery segmentation algorithm in the second stage.

2.4 Artery Segmentation and AIF Determination

The detected artery is then segmented using a region growing technique. The slope is recalculated using the refined time-to-peak t_p". A refined slope filter using a slightly lower slope threshold (θ_2) is conducted to ensure that the entire major artery is segmented.

Then on the middle axial slice we run the region growing algorithm using the seed obtained in the detection stage to segment the artery. The region growing is then propagated to every other axial slice using the center of the segmented artery on the previous slice as the seed. The segmented main artery is shown in Fig 2d.

For each axial slice of the object, the average time-intensity curve of voxels in the artery is computed as the AIF. To accommodate for possible flow artifacts, the AIF in the axial slice with the highest peak is omitted and the AIF that has the second highest peak is used for calculation in the pharmacokinetic models.

2.5 Setting the Parameters and Thresholds

There are several parameters in our method. The first one is time-to-peak t_p. t_p is the time over which to calculate the uptake slope. This parameter is initially set depending on the image protocol used. Initially t_p=6, 4, 9 and 7 for breast, liver, brain and prostate respectively. t_p is later adaptively refined twice using the detected blobs and arteries.

The next parameter is the artery size threshold. A 2d blob region can not be too big or too small to be considered as potentially being part of the artery. The aorta near the breast and liver is larger than the superior sagittal sinus in the brain and iliac artery near the prostate so the breast and liver images are set to have a higher size threshold. The minimum size threshold is set to 50, 50, 30, and 20 voxels for the breast, liver, brain, and prostate respectively. The max size threshold is set to 1500 voxels.

The other 2 parameters are the slope thresholds used in the two stage slope filters. The first slope threshold θ_1 is used to remove unwanted voxels in the artery detection phase. The second slope threshold θ_2 is set lower than the first one to ensure the whole artery is segmented. The breast and liver DCE-MRI are set to a higher slope threshold than the brain and prostate. The reason for this is the breast and liver have a bigger artery (aorta) and more blood flow which allows faster contrast uptake in the breast and liver compared to the iliac artery near the prostate and the superior sagittal sinus in the brain. The default value of θ_1 = 0.6, 0.9, 0.2 and 0.2 breast, liver, brain and prostate respectively, and that of θ_2 = 0.6, 0.9, 0.2 and 0.1

3 Experiments and Results

3.1 Data Sets

We have randomly selected 10 DCE-MRI studies for each body part in our experiments. Table 1 lists the study specifications, including number of axial slices, number of time points, time interval between images, and injection rate. Among the 10 breast studies, 5 have invasive breast cancer, 2 are invasive ductal carcinoma cases and 3 are some type of cancerous tumor.

3.2 Segmentation Success Rate

We conducted experiments to evaluate the segmentation success rate. We checked the automatic artery segmentation on every axial slice and compared it with an operator

Table 1. DCE-MRI data

DCE-MRI scan	Studies	Slices	Time Points	Interval (sec).	Injection Rate
Breast	10	30	16/18	30	.3 cc/sec & 2cc/sec
Prostate	10	10 & 12	56	5	.3 cc/sec & 2cc/sec
Liver	10	12	23	23	.3 cc/sec & 2cc/sec
Brain	10	12	30	30	.3 cc/sec

Table 2. Segmentation success rate

	Success rate (%)	Std (%)	Worst (%)	Best (%)
Breast	95.5	11.5	70	100
Prostate	82.9	18.9	40	100
Liver	98.3	3.5	91.7	100
Brain	81.3	18.9	50	100
Average	89.5	13.2	62.9	100

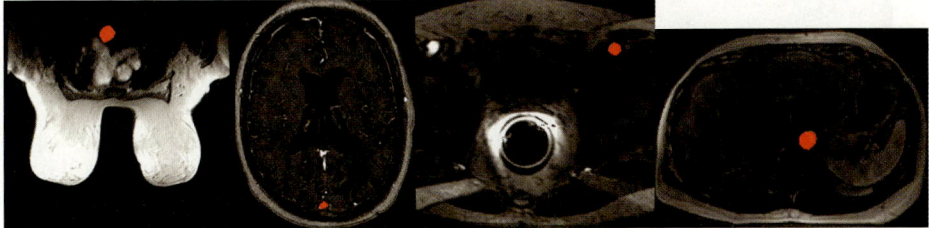

Fig. 3. Automatic artery segmentation colored in red on DCE-MRI of **(a)** breast, **(b)** brain, **(c)** prostate, and **(d)** liver

manual segmentation. The automatic artery segmentation is determined to be a success if more than 80% of the artery segmentation agrees with each other. Table 2 shows the summary of success rate for the 4 different DCE-MRI studies. Examples of successful segmentation are shown in Figure 3.

3.3 Comparison of Pharmacokinetic Parameters

To further validate our method, we used the automatically determined AIF to compute pharmacokinetic parameters (K_{trans}, k_{ep}, and ve) of the Generic Kinetic Model using a software called Cine Tool (GE Medical Systems) [4]. In addition to the automatically determined AIF, we also obtained AIFs from a manual segmentation of the artery on the same slice and two semi-automatic segmentations of the artery on the same and a different slice. For manual segmentation, the user manually traces the border of the artery. For semiautomatic segmentation, the user picks a seed point inside the artery and a region growing algorithm is run to segment the entire vessel (Cine Tool). Figure 4 shows examples of the four vessel segmentations, AIFs, and parameter maps. We used the 10 breast DCE-MRI cases for this experiment. For each case, we selected a biopsy-verified tumor region and evaluated the K_{trans}, k_{ep}, and ve values of the tumor. Table 3 summarizes the differences between the tumor permeability kinetics values calculated using the four AIFs.

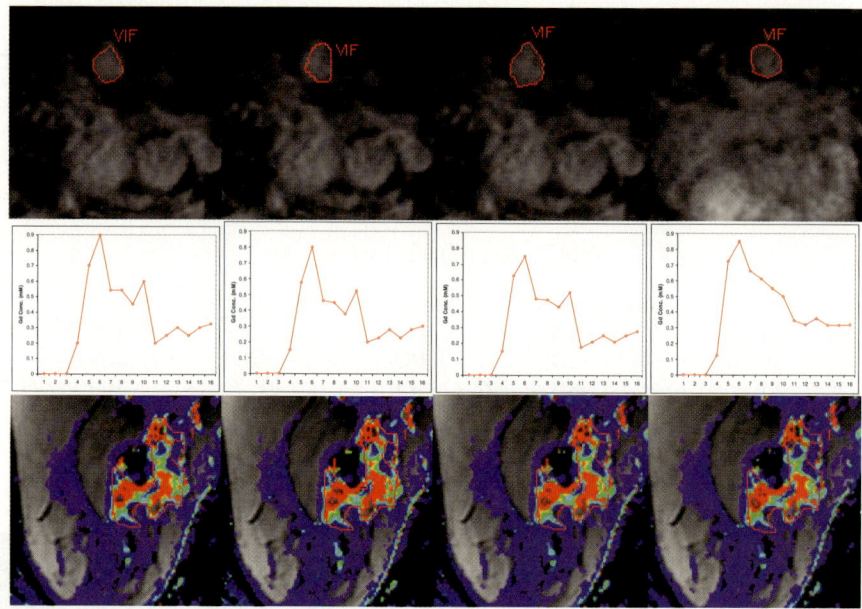

Fig. 4. For each Row: **(1st Row)** Aorta segmentation, **(2nd Row)** AIF, **(3rd Row)** Color map of K_{trans} values of a tumor ROI. Each Column: **(a)** Automatic segmentation on axial slice 11, **(b)** Manual Segmentation on axial slice 11, **(c)** Semi-Automatic Segmentation on axial slice 11 using Cine Tool, **(d)** Semi-Automatic Segmentation on axial slice 15 using Cine Tool.

Table 3. Average percentage difference in GKM values compared to GKM values calculated using the semi-automatically determined AIF

% Difference	Manual	Automatic	Semi-Auto on different axial slices
K_{trans}	13.6±15.1	16.7±8.7	15.8±18.1
k_{ep}	11.9±9.6	9.08±10.4	18.9±10.9
ve	6.2±8.0	9.0±8.5	9.4±9.5

Table 4. Comparison of K_{trans} values of one tumor, chi-squared and t-test

Correlation	Manual vs. Auto	Semi-Auto vs. Auto	Semi-Auto on different slices
R^2	0.89	0.98	0.95
P(T<=t)	0.19	0.01	0.02

We further conducted paired t-tests comparing the average GKM K_{trans} of the tumor region shown in Figure 4. Table 4 summarizes the comparison. The K_{trans} values from the automatic AIF and the manually derived AIF are correlated though without statistical significance which is likely due to one outlier in the data set, giving validity that using the automated AIF can accurately calculate pharmacokinetic parameters. Comparison of K_{trans} values derived from our automatic method and the semi-automatic AIF are statistically similar. The K_{trans} values calculated from semi-automatic AIFs on different slices are also statistically similar (P=0.02); however, their difference is bigger than the difference between automatic AIF and the semi-auto on the same slice (P=0.01). This indicates that there is more variation when a different slice is used to generate the AIF than when picking a slightly different AIF on the same slice. Our automatic method will pick the same axial slice every time when choosing the AIF, making it more consistent than when two different operators possibly pick different axial slices to get the AIF on the same study.

4 Conclusion and Discussion

We have proposed a versatile and robust method to automatically segment a major artery in various parts of the body to generate an AIF in DCE-MRI.

The manual and automatic artery segmentations are similar; however, small deviations in voxels used for the AIF can cause a change of GKM values up to 45%. Although there is variability, the GKM values calculated from the automatically derived AIF still reflect an estimate of the expected high tumor permeability. This shows validity that the automatically derived AIF can be used to calculate important values of pharmacokinetic models to assess tumors.

Our automatic method performed well in segmenting the aorta near the breast and liver. In some studies there was some over-segmentation when the aorta is close to the heart. The method had errors segmenting the major vessel in the brain in 3 out of the 10 studies due to over-segmentation of the branches off the main vessel. The prostate images were of worse quality and when the ureter runs adjacent to the iliac arteries, the method has a higher chance of failing by also segmenting the ureter. In the liver cases our method had the least problems in segmenting the artery. This is due to various factors; there were almost no motion artifacts; the aorta does not move even though surrounding organs may be moving, the aorta does not bend next to the liver; and there are no enhancing anatomical structures adjacent to the aorta.

We must point out that our method is not yet completely automatic for some cases. The two slope filter thresholds may needed to be adjusted manually to achieve optimal results. We are investigating adaptive techniques to fully automate these parameter settings.

References

1. Cancer Facts & Figures 2008 – American Cancer Society (2008)
2. Kety, S.: Cerebral circulation. In: Magoun, H. (ed.) Neurophysiology. Handbook of physiology, vol. III, sec. 1, pp. 1751–1760. American Physiological Society (1960)
3. Tofts, P., et al.: Estimating kinetic parameters from dynamic contrast-enhanced T1-weighted MRI of diffusible tracer: Standardized quantities and symbols. Journal of Magnetic Resonance Imaging (10), 223–232 (1999)
4. Thukral, A., et al.: Inflammatory Breast Cancer: Dynamic Contrast-enhanced MRI in Patients Receiving Bevacizumab-Initial Experience. Radiology 2007 244, 727–735 (2007)
5. Harrer, J.U., Parker, G.J., et al.: Comparative study of methods for determining vascular permeability and blood volume in human gliomas. J. Magn. Reson. Imaging 20(5), 748–757 (2004)
6. Choyke, P., Dwyer, A., Knopp, M.: Functional Tumor Imaging With Dynamic Contrast-Enhanced Magnetic Resonance Imaging. J. Magn. Reson. Imaging 17, 509–520 (2003)
7. Morris, E.D., et al.: Automated Determination of the Arterial Input Function for MR Perfusion Analysis. In: 8th ISMRM, Denver, CO, April 3-7 (2000)
8. Parker, G.J., Jackson, A., Waterton, J.C., Buckley, D.L.: Automated Arterial Input Function Extraction for T1-Weighted DCE-MRI. In: ISMRM (2003)

Robust Vessel Tree Modeling

M. Akif Gülsün and Hüseyin Tek

Imaging and Visualization, Siemens Corporate Research, Princeton, NJ, USA
akif.gulsun@siemens.com, Huseyin.Tek@siemens.com

Abstract. In this paper, we present a novel method for extracting center axis representations (centerlines) of blood vessels in contrast enhanced (CE)-CTA/MRA, robustly and accurately. This graph-based optimization algorithm which employs multi-scale medialness filters extracts vessel centerlines by computing the *minimum-cost* paths. Specifically, first, new medialness filters are designed from the assumption of circular/elliptic vessel cross-sections. These filters produce contrast and scale independent responses even the presence of nearby structures. Second, they are incorporated to the minimum-cost path detection algorithm in a novel way for the computational efficiency and accuracy. Third, the full vessel centerline tree is constructed from this optimization technique by assigning a *saliency measure* for each centerline from their length and radius information. The proposed method is computationally efficient and produces results that are comparable in quality to the ones created by experts. It has been tested on more than 100 coronary artery data set where the full coronary artery trees are extracted in 21 seconds in average on a 3.2GHz PC.

1 Introduction

Modeling of vascular structures from contrast enhanced (CE) Computer Tomography Angiography(CTA) and Magnetic Resonance Angiography (MRA) is often a necessary task for diagnosis, treatment planning and follow-up studies in clinical applications. While recent technological advances in image acquisition devices *e.g.*, new multi-detector CT machines, increase the spatial resolution of image data significantly, *accurate* and *timely* modeling of blood vessels is a still challenging task in many applications. Specifically, (*i*) intensity contrast may change drastically along a single vessel; (*ii*) vessels may touch nearby bright structures such as bone or other vessels; (*iii*) a single vessel tree can have large and small vessels *i.e.*, significant scale change; (*iv*) local vessel structure may deviate from a tubular structure due to the presence of pathologies such as stenosis. In clinical applications, a vessel modeling algorithm must be able to handle these imaging issues and still produce robust and accurate results in *short time e.g.* in few seconds for a single vessel, which are the main goals of our work. Some of the previous work on vessel centerline modeling methods include vesselness-based methods [6,5,12,11] and medialness filters based methods [2,1,11,8].

In this paper, we propose a new framework for the extraction of center-axis representation of vessels from CTA, MRA and 3D-X ray. Specifically, first, a novel *medialness* measure based on 2D multi-scale cross-sectional models is introduced. This new measure is contrast and scale independent and it works well in the presence of nearby bright structures such as bones or other vessels. Second, we present a minimal path detection method working on a discrete grid where the cost of graph edges are computed from multi-scale medialness filters. Third, the full vessel centerline tree from a single seed is extracted by a post-processing algorithm which uses the length and scale of vessel centerlines. In general, the proposed method can produce centerline model(s) for a vessel segment as well as the full vessel tree. In addition, it is capable of capturing different size of vessel branches, crossing over stenosis. Moreover, it is computationally efficient, i.e., it takes less than 21 seconds in average on a typical PC to obtain the centerlines of the full coronary artery trees including smaller branches. Furthermore, it works well for different types of vessels such as carotid, peripheral, aorta obtained from different imaging modalities such as CTA, MRA and 3D-X ray. We have tested it on more than 100 coronary CTA data as well as on several other types of vessels and the computed results were comparable to the expert created ones.

2 Medialness Measure from 2D Cross-Sectional Models

In this paper, our goal is to obtain the centerline representations of vessels directly from images without creating a binary vessel mask. Specifically, we propose a novel technique for computing medialness measure which is based on multi-scale cross-sectional vessel modeling. Blood vessels in CTA/MRA have typically circular/elliptic shapes in cross-sectional views even though local variations on them are not too uncommon due to the presence of nearby vessels or pathologies. Ideally, 2D cross-sectional vessel profile consists of a circular/elliptic bright disk and darker ring around it. Our medialness measure uses this circularity assumption and edge responses obtained from multi-scale filters. Specifically, our medialness response, $m(\boldsymbol{x_0})$ at $\boldsymbol{x_0}$, is computed from a circle $C(\boldsymbol{x_0}, R)$ centered at $\boldsymbol{x_0}$, with radius R, and is given by

$$m(\boldsymbol{x_0}) = \max_R \{ \frac{1}{N} \sum_{i=0}^{N-1} E(\boldsymbol{x_0} + R\boldsymbol{u}(2\pi i/N)) \} \quad (1)$$

where $\boldsymbol{u}(\alpha) = sin(\alpha)\boldsymbol{u_1} + cos(\alpha)\boldsymbol{u_2}$ and $\boldsymbol{u_1}$ and $\boldsymbol{u_1}$ defines a 2D plane. E measures the normalized edge response which is described below. Krissian *et. al.*, [7] proposed a similar medialness measure where the cross-sectional plane is computed from the eigenvectors of Hessian matrix.

Let us consider a 1-D intensity profile $I(x)$ along a ray $\boldsymbol{u_\alpha}$ on a cross-sectional plane of a vessel starting from the location $\boldsymbol{x_0}$. Suppose that $\boldsymbol{x_0}$ is the center of the vessel with a radius R. Then the cross-sectional boundary of the vessel along the ray should occur at $(\boldsymbol{x_0} + R\boldsymbol{u_\alpha})$ where the gradient of $I(x)$ has a maxima and the second derivative of $I(x)$ has a zero-crossing. We propose to use the gradient, $\nabla_\sigma I(x)$ for measuring responses at vessel boundaries, in which σ corresponds to the spatial scale of the vessel boundary. These gradients are normalized based on their filter sizes, σ to obtain comparable results between different scales. In general, filter sizes are often selected from the size of vessels for computing gradient responses [7], *i.e.*, larger spatial filters for large vessels. It should be noted that vessel scale, namely R and boundary scale, σ are not always related. For example, the boundary of a large vessel can be detected *better* with small size filters when such vessels are surrounded by other bright structures. Similarly, it is possible that small scale vessels can have long diffused boundaries which cannot be accurately detected via small scale filters.

Let us now define the boundary measure along a ray $\boldsymbol{u_\alpha}$ at the location x,

$$b(x) = max_\sigma\{(|\nabla_\sigma I(x)|)\} sign(\nabla_\sigma I(x)) \tag{2}$$

where $sign(x)$ is used to distinguish the rising (dark to bright changes) and falling edges (bright to dark changes). Observe that this boundary measure, $\nabla_\sigma I$ is contrast dependent, *i.e.*, it obtains higher values from high contrast vessels and lower values from low contrast vessels, respectively. Unfortunately, vessels may have significant intensity variations on them - especially vessels in MRA and small size vessels in CTA. In addition, boundaries of bones, calcifications in CTA and vessels next to airways can have strong gradients which usually effect the response of medialness filters. We, in fact, believe that medialness responses should be contrast independent, which can be accomplished by normalizing the boundary measure via the highest gradient obtained for different R values along the ray. Mathematically, we define a normalized boundary measure as $\hat{b}(x) = b(x)/b_{max}$ where b_{max} is the maximum falling edge response along $I(x)$ for $x = \{\boldsymbol{x_0} + R_{min}\boldsymbol{u_\alpha}, .., \boldsymbol{x_0} + R_{max}\boldsymbol{u_\alpha}\}$ and R_{min} and R_{max} are the minimum and maximum vessel scales, respectively.

Since the size of vessels to be modeled is not known a priori, our method searches for strong edge responses at the different locations along the ray u_α with different R, $R \in [R_{min}, R_{max}]$. However, observe that for large values of R this produces strong boundary responses at locations which are outside the vessel. In general, there should not be any strong rising edge between $\boldsymbol{x_0}$ and $\boldsymbol{x_0} + R\boldsymbol{u_\alpha}$ where the boundary is searched. If there exists such a strong rising edge, it probably means that the point $\boldsymbol{x_0}$ is outside the vessel, thus it should have a lower medialness measure. This is accomplished by first computing the maximum rising boundary response up to the location $\boldsymbol{x_0} + R\boldsymbol{u_\alpha}$ along the ray and then subtracting this value from the response obtained at $\boldsymbol{x_0} + R\boldsymbol{u_\alpha}$. Based on these modifications, the final edge response along a ray, $\boldsymbol{u_\alpha}$, starting from at $\boldsymbol{x_0}$, $E(\boldsymbol{x_0} + R\boldsymbol{u_\alpha})$ is given as

$$E(\boldsymbol{x_0} + R\boldsymbol{u_\alpha}) = \frac{max(-b(\boldsymbol{x_0} + R\boldsymbol{u_\alpha}) - min_{x \in \{\boldsymbol{x_0}, \boldsymbol{x_0}+R\boldsymbol{u_\alpha}\}}(b(x), 0), 0)}{max_{x \in (\boldsymbol{x_0}+R_{min}\boldsymbol{u_\alpha}, \boldsymbol{x_0}+R_{max}\boldsymbol{u_\alpha})}(-b(x), 1)} \tag{3}$$

Observe that our medialness measure integrates edge responses along different size circles, thus, it is not sensitive to the isolated noise on a particular location. In general, this proposed technique has two major contributions: First, its response characteristics are very close to the ones that may be expected from an ideal medialness filter. Specifically, the proposed medialness measure gives strong responses at the center of a vessel and responses drop rapidly towards vessel boundaries and very small responses are obtained in non-vascular areas, Figure 1. Also, the presence of bright structures does not have strong impact on

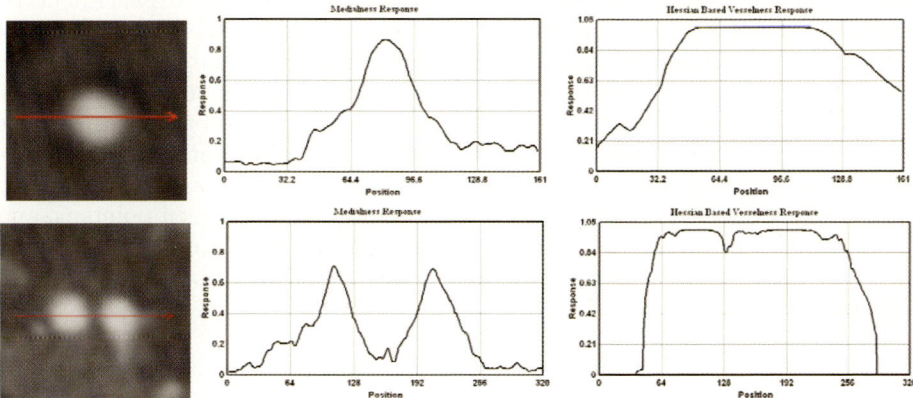

Fig. 1. This figure illustrates the medialness responses along a ray on two different examples obtained from our method (middle column) and the Hessian-based method (right column). Observe that unlike Hessian based methods, our technique gives low responses between two nearby vessels.

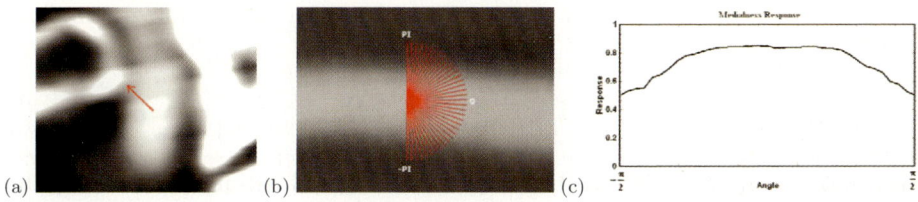

Fig. 2. (a) This figure illustrates the vessel direction obtained from the Hessian-based method. Observe that the presence of bone erroneously effects the direction of the vessel. (b) and (c) Medialness measure of a point when our medialness filters are applied on different orientations.

the responses. In fact, unlike Hessian based techniques [6,5,12,11], our approach gives low response between two nearby vessels, Figure 1. Second, our technique does not require the estimation of the vessel direction. Other techniques often uses the eigenvectors of the Hessian matrix to determine the vessel direction. However, bright structures such as bone, vessels, calcification, which are close to the vessel of interest can erroneously effect the direction of the vessel, thus medialness measure, as well, Figure 2a. Our proposed filtering technique produces higher responses when they are computed from orthogonal planes and lower responses when they are computed from oblique planes, Figure 2b, c.

3 Local Center-Axis from Graph-Based Optimization

Medialness map of an image alone cannot be used in analyzing vessels without additional post-processing. Instead, they are constructed to obtain vessel center axis representations which are very useful in visualizing vessels in curved (or ribbon - flattened) multi-planar reformatting (MPR), in quantification of pathologies, in navigation during endovascular interventional treatments, etc. Local vessel center axis between two user selected points is often sufficient for analyzing a segment of a vessel quickly in clinical applications. Thus, in this section, we propose a method for extracting such local center axis representations by integrating the medialness map in a discrete optimization framework. Specifically, we seek to obtain a curve $C(s)$ (center axis) between points p_0 and p_1 which travels through the center of a vessel. This problem can be successfully solved by the *minimum-cost* path detection algorithms [3,8,10]: Let $E(C)$ be the total energy along a curve C

$$E(C) = \int_\Omega (P(C(s)) + w) ds \qquad (4)$$

where $P(C)$ is called potential, w is the regularization term and s is the arch length, *i.e.*, $||C(s)||^2 = 1$. In vessel centerline extraction methods, potential $P(x)$ at x corresponds to the inverse of a medialness measure at that location, namely, $P(x) = \frac{1}{m(x)}$. Let A_{p_0,p_1} represents the set of all curves between p_0 and p_1. The curve with total minimum energy can be computed from the *minimum-accumulative cost*, $\phi(p)$ which measures the minimal energy at p integrated along a curve starting from the point p_0:

$$\phi(p) = \inf_{A_{p_0,p_1}} \{E(C)\} \qquad (5)$$

This type of minimization problems has been studied extensively in computer vision for different problems, *e.g.*, segmentation. They are usually solved by either Dijkstra's algorithm [4] or Fast Marching methods [9]. In this paper, we propose to use Dijkstra's algorithm for solving equation (5) in a discrete domain. Specifically, let $G = (N, E)$ be a discrete graph where N and E represent nodes and edges, respectively. The minimum-accumulative cost at the node P_{ij} for a four connected 2D graph is then given by

$$\phi(P_{ij}) = min(\phi(P_{i-1j}) + C^{ij}_{(i-1)j}, \phi(P_{i+1j}) + C^{ij}_{(i+1)j}, \phi(P_{ij-1}) + C^{ij}_{i(j-1)}, \phi(P_{ij+1}) + C^{ij}_{i(j+1)}) \qquad (6)$$

where, for example, $C^{ij}_{(i-1)j}$ corresponds to the cost of propagation from point $P_{(i-1)j}$ to P_{ij} which is obtained from the inverse of medialness measure. This above algorithm can be easily implemented by first setting minimum-accumulative cost of all nodes to infinity (or a large value) and then using an explicit discrete front propagation method where propagation always takes places from the minimum value to its neighboring nodes. In our implementation, we use 27-connected lattice in 3D, *i.e.*, diagonal propagations are also included for better accuracy. In addition, the medialness measure is computed orthogonal to the direction of propagation instead of computing at nodes. The discrete path (curve) from a point P_{ij} to source P_0 can then be easily obtained by traversing (backtracking) along the propagation.

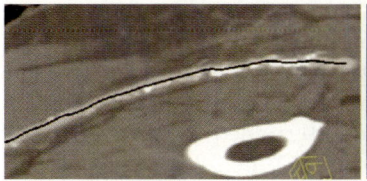 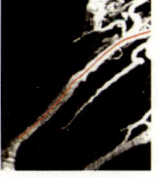 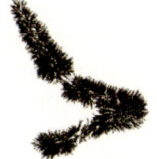 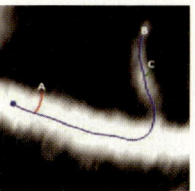

Fig. 3. This figure illustrates the local center axis models of vessels from CTA and MRA. Our algorithm works well even in the presence of nearby vessels, strong calcification and strong contrast change along a vessel.

Fig. 4. (left) The discrete front and centerlines from these front points. (right) The branch removal process. Observe that front point B is kept while front points A are C are removed.

Our major contribution of this minimum-cost path finding algorithm is the use of medialness measure as the cost of a graph edge and its *orthogonal computation* to the graph edge during propagations. In fact, this orthogonal computation is the key factor for accuracy and increased computational efficiency since the costs obtained on vessel cross-sections are small, *i.e.*, high medialness response. In other words, fronts propagates much faster in the center of vessels and much slower to towards vessel walls due to this fact. In fact, the proposed centerline extraction algorithm may also be viewed as the minimum-cost cross-sectional plane estimation algorithm since the propagation prefers directions which produce better cross-sections. Figure 3 illustrates some centerlines obtained between two seeds from this algorithm. This algorithm works well even in the presence of nearby vessels, strong calcification and strong contrast change along a vessel and it is computationally efficient. For example, a centerline segment of a coronary artery can be obtained from this algorithm in 3 seconds via two seed placements.

4 Vessel Centerline Tree Extraction

In this section, we extend the local centerline detection algorithm to recover the full vessel tree from a single point, a *source* which may be initialized by an user or another process. Recall that the above algorithm terminates when the front propagation reaches to a *sink*, an end point. When there is no sink point defined for an explicit stopping, the propagation should continue until it reaches to all the branches. The stopping criteria that we choose in our algorithm is based on the medialness measure along a discrete front. Specifically, propagation is forced to stop when the minimum medialness measure along a discrete front at any time drops below a threshold. In our experiments, we found this stopping criteria to be very reliable in clinical applications since our medialness measure is designed to be very low outside vessels. However, the total occlusion cases, where piece of a vessel is totally closed, require starting the propagation on the other side of an occlusion, manually or automatically. We first illustrate how to determine the *correct* vessel centerline tree from the converged propagation.

Suppose that the propagation has converged at time t_f with a set of graph nodes, $F = (P_1, ..., P_K)$, representing a discrete front F, Figure 4. A minimum-cost path between each point P_i of a discrete front, F and the source P_0 can be computed from the minimum accumulative cost map, ϕ, resulting in K different paths. It is obvious that most of these paths are redundant, i.e., a single vessel branch should represented by a single centerline or a single front point. In addition, the existence of a vessel branch can be determined by its length, L_B and its approximate radius, R_B along its centerline, C, i.e., $L_B >> R_B$ [1]. Let us illustrate the basic idea of selecting one centerline for each vessel branch via an example, in Figure 4b which depicts three points A, B, C on a vessel boundary and their corresponding minimum-cost paths. It is clear that the point B with its path C_B represents a branch while the front point A does not since the length of its path is similar to its radius. The front point C may be considered as representing a vessel branch since the length of its minimal path to the source P_0 is significant relative to its average radius. However, the path C_B represents the vessel branch better than the path C_C starting from C. These observations suggest that a front point with the longest path represents a vessel branch better when there are several front points on the same vessel boundary, which is the case after stopping the propagation. This can be implemented very efficiently with the following algorithm:

1. compute the minimum-cost path C_i and the length L_i for each point P_i in the discrete front set F.
2. compute the average radius, R_C along the each path C_i from the scale information contained in the medialness filters.
3. order the paths based on their length and store them in a queue, Q_C, i.e., maximum is on top.
4. continue until the queue, Q_C is empty
    (a) select the path C from the top of the queue and remove it from the queue.
    (b) recompute the path by backtracking until the source, P_0 or the previously computed path on the minimum-accumulative cost map is encountered
    (c) mark the path in the minimum-accumulative cost map during the tracking process
    (d) recompute the length of the new path, L_C
    (e) set the saliency of the path C or its corresponding front point, P as L_C/R_C
5. delete the paths whose saliency is less than a user-defined threshold,

In our experiments, the saliency threshold is set to 2.0, which means that length of a vessel branch should be two times greater than its average radius along its centerline, otherwise it does not appear to be a significant vessel branch. Figure 5 illustrates some examples of vessel centerline tree for coronary arteries and cerebral vessels and others.

5 Results and Validations

We have tested our centerline detection algorithm on coronary, carotid, aorta, peripheral, cerebral, and other vessels obtained from CTA, MRA and 3D rotational angiography data. Figure 5 illustrates some of the results which are

---
[1] The length of a centerline, C, is given by $L_C = \int_C ds$ where s is the arc length.

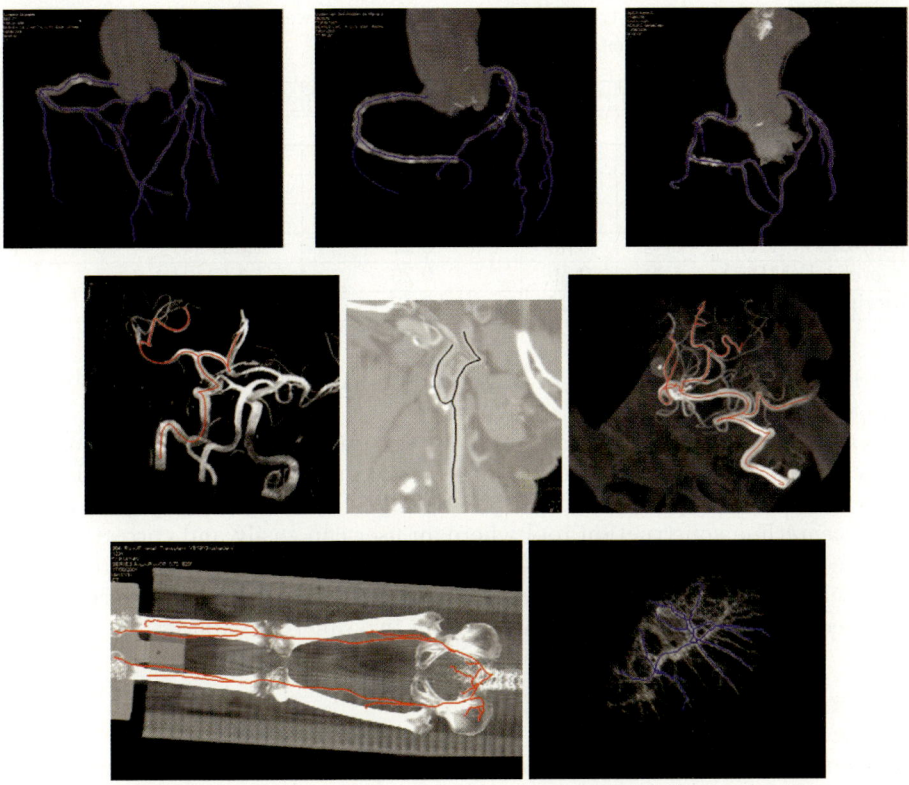

Fig. 5. This figure illustrates the results obtained from our algorithm. Top row: coronary arteries obtained from CTA. Centerlines are drawn in blue and coronary vessel masks are created by using the scales contained in centerline trees. Middle row: cerebral vessels from MRA, CTA and 3D rotational angiography Bottom row: peripheral vessels from CTA and liver vessels after liver segmentation.

obtained by initializing a single seed on a vessel. In our validation studies, coronary arteries from CTA were our main focus where the accuracy of vessel detection (structural validation) was measured and the computed centerline locations were compared with the expert created ground-truth. Specifically, there were 100 coronary artery CTA data in the experiment. The centerline tree extraction algorithm started from the ostia points, namely the beginning of coronary arteries from aorta, which were automatically determined by an aorta detection algorithm. If there were errors in the locations of such ostia points, the user were given tools to correct them. In the structural validations, an expert visualized the detected centerlines on original data and quantified the number of correctly detected arteries. The following detection ratios were obtained: left coronary artery (LCA) %100, right coronary artery (RCA) %100, left anterior descending artery (LAD) %95, left circumflex branch (LCX) %93, Left Acute Marginal %94, Obtuse Marginal, %92, where a failure is marked when a centerline went outside a certain artery or it was not able to reach to the end of a branch. It should be

Table 1. This table illustrates the error (mm) between computed and expert-constructed vessel centerlines

Vessel Type - Error (mm)	Average	Standard Deviation	Maximum	No of Data Set
Coronary: LCA (CTA)	0.33	0.14	0.74	8
Coronary: RCA (CTA)	0.30	0.12	0.55	8
Coronary: LCX (CTA)	0.28	0.15	0.59	8
Coronary: LAD (CTA)	0.31	0.16	0.67	8
Carotid (CTA)	0.45	0.21	1.08	3
Cerebral (MRA)	0.49	0.29	1.13	3
peripheral (CTA)	0.64	0.42	3.59	3

noted that it took an average of 21 seconds to construct such trees from CTA data sets on a 3.2 GHz PC.

In addition to these validations, we have also quantified the errors between expert created centerlines and the computed centerlines by measuring the distances between each corresponding centerline. Specifically, we first designed a manual vessel centerline construction tool where an user can easily and correctly create vessel centerlines. Table 1 illustrates the quantitative results on different types of vessels obtained from both CTA and MRA. Interestingly, similar errors were observed between the results obtained from two different experts.

6 Conclusions

In this paper, we presented a novel algorithm for the extraction of center axis representations for the blood vessels found in different imaging modalities such as CTA, MRA and 3D X-Ray data. The algorithm is suitable for clinical applications for diagnosis, treatment planning and follow-up studies of vascular structures.

References

1. Aylward, S., Eberly, E.: Initialization, noise, singularities, and scale in height-ridge traversal for tubular object centerline extraction. TMI 21(2), 61–75 (2002)
2. Aylward, S., Pizer, S., Bullitt, E., Eberly, D.: Intensity ridge and widths for 3d object segmentation and description. In: IEEE Proc. Workshop MMBIA, pp. 131–138 (1996)
3. Deschamps, T., Cohen, L.: Fast extraction of minimal paths in 3d images and applications to virtual endoscopy. Medical Image Analysis 5(4), 281–299 (2001)
4. Dijkstra, E.W.: A note on two problems in connections with graphs. Numerische Mathematic 1, 269–271 (1959)
5. Frangi, A.F., Niessen, W.J., Vincken, K.L., Viergever, M.A.: Multiscale vessel enhancement filtering. In: Wells, W.M., Colchester, A.C.F., Delp, S.L. (eds.) MICCAI 1998. LNCS, vol. 1496, pp. 82–89. Springer, Heidelberg (1998)
6. Koller, T.M., Gerig, G., Szekely, G., Dettwiler, D.: Multiscale detection of curvilinear structures in 2-D and 3-D image data. In: ICCV, pp. 864–869 (1995)
7. Krissian, K., Malandain, G., Ayache, N., Vaillant, R., Trousset, Y.: Model based multiscale detection of 3D vessels. In: IEEE Conf. CVPR, pp. 722–727 (1998)

8. Li, H., Yezzi, A.J.: Vessels as 4-D curves: Global minimal 4-D paths to extract 3-D tubular surfaces and centerlines. IEEE Trans. Med. Imaging 26(9), 1213–1223 (2007)
9. Sethian, J.A.: Level Set Methods. Cambridge University Press, New York (1996)
10. Siddiqi, K., Vasilevskiy, A.: 3D flux maximizing flows. In: International Workshop on Energy Minimizing Methods In Computer Vision (2001)
11. Tyrrell, J.A., di Tomaso, E., Fuja, D., Tong, R., Kozak, K., Brown, E.B., Jain, R., Roysam, B.: Robust 3-D modeling of vasculature imagery using superellipsoids. IEEE Transactions on Medical Imaging (2006)
12. Wink, O., Niessen, W.J., Viergever, M.A.: Multiscale vessel tracking. IEEE Trans. on Medical Imaging 23(1), 130–133 (2004)

Exploratory Identification of Image-Based Biomarkers for Solid Mass Pulmonary Tumors

Ifeoma Nwogu and Jason J. Corso

Department of Computer Science and Engineering, University at Buffalo, SUNY
201 Bell Hall - Buffalo, New York 14260
{inwogu,jcorso}@cse.buffalo.edu

Abstract. If imaging is to serve as a valid biomarker in the assessment of the response of cancer to therapies, a reproducible and predictive radiologic metric is required. A biomarker is an indicator of a biological property that can be used to measure the progress of disease. While current size-based, quantitative techniques provide numerical representations of tumors, they are not necessarily indicative of disease progression for advanced cancers. In this paper, we present an end-to-end process to explore the use of other image-based features especially statistical textural features for cancer change detection. We exploit the earth mover's distance metric for measuring the change in the tumor burden over a period, between the time the baseline scans were taken, and the time the therapy response scans were taken. The time-to-progression (TTP) of the disease is our known patient outcome. We analyze the correlations between TTP and our change measurements and discover that the local texture energy feature is most predictive of disease progression, more so than the tumor burden size on which current quantitative measures are made.

1 Introduction

Lung cancer is the leading cause of cancer deaths in North America and results in more deaths than breast, prostrate and colon cancer combined [1]. It is often diagnosed in late stages when surgery is no longer a viable treatment option and at this stage alternative therapies are required to manage the disease. As novel therapies become available, it is critical to rapidly assess their effectiveness for lung cancer treatment.

Imaging holds the promise of serving as an earlier, more accurate indicator of patient outcome than serologic or clinical parameters [2][3]; it can be non-invasive, is comparatively cheap, requires no extensive lab time, is nearly ubiquitous, and contains rich information describing the underlying cancer. But the large oncology groups and the Food and Drug Administration (FDA) require a reproducible radiologic metric to assess patient response to drug therapy if imaging is to serve as a biomarker [3][4]. A *biomarker* is an indicator of a specific biological property that can be used to measure the progress of disease or the effects of treatment.

The primary contribution of this study is to present an outcomes-driven process for evaluating image-based features that can potentially serve as image-based biomarkers for quantifying and qualifying the extent of different cancers in the thoracic region. We also introduce the use of a robust method to compare tumor changes over time, and lastly, we show quantitatively that for advanced cancers, size might not be the optimal measure to assess disease progression.

The remainder of this section discusses the motivation and background of the study and section 2 discusses the materials used as well as the approach taken. Section 3 provides the results of our analysis as well as some observations and issues encountered during the study. Lastly, section 4 discusses our conclusions and directions for future work.

1.1 Motivation

CT is currently a very widely used imaging modality to assess the change in patient tumor burden. The tumor burden size is typically represented by basic quantitative values such as the two dimensional World Health Organization (WHO) [5] criterion or the Response Assessment Criteria for Solid Tumors (RECIST) one dimensional criterion [6]. From a dataset of 18 patients with advanced lung cancer, based on the RECIST measurements taken by four expert clinicians, 14 of the patients were classified as having *stable disease* with little or no disease progression over a given period of time. Of the 14, eight of the patients did not survive for more than twelve months after their progression date. One patient was recorded as having *complete response*, where the tumor burden has significantly reduced in size, but the patient only survived for about 3 months after the follow-up date.

These figures (though not statistically significant) present a snapshot of the current state of lung cancer tumor burden quantification - expert human readers currently using only size-based qualitative measurements such as RECIST, often give inaccurate prognosis for advanced cancers. We therefore investigate the correlations of additional features (texture and size) with the patient-outcome, time-to-progression (TTP), discussed in more detail in section 2.

1.2 Background and Related Past Work

A large percentage of published computer-aided diagnosis (CAD) research is focused on detecting lung cancer, where the main focus is the detection of lung nodules. Some successful nodule detection methods are given in [7], although this citation list is by no means exhaustive. In recent years, the FDA has approved several commercial CAD systems for nodule detection in the clinic and this research area appears stable today.

Typically, lung nodules are defined as pulmonary disorders less than 20mm in diameter, and are always located in the lungs away from the hilar or root of the lungs, whereas solid mass lung tumors are about 200mm or larger and can be located anywhere in the thoracic region. They can be buried in pleural effusion (fluid in the lungs), they can be located amidst blood vessels or as enlarged lymph

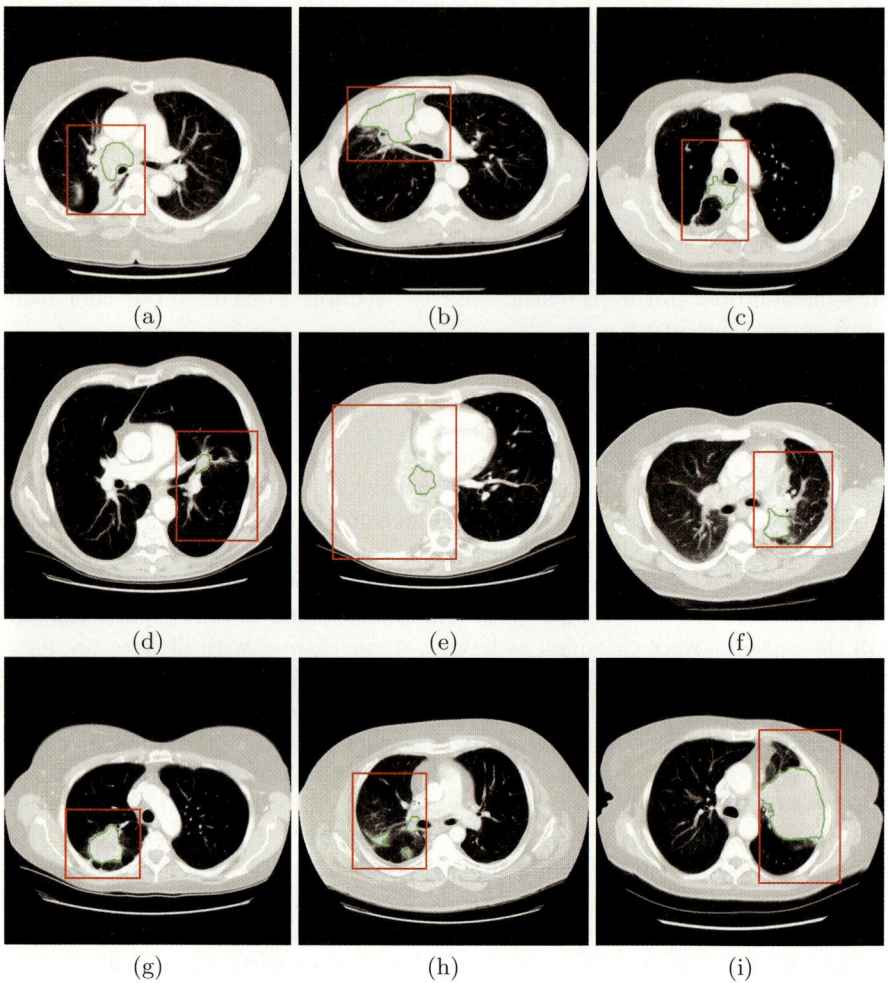

Fig. 1. CT slice images showing the ROI and contours of solid mass tumors in the thoracic region, highlighting the diversity in the tumor structures and locations

nodes, or in the mediastinum, etc. as shown in Figure 1. The most important characteristics for qualifying nodules appear to be size and growth rate, whereas there are no similar clear qualifiers for solid mass tumors. Also, lung nodules are structurally distinct in the thoracic region but solid mass tumors are very structurally diverse again as seen in Figure 1.

Hence, although CAD for early detection of lung cancer via lung nodules has been studied extensively, research in developing CAD techniques for solid mass chest tumors is still in its very early stages[7]. We are investigating the use of size and texture-based measurement techniques for quantifying lung cancer change detection.

2 Materials and Methods

Our data set consists of two series of CT scans from eighteen patients with advanced lung cancer. One series of scans is the baseline taken before a particular therapy is administered to the patient, and the other series, the therapy response scans, are recorded after the patients is taken off the therapy. The response dates are recorded for each patient that survived beyond the duration of the treatment and this time period is recorded as the time-to-progression (in general, TTP is recorded when the disease is shown to change significantly). Also, the extent of survival for the patients is recorded. Hence, the known patient outcomes for this study are TTP and survival. Four expert radiologists also predicted the patient responses based on RECIST measurements. We restrict our analysis, in this study, to the primary tumor in each CT scan series.

Images are acquired using the 3-D CT scanner, GE Medical System LightSpeed QX/i helical, yielding 16-bit slices of 512 x 512 pixel arrays. The image values are recorded as Hounsfield Unit(HU) values, representing the densities of different human tissues. Because the tumors being investigated are very different in many of the cases (as shown in Figure 1), both manual and automatic processes are required to isolate the tumor regions-of-interest (ROI) and demarcate the tumor contours. The localization and demarcation results are then verified by our collaborating radiologists, to ensure the tumor regions and contours agreed with their findings. Computer-assisted localization and demarcation of solid mass lung tumor regions and contours is still an open area of research, essential for developing image-based biomarkers. We hypothesize that tracking density and vasculature changes in a tumor through its exhibited texture patterns, as well as tracking changes in the tumor burden size will provide deeper insight into detecting meaningful changes in the advanced cancer over time.

2.1 Preprocessing

Since the tissue densities we are currently interested in only extend over a fairly narrow range (or window), we shift the pixel values based on a window-level setting into the interval [0, 255]. This shift is necessary not only for improved visualization, but to better perform the texture analysis. The mean density level of the window is set in such a way as to highlight tissue in the lungs as well as in the mediastinum and the width of the window affects the contrast of the resulting images. All CT slice images displayed in this paper result from the same window-level adjustments.

2.2 Feature Extraction

In most of the cases we evaluated, the tumor burden only occupied a small portion of the ROI. We therefore use a local texture analysis process based the construction of local gray-level co-occurrence matrices (GLCM). As mentioned in section 2.1, the CT slice image is down-scaled since the processing required to calculate a GLCM for the full dynamic range of a CT slice image is prohibitive.

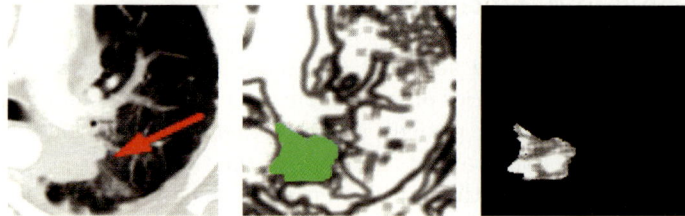

Fig. 2. Left: an example of an ROI indicating the tumor burden in 2D; center: the textured image (local energy) with the tumor mask applied; right: the input to the tumor signature

The statistical measurements we use are homogeneity, correlation, contrast and energy as defined by Haralicks's texture approaches [8], and implemented using the MATLAB Image Processing Toolbox.

Each ROI image is divided into overlapping 7x7 windows, the statistical texture values are computed on each window in four different directions and then averaged for rotational invariance. A mask of the specific tumor burden is then applied to the texture images resulting in texture representations of the tumor burden only. The tumor from each series therefore forms the input to the specific tumor *signature*. A signature is any variable length representation of a signal and is explained in more detail in section 2.3. Figure 2 shows how the texture image of a tumor is obtained. The size features are obtained as pixel count of the tumors within the demarcation contours. The tumor annotations were provided/validated by the expert clinicians, and they currently represent our best estimates of the tumor burden.

2.3 Change Measurement Computation

The *Earth Mover's Distance* is a metric function that measures the distance between two distributions [9]. EMD computes the minimal cost that must be paid in order to transform one distribution to the other. The EMD method is more robust than histogram matching techniques such as histogram intersection, the Kullback-Leibler divergence, Niblack quadratic-form distance and Kolmogorov-Smirnov distance, as shown by Rubner et al. in [9]. EMD operates on variable length representations (or signatures) and naturally allows for partial matching.

Our representative signature $\{s_j = (\mathbf{m}_j, w_{\mathbf{m}_j})\}$ is a set of feature clusters where each cluster is represented by its mean $\mathbf{m}_j$ and by $w_{\mathbf{m}_j}$, the fractional weight of that cluster. Our specific signature is made of histograms whose clusters are pre-determined by the binning size and whose weights are fractional values of the normalized histogram.

Given two signatures $P = (\mathbf{p}_1, w_{\mathbf{p}_1}), \ldots (\mathbf{p}_m, w_{\mathbf{p}_m})$ with m clusters and $Q = (\mathbf{q}_1, w_{\mathbf{q}_1}), \ldots (\mathbf{q}_m, w_{\mathbf{q}_m})$ with n clusters; and $\mathbf{D} = [d_{ij}]$ where d_{ij} the Euclidean distance between $\mathbf{p}_i$ and $\mathbf{q}_j$. We want to find a flow $\mathbf{F} = [f_{ij}]$ so that the cost equation 2 can be minimized subject to a given set of constraints given in detail in [9].

$$\text{WORK}(P, Q, \boldsymbol{F}) = \sum_{i=1}^{m}\sum_{j=1}^{n} d_{ij} f_{ij} \quad (1)$$

so that

$$\text{EMD}(P, Q) = \frac{\sum_{i=1}^{m}\sum_{j=1}^{n} d_{ij} f_{ij}}{\sum_{i=1}^{m}\sum_{j=1}^{n} f_{ij}} \quad (2)$$

Equation 2 defines the earth movers distance as the resulting work normalized by the total flow computed.

At the end of this process, we have eight signatures for each patient, four from the baseline scan and four from the therapy response scan. The four signatures represent the four local texture features. The EMD is then computed for each pair of texture feature signatures (one from baseline, one from therapy response) to obtain the measures of local texture change. To compute size changes, we take the absolute difference between the tumor burden size at baseline and at therapy response and divide by the value at baseline, yielding a fractional size change value.

3 Experimental Results

In this section we provide some numerical indicators and qualitative analysis to demonstrate the usefulness of the features investigated as potential candidates for image-based biomarker feature measures. We display five scatter plots in

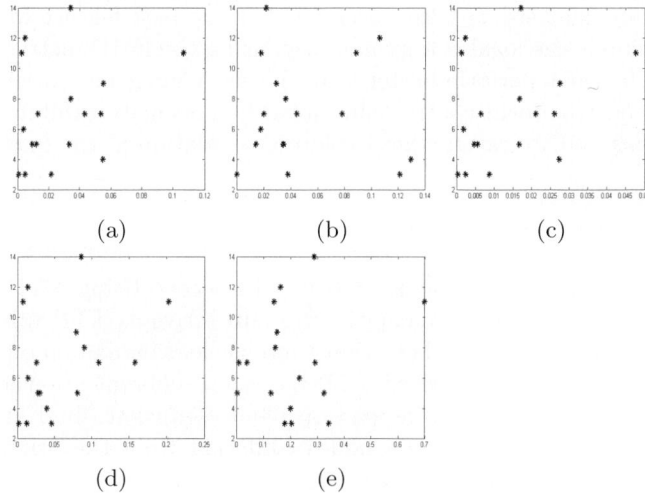

Fig. 3. (a)-(d) show the scatter plots of TTP (y-axis) versus the earth mover's distance between the texture features of a tumor taken at two different periods - local contrast, local texture correlations, local texture homogeneity and local energy (x-axis). (e) shows the scatter plot of TTP versus the fractional change in 2D tumor size.

Table 1. The first four rows display the correlation coefficients for TTP values and the feature distance measures between the two readings obtained at two different time periods for each tumor. The last row shows the correlation coefficient for TTP and the fractional change in the tumor size, for readings obtained at two different time periods.

Feature change measure	Low	Medium	High
EMD for local contrast	-	0.3037	-
EMD for local correlations	0.0817	-	-
EMD for local homogeneity	0.2968	-	-
EMD for local energy	-	0.3356	-
Fractional change in size	0.1614	-	-

Figure 3 to show the trend of the relationships between the measurements of feature changes (between baseline and therapy response times) and the patient outcomes, TTP. We also compute the correlation coefficients between the patient outcomes, TTP, and the feature changes to discover the degree of the linear relationship between them, and the resulting values are provided in Table 1.

3.1 Observations

From reviewing the qualitative results in Figure 3, there is clearly a positive trend between the changes in the texture measurements and disease progression, although the correlations are not very strong. As expected, our analysis show that size, the current measurement standard, might not be a very good indicator of disease progression when the cancer is in its advanced stages.

Based on our analysis, we also observed that the best feature for measuring change detection is the local energy measure, using the EMD metric, and all the other texture features perform better than the size change measurement. Lastly, we observed that the local contrast and local homogeneity exhibit very similar change patterns and we can further explore this relation in the future.

3.2 Issues with the Process

Can TTP be reliably measured for advanced cancer? Using TTP as the primary patient outcomes measurement is very subjective as TTP values are only recorded when the clinicians believe that there is clear indication of disease progression. Different clinicians record TTP based on different criteria such as an increase in sum of tumor sizes, increase in pleural effusion (fluid in the lungs), enlargement of surrounding lymph nodes (different from the primary tumor), increase in the number of lesions present. In addition, TTP requires very careful follow-up.

Registration and delineation of the tumor are done on 2D slices limiting the spatial relationship measures between the pixels in a tumor, hence the texture and size feature measurements are not as accurate as they would be in a 3D model.

In order to develop fully reproducible and repeatable biomarkers, there is a need for a semi- (or fully-)automated solid mass tumor detection procedure, but this is not the subject of this stage of the study.

4 Discussion

We presented an end-to-end outcomes-driven process for evaluating image-based features that can potentially serve as CT image-based biomarkers. We also highlighted some of the challenges involved in CAD for solid mass tumors in the thoracic region, a problem that needs to be sufficiently addressed in the development computer-generated image-based biomarkers for cancer change detection. Lastly, we provided some numerical indicators and qualitative analysis to demonstrate the usefulness of features investigated as potential candidates for image-based biomarker feature measures.

We intend to address the issues highlighted in section 3.2 and in addition, perform an even more thorough study to evaluate the role of the local windowing function for the GLCM texture analysis as well the use of other distance metrics including EMD with other methods of clustering.

Acknowledgements. The authors gratefully acknowledge the support provided by Drs. Ronald Gottlieb and Alan Litwin from the Radiology department at Roswell Park Cancer Institute; Janhavi Athale for her assistance in labeling the CT images. Ifeoma Nwogu was funded by the NSF award DGE-0333417.

References

1. Jemal, A., Tiwari, R.C., Murray, T., Ghafoor, A., Samuels, A., Ward, E., Feuer, E.J., Thun, M.J.: Cancer statistics, 2004. Cancer J. Clin. 54(8), 8–29 (2004)
2. Smith, J.J., Sorensen, A.G., Thrall, J.H.: Biomarkers in imaging: Realizing radiology's future. Radiology 227, 633–638 (2003)
3. El-Deiry, W., Sigman, C., Kelloff, G.: Imaging and oncologic drug development. J. Clin. Oncol. 24(20), 3261–3273 (2006)
4. Johnson, J.R., Williams, G., Richard, P.: End points and United States Food and Drug Administration approval of oncology drugs. J. Clin. Oncol. 21, 1404–1411 (2003)
5. World Health Organization: WHO Handbook for reporting results of cancer treatment (1979)
6. Therasse, P., Arbuck, S.G., Eisenhauer, E.A., Wanders, J., Kaplan, R.S., Rubinstein, L., Verweij, J., Van Glabbeke, M., van Oosterom, A.T., Christian, M.C.: New guidelines to evaluate the response to treatment in solid tumors. J. Natl. Cancer Inst. 92, 205–216 (2000)
7. Sluimer, I., Schilham, A., Prokop, M., van Ginneken, B.: Computer analysis of computed tomography scans of the lung: A survey. IEEE Trans. Med. Img. 25(4), 385–405 (2006)
8. Haralick, R.M.: Statistical and Structural Approaches to Texture. IEEE 67(5), 786–804 (1979)
9. Rubner, Y., Tomasi, C., Guibas, L.J.: The earth mover's distance as a metric for image retrieval. Int. J. Comp. Vis. 40(2), 99–121 (2000)

Measuring Brain Lesion Progression with a Supervised Tissue Classification System

Evangelia I. Zacharaki, Stathis Kanterakis, R. Nick Bryan, and Christos Davatzikos

Department of Radiology, University of Pennsylvania, Philadelphia, PA 19104, USA
{Eva.Zacharaki,Efstathios.Kanterakis,R.Nick.Bryan,
Christos.Davatzikos}@uphs.upenn.edu

Abstract. Brain lesions, especially White Matter Lesions (WMLs), are associated with cardiac and vascular disease, but also with normal aging. Quantitative analysis of WML in large clinical trials is becoming more and more important. In this paper, we present a computer-assisted WML segmentation method, based on local features extracted from conventional multi-parametric Magnetic Resonance Imaging (MRI) sequences. A framework for preprocessing the temporal data by jointly equalizing histograms reduces the spatial and temporal variance of data, thereby improving the longitudinal stability of such measurements and hence the estimate of lesion progression. A Support Vector Machine (SVM) classifier trained on expert-defined WML's is applied for lesion segmentation on each scan using the AdaBoost algorithm. Validation on a population of 23 patients from 3 different imaging sites with follow-up studies and WMLs of varying sizes, shapes and locations tests the robustness and accuracy of the proposed segmentation method, compared to the manual segmentation results from an experienced neuroradiologist. The results show that our CAD-system achieves consistent lesion segmentation in the 4D data facilitating the disease monitoring.

Keywords: white matter lesions, classification, segmentation, MRI, SVM, CAD, lesion progression.

1 Introduction

Population studies have shown that brain lesions, especially WMLs, are associated with several diseases, such as arterial fibrillation, arterioscleroses, impaired cognition and others [1,2]. The increased interest in brain lesion research may improve diagnosis and prognosis possibilities for patients with cardiovascular symptoms. Since brain lesion patterns are very heterogeneous, ranging from punctuate lesions in the deep white matter to large confluent periventricular lesions, the scoring of such lesions is complicated. For longitudinal studies aiming to capture relatively small changes in brain lesion patterns, accurate information of lesion volume and location is essential. It is known that expert-based delineation of brain lesions is difficult to reproduce across raters, or even within the same rater, and that combination of readings from independent reader may be necessary in a longitudinal study.

The use of an automated segmentation method that detects brain lesions with a high sensitivity and specificity could be advantageous. Most of the methods in the literature have been developed for the detection of Multiple Sclerosis (MS) lesions by combining multi-parametric MR images, i.e. images obtained via different MR protocols. The advantage of integrating information from multiple sequences is that it can reduce the uncertainty and increase the accuracy of the segmentation. They usually apply supervised voxel-wise classification in which the desired segmentation is known (expert manual delineation) and used as a training set to build the segmentation model [3,4,5,6]. However, relatively less attention has been given to brain lesion segmentation in elderly individuals, and AD or diabetic patients. Since MS lesions present different characteristics from lesions in elderly and/or diabetic individuals, those methods are not directly applicable to our studies, albeit they have formed the foundation for our development. Because of the decreased contrast between white matter (WM) and gray matter (GM) in MRI in elderly, techniques that require the segmentation of WM and GM for the extraction of the WMLs perform moderately well when applied to geriatric patients, especially when they were originally designed and trained to extract lesions in MS patients. Mohamed et al. [7] presented a method for differentiating WMLs using a supervised classification method with relatively good sensitivity but somewhat limited specificity to lesions.

Moreover, only a few methods have combined space and time into the lesion characterization process [8,9]. These approaches focused primarily on quantifying the temporal variations of MS lesions, important in differentiating active from chronic lesions. In contrast to the complicated MRI dynamics of lesions in MS, the monitoring of WMLs does not require spatiotemporal modeling, since the effects in WMLs are irreversible.

In this paper, we present a computer-assisted WML segmentation approach that has been designed to process longitudinal MR scans of elderly diabetes patients [10]. Our method uses a combination of image analysis and pattern classification using SVM. Image intensities from multiple MR acquisition protocols, after co-registration, are used to form a voxel-wise feature vector that helps to discriminate lesion from various normal tissue image profiles during segmentation. In general, there are three steps in our approach. First, we jointly preprocess baseline and follow-up data. The preprocessing step includes co-registration of different MR modalities of the same patient, skull-stripping, intensity normalization, as well as inhomogeneity correction. Second, a set of training samples is manually delineated by an expert reader on the baseline images, and then used to build a classification model via SVM [11] and the AdaBoost algorithm [12]; this step is applied only once, during training. Third, the SVM model is used to perform the voxel-wise segmentation of the longitudinal data. The methodology is validated against the expert human readings. In the current study we present results obtained using training samples defined by a single expert. However, we have also performed experiments using samples defined by two different experts, which have shown that the lesion load detected by the proposed method showed high correlation across experts.

2 Methods

MRI's used herein were obtained from individuals with diabetes, with an inter-scan period of approximately 3 years. All 42 participants' exams consisted of transaxial T1-w, T2-w, PD and FLAIR scans with 23 of the participants having currently a follow-up study. All scans except T1-w were performed with a 3 mm slice thickness, no slice gap, a 240 × 240 mm FOV and a 256 × 256 scan matrix. T1-w scans were performed with a 1.5mm slice thickness, same slice gap, FOV and scan matrix. The data are preprocessed and features are extracted in order to train an SVM classifier, as explained next.

2.1 Data Preprocessing and Feature Extraction

Preprocessing: The multiple images acquired from the same individual are co-registered, in order to compensate for possible motion between scans. Using as similarity metric the correlation ratio and normalized mutual information, affine registration [13] implemented in FSL [14] is employed for co-registration of multi-modality images. The FLAIR image of each subject is used as reference space, to which all other sequences are transformed. Then each sequence of the follow-up data is co-registered with the corresponding aligned baseline sequence. The intra-modal registration can generally achieve better accuracy. After co-registration, a deformable model based skull-stripping algorithm called BET [15], implemented in FSL [14], is used to generate an initial brain tissue mask from the co-registered T1-w image, and then this brain tissue mask is used to extract the brain region from all other modality images. Finally, for each image volume, inhomogeneities are corrected by N3 [16].

A fundamentally important step in our segmentation algorithm, as well as in most supervised classification methods, is the standardization of the image histograms. To this end, a linear transformation (translation and scaling) is calculated, that minimizes the L_2-norm of the histogram difference between transformed image and template image, and reverse. The histograms are first smoothed and the bin representing the background is excluded from the least-squares error minimization. In order to achieve high temporal stability in the histogram normalization, we constrain the baseline and the follow-up histograms to be normalized to the template used in the study in exactly the same way. Follow-up histograms are normalized to their respective - standardized to the template - baselines, a problem that is relatively easy to solve, since baseline and follow-up images belong to the same individual. Thus, histograms between images of the same subject get aligned consistently, and the temporal variance is reduced. We will refer to this approach of histogram equalization using (intra-subject) 4D data as *TVR* (temporal variance reduction), as opposed to the standard 3D approach aligning baseline and follow-up images independently to the template histogram. This second approach aims at reducing the inter-subject variance, and will be refer to as *IVR*. Since the inter-subject variability (between subject and template) is much larger than the intra-subject temporal variability, a global histogram matching based on *IVR* fails, and tends to produce inconsistent 4D WML segmentation. We will show the proposed *TVR* approach is more appropriate for measuring temporal WML change.

Feature extraction: In general, the amount of intensity overlap between WMLs and normal tissue varies greatly across different modalities. In T1-w images, WMLs have intensities similar to GM, and in T2-w and PD images, WMLs look very similar to CSF. Although the FLAIR image has the least intensity overlap between WMLs and normal tissues, it has been suggested in the literature that FLAIR is less sensitive in the posterior fossa [17], may lead to "overestimation" of lesion load, and has a higher inter-vendor variability [18]. Furthermore, FLAIR may present hyperintensity artifacts [19] that might lead to false positives, thereby rendering it difficult to use only the FLAIR images to segment WMLs. Therefore, it is important to integrate information from different modalities, in order to minimize the ambiguity in identifying WMLs from using only a single modality image. A feature vector is computed for each non-background voxel in a 3D reference space for each subject. In order to make the features robust to noise, each sequence is smoothed by a Gaussian filter with a very small kernel (0.5mm).

2.2 Lesion Segmentation (Training and Testing)

SVM has been shown to be a powerful technique for learning from data and in particular, for solving binary classification problems [11]. In a binary classification task like the one in our study (normal tissue/lesion tissue), the aim is to find an optimal separating hyperplane between the two data sets. In our application we use linear SVM.

Training SVM via AdaBoost: A nonlinear pattern classifier is constructed from the entire training set, i.e. by using all lesion voxels of all training scans as examples of imaging profiles to be recognized in new scans, along with a large number of normal tissue voxels. Because the number of normal tissue voxels is far higher than the number of lesion voxels, it is essential to select only a representative set of normal tissue voxels comparable to the number of lesion voxels. This selection is not random, but it is rather guided by the classification results themselves, using the AdaBoost algorithm [12]. This approach is based on a sequence of classifiers that rely increasingly on misclassified voxels, since those are presumably the voxels on which the classifier must focus. During this adaptive boosting procedure, each sample receives a weight that determines its probability of being selected in a training set for the next iteration. If a training sample is accurately classified, then its likelihood of being used again in subsequent iterations is reduced; conversely, if a training sample is inaccurately classified, then its likelihood of being used again is increased.

Segmentation (testing): In the testing stage, T1-w, T2-w and PD images of a new (not in the training set) subject are firstly preprocessed (co-registered etc.) by the procedure described before, and then the pseudo-likelihood of each voxel being WML is measured by the generated SVM classifier. The output of SVM is a scalar measure of abnormality (as shown in Fig.1), which is further binarized by an optimal threshold to produce the WML segmentation.

Subsequently, two post-processing steps are applied in order to remove remaining false positives. Extra-axial hyperintense regions, like fat in the orbits, can not always be completely removed by the skull-stripping algorithm used in preprocessing stage.

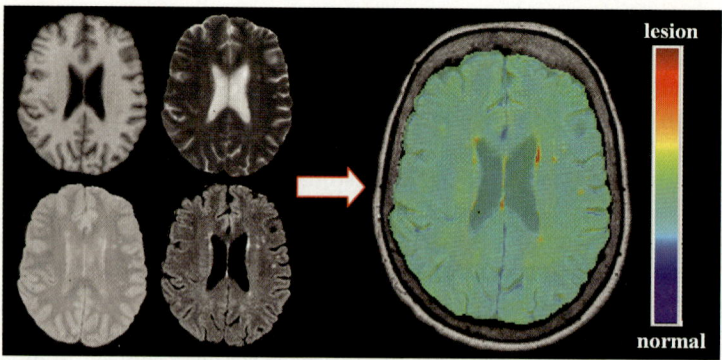

Fig. 1. Integration of multi-parametric MRI for creation of voxel-wise abnormality maps based on SVM classifier. From left to right and top to bottom T1-w, T2-w, PD, FLAIR image and generated abnormality map (shown in color scale). The color scale is only relative, i.e. appropriate (non-linear) scaling is required, such as fitting a sigmoid function using Platt's method [20], to represent actual (pseudo)probabilities.

Imaging profiles belonging to these regions are more similar to WMLs than that of normal tissue and therefore they are eliminated from the segmentation mask after SVM classification. This is done by morphological operations combined by adaptive thresholding in skull-stripped FLAIR image. Finally, remaining false positives are further reduced by applying spatial constraints using an unsupervised clustering technique. Specifically, the automated segmentation tool FAST [21] was applied to segment the FLAIR image into 6 classes. The 6th class includes hyperintense regions in FLAIR, such as bright GM regions and lesions, and was used as a mask to constraint the segmentation.

It should be noted that all steps in the WML segmentation procedure are automated and the same parameters are used for all subjects. Only one parameter has been shown to be important and vary across subjects, which is the threshold for binarizing the abnormality map generated by the SVM classifier. This threshold is optimized for each subject in the training set by maximizing the *Jaccard score* (*Jac*) [12]. The average threshold maximizing the *Jaccard score* is then used as the default value for segmenting new data. The *Jaccard score* is defined as $Jac = TP / (TP + FP + FN)$, where *TP*, *FP* and *FN* stand for true positive, false positive, and false negative, respectively.

3 Results

The dataset consisted of 23 subjects having baseline and follow-up data and 19 subjects having only baseline data. We used one subset to train a linear SVM classifier for lesion segmentation, a second subset to optimize the threshold (based on the *Jaccard score*) for generating a binary lesion mask from the abnormality map and the remaining subjects ($N=16$) to assess the 4D the segmentation method. In the future we plan to perform leave-one-out cross validation for training and testing in order to exploit more effectively the dataset.

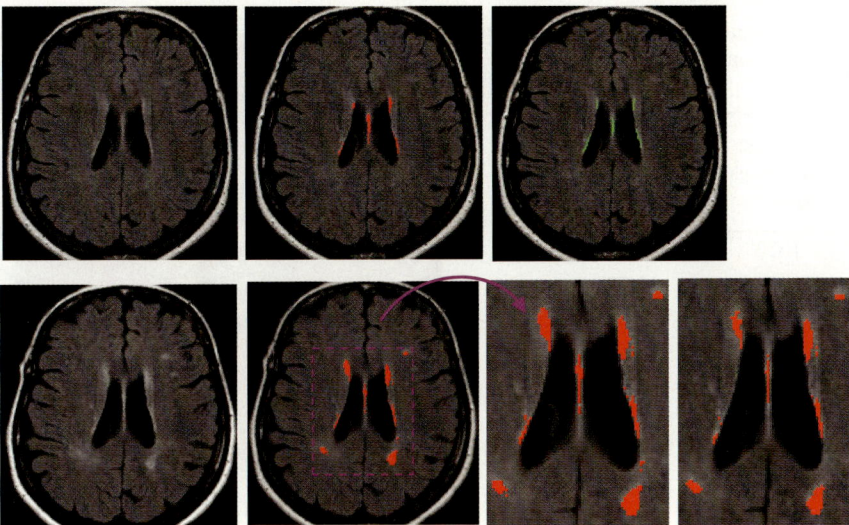

Fig. 2. Evaluation of 4D WML segmentation. The 1st row shows the baseline and the 2nd row the follow-up images. The automatic WML segmentation (red) in baseline is very similar to the expert-defined WML (green). The zoomed figures in 2nd row show the result of two histogram equalization approaches: the proposed *TVR* (left) versus the standard *IVR* (right).

Fig. 2 shows the progression of white matter lesions in an elderly subject. The first row illustrates the baseline image and the corresponding lesion segmentation (red for our method and green for the expert-defined WML). It can be noticed the 3D WML segmentation has high sensitivity and specificity. The second row shows the follow-up image and the segmentation produced by our method by either aligning the histogram of the follow-up image to the intensity-normalized baseline image (proposed approach, shown on the left) or, as usually performed, by aligning the histogram of the follow-up image independently to the template image (usual approach, shown on the right). The proposed approach has higher sensitivity in WML segmentation.

Since expert-defined ground truth is not available for the follow-up studies, the segmentation in the follow-up cannot be directly assessed. However, we calculate the lesion volume in baseline and follow-up studies and assess the rate of change by the gradient of the time function. Since only disease progression (increasing lesion load) is expected, the temporal consistency of the multi-parametric segmentation scheme can be easily evaluated. The lesion load for baseline and follow-up data is shown in Table 1. The results show that the proposed *TVR* approach for jointly normalizing the histograms of baseline and follow-up images, gives increasing lesion volume for all subjects. On the contrary, the alignment of histograms of each baseline and follow-up images independently to the template applying a global transformation, does not optimally estimate the MRI dynamics for each subject and therefore false reduction in lesion load is observed. An example is shown in Fig. 3 (bottom right) where the follow-up images are processed independently of the baseline using the *IVR* approach. It can be seen that one of the lesions has not been detected in the follow-up study.

Table 1. Evaluation of WML progression in 16 participants

Volume in baseline (mm³)	Volume increase in follow-up (%)	
	TVR	IVR
1622	91.22	38.05
1371	11.73	-4.81
654	375.00	340.32
2716	63.69	55.15
427	142.59	116.05
1113	7.58	-11.14
3533	15.52	27.16
2078	170.43	132.74
272	20.39	-18.45
3987	42.79	27.84
1192	90.27	27.21
1553	144.99	53.65
1830	42.80	18.88
1972	78.74	28.61
308	44.44	-56.41
198	8.00	5.33

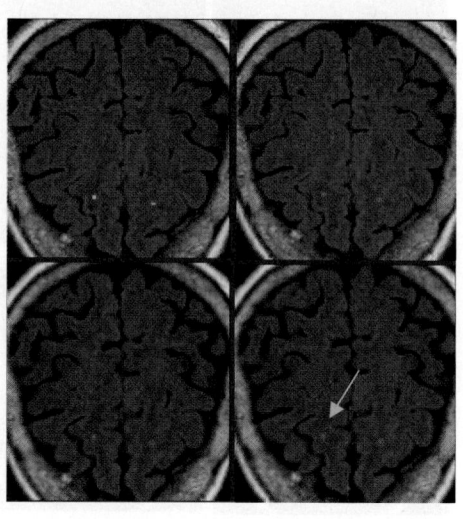

Fig. 3. Example illustrating misleading disease regression when using the *IVR* approach. 1st row: expert-defined WML (green) and WML segmentation in baseline. 2nd row: WML segmentation in follow-up with *TVR* approach (left) and *IVR* approach (right). The *TVR* approach is more consistent, whereas the *IVR* approach misses a lesion in the follow-up that was there in the baseline.

4 Discussion and Conclusions

The objective, quantitative, and reproducible evaluation of WMLs has been a challenge in many neuroimaging studies. Although qualitative readings have been employed by many studies, the relatively limited sensitivity and inter-rater agreement is an obstacle, particularly in longitudinal studies or in studies seeking to detect subtle effects. This paper presents a CAD-system for monitoring the progression of WMLs that is based on the integration of different MR acquisition protocols and training of a nonlinear pattern classification algorithm. Our experiments show that the proposed system segments WML accurately even when the load is small. More important, by jointly normalizing the histogram of baseline and follow-up images, lesion load increase was consistently observed for all subjects.

We are currently in the process of applying this method to data from different centers in multi-site studies seeking to quantify vascular disease.

Acknowledgments. The authors would like to thank the committee of ACCORD-MIND project, which is funded by the NIA through an intra-agency agreement with NIHLBI [Y3-HC-3065], for providing the datasets, valuable comments and giving us permissions to publish this paper. This work was also supported, in part, by R01-14973.

References

1. de Groot, J.C., et al.: Cerebral white matter lesions and cognitive function: the Rotterdam Scan Study. Annals of Neurology 47(2), 145–151 (2000)
2. Longstreth Jr., W.T., et al.: Clinical correlates of white matter findings on cranial magnetic resonance imaging of 3301 elderly people. The Cardiovascular Health Study, Stroke 27(8), 1274–1282 (1996)
3. Zijdenbos, A.P., Forghani, R., Evans, A.C.: Automatic "pipeline" analysis of 3-D MRI data for clinical trials: application to multiple sclerosis. IEEE Trans. on Medical Imaging 21(10), 1280–1291 (2002)
4. Wei, X., et al.: Quantitative Analysis of MRI Signal Abnormalities of Brain White Matter With High Reproducibility and Accuracy. Journal of Magnetic Resonance Imaging 15(2), 203–209 (2002)
5. Anbeek, P., et al.: Probabilistic segmentation of white matter lesions in MR imaging. NeuroImage 21(3), 1037–1044 (2004)
6. Admiraal-Behloul, F., et al.: Fully automatic segmentation of white matter hyperintensities in MR images of the elderly. NeuroImage 28(3), 607–617 (2005)
7. Mohamed, F.B., et al.: Increased differentiation of intracranial white matter lesions by multispectral 3D-tissue segmentation: preliminary results. Magnetic Resonance Imaging 19(2), 207–218 (2001)
8. Gerig, G., et al.: Exploring the discrimination power of the time domain for segmentation and characterization of lesions in serial MR data. In: Taylor, C., Colchester, A. (eds.) MICCAI 1999. LNCS, vol. 1679. Springer, Heidelberg (1999)
9. Meier, D.S., Guttmann, C.R.G.: MRI time series modeling of MS lesion development. NeuroImage 32(2), 531–537 (2006)
10. Williamson, J., et al.: The Action to Control Cardiovascular Risk in Diabetes Memory in Diabetes Study (ACCORD-MIND): Rationale, Design, and Methods. American Journal of Cardiology (2007)
11. Vapnik, V.N.: Statistical Learning Theory, p. 736. Wiley, New York (1998)
12. Tan, P.-N., Steinbach, M., Kumar, V.: Introduction to Data Mining (2005)
13. Jenkinson, M., Smith, S.M.: A global optimisation method for robust affine registration of brain images. Medical Image Analysis 5(2), 143–156 (2001)
14. Smith, S.M., et al.: Advances in functional and structural MR image analysis and implementation as FSL. NeuroImage 23(S1), 208–219 (2004)
15. Smith, S.M.: BET: Brain Extraction Tool. FMRIB technical report TR00SMS26
16. Sled, J., Zijdenbos, A., Evans, A.: A nonparametric method for automatic correction of intensity nonuniformity in MRI data. IEEE Trans. on Medical Imaging 17(1), 87–97 (1998)
17. Gawne-Cain, M.L., et al.: MRI lesion volume measurement in multiple sclerosis and its correlation with disability: a comparison of fast fluid attenuated inversion recovery (fFLAIR) and spin echo sequences. J. Neurol. Neurosurg. Psychiatry 64, 197–203 (1998)
18. Rovaris, M., et al.: Relevance of Hypointense Lesions on Fast Fluid-Attenuated Inversion Recovery MR Images as a Marker of Disease Severity in Cases of Multiple Sclerosis. Am. J. Neuroradiology 20(5), 813–820 (1999)
19. Bakshi, R., et al.: Intraventricular CSF Pulsation Artifact on Fast Fluid-Attenuated Inversion-Recovery MR Images: Analysis of 100 Consecutive Normal Studies. Am. J. Neuroradiology 21(3), 503–508 (2000)
20. Platt, J.: Probabilistic outputs for support vector machines and comparison to regularized likelihood methods. In: Schuurmans, D. (ed.) Advances in Large Margin Classifiers. MIT Press, Cambridge (2000)
21. Zhang, Y., Brady, M., Smith, S.: Segmentation of brain MR images through a hidden Markov random field model and the expectation maximization algorithm. IEEE Trans. on Medical Imaging 20(1), 45–57 (2001)

Regularized Discriminative Direction for Shape Difference Analysis

Luping Zhou[1], Richard Hartley[1,2], Lei Wang[1], Paulette Lieby[2], and Nick Barnes[2]

[1] RSISE, The Australian National University
[2] Embedded Systems Theme, NICTA*

Abstract. The "discriminative direction" has been proven useful to reveal the subtle difference between two anatomical shape classes. When a shape moves along this direction, its deformation will best manifest the class difference detected by a kernel classifier. However, we observe that such a direction cannot maintain a shape's "anatomical" correctness, introducing spurious difference. To overcome this drawback, we develop a *regularized* discriminative direction by requiring a shape to conform to its population distribution when it deforms along the discriminative direction. Instead of iterative optimization, an analytic solution is provided to directly work out this direction. Experimental study shows its superior performance in detecting and localizing the difference of hippocampal shapes for sex. The result is supported by other independent research in the same domain.

1 Introduction

It is critical to identify and understand the difference between two anatomical shape classes, such as normal/abnormal or male/female hippocampi. To differentiate linearly non-separable classes, kernel classifiers, such as SVMs, have been widely used. The class difference is identified in a high dimensional feature space $\mathcal{F}$ induced by a kernel function. While such difference is *mathematically* meaningful, it needs to be projected back to the shape descriptor space $\mathbb{R}^d$ to be explained in an *anatomically* meaningful way. For this purpose, Golland et al. proposed a "discriminative direction" method to isolate and visualize the subtle class difference in the shape descriptor space ([1,2]). As in Figure 1, when a shape deforms along the discriminative direction towards the opposite class, the movement of its image in $\mathcal{F}$ will follow the direction **w** which best discriminates the two classes in $\mathcal{F}$. Hence the deformation can localize the class difference by ignoring the within-class variability. This method has been used to analyze the hippocampal shape difference between normal controls and patients [2]. In our

---

* National ICT Australia is funded by the Australian Government's Backing Australia's Ability initiative, in part through the Australia Research Council. The authors thank the PATH research team at the Centre for Mental Health Research, ANU, Canberra, and the Neuroimaging Group (Neuropsychiatric Institute), Prince of Wales Hospital, Sydney, for providing the original MR and segmented data sets.

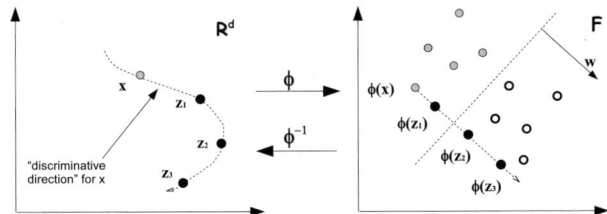

Fig. 1. Discriminative direction for a point, $\mathbf{x}$. A nonlinear mapping Φ maps the shape descriptor space $\mathbb{R}^d$ onto a feature space $\mathcal{F}$, where the two classes (gray and white dots) become linearly separable. The $\mathbf{w}$ is the normal of a hyperplane found in $\mathcal{F}$ to best discriminate the two classes. Move $\Phi(\mathbf{x})$ along $\mathbf{w}$ to a new position $\Phi(\mathbf{z}_1)$, and project $\Phi(\mathbf{z}_1)$ back to $\mathbb{R}^d$ as $\mathbf{z}_1$. The vector $\mathbf{z}_1 - \mathbf{x}$ is the "discriminative direction" of $\mathbf{x}$. Similar results can be obtained for $\Phi(\mathbf{z}_2)$ and $\Phi(\mathbf{z}_3)$.

previous work [3] we proposed a different way to calculate this discriminative direction and obtained the result similar to that of Golland's method.

However, we observed that simply deforming along this discriminative direction may introduce spurious shape differences. This is because the deformed shapes deviate from the underlying distribution of a shape class and untrue shapes are generated. That is, the intrinsic characteristic of a shape which makes it belong to a particular shape class (called "anatomical correctness" in this paper) is no longer maintained. In such cases, comparing the shapes before and after the deformation will lead to artifact differences, as shown later in the experiments. To remedy this, we argue that the shape distribution should not be ignored because (i) the shapes may only reside in a sub-dimensional manifold though the shape descriptor space has high dimensionality, and (ii) the deformation of an organ may be spatially restricted by its surroundings.

Our contributions are: (i) We identify the cause of the spurious difference as that deforming along the discriminative direction ignores the underlying shape distribution; (ii) We propose a regularized discriminative direction by requiring a shape to conform to the distribution when it deforms, and this is formulated as a penalized optimization problem; (iii) We derive an analytical solution for this optimization problem. It avoids performing optimization in a possibly high-dimensional shape descriptor space and directly works out the direction; (iv) After verifying our approach with controlled experiments, we analyze the shape difference of hippocampi for sex and compare it with that using the approach in [1]. We found our result agrees better with a published work about sex difference in hippocampal shapes [4] studied by a different approach.

2 Review of Discriminative Direction Methods

Let $\mathcal{D} = \{\mathbf{x}_1, \cdots, \mathbf{x}_n\}$ ($\mathbf{x}_i \in \mathbb{R}^d$) be a set of n training samples from two classes. A kernel classifier implicitly performs a mapping $\Phi(\cdot)$ from the input space $\mathbb{R}^d$ to the feature space $\mathcal{F}$. An optimal separating hyperplane is obtained in $\mathcal{F}$ as

$f(\mathbf{x}) = \mathbf{w}^\top \Phi(\mathbf{x}) + b$ where $\mathbf{w}$ is the normal and b is a bias. The vector $\mathbf{w}$ indicates the direction that best discriminates the two classes. Ideally $\Phi(\mathbf{x})$ should move along $\mathbf{w}$ strictly to reflect only the class difference. However there is a dilemma. If $\Phi(\mathbf{x})$ moves strictly along $\mathbf{w}$, the resulting images in $\mathcal{F}$ might not have a pre-image in $\mathbb{R}^d$. On the other hand, by enforcing that the pre-image of $\Phi(\mathbf{x})$ does exist, $\Phi(\mathbf{x})$ cannot move strictly along $\mathbf{w}$. Two different solutions to this problem are given in [1,2] and in our previous paper [3]. In [1,2], Golland's method searched for the direction $d\mathbf{x}$ in $\mathbb{R}^d$ under the constraint $\|d\mathbf{x}\| = \epsilon$. When $\mathbf{x}$ moves along $d\mathbf{x}$, the divergence of the displacement $d\mathbf{z} = \Phi(\mathbf{x} + d\mathbf{x}) - \Phi(\mathbf{x})$ from $\mathbf{w}$ will be minimized in $\mathcal{F}$. Note that the constraint of $\|d\mathbf{x}\| = \epsilon$ allows $d\mathbf{x}$ to be searched identically along *all* directions in $\mathbb{R}^d$. Clearly the underlying distribution of $\mathbf{x}$ is not taken into account. From a different perspective, our previous work makes the movement of $\Phi(\mathbf{x})$ strictly follow $\mathbf{w}$, and approximates the corresponding pre-images in $\mathbb{R}^d$ by minimizing the reconstruction error $\rho(\mathbf{z}) = \| \Phi(\mathbf{x}) + s\mathbf{w} - \Phi(\mathbf{z}) \|^2$. Here $\mathbf{z} \in \mathbb{R}^d$ denotes the estimated pre-image and s denotes the step of movement in $\mathcal{F}$. Our previous work also allows $\mathbf{z}$ to freely move in all directions in $\mathbb{R}^d$.

3 Our Approach - Regularized Discriminative Direction

The key idea of our new approach is that, when seeking for the pre-image of a point in $\mathcal{F}$, the possible solutions are restricted into a certain region rather than the whole $\mathbb{R}^d$ as in [1,2,3]. Without loss of generality, assume that $\mathbf{w}$ has been normalized as a unit vector. Let $\hat{\mathbf{x}}$ denote a particular shape to be deformed. Moving $\Phi(\hat{\mathbf{x}})$ along $\mathbf{w}$ in $\mathcal{F}$ for a step s arrives at a new position $\Phi(\hat{\mathbf{x}}) + s\mathbf{w}$. Let $\mathbf{z}$ be the pre-image of $\Phi(\hat{\mathbf{x}}) + s\mathbf{w}$, representing the new shape of $\hat{\mathbf{x}}$ after deformation. The estimation of $\mathbf{z}$ is elaborated below.

We argue that to ensure "anatomical correctness", the pre-image $\mathbf{z}$ should comply with the probability distribution of $\mathbf{x}$. For example, if $\mathbf{x}$ resides in a low-dimensional manifold, $\mathbf{z}$ should reside in it too. Let $\epsilon(\hat{\mathbf{x}}) = \|\mathbf{x} - \hat{\mathbf{x}}\| \leq \epsilon_0$ be a neighborhood of $\hat{\mathbf{x}}$ and $p(\mathbf{x}| \mathbf{x} \in \epsilon(\hat{\mathbf{x}}))$ be an empirical probability density function of $\mathbf{x}$ in $\epsilon(\hat{\mathbf{x}})$ estimated from the training shapes. We model $p(\mathbf{x}| \mathbf{x} \in \epsilon(\hat{\mathbf{x}}))$ as a normal distribution [1] with mean $\boldsymbol{\mu} = \hat{\mathbf{x}}$ and covariance matrix $\boldsymbol{\Sigma}$. For an RBF kernel $k(\mathbf{x}_i, \mathbf{x}_j) = \exp(-\|\mathbf{x}_i - \mathbf{x}_j\|^2/2\sigma^2)$, moving $\Phi(\mathbf{x})$ with a sufficiently small step s in $\mathcal{F}$ can always ensure that $\mathbf{z}$ stays in $\epsilon(\hat{\mathbf{x}})$. Hence we require that $p(\mathbf{z})$ should be large enough, or equally $(\mathbf{z} - \boldsymbol{\mu})^\top \boldsymbol{\Sigma}^{-1}(\mathbf{z} - \boldsymbol{\mu})$ be adequately small, provided that $\boldsymbol{\Sigma}$ has full rank. In this way, the optimal $\mathbf{z}$ is defined as

$$\mathbf{z}^* = \arg\min_{\mathbf{z} \in \mathbb{R}^d} \rho(\mathbf{z}) + 2\eta \cdot (\mathbf{z} - \boldsymbol{\mu})^\top \boldsymbol{\Sigma}^{-1}(\mathbf{z} - \boldsymbol{\mu}) \quad (1)$$

where $\rho(\mathbf{z})$ is defined in Section 2, and η ($\eta \geq 0$) is the regularization parameter. When η is 0, this problem reduces to that in our previous work in [3]. According to our observation, our algorithm is insensitive to η in a reasonably large range.

---

[1] Using a more complicated model may be dangerous in the sense that its parameters may not be reliably estimated because the number of training samples in $\epsilon(\hat{\mathbf{x}})$ is quite limited in practice.

Consider the case when the shapes reside in a sub-dimensional manifold, causing Σ to be rank-deficient. Decompose Σ as $\Sigma = \Gamma \Lambda \Gamma^\top$, where each column of Γ is an eigenvector and Λ is $\mathrm{diag}\{\lambda_1, \cdots, \lambda_k, 0, \cdots, 0\}$. The λ_i is the i-th positive eigenvalue and k is the rank of Σ. An optimal solution $\mathbf{z}^\star$ should satisfy:

$$\mathbf{z}^\star \in \{\mathbf{z}|(\Gamma^\top(\mathbf{z}-\boldsymbol{\mu}))_i = 0 \text{ for } i = k+1, \cdots, d\} = \{\mathbf{z}|\mathbf{z} = \boldsymbol{\mu} + \hat{\Gamma}\hat{\Lambda}^{\frac{1}{2}}\mathbf{u}\} \quad (2)$$

where $\mathbf{u} \in \mathbb{R}^k$, the $\hat{\Lambda}$ is $\mathrm{diag}\{\lambda_1, \cdots, \lambda_k\}$, and $\hat{\Gamma}$ contains the corresponding eigenvectors. This optimization problem is explained as follows. Let $\mathcal{M}$ be the manifold where the shapes reside, and $T_{\boldsymbol{\mu}}(\mathcal{M})$ be a tangent plane of $\mathcal{M}$ at $\boldsymbol{\mu}$. This tangent plane is spanned by the eigenvectors in $\hat{\Gamma}$. Since a manifold can be approximated locally by its tangent plane, the result in (2) can be thought of as confining the solution $\mathbf{z}$ to the manifold $\mathcal{M}$. Moreover noting that the shapes do not necessarily isometrically distribute in $T_{\boldsymbol{\mu}}(\mathcal{M})$, our regularized method naturally incorporates such distribution information via the $\hat{\Lambda}^{\frac{1}{2}}$ in (2). This makes it achieve better performance than merely projecting $\mathbf{z}$ which maximizes $\rho(\mathbf{z})$ onto the tangent plane [2], as shown later in experiments. Finally, the problem in (1) can be simplified by optimizing $\mathbf{u}$ as:

$$\mathbf{u}^\star = \arg\min_{\mathbf{u} \in \mathbb{R}^k} \rho(\boldsymbol{\mu} + \hat{\Gamma}\hat{\Lambda}^{\frac{1}{2}}\mathbf{u}) + 2\eta \cdot \mathbf{u}^\top \mathbf{u} \quad (3)$$

and $\mathbf{z}^*$ is computed by (2). This greatly reduces the number of parameters to estimate compared with directly optimizing over $\mathbf{z}$. Iterative optimization methods can be used to estimate $\mathbf{u}$. However, when k is large, optimizing $\mathbf{u}$ is still cumbersome. Below we propose a new differential equation based solution so that for a given step s, first $\mathbf{u}^\star$ and then $\mathbf{z}^\star$ can be directly worked out.

3.1 An Analytic Solution to the Pre-image $\mathbf{z}^\star$

The problem in (3) is equivalent to maximizing $\langle \Phi(\hat{\mathbf{x}}) + s\mathbf{w}, \Phi(\boldsymbol{\mu} + \hat{\Gamma}\hat{\Lambda}^{\frac{1}{2}}\mathbf{u}) \rangle - \eta \cdot \mathbf{u}^\top \mathbf{u}$ provided $\langle \Phi(\mathbf{x}), \Phi(\mathbf{x}) \rangle$ is a constant, such as for an RBF kernel. Noting that $\mathbf{w}$ lies in a space spanned by the training samples: $\mathbf{w} = \sum_i \alpha_i \Phi(\mathbf{x}_i)$, $\alpha_i \in \mathbb{R}$, we maximize the expression below. Note that k indicates the kernel function.

$$\begin{aligned} f(s, \mathbf{u}) &= \langle \Phi(\hat{\mathbf{x}}) + s\mathbf{w}, \Phi(\boldsymbol{\mu} + \hat{\Gamma}\hat{\Lambda}^{\frac{1}{2}}\mathbf{u}) \rangle - \eta \cdot \mathbf{u}^\top \mathbf{u} \\ &= k(\hat{\mathbf{x}}, \boldsymbol{\mu} + \hat{\Gamma}\hat{\Lambda}^{\frac{1}{2}}\mathbf{u}) + s \sum_i \alpha_i k(\mathbf{x}_i, \boldsymbol{\mu} + \hat{\Gamma}\hat{\Lambda}^{\frac{1}{2}}\mathbf{u}) - \eta \cdot \mathbf{u}^\top \mathbf{u} \\ &\triangleq g(\mathbf{u}) + s \cdot h(\mathbf{u}) - \eta \cdot l(\mathbf{u}). \end{aligned}$$

For each given s, there will be a $\mathbf{u}^*$ which maximizes $f(s, \mathbf{u})$. This optimization problem is not convex and has multiple local maxima. We propose an approach which does not directly solve the optimization over $\mathbf{u}$ for a given s. Instead it makes use of the fact that $(0, \mathbf{0})$ is a global maximum of $f(s, \mathbf{u})$ and traces the

---

[2] This approach is called "tangent plane projection" later in our experiments.

change of the global maximum with respect to s. As long as $\mathbf{u}^*(s)$ is continuous and differentiable, our solution remains the global or at least local maximum. The change of $\mathbf{u}^*$ with respect to s can be considered as a curve $\mathbf{u}^*(s)$ in $\mathbb{R}^k$ parametrized by s, passing through $(0, \mathbf{0})$. The curve can be traced out by computing its tangent $\frac{d\mathbf{u}^*}{ds}$. We approximate f by a second order Taylor expansion

$$\begin{aligned} f(s, \mathbf{u}) \approx & g(\mathbf{u}_0) + \mathbf{J}_g(\mathbf{u} - \mathbf{u}_0) + \frac{1}{2}(\mathbf{u} - \mathbf{u}_0)^\top \mathbf{H}_g(\mathbf{u} - \mathbf{u}_0) \\ & + sh(\mathbf{u}_0) + s\mathbf{J}_h(\mathbf{u} - \mathbf{u}_0) + s\frac{1}{2}(\mathbf{u} - \mathbf{u}_0)^\top \mathbf{H}_h(\mathbf{u} - \mathbf{u}_0) \\ & - \eta l(\mathbf{u}_0) - \eta \mathbf{J}_l(\mathbf{u} - \mathbf{u}_0) - \eta \frac{1}{2}(\mathbf{u} - \mathbf{u}_0)^\top \mathbf{H}_l(\mathbf{u} - \mathbf{u}_0), \end{aligned} \quad (4)$$

where $\mathbf{J}$ and $\mathbf{H}$ are the Jacobian and Hessian of the functions g, h and l with respect to $\mathbf{u}$, evaluated at $\mathbf{u}_0$. Here $\mathbf{u}_0$ maximizes $f(s, \mathbf{u})$ when $s = s_0$. The first order derivative of f with respect to $\mathbf{u}$ vanishes at $\mathbf{u}_0$ and other extrema $\mathbf{u}^*$. Since $\frac{\partial f}{\partial \mathbf{u}}\big|_{\mathbf{u}_0} = 0$, we have $s_0 \mathbf{J}_h = -\mathbf{J}_g + \eta \mathbf{J}_l$. Combining it in $\frac{\partial f}{\partial \mathbf{u}}\big|_{\mathbf{u}^*} = 0$ gives

$$\frac{d\mathbf{u}^*}{ds}\bigg|_{s=s_0} = -(\mathbf{H}_g + s_0 \mathbf{H}_h - \eta \mathbf{H}_l)^{-1} \mathbf{J}_h. \quad (5)$$

The curve of $\mathbf{u}^*(s)$ can be therefore traced out by

$$\mathbf{u}^{*(t)} = \mathbf{u}^{*(t-1)} + \frac{d\mathbf{u}^{*(t-1)}}{ds}\bigg|_{s=0}(s_t - s_{t-1}); \quad \mathbf{z}^{*(t)} = \boldsymbol{\mu}^{(t-1)} + \hat{\boldsymbol{\Gamma}}^{(t-1)}[\hat{\boldsymbol{\Lambda}}^{(t-1)}]^{\frac{1}{2}} \mathbf{u}^{*(t)}$$

where $\mathbf{u}^{*(0)} = \mathbf{0}$, $\hat{\boldsymbol{\Gamma}}^{(t-1)}$ and $\hat{\boldsymbol{\Lambda}}^{(t-1)}$ are estimated from $\mathbf{z}^{*(t-1)}$, and $\mathbf{z}^{*(0)} = \hat{\mathbf{x}}$. A four-stage Runge Kutta method is integrated to suppress the lower-order error terms of this ordinary differential equation. Our algorithm is summarized below.

■ **Algorithm 1**

1. $\mathbf{z}_0 \equiv \hat{\mathbf{x}}$, $s_0 \equiv 0$, $\mathbf{u}_0 \equiv \mathbf{0}$
2. Estimate $\hat{\boldsymbol{\Gamma}}$ and $\hat{\boldsymbol{\Lambda}}$ at $\mathbf{z}_0$; Evaluate $\mathbf{J}_h$, $\mathbf{H}_g$, $\mathbf{H}_h$ at $\mathbf{u}_0$ with an RBF kernel.
3. Compute $\mathbf{u}$ and the new position $\mathbf{z}$ using a four-stage Runge Kutta method.
   (1) $\mathbf{u}_1 \longleftarrow \mathbf{u}_0$, $s_{u1} \longleftarrow s_0$, compute $\mathbf{t}_1 = \frac{d\mathbf{u}^*}{ds}\big|_{s=s_{u1}, \mathbf{u}=\mathbf{u}_0}$.
   (2) $\mathbf{u}_2 \longleftarrow \mathbf{u}_1 + \mathbf{t}_1 \Delta s/2$, $s_{u2} \longleftarrow s_0 + \Delta s/2$, compute $\mathbf{t}_2 = \frac{d\mathbf{u}^*}{ds}\big|_{s=s_{u2}, \mathbf{u}=\mathbf{u}_0}$
   (3) $\mathbf{u}_3 \longleftarrow \mathbf{u}_1 + \mathbf{t}_2 \Delta s/2$, $s_{u3} \longleftarrow s_0 + \Delta s/2$, compute $\mathbf{t}_3 = \frac{d\mathbf{u}^*}{ds}\big|_{s=s_{u3}, \mathbf{u}=\mathbf{u}_0}$
   (4) $\mathbf{u}_4 \longleftarrow \mathbf{u}_1 + \mathbf{t}_3 \Delta s/2$, $s_{u4} \longleftarrow s_0 + \Delta s$, compute $\mathbf{t}_4 = \frac{d\mathbf{u}^*}{ds}\big|_{s=s_{u4}, \mathbf{u}=\mathbf{u}_0}$
   (5) Compute $\mathbf{u} = \mathbf{u}_0 + \Delta s \times (1/6 \mathbf{t}_1 + 1/3 \mathbf{t}_2 + 1/3 \mathbf{t}_3 + 1/6 \mathbf{t}_4)$
   (6) Compute the new position $\mathbf{z}$: $\mathbf{z} = \boldsymbol{\mu} + \hat{\boldsymbol{\Gamma}} \hat{\boldsymbol{\Lambda}}^{\frac{1}{2}} \mathbf{u}_0$
4. $\hat{\mathbf{x}} \longleftarrow \mathbf{z}$
5. Repeat step 1 $\sim$ 4 to get the pre-images of the movement along $\mathbf{w}$ in $\mathcal{F}$.

---

4 Experiment Result

Our main purpose is to use the regularized discriminative direction to localize the class difference for human hippocampal shapes between sexes. This remains an open problem and lacks ground truth. Hence, first we have to perform a

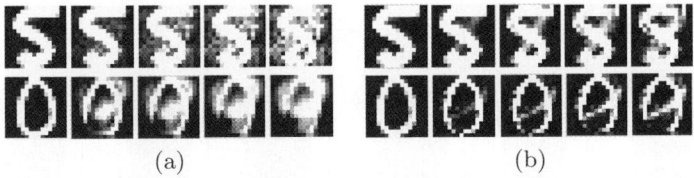

(a)　　　　　　　　　(b)

Fig. 2. Sanity check on the USPS data by (a) Golland's method and (b) the regularized method. The top row shows the deformation from digit 5 to digit 8. The bottom row shows the deformation from digit 0 to digit 9.

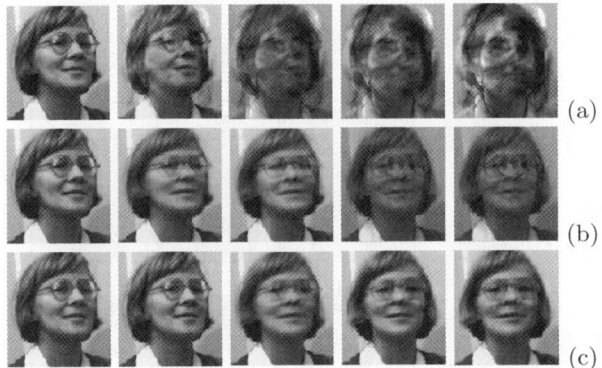

(a)

(b)

(c)

Fig. 3. Sanity check on UMIST data. (a) Golland's method, (b) the tangent plane projection (see footnote 3), (c) the regularized method. During the deformation, a right-side view face (the leftmost image) gradually turns towards the left (keeping adding class difference) while remaining a face image of the same person (filtering individual variability) in (b) and (c). However Golland's method in (a) cannot guarantee this.

sanity check on our proposed method with data for which we know what kind of deformations to expect, and compare it with Golland's method.

The sanity check is taken on the USPS handwritten digit image database and the UMIST facial image database [5]. Each image is represented by a high-dimensional feature vector comprising all pixels, analogic to the landmark representation of shapes. The images have been known to only reside in a low-dimensional manifold [6]. We aim to discriminate (i) the shapes of two groups of digits, and (ii) two classes of human faces (8 individuals): left-side view and right-side view. In experiments, a particular feature vector is moved from one class towards the other along the discriminative direction. Note that the resulting generated images do not exist in the database. Fig. 2 is the result on USPS. As shown, Golland's method introduces much more noise (spurious difference), while our regularized method well localizes the discrimination, adding the minimum necessary shape changes. The advantages of the regularized method are more obvious on UMIST shown in Fig. 3. During deformation, it only introduces the class difference (the change of view), leaving the individual variability (the owner of the face) unchanged (Fig. 3 (c)). Most importantly, the newly

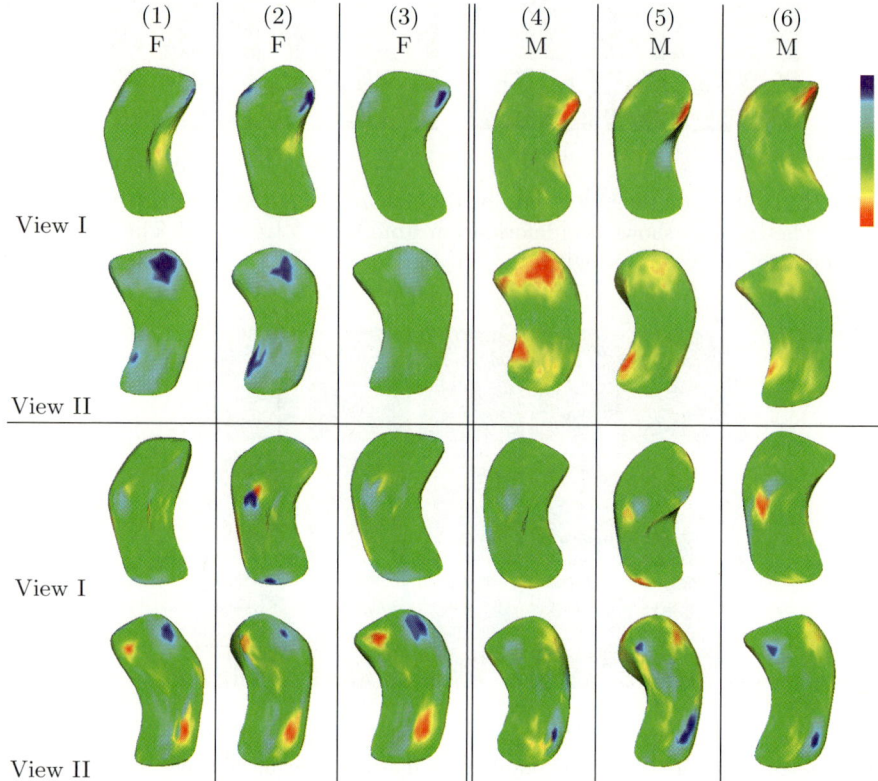

Fig. 4. Localized discrimination for sex on hippocampi of 6 individuals (three females on the left, three males on the right) from two perspective of views. The top two rows are generated by our regularized method, while the bottom two rows are generated by Golland's method. The color code indicates the deformation that a female/male hippocampus undergoes to become a male-like/female-like one. Green indicates small shape change. From green to red, the amount of protrusion increases. From green to blue, the amount of shrinkage increases.

generated images remain faces. However Golland's method cannot guarantee this (Fig. 3 (a)), and the authentic difference is overwhelmed by noise. Fig. 3 (b) shows the result obtained by the "tangent plane projection" (see footnote 2). It is better than Golland's method, but still worse than the regularized method (see the ghost around the glasses). This demonstrates the benefit of using $\hat{\Lambda}$ in the regularized method.

After the sanity check, we analyze the class difference of hippocampal shapes for sex. This is part of a longitudinal study in mental health research in Australian National University. Hand-traced left hippocampi of healthy individuals is used, which comprise 219 females and 181 males in an age span of 40-44. Each shape is normalized with respect to volume and represented by 642 landmarks generated by spherical harmonics (SPHARM) [7] with degree 5. An SVM classifier with the

RBF kernel is employed for classification. The localized discrimination is shown in Fig. 4. These hippocampi belong to 6 individuals (a column for each one), 3 females and 3 males. The color code indicates the nature of deformation that an actual hippocampal shape undergoes to become a shape akin to the opposite class. Take the leftmost hippocampus in Fig. 4 for example. To make this female hippocampus to be male-like, the blue areas should shrink. As observed, the shape changes are not uniform over the whole hippocampus: small changes (either compression or expansion, in green color) occur on most of the shape, while sharp changes are localized on the head and the tail. Comparing the deformations in both ways (female to male and vice versa), the regularized method consistently captures the compression in the lateral parts at the head and the tail for male hippocampi. Compared with Golland's method which shows a different pattern (a compression next to an expansion in the head), our results are also more compact, with changes concentrated in fewer regions but at greater magnitude. Interestingly, the work in [4] has reported findings similar to that of our method. In [4], the hippocampal shapes are represented by medial models, totally different from our SPHARM-based shape descriptors. Shape difference for sex is observed and found that it is mostly due to the volume loss in males with age in young adulthood in the lateral areas of the hippocampus head and tail, which is not observed for females. This finding supports that of our regularized method.

5 Conclusion

Our research demonstrates the importance and benefit of incorporating the shape distribution in identifying the essential difference between two shape classes. The proposed regularized discriminative direction is applied to studying the sex difference in hippocampal shapes, localizing the key difference at the lateral parts of the head and tail. More applications are expected in our future work.

References

1. Golland, P.: Discriminative direction for kernel classifiers. In: Advances in Neural Information Processing Systems (NIPS), pp. 745–752 (2001)
2. Golland, P., Grimson, W.E., Shenton, M.E., Kikinis, R.: Detection and analysis of statistical differences in anatomical shape. Med. Image Analysis 9(1), 69–85 (2005)
3. Zhou, L., Hartley, R., Lieby, P., Barnes, N., Anstey, K., Cherbuin, N., Sachdev, P.: A study of hippocampal shape difference between genders by efficient hypothesis test and discriminative deformation. In: Ayache, N., Ourselin, S., Maeder, A. (eds.) MICCAI 2007, Part I. LNCS, vol. 4791, pp. 375–383. Springer, Heidelberg (2007)
4. Bouix, S., Pruessner, J.C., Collins, D.L., Siddiqi, K.: Hippocampal shape analysis using medial surfaces. NeuroImage 25, 1077–1089 (2005)
5. Graham, D.B., Allinson, N.M.: Face recognition: From theory to applications. NATO ASI Series F, Computer and Systems Sciences 163, 446–456 (1998)
6. Tenenbaum, J.B., de Silva, V., Langford, J.C.: A global geometric framework for nonlinear dimensionality reduction. Science 290, 2319–2323 (2000)
7. Kelemen, A., Szekely, G., Gerig, G.: Elastic model-based segmentation of 3-D neuroradiological data sets. IEEE Trans. on Medical Imaging 18(10), 828–839 (1999)

LV Motion and Strain Computation from tMRI Based on Meshless Deformable Models

Xiaoxu Wang[1], Ting Chen[2], Shaoting Zhang[1], Dimitris Metaxas[1], and Leon Axel[2]

[1] Rutgers University, Piscataway, NJ, 08854, USA
[2] New York University, New York, NJ, 08854, USA

Abstract. We propose a novel meshless deformable model for *in vivo* Left Ventricle (LV) 3D motion estimation and analysis based on tagged MRI (tMRI). The meshless deformable model can capture global deformations such as contraction and torsion with a few parameters, while track local deformations with Laplacian representation. In particular, the model performs well even when the control points (tag intersections) are relatively sparse. We test the performance of the meshless model on a numeric phantom, as well as *in vivo* heart data of healthy subjects and patients. The experimental results show that the meshless deformable model can fully recover the myocardial motion and strain in 3D.

1 Introduction

The primary function of heart is mechanical pumping, and the strain fields are one of the basic measures of myocardial mechanics. The alteration of myocardial motion is a sensitive indicator of heart diseases such as ischemia and infarction. Usually infarcted myocardium and the myocardium adjacent to ischemia display abnormal motion pattern and smaller systolic strain. The motion and strain analysis can also contribute in the research on the development of some cardiac diseases, such as hypertrophy. In this paper, we will compare 3D strain field of normal hearts and hypertrophic hearts quantitatively.

Tagged Magnetic Resonance Imaging (tMRI) is a non-invasive way to track the *in vivo* myocardial motion during cardiac cycles. Compared to conventional MRI, tMRI provides more landmarks in myocardium. Myocardial motion in one direction can be quantitatively measured by tracking the deformation of tags that are initially in the perpendicular direction. In heart studies, usually tags are created in three sets of mutually orthogonal tag planes, two of which are perpendicular to the short axis (SA) image plane and one to the long axis (LA). Constructing a volumetric model with higher resolution from 2D tMRI slices can help with comprehensive understanding of myocardial motion and conducting quantitative analysis on 3D displacement fields and strain fields.

Spline models have been used to reconstruct cardiac motion [1] [2]. Denny and McVeigh [3] gave a discrete finite difference analysis method to reconstruct displacement and strain fields. FEM models have been used on volumetric motion reconstruction. Young [4] built a cubic polynomial model driven by FEM, fit it to the human tMRI data, and gave qualitative motion fields and strain fields. Deformable models have been used for the cardiac motion reconstruction from tagged MRI for years. Park et al. [5] presented deformable models combining spatially varying parameter functions to track the LV motion. Haber et al. [6] and Park et al. [7] further extended parameter functions to recover the right ventricle (RV) motion and conducted 4D cardiac functional analysis using Finite Element Methods (FEM).

As a comparably new technique tMRI is still under intensive research, and the imaging quality and resolution has been improved dramatically since it was firstly introduced. We propose a new meshless deformable model integrating meshless methods into the framework of deformable models developed by Metaxas et al [8]. The meshless deformable model can model global motion pattern such as contraction and twisting and recover local deformation with intrinsic Laplacian representation. It also avoids time-consuming remeshing procedure required in FEM, which used as local deformation method in the previous cardiac deformable models. When the size of the finite elements is close to the scale of deformation, the elements tend to degenerate into irregular shape and cause singularity problem in numerical computation. As we increase the resolution of deformable meshes by incrementally subdividing elements into small size, element degeneration and remeshing become inevitable. With meshless methods, the remeshing can be replaced by a simple point-resampling procedure with much lower cost. Strain fields are calculated on the displacement fields with the Moving Least Square (MLS) method.

Our paper is organized as follows: section 2 introduces the framework of the new meshless deformable model; section 3 presents the deformation results on a numerical phantom and then elaborates its medical application on tagged MRI analysis; in section 4 we draw the conclusions.

2 Methology

2.1 Data Description and Prepossessing

Tagged MR images were obtained from a Siemens Trio 3T MR scanner with 2D grid tagging. The 3D tagged MR image set we used consisted of a stack of 5 SA image sequence equally spaced from the base to the apex of the LV, and 3 LA images which are parallel to the LA and with 60 degree angles in between, as shown in Figure 1 (a).

The LA and SA tag MR images were aligned with the spatial information in the dicom header file. The heart wall around the LV is segmented semi-automatically using a machine-learning based approach as in [9]. We detected hundreds of landmarks on the myocardial contours based on local curvature. The landmarks were then matched between image contours and the corresponding slices of the model. The matched point pairs provided long range external forces for the convergence of the meshless deformable model and the image data. The boundary of the registered heart is displayed in Figure 1(b).

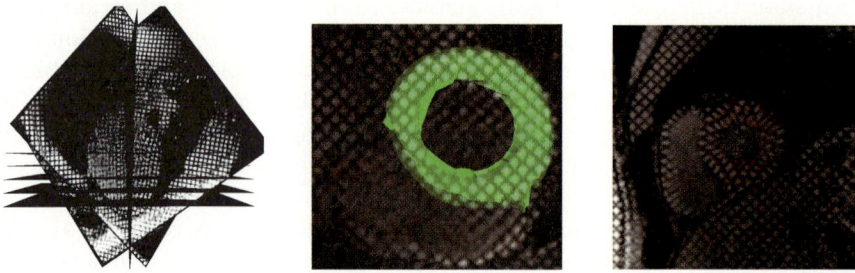

Fig. 1. (a)The setting of MR Images: 5 SA parallel images are placed with equal space from apex to base. 3 rotated LA images are taken with 60 degree angles in between. (b)Registered LV on SA images. (c) The intersections of grid tagging lines tracked by gabor filters.

The automatic tracking of tag intersections provided the external forces for the meshless deformable model. As introduced in Chen et al. [10][11], a Gabor filter bank was implemented to generate corresponding phase maps for tMRI images. A Robust Point Matching (RPM) module has been integrated into the approach to avoid false tracking results caused by through-plane motion and irregular tag spacing. Tracked tag intersections are shown in Figure 1(c).

2.2 Motion Reconstruction by Meshless Deformable Models

Different from previous works on LV motion reconstruction with deformable models, an object is represented as a point cloud inside the object boundary in meshless deformable models. The interaction of points are mechanized with radius based kernels. A point and its neighboring points are grouped into a phyxel with a kernel function.

Global Deformation. An object is represented by parameterized point clouds in meshless deformable models. The world coordinates of model points are transformed to model centered polar coordinates and controlled by a set of global parameters. The coordinates of points in the world coordinate system are transformed into a model-centered coordinate system as $x = c + Rp$, where c is the world coordinates of the model centroid, and R is the rotation matrix. Model-centered coordinates $p = s + d$ can be further decomposed into two parts to incorporate global and local deformations, which will be introduced in the following two subsections. The contraction and torsion of LV myocardium can be taken as global deformation. We interpret the model centered coordinates $s = f(q_s) = f(a_0, a_1, a_2, a_3, \tau)$ in a polar geometry with coordinates (α, β, w).

$$e = wa_0 \begin{pmatrix} a_1 cos(\alpha)cos(\beta) \\ a_2 cos(\alpha)sin(\beta) \\ a_3 sin(\alpha) \end{pmatrix}, \quad s = \begin{pmatrix} e_1 cos(\varphi) - e_2 sin(\varphi) \\ e_1 sin(\varphi) + e_2 cos(\varphi) \\ e_3 \end{pmatrix} \quad (1)$$

Parameters q_s include a scaling factor a_0, radiuses in three directions a_1, a_2, a_3, and a twisting factor τ. In the LV reconstruction, usually we define $\alpha \in [-\frac{\pi}{2}, \frac{\pi}{4}]$ runs from apex to the base. $\beta \in [-\pi, \pi)$ is horizontal, starting and ending at the inferior junction. The transmural factor $w \in [0, 1]$ is defined in a way that it equals to 1 on model's epi-surface, and 0 at model's centroid. Twisting angle $\varphi = \pi \tau \sin(\alpha)$.

We calculate the displacements of points by integrating velocities over time. The velocity can be derived from external force by dynamics equation

$$\dot{x} = f \qquad (2)$$

The global deformation of the model is captured by applying small displacements on global parameters. The velocity of points can be deduced from the velocity of global parameters via Jacobian matrix $\mathbf{L}$.

$$\dot{x} = \mathbf{L}\dot{q}_s \qquad (3)$$

The dynamics equation 2 can also be used on global variables q_s. The velocity of global variables q_s can be calculated by combining formula 2 and formula 3 and applying the Lagrangian equation. The external forces on global parameters f_{q_s} are integrated over the object volume

$$\dot{q}_s = f_{q_s} = \int_\Omega f\mathbf{L} \qquad (4)$$

The integration over the volume can be interpreted as the sum of the integrals over each phyxel in the volume.

Local Laplacian Editing. We encode each point in the meshless deformable models into a Laplacian representation to keep the intrinsic geometric detail of myocardium. The Laplacian of a mesh is enhanced to be invariant to locally linearized rigid transformations and scaling in Sorkine et al. [12]. We further extend it from a surface editing tool to a method for tracking geometric details of a volume.

The geometry of points in the model can be described as a set of differentials $\Delta = \{\delta_i\}$. The Laplacian coordinate of a point as introduced in Desbrun et al. ([13]), is the difference between and the average of its neighbors.

$$\delta = \mathscr{L}(x_0) = x_0 - \frac{1}{d} \sum_{|x-x_0|<h} x \qquad (5)$$

The transformation can be described in a matrix form $\Delta = LX$, where $L = I - D^{-1}A$. A is the mesh adjacency matrix and $D = \{d_1, d_2, ..., d_n\}$ is the degree matrix. We combine landmarks and sampled points together to make a point set. Fixing the landmarks at the target locations $\{v_i\}$ obtained from the next MRI frame, the rest free points deform to minimize the following error function.

$$E(X') = \sum_{i=1}^{n} ||T_i\delta_i - \mathscr{L}(x')||^2 + \sum_{i=1}^{m} ||x'_i - v_i||^2 \qquad (6)$$

where transformation T_i on each point is the unknown matrix and can be written as a linear function of X'. X' can be solve by minimize the quadratic function. As a 3D transformation matrix with only rotation and uniform scaling on homogeneous coordinate, T_i can be written as

$$T_i = \begin{pmatrix} s & -h_3 & h_2 & t_x \\ h_3 & s & h_1 & t_y \\ -h_2 & h_1 & s & t_z \\ 0 & 0 & 0 & 1 \end{pmatrix} \tag{7}$$

Let vector$(s_i, \mathbf{h_i}^T, \mathbf{t_i}^T)^T$ be the unknowns in T_i. The first term for each point in equation (6) can be rewrite as $||A_i((s_i, \mathbf{h_i}^T, \mathbf{t_i}^T)^T - b_i||^2$, where

$$A_i = \begin{pmatrix} x_{k_1} & 0 & x_{k_3} & -x_{k_2} & 1 & 0 & 0 \\ x_{k_2} & -x_{k_3} & 0 & x_{k_1} & 0 & 1 & 0 \\ x_{k_3} & x_{k_2} & -x_{k_1} & 0 & 0 & 0 & 1 \\ \vdots & & & & & & \end{pmatrix}, \mathbf{b}_i = \begin{pmatrix} x'_{k_1} \\ x'_{k_2} \\ x'_{k_3} \\ \vdots \end{pmatrix}, k \in i \cup \text{Neighbor}(i) \tag{8}$$

The above least-squares problem can be solved by

$$(s_i, \mathbf{h_i}^T, \mathbf{t_i}^T)^T = (A_i^T A_i)^{-1} A_i^T \mathbf{b}_i \tag{9}$$

As long as T_i is solved, we can update $X'_i = T_i X_i$ accordingly. When X' converge, this error minimization problem is solved.

Transformation T_i is an approximation of the isotropic scaling and rotations when the rotation angle is small. In our model, the major rotation is handled in the global deformation part. The small rotation angle of local deformation fits the small angle assumption of Laplacian edition.

2.3 Strain Computation by Moving Least Squares

After the displacements of points are computed, we want to compute the strain tensor at each point. Without a point set as a structured 3D grid, the strain tensor cannot be obtained by the definition. The deformation gradient is approximated with MLS (Lancaster and Salkauskas [14]). The MLS minimized the weighted difference between the observed displacement of a point and the displacement approximated by its neighbors with first order accuracy

$$e = \sum_j (\tilde{u}_j - u_j)^2 w_{ij}, \text{ where } \tilde{u}_j \text{ is } u_j\text{'s neighbor} \tag{10}$$

Components of the displacement gradient ∇u at node i can be computed as (for example, the x component):

$$\nabla u|_{x_i} = A^{(-1)} \sum_j (u_x(j) - u_x(i)) x_{ij} w_{ij}, \text{where } A = \sum_j x_{ij} x_{ij}^T w_{ij} \tag{11}$$

Given the initial position of a phyxel $x_0 = (x, y, z)$ in a world coordinate and the displacement $u(t) = (u_x, u_y, u_z)$ at time t, the current position of the phyxel in the deformed model is $x(t) = x_0 + u(t)$. The Jacobian of this mapping is

$$J = I + \nabla u^T = \begin{bmatrix} 1 + u_{x,x} & u_{x,y} & u_{x,z} \\ u_{y,x} & 1 + u_{y,y} & u_{y,z} \\ u_{z,x} & u_{z,y} & 1 + u_{z,z} \end{bmatrix} \quad (12)$$

Given the Jacobian J, the Lagrangian strain tensor ε of the phyxel is

$$\varepsilon = \frac{1}{2}(J^T J - I) = \frac{1}{2}(\nabla u + \nabla u^T + \nabla u \nabla u^T) \quad (13)$$

3 Experimental Result

3.1 Test on a Phantom

We tested the meshless deformable model and MLS strain computation with a numeric phantom. To test the performance of the meshless deformable model with sparse external forces, we reconstruct the motion using 10% of control points. The model still converges to the target state in the same accuracy. The strain field computed based on the deformation results are displayed in Figure 2. Given a phantom in the similar size of LV, the MAE of the strain calculated by MLS is 0.0076.

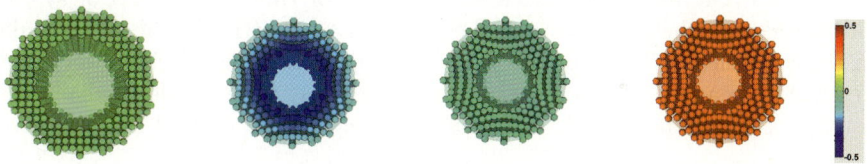

Fig. 2. The top view of strain field on a phantom(from left to right): initial, circumferential strain, longitudinal strain and radial strain

3.2 LV Deformation and Strain Analysis

After getting the deformation of the LV with meshless methods, we compute strain based on the deformation. Some videos on the strain field and deformations are submitted as supplemental materials.

The global deformation of the LV can be described as radial contraction, longitudinal shortening and torsion along the LA. The longitudinal strain in the middle ventricle is negative. Circumferential strains reveal larger contraction near the endocardium than near the epicardium. In the circumferential and longitudinal strain fields, we can observe that a high strain area starts from the apical endocardium and passes quickly toward the base, which can be explained by the activation of myocardium. The radial strain in the middle ventricle is

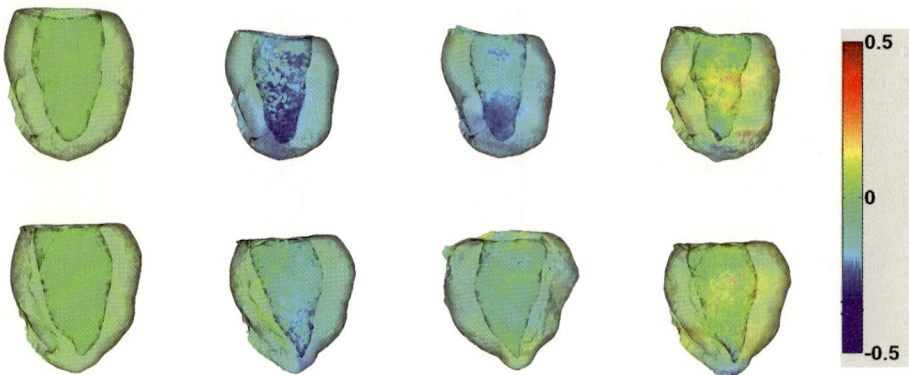

Fig. 3. The first row is a healthy heart and the second row is a hypertrophic heart. The first column shows the LV shape at the end of diastolic, The rest columns show the LV at the end of systolic. The colors show the initial strain, circumferential strain, longitudinal strain and radial strain at the end of systolic from left to right.

mostly positive. Due to the fact that there is less tag information along the radial direction, the strain obtained along the radial direction is less reliable than the other two directions.

We divide each LV into 17 parts and compute the average strain of each part. From the strain time series in the middle anterior calculated from 5 subjects in each group shown in Figure 4, we observe that a healthy heart contracts early in a cardiac cycle, and holds for a short period of time at the end of systolic before it relaxes. The magnitude of the strain in a hypertrophic heart is smaller than a normal heart. The motion of a hypertrophic heart is much slower, hence the contraction and relaxation procedure almost last for a whole cardiac cycle. The tense stage at the end of systolic is not as clear as a normal heart either.

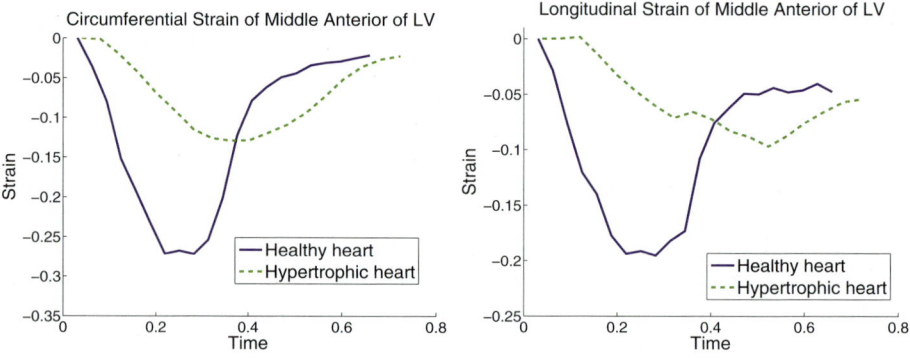

Fig. 4. The strain of the middle anterior of a healthy heart and hypertrophic heart. (a) Circumferential strain (b)Longitudinal strain.

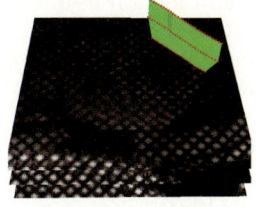 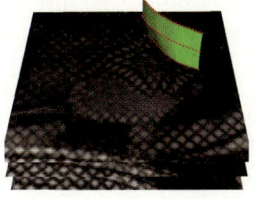

Fig. 5. (a) is a tag plane in the initial state when the LV is at the end of diastolic. (b) is a tag plane at the end of systolic.

3.3 Validation

In meshless deformable models, we can track the deformation of an arbitrary point inside the myocardium. We tracked the deformation of a tagging plane with our model for a whole cardiac cycle and projected the tagging plane onto the tMRI at the end of systolic. The projections of the deformed tagging plane align very well with the tagging lines in images. We evaluate the difference between the projections and the tagging lines on 156 tag planes, the MAE is 1.383mm (The pixel spacing in tMRI is 1.0938mm). The projections lie in the 95% confidence interval of the semi-automatically tracked tagging line ground truth. This experiment demonstrated that our model can reconstruct the 3D deformation field accurately.

4 Conclusion

We have proposed a meshless deformable model for *in vivo* LV 3D motion tracking and strain analysis based on tMRI. The model can fully recover the 3D deformation of LV with sparse tMRI slices, while keep the intrinsic geometric details of the myocardium. The meshless approach avoids tedious remeshing procedures in mesh based approaches. The experiments prove the strength of the model against motion complexity, image artifacts, and noises. The strain analysis based on this model can help early diagnosis of cardiac deceases like hypertrophic cardiomyopathy.

References

1. Huang, J., Abendschein, D., Davila-Roman, V., Amini, A.: Spatio-temporal tracking of myocardial deformations with a 4D b-spline model from tagged MRI. IEEE Transactions Medical Imaging 18, 957–972 (1999)
2. Declerck, J., Feldmar, J., Ayache, N.: Definition of a 4D continuous planispheric transformatin for the tracking and the analysis of the LV motion. Medical Image Analysis, 197–213 (1998)
3. Jr, T., McVeigh, E.: Model-free reconstruction of three-dimensional myocardial strain from planar tagged mr images. Journal Magnetic Resonance Imaging 7, 799–810 (1997)

4. Young, A.: Model tags: direct 3d tracking of heart wall motion from tagged magnetic resonance images. Medical Image Analysis, 361–372 (1999)
5. Park, J., Metaxas, D., Axel, L.: Volumetric deformable models with parameter functions: A new approach to the 3D motion analysis of the LV from MRI-SPAMM. In: ICCV, pp. 700–705 (1995)
6. Haber, E., Metaxas, D.N., Axel, L.: Motion analysis of the right ventricle from the MRI images. In: Wells, W.M., Colchester, A.C.F., Delp, S.L. (eds.) MICCAI 1998. LNCS, vol. 1496, pp. 177–188. Springer, Heidelberg (1998)
7. Park, K., Metaxas, D.N., Axel, L.: A finite element model for functional analysis of 4D cardiac-tagged MR images. In: Ellis, R.E., Peters, T.M. (eds.) MICCAI 2003. LNCS, vol. 2878, pp. 491–498. Springer, Heidelberg (2003)
8. Metaxas, D.N., Terzopoulos, D.: Dynamic 3D models with local and global deformations: Deformable superquadrics. IEEE Transaction on Pattern Analysis Machine Intelligence 13(7), 703–714 (1991)
9. Qian, Z., Metaxas, D.N., Axel, L.: Boosting and noparametric based tracking of tagged MRI cardiac boundaries. In: Larsen, R., Nielsen, M., Sporring, J. (eds.) MICCAI 2006. LNCS, vol. 4190, pp. 636–644. Springer, Heidelberg (2006)
10. Chen, T., Chung, S., Axel, L.: 2D motion analysis of long axis cardiac tagged MRI. In: Ayache, N., Ourselin, S., Maeder, A. (eds.) MICCAI 2007, Part II. LNCS, vol. 4792, pp. 469–476. Springer, Heidelberg (2007)
11. Chen, T., Chung, S., Axel, L.: Automated tag tracking using gabor filter bank, robust point matching, and deformable models. In: Sachse, F.B., Seemann, G. (eds.) FIHM 2007. LNCS, vol. 4466, pp. 22–31. Springer, Heidelberg (2007)
12. Sorkine, O., Lipman, Y., Cohen-Or, D., Alexa, M., Rössl, C., Seidel, H.P.: Laplacian surface editing. In: Proceedings of the Eurographics/ACM SIGGRAPH Symposium on Geometry Processing, pp. 179–188. Eurographics Association (2004)
13. Desbrun, M., Meyer, M., Schroder, P., Barr, A.H.: Implicit fairing of irregular meshes using diffusion and curvature flow. In: ACM SIGGRAPH, pp. 317–324 (1999)
14. Lancaster, P., Salkauskas, K.: Surfaces generated by moving least squares methods. In: Mathematics of Computation, pp. 141–158 (1981)

Surface-Based Texture and Morphological Analysis Detects Subtle Cortical Dysplasia

Pierre Besson[1], Neda Bernasconi[1], Olivier Colliot[2], Alan Evans[1], and Andrea Bernasconi[1]

[1] McConnell Brain Imaging Centre, Montreal Neurological Institute,
Montreal, Canada
[2] Cognitive Neuroscience and Brain Imaging Laboratory, CNRS UPR 640-LENA,
Université Pierre et Marie Curie - Paris 6,
Hôpital de la Pitié-Salpêtrière, Paris, France

Abstract. Focal cortical dysplasia (FCD), a malformation of cortical development, is an important cause of pharmacoresistant epilepsy. Small FCD lesions are difficult to distinguish from normal cortex and remain often overlooked on radiological MRI inspection. This paper presents a method to detect small FCD lesions on T1-MRI relying on surface-based features that model their textural and morphometric characteristics. The automatic detection was performed by a two step classification. First, a vertex-wise classifier based on a neural-network bagging trained on manual labels. Then, a cluster-wise classification designed to remove false positive clusters. The method was tested on 19 patients with small FCD. At the first classification step, 18/19 (95%) lesions were detected. The second classification step kept 13/19 (68%) lesions and decreased efficiently the amount of false positive. This new approach may assist the presurgical evaluation of patients with intractable epilepsy, especially those with unremarkable MRI findings.

1 Introduction

Malformations of cortical development have been increasingly recognized as an important cause of pharmacoresistant epilepsy. Focal cortical dysplasia (FCD) [1], a malformation due to abnormal neuroglial proliferation, is the most frequent form in patients with intractable epilepsy [2]. Epilepsy surgery, consisting in the removal of the FCD lesion, is an effective treatment for these patients and magnetic resonance images (MRI) play a pivotal role in presurgical evaluation [3].

Previous automated image analysis techniques to detect FCD on MRI relied on various types of voxel-wise analyses [4,5,6]. In particular, computational models of FCD characteristics were developed to highlight the lesion [7] and a Bayesian classifier used for lesion detection [4]. While these approaches successfully identified FCD in a majority of patients, most of the lesions included in these studies were detected on routine radiological evaluation. On the other hand, the detection of small FCD lesions, overlooked in more than 80% of cases [8], is a much more challenging task and has never been addressed.

Recently, robust and automatic methods have been developed to reconstruct the inner and outer cortical surfaces [9,10]. These techniques have enabled the identification of *subtle* variations in cortical thickness in the healthy [11] and diseased brain [12], and were also used for morphometric analysis of the cortex [13]. Moreover, cortical matching techniques align corresponding cortices across individuals using morphological measurement such as specific sulci [14] or cortical surface curvature [15], thus allowing a precise vertex-wise comparison.

This paper presents a new method for detecting small FCD lesions on T1-weighted MRI that relies on surface-based features. To that purpose, we modeled morphological and textural characteristics of FCD at each vertex of the cortical surface. To our knowledge, this is the first application of surface-based analysis to the detection of cortical malformations.

2 Methods

2.1 Image Acquisition and Preprocessing

3D MR images were acquired on a 1.5T scanner using a T1-fast field echo sequence (TR=18, TE=10, 1 acquisition average pulse sequence, flip angle=30, matrix size=256×256, FOV=256, thickness=1mm) with an isotropic voxel size of 1mm3. All images underwent automated correction for intensity non-uniformity and intensity standardization [16], automatic registration into stereotaxic space [17], automatic tissue classification [18] and brain extraction.

2.2 FCD Features Extraction

Five features were extracted from the MR images. These features correspond to morphometric and textural characteristics specific to small FCD lesions: cortical thickening, blurred grey matter (GM) / white matter (WM) transition, hyperintense T1 signal, deep beneath the outer cortical surface and located at concavely curved cortical surface [8].

In each hemisphere, the inner and outer-cortical surfaces were computed using the CLASP (Constrained Laplacian Anatomical Segmentation using Proximities) algorithm [9]. The inner-cortical surface was extracted by inflating a sphere polygon model to the boundary between GM and WM. The outer-cortical surface was obtained by expanding the inner-cortical surface to match the boundary between GM and cerebrospinal fluid (CSF). These two surfaces are formed of 81920 corresponding vertices.

The *cortical thickness* was measured using the t-link method, defined as the distance between corresponding vertices [19].

The *blurred WM/GM interface* was modeled by applying a gradient operator on the MR image. The gradient magnitude was then interpolated at each vertex of the inner cortical surface to obtain the gradient surface map (Fig. 1A).

To model *hyperintensity* of the lesion with respect to healthy cortex, we constructed three equidistant intra-cortical surfaces by placing three uniformly

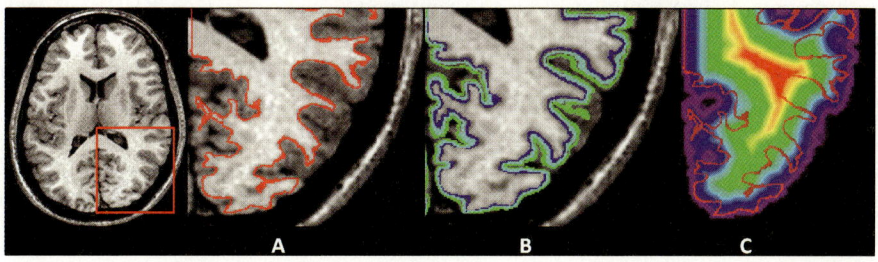

Fig. 1. Projection of the features on cortical surfaces. **A.** Inner cortical surface onto which the gradient was projected to model the blurred WM/GM transition. **B.** Three equidistantly placed intra-cortical surfaces between WM and GM surfaces on which T1 signal intensity was projected and averaged. **C.** Depth calculated as the distance between the WM surface and the boundary of the cortical mask.

spaced vertices between linked vertices of inner and outer cortical surfaces. The intensity of the underlying MR image was then interpolated at each vertex of the intra cortical surfaces. The intensity feature was modeled by the mean intensity of the three corresponding vertices of the intra-cortical surfaces (Fig. 1B).

The *depth* was defined as the shortest distance between each vertex of the WM surface and the boundary of the brain mask obtained with the brain extraction tool (BET) (Fig. 1C).

The *curvature* was calculated at each vertex using area-minimizing flows to define a deviation from the cortical surface to a sphere [15].

2.3 Vertex-Based Analysis

In the normal brain, feature values vary depending on the anatomical location. To take into account these regional variations, we proposed to use a vertex-based analysis (VBA) of the features by applying vertex-wise comparison between a group of healthy controls and a given patient. VBA included the following steps: 1) blurring of the features using a 5 mm FWHM Gaussian surface kernel [19]; 2) registration of the surface features to a template [15]; 3) computation of the mean and standard deviation (SD) at each vertex within the group of healthy controls; 4) deviation from normal is obtained using vertex-wise z-score transform for each patient with respect to the healthy controls mean and SD. We computed the VBA on cortical thickness, gradient, intensity and depth maps.

To classify small FCD lesions, we used the following features: VBA of the gradient and VBA of the intensity (to model the textural characteristics of the lesions); cortical surface curvature and depth, VBA of the cortical thickness and VBA of depth (to model the morphometric characteristics of the lesions).

2.4 Automatic FCD Detection

The automatic detection was performed using two classification steps. The first step was designed to recognize lesional vertices with the highest detection rate.

The purpose of the second step was to remove the false positives (FP) generated by the first classifier using a cluster-wise classification.

Lesions were manually segmented on 3D MRI by trained raters and interpolated at each vertex of the cortical surfaces. Since the small FCD lesions are difficult to distinguish on T1-MRI, the rater made use of other image sequences such as T2, proton density (PD) and fluid-attenuated inversion recovery (FLAIR), when available. The spatial extent of the lesions being difficult to define [20], the labels were considered as silver standard.

Vertex-Wise Classification. For vertex-wise classification, we chose to use four layer feed forward neural networks with the following number of neurons in each layer: (6-4-4-1); tan-sigmoid function was used at each neuron and the output node resulted in a number between 0 and 1 representing the probability of being lesional. To avoid over fitting, we used a cross-validation method to optimize the nets. From all patients, we obtained a database constituted of about $2.8 \cdot 10^2 6$ non-lesional and 1841 lesional instances in which we randomly picked 200 vertices (80 lesional, 120 non-lesional) to construct the training set and 200 different vertices (80 lesional, 120 non-lesional) for the validation set. The neural network was optimized on the training set until the error on validation set started increasing. To avoid poorly performing nets, we used a bagging approach: we created 200 nets and kept only the best 100 (i.e. having the lowest validation error). The proportion of lesional instances in the training and validation sets and the ratio of discarded nets were ad hoc choices obtained from experiments. The final output of the networks bagging was the average of the 100 nets.

The lesional probability maps obtained from the classifier were binarized by thresholding them to keep a high detection rate and an acceptable amount of false positives (FP).

Cluster-Wise Classification. Clusters (defined by the 6-connected neighbours of the triangulated cortical surface) generated by the vertex-wise classifier were further separated into FP or lesional based on their global features as explained below.

Each cluster was characterized by 13 features: size, mean and SD of the 6 features used for vertex-wise classification. The classification step was performed using a fuzzy k-Nearest Neighbor classifier (fkNN) that determines the membership value to the lesional class. A leave-one-out scheme was used to construct the training set. The clusters of all the patients but one were compared to the corresponding manual label and identified as FP or lesional. They constituted the training set for the classification of the excluded patient. On the other hand, the classification of the healthy controls was performed using a training set formed by all patients.

To find the best trade-off between the lesional detection rate and the amount of FP in healthy controls, we plotted the lesional membership value threshold against the detection rate and the number of false positives clusters in controls.

3 Experiment and Results

3.1 Subjects

We studied 41 consecutive patients with FCD. The volume of the lesions ranged from 128 to 94620 mm3 (mean ± SD = 7731 ± 14891 mm3).

Using an entropy index based on their size and visibility on routine clinical MRI examination (89% of small FCD – volume smaller than 3093mm^3 – were overlooked, as opposed to 0% of FCD larger than 3093mm^3) [8], 19 patients had a lesion defined as small and therefore were included in the study (mean age = 24.9 ± 10.9). Their mean volume was 1380 ± 808 mm3 (range: 128 - 3093 mm3), 17/19 (89%) had been overlooked on routine clinical MRI examination. The extent of the manual labels on the cortical surface was 96 ± 66 vertices (range: 14 - 236).

We used 48 healthy controls (mean age = 27.3 ± 7.8) to construct the VBA models 11 additional healthy controls (mean age = 29.8 ± 10.1; 59 healthy controls in total) for the evaluation of the FP rate generated by the classification steps.

3.2 Results

The results of the two classifiers are summarized in Table 1.

For vertex-wise classification, we set the threshold to 0.87 and detected the FCD in 18/19 (95%) patients. The size of the lesional clusters was 39.9 ± 58.9 vertices (range: 1 - 226). On average, 23.1 ± 19.8 (range: 1 - 79) FP clusters were generated in all patients. Their size was 7.4 ± 11.5 vertices (range: 1 - 99 vertices). In healthy controls, the vertex-wise classifier produced 7.1 ± 5.7 FP clusters (size: 10.0 ± 9.9 vertices) in 57/59 (96%) healthy controls.

Table 1. Summary of the results obtained by the two step classification. Detection rate and size (mean ± SD vertices) of the lesional clusters. Size and amount (number of FP clusters) of false positive clusters in patients and in healthy controls (HC).

Step	Lesional Clusters		False positive clusters in patients		False Potive Clusters in HC	
	Detection Rate	Size	Size	Quantity	Size	Quantity
Vertex-wise Classifier	18/19 (95%)	39.9 ± 58.9	7.4 ± 11.5	23.1 ± 19.8	10.0 ± 9.9	7.1 ± 5.7
Cluster-wise Classifier	13/19 (68%)	82.2 ± 71.6	30.2 ± 25.2	2.8 ± 2.2	27.2 ± 21.3	1.4 ± 0.8

For the cluster-wise classification, we chose k=20 for the fkNN classifier because of the large number of FP clusters relatively to the lesional clusters in patients. We chose a lesional membership value threshold of 0.13 (Figure 2) to achieve the best trade-off between FCD detection and the amount of FP in healthy controls. Using these parameters, 13/19 (68%) lesions were detected. The size of the lesional clusters was 82.2 ± 71.6 vertices (range: 8 - 126 vertices).

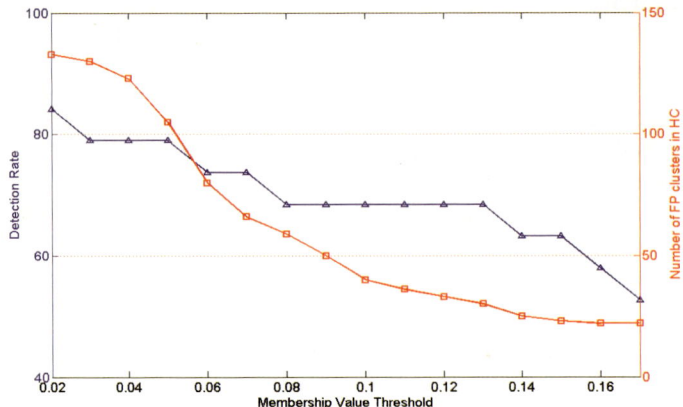

Fig. 2. Detection rate and amount of FP clusters in healthy controls (HC) (y-axis) plotted against the membership value threshold. We set the threshold to 0.13.

In 12/19 (63%) patients, we found 2.8 ± 2.2 FP clusters (range: 1 - 8) and their size was 30.2 ± 25.2 vertices (range: 1 - 99 vertices). In healthy controls, 1.4 ± 0.8 FP clusters were generated in 21/59 (35%) individuals. Their size was 27.2 ± 21.3 vertices (range: 3 - 66 vertices). Examples are presented in Figure 2.

To evaluate the efficacy of our two-step classification, we changed the threshold of the vertex-wise classifier from 0.87 to 0.94 and obtained on average 1.85 ± 1.66 FP clusters in healthy controls. This rate is comparable to the amount of FP clusters kept by the above cluster-wise classification. However, at this threshold, only 9/19 (47%) lesions were detected. This demonstrates that the cluster-wise classification is an efficient step in the removal of FP, while most of the lesional clusters are maintained.

4 Discussion

The purpose of this study was to develop an automatic method for small FCD detection, a challenging and clinically valuable task that has not been addressed previously. We included features derived from textural and morphometric characteristics specific to small FCD lesions. To increase the sensitivity of our model, we introduced for the first time the concept of vertex-based analysis that allowed us to compute vertex-wise deviation from a group of healthy controls. We performed a two step classification combining vertex-wise and cluster-wise classification.

The vertex-wise classifier successfully identified 95% of small FCD lesions. Furthermore, the cluster-wise classifier efficiently removed false positive clusters, while retaining high detection rate of 68%. This represents a 6.5 times higher detection rate that conventional radiological visual inspection, which allowed identifying only about 10% of the cases.

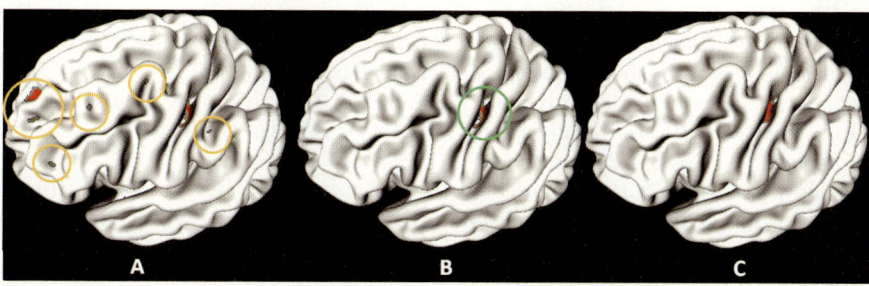

Fig. 3. A. Result of the vertex-wise classification. **B.** Result of the cluster-wise classification. **C.** Manual label. The vertex-wise classification step (A) successfully identified the FCD lesion, but generated FP clusters (yellow circles). However, they were suppressed by the cluster-wise classification step (B) and only the lesional cluster remained (green circle).

The average size of the false positive clusters was similar in patients and healthy controls. However, in the patients the cluster-wise classifier revealed some unusually large clusters with high lesional membership value located in areas distant from the primary FCD lesion. These clusters may indicate structurally abnormal regions, as previously suggested in a voxel-based study of FCD [6]. In some cases, due to hyperintense GM, part of the lesion may be classified as WM leading to a displacement of the WM surface. Thus, the gradient, measured on the WM surface, will be low because positioned within lesional GM compensating for the erroneous GM thinning.

This new surface-based analysis may become a useful clinical tool to assist the detection of subtle FCD lesions that are frequently overlooked by conventional means of analysis. We designed our protocol to attain high specificity, which is critical in the management of patients who undergo presurgical evaluation for medically intractable seizures.

References

1. Taylor, D.C., Falconer, M.A., Bruton, C.J., Corsellis, J.A.N.: Focal Dysplasia of the Cerebral Cortex in Epilepsy. J. Neurol. Neurosurg. Psychiatry 34, 369–387 (1971)
2. Sisodiya, S.M.: Surgery for Malformations of Cortical Development Causing Epilepsy. Brain 123, 1075–1091 (2000)
3. Tassi, L., Colombo, N., Garbelli, R., Francione, S., Lo, R.G., Mai, R., Cardinale, F., Cossu, M., Ferrario, A., Galli, C., Bramerio, M., Citterio, A., Spreafico, R.: Focal Cortical Dysplasia: Neuropathological Subtypes, EEG, Neuroimaging and Surgical Outcome. Brain 125, 1719–1732 (2002)
4. Antel, S.B., Collins, D.L., Bernasconi, N., Andermann, F., Shinghal, R., Kearney, R.E., Arnold, D.L., Bernasconi, A.: Automated Detection of Focal Cortical Dysplasia Lesions Using Computational Models of their MRI Characteristics and Texture Analysis. Neuroimage 19, 1748–1759 (2003)

5. Wilke, M., Kassubek, J., Ziyeh, S., Schulze-Bonhage, A., Huppertz, H.J.: Automated Detection of Gray Matter Malformations Using Optimized Voxel-Based Morphometry: a Systematic Approach. Neuroimage 20, 330–343 (2003)
6. Colliot, O., Bernasconi, N., Khalili, N., Antel, S.B., Naessens, V., Bernasconi, A.: Individual Voxel-Based Analysis of Gray Matter in Focal Cortical Dysplasia. Neuroimage 29, 162–171 (2006)
7. Colliot, O., Antel, S.B., Naessens, V.B., Bernasconi, N., Bernasconi, A.: In Vivo Profiling of Focal Cortical Dysplasia on High-Resolution MRI with Computational Models. Epilepsia 47, 134–142 (2006)
8. Besson, P., Bernasconi, A.: Small FCD Lesions are Located at the Bottom of a Sulcus. Epilepsia 47, 16 (2006)
9. Kim, J.S., Singh, V., Lee, J.K., Lerch, J., Ad-Dab'bagh, Y., MacDonald, D., Lee, J.M., Kim, S.I., Evans, A.C.: Automated 3-D Extraction and Evaluation of the Inner and Outer Cortical Surfaces Using a Laplacian Map and Partial Volume Effect Classification. NeuroImage 27, 210–221 (2005)
10. Dale, A.M., Fischl, B., Sereno, M.I.: Cortical Surface-Based Analysis. I. Segmentation and Surface Reconstruction. Neuroimage 9, 179–194 (1999)
11. Salat, D.H., Buckner, R.L., Snyder, A.Z., Greve, D.N., Desikan, R.S.R., Busa, E., Morris, J.C., Dale, A.M., Fischl, B.: Thinning of the Cerebral Cortex in Aging. Cereb. Cortex 14, 721–730 (2004)
12. Lerch, J.P., Pruessner, J.C., Zijdenbos, A., Hampel, H., Teipel, S.J., Evans, A.C.: Focal Decline of Cortical Thickness in Alzheimer's Disease Identified by Computational Neuroanatomy. Cereb. Cortex 15, 995–1001 (2005)
13. Luders, E., Narr, K.L., Thompson, P.M., Rex, D.E., Jancke, L., Steinmetz, H., Toga, A.W.: Gender Differences in Cortical Complexity. Nat. Neurosci. 7, 799–800 (2004)
14. Thompson, P.M., Woods, R.P., Mega, M.S., Toga, A.W.: Mathematical/Computational Challenges in Creating Deformable and Probabilistic Atlases of the Human Brain. Hum. Brain Mapp. 9, 81–92 (2000)
15. Lyttelton, O., Boucher, M., Robbins, S., Evans, A.: An Unbiased Iterative Group Registration Template for Cortical Surface Analysis. NeuroImage 34, 1535–1544 (2007)
16. Sled, J.G., Zijdenbos, A.P., Evans, A.C.: A Nonparametric Method for Automatic Correction of Intensity Nonuniformity in MRI Data. IEEE Trans. Med. Imaging 17, 87–97 (1998)
17. Collins, D.L., Neelin, P., Peters, T.M., Evans, A.C.: Automatic 3D Intersubject Registration of MR Volumetric Data in Standardized Talairach Space. J. Comput. Assist. Tomogr. 18, 192–205 (1994)
18. Zijdenbos, A.P., Forghani, R., Evans, A.C.: Automatic Quantification of MS Lesions in 3D MRI Brain Data Sets: Validation of INSECT. In: Wells, W.M., Colchester, A.C.F., Delp, S.L. (eds.) MICCAI 1998. LNCS, vol. 1496, pp. 439–448. Springer, Heidelberg (1998)
19. Lerch, J.P., Evans, A.C.: Cortical Thickness Analysis Examined through Power Analysis and a Population Simulation. NeuroImage 24, 163–173 (2005)
20. Colliot, O., Mansi, T., Bernasconi, N., Naessens, V., Klironomos, D., Bernasconi, A.: Segmentation of Focal Cortical Dysplasia Lesions on MRI Using Level Set Evolution. Neuroimage 32, 1621–1630 (2006)

Multi-Attribute Non-initializing Texture Reconstruction Based Active Shape Model (MANTRA)

Robert Toth[1], Jonathan Chappelow[1], Mark Rosen[2], Sona Pungavkar[3], Arjun Kalyanpur[4], and Anant Madabhushi[1]

[1] Rutgers, The State University of New Jersey, New Brunswick, NJ, USA
[2] University of Pennsylvania, Philadelphia, PA, USA
[3] Dr. Balabhai Nanavati Hospital, Mumbai, India
[4] Teleradiology Solutions, Bangalore, India

Abstract. In this paper we present MANTRA (Multi-Attribute, Non-Initializing, Texture Reconstruction Based Active Shape Model) which incorporates a number of features that improve on the the popular Active Shape Model (ASM) algorithm. MANTRA has the following advantages over the traditional ASM model. (1) It does not rely on image intensity information alone, as it incorporates multiple statistical texture features for boundary detection. (2) Unlike traditional ASMs, MANTRA finds the border by maximizing a higher dimensional version of mutual information (MI) called combined MI (CMI), which is estimated from kNN entropic graphs. The use of CMI helps to overcome limitations of the Mahalanobis distance, and allows multiple texture features to be intelligently combined. (3) MANTRA does not rely on the mean pixel intensity values to find the border; instead, it reconstructs potential image patches, and the image patch with the best reconstruction based on CMI is considered the object border. Our algorithm was quantitatively evaluated against expert ground truth on almost 230 clinical images (128 1.5 Tesla (T) T2 weighted *in vivo* prostate magnetic resonance (MR) images, 78 dynamic contrast enhanced breast MR images, and 21 3T *in vivo* T1-weighted prostate MR images) via 6 different quantitative metrics. Results from the more difficult prostate segmentation task (in which a second expert only had a 0.850 mean overlap with the first expert) show that the traditional ASM method had a mean overlap of 0.668, while the MANTRA model had a mean overlap of 0.840.

1 Introduction

The Active Shape Model (ASM) [1] and Active Appearance Model (AAM) [2] are both popular methods for segmenting known anatomical structures. The ASM algorithm involves an expert initially selecting landmarks to construct a statistical shape model using Principal Component Analysis (PCA). A set of intensity values is then sampled along the normal in each training image. During segmentation, any potential pixel on the border also has a profile of intensity values sampled. The point with the minimum Mahalanobis distance between the mean training intensities and the sampled intensities presumably lies on the object border. Finally, the shape model is updated to fit these landmark points, and the process repeats until convergence. However, there are several limitations with traditional ASMs with regard to image segmentation. (1) ASMs require an accurate initialization and final segmentation results are sensitive to the user defined initialization. (2) The border detection requires that the distribution of intensity values in the training data is Gaussian, which need not necessarily be the case. (3) Limited training data could result a near-singular covariance matrix, causing the Mahalanobis distance to not be defined.

Alternatives and extensions to the traditional ASM algorithm have been proposed [3,4,5]. An interesting alternative classifier-based method was proposed in [3] where Taylor-series gradient features are calculated and the features that improve classification accuracy during training are used during segmentation. Then, the classifier is used on the features of the test image to determine border landmark points. The classifier approach provides an alternative to the Mahalanobis distance for finding landmark points, but requires an offline feature selection stage. The segmentation algorithm presented in [5] gave very promising results as it implemented a multi-attribute based approach and also allowed for multiple landmark points to be incorporated; however, it still relies on the Mahalanobis distance for its cost function which might not be optimal.

MANTRA differs from the traditional AAM in that AAMs employ a global texture model of the entire object, which is combined with the shape information to create a general appearance model. For several medical image tasks however, local texture near the object boundary is more relevant to obtaining an accurate segmentation instead of global object texture, and MANTRA's approach is to create a local texture model for each individual landmark point.

In this paper we present a novel segmentation algorithm: Multi-Attribute Non-Initializing Texture Reconstruction Based ASM (MANTRA). MANTRA comprises of a new border detection methodology, from which a statistical shapes model can be fitted. In the following page we briefly describe several novel aspects of MANTRA and several ways it overcomes limitations associated with the traditional approach.

(a) Local Texture Model Reconstruction: To overcome the limitations associated with using the Mahalanobis distance, MANTRA performs PCA on pixel neighborhoods surrounding the object borders of the training images to create a local texture model for each landmark point. Any potential border landmark point of the test image has a neighborhood of pixels sampled, and the PCA-based local texture model is used to reconstruct the sampled neighborhood in a manner similar to AAMs [2]. These training reconstructions are compared to the original pixels values to detect the object border, where the location with the best reconstruction is presumably the object border.

(b) Use of Multiple Attributes with Combined Mutual Information: Since mutual information (MI), a metric that quantifies the statistical interdependence of multiple random variables, operates without assuming any functional relationship between the variables [6], we employ it as a robust image similarity measure to compare the reconstructions to the original pixel values. In order to overcome the limitations of using image intensities to represent the object border, 1st and 2nd order statistical features [7,8] are generated from each training image. These features have been previously shown to be useful in both computer aided diagnosis systems and registration tasks [7,8,9,10]. To integrate multiple image attributes, we utilize Combined MI (CMI) because of its property to incorporate non-redundant information from multiple sources, and its previous success in complementing similarity measures with information from multiple feature calculations [10,11,12]. Since CMI operates in higher dimensions, histogram-based estimation approaches would become too sparse when more than 2 features are used. Therefore, we implement the k nearest neighbor (kNN) entropic graph technique to estimate the CMI [13]. The values are plotted in a high dimensional graph, and the entropy is estimated from the distances to the k nearest neighbors, which is subsequently used to estimate the MI value.

(c) Non-requirement of Model Initialization: Similarly to several other segmentation schemes, MANTRA is cast within a multi-resolution framework, in which the shape is updated in an iterative fashion and across image resolutions [14]. At each resolution increase, the area of the search neighborhood decreases, allowing only fine adjustments to be made in the higher resolution. This overcomes the problem of noise near the object boundary and makes MANTRA robust to different initializations.

The experiments were performed on nearly 230 images comprising 3 MR protocols and 2 body regions. Three different 2D models were tested: MANTRA, the traditional ASM, and ASM+MI (a hybrid with aspects of both MANTRA and ASM). Quantitative evaluation was performed against expert delineated ground truth via 6 metrics.

2 Brief Overview of MANTRA

MANTRA comprises of a distinct training and segmentation step (Figure 1).

Training
1. *Select Landmark Points* of object border on each training image.
2. *Generate Shape Model Using PCA* as in traditional ASMs [1].
3. *Generate Texture Features*: K statistical texture feature scenes are generated for each of the N training images, which include gradient and second order co-occurrence features [7,8]. Then, a neighborhood surrounding each landmark point is sampled from each of the K feature scenes for all N training images.
4. *Generate Texture Model Using PCA*: Each landmark point has K texture models generated by performing PCA on all N neighborhood vectors for each given feature.

Segmentation
5. *Overlay Mean Shape* on test image to anchor the initial landmark points.
6. *Generate Texture Features*: The same texture features used for training (gradient and second order co-occurrence [7,8]) are generated from the test image.
7. *Reconstruct Patches Using Texture Model*: A neighborhood is searched near each landmark point, and the search area size is inversely related to the resolution, so that only fine adjustments are made at the highest resolution. For any potential border landmark point, its surrounding values are reconstructed from the training PCA models.
8. *Use kNN Entropic Graphs to Maximize CMI*: kNN entropic graphs [13] are used to estimate entropy, and then CMI. The location with the highest CMI value between its reconstructed values and its original values is the new landmark point.
9. *Fit Shape Model To New Landmark Points*: Once a set of new landmarks points have been found, the current shape is updated to best fit these landmark points [1], and

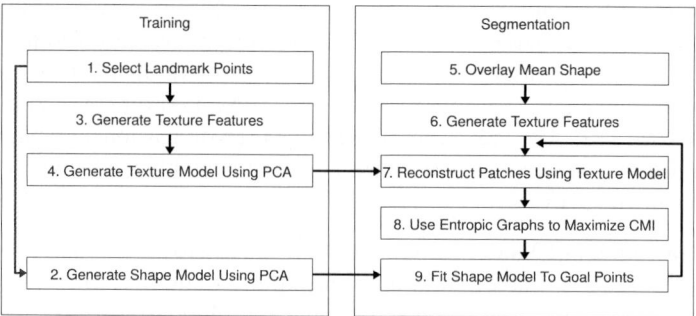

Fig. 1. The modules and pathways comprising MANTRA, with the training module on the left and the testing module on the right

constrained to +/- 2.5 standard deviations from the mean shape. The resolution is then doubled at each iteration until convergence is obtained.

3 Methodology

This section is focused on Steps 4, 6-9 of the MANTRA scheme, as Steps 1-3, 5 are identical to corresponding steps in [1].

3.1 Generating Texture Models

We define the set of N training images as $S_{tr} = \{C^\alpha \mid \alpha \in \{1, \ldots, N\}\}$, where $C^\alpha = (C, f^\alpha)$ is an image scene where $C \in \Re^2$ represents a set of 2D spatial locations and $f^\alpha(c)$ represents a function that returns the intensity value at any $c \in C$. For $\forall C^\alpha \in S_{tr}, X^\alpha \subset C$ is a set of M landmark points manually delineated by an expert, where $X^\alpha = \{c_m^\alpha \mid m \in \{1, \ldots, M\}\}$. For $\forall C^\alpha \in S_{tr}, K$ features scenes $\mathcal{F}^{\alpha,k} = (C, f^{\alpha,k}), k \in \{1, \ldots, K\}$ are then generated. For our implementation, we used the gradient magnitude, Haralick inverse difference moment, and Haralick entropy texture features [7,8]. For each training image C^α, and each landmark point c_m^α, a κ-neighborhood $\mathcal{N}_\kappa(c_m^\alpha)$ (where for $\forall d \in \mathcal{N}_\kappa(c_m^\alpha), \| d - c_m^\alpha \|_2 \leq \kappa, c_m^\alpha \notin \mathcal{N}_\kappa(c_m^\alpha)$) is sampled on each feature scene $\mathcal{F}^{\alpha,k}$ and normalized. For each landmark point m and each feature k, the normalized feature values for $\forall d \in \mathcal{N}_\kappa(c_m^\alpha)$ are denoted as the vector $\mathbf{g}_m^{\alpha,k} = \left[f^{\alpha,k}(d) / \sum_d f^{\alpha,k}(d) \mid d \in \mathcal{N}_\kappa(c_m^\alpha) \right]$. The mean vector for each landmark point m and each feature k is given as $\bar{\mathbf{g}}_m^k = \left[\frac{1}{N} \sum_\alpha f^{\alpha,k}(d) \mid \alpha \in \{1, \ldots, N\}, d \in \mathcal{N}_\kappa(c_m^\alpha) \right]$ and the covariance matrix of $\mathbf{g}_m^{\alpha,k}$ over $\forall \alpha \in \{1 \ldots N\}$ is denoted as φ_m^k. Then, PCA is performed by calculating the Eigenvectors of φ_m^k and retaining the Eigenvectors that account for most ($\sim 98\%$) of the variation in the training data, denoted as $\mathbf{\Phi}_m^k$.

3.2 Reconstructing Local Image Texture

We define a test image as the scene $\mathcal{C}_{te}$, where $\mathcal{C}_{te} \notin S_{tr}$, and its corresponding K feature scenes as $\mathcal{F}^k, k \in \{1, \ldots, K\}$. The M landmark points for the current iteration

j are denoted as the set $X_{te} = \{c_m \mid m \in \{1, \ldots, M\}\}$. A γ-neighborhood $\mathcal{N}_\gamma$ (where $\gamma \neq \kappa$) is searched near each current landmark point c_m to identify a landmark point $\tilde{c}_m$ which is in close proximity to the object border. For $j = 1$, c_m denotes the initialized landmark point, and for $j \neq 1$, c_m denotes the result of deforming to $\tilde{c}_m$ from iteration $(j-1)$ using the statistical shape model [1]. For $\forall e \in \mathcal{N}_\gamma(c_m)$, we sample a κ-neighborhood $\mathcal{N}_\kappa(e)$ on each feature scene $\mathcal{F}^k$ and normalize, denoted as the vector $\mathbf{g}_e^k = \{f^k(d)/\sum_d f^k(d) \mid d \in \mathcal{N}_\kappa(e)\}$. Then, for each e (which is a potential location for $\tilde{c}_m$), the K vectors $\mathbf{g}_e^k, k \in \{1, \ldots, K\}$ are reconstructed from the training PCA models, where the vector of reconstructed pixel values for feature k is given as

$$\mathcal{R}_e^k = \bar{\mathbf{g}}_m^k + \mathbf{\Phi}_m^k \cdot (\mathbf{\Phi}_m^k)^T \cdot (\mathbf{g}_e^k - \bar{\mathbf{g}}_m^k). \tag{1}$$

3.3 Identifying New Landmarks in 3 Models: ASM, ASM+MI, and MANTRA

We wish to compare three different methods for finding new landmark points. The first is the traditional ASM method, which minimizes the Mahalanobis distance. The remaining 2 methods utilize the Combined Mutual Information (CMI) metric to find landmark points. The MI between 2 vectors is a measure of how predictive they are of each other, based on their entropies. CMI is an extension of MI, where 2 sets of vectors can be compared intelligently by taking into account the redundancy between the sets [10]. For 2 sets of vectors $\{\mathbf{A}_1, \ldots, \mathbf{A}_n\}$ and $\{\mathbf{B}_1, \ldots, \mathbf{B}_n\}$, where each $\mathbf{A}$ and $\mathbf{B}$ is a vector of the same dimensionality, the MI between them is given as $I(\mathbf{A}_1 \cdots \mathbf{A}_n, \mathbf{B}_1 \cdots \mathbf{B}_n) = H(\mathbf{A}_1 \cdots \mathbf{A}_n) + H(\mathbf{B}_1 \cdots \mathbf{B}_n) - H(\mathbf{A}_n \cdots \mathbf{A}_n \mathbf{B}_1 \cdots \mathbf{B}_n)$ where H denotes the joint entropy [10,12]. To estimate this joint entropy, we utilize k-nearest-neighbor (kNN) entropic graphs, where H is estimated from average kNN distance, the details of which can be found in [13].

1. ASM: To use the Mahalanobis distance with features, we averaged the Mahalanobis distance for each feature, which yields the mth landmark point of the ASM method as

$$\tilde{c}_m = \underset{e \in \mathcal{N}_\gamma(c_m)}{\operatorname{argmin}} \frac{1}{K} \sum_{k=1}^{K} \left[(\mathbf{g}_e^k - \bar{\mathbf{g}}_m^k)^T \cdot (\varphi_m^k)^{-1} \cdot (\mathbf{g}_e^k - \bar{\mathbf{g}}_m^k) \right]. \tag{2}$$

2. MANTRA: The MANTRA method maximizes the CMI between the reconstructions and original vectors to find landmark points, so that the mth landmark point is given as

$$\tilde{c}_m = \underset{e \in \mathcal{N}_\gamma(c_m)}{\operatorname{argmax}} I(\mathcal{R}_e^1 \ldots \mathcal{R}_e^K, \mathbf{g}_e^1 \ldots \mathbf{g}_e^K). \tag{3}$$

3. ASM+MI: Finally, to evaluate the effectiveness of using the reconstructions, the ASM+MI method [4] maximizes the CMI between $\mathbf{g}_e$ and $\bar{\mathbf{g}}_m$ instead of between $\mathbf{g}_e$ and $\mathcal{R}_e$, so that the mth landmark point is defined as

$$\tilde{c}_m = \underset{e \in \mathcal{N}_\gamma(c_m)}{\operatorname{argmax}} I(\bar{\mathbf{g}}_m^1 \ldots \bar{\mathbf{g}}_m^K, \mathbf{g}_e^1 \ldots \mathbf{g}_e^K). \tag{4}$$

Table 1. Quantitative results for all test performed (ASM, ASM+MI, MANTRA) as mean ± standard deviation

Object	Method	Overlap	Sensitivity	Specificity	PPV	MAD	Hausdorff
Prostate with Intensities	MANTRA	.752±.118	.880±.115	.765±.131	.849±.113	4.3±2.1	11.6±5.0
	ASM+MI	.731±.128	.831±.130	.813±.151	.879±.139	4.5±2.2	12.3±5.8
	ASM	.668±.165	.737±.187	.855±.149	.903±.134	5.6±3.1	13.7±6.8
Prostate with Features	MANTRA	.840±.096	.958±.041	.784±.098	.873±.106	2.6±1.1	8.1±3.3
	ASM+MI	.818±.094	.925±.055	.796±.113	.881±.111	2.9±1.2	8.7±3.4
	ASM	.766±.144	.814±.163	.888±.087	.933±.099	3.6±1.9	10.0±3.8
Prostate	Expert 2	.858±.101	.961±.089	.778±.119	.886±.083	2.4±1.7	7.7±5.1
Breast	MANTRA	.925±.102	.952±.102	.935±.044	.970±.022	4.9±6.7	16.3±11.6
	ASM+MI	.925±.098	.954±.098	.930±.042	.968±.021	4.9±6.6	16.6±11.3
	ASM	.924±.104	.952±.104	.934±.041	.970±.020	5.0±7.1	16.9±12.3

4 Results

Our data consisted of 128 1.5 Tesla (T), T2-weighted *in vivo* prostate MR slices, 21 3T T1-weighted DCE *in vivo* prostate MR slices, and 78 1.5T T1-weighted DCE MR breast images. To evaluate our methods, a 10-fold cross validation was performed on each of the datasets for the MANTRA, ASM+MI, and ASM methods, in which 90% of the images were used for training, and 10% were used for testing, which was repeated until all images had been tested.

4.1 Quantitative Results

For nearly 230 clinical images, MANTRA, ASM, and ASM+MI were compared against expert delineated segmentations (Expert 1) in terms of 6 error metrics [7,15], where PPV and MAD stand for Positive Predictive Value and Mean Absolute Distance respectively. The segmentations of an experienced radiologist (Expert 1) were used as the gold standard for evaluation. Also shown in Table 1 is the segmentation performance of a radiologist resident (Expert 2) compared to Expert 1. Note that MANTRA performs comparably to Expert 2, and in 78% of the 18 scenarios (6 metrics, 3 tests), MANTRA performs better than ASM and ASM+MI. The scenarios in which it failed (specificity and PPV of the prostate) did not take into account false negative area. Using the proposed ASM+MI algorithm performed better than the ASM method but worse than the MANTRA method, suggesting that MI is a more effective metric than the Mahalanobis distance for border detection, but also justifying the use of the reconstructions in MANTRA. In addition, using statistical texture features improved the performance of all results, showing the effectiveness of the multi-attribute approach. For breast segmentation task, all 3 methods performed equivalently, indicating that our new method is as robust as the traditional ASM method in segmenting a variety of medical images.

4.2 Qualitative Results

In Figure 2 are shown the results of qualitatively comparing the ground truth in the first column (Figures 2 (a), (e), (i), and (m)), MANTRA in the second column (Figures 2 (b),

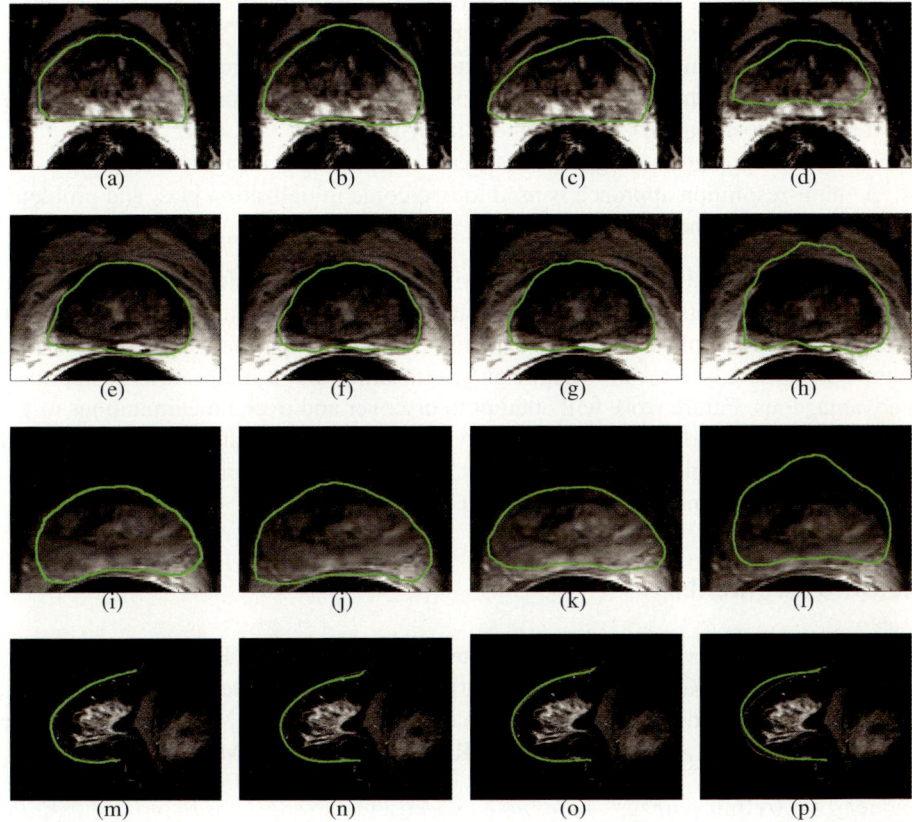

Fig. 2. The ground truth is shown in (a), (e), (i), and (m), MANTRA in (b), (f), (j), and (n), ASM+MI in (c), (g), (k), and (o), and ASM in (d), (h), (l), and (p). (a)-(h) show the results of the models on 1.5T T2-weighted prostate slices, in (i)-(l) are shown 3T T1-weighted prostate slices results, and finally in (m)-(p) are shown 1.5T DCE breast results.

(f), (j), and (n)), ASM+MI in the third column (Figures 2 (c), (g), (k), and (o)), and ASM in the fourth column (Figures 2 (d), (h), (l), and (p)). Figures 2 (a)-(h) show the results of the models on 1.5T T2-weighted prostate slices, Figures 2 (i)-(l) show 3T T1-weighted prostate slices results, and finally Figures 2 (m)-(p) show 1.5T DCE breast results. In all the cases, the MANTRA segmentation is most similar to the ground truth segmentation. The false edges that sometimes cause the models to deviate from the true prostate edge can be seen in Figures 2 (c) and (d), and in Figures 2 (i)-(l) the lack of a clear prostate edge at the top prevents the ASM+MI and ASM from finding the correct object border.

5 Concluding Remarks

We have presented a Multi-Attribute, Non-Initializing, Texture Reconstruction Based Active Shape Model (MANTRA) with the following strengths:

1. PCA-based texture models are used to better represent the border instead of simply using mean intensities as in the traditional ASM.
2. CMI is used as an improved border detection metric to overcome several inherent limitations with the Mahalanobis distance. The use of kNN entropic graphs makes it possible to compute CMI in higher dimensions.
3. Using multiple attributes gives better results than simply using intensities.
4. A multi-resolution approach is used to overcome initialization bias, and problems with noise at higher resolutions.

MANTRA was tested on over 230 clinical images, and outperformed the traditional ASM method. In addition, MANTRA was successful with different field strengths (1.5T and 3T) and on multiple protocols (DCE and T2). The incorporation of multiple texture features also increased results significantly, indicating that a multi-attribute approach is advantageous. Future work will attempt to discover and overcome limitations of the choice of features, and to extend MANTRA to be 3D (our tests show that a single CMI calculation for 2 neighborhoods of 64x64x10 pixels is on the order of 10^{-3} seconds, indicating that a 3D model can work in real time).

Acknowledgments

Work made possible via grants from Coulter Foundation (WHCF 4-29368), New Jersey Commission on Cancer Research, National Cancer Institute (R21CA127186-01, R03CA128081-01), and the Society for Imaging Informatics in Medicine (SIIM). The authors would like to acknowledge the ACRIN database for the MRI/MRS data.

References

1. Cootes, T., Taylor, C., Cooper, D., Graham, J.: Active shape models - their training and application. Computer Vision and Image Understanding 61(1), 38–59 (1995)
2. Cootes, T.F., Edwards, G.J., Taylor, C.J.: Active appearance models. In: Burkhardt, H., Neumann, B. (eds.) ECCV 1998. LNCS, vol. 1407, pp. 484–498. Springer, Heidelberg (1998)
3. van Ginneken, B., Frangi, A.F., Staal, J.J., et al.: Active shape model segmentation with optimal features. IEEE Trans. Med. Imag. 21(8), 924–933 (2002)
4. Toth, R., Tiwari, P., Rosen, M., Kalyanpur, A., Pungabkar, S., Madabhushi, A.: A multi-modal prostate segmentation scheme by combining spectral clustering and active shape models. In: SPIE, vol. 6914, pp. 69144S1–69144S12 (2008)
5. Seghers, D., Loeckx, D., Maes, F., Vandermeulen, D., Suetens, P.: Minimal shape and intensity cost path segmentation. IEEE Trans. Med. Imag. 26(8), 1115–1129 (2007)
6. Pluim, J.P.W., Maintz, J.B.A., Viergever, M.A.: Mutual-information-based registration of medical images: a survey. IEEE Trans. Med. Imag. 22(8), 986–1004 (2003)
7. Madabhushi, A., Feldman, M., Metaxas, D., Tomaszeweski, J., Chute, D.: Automated detection of prostatic adenocarcinoma from high-resolution ex vivo MRI. IEEE Trans. Med. Imag. 24(12), 1611–1625 (2005)
8. Doyle, S., Madabhushi, A., Feldman, M., Tomaszewski, J.: A boosting cascade for automated detection of prostate cancer from digitized histology. In: Larsen, R., Nielsen, M., Sporring, J. (eds.) MICCAI 2006. LNCS, vol. 4191, pp. 504–511. Springer, Heidelberg (2006)

9. Viswanath, S., Rosen, M., Madabhushi, A.: A consensus embedding approach for segmentation of high resolution in vivo prostate magnetic resonance imagery. In: SPIE (2008)
10. Chappelow, J., Madabhushi, A., Rosen, M., Tomaszeweski, J., Feldman, M.: A combined feature ensemble based mutual information scheme for robust inter-modal, inter-protocol image registration. In: ISBI 2007, pp. 644–647 (April 2007)
11. Tomazevic, D., Likar, B., Pernus, F.: Multifeature mutual information. In: Fitzpatrick, J.M., Sonka, M. (eds.) Proceedings of SPIE: Medical Imaging, vol. 5370, pp. 143–154 (2004)
12. Matsuda, H.: Physical nature of higher-order mutual information: Intrinsic correlations and frustration. Phys. Rev. E 62(3), 3096–3102 (2000)
13. Kraskov, A., Stögbauer, H., Grassberger, P.: Estimating mutual information. Phys. Rev. E 69(6), 066138 (2004)
14. Cootes, T., Taylor, C., Lanitis, A.: Evaluating of a multi-resolution method for improving image search. In: Proc. British Machine Vision Conference, pp. 327–336 (1994)
15. Madabhushi, A., Metaxas, D.N.: Combining low-, high-level and empirical domain knowledge for automated segmentation of ultrasonic breast lesions. IEEE Trans. Med. Imag. 22(2), 155–170 (2005)

A Comprehensive Segmentation, Registration, and Cancer Detection Scheme on 3 Tesla *In Vivo* Prostate DCE-MRI

Satish Viswanath[1], B. Nicolas Bloch[2], Elisabeth Genega[2], Neil Rofsky[2], Robert Lenkinski[2], Jonathan Chappelow[1], Robert Toth[1], and Anant Madabhushi[1]

[1] Department of Biomedical Engineering, Rutgers University, NJ, USA
anantm@rci.rutgers.edu
[2] Department of Radiology, Beth Israel Deaconess Medical Center, MA, USA*

Abstract. Recently, high resolution 3 Tesla (T) Dynamic Contrast-Enhanced MRI (DCE-MRI) of the prostate has emerged as a promising modality for detecting prostate cancer (CaP). Computer-aided diagnosis (CAD) schemes for DCE-MRI data have thus far been primarily developed for breast cancer and typically involve model fitting of dynamic intensity changes as a function of contrast agent uptake by the lesion. Comparatively there is relatively little work in developing CAD schemes for prostate DCE-MRI. In this paper, we present a novel unsupervised detection scheme for CaP from 3 T DCE-MRI which comprises 3 distinct steps. First, a multi-attribute active shape model is used to automatically segment the prostate boundary from 3 T *in vivo* MR imagery. A robust multimodal registration scheme is then used to non-linearly align corresponding whole mount histological and DCE-MRI sections from prostatectomy specimens to determine the spatial extent of CaP. Non-linear dimensionality reduction schemes such as locally linear embedding (LLE) have been previously shown to be useful in projecting such high dimensional biomedical data into a lower dimensional subspace while preserving the non-linear geometry of the data manifold. DCE-MRI data is embedded via LLE and then classified via unsupervised consensus clustering to identify distinct classes. Quantitative evaluation on 21 histology-MRI slice pairs against registered CaP ground truth estimates yielded a maximum CaP detection accuracy of 77.20% while the popular three time point (3TP) scheme yielded an accuracy of 67.37%.

1 Introduction

Prostatic adenocarcinoma (CaP) is the second leading cause of cancer related deaths among males in the United States, with an estimated 186,000 new cases

---

* This work is made possible via grants from the Wallace H. Coulter Foundation, New Jersey Commission on Cancer Research, National Cancer Institute (R21CA127186-01,R03CA128081-01), the Department of Defense, and the Society for Imaging Informatics in Medicine (SIIM).

in 2008 (Source: *American Cancer Society*). Recently, high resolution 3 Tesla (T) endorectal *in vivo* prostate Dynamic Contrast-Enhanced MRI (DCE-MRI) has been shown to discriminate effectively between normal and cancerous regions [1].

Most current efforts in computer-aided diagnosis of CaP from DCE-MRI involve pharmacokinetic curve fitting such as in the 3 Time Point (3TP) scheme [2]. Based on the curve/model fits these schemes attempt to identify wash-in and wash-out points, i.e. time points at which the lesion begins to take up and flush out the contrast agent. Lesions are then identified as benign, malignant or indeterminate based on the rate of the contrast agent uptake and wash out. Vos et al. [3] described a supervised CAD scheme for analysis of the peripheral zone of the prostate. Pharmacokinetic features derived from curve fitting were used to train the model and coarse quantitative evaluation was performed based on a roughly registered spatial map of CaP on MRI. Area under the Receiver Operating Characteristic (ROC) curve (AUC) was used as a measure of accuracy. A mean AUC of 0.83 was reported. Due to the lack of perfect slice correspondences between MRI and histology data and the large difference in the number of slices between the two modalities, we suggest training a supervised classification system based on such labels would be inappropriate.

The 3TP and pharmacokinetic modeling approaches assume linear changes in the dynamic MR image intensity profiles. We have previously shown that such data suffers from intensity non-standardness [4] wherein MR image intensities do not have fixed tissue-specific meaning within the same imaging protocol, body region, and patient. Figures 1(a), (b), and (c) show the image intensity histograms for the non-lesion areas within 7 3 T *in vivo* DCE-MRI prostate studies for timepoints $t = 2$, $t = 4$, and $t = 6$ respectively. An obvious intensity drift in the MR images can be seen in the apparent mis-alignment of the intensity histograms. Non-linear dimensionality reduction methods such as locally linear embedding (LLE) [5] have been shown to faithfully preserve relative object relationships in biomedical data from the high- to the low-dimensional representation. Varini et al. [6] performed an exploratory analysis of breast DCE-MRI data via different dimensionality reduction methods. LLE was found to be more robust and accurate in differentiating between benign and malignant tissue classes as compared to linear methods such as Principal Component Analysis (PCA).

In this paper we present a comprehensive segmentation, registration and detection scheme for CaP from 3 T *in vivo* DCE-MR imagery that has the following main features: (1) a multi-attribute active shape model [7] is used to automatically segment the prostate boundary, (2) a multimodal non-rigid registration scheme [8] is used to map CaP extent from whole mount histological sections onto corresponding DCE-MR imagery, and (3) an unsupervised CaP detection scheme involving LLE on the temporal intensity profiles at every pixel location followed by classification via consensus clustering [9]. Our proposed methodology is evaluated on a per-pixel basis against registered spatial maps of CaP on MRI. Additionally, we quantitatively compare our results with those obtained from the 3TP method for a total of 21 histology-MRI slice pairs.

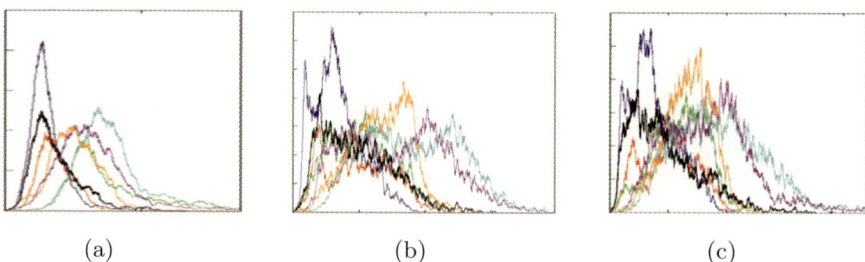

(a)   (b)   (c)

Fig. 1. Image intensity histograms for non-cancerous regions in 7 *in vivo* 3 T DCE-MRI prostate studies at time points (a) $t = 2$, (b) $t = 4$, and (c) $t = 6$. A very obvious misalignment between the MR intensity histograms across the 7 DCE-MRI studies is apparent at multiple time points.

2 Experimental Design

2.1 Data Description and Notation

A total of 21 3 T *in vivo* endorectal MR (T2-weighted and DCE protocols) images with corresponding whole mount histological sections (WMHS) following radical prostatectomy were obtained from 6 patient datasets from the Beth Israel Deaconess Medical Center. The DCE-MR images were acquired during and after a bolus injection of 0.1 mmol/kg of body weight of gadopentetate dimeglumine using a 3-dimensional gradient echo sequence (3D-GE) with a temporal resolution of 1 min 35 sec. Following radical prostatectomy, whole-mount sections of the prostate were stained via Haemotoxylin and Eosin (H & E) and examined by a trained pathologist to accurately delineate the presence and extent of CaP.

We define a 2D DCE-MR image $\mathcal{C}^{D,t} = (C, f^{D,t})$ where C is a set of spatial locations $c_i \in C, i \in \{1, \ldots, |C|\}$, $|C|$ is the cardinality of C and $t \in \{1, \ldots, 7\}$. $f^{D,t}(c)$ then represents the intensity value at location $c \in C$ at timepoint t. We define a 2D T2-weighted (T2-w) MR image as $\mathcal{C}^{T2} = (C, f^{T2})$ and the corresponding WMHS as $\mathcal{C}^H$. $G(\mathcal{C}^H)$ is defined as the set of locations in the WMHS $\mathcal{C}^H$ that form the spatial extent of CaP ("gold standard").

2.2 Automated Boundary Segmentation on *in vivo* MR Imagery

We have recently developed a Multi-Attribute, Non-initializing, Texture Reconstruction based Active shape model (MANTRA) [7] algorithm. Unlike traditional ASMs, MANTRA makes use of local texture model reconstruction to overcome limitations of image intensity, as well as multiple attributes with a combined mutual information metric. MANTRA also requires only a rough initialization (such as a bounding-box) around the prostate to be able to segment the boundary accurately.

Step 1 (Training): PCA is performed on expert selected landmarks along the prostate border to generate a statistical shape model. A statistical texture model is calculated for each landmark point by performing PCA across patches of pixels sampled from areas surrounding each landmark point in each training image.

Step 2 (Segmentation): Regions within a new image are searched for the prostate border and potential locations have patches of pixels sampled from around them. The pixel intensity values within a patch are reconstructed from the texture model as best possible, and mutual information is maximized between the reconstruction and the original patch to test for a border location. An active shape model (ASM) is fit to such locations, and the process repeats until convergence. Figure 2(a) shows an original sample T2-w image $\mathcal{C}^{T_2}$. The final segmentation of the prostate boundary via MANTRA is seen in Figure 2(b) in green. MANTRA is applied to segment the prostate boundary for all images $\mathcal{C}^{T_2}$ and $\mathcal{C}^{D,t}, t \in \{1, \ldots, 7\}$.

2.3 Establishment of CaP Ground Truth on DCE-MRI Via Elastic Multimodal Registration of Histology, T2-w, and DCE-MRI

This task comprises the following steps:

1. Affine alignment of $\mathcal{C}^H$ to corresponding $\mathcal{C}^{T_2}$ is done using our Combined Feature Ensemble Mutual Information (COFEMI) scheme, previously presented in [8]. This is followed by elastic registration using thin plate splines (TPS) warping based of $\mathcal{C}^H$ (Figure 2(c)) to correct for non-linear deformations from endorectal coil in $\mathcal{C}^{T_2}$ (Figure 2(b)) and histological processing.
2. Having placed $\mathcal{C}^{T_2}$ and $\mathcal{C}^H$ in spatial correspondence, the histological CaP extent $G(\mathcal{C}^H)$ is mapped onto $\mathcal{C}^{T_2}$ to obtain $G^r(\mathcal{C}^{T_2})$ via the transformation r determined in step 1.
3. MI-based affine registration of $\mathcal{C}^{T_2}$ to $\mathcal{C}^{D,5}$ (chosen due to improved contrast) is done to correct for subtle misalignment and resolution mismatch between the MR protocols. It is known that the individual DCE time point images $\mathcal{C}^{D,t}, t \in \{1, \ldots, 7\}$ are in implicit registration, hence requiring no alignment.
4. Mapping of histology-derived CaP ground truth $G^r(\mathcal{C}^{T_2})$ (Figure 2(d)) onto $\mathcal{C}^{D,5}$ to obtain $G^R(\mathcal{C}^{D,5})$ via the transformation R determined in step 3.

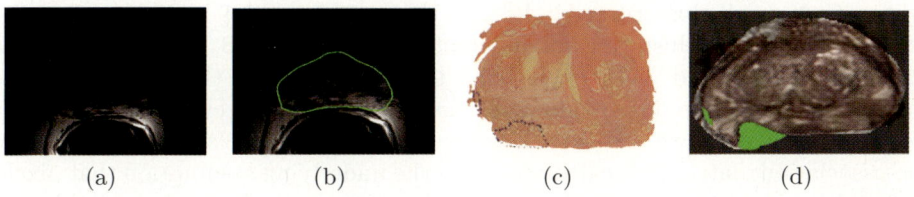

(a) (b) (c) (d)

Fig. 2. (a) Original 3 T *in vivo* endorectal T2-w prostate MR image $\mathcal{C}^{T_2}$, (b) prostate boundary segmentation via MANTRA in green, (c) corresponding WMHS $\mathcal{C}^H$ with CaP extent $G(\mathcal{C}^H)$ outlined in blue by a pathologist, (d) result of registration of $\mathcal{C}^H$ and $\mathcal{C}^{T_2}$ via COFEMI visualized by an overlay of $\mathcal{C}^H$ onto $\mathcal{C}^{T_2}$. The mapped CaP extent $G^r(\mathcal{C}^{T_2})$ is highlighted in green.

2.4 Classification of DCE-MRI Via LLE and Consensus Clustering

Locally Linear Embedding (LLE): For each pixel c within each DCE-MR image $\mathcal{C}^{D,t}, t \in \{1,\ldots,7\}$, there is an associated intensity feature vector $F(c_i) = [f^{D,t}(c_i)|t \in \{1,\ldots,7\}], c_i \in C, i \in \{1,\ldots,|C|\}$. LLE [5] is used to embed the set $\mathcal{F} = \{F(c_1), F(c_2),\ldots, F(c_p)\}, p = |C|$ to result in the set of lower dimensional embedding vectors $\mathcal{X} = \{X_{LLE}(c_1), X_{LLE}(c_2),\ldots, X_{LLE}(c_p)\}$. Let $\{c_{\eta_i(1)},\ldots, c_{\eta_i(m)}\}$ be the m nearest neighbors (mNN) of c_i where $\eta_i(m)$ is the index of the mth neighbor of $c_i \in C$. $F(c_i)$ is then approximated by a weighted sum of its own mNN, $F(c_{\eta_i(1)}), F(c_{\eta_i(2)}),\ldots, F(c_{\eta_i(m)})$ by assuming local linearity, thus allowing us to use Euclidean distances between the neighbors. The optimal reconstruction weights are given by the sparse matrix $W_{LLE} \in \Re^{|C| \times |C|}$:

$$\psi_1(W_{LLE}) = \sum_{i=1}^{p} \left\| F(c_i) - \sum_{j=1}^{m} W_{LLE}(i, \eta_i(j)) F(c_{\eta_i(j)}) \right\|_2, \quad (1)$$

subject to the constraints $W_{LLE}(i,j) = 0$ if c_j does not belong to the mNN of c_i and $\sum_j W_{LLE}(i,j) = 1, c_i, c_j \in C$. The low-dimensional projection of the points in $\mathcal{F}$ that preserves the weighting in W_{LLE} is determined by approximating each projection $X_{LLE}(c_i)$ as a weighted combination of its own mNN. The optimal $\mathcal{X}_{LLE}$ in the least squares sense minimizes

$$\psi_2(\mathcal{X}_{LLE}) = \sum_{i=1}^{p} \left\| X_{LLE}(c_i) - \sum_{j=1}^{p} W_{LLE}(i,j) X_{LLE}(c_j) \right\|_2 = \text{tr}\left(\mathcal{X}_{LLE} L \mathcal{X}_{LLE}^{\mathsf{T}}\right), \quad (2)$$

where tr is the trace operator, $\mathcal{X}_{LLE} = [X_{LLE}(c_1), X_{LLE}(c_2),\ldots, X_{LLE}(c_p)]$, $L = (I - W_{LLE})(I - W_{LLE}^{\mathsf{T}})$ and I is the identity matrix. The minimization of (2) subject to the constraint $\mathcal{X}_{LLE} \mathcal{X}_{LLE}^{\mathsf{T}} = I$ (a normalization constraint that prevents the solution $\mathcal{X}_{LLE} \equiv \mathbf{0}$) is an Eigenvalue problem whose solutions are the Eigenvectors of the Laplacian matrix L.

Unsupervised classification via consensus k-means clustering: To overcome the instability associated with centroid based clustering algorithms, we generate N weak clusterings $\tilde{V}_n^1, \tilde{V}_n^2,\ldots, \tilde{V}_n^k, n \in \{0,\ldots, N\}$ by repeated application of k-means clustering for different values of $k \in \{3,\ldots,7\}$ on the low dimensional manifold $X_{LLE}(c)$, for all $c \in C$, and combine them via consensus clustering [9]. As we do not know *a priori* the number of classes (clusters) to look for in the data, we vary k to determine upto 7 possible classes in the data. A co-association matrix H is calculated with the underlying assumption that pixels belonging to a *natural* cluster are very likely to be co-located in the same cluster for each iteration. $H(i,j)$ thus represents the number of times $c_i, c_j \in C, i \neq j$ were found in the same cluster $\tilde{V}_n^k$ over N iterations. If $H(i,j) = N$ then there is a high likelihood that c_i, c_j do indeed belong to the same cluster. We apply multidimensional scaling [10] (MDS) to H, which finds optimal positions for the data points c_i, c_j in lower-dimensional space through minimization of the least squares error in the input pairwise similarites in H. A final unsupervised classification via k-means is used to obtain the stable clusters $V_k^1, V_k^2, \ldots, V_k^q, q = k$ for all $k \in \{3, \ldots, 7\}$.

3 Results

3.1 Qualitative Results

Representative results from experiments on 21 DCE-histology slice pairs are shown in Figure 3 with each row corresponding to a different dataset. Corresponding histology sections (not shown) were registered to DCE-MRI data ($\mathcal{C}^{D,5}$) to obtain the ground truth estimate $G^R(\mathcal{C}^{D,5})$ shown in Figures 3(a), 3(e), and 3(i) highlighted in green. Figures 3(b), 3(f) and 3(j) show the RGB scaled values of $X_{LLE}(c)$ at every $c \in C$ by representing every spatial location on the image by its embedding co-ordinates and scaling these values to display as an RGB image. Similar colors in Figures 3(b), 3(f) and 3(j) represent pixels embedded close together in the LLE-reduced space. Each of the clusters $V_k^1, V_k^2, \ldots, V_k^q$ for each value of $k \in \{3, \ldots, 7\}$ are evaluated against $G^R(\mathcal{C}^{D,5})$ and the cluster showing the most overlap is considered to be the cancer class. Figures 3(c), 3(g), and 3(k) show the result of plotting this cluster back onto the slice (in red). Figures 3(d), 3(h) and 3(l) show 3TP results based on the DCE images $\mathcal{C}^{D,t}, t \in \{1, \ldots, 7\}$ in Figures 3(a), 3(e), and 3(i). Red, blue and green colors are used to represent different classes based on the ratio $w = \frac{\text{Rate of wash-in}}{\text{Rate of wash-out}}$ of the contrast agent uptake. When w is close to 1, the corresponding pixel is identified as cancerous area (red), when w is close to zero, the pixel is identified as benign (blue), and green pixels are those are identified as indeterminate.

3.2 Quantitative Evaluation against Registered CaP Ground Truth Estimates on DCE

For each of 21 slices, labels corresponding to the clusters $V_k^1, V_k^2, \ldots, V_k^q, q = k$, for each $k \in \{3, 4, 5, 6, 7\}$ are each evaluated against the registered CaP extent on DCE-MRI ($G^R(\mathcal{C}^{D,5})$). The cluster label showing the largest overlap with this ground truth is then chosen as the cancer class. This class is used to calculate the sensitivity, specificity, and accuracy of our CAD system at a particular k value for the slice under consideration. These values are then averaged across all 21 slices and are summarized in Table 1. The maximum sensitivity observed is 60.64% ($k = 3$), the maximum specificity is 84.54% ($k = 7$), and the maximum accuracy is 77.20% ($k = 7$). We see a reduction in sensitivity as k increases from 3 to 7, with a corresponding increase in specificity and accuracy. Using the 3TP technique (which assumes that only 3 classes can exist in the data), we achieve a sensitivity of 41.53% and sensitivity of 70.04%. It can be seen that our proposed technique has an improved performance as compared to the popular state-of-the-art 3TP method across $k \in \{3, 4, 5, 6, 7\}$.

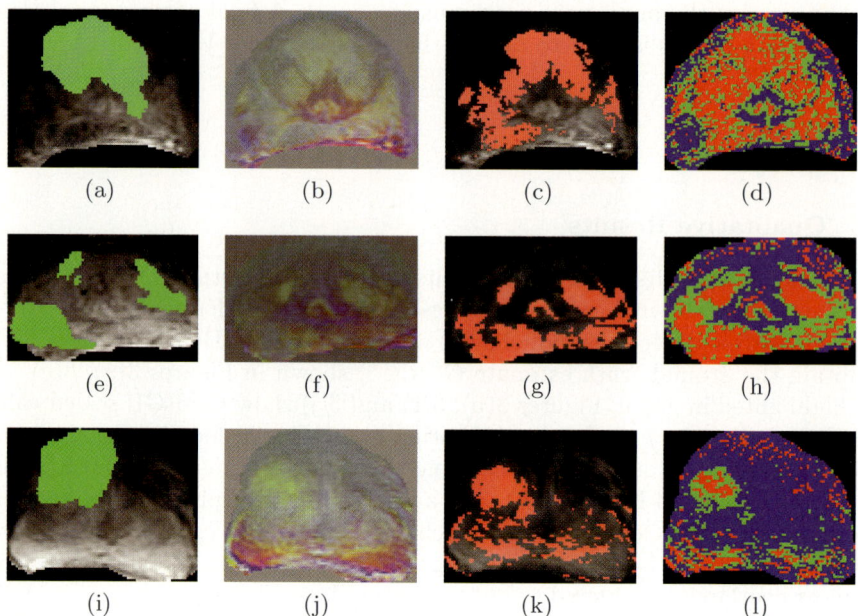

Fig. 3. (a), (e), (i) showing the CaP extent $G^R(\mathcal{C}^{D,5})$ on the DCE-MRI slice $\mathcal{C}^{D,5}$ highlighted in green via registration with corresponding histology (not shown), (b), (f), (j) RGB visualization of the embedding coordinates from X_{LLE} onto the slice, (c), (g), (k) classification result from plotting the cluster in $V_k^1, V_k^2, \ldots, V_k^q, q=k$ (for $k=3$) that shows the highest overlap with the ground truth $G^R(\mathcal{C}^{D,5})$ back onto the slice in red, (d), (h), (l) results from using the 3TP method on the DCE data. The improved correspondence of the red regions in (c), (g), (k) with the ground truth over the red regions in the 3TP results in (d), (h), (l) can be seen.

Table 1. CaP detection sensitivity and specificity at the pixel resolution averaged over 21 3 T DCE-MRI datasets. These are compared for different values of k within consensus clustering, as well as for the 3TP method.

	k=3	k=4	k=5	k=6	k=7	3TP
Sensitivity	60.64	51.77	49.06	42.33	41.73	41.53
Specificity	65.80	76.24	79.60	83.30	84.54	70.04
Accuracy	64.54	71.30	74.20	76.65	77.20	67.37

Comparison against existing prostate DCE CAD: Analyzing the results by Vos et al. [3] in differentiating between non-malignant suspicious enhancing and malignant lesions in the prostate, reveal that their sensitivity of 83% corresponds to a 58% specificity. These values were obtained by only considering the peripheral zone of the prostate. Comparatively our metrics (60.64% sensitivity, 84.54% specificity, and 77.20% accuracy) have been achieved when examining the *whole* of the prostate while utilizing a more rigorously registered CaP extent for evaluation. We may hypothesize that had we similarly limited our analysis to the peripheral zone alone, our results would have been markedly superior compared to those reported in [3].

4 Concluding Remarks

In this paper we have presented a novel comprehensive methodology for segmentation, registration, and detection of prostate cancer from 3 Tesla *in vivo* DCE prostate MR images. A multi-attribute active shape model based segmentation scheme (MANTRA) was used to automatically segment the prostate from *in vivo* DCE and T2-w images, following which a multimodal registration algorithm, COFEMI, was used to map spatial extent of CaP from corresponding whole mount histology to the DCE-MRI slices. Owing to the presence of MR image intensity non-standardness we utilized a non-linear DR scheme (LLE) coupled with consensus clustering to identify cancerous image pixels. Our CaP detection results, 60.72% sensitivity, 83.24% specificity, and 77.20% accuracy compare very favourably with results obtained by Vos et al [3] and were superior compared to those obtained via the 3TP method (41.53% sensitivity, 70.04% specificity, 67.37% accuracy). Future work will focus on validating our methodology on a much larger cohort of data.

References

1. Padhani, A., Gapinski, C., et al.: Dynamic Contrast Enhanced MRI of Prostate Cancer: Correlation with Morphology and Tumour Stage, Histological Grade and PSA. Clinical Radiology 55(2), 99–109 (2000)
2. Degani, H., Gusis, V., et al.: Mapping pathophysiological features of breast tumours by MRI at high spatial resolution. Nature Medicine 3(7), 780–782 (1997)
3. Vos, P., Hambrock, T., et al.: Computerized analysis of prostate lesions in the peripheral zone using dynamic contrast enhanced MRI. Medical Physics 35(3), 888–899 (2008)
4. Madabhushi, A., Udupa, J.: New Methods of MR Image Intensity Standardization via Generalized Scale. Medical Physics 33(9), 3426–3434 (2006)
5. Roweis, S., Saul, L.: Nonlinear Dimensionality Reduction by Locally Linear Embedding. Science 290(5500), 2323–2326 (2000)
6. Varini, C., Degenhard, A., et al.: Visual exploratory analysis of DCE-MRI data in breast cancer by dimensional data reduction: a comparative study. Biomedical Signal Processing and Control 1(1), 56–63 (2006)
7. Toth, R., Tiwari, P., et al.: A multi-modal prostate segmentation scheme by combining spectral clustering and active shape models. In: SPIE Medical Imaging, pp. 69144S1–69144S12 (2008)
8. Chappelow, J., Madabhushi, A., et al.: A combined feature ensemble based mutual information scheme for robust inter-modal, inter-protocol image registration. In: International Symposium on Biomedical Imaging, pp. 644–647 (2007)
9. Fred, A., Jain, A.: Combining Multiple Clusterings Using Evidence Accumulation. IEEE Transactions on Pattern Analysis and Machine Intelligence 27(6), 835–850 (2005)
10. Venna, J., Kaski, S.: Local multidimensional scaling. Neural Networks 19(6), 889–899 (2006)

A New Method for Creating Electrophysiological Maps for DBS Surgery and Their Application to Surgical Guidance

Srivatsan Pallavaram[1], Pierre-Francois D'Haese[1], Chris Kao[2], Hong Yu[2], Michael Remple[2], Joseph Neimat[2], Peter Konrad[2], and Benoit Dawant[1]

[1] Dept. Of Electrical Eng. & Computer Science, Vanderbilt University, Nashville, TN, USA
[2] Dept. Of Neurosurgery, Vanderbilt University Medical Center, Nashville, TN, USA
{sri.pallavaram, pierre-francois.dhaese, chris.kao, hong.yu, mike.remple, joseph.neimat, peter.konrad, benoit.dawant}@vanderbilt.edu

Abstract. Electrophysiological maps based on a Gaussian kernel have been proposed as a means to visualize response to stimulation in deep brain stimulation (DBS) surgeries. However, the Gaussian model does not represent the underlying physiological phenomenon produced by stimulation. We propose a new method to create physiological maps, which relies on spherical shell kernels. We compare our new maps to those created with Gaussian kernels and show that, on simulated data, this new approach produces more realistic maps. Experiments we have performed with real patient data show that our new maps correlate well with the underlying anatomy. Finally, we present preliminary results on an ongoing study assessing the value of these maps as pre-operative planning and intra-operative guidance tools.

Keywords: Deep brain stimulation, electrophysiological efficacy maps, pre- and intra-operative guidance, surgical navigation.

1 Introduction

Deep brain stimulation (DBS) is widely used to provide symptomatic relief in patients with movement disorders like Parkinson's disease. Electrodes are placed in specific targets deep within the brain. Such functional neurosurgical procedures require precise targeting. Traditionally, such targeting is performed in two steps. An approximate target location is first selected preoperatively by a neurosurgeon based on preoperative imaging. The target position is then adjusted intra-operatively using multiple electrodes to map the electrophysiology of the brain around the planned target. The intra-operative adjustment is based on micro-electrode recordings and response to stimulation. The goal is to find a location where symptom reduction (efficacy) occurs at a low stimulation voltage, while any side effects occur at much higher voltage.

It has been reported [1] that there are multiple regions in the brain where efficacy for a given movement disorder can be achieved by DBS. For instance, for Parkinson's disease it is reported that both the dorsal part of the subthalamic nucleus (STN) and zona inserta (ZI) provide symptom relief. Unfortunately, these areas are not easily visualized on pre-operative imaging. Targeting could be facilitated by a map containing the high efficacy locations in a particular patient.

One way to provide the surgical team with such information is to create probabilistic maps that show the efficacy zones based on intra-operative data recorded in a population of patients. D'Haese et al [2] and Guo et al [3] have used a truncated Gaussian (referred in this document as trunc-Gaussian) function as an approximation to the distribution of the electric field around a point of stimulation. They have also used this as the basis to generate maps of stimulation efficacy and side effects. We note that such a function may be appropriate as an approximation to the electric field but is not the appropriate kernel to represent the underlying physiological phenomenon caused by stimulation. The problem at hand can be considered as an inverse problem where the objective is to find loci of points that are likely to have caused the observed stimulation response. We propose the use of a new kernel; a spherical shell, that is representative of this cause and effect relationship between stimulation and the response observed. We present results we have obtained with a total of 95 stimulation points obtained from 19 patients and we show that the areas of high efficacy we identify with our method correspond to or are proximal to target points selected intra-operatively.

2 Method

2.1 Registration

A key component of the method is our ability to map information acquired from a population of patients onto one reference image volume, termed the atlas. Two types of registration algorithms are needed to perform such mapping; rigid and non-rigid. The rigid registration algorithm is required to register preop MRI and preop CT (preop CT scans are acquired at our institution because the stereotactic frame we use, which is described in section 2.2, requires it). Non-rigid registration is required to register each patient's data to an MRI atlas, which serves as a repository of information from a population of patients. In this study, non-rigid registration is always performed on MRI volumes using the adaptive bases algorithm proposed by Rhode et al [4]. Briefly, this algorithm computes a deformation field that is modeled as a linear combination of radial basis functions with finite support. This results in a transformation with several thousands of degrees of freedom. Two transformations (one from the atlas to the subject and the other from the subject to the atlas) that are constrained to be inverses of each other are computed simultaneously. Both the rigid and non-rigid registration algorithms are mutual information based.

2.2 Data Preparation

At our institution DBS is performed with a miniature stereotactic frame, the StarFix microTargeting Platform® (501(K), Number K003776, Feb. 23, 2001, FHC, INC; Bowdoin, ME). During surgery, a micropositioning drive (microTargeting® drive system, FHC Inc., Bowdoin, ME) is mounted on the platform. Recording and stimulating leads are then inserted using the microdrive. Details on the platform, including a study of its accuracy demonstrating it to be at least as accurate as standard frames can be found in [5]. The depth of the electrode is read from the micropositioning device and converted into X, Y, and Z coordinates in preop CT coordinates .

A set of pre-operative CT and MRI scans is acquired for each patient. CT and MRI volumes are acquired with the patient anesthetized and head taped to the table to minimize motion. Typical CT images were acquired at 120 kVp, exposure time of 350mAs and 512x512x256 voxels. In-plane resolution and slice thickness were approximately 0.5mm and 0.75mm respectively. 3D-SPGR MRI images (TR 12.2ms and TE 2.4ms) were acquired with a 1.5T Philips scanner. Typical MRI volumes consist of 256x256x170 voxels, with voxel resolution 1x1x1 mm³.

Intra-operative stimulation data used in this study include efficacy assessment by a neurologist (expressed in percentage) at various points in the brain and the voltage at which the efficacy was observed. We used a total of 95 stimulation data points from 19 patients to build the maps shown in this study.

2.3 Justification for a Spherical Shell Kernel

Butson et al [6, 7] have used diffusion tensor based finite element models (FEM) of electric field, coupled to multi-compartment cable axon models, to predict the volume of tissue activated by DBS as a function of the stimulation parameter settings. However, in the absence of diffusion tensor imaging data and sophisticated FEM solver software, a three dimensional Gaussian can be used to approximate the electric field. This is the model we have used in this work to generate field maps.

At a point where stimulation response is evaluated, the stimulating voltage is increased from zero until a response is observed. The observation and the corresponding voltage are recorded. As voltage increases, the region affected by the electric field also grows. Therefore, a response that was observed at a certain voltage V_2 but not at the previously tested lower voltage V_1 occurs due to the activation of tissue in the region that was not activated by V_1 but activated by V_2. For example, in Fig. 1(b), Q is a point whose activation causes efficacy. With the electrode at P, the electric field does not reach Q at 1V or 2V and thus no efficacy is observed. But, at 3V the electric field activates Q to produce efficacy. Assuming isotropic tissue properties and the tip of the electrode as a point source, Q would exist on a circle whose radius is a function of the stimulation voltage. Therefore, all points inside this circle; including the point where the electrode is placed should have almost zero (if not zero) probability of causing the response. On the contrary, a Gaussian kernel centered at P, assigns the highest probability value to P itself and a smaller value to Q. Furthermore, in the absence of additional information, all points on the circle where Q lies can be considered to be equally likely to have caused the response and therefore should have equal probability. In 2D discrete space, Q would lie on an annulus kernel. In 3D space, the equivalent kernel can be visualized as the region between two concentric spheres; or as a spherical shell. Since intra-operative stimulation at our institution is provided using the tip of the cannula that holds the recording micro electrodes it is considered a point source suggesting isotropic field distribution in all three directions.

A comparison of the two kernels in discrete 2D space is shown in Fig. 2. Both the kernels are normalized such that their values sum to 1 so that they represent a

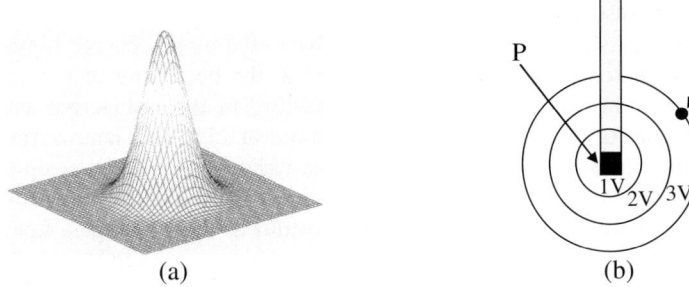

Fig. 1. (a.) A two dimensional Gaussian function, (b.) Diagrammatic representation of the extent of the electric field around a stimulating electrode for different stimulation voltages (1V, 2V and 3V). The electrode tip (located at the point P being tested) is assumed to be a point source. Stimulation of point Q results in reductions in symptoms (efficacy).

probability density function (pdf). All the values on the annulus (Fig. 2(b)) have equal probability. The radius of the outer circle of the annulus is the same as that for the trunc-Gaussian kernel (r_1) and corresponds to stimulation voltage V Volt. The radius of the inner circle (r_2) of the annulus corresponds to voltage (V − 1) Volt. Computing a precise relationship between the stimulation voltage (V Volt) and the distance (r mm) from the electrode up to which this voltage causes activation is difficult and requires knowledge of material conductivity, which varies from patient to patient.

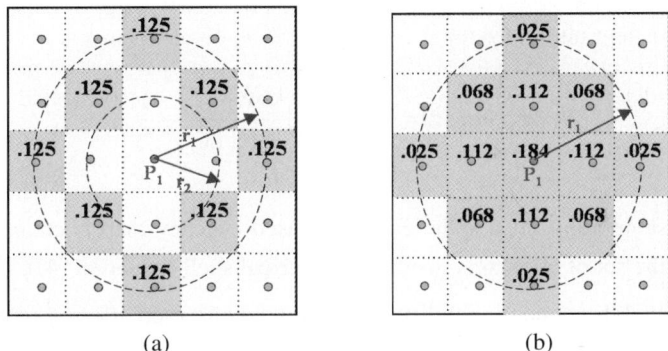

Fig. 2. Example of (a) Annulus pdf kernel (b) Truncated Gaussian (trunc-Gaussian) pdf kernel

Here we rely on a heuristic approach, i.e., we define r = k*V, where k is some proportionality constant. By using various values of k from 0.25 to 3, we determined that k = 1 produced maps that correlated the best with the underlying anatomy.

2.4 Creation of Field and Efficacy Maps

In order to minimize the variability among neurologists in their subjective assessment of efficacy, we included only those data points that recorded efficacies of at least 75% at 4V or less. Let P_1 be a stimulation point with image coordinates (X, Y, Z) be one such point. At our institution the assessment of efficacy by neurologists during DBS surgery is a personal subjective measure. It is expressed as percentage improvement in symptoms compared to the baseline measured at the beginning of the surgery or evaluation process. In order to reduce the variability in this subjective assessment across various neurologists, we have used a threshold of 75%. Our neurosurgical team agreed that a minimum assessment of 75% across various neurologists would in general represent good symptomatic relief. The 4V cutoff is used because the linear relationship assumed between V and r may not be valid at high voltages. Let *Efficacy* represent the percentage efficacy observed at P_1 by applying voltage V.

For the creation of a Gaussian kernel based field map, a truncated 3D Gaussian is placed at P_1. Let Ω_1 be the set of all points inside a sphere centered at P_1 having a radius r_1 mm (equation (1)). The value of the Gaussian kernel based map at any point with coordinates (x, y, z) in the image due to the observation at P_1 is $F_{P1}(x, y, z)$ defined in equation (2). The map values $F_{P1}(x, y, z)$ are normalized so that they result in a probability density function (equation (3)).

$$Let\ \Omega_1 = \{(x,y,z) \in \mathbb{N}^3 \mid (x-X)^2 + (y-Y)^2 + (z-Z)^2 \leq r_1^2\}, where\ r_1 = V \qquad (1)$$

$$F_{P_1}(x,y,z) = \begin{cases} \dfrac{1}{\sigma * \sqrt{2*\pi}} * \exp\left(\dfrac{-\{(x-X)^2 + (y-Y)^2 + (z-Z)^2\}}{2*\sigma^2}\right), \\ when\ (x,y,z) \in \Omega_1 \\ 0, otherwise \end{cases} \qquad (2)$$

$$\overline{F}_{P_1}(x,y,z) = \dfrac{F_{P_1}(x,y,z)}{\sum\limits_{(x',y',z') \in \Omega_1} F_{P_1}(x',y',z')} \qquad (3)$$

For the same point P_1, a spherical shell based efficacy map is created as follows. Let Ω_2 be the set of all voxels inside the spherical shell (equation (4)). Every point in Ω_2 is assigned the same probability of causing the observed efficacy (equation (5)).

$$\Omega_2 = \{(x,y,z) \in \mathbb{N}^3 \mid r_2^2 < (x-X)^2 + (y-Y)^2 + (z-Z)^2 \leq r_1^2\}$$
$$where\ r_1 = V\ and\ r_2 = r_1 - 1 \qquad (4)$$

$$\overline{F}_{P_1}(x,y,z) = \begin{cases} \dfrac{1}{n(\Omega_2)} & when\ (x,y,z) \in \Omega_2 \\ 0, otherwise \end{cases} \qquad (5)$$

where $n(\Omega_2)$ is the number of elements in the set Ω_2

When multiple points $P_1, P_2... P_N$ are used in building a map, the overall efficacy map is defined as in equation (6). For any point with coordinates (a, b, c) in the image:

$$F(a,b,c) = \frac{1}{N} * \left(\sum_{i=1}^{N} \overline{F}_{P_i}(a,b,c) \right) \qquad (6)$$

Efficacy maps attain greater significance when they can be created for a new patient using data from a number of other patients. To create such a map for a new patient, efficacy data from a population of previously treated patients is first projected onto an atlas using non-rigid registration between each patient and the atlas. This data is then projected onto the new patient using non-rigid registration between the atlas and the new patient. Using these projected data points a map can be created on the new patient by the method described above.

3 Validation Results and Discussion

We simulated both Gaussian field maps and annulus based efficacy maps. The results are shown in Fig. 3. On a grid with voxel dimensions 0.5x0.5 mm^2, Gaussian and annulus kernels were placed at measurement points (marked by gray circles) as shown in Fig. 3(a) and Fig. 3(b) respectively. Let the stimulation voltage at all the points be 2V. Thus, the radius of the Gaussian kernel was 2 mm (4 pixels). The outer radius of the annulus kernel was also 4 pixels while the inner radius was 2 pixels (equivalent to 1V). The two maps were created using the procedure described in section 2.4. Low probability values are represented by dark pixels while higher probability values are represented by brighter pixels. It would be expected from the positions of the points that stimulation response observed at each of the points is likely due to stimulation of the common region enclosed by the points (shown by large dotted circle). This is exactly what the annulus map suggests. The figure also shows that the field map does not permit localizing this point easily.

On a number of real patient datasets (not shown here for lack of space), our neurosurgical team has validated the spherical shell based maps and concluded that their locations are anatomically valid.

We have also started a prospective study where we create an efficacy map for a patient undergoing surgery and validate it as the surgery progresses. Two such maps created for recent surgeries are shown in Fig. 4. Low probability of efficacy values are represented by dark pixels while higher probability values are represented by brighter pixels. It can be seen that these spherical shell efficacy maps overlap well with the location where the implant was placed. The four contacts of the Medtronic 3389 implant are shown as four squares with the center of the implant (mid-point of the four contacts) labeled as the *final electrode position* (FEP). The point marked *planned target* refers to the target selected manually by the neurosurgeon preoperatively based on anatomical information (the efficacy map was not presented to the surgeon at the time of planning). *Atlas predicted target* refers to the point selected by the atlas using the method proposed by D'Haese et al [8].

It can be seen that at least two contacts of the implant are inside the hot zone (brighter areas) of the efficacy maps. In Fig. 4(b), it can be seen clearly that the planned target was outside the efficacy zones in the map, but intraop adjustment moved the final implant position inside the map. Similar results are shown in

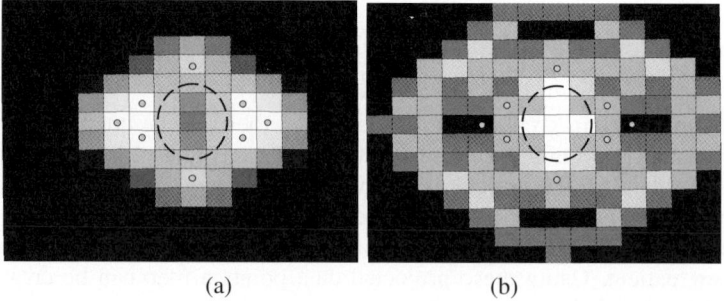

Fig. 3. Simulation of maps using (a) Gaussian kernel, (b) annulus kernel; on a grid with voxel dimensions 0.5x0.5 mm². At each measurement point (marked by a gray circle) efficacy is assumed to be recorded at 2V. The maps are created using the method described in section 2.4. Low probability values in the map are in dark while higher probability values are brighter.

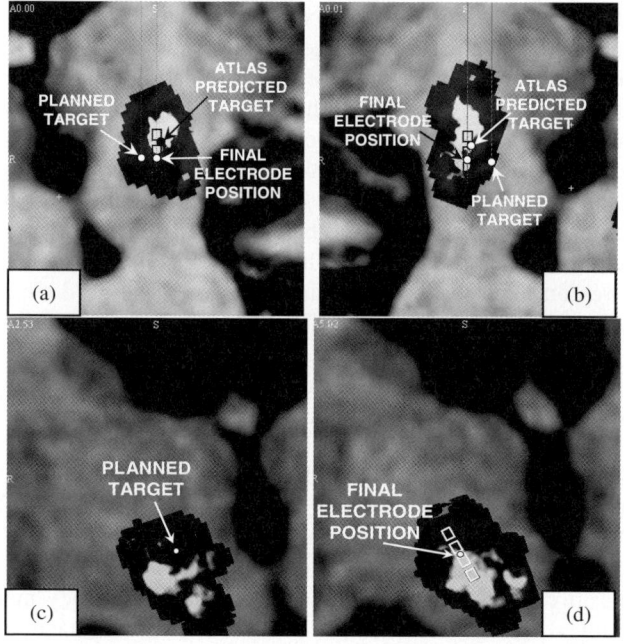

Fig. 4. Spherical shell efficacy maps overlaid on patient MRI T1 coronal slices aligned to the axis of the Medtronic 3389 implant. The center of the implant (final electrode position - FEP), the planned target and the atlas predicted target are marked. (a) Left STN, (b) Right STN for one patient. For right STN on another patient (c) planned target, (d) FEP. Low probability values in the map are shown as dark while higher probability values are brighter.

Figs. 4(c) and 4(d) for another patient. However, it can be seen that the FEPs in the figures are still not centered on the efficacy maps. One of the reasons is that the final implant is placed at a location where efficacy is high at low voltage but also where side effects occur (if any) at higher voltages. Therefore, we are generating side effect maps using the same method described in this paper to use them in combination with the efficacy maps. Another reason could be intra-op brain shift. We are evaluating its significance and working on accounting for it while generating such maps. Submission rules for the conference required us to submit the manuscript in black and white. On a color scale the maps present more detailed information on the locations and topologies of high efficacy spots. These results, albeit preliminary, show that accurate efficacy maps superimposed to anatomic images could be of value when planning DBS surgery.

4 Conclusion

In this work, we have shown that Gaussian kernels are not the best choice to create electrophysiological maps from discrete stimulation data points recorded during surgery. We have proposed a new spherical shell kernel consistent with the cause and effect relationship between stimulation and the response observed. Our simulation results confirm that spherical shell kernels are better than Gaussian kernels. On a number of real patient datasets, our neurosurgical team has validated the spherical shell based maps and concluded that their locations are anatomically valid. We also show the performance of our new maps on real patient data and report on a prospective study we have started to further validate our maps and to test their value as pre-operative planning and intra-operative guidance tools. The framework provided here can also be used to create side effect maps, which are under construction. If accurate and patient-specific efficacy and side effect maps can be produced, the selection of the optimal DBS target will be greatly facilitated.

References

1. Plaha, P., et al.: Stimulation of the caudal zona incerta is superior to stimulation of the subthalamic nucleus in improving contralateral parkinsonism. Brain 129(7), 1732–1747 (2006)
2. D'Haese, P.-F., et al.: Deformable Physiological Atlas-Based Programming of Deep Brain Stimulators: A Feasibility Study. In: Pluim, J.P.W., Likar, B., Gerritsen, F.A. (eds.) WBIR 2006. LNCS, vol. 4057, pp. 144–150. Springer, Heidelberg (2006)
3. Guo, T., Parrent, A.G., Peters, T.M.: Automatic target and trajectory idetification for deep brain stimulation (DBS) procedures. In: Ayache, N., Ourselin, S., Maeder, A. (eds.) MICCAI 2007, Part I. LNCS, vol. 4791, pp. 483–490. Springer, Heidelberg (2007)
4. Rhode, G.K., Aldroubi, A., Dawant, B.M.: The adaptive bases algorithm for intensity-based nonrigid image registration. IEEE Trans. On Medical Imaging 22(11), 1470–1479 (2003)
5. Fitzpatrick, J.M., et al.: Accuracy of Customized Miniature Stereotactic Platforms. Stereotactic and Functional Neurosurgery 83, 25–31 (2005)
6. Butson, C.R., McIntyre, C.C.: Role of electrode design on the volume of tissue activated during deep brain stimulation. Neural Eng. 3, 1–8 (2006)
7. Butson, C.R., McIntyre, C.C.: Current steering to control the volume of tissue activated during deep brain stimulation. Brain Stimulation 1, 7–15 (2008)
8. D'Haese, P.-F., et al.: Computer-Aided Placement of Deep Brain Stimulators: From Planning to Intraoperative Guidance. IEEE Trans. on Medical Imaging 24(11), 1469–1478 (2005)

Cardiac Electrophysiology Model Adjustment Using the Fusion of MR and Optical Imaging

D. Lepiller[1], M. Sermesant[1], M. Pop[2], H. Delingette[1], G.A. Wright[2], and N. Ayache[1]

[1] ASCLEPIOS Research Project, INRIA, Sophia Antipolis, France
[2] Department of Medical Biophysics, University of Toronto, Sunnybrook Health Sciences Centre, Toronto, Canada

Abstract. Despite important recent efforts in cardiac electrophysiology modelling, there is still a strong need for validating macroscopic models, that are well suited for diagnosis and treatment planning. In this paper we present a method to adjust the parameters of a macroscopic electrophysiology model on depolarisation and repolarisation maps obtained *ex-vivo* from optical imaging. With this imaging technique, optical fluorescence data are recorded with high spatial and temporal resolution on a large healthy porcine heart. A model of the myocardium is built from the MR images of the same heart, which also integrates the myocardial fibre orientation measured with DTI. We then present the first quantitative adjustment of a personalised volumetric model of the myocardium.

1 Introduction

In order to provide a better understanding of the mechanisms involved in cardiac arrhytmias, a variety of mathematical models have been developed for several decades to numerically simulate the cardiac electrophysiology at different scales. There are three main categories of such models. Ionic models [1] of the cardiac electrical activity describe the variation of ion concentrations across the membrane of cardiac cells. They may include a large number of variables and parameters. Their relative complexity usually leads to large computation times, but they can be precisely validated at the cell level. Far more simple are the Eikonal-based models [2], which only describe the time at which a depolarisation wave reaches a given point. At an intermediate level of complexity, we chose to use phenomenological models based on the transmembrane potential but without the different ion concentrations. They are based on PDEs that can describe with very few variables the coupled depolarisation and repolarisation processes.

This paper tackles the important issue of creating personalised electrophysiology models of the heart. Estimating the parameters of a model in order to decrease the error between the simulated variables and the observed ones is typically an inverse problem. Authors [3] focused recently on parameter estimation of the 63 variables Beeler-Reuter model at the cell level, but ionic models are not well suited for macroscopic model inversion due to the high number of parameters and variables to estimate. Theoretical results were recently demonstrated on the estimation of the bidomain model parameters and anisotropy, but only on a 2D surface, and with synthetic data [4]. On the other hand, the estimation of apparent electrical conductivity has been reported from clinical or experimental data based on Eikonal [5] and phenomenological models [6]. Although those pioneering works have reported good agreement between simulation and observations, they are somewhat limited since they only consider the depolarisation propagation on a surface and in some case [6] without taking into account the fibre orientation.

The objective of our work is to create a volumetric personalised electrophysiology model of the myocardium that takes into account the fibre orientation. Our approach relies on a tetrahedral mesh of the myocardium and estimates regionally two parameters in order to fit both the depolarisation and repolarisation isochrone maps. The parameter estimation is based on a calibration stage that takes advantage of existing analytical relationships in 1D between parameters and data. Furthermore, we rely on state of the art optical fluorescence imaging techniques to acquire *ex-vivo* isochrone maps on a pig heart. After applying different signal processing algorithms, dense maps can be retrieved. We then describe the creation of a computational personalised electrophysiology model from anatomical MR images, fibre orientation being extracted from subject specific Diffusion Tensor Imaging. Finally, we show the results of the estimation and discuss about the relevance of a synthetic model of fibre orientations.

2 Simulation of the Transmembrane Potential

The contraction of the heart muscle, the myocardium, is triggered by the depolarisation of the transmembrane potential. After depolarisation, a plateau phase begins during which the contraction develops ; this is the action potential duration (*apd*). The transmembrane potential then returns to a non-excited state (step called repolarisation). We use a phenomenological reaction-diffusion type model designed by Aliev-Panfilov [7], based on the transmembrane potential, to describe this propagation. It also takes into account the restitution phenomenon, *i.e.* the relation between heart rate and action potential duration. However, since we simulate and observe only one single cardiac cycle, a simplified repolarization equation, which neglects the description of the restitution curve, is used:

$$\begin{cases} \partial_t u = div(D\nabla u) + ku(1-u)(u-a) - uz \\ \partial_t z = -\epsilon(ku(u-a-1) + z) \end{cases} \quad (1)$$

In this formulation, u is a normalised transmembrane potential, and z is a variable modelling the repolarisation. The diffusion term is controlled by the diffusion tensor D which is similar to a physical conductivity. In the main direction of the tensor, this pseudo-conductivity is set to d which is one of the parameters we adjust, and to $d/2.5^2$ in the orthogonal directions [8]. Parameter k controls the repolarization, a the reaction phenomenon and ϵ the coupling between the transmembrane potential and the repolarization variable. This system is solved over a volumetric tetrahedral mesh of the left and right ventricles using the finite elements method. The excitation is generated by imposing a potential on a small set of vertices for a few milliseconds. The time integration of the system is done with an explicit Euler scheme.

3 Data Acquisition, Processing, and Fusion

Optical Imaging. It is very challenging to acquire quantitative data that precisely reveals *in vivo* physiology. However, useful data can still be extracted from electrical or, as it is the case here, optical recordings. They consist of the instants when the depolarisation (and the repolarisation) occurs at specific locations of the heart. These data, called activation times, are enough to estimate the speed of the depolarisation front, and thus to adjust the pseudo-conductivity d, and to calibrate the parameter a regarding the action potential duration, i.e. the difference between repolarisation and depolarisation times.

In this paper we performed the adjustments using optical recordings obtained in a healthy porcine heart. Large hearts are preferred for this work as they are close in size to human hearts. The explanted hearts were attached to a Langendorff perfusion system which permits to maintain the electrophysiological integrity of the hearts over 1-2 hours. The fluorescence dye (reflecting directly the changes of transmembrane potential) and the electromechanical uncoupler were injected into the perfusion line (more details are given in [9]). The hearts were paced with an electrode near the apex for 5 ms. The fluorescence signals are captured with high temporal (270 fps) and spatial ($<1~mm$) resolution, using a pair of CCD cameras (BrainVision, Jp). The signals giving the action potential waves at each pixel (Fig. 2a) were then filtered and further analysed to get a consistent map of activation times. The signal is scaled for each pixel between its baseline value and its maximum, cropping under the baseline which we got from segmenting the values into two clusters: the baseline being defined as the mean value of the lowest cluster. The scaled recording was then blurred by convolution with a 3D Gaussian, isotropic through space but wider in time (Fig. 2b). The depolarisation time is computed with the first derivative of each pixel signal, which presents a large peak when the depolarisation occurs. The repolarisation time is detected when the signal decreases 90% from its maximal value after depolarisation. Finally, the time maps for each cycle are reconstructed, stored as images and rectified based on the cameras calibration and stereoscopic parameters.

Optical and MR Data Fusion. At the end of the optical image acquisition, markers were put on the surfaces of the hearts, imaged with the CCD cameras, and the pig hearts scanned with a 1.5T Signa GE MR scanner. It can provide a detailed anatomical description of both the geometry and the fibre orientation (Fig. 1a,b). The surfaces of the hearts were created using classical segmentation algorithms (thresholding, mathematical morphology, isosurface extraction) and volumetric meshes were generated with a meshing software (GHS3D, developed at INRIA) resulting in tetrahedral geometries of approximatively 75 000 elements, with fibre orientation (Fig. 1c). Several hearts were imaged this way.

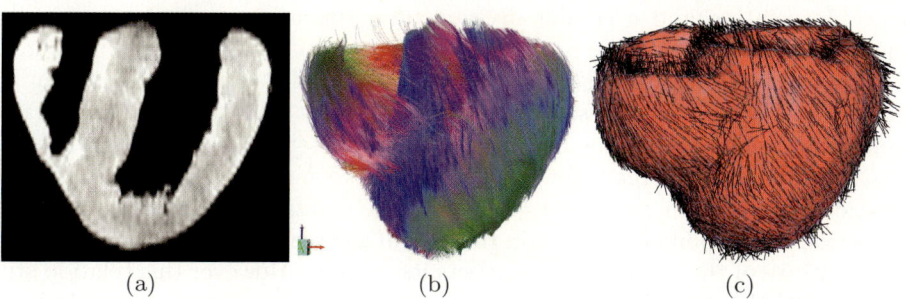

Fig. 1. MRI Data: **(a)** slice of the 3D volume used to create the myocardial mesh, **(b)** DTI fibre tracking, **(c)** generated volumetric mesh with assigned fibres (lateral views)

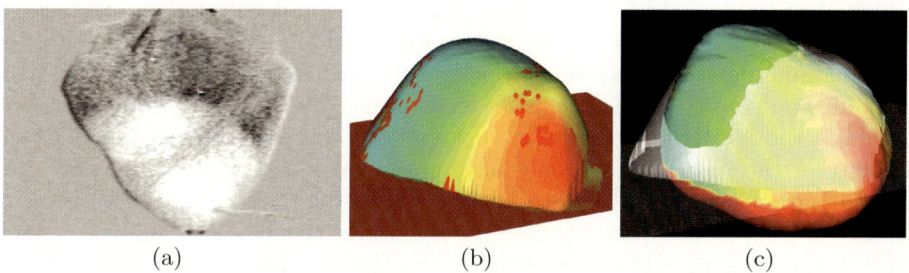

Fig. 2. Activation times measurement: **(a)** raw signal (anterolateral view) **(b)** isochrones computed from filtered signal on stereoscopic surface, **(c)** projection of the depolarisation times onto the MR derived mesh using registration (stereoscopic surface in transparency)

However, due to the complexity of the overall process, the full adjustment process was only done on one dataset.

The optical images recorded by the 2 CCD cameras were used to reconstruct the 3D surface of the heart using stereoscopy. Moreover, several opaque markers were glued onto the epicardium to provide a way to register the optical images with the MR images. We estimated a rigid transformation between the markers' optical and MR coordinates by minimizing the least-square difference. Each pixel of the optical recording corresponds to a vertex on the grid mesh which results from the stereoscopic reconstruction of the surface of the pig heart (further details can be found in [10]). Therefore the depolarisation front was spatially reconstructed, discretised on the mesh. We then projected these data onto the surface of the registered volumetric mesh from MR Imaging (results at Fig. 2c).

4 Parameter Estimation

Preparations. Setting constant parameters on the whole mesh would not allow us to take into account the local variations of the conduction velocity we observe. The left ventricle is therefore divided into 17 zones as defined by the American

Heart Association and a similar division into 9 zones is applied to the right ventricle.

From the one dimensional analysis of the Aliev and Panfilov model, it can be shown that planar waves are solutions, and it provides a relationship between the conduction velocity c and the first equation parameters [2] : $c = \sqrt{2kd}\,(0.5 - a)$. The same analysis was made for the relation between a and the action potential duration (apd), which gives: $apd = (a - 1)^2 / 4a$. Again, this formula is only the restriction to one dimension since in the case of a three dimensional propagation, the curvature of the diffusion front affects its velocity. However this relation still tells us that the diffusion speed depends on several parameters and provides a probable relationship.

It seems more appropriate to first adjust the parameter a from the action potential duration, since it does not depend on any other parameter, and then adjust the pseudo-conductivity parameter which would reflect the differences in conduction velocity in the tissue. In the Aliev-Panfilov model, d and k are the main parameters that affect this propagation speed. The d parameter represents the diffusion properties of the myocardial tissue whereas k accounts for the reaction of the ionic channels. Both can represent the variations of the electrical velocity of the tissue. As we only have one measure to adjust this speed, the depolarisation time, we chose to locally adjust the value of the parameter d, which represents this pseudo-conductivity, while keeping k globally constant. Due to the imaging and registration errors, the activation times could present local variations. To avoid the amplification of this noise by the spatial derivatives of these depolarisation times, we smoothed the local speed computation by averaging it over a neighbouring area, weighted by the Euclidean distance between the vertices and the point where the speed is computed.

Calibration. The calibration method involves simulating several propagations on the mesh using a range of values for d (resp. a), and to look at the corresponding speeds (resp. action potential duration). Then a function is fitted in the least square sense to these points in order to extract an analytical relationship between d and c (resp. a and apd), selected from the one dimensional analysis:

$$c(d) = \alpha\sqrt{d} + \beta \quad \text{and} \quad apd(a) = \frac{\gamma a^2 + \delta a + \mu}{a} \qquad (2)$$

We added a constant β to the relationship between d and c in order to better fit the numerical simulations. The idea of the calibration is also to take into account the numerical diffusion and discretisation errors in the calibration function.

This approximation is determined by computing the median conduction velocity (resp. apd) of each zone for each value of the parameter d (resp. a) throughout a range of values. Then we minimise the least square difference to estimate the function parameters. Once this relationship is estimated, we can use it to initialise the value of each parameter d_i (resp. a_i) for each zone, using the mean conduction velocity of each zone $\bar{c}_i$ (resp. the mean action potential duration $\bar{apd}_i$) computed with the measured activation times:

$$d_i = \left(\frac{\bar{c}_i - \beta}{\alpha}\right)^2 \quad \text{and} \quad a_i = \frac{(a\bar{p}d_i - \delta) \pm \sqrt{(a\bar{p}d_i - \delta)^2 - 4\gamma\mu}}{2\gamma} \quad (3)$$

Regarding the *apd*, since there are usually two solutions, we choose the one within the range of acceptable values for parameter a.

Iterative adjustment. After the initialisation of the chosen parameter, we iteratively improve the model fitting, with a simple gradient descent algorithm. We minimise the following criteria on each zone: $J(d_i) = (\bar{c}_i - \hat{c}(d_i))^2$ and $J(a_i) = (a\bar{p}d_i - a\hat{p}d(a_i))^2$ where $\hat{c}(d_i)$ is the median value of the simulated speed on the given zone using the parameter d_i ($a\hat{p}d(a_i)$ defined alike). By minimising the differences between the simulated and measured depolarisation speeds for each zone instead of using the depolarisation times, we adjust all zones at the same time and thus considerably reduce the number of simulations to compute the gradient descent algorithm. Indeed, we can simplify the problem by assuming that the conduction velocity (and the action potential duration) of a zone is not strongly influenced by their neighbouring velocities.

5 Results

Action potential duration. Even if the initial value for a was rather close to the measured values, the mean error on *apd* was still 44.6 *ms* ($\approx$15% of APD) (Fig. 3b) before the adjustment process, 28.1 *ms* ($\approx$9%) after calibration, and 21.5 *ms* ($\approx$7%) after adjustment (Fig. 3c). The histograms of errors (Fig. 3a) clearly show this decrease. We find a shorter action potential duration on the right ventricle, as described in the literature.

Depolarisation times. Before calibrating the model, the mean absolute error on depolarisation times was 30.6 *ms* ($\approx$17% of the depolarisation duration)

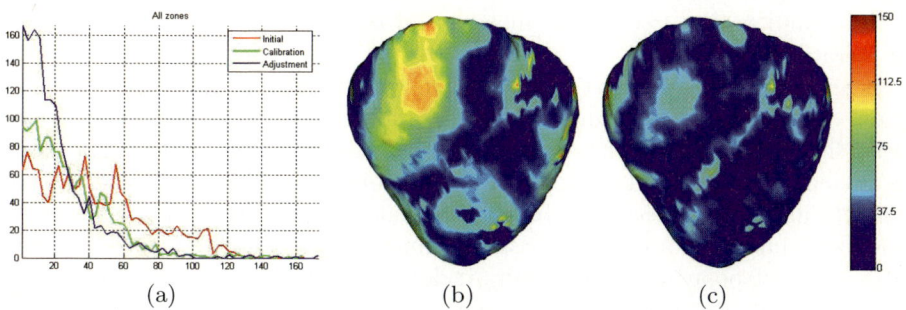

Fig. 3. (a) Histogram of errors on action potential duration across vertices (abscissa : error values in *ms*) and map of the error (b) before and (c) after adjustment (times in *ms*, anterolateral views)

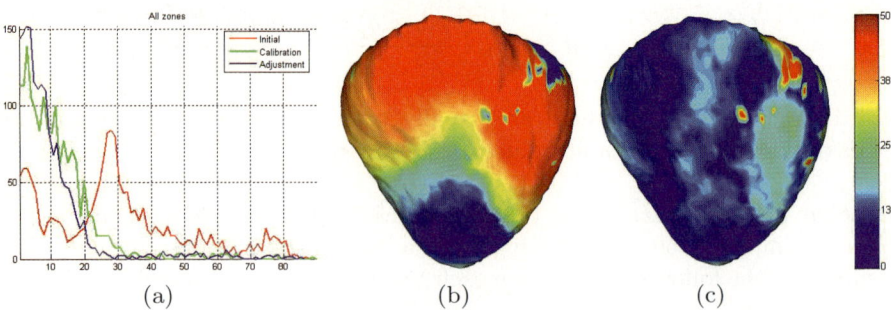

Fig. 4. (a) Histogram of errors on depolarisation time across vertices (abscissa : error values in ms) and map of the error (b) before and (c) after adjustment (times in ms, anterolateral views)

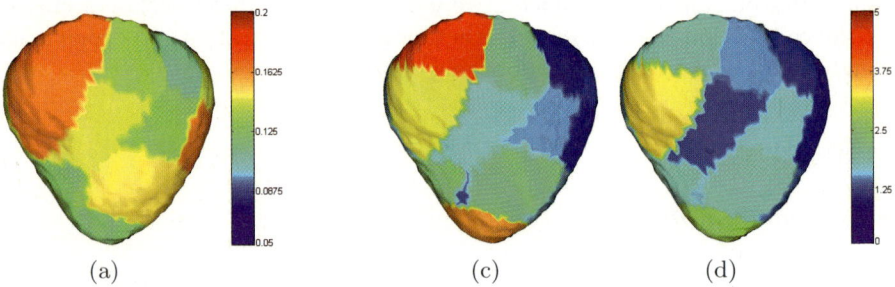

Fig. 5. Values of parameters after adjustment (a) of parameter a (c) of pseudo-conductivity d with measured fibre directions, (d) of pseudo-conductivity d with synthetic model of fibres (anterolateral views)

(Fig. 4b). After the initial step of calibration, it decreased to 12.0 ms ($\approx 7\%$) and the gradient descent algorithm further reduced it to 10.0 ms ($\approx 5.5\%$) (Fig. 4c). With an error nearly divided by three, the calibration clearly improved the model accuracy and proved itself to be more useful than just an initialisation step of the iterative adjustment.

As in-vivo DTI is not yet available, we tested the relevance of a synthetic model of the fibre orientation, for clinical applications. The generation of synthetic fibres is based on the assumption that the elevation angle of the fibres on the endocardium and the epicardium is constant ($+90°$ and $-60°$ respectively, to match the measured fibres), and that it varies linearly in between. Although the initial error on depolarisation times was higher than before (37.9 ms, $\approx 21\%$ of the depolarisation duration), it decreased at nearly the same level than the previous adjustment final result with 10.7 ms ($\approx 6\%$), showing that in this healthy case, the synthetic fibres provide a good alternative. Moreover, we can see with the comparison of estimated pseudo-conductivity maps with natural and synthetic fibres (Fig. 5c and 5d) that synthetic fibres provide a smoother variation.

6 Conclusion

In this work we have verified that phenomenological models having a small number of parameters are well suited for personalisation, while keeping their ability to match the main characteristics of the action potential propagation: duration, speed, anisotropy. The processing of the activation times gives good results and the stereoscopic reconstruction and registration are accurate enough to convert the optical measurements into a smooth dataset of epicardial activation times. This leads to an estimation of parameters which considerably decreases the final error between model predictions and experimental measurements. Finally, the relevance of a synthetic anisotropy model was demonstrated. In the future, a multi-resolution scheme with an automatic recursive zone splitting should help the parameter optimisation process in convergence and provide a better segmentation of the locations where the conductivity varies significantly.

References

1. Noble, D.: A modification of the hodgkin–huxley equations applicable to purkinje fibre action and pace-maker potentials. J. Physiol. 160, 317–352 (1962)
2. Keener, J., Sneyd, J.: Mathematical Physiology. Springer, Heidelberg (1998)
3. Dokos, S., Lovell, N.H.: Parameter estimation in cardiac ionic models. Progress in Biophysics and Molecular Biology 85(2-3), 407–431 (2004)
4. Sadleir, R., Henriquez, C.: Estimation of cardiac bidomain parameters from extracellular measurement: two dimensional study. Annals of Biomedical Engineering 34(8), 1289–1303 (2006)
5. Chinchapatnam, P., Rhode, K., King, A., Gao, G., Ma, Y., Schaeffter, T., Hawkes, D., Razavi, R., Hill, D., Arridge, S., Sermesant, M.: Anisotropic wave propagation and apparent conductivity estimation in a fast electrophysiological model: Application to XMR interventional imaging. In: Ayache, N., Ourselin, S., Maeder, A. (eds.) MICCAI 2007, Part I. LNCS, vol. 4791, pp. 575–583. Springer, Heidelberg (2007)
6. Moreau-Villéger, V., Delingette, H., Sermesant, M., Ashikaga, H., McVeigh, E., Ayache, N.: Building maps of local apparent conductivity of the epicardium with a 2D electrophysiological model of the heart. IEEE Transactions on Biomedical Engineering 53(8), 1457–1466 (2006)
7. Aliev, R., Panfilov, A.: A simple two-variable model of cardiac excitation. Chaos, Solitons & Fractals 7(3), 293–301 (1996)
8. Hsu, E., Muzikant, A., Matulevicius, S., Penland, R., Henriquez, C.: Magnetic resonance myocardial fiber-orientation mapping with direct histological correlation. American Journal of Physiology 274, 1627–1634 (1998)
9. Pop, M., Sermesant, M., Chung, D., Liu, G., McVeigh, E., Crystal, E., Wright, G.: An experimental framework to validate 3D models of cardiac electrophysiology via optical imaging and MRI. In: Sachse, F.B., Seemann, G. (eds.) FIHM 2007. LNCS, vol. 4466, pp. 100–109. Springer, Heidelberg (2007)
10. Chung, D., Pop, M., Sermesant, M., Wright, G.: Stereo reconstruction of the epicardium for optical fluorescence imaging. In: MICCAI Workshop on Biophotonics Imaging for Diagnostics and Treatment, pp. 33–40 (2006)

Dynamic Model-Driven Quantitative and Visual Evaluation of the Aortic Valve from 4D CT*

Razvan Ioan Ionasec[1,2,**], Bogdan Georgescu[1], Eva Gassner[3], Sebastian Vogt[4], Oliver Kutter[2], Michael Scheuering[4], Nassir Navab[2], and Dorin Comaniciu[1]

[1] Integrated Data Systems, Siemens Corporate Research, Princeton, USA
[2] Computer Aided Medical Procedures, Technical University Munich, Germany
[3] Department of Radiology, Medical University of South Carolina, Charleston, USA
[4] Siemens Medical Solutions, Computed Tomography, Forchheim, Germany
razvan_ionasec.ext@siemens.com

Abstract. Aortic valve disease is an important cardio-vascular disorder, which affects 2.5% of the global population and often requires elaborate clinical management. Experts agree that visual and quantitative evaluation of the valve, crucial throughout the clinical workflow, is currently limited to 2D imaging which can potentially yield inaccurate measurements. In this paper, we propose a novel approach for morphological and functional quantification of the aortic valve based on a 4D model estimated from computed tomography data. A physiological model of the aortic valve, capable to express large shape variations, is generated using parametric splines together with anatomically-driven topological and geometrical constraints. Recent advances in discriminative learning and incremental searching methods allow rapid estimation of the model parameters from 4D Cardiac CT specifically for each patient. The proposed approach enables precise valve evaluation with model-based dynamic measurements and advanced visualization. Extensive experiments and initial clinical validation demonstrate the efficiency and accuracy of the proposed approach. To the best of our knowledge this is the first time such a patient specific 4D aortic valve model is proposed.

1 Introduction

Aortic valve disease represents the most common valvular disease in developed countries [1], and shows the second highest incidence among congenital valvular defects [2]. Although, aortic root preserving surgery [3] along with minimally invasive procedures are emerging, the management of patient with valvular heart disease (VHD) has remained challenging. Precise knowledge and reliable display of the four-dimensional valve characteristics are requested by clinicians.

To date, most data on geometry and dynamics were obtained by experimental studies on explanted valves or using animal models [4], with small numbers of

---

* This work was initiated as a joint diploma thesis between Friedrich-Alexander-University of Erlangen-Nuremberg and Siemens Corporate Research. We acknowledge the advice of Prof. Joachim Hornegger and Dr. Martin Huber.
** Corresponding author.

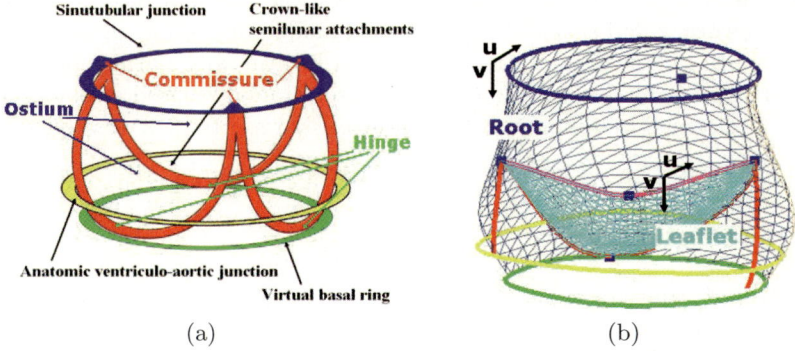

Fig. 1. (a) A generic aortic valve model in perspective view. Reproduced with permission of the author and the European Association for Cardio-Thoracic Surgery from: Anderson RH (doi:10.1510/mmcts.2006.002527). (b) The proposed aortic valve model in perspective view, where u and v are the circumferential and height parametric direction, respectively, of the root and leaflets.

cases across publications. Standard dimensions of the aortic root are given in literature, though considerable variations in the geometry are recognized [5]. Quantitative and visual evaluation methods are limited to 2D images and are potentially affected by measurement inaccuracies [6].

Computed tomography is a rapidly evolving modality for non-invasive imaging of the heart which enables dynamic four-dimensional evaluation of cardiac structures throughout the cardiac cycle. However, quantification of the aortic valve is impaired by the need to translate the four-dimensional data set into a set of 2D planes in order to obtain measurements. This gives potentially erroneous results for the curved anatomy of the basal aorta. A four dimensional model derived from CT data sets offers the unique possibility to non-invasively visualize and quantify the dynamics of the human aortic root and leaflets in healthy and diseased valves.

Existent valve models presented in the literature [7,8] are either used for hemodynamic studies or for analysis of various prosthetic valves. Although some of them are generated from volumetric data, these models are generic and obviously not applicable for the evaluation of individual patients.

In this paper we introduce a new modeling framework for the aortic valve from 4D cardiac CT data. A dynamic model of the valve is constructed from anatomic structures together with physiology driven geometrical and topological constraints (Section 2.1). The patient specific parameters of the model are estimated from CT data by combining learning-based technologies into a three-stage, coarse-to-fine parameter estimation algorithm (Section 2.2): landmark detection, full model fitting and model dynamics estimation.

The estimated model enables for the first time precise morphological and functional quantification as well as enhanced visualization of the aortic valve. This novel model-based evaluation paradigm has the potential to significantly advance the management of valvular heart disease.

Extensive experiments on 37 patients with various valvular disorders demonstrate the accuracy and speed of the proposed model estimation algorithm (Section 3.1). Initial clinical validation on various healthy and pathological valves shows a strong correlation among a proposed set of model-based measurements, manually performed measurements and previously reported aortic valve dimensions (Section 3.2).

2 Physiological Valve Modeling

The morphology and function of the aortic valve is very complex, which is underlined by the lack of consensus regarding its optimal physiological description [9]. The central anatomical structures of the aortic valve are the leaflets and the root. Its function is to regulate the blood flow between the left ventricle and aorta.

2.1 Model Representation

We propose a physiology driven parametric 4D model capable to express a large spectrum of morphological and pathological variations of the aortic valve. A set of well-defined landmarks, which includes hinges, commissures, leaflet tips and coronary ostia, describe key anatomical locations of the valve (see Fig. 1(a)). The aortic root and leaflets form the central anatomic structures and their geometries are represented by Non uniform rational B-splines (NURBS), which is the de facto standard in computational modeling. These components together with topological and geometrical constraints define a physiologically compliant model of the aortic valve, capable to implicitly handle bicuspid malformations.

The aortic root connects the left ventricular outflow tract to the ascending aorta and provides the supporting structures for the leaflets. This is represented by a NURBS surface $C^{root}(u,v)$ closed in the u parametric direction and can be imagined as a deformed cylinder constrained by the hinge, commissure and ostia points:

$$\underbrace{C^{root}(u,v)}_{u,v \in [0,1]} = \frac{\sum_{i=0}^{n}\sum_{j=0}^{m} N_{i,d}(u)N_{j,e}(v)w_{i,j}\boldsymbol{P}_{i,j}^{root}}{\sum_{i=0}^{n}\sum_{j=0}^{m} N_{i,d}(u)N_{j,e}(v)w_{i,j}} \quad \begin{aligned} C^{root}(u_k^h, v_k^h) &= \boldsymbol{L}_k^h, 0 \leq k < 3 \\ C^{root}(u_k^c, v_k^c) &= \boldsymbol{L}_k^c, 0 \leq k < 3 \\ C^{root}(u_k^o, v_k^o) &= \boldsymbol{L}_k^o, 0 \leq k < 2 \end{aligned}$$

$$\boldsymbol{P}_{l,j}^{root} = \boldsymbol{P}_{l-n,j}^{root}, 0 \leq l \leq d, 0 \leq j \leq m$$

(1)

where $\boldsymbol{P}_{i,j}^{root}$ are the control points, $w_{i,j}$ are the corresponding weights, $N_{i,d}(u)$ and $N_{j,e}(u)$ are the dth and e^{th} degree B-splines basis functions defined on the non-periodic knot vector U and V, respectively. The root surface C^{root} passes through the hinges ($\boldsymbol{L}_h^r$), commissures ($\boldsymbol{L}_c^r$) and ostia ($\boldsymbol{L}_o^r$) landmarks at parametric location (u_k^h, v_k^h), (u_k^c, v_k^c) and (u_k^o, v_k^o), respectively. A comprehensive description of NURBS is given in [10].

The three valvular leaflets, expressed as NURBS paraboloids, are fixed to the root on an attachment crown delineated by the hinges and commissures, while the remaining free edge of the leaflets is constrained by the corresponding tip point. These open and close during the cardiac cycle allowing one way blood flow during systole, from the left ventricle to the aorta:

$$\underbrace{C^{leaf^l}(u,v)}_{u,v \in [0,1]} = \frac{\sum_{i=0}^{n}\sum_{j=0}^{m} N_{i,d}(u)N_{j,e}(v)w_{i,j}\boldsymbol{P^{leaf^l}}_{i,j}}{\sum_{i=0}^{n}\sum_{j=0}^{m} N_{i,d}(u)N_{j,e}(v)w_{i,j}}$$

$$C^{leaf^l}(u_l^h, v_l^h) = \boldsymbol{L}_l^h$$
$$C^{leaf^l}(u_l^t, v_l^t) = \boldsymbol{L}_l^t$$
$$C^{leaf^l}(u, 0) = C^{root}(u_k^l, v_k^l)$$

$$\boldsymbol{P^{leaf^l}}_{0,0} = \boldsymbol{P^{leaf^l}}_{0,j} = \boldsymbol{L}_l^c, 0 \leq j \leq m$$
$$\boldsymbol{P^{leaf^l}}_{n,0} = \boldsymbol{P^{leaf^l}}_{n,j} = \boldsymbol{L}_{l+1}^c, 0 \leq j \leq m$$

(2)

where C^{leaf} stands for the lth leaflet surface and $\boldsymbol{P^{leaf^l}}_{i,j}$, $w_{i,j}$, $N_{i,d}(u)$ and $N_{j,e}(u)$ are defined analogous to equation (1). The surface converges into the adjacent commissures ($\boldsymbol{L}_l^c$ and $\boldsymbol{L}_{l+1}^c$), passes through the corresponding hinge ($\boldsymbol{L}_l^h$) and tip ($\boldsymbol{L}_l^t$), and the $0 - isocurve$ lies on the root at parametric locations (u_k^l, v_k^l).

It is straightforward within the NURBS framework to extend the above presented 3D model to a dynamic model (4D) using the tensor product, which introduces a temporal parametric direction t to the model representation [10].

2.2 Model Estimation

The parameters of the valve model proposed in section 2.1 are estimated for each patient from 4D cardiac CT data. A specific instance of the model is exactly determined by the landmarks and NURBS control points in a four-dimensional Euclidean space (3D+time), which cumulates into $3T(11 + 300)$ parameters[1]. Due the high dimension of the parameter vector, direct estimation in the original space is very difficult. We propose a three-step approach to estimate the parameters of the dynamic valve model, which are: landmarks detection, full model fitting and model dynamics estimation.

Landmark Detection. Recent advances in discriminative learning and incremental searching techniques are applied to automatically determine the landmarks locations ($\boldsymbol{L}_h^r$, $\boldsymbol{L}_c^r$, $\boldsymbol{L}_o^r$ and $\boldsymbol{L}_t^r$) from an input volume. A training set, which contains positive and negative samples of the landmarks positions, is created from a manually annotated database. We train a discriminative classifier $H(x, y, z)$ based on the Probabilistic Boosting Tree (PBT) [11], which learns the target distribution by exploiting a divide-and-conquer strategy:

$$p(\boldsymbol{L}_i|x_s, y_s, z_s) = H_i(x_s, y_s, z_s), x_s, y_s, z_s \in D_i \qquad (3)$$

---

[1] T represents the number of discrete samples in the time dimension (10 for a regular 4D cardiac CT acquisitions), 11 and 300 the number of landmarks and control points, respectively.

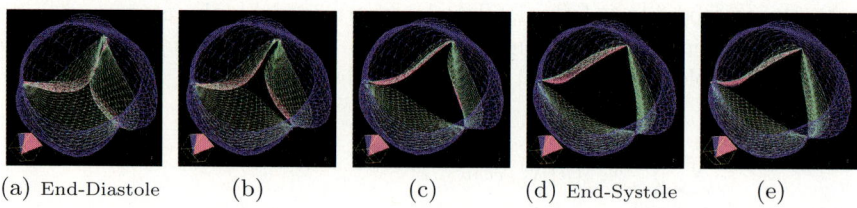

Fig. 2. (a-e) Five frames of the dynamic valve model obtained from a CT sequence

where $p(\boldsymbol{L_i}|x_s, y_s, z_s)$ is the probability of landmark $\boldsymbol{L_i}$ at location (x_s, y_s, z_s), H_i the strong classifier trained for $\boldsymbol{L_i}$ and D_i the search domain obtain from the training set. The detection is performed in a coarse-to-fine manner as well as in incrementally increasing parameter spaces similar to the marginal space learning (MSL) [12] concept.

A thin-plate-spline (TPS) transformation [13,14] is computed from the detected set of corresponding points, $K = \{(\boldsymbol{L_i^m}, \boldsymbol{L_i^I}), \boldsymbol{L_i^m} \in M, \boldsymbol{L_i^I} \in I, 0 < i \leq N\}$, which maps each control point of previously computed mean shape M at the corresponding location in the image I and provides an initial model estimation.

Full Model Fitting. The initial estimation obtained through landmark detection and TPS transformation provides a quite accurate global fitting of the model, however it requires further local processing for precise object delineation. A boundary detector is trained using the PBT algorithm in combination with steerable features, proposed in [12]. This is applied locally at a set of discrete boundary locations and is used to evolve the shape towards high probability responses of the boundary detector. The final estimation is obtained by fitting the parametric model to the refined samples by solving a linear least squares problem [15].

Model Dynamics Estimation. The estimation of the dynamic valve model follows a physiology-driven strategy and is more accurate and efficient compared to a sequential computation of the input sequence. Parameter estimation is initially performed for the dominant shapes observed in the end-diastolic (valve is completely closed) and end-systolic (valve is completely opened) cardiac phases, according to the algorithm described above. The estimation for the remaining frames exploits a prior model constructed as a linear combination of the two reference shapes, leading to a significant performance boost. Fig. 2 illustrates the dynamic model of the aortic valve estimated from a CT cardiac sequence.

3 Results

3.1 Results on Valve Model Estimation

We demonstrate the performance of the proposed algorithm on 37 4D cardiac CT data set, which consist of 364 CT volumes. The scans are acquired from

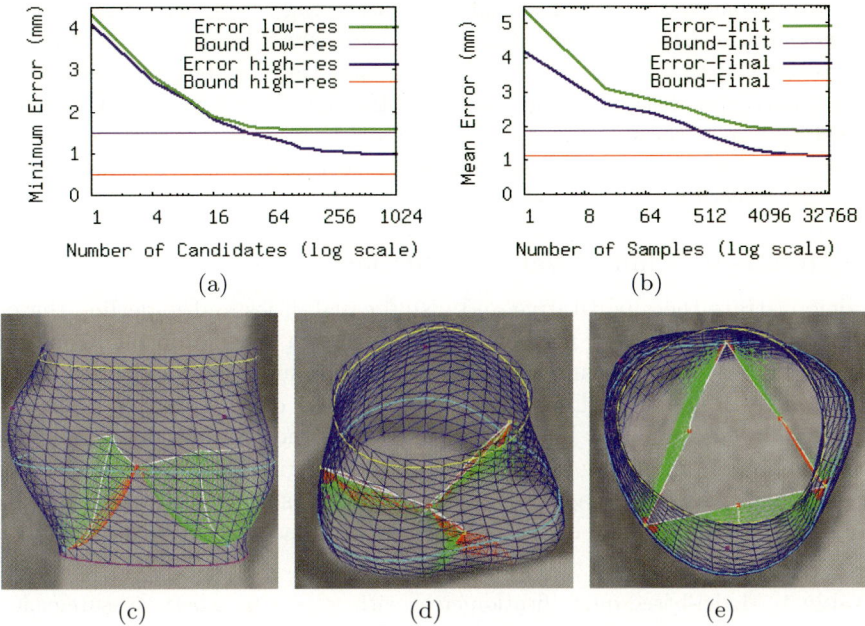

Fig. 3. (a) The detection error for the landmarks with respect to the cardinality of the candidates set. (b) The error curve for model estimation with respect to the number of samples. (c-e) Model estimation results in fused visualization.

different patients with various cardiovascular diseases using heterogeneous protocols, resulting in significant resolution and capture range variation (80 to 350 slices with sizes from 512x 512 to 153x153 pixels and resolution from 0.28 mm to 2.0 mm). Each volume in the data set is associated to an annotation, which was manually generated and is considered to be the ground truth. Three-fold cross validation is performed in order to evaluate our algorithm.

Performance of Landmark Detection. The landmark detection is evaluated by the Euclidean distance between the ground truth and detected positions. Initially, the detection is performed in low-resolution images and generates a set of position hypotheses for each landmark. Fig. 3(a) shows the error of the most accurate hypothesis, averaged over all landmarks, with respect to the cardinality of the hypotheses set. An optimal trade-of between speed and accuracy is achieved by keeping 100 candidates with an error of 1.59 mm. Detection is refined in high resolution images (1mm), which enables 10% increase in accuracy for 30% hypothesis. Averaging over the candidates set results in the final detection error of 2.28 mm.

Performance of Model Estimation. The model estimation accuracy is evaluated by the point-to-mesh measurement, which computes the average distance between sample pairs of the detected and ground-truth model. The accuracy of the initial model estimation relative to the rendering and computation resolution used within the system (2500 samples) is on average 2.00 mm. The model refinement improves the estimation accuracy by nearly 40% (see Fig. 3(b)), equivalent to an error of 1.33 mm. The computation time of the proposed method was evaluated on a standard desktop machine (3.0 GHz CPU, 2.0 GB RAM). The estimation of the full dynamic valve model from a regular CT sequence (10 volumes), is computed in 21.3 seconds with 70% of the time required for the landmark detection.

3.2 Results on Clinical Valve Evaluation

We demonstrate the quantitative and visual capabilities and underline the performance of the proposed method by comparing a set of morphological and dynamic model-based measurements to expert measurements and literature reported valve dimensions. Evaluation is performed on CT images of healthy, stenotic, dilated aorta and bicuspid valves, while the ground truth is provided by measurements manually performed by a radiologist with five years of experience in cardiovascular imaging. Table 1 summarizes the evaluation results and demonstrates the precision of the proposed model-based quantification method.

Table 1. Model-based quantification error with respect to expert measurements

	VAJ (cm)	SV (cm)	STJ (cm)	AVA (cm^2)	LCT (mm)	RCT (mm)	NCT (mm)
Mean	0.137	0.166	0.098	0.120	2.211	1.951	2.352
STD	0.017	0.043	0.029	0.380	0.866	0.936	1.162

The root diameter, important in surgical treatment of dilated and stiff anatomies [4] is computed at three levels: ventricular-arterial junction (VAJ), sinus of valsalva (SV) and sinotubular junction (SJ). Severity assessment in patients with degenerative aortic stenosis is supported through the aortic valve area (AVA) measurement [6]. The mean AVA derived from the model was $3.74 \pm 1.34 cm^2$, correlation with respect to manual planimetry $r = 0.963$ and $p < 0.0001$, and Bland-Altman systematic bias $0.12 \pm 0.38 cm^2$. Left-coronary tip (LCT), non-coronary tip (NCT) and right-coronary tip (RCT) orthogonal excursion is proposed for the evaluation of valve's function and motion characteristic after surgery. Measurements variation in healthy and diseased valves is illustrated in Fig. 4.

Fused visualization of direct volume rendering (DVR) of the 4D CT dataset and the estimated model provides further anatomical insight. Advanced techniques [16] enable visualization via post color-attenuated transfer functions [17] of the aortic lumen from CTA and integration of the valve model geometry into the DVR. Combination of CT data and model geometry can be directly used for visual validation of the estimated parameters with respect to the anatomy and visual quantification of pathological valves. For real-time 4D rendering of the sequence we use GPU Raycasting to efficiently stream the volume and geometry data to the graphics card. The combination of these techniques is capable of rendering high quality images, at interactive frame rates (Fig. 4(a), 4(b)).

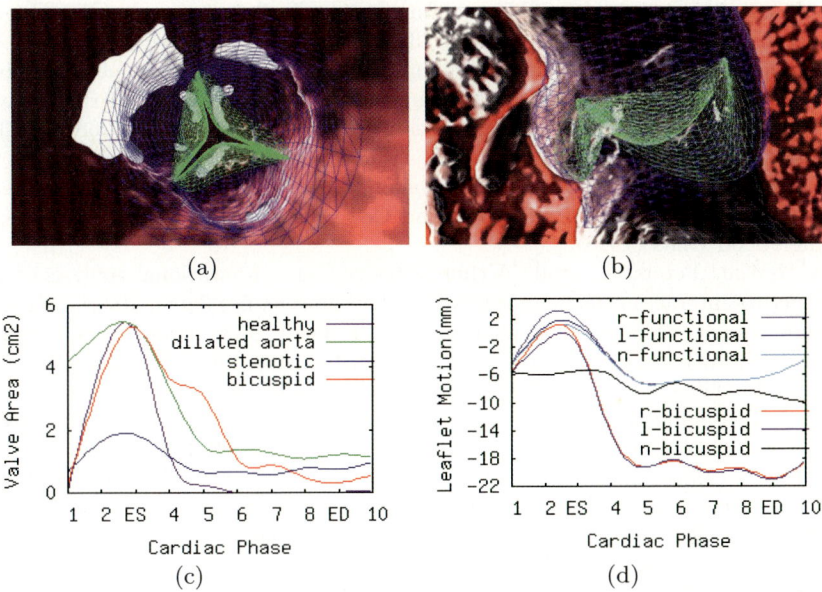

Fig. 4. Advanced visualization of (a) calcified aortic valve in endoscopic view and (b) bicuspid valve in long axis view. (c,d) Valve area and leaflet motion variation in different pathologies.

4 Discussion

This paper proposes a novel quantitative and visual evaluation approach of the aortic valve, based on a dynamic model estimated from 4D CT sequences. A robust and computationally efficient algorithm, which combines learning-based technologies into a coarse-to-fine approach, was proposed for estimating a patient specific valve model from imaging data. Automatic model-based measurements provide a significant advance in morphological and functional clinical evaluation of the aortic valve, currently limited to 2D imaging methods, operator-dependent and potentially inaccurate measurements. Future research will include high-level information provided by soft tissue composition and mechanical constrains, as well as investigations for other modalities (e.g. Ultrasound and MRI).

References

1. Nkomo, V., Gardin, J., et al.: Burden of valvular heart diseases: a population-based study. Lancet. 368(10), 1005–1011 (2006)
2. Hoffman, J., Kaplan, S.: The incidence of congenital heart disease. J. Am. Coll. Cardiol. 39(12), 1890–1900 (2002)
3. Yacoub, M.: Late results of a valve-preserving operation in patients with aneurysms of the ascending aorta and root. J. Thorac. Cardiovasc. Surg. 115, 1080–1090 (1998)
4. Dagum, P., Green, G., et al.: Deformational dynamics of the aortic root: modes and physiologic determinants. J. Thorac. Cardiovasc. Surg. 100(19), II54–62 (1999)

5. Labrosse, M.: Geometric modeling of functional trileaflet aortic valves: development and clinical applications. J. Biomech. 39(14), 2665–2672 (2006)
6. Vahanian, A., Baumgartner, H., et al.: Guidelines on the management of valvular heart disease: The task force on the management of valvular heart disease of the european society of cardiology. European heart journal 28(2), 230–268 (2007)
7. Peskin, C.S., McQueen, D.M.: Fluid dynamics of the heart and its valves. In: Othmer, H.G., Adler, F.R., Lewis, M.A., Dallon, J.C. (eds.) Case Studies in Mathematical Modeling: Ecology, Physiology, and Cell Biology, pp. 309–337. Prentice-Hall, Englewood Cliffs (1996)
8. De Hart, J., Peters, G., et al.: A three-dimensional computational analysis of fluid–structure interaction in the aortic valve. J. Biomechanics 36(1), 103–110 (2002)
9. Anderson, R.: The surgical anatomy of the aortic root. Multimedia Manual of Cardiothoracic Surgery (MMCTS) (2006)doi:10.1510/mmcts.2006.002527
10. Piegl, L., Tiller, W.: The NURBS book. Springer, London (1995)
11. Tu, Z.: Probabilistic boosting-tree: Learning discriminative methods for classification, recognition, and clustering. In: ICCV 2005, pp. 1589–1596 (2005)
12. Zheng, Y., Barbu, A., et al.: Fast automatic heart chamber segmentation from 3D ct data using marginal space learning and steerable features. In: ICCV (2007)
13. Duchon, J.: Interpolation des fonctions de deux variables suivant le principe de la flexion des plaques minces. RAIRO Analyse Numerique 10, 5–12 (1976)
14. Bookstein, F.L.: Principal warps: Thin-plate splines and the decomposition of deformations. IEEE PAMI 11(6), 567–585 (1989)
15. DeBoor, H.: A Practical Guide to Splines. Springer, New York (1978)
16. Scharsach, H., Hadwiger, M., Neubauer, A., Wolfsberger, S., Buhler, K.: Perspective Isosurface and Direct Volume Rendering for Virtual Endoscopy Applications. In: Proceedings of Eurovis/IEEE-VGTC Symposium on Visualization 2006, pp. 315–322 (2006)
17. Zhang, Q., Eagleson, R., Peters, T.: Rapid Voxel Classification Methodology for Interactive 3D Medical Image Visualization. In: Ayache, N., Ourselin, S., Maeder, A. (eds.) MICCAI 2007, Part II. LNCS, vol. 4792, pp. 86–93. Springer, Heidelberg (2007)

Interactive Simulation of Embolization Coils: Modeling and Experimental Validation

Jérémie Dequidt[1], Maud Marchal[1], Christian Duriez[1], Erwan Kerien[2], and Stéphane Cotin[1]

[1] Project-Team Alcove, INRIA Nord-Europe, France
{jeremie.dequidt,maud.marchal,christian.duriez,stephane.cotin}@lifl.fr
[2] Project-Team Magrit, INRIA Lorraine, France
erwan.kerrien@loria.fr

Abstract. Coil embolization offers a new approach to treat aneurysms. This medical procedure is namely less invasive than an open-surgery as it relies on the deployment of very thin platinum-based wires within the aneurysm through the arteries. When performed intracranially, this procedure must be particularly accurate and therefore carefully planned and performed by experienced radiologists. A simulator of the coil deployment represents an interesting and helpful tool for the physician by providing information on the coil behavior. In this paper, an original modeling is proposed to obtain interactive and accurate simulations of coil deployment. The model takes into account geometric nonlinearities and uses a shape memory formulation to describe its complex geometry. An experimental validation is performed in a contact-free environment to identify the mechanical properties of the coil and to quantitatively compare the simulation with real data. Computational performances are also measured to insure an interactive simulation.

1 Introduction

Interventional radiology offers a new alternative for the treatment of brain aneurysms. An aneurysm often consists in an abnormal bulge that appears close to branching arteries. Detachable coil embolization is a minimally invasive procedure that uses the vascular network to reach the diseased vessel. The interventional radiologist starts by inserting a catheter (a long, thin and flexible tube) into the femoral artery. This catheter is then manipulated through the arterial system until the aneurysm location is reached. Once in position, the physician places one or more small coils through the catheter into the aneurysm. The body responds by forming a blood clot around the coil, thus blocking off the aneurysm and considerably reducing the risk of rupture.

Although coil embolization is less invasive than open surgery, and allows treatment of cerebral aneurysms that previously were considered inoperable, such procedures are very difficult to perform and require an important experience from the interventional radiologist. This is particularly true when treating brain aneurysms, where any mistake occurring during the coil deployment or when

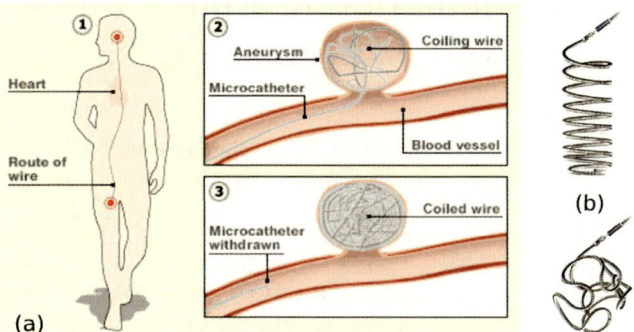

Fig. 1. (a): Coil embolization procedure: a catheter is inserted into the femoral artery to reach the brain (1) then a micro-catheter is placed near the diseased vessel and coils are inserted in the aneurysm (2). Finally, the micro-catheter is withdrawn and the body starts forming a blood clot around the coils (3). (b): two examples of coils with very different shapes: an helical shape (up) and a bird cage coil (bottom).

reaching the aneurysm could lead to a brain hemorrhage. Yet, even in the case of a successfully performed procedure, the choice of the coil (shape, length, diameter) plays a key role in the long term success of the procedure. In this context, the development of training systems or interactive planning systems, where the physician could select different coils and test their behavior in a patient-specific environment, could be very helpful. Previous work in the area of real-time or near real-time simulation for interventional radiology has mainly focused on training. For instance, Nowinski *et al.* [1], Hoefer *et al.* [2], Alderliesten *et al.* [3], or Duriez *et al.* [4] have proposed different approaches for modeling either catheter deformation and more generally catheter navigation in vascular networks. However, besides [3] none of these method has been validated, and currently, no real-time simulation of coils has been proposed nor validated.

In this paper, we introduce in section 2 a model for simulating very thin and flexible devices such as coils. We then show how to solve in real-time the dynamic equations derived from the model by using an optimized block matrix inverse method. An original approach is also proposed for describing the complex rest shape of coils. Co-axial combinations of endovascular devices (coil inside a micro-catheter for instance) are achieved using a *composite model*, which is based on a geometric combination of the characteristic rest shapes of each model. Section 3 presents the results of a quantitive validation study, based on a series of real coil deployments, which was performed to estimate the accuracy of our model.

2 Real-Time Model of Embolization Coil

2.1 Coil Model

Different types of coils can be used for embolization. Most of them have a core made of platinum, and are sometimes coated with another material or a biologically active agent. All types are made of soft platinum wire of less than a millimeter diameter and therefore are very soft. The softness of the platinum allows the coil to conform to the often irregular shape of the aneurysm, while the diameter, length and shape of the coil are chosen based on the shape and volume of the aneurysm, as well as the size of the neck of the aneurysm. In most cases, several coils are required to completely fill the aneurysm and maximize the chances to clot (see figure 1.

The proposed coil model uses a series of serially linked beam elements, similarly as proposed by Duriez et al. [4] for simulating catheters and guidewires. However, we introduce several modifications to take into account for the particular nature of coils. A different approach for solving the mechanical system of connected beams is also proposed. To model the deformation of the coil, a representation based on three-dimensional beam theory [4], [5] is used. Since coils exhibit a more important dynamic behavior during their deployment than catheter or guidewires during navigation, we additionally present a dynamic formulation of the model. For the entire structure describing a catheter or guidewire, the global stiffness matrix $\mathbf{K}$ is recomputed, at each time stetp, by summing the contributions of each beam element, through its elementary stiffness matrix $\mathbf{K_e}$. Assuming lumped masses at the nodes, the mass matrix $\mathbf{M}$ is a diagonal matrix. A damping matrix $\mathbf{D}$ is also introduced, thus leading to the following equilibrium equation:

$$\mathbf{M\ddot{x}} + \mathbf{D\dot{x}} + \mathbf{Kx} = \mathbf{f} \tag{1}$$

where $\mathbf{K}$ is a band matrix due to the serial structure of the model, and $\mathbf{\ddot{x}}$, $\mathbf{\dot{x}}$, and $\mathbf{x}$ represent, respectively, the vector of accelerations, velocities and positions of the nodes, while $\mathbf{f}$ represents the external forces applied to the coil. The damping matrix $\mathbf{D}$ is defined as a linear combination of the stiffness and mass matrices $\mathbf{D} = \alpha \mathbf{M} + \beta \mathbf{K}$, known as Raleigh damping. Note that each node is described by six degrees of freedom, three of which correspond to the spatial position, and three to the angular position of the node in a global reference frame (see figure 2a). The elementary stiffness matrix $\mathbf{K_e}$ introduced above is a 12×12 symmetric matrix that relates spatial and angular positions of each end of a beam element to the forces and torques applied to it (see [4] or [5] for more details). Each beam stiffness matrix is initially calculated in local coordinates, defined by a reference frame associated to the first node of the beam. In this reference frame, only deformations (bending, torsion, elongation) are measured. A transformation matrix $\mathbf{\Lambda}$ is then defined to change the local frame of reference to a global coordinate system. This leads to the following relationship between $\mathbf{\overline{K}_e}$ in local coordinates and $\mathbf{K_e}$ in a global frame: $\mathbf{K_e} = \mathbf{\Lambda}^T \mathbf{\overline{K}_e} \mathbf{\Lambda}$ As the beam deforms, only $\mathbf{\Lambda}$ changes and needs to be recomputed, while $\mathbf{\overline{K}_e}$ remains constant, as long as the deformation of the beam in its local frame remains small. To model a complex structure such as a coil, which undergoes large displacements, we need to discretize it as a series of beam elements to ensure that each beam deformation will remain small.

Boundary conditions are specified by defining a particular translation or rotation for the first node of the model to represent user control of the device (the coil is manipulated by pushing and twisting a wire). Since the first node

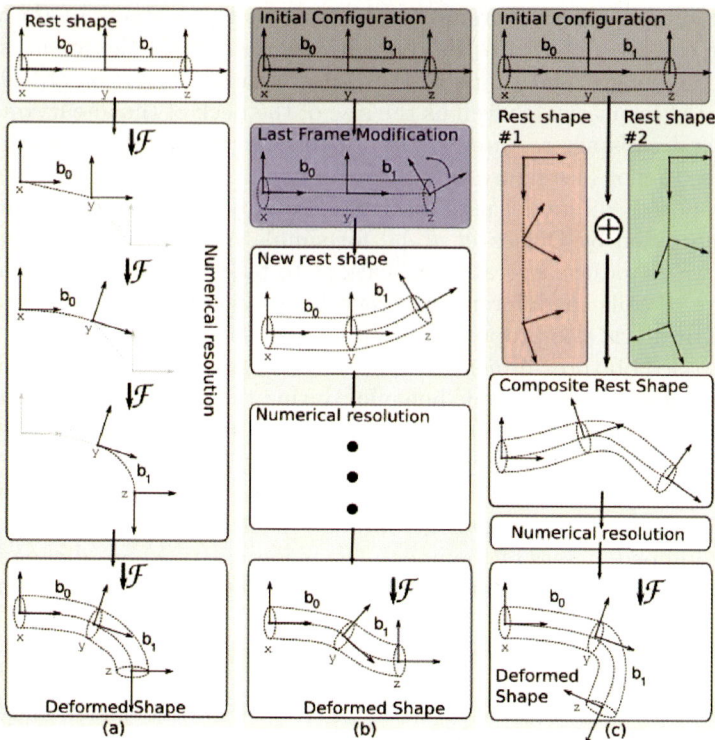

Fig. 2. Modeling of a wire using linked beam elements. (a) Given an initial rest shape and forces applied on DOFs, internal forces are computed using a local reference frame to handle large deformations. Starting from the first beam, reference frames are updated to suppress rigid transformation from the expression of the beam deformation. (b) Modification of the initial shape by moving frames or positions allows the generation of various deformed shapes. (c) A composite model (co-axial combination of two wires) is obtained by geometrically mixing different rest shapes on one geometric model.

of the model is constrained, the first beam equation will be used to update the local frame for the second node, thus allowing the second beam to be computed in a reference frame where no rigid transformation occurs. By repeating this process through the whole structure, we can compute $\mathbf{\Lambda}$ for each beam element and therefore determine $\mathbf{K_e}$. This method is closer to the co-rotational approach [6] than the incremental approach proposed in [4] and permits to model the geometric non-linearities that occur during the deformation of the coil.

2.2 Real-Time Computation

Equation (1) is integrated in time using a implicit integration scheme (Euler implicit) and then solved using an optimized linear solver that takes advantage of the nature of our model. All beam elements being serially connected, the resulting stiffness matrix $\mathbf{K}$ is a tridiagonal matrix with a band size of 12 (since each $\mathbf{K_e}$ is a 12×12 matrix). Since the mass and damping matrices are also diagonal, we solve the linear system using the algorithm proposed by Kumar *et al.* [7]. The solution can be obtained in $O(n)$ operations instead of $O(n^3)$. This allows computation times of less than 10 ms for a coil composed of 100 beam elements on a computer with a Core2Duo processor running at 2.66GHz.

2.3 Shapes Alteration and Composite Model

Devices such as catheters, guidewires and coils are not subject to elongation but mainly bending and twisting. They are also characterized by their rest shape, which plays a very important role in the delivery of the therapy. We model these complex shapes by changing the local frame at each node of the model, as illustrated in figure 2b. Obviously, an important feature is to dynamically modify theses frames at run-time to describe more complex behaviors. For instance, to simulate a coil being deployed from a micro-catheter, we avoid computing the complex interactions the take place between the coil and the micro-catheter. Instead we propose to simulate this behavior by using a composite model. The Halpin-Tsai [8] equations provide a framework to update mechanical properties of a reinforced fiber. This approach was applied to the simulation of catheters and guidewires by Lenoir *et. al.* [9]. In this paper, we propose an extension of this framework to take into account two or more local frames and combine them using weighted ponderation (see figure 2c) : $q_{cmp} = q_1 E_1/(E_1+E_2) + q_2 E_2/(E_1+E_2)$ where each q_i is the quaternion representing the transfomation from local frame global frame and E_i represents the beam Young modulus of the considered rest shape. As a consequence, such ponderation will give more influence on the final composite shape to stiff materials.

2.4 Parameter Identification

Exact mechanical properties of coils are difficult to obtain since they are not shared by device manufacturers. Among the parameters required to simulate our coil model, some of them are usually provided, such as coil length, diameter of the cross section and possibly some hints about the rest shape (circle diameter for helical-shaped coil for instance). Other parameters such as volumic mass, Young modulus and Poisson ratio can be found in mechanical engineering handbooks. Coils are made of platinum and other materials such as titanium, giving us an initial guess for what Young modulus and Poisson ratio values to use. Eventually, the rest shape is the decisive parameter we need to identify because this feature is very important for embolization coils. An optimization algorithm was used to determine the Young modulus, Poisson ratio and to adapt the rest shape of the coil given some datasets of a real coil.

3 Validation Experiment and Results

Qualitative and quantitative validations have been performed in order to verify the behavior of our coil modeling. A series of volumetric angiographic datasets of a coil deployment were used for our experimental validation. Simulations of a coil submitted to the same forces and constraints were computed and compared to the actual coil data. Through our optimization method, the unknown parameters were determined.

3.1 Experimental Setup

Our experimental setup consists of a box filled with water and a transversal fixed guide, defining the path for the catheter. The catheter is first introduced, followed by the helical coil as in the real procedure. The three-dimensional shape of the coil at different stages of the deployment is obtained from 3DXA (3D X-ray angiography) images using a marching cubes algorithm. The different steps of the experiment are illustrated in figure 3. In the following section, a validation of the coil simulations is reported for three different stages of the deployment. In these experiments, the coil is only subject to a gravity force, and contacts with the box were avoided.

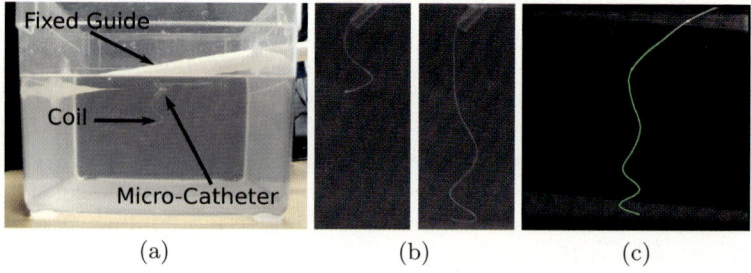

Fig. 3. Experimental setup: (a) the coil is deployed in a contact-free environment. (b) Volumetric data is obtained by 3DXA and a marching cube is performed to get a mesh of the real coil. (c) Central line of the coil is extracted and a continuous formulation is built using splines.

Table 1. Error measurement. The average and the standard deviation (SD) of the relative energy norm error are given in percentage in the first column. The second column contains the mean displacement of the coil for the three different steps.

	Relative Energy norm error	Mean total displacement
	Average % (SD)	(mm)
Stage 1	9.80% (4.05)	18.2
Stage 2	6.19 % (5.05)	24.99
Stage 3	4.17 % (1.42)	39.11

3.2 Coil Parameters

A helical coil *Micrus MicroCoil Platinum* is used for the validation. The parameters given by the manufacturer or those which can simply deducted are: mass: 1.28 g, length: 150 mm , radius: 0.3556 mm, helix diameter: 7 mm. This coil has

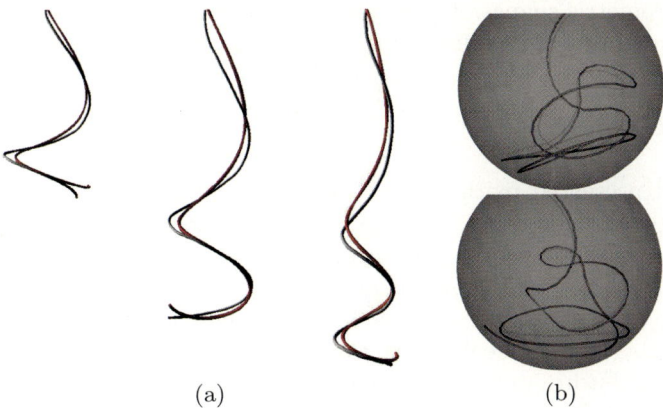

Fig. 4. (a) Visual comparison of our coil simulation (in red) with the reconstructed coil model from our experiments (in yellow) at different stages of the deployment. (b) Simulation of the deployment of a bird-cage coil in a simple virtual aneurysm using the same parameters as for the helical coil but a different rest shape.

an helical rest shape and it is therefore easy to create a good *initial guess* for our optimization method. The algorithm was applied for different datasets and the obtained parameters are: Young modulus $E = 7.5$ GPa, Poisson ratio $\nu = 0.39$ and the distance between two coils of the helix is equal to 0.25 mm. The value of those parameters are consistant with the values given in the handbooks.

3.3 Error Measurement

Figure 4 shows a visual comparison between our simulated coil deployment and a reconstructed model from experimental data. Once the real coil positions have been tracked and the shape segmented for three different stages of the coil deployment, an algorithm using a B-spline formulation was applied to the real coil data to obtain a continuous description of the shape. Then, simulations of the coil were performed using the same boundary conditions as measured during the actual coil deployment. In order to compare our simulation with the actual data, the B-spline curve was descretized using the same number of points as the number of nodes in the simlation. The error metric used to validate the coil simulation is the relative energy norm error [10]. The metric is defined as the ratio of the displacement between the simulated and the real coil and the real displacement. The error is computed for each node and for the three different steps of the deployment. The results are given in table 1. The relative energy norm error is small and exhibits that our simulation is close from real data. The absolute mean distance between simulated and real positions after deployment is equal to $1mm$ for each stage, explaining why the error increases if the coil is deployed on a small length.

3.4 Simulation of Other Coils

Given the parameters found for the helical coil, we can simulate the behavior or other types of coil as our rest-shape formulation allows an easy way to generate complex geometric shapes. Figure 4b illustrates this in the case of a "bird-cage" coil deployed inside a simplified aneurysm shape.

4 Conclusion

The model presented in this paper offers a computationnaly efficient simulation of surgical microcoils. The experimental validation against real data and the errors measured proves the accuracy of our model. Results are provided to demonstrate that our model is generic and can handle different rest shapes allowing to simulate different types of coils available from medical device manifacturers. This work is the first step towards building a realistic simulator for coil embolization. Future work will extend this experimental validation to the study of contacts between the coil and aneurysm wall and the influence of turbulent blood flow in the aneursym during coil deployment.

References

1. Nowinski, W., Chui, C.: Simulation of interventional neuroradiology procedures. In: MIAR, pp. 87–94 (2001)
2. Hoefer, U., Langen, T., Nziki, J., Zeitler, F., Hesser, J., Mueller, U., Voelker, W., Maenner, R.: Cathi - catheter instruction system. In: Computer Assisted Radiology and Surgery (CARS), Paris, France, pp. 101–106 (2002)
3. Alderliesten, T.: Simulation of Minimally-Invasive Vascular Interventions for Training Purposes. PhD dissertation, Utrecht University (2004)
4. Duriez, C., Cotin, S., Lenoir, J., Neumann, P.F.: New approaches to catheter navigation for interventional radiology simulation. Computer Aided Surgery 11, 300–308 (2006)
5. Przemieniecki, J.: Theory of Matrix Structural Analysis. McGraw-Hill, New York (1968)
6. Felippa, C.A.: A systematic approach to the element independent corotational dynamics of finite elements. Technical Report CU-CAS-00-03, Center for Aerospace Structures (2000)
7. Kumar, S., Petho, A.: An algorithm for the numerical inversion of a tridiagonal matrix. Communications in Numerical Methods in Engineering 9(4), 353–359 (1993)
8. Halpin, J., Kardos, J.: The halpin-tsai equations: a review. Polymer Engineering Science 16, 344–352 (1976)
9. Lenoir, J., Cotin, S., Duriez, C., Neumann, P.: Interactive physically-based simulation of catheter and guidewire. In: Second Workshop in Virtual Reality Interactions and Physical Simulations (VRIPHYS), Pisa, Italy (November 7, 2005)
10. Zienkiewicz, O., Taylor, R.: The Finite Element Method, 5th edn. Butterworth-Heinermann (2000)

Modelling Anisotropic Viscoelasticity for Real-Time Soft Tissue Simulation

Zeike A. Taylor[1], Olivier Comas[2], Mario Cheng[2], Josh Passenger[2], David J. Hawkes[1], David Atkinson[1], and Sébastien Ourselin[1]

[1] Centre for Medical Image Computing, University College London, Gower St, London, WC1E 6BT, UK
[2] BioMedIA Lab, e-Health Research Centre, CSIRO ICT Centre, Level 20, 300 Adelaide St, Brisbane, QLD, 4000, Australia
z.taylor@cs.ucl.ac.uk

Abstract. Previously almost all biomechanically-based time-critical surgical simulation has ignored the well established features of tissue mechanical response of anisotropy and time-dependence. We address this issue by presenting an efficient solution procedure for anisotropic visco-hyperelastic constitutive models which allows use of these in nonlinear explicit dynamic finite element algorithms. We show that the procedure allows incorporation of both anisotropy and viscoelasticity for as little as 5.1% additional cost compared with the usual isotropic elastic models. When combined with high performance GPU execution the complete framework is suitable for time-critical simulation applications such as interactive surgical simulation and intraoperative image registration.

1 Introduction

In recent years there has been growing interest in the use of computational biomechanics as a basis for simulation of soft tissues deformation. Example applications include interactive simulation environments [1,2,3] and biomechanically driven image registration [4,5,6]. Both such applications may be subject to stringent solution time constraints; interactive simulation requires solutions to be obtained at visual, or even haptic feedback rates ($>$500Hz), while *intraoperative* image registration must be fast enough that the work flow of the surgical procedure is not interrupted. Therefore viable simulation procedures for these applications are necessarily those that yield rapid solutions.

While progress has been made with respect to inclusion of constitutive and kinematic nonlinearities, virtually all previous work in this area has ignored the well established phenomena of anisotropy and time-dependence (predominantly manifested as stress relaxation, creep, hysteresis, and strain rate-dependence) of tissue mechanical response [7]. Notable exceptions include [2,8], in which liver and facial muscles were treated as transversely isotropic, and [9,10], in which viscoelastic effects were included. Of these, only [2] reported real-time solution speeds, and to the best of our knowledge no authors have included both anisotropy and viscoelasticity in time-critical applications. In light of the abundant experimental evidence testifying the importance of these phenomena [11,7] and the comprehensive modelling approaches developed for their analysis [12], the issue appears to be one of computational complexity and the mentioned time-constraints.

We address this issue by presenting a constitutive update procedure for visco-hyperelastic materials suitable for use in explicit finite element algorithms. Material models of this type have been shown to very accurately reproduce the phenomena described above [11,7]. The formulation is general in the sense that any underlying elastic response may be included. In particular we show that kinematically consistent anisotropic formulations valid for large deformations are naturally accommodated. We demonstrate the validity and efficiency of the procedure within a graphics processor (GPU) -based finite element solver (specifically, a total Lagrangian explicit dynamic (TLED) solver [13,14,15]), and show that the framework is suitable for use in time-critical applications.

2 TLED Finite Element Algorithm

A complete description of the TLED algorithm is available in previous publications [13,15], where it has been shown to allow very rapid nonlinear analysis of soft tissues. Briefly, the algorithm consists of a precomputation phase in which various element and system quantities are calculated, followed by a time-loop in which incremental solutions for the node displacements $\mathbf{u}$ are found. During each step of the time-loop we

1. Apply loads (displacements and/or forces) and boundary conditions to relevant nodal degrees of freedom
2. For each element compute
   (a) deformation gradient $\mathbf{F}$ and right Cauchy-Green deformation tensor $\mathbf{C}$
   (b) linear strain-displacement matrix $\mathbf{B}_L$
   (c) 2nd Piola-Kirchhoff stress $\mathbf{S}$
   (d) element nodal forces $\tilde{\mathbf{f}}$, and add these to the total nodal forces $\mathbf{f}$
3. For each node compute new displacements $\mathbf{u}$ using the central difference method.

For under-integrated 8-node hexahedral elements the nodal force contributions from each element are obtained (via Gaussian quadrature) from $\tilde{\mathbf{f}} = 8\,\mathbf{B}_L^T \check{\mathbf{S}} \det \mathbf{J}$, where $\mathbf{J}$ is the precomputed element Jacobian matrix and $\check{\mathbf{S}}$ is the vector form of the stress tensor $\mathbf{S}$. This equation makes no assumption concerning the constitutive model employed. In the subsequent sections we describe a general formulation for anisotropic viscoelasticity, particular cases of which have been shown to be excellent models of the mechanical response of many soft tissues.

3 Anisotropic Visco-hyperelastic Constitutive Equations

In continuum mechanics the Helmholtz free energy (strain energy) function Ψ encapsulates the energy per unit volume associated with deformation of a material, and is the standard representation of the material's constitutive response. For hyperelastic materials Ψ is a function of the current deformation only, whereas for visco-hyperelastic materials it is a function of the entire deformation history. A complete visco-hyperelastic response may be obtained by augmenting hyperelastic strain energy functions with time dependent relaxation terms and expressing in convolution integral form. This affords generality since any underlying hyperelastic form may be used. In particular the formulation naturally accommodates anisotropic hyperelastic terms. We present equations for the case of transverse isotropy, which is the simplest class of anisotropy.

3.1 Hyperelastic Response

Transversely isotropic (TI) materials are characterised by a single preferred direction $\mathbf{a}$; the mechanical response is isotropic in the plane orthogonal to $\mathbf{a}$. In the present work we consider TI strain energy functions with separated isochoric (volume-preserving) and volumetric terms [12]: $\Psi(\mathbf{C}, \mathbf{a}) = \Psi^{\text{iso}}(\bar{I}_1, \bar{I}_2, \bar{I}_4, \bar{I}_5) + \Psi^{\text{vol}}(J)$, where $J = \det \mathbf{F}$. Here $\bar{I}_1 = \operatorname{tr} \bar{\mathbf{C}}$ and $\bar{I}_2 = [(\operatorname{tr} \bar{\mathbf{C}})^2 - \operatorname{tr}(\bar{\mathbf{C}}^2)]/2$ are the first two invariants of the modified right Cauchy-Green deformation tensor $\bar{\mathbf{C}} = J^{-2/3} \mathbf{F}^T \mathbf{F}$, while $\bar{I}_4 = \mathbf{a} \cdot \bar{\mathbf{C}} \mathbf{a}$ and $\bar{I}_5 = \mathbf{a} \cdot \bar{\mathbf{C}}^2 \mathbf{a}$ are pseudo-invariants of both $\bar{\mathbf{C}}$ and $\mathbf{a}$. It may be observed that $\bar{I}_{1,2}$ are functions of deformation $\bar{\mathbf{C}}$ only, and therefore produce isotropic strain energy terms. In contrast $\bar{I}_{4,5}$ are direction-dependent, and produce strain energy terms associated with deformation in the direction $\mathbf{a}$ only – effectively producing a different stiffness in this direction.

The stresses are obtained by differentiation of Ψ: $\mathbf{S} = 2 \partial_\mathbf{C} \Psi = \mathbf{S}^{\text{iso}} + \mathbf{S}^{\text{vol}}$, where ∂_x denotes differentiation with respect to x. $\mathbf{S}^{\text{iso}}$ and $\mathbf{S}^{\text{vol}}$ are stresses obtained from differentiation of isochoric and volumetric strain energy terms, respectively, and may be shown to be [12]

$$\mathbf{S}^{\text{vol}} = 2\, \partial_\mathbf{C} \Psi^{\text{vol}} = Jp\mathbf{C}^{-1}, \qquad \mathbf{S}^{\text{iso}} = 2\, \partial_\mathbf{C} \Psi^{\text{iso}} = J^{-2/3} \operatorname{Dev} \bar{\mathbf{S}}, \qquad (1)$$

where

$$\bar{\mathbf{S}} = \bar{\gamma}_1 \mathbf{I} + \bar{\gamma}_2 \bar{\mathbf{C}} + \bar{\gamma}_4 \mathbf{a} \otimes \mathbf{a} + \bar{\gamma}_5 (\mathbf{a} \otimes \bar{\mathbf{C}} \mathbf{a} + \bar{\mathbf{C}} \mathbf{a} \otimes \mathbf{a}). \qquad (2)$$

Here $\bar{\gamma}_1 = 2\left(\partial_{\bar{I}_1} \Psi^{\text{iso}} + \bar{I}_1 \partial_{\bar{I}_2} \Psi^{\text{iso}}\right)$, $\bar{\gamma}_a = -2 \partial_{\bar{I}_a} \Psi^{\text{iso}}$ $(a = 2, 4, 5)$, $p = \mathrm{d}\Psi^{\text{vol}}/\mathrm{d}J$ is the hydrostatic pressure, and $\operatorname{Dev}(\bullet) = (\bullet) - (1/3)[(\bullet) : \mathbf{C}]\mathbf{C}^{-1}$ is the referential configuration deviatoric operator for a second order tensor.

Eqns. (1) and (2) are the general form of a TI hyperelastic stress response, defined in terms of invariants. They represent a kinematically consistent framework valid for large deformations. Specification of particular forms for Ψ^{iso} and Ψ^{vol} would be motivated by the particular tissue under analysis, and may stem from phenomenological or microstructural considerations.

3.2 Viscoelastic Response

As mentioned, viscoelastic energy functions $\hat{\Psi}(\mathbf{C}, \mathbf{a}, t)$ valid for large deformations may be formulated by including relaxation functions $\alpha(t) = 1 - \sum_{i=1}^{N} \alpha_i (1 - \exp(-t/\tau_i))$, where N, α_i and τ_i are constants, and t is time, and expressing the strain energy function in convolution integral form: $\hat{\Psi}(\mathbf{C}, \mathbf{a}, t) = \int_0^t \alpha(t - \tau) \partial_\tau \Psi(\mathbf{C}, \mathbf{a}) \, d\tau$. Such a form views the stress response at any time t as the sum of responses to excitations at all previous times – the mentioned deformation history-dependence. If separated isochoric and volumetric terms are used, as above, relaxation functions may be applied to either or both independently. Stresses are then obtained as

$$\mathbf{S}^{\text{iso}} = 2 \, \partial_\mathbf{C} \hat{\Psi}^{\text{iso}} = \int_0^t \alpha^{\text{iso}}(t - \tau) \, \partial_\tau \boldsymbol{\Phi}^{\text{iso}} \, d\tau, \tag{3}$$

$$\mathbf{S}^{\text{vol}} = 2 \, \partial_\mathbf{C} \hat{\Psi}^{\text{vol}} = \int_0^t \alpha^{\text{vol}}(t - \tau) \, \partial_\tau \boldsymbol{\Phi}^{\text{vol}} \, d\tau, \tag{4}$$

where $\boldsymbol{\Phi}^{\text{iso}} = 2 \partial_\mathbf{C} \Psi^{\text{iso}}$ and $\boldsymbol{\Phi}^{\text{vol}} = 2 \partial_\mathbf{C} \Psi^{\text{vol}}$ are the instantaneous hyperelastic stress responses (Eqns. (1)). Compared with use of purely hyperelastic models, in which stress may be computed directly from the (known) current deformation, use of visco-hyperelastic models within the TLED algorithm requires a constitutive update scheme involving time integration of the stress Eqns. (4).

4 Constitutive Update Procedure for Explicit Analyses

In the following we derive equations based on $\mathbf{S}^{\text{iso}}$, and note that an equivalent procedure may be applied for the volumetric term, if applicable. Referring to Eqn. (4) we note that $\mathbf{S}^{\text{iso}}$ may be restated as $\mathbf{S}^{\text{iso}} = \boldsymbol{\Phi}^{\text{iso}} - \sum_{i=1}^{N^{\text{iso}}} \boldsymbol{\Upsilon}_i^{\text{iso}}$, where

$$\boldsymbol{\Upsilon}_i^{\text{iso}} = \int_0^t \alpha_i^{\text{iso}} \left(1 - \exp((\tau - t)/\tau_i^{\text{iso}})\right) \partial_\tau \boldsymbol{\Phi}^{\text{iso}} d\tau, \quad i \in [1, N^{\text{iso}}] \tag{5}$$

are rate-dependent terms associated with each term in the relaxation functions. In an incremental analysis we require the stress at the current increment given the deformation state and history of the material. Adding subscripts to indicate time increments the isochoric stress may be updated using

$$\mathbf{S}_n^{\text{iso}} = \boldsymbol{\Phi}_n^{\text{iso}} - \sum_{i=1}^{N^{\text{iso}}} (\boldsymbol{\Upsilon}_i^{\text{iso}})_n. \tag{6}$$

As mentioned, instantaneous terms $\boldsymbol{\Phi}_n^{\text{iso}}$ may be computed from the current deformation $\mathbf{C}_n$ (Eqn. (1)$_2$). The main difficulty then is computation of the incremental rate-dependent terms $(\boldsymbol{\Upsilon}_i^{\text{iso}})_n$. Our strategy is to maintain each $\boldsymbol{\Upsilon}_i^{\text{iso}}$ as a state variable to be updated at each increment also. For clarity hereafter we consider only a single Prony term, but note that more terms may be added without difficulty.

Our approach is to convert the integral equation (5) into a rate form which may then be numerically integrated to produce an incremental update formula for $\boldsymbol{\Upsilon}^{\text{iso}}$. It may be shown that such a rate form is given by

$$\dot{\boldsymbol{\Upsilon}}^{\text{iso}} = \frac{1}{\tau^{\text{iso}}} \left(\alpha^{\text{iso}} \boldsymbol{\Phi}^{\text{iso}} - \boldsymbol{\Upsilon}^{\text{iso}} \right). \tag{7}$$

Integration of (7) using the backward Euler method yields a formula for Υ_n^{iso}:

$$\Upsilon_n^{\text{iso}} = A\Phi_n^{\text{iso}} + B\Upsilon_{n-1}^{\text{iso}}, \tag{8}$$

where $A = \Delta t \alpha^{\text{iso}} / (\Delta t + \tau^{\text{iso}})$ and $B = \tau^{\text{iso}} / (\Delta t + \tau^{\text{iso}})$ are constant coefficients, and Δt is the time step size. A similar expression may be obtained for volumetric terms.

The constitutive update procedure thus consists of (a) updating state variables (one for each Prony term) via Eqn. (8), and (b) updating stresses via Eqn. (6). We note in particular that when used with reduced integration hexahedra or linear tetrahedra the present scheme introduces only $12N_P$ ($N_P = N^{\text{iso}} + N^{\text{vol}}$) extra multiplications per element per time step compared with an equivalent hyperelastic formulation. Additional storage requirements are also minimal since only state variables (6-vectors) are retained between increments.

5 Algorithm Performance

The procedure was implemented (within the TLED algorithm) for GPU execution using the CUDA API [16], however the arrangement of kernel computations was essentially the same as that of our earlier OpenGL-based implementation [15]. We used reduced integration 8-node hexahedral elements which are preferable to the 4-node tetrahedra used in our previous implementation [15], both in terms of solution accuracy and computational efficiency.

We present examples based on compression and shear of cube models to demonstrate the validity and performance of the constitutive update procedure. We emphasise that these geometrically simple examples are aimed at verifying the numerical solution method (being the contribution of this paper), not at validating any particular constitutive model itself. In each case we used a TI visco-hyperelastic model with elastic strain energy components defined by

$$\Psi^{\text{iso}} = \frac{\mu}{2}(\bar{I}_1 - 3) + \frac{\eta}{2}(\bar{I}_4 - 1)^2, \qquad \Psi^{\text{vol}} = \frac{\kappa}{2}(J - 1)^2, \tag{9}$$

where μ is the small strain shear modulus, κ is the bulk modulus, and η is a material parameter with units of Pa. $\bar{I}_5$-dependent terms were omitted for simplicity. We used viscoelastic isochoric terms only, with $N^{\text{iso}} = 1$. Material parameters $\mu = 6568\text{Pa}$, $\kappa = 326\,210\text{Pa}$, $\alpha_1 = 0.5$, and $\tau_1 = 0.58\text{s}$ were chosen based on recent results for the viscoelastic response of human liver in vivo [17][1]. In the absence of appropriate experimental data for liver we selected $\eta = 2\mu$. Since η and μ are similarly dimensioned parameters, this ensures η is of an appropriate order of magnitude.

We first assessed the effects of anisotropy on the deformation response. A cube model with preferred direction $\mathbf{a} = [0\ \frac{1}{\sqrt{2}}\ \frac{1}{\sqrt{2}}]$ was compressed by 30% along the x−axis. The deformed shape is shown in Fig. 1 along with that of an isotropic

---

[1] In [17] an estimate of $\mu = 19\,704\text{Pa}$ is given, but it is also noted that the parenchyma itself is likely to be up to 3× less stiff.

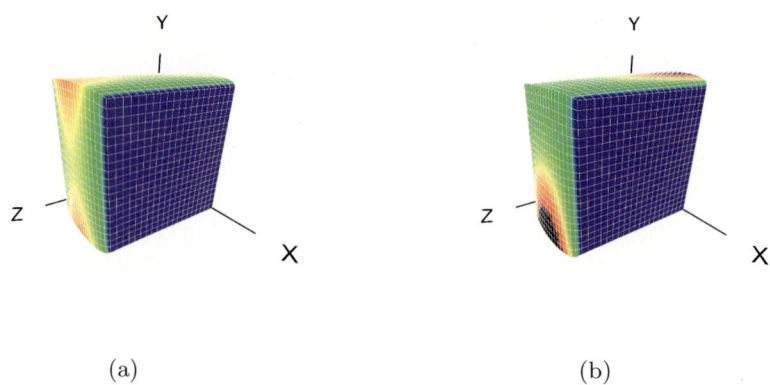

Fig. 1. Deformation pattern of (a) an isotropic model compared with (b) that of a TI model. Colour maps indicate magnitude of lateral displacement ($(u_y^2 + u_z^2)^{1/2}$)

model (with $\eta = 0$). With no preferred direction the expansion of the middle section was uniform (Fig. 1(a)). For the anisotropic model the direction defined by $y = z$ was stiffened, and Fig. 1(b) shows the resulting reduced expansion along this axis and the increased orthogonal expansion.

Next we confirmed the validity of the solution procedure by modelling a pure shear loading on the cube. Under such conditions an analytical solution for the stresses is available (omitted for brevity) and is compared with the numerical solutions in Fig. 2(a) for various loading speeds. The strain rate-dependence introduced by the model (and commonly observed in biological tissues) is clearly shown. Additionally the close match between the analytic and numerical solutions demonstrates the validity of the developed constitutive update scheme.

Finally we assessed the computational efficiency of the constitutive update scheme by measuring computation times for various constitutive models over a range of mesh densities. Using the cube geometry as above we generated models with mesh sizes between 3993 DOF and 177 957 DOF. Three constitutive models were considered: the TI viscoelastic model (TIV), TIV minus the viscoelastic terms (TIE), and TIE minus the anisotropy terms (NHE – since this represents a neo-Hookean model). The test machine included an Intel Core2Duo 2.4GHz CPU, 2GB RAM, and an NVIDIA GeForce 8800GTX GPU.

Fig. 2(b) indicates that solution times are little affected by the introduction of the more complex constitutive models, and importantly by the use of the developed constitutive update scheme. We observe that the maximum solution time ratio for model TIE to model NHE (anisotropic vs isotropic) was 1.013, and that of model TIV to model TIE (viscoelastic vs elastic) was 1.043. The largest *total* solution time increase for an anisotropic viscoelastic model compared with an isotropic elastic one was 5.1%. We conclude that the key features of anisotropy and viscoelasticity may be included in simulations at very little additional computational cost. Moreover, using the present material parameters

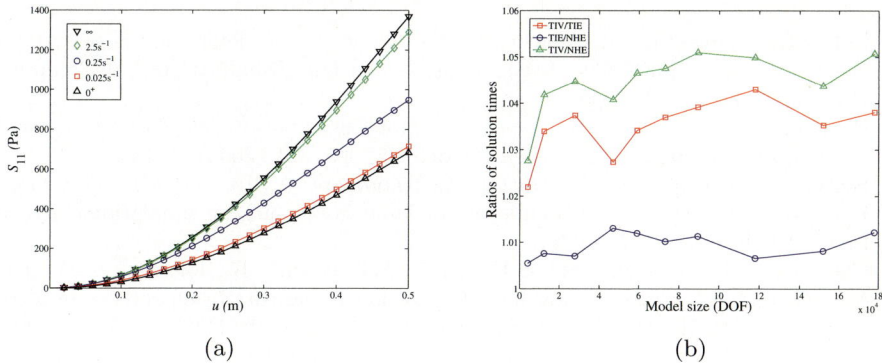

Fig. 2. (a) S_{11} curves for pure shear deformation at varying strain rates. Curves for strain rates of $2.5\mathrm{s}^{-1}$, $0.25\mathrm{s}^{-1}$, and $0.025\mathrm{s}^{-1}$ are given, along with the bounding instantaneous and equilibrium responses, labelled ∞ and 0^+, respectively. Solid lines correspond to analytical solutions, while markers indicate the numerical solution. (b) ratios of solution times for the constitutive models: TIV to TIE, TIE to NHE, and TIV to NHE.

and GPU implementation models of up to approx. 10 000 DOF may be solved in real-time. For more compliant tissues such as brain (for which the critical solution time step is larger) models of up to 55 000 DOF may be solved in real-time.

6 Conclusion

There is abundant evidence that most biological tissues exhibit time-dependent mechanical responses, and that even non-load bearing organs exhibit direction-dependence. These phenomena may be modelled using viscoelastic and anisotropic constitutive formulations. We presented a constitutive update scheme which allows use of such models within explicit finite element procedures for as little as 5.1% additional computational cost compared with isotropic elastic models. The scheme was general in the sense that any strain energy function (e.g. specific to particular organs) may be incorporated. Combined with GPU execution the presented scheme is suitable for real-time applications.

Explicit procedures have recently been shown to allow very rapid soft tissue simulation whilst retaining physically consistent kinematic nonlinearities. The present contribution expands the utility of such procedures and should find applications in time-critical simulation applications.

Acknowledgements

The financial support of the EPSRC (Grant reference: EP/F01144X/1) and the CSIRO Preventative Health Flagship is gratefully acknowledged.

References

1. Cotin, S., Delingette, H., Ayache, N.: Real-time elastic deformations of soft tissues for surgery simulation. IEEE Transactions On Visualization and Computer Graphics 5(1), 62–73 (1999)
2. Picinbono, G., Delingette, H., Ayache, N.: Non-linear anisotropic elasticity for real-time surgery simulation. Graphical Models 65, 305–321 (2003)
3. Szekely, G., Brechbühler, C., Hutter, R., Rhomberg, A., Ironmonger, N., Schmid, P.: Modelling of soft tissue simulation for laparscopic surgery simulation. Medical Image Analysis 4, 57–66 (2000)
4. Clatz, O., Delingette, H., Talos, I.F., Golby, A.J., Kikinis, R., Jolesz, F.A., Ayache, N., Warfield, S.K.: Robust nonrigid registration to capture brain shift from intra-operative MRI. IEEE Transactions on Medical Imaging 24(11), 1417–1427 (2005)
5. Ferrant, M., Warfield, S.K., Nabavi, A., Macq, B., Kikinis, R.: Registration of 3D intraoperative MR images of the brain using a finite element biomechanical model. In: 3rd International Conference on Medical Image Computing and Computer Assisted Intervention, Pittsburgh, USA, pp. 19–28 (2000)
6. Miga, M.I., Paulsen, K.D., Hoopes, P.J., Kennedy Jr., F.E., Hartov, A., Roberts, D.W.: In vivo quantification of a homogeneous brain deformation model for updating preoperative images during surgery. IEEE Transactions on Biomedical Engineering 47(2), 266–273 (2000)
7. Humphrey, J.D.: Continuum biomechanics of soft biological tissues. Proceedings Of The Royal Society Of London Series A-Mathematical, Physical and Engineering Sciences 459, 3–46 (2003)
8. Chabanas, M., Luboz, V., Payan, Y.: Patient specific finite element model of the face soft tissues for computer-assisted maxillofacial surgery. Medical Image Analysis 7(2), 131–151 (2003)
9. Hu, J., Jin, X., Lee, J.B., Zhang, L., Chaudhary, V., Guthikonda, M., Yang, K.H., King, A.I.: Intraoperative brain shift prediction using a 3D inhomogeneous patient-specific finite element model. Journal of Neurosurgery 106(1), 164–169 (2007)
10. Wittek, A., Miller, K., Kikinis, R., Warfield, S.K.: Patient-specific model of brain deformation: Application to medical image registration. Journal of Biomechanics 40, 919–929 (2007)
11. Fung, Y.C.: Biomechanics: mechanical properties of living tissues, 2nd edn. Springer, New York (1993)
12. Holzapfel, G.A.: Nonlinear Solid Mechanics: A Continuum Approach for Engineering. John Wiley & Sons, Chichester (2000)
13. Miller, K., Joldes, G., Lance, D., Wittek, A.: Total Lagrangian explicit dynamics finite element algorithm for computing soft tissue deformation. Communications in Numerical Methods in Engineering 23(2), 121–134 (2007)
14. Taylor, Z.A., Cheng, M., Ourselin, S.: Real-time nonlinear finite element analysis for surgical simulation using graphics processing units. In: 10th International Conference on Medical Image Computing and Computer Assisted Intervention, Brisbane, Australia, pp. 701–708 (2007)
15. Taylor, Z.A., Cheng, M., Ourselin, S.: High-speed nonlinear finite element analysis for surgical simulation using graphics processing units. IEEE Transactions on Medical Imaging 27(5), 650–663 (2008)
16. NVIDIA Corporation: NVIDIA CUDA Programming Guide Version 1.1 (2007)
17. Nava, A., Mazza, E., Furrer, M., Villiger, P., Reinhart, W.H.: In vivo mechanical characterization of human liver. Medical Image Analysis 12(2), 203–216 (2008)

3D Ultrasound-Guided Motion Compensation System for Beating Heart Mitral Valve Repair

Shelten G. Yuen[1], Samuel B. Kesner[1], Nikolay V. Vasilyev[2], Pedro J. Del Nido[2], and Robert D. Howe[1,3]

[1] Harvard School of Engineering and Applied Sciences, Cambridge, MA
[2] Department of Cardiovascular Surgery, Children's Hospital Boston, MA
[3] Harvard-MIT Division of Health Sciences & Technology, Cambridge, MA

Abstract. Beating heart intracardiac procedures promise significant benefits for patients, however, the fast motion of the heart poses serious challenges to surgeons. We present a new 3D ultrasound-guided motion (3DUS) compensation system that synchronizes instrument motion with the heart. The system utilizes the fact that the motion of some intracardiac structures, including the mitral valve annulus, is largely constrained to translation along one axis. This allows the development of a real-time 3DUS tissue tracker which we integrate with a 1 degree-of-freedom actuated surgical instrument, real-time 3DUS instrument tracker, and predictive filter to devise a system with synchronization accuracy of 1.8 mm RMSE. User studies involving the deployment of surgical anchors in a simulated mitral annuloplasty procedure demonstrate that the system increases success rates by over 100%. Furthermore, it enables more careful anchor deployment by reducing forces to the tissue by 50% while allowing instruments to remain in contact with the tissue for longer periods.

1 Introduction

Beating heart intracardiac repairs are now feasible with the use of real-time 3D ultrasound (3DUS) guidance [1]. These procedures avoid the need for cardiopulmonary bypass, which has a number of adverse effects including increased stroke risk and cognitive impairment [2]. Operating on the beating heart has the added advantage of allowing the surgeon to evaluate the status of the repair while the heart continues to function. Although beating heart procedures have many clear benefits, heart motion can make the safe manipulation of its tissues extremely challenging. This is particularly the case for the mitral valve, which is comprised of fast-moving and delicate tissues.

A promising solution to these problems is to employ a robotic motion compensation system to synchronize instrument motion with the heart. This approach has been studied extensively for coronary artery bypass graft procedures using multiple degree-of-freedom (DOF) robots and exploiting near periodicity in heart motion to synchronize with the external surface of the heart [3][4]. Operating on the mitral valve, though, provides additional challenges from working inside the heart. First, the restricted confines make using a multi-DOF robot difficult.

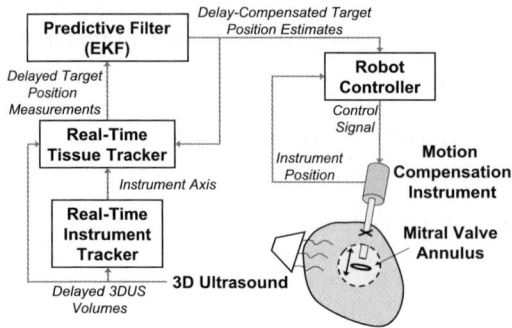
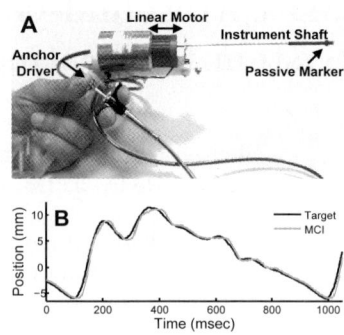

Fig. 1. Motion compensation system

Fig. 2. (A) MCI hardware prototype. (B) MCI tracking recorded mitral valve annulus motion.

Second, 3DUS must be used for guidance because it is currently the only real-time volumetric imaging technique that can image tissue through blood. Its use introduces time delays [5] and can make tracking of the tissue target difficult due to poor shape definition [1].

In this work, we present a 3DUS-guided motion compensation system that overcomes these challenges to beating heart intracardiac procedures. The design of the system is guided by the clinical observation that the rapid motion of the annulus is dominated by translation along a single axis between the left atrium and left ventricle [6]. This allows the use of a simplified 1 DOF motion compensation system that can be used for surgical procedures like the anchor driving found in mitral annuloplasty. In the following we describe this system and its components, then validate its performance in a user study.

2 Motion Compensation System

In previous work we developed a real-time 3DUS instrument tracker [5], motion compensation instrument [6], and quasiperiodic predictive filter [7] for beating heart intracardiac surgery. Here we develop a real-time 3DUS tissue tracking technique and integrate these technologies into a system for 3DUS-guided motion compensation (Fig. 1). The resulting system enables beating heart procedures on intracardiac structures that undergo rapid translational motions primarily along one axis, like the mitral valve annulus [6]. The system comprises an actuated 1 DOF instrument commanded by a predictive filter that is in turn fed time-delayed, noisy measurements from a real-time 3DUS tissue segmentation algorithm. The filter used to command the actuator, an extended Kalman filter (EKF), accurately estimates and predicts the annulus trajectory by exploiting quasiperioidicity in its motion. In addition to being used to feed-forward the trajectory of the cardiac target to the instrument controller for motion synchronization, it is fed back to the tissue tracker to assist in detecting the target.

2.1 Motion Compensation Instrument

The motion compensation instrument (MCI) is a handheld anchor deployment device that actively cancels the dominant 1D motion component of the mitral valve annulus (Fig. 2A). It incorporates a voice coil linear motor (NCC10-15-023-1X, H2W Technologies, Valencia, CA, USA) for actuation of the anchor deployment stage up to speeds and accelerations of 1490 mm/s and 103000 mm/s^2. The instrument is controlled with a slightly underdamped response by a 1 kHz PID servo loop and has a -3 dB point of 35.0 Hz (-40 dB/dec roll off rate). The resulting instrument is capable of following the fast motion of the mitral annulus with an effective delay of 10 ms, as depicted in Fig. 2B. A detailed description of the MCI design is given in [6].

2.2 Quasiperiodic Predictive Filter: Extended Kalman Filter

The intrinsic time delays in 3DUS make direct visual servoing of the MCI potentially dangerous. We estimate delays of $\approx$70 ms in the acquisition, transmission, and computation times associated with 3DUS [5] - sufficient time for the mitral valve annulus to traverse the majority of its path at end systole [6]. Left uncompensated, these delays would lead to collisions between the instrument and annulus that would result in tissue damage. To avoid this outcome, we exploit the near periodicity of the mitral valve trajectory to predict its path and hence compensate for time delay.

Prior research in motion compensated coronary artery bypass graft has investigated prediction using an adaptive filter bank [4], an estimator based on Takens theorem [8], and a vector autoregressive least squares estimator [9]. In this work, we employ an extended Kalman filter (EKF) with an explicity quasiperiodic model, which is effective for 3DUS-guided mitral valve motion compensation [7]. To model quasiperiodic heart motion, we consider the following m-order time-varying Fourier series with an offset

$$y(t) = c(t) + \sum_{i=1}^{m} r_i(t) \sin \theta_i(t), \qquad (1)$$

where $y(t)$ is the target position in ultrasound coordinates, $c(t)$ is the offset, $r_i(t)$ are the harmonic amplitudes, and $\theta_i(t) \triangleq i \int_0^t \omega(\tau) d\tau + \phi_i(t)$, with heart rate $\omega(t)$ and harmonic phases $\phi_i(t)$. This parameterization was introduced in [10] and shown to be a robust model for mitral annulus tracking with $m = 8$ harmonics [7].

Defining the state vector $\boldsymbol{x}(t) \triangleq [c(t), r_i(t), \omega(t), \theta_i(t)]^\mathrm{T}$, $i \in (1, \ldots, m)$ and assuming that $c(t), r_i(t), \omega(t),$ and $\phi_i(t)$ evolve through a random walk, the state space model for this system is

$$\begin{aligned}\boldsymbol{x}(t+\Delta t) &= \boldsymbol{F}(\Delta t)\boldsymbol{x}(t) + \boldsymbol{\mu}(t), \\ z(t) &= h(\boldsymbol{x}(t)) + \nu(t),\end{aligned} \qquad \boldsymbol{F}(\Delta t) = \begin{bmatrix} \boldsymbol{I}_{m+1} & & & & \boldsymbol{0} \\ & 1 & & & \\ & \Delta t & 1 & & \\ \boldsymbol{0} & 2\Delta t & 0 & 1 & \\ & \vdots & & & \ddots \\ & m\Delta t & & & 1 \end{bmatrix},$$

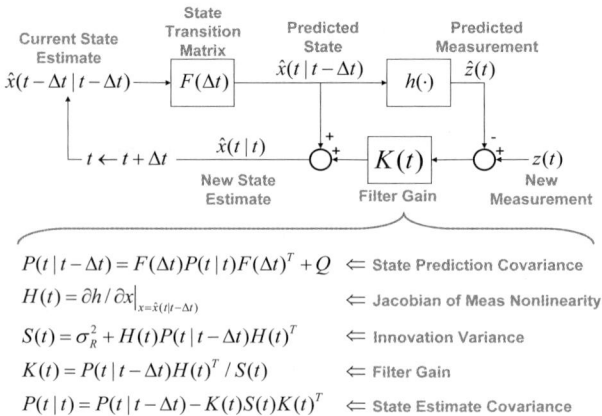

Fig. 3. Extended Kalman filter recursion

where $h(\boldsymbol{x}(t)) \triangleq y(t)$ from (1), $\nu(t) \sim \mathcal{N}(0, \sigma_R^2)$ is zero mean Gaussian noise, and $\boldsymbol{\mu}(t) \sim \mathcal{N}(\boldsymbol{0}, \boldsymbol{Q})$ is the random step of the states assumed to be drawn from a zero mean multivariate normal distribution with covariance matrix $\boldsymbol{Q}$.

Prediction with this model requires estimation of $\boldsymbol{x}(t)$; a nonlinear estimation problem owing to the measurement function, $h(\boldsymbol{x}(t))$. We employ the EKF, a nonlinear filtering method that approximates the Kalman filter through linearization about the state estimate $\hat{\boldsymbol{x}}(t - \Delta t | t - \Delta t)$. The EKF is computed in real-time using the recursion given in Fig. 3. Details may be found in [7].

2.3 Real-Time Tissue Tracking

Automatic, real-time segmentation of a tissue target in 3DUS is challenging due to poor shape definition and the number of computations required to process volumes at 28 Hz (the 3DUS sampling rate). In this work we achieve real-time tissue tracking in 3DUS by making use of the instrument to designate a tissue target in the 3DUS volumes, essentially by pointing at it. Tracking is then reduced to detecting the tissue that is along the instrument axis.

This approach first requires locating the instrument in 3DUS. We accomplish this with a GPU-based Radon transform algorithm that finds the instrument axis in real-time 3DUS [5]. When the instrument is stationary and not in contact with the tissue, both are readily detected by peaks in an intensity-based objective function that is calculated on a 2D image slice through the instrument shaft. An example of this is shown in Figs. 4A and C, where *a priori* knowledge of the 3DUS probe placement relative to the instrument allows the identification of the left-most peak in the objective as the passive marker on the instrument. The peak immediately following it to the right is the tissue target.

Complications in the segmentation of the passive marker can arise when the instrument moves to compensate target motion or comes into contact with the target. Specularities on the shaft can be confused with the passive marker and it can be difficult to distinguish the instrument tip when it may in fact be embedded

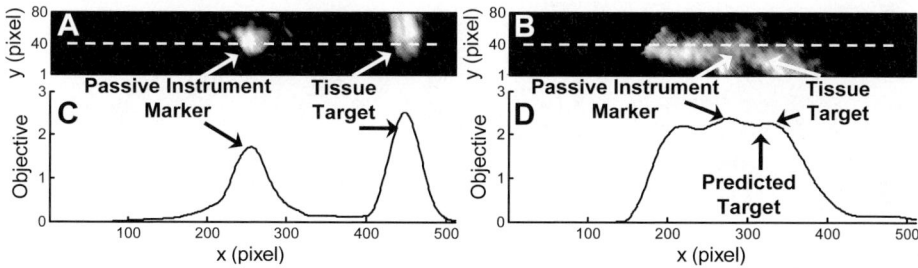

Fig. 4. Example ultrasound slices along instrument shaft when instrument is not in contact with target (A) and when it is in contact with target (B). The corresponding intensity-based objective functions are shown in (C) and (D), with the EKF-predicted target location shown in (D). The x axis is parallel to instrument axis (white dash).

in the tissue (Figs. 4B and D). These challenges are overcome by using the EKF to predict the location of the target in the current frame, in an analogous manner to *gating* in radar target tracking. The peak in the objective that is nearest to the predicted location is taken as the target peak, thereby obviating the need to further segment the instrument marker.

3 Performance in a Surgical Task

The accuracy and benefits of the proposed motion compensation system were assessed through a study of user performance in an *in vitro* beating heart surgical task. Ten subjects (seven male, three female, ages 20–34) were instructed to use the MCI to drive surgical anchors (similar to staples, deployed from the tip of the instrument shaft) into a tissue phantom that simulated the motion of the mitral valve annulus in a water tank. The MCI either provided motion compensation through the system described in the preceding section or the MCI was set to act as a solid, noncompensating instrument.

3.1 Experimental Setup

The user trials were conducted in conditions that mimic those expected in a beating heart mitral valve annuloplasty procedure. Fig. 5 depicts the setup. Valve motion was simulated by a cam follower mechanism that replicates the dominant 1D motion component of the human mitral valve (Fig. 2B), as determined in [6]. A tissue phantom of 2 cm thick polyethylene foam was affixed to a load cell (Kistler, Spartanburg, SC, USA) that measured the forces applied by the MCI during the task, then mounted to the cam and positioned in a water tank. The cam simulated a heart beat of 60 beats per minute. The MCI was aligned at roughly 15 deg to the motion axis of the target and contrained to move in 1 DOF by a linear bearing guide rail. Subjects viewed the task through the monitor of the 3DUS machine (SONOS 7500, Philips Medical, Andover, MA, USA), which

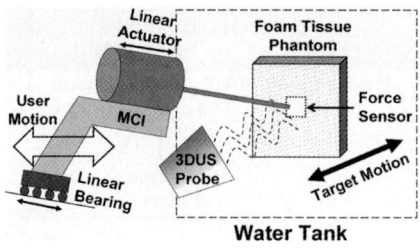
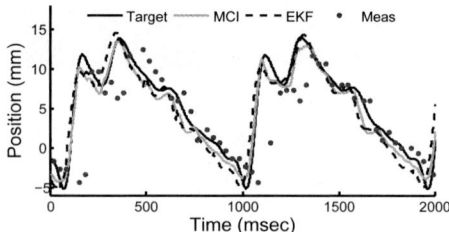

Fig. 5. Experimental setup for user trials

Fig. 6. Example of MCI tracking the mitral annulus target. Measurements from the tissue tracker and EKF predictions are shown.

was set up to image the target and instrument simultaneously. A potentiometer measured target position for off-line assessment of system accuracy.

The motion compensation system used a dual CPU AMD Opteron 285 2.6 GHz PC with 4 GB of RAM to process the ultrasound data, control the MCI, and record the force readings from the load cell. The 3DUS machine streamed volumes to the PC over a 1 Gb LAN using TCP/IP. A program written in C++ retrieved the ultrasound volumes and loaded them onto a GPU (7800GT, nVidia Corp, Santa Clara, CA) for real-time instrument axis detection. Subsequent tissue tracking, predictive filtering, and control algorithms were implemented in C++ on the CPU.

3.2 Testing Protocol

The subjects were instructed to deploy anchors into the moving tissue phantom with the MCI in a series of trials. They were informed that the dual criteria for a successful trial were that the anchor be securely deployed in the target and that the forces applied to the target by the MCI during the task not exceed 15 N (the puncture force as determined in pilot studies on excised porcine mitral valve annulus). The subjects were taught to use the MCI's anchor driver mechanism and trained to recognize the "feeling" of forces up to 15 N when pushing the MCI into a stationary target. When the subjects became confident in their sense of the forces applied, they were given six practice anchoring trials with the moving target: three with motion compensation and three with a solid instrument. After training, the subjects proceeded to perform the task in ten trials (five with motion compensation and five with a solid instrument) in randomized order. The outcome of each stapling attempt and the amount of force applied was shared with the subject directly after each trial.

3.3 Results

The motion compensation system provided instrument synchronization to the target with 1.8 mm RMS error. A representative example from a user trial is shown in Fig. 6. Position measurements from the tissue tracker had RMS errors

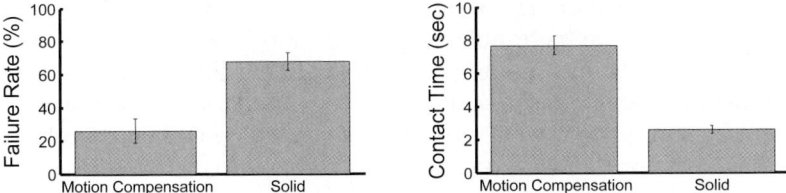

Fig. 7. Mean failure rates (A) and mean continuous contact time (B) with motion compensation and with a solid instrument. Error bars indicate standard error.

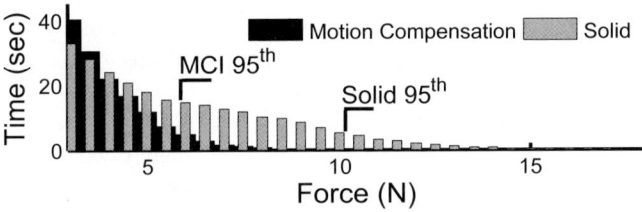

Fig. 8. Histogram of applied forces over all user trials. 95th percentiles are shown.

of 2.5 mm and were delayed by 68 ms. Both error and time delay were mitigated by the EKF, which had RMS prediction errors of 1.7 mm.

Motion compensated anchor driving provided a mean failure rate that was roughly 60% less than that observed for a solid instrument (Fig. 7A). A statistically significant difference between the means ($26.0 \pm 7.3\%$ for motion compensation and $68.0 \pm 5.3\%$ for a solid instrument, mean $\pm$ standard error) was apparent using a two-sided t-test ($p = 0.0002$). It should be noted that a subset of four subjects obtained 0% failure rates with motion compensation and $70.0 \pm 12.9\%$ without. The three engineers participating in the study belonged to this subset.

Motion compensation also enabled the subjects to place the instrument in continuous contact with the target for nearly three times longer than with a solid instrument (Fig. 7B). On average, subjects kept constant contact on the target for 7.7 ± 0.6 sec with motion compensation and 2.6 ± 0.2 sec without. This difference between the means is statistically significant ($p < 0.0001$). The range of continuous contact times observed over all motion compensation trials was 2.0 – 17.5 sec while the range for the solid instrument was 0.7 – 7.9 sec.

The forces applied to the target were reduced for trials using motion compensation. Fig. 8 shows a histogram of force samples for all trials for the motion compensated and solid instrument cases. The 95th percentile of forces for the solid instrument (10.2 N) is nearly twice that seen for motion compensation (5.8 N).

4 Discussion and Conclusions

These results demonstrate that the 3D ultrasound-guided motion compensation system described here provides substantial performance gains for surgical tasks on beating mitral valve targets. By exploiting the predominantly 1 DOF motion of the mitral valve, we were able to develop novel solutions to actuating an instrument within the confines of the heart and tracking tissue targets in real-time 3D ultrasound. A quasiperiodic predictive filter enabled compensation for the time delays in the system so that the instrument could be actuated to track fast-moving tissue without lag, as evidenced in our *in vitro* experiments.

To the knowledge of the authors, this is the first demonstration of a fully integrated surgical motion compensation system based on real-time volumetric image data that can interact with the beating heart. Using the system, subjects achieved success rates for a surgical anchor deployment task that were more than double those achieved with a non-compensated instrument. Furthermore, the system permitted more careful placement of the anchors by reducing the forces applied and prolonging the amount of continuous contact between the instrument and the target.

While motion compensated anchor driving had relatively low failure rates in our study, we anticipate that it can be driven to nearly zero with additional user training and a small modification to the instrument. The flawless performance of users with technology experience (e.g., engineers) suggests that the other users could benefit from more practice. Indeed, several users were confused by ultrasound visualization and impaired by the inertial forces resulting from the actuator's moving mass, which could be difficult to distinguish from contact forces. This led to cases where the user would not push the instrument firmly into contact with the target. Modification of the instrument to include a counterbalancing mass will mitigate the loss in haptic feedback due to inertial effects. Further research is underway to evaluate the efficacy and usability of this motion compensating system in *in vivo* beating heart mitral annulus repair.

Acknowledgements

This work is supported by the US National Institutes of Health under grant NIH R01 HL073647-01.

References

1. Cannon, J., et al.: Real-time three-dimensional ultrasound for guiding surgical tasks. Computer Aided Surgery 8(2), 82–90 (2003)
2. Murkin, J., et al.: Beating heart surgery: why expect less central nervous system morbidity? Annals of Thoracic Surgery 68, 1498–1501 (1999)
3. Nakamura, Y., Kishi, K., Kawakami, H.: Heartbeat synchronization for robotic cardiac surgery. In: Proc. ICRA, Seoul Korea, pp. 2014–2019 (May 2001)
4. Ginhoux, R., et al.: Active filtering of physiological motion in robotized surgery using predictive control. IEEE Transactions on Robotics 21(1), 67–79 (2006)
5. Novotny, P., et al.: GPU based real-time instrument tracking with three-dimensional ultrasound. Medical Image Analysis 11, 458–464 (2007)
6. Kettler, D., et al.: An active motion compensation instrument for beating heart mitral valve surgery. In: Proc. IEEE IROS, San Diego, USA (October 2007)

7. Yuen, S., Novotny, P., Howe, R.: Quasiperiodic predictive filtering for robot-assisted beating heart surgery. In: Proc. IEEE ICRA, Pasadena, USA (May 2008)
8. Ortmaier, T., et al.: Motion estimation in beating heart surgery. IEEE Transactions on Biomedical Engineering 52(10), 1729–1740 (2005)
9. Franke, T., Bebek, O., Cavusoglu, C.: Improved prediction of heart motion using an adaptive filter for robot assisted beating heart surgery. In: Proc. IEEE IROS, San Diego, USA, pp. 509–515 (October-November 2007)
10. Parker, P., Anderson, B.: Frequency tracking of nonsinusoidal periodic signals in noise. Signal Processing 20, 127–152 (1990)

A Novel Algorithm for Heart Motion Analysis Based on Geometric Constraints

Mingxing Hu[1], Graeme Penney[2], Daniel Rueckert[3], Philip Edwards[4], Michael Figl[4], Philip Pratt[4], and David Hawkes[1]

[1] Centre for Medical Image Computing, University College London
[2] Department of Imaging Sciences, King's College London
[3] Visual Information Processing, Department of Computing, Imperial College
[4] Department of Surgical Oncology and Technology, Imperial College
London, United Kingdom
{mingxing.hu,d.hawkes}@ucl.ac.uk, graeme.penney @kcl.ac.uk,
{d.rueckert,eddie.edwards,m.figl,p.pratt}@imperial.ac.uk

Abstract. Recently, much attention has been focused on heart motion analysis for minimally invasive beating-heart surgery. Unfortunately existing techniques usually require the camera(s) to be fixed during the motion analysis, which can restrict its usefulness during surgery. In this paper we present a novel method for heart motion analysis using geometric constraint, which can estimate the motion from a moving camera and employ multiple image features to improve robustness to noise. Our approach combines the benefits of geometry estimation for obtaining an accurate and robust solution with the proper treatment of respiratory motion. The proposed method can be applied to not only beating heart surgery, but also to other procedures involving periodic organ motion, such as lung and liver.

1 Introduction

Totally endoscopic coronary artery bypass (TECAB) surgery offers substantial benefits to the patient in terms of reduced trauma and blood loss, shorter hospitalisation time and lower risk of cardiac arrest [1]. Nevertheless, operating on a beating heart can be problematic, which slows down the surgical procedures, and demands high concentration from the surgeon. Motion analysis has received a lot of attention from both the research and clinical community over the last decade. It appears to be key to more accurate and safer TECAB surgery and an essential prior step for 2D-3D registration [1], surface reconstruction [2] and robot control [3-9].

In earlier studies, Nakamura et al. proposed a heartbeat synchronization method using a high speed camera to precisely sample heart motion [3]. An artificial marker was put on heart surface for motion tracking and the amplitude of the motion was evaluated based on the variations of the marker's coordinates. Thakral also investigated the use of a fiber-optic laser sensor to measure Z-axis motion and tested their method using a surgically prepared rodent [4]. Groeger et al. employed an affine model to measure the local motion of a beating heart and performed analysis of measured trajectories for motion estimation and global prediction [5, 6]. Around the same time, Ginhoux et al. reported their in-vivo results of beating heart tracking and proposed two different predictive-control schemes for the compensation of respiratory and cardiac motion respectively [7, 8]. More recently, a model-based motion estimation was proposed by Bader et al., which describes motion behaviour using a partial differential equation and obtains the measurement by reconstructing 3D positions of markers from a stereo camera system [9].

However, as maybe observed, a common trait shared by all these methods is that they can only use image sequence from fixed camera(s). That is, the position and orientation of the camera(s) must be fixed during the video capture, allowing feature values in X, Y or Z directions to be measured in order to analyze the heart motion. In addition, these methods usually rely on only one image feature for the motion analysis, so it is difficult to employ some robust techniques to deal directly with image noise problem.

Therefore in this paper we seek a new heart motion analysis approach that works for moving camera systems and makes the following contributions: (1) The heart motion is estimated by employing the geometry distance between images, rather than insisting on using directly the feature values in X, Y or Z positions. Epipolar geometry encapsulates camera information (intrinsic and extrinsic parameters) and so it can handle the movement of the camera and even the change of the internal geometry. (2) The estimation is based on multiple feature points tracked in the image sequence, which make the proposed method more robust to image noise. If there are enough features present, some robust techniques can also be applied to solve the outlier problem. (3) With this robust technique, it is possible to extract images from the same position within each beating heart cycle automatically, and to convert the difficult 4D (3D+time) dynamic reconstruction problem back to 3D static reconstruction problem, which is easier to solve.

2 Materials and Methods

2.1 Epipolar Geometry

Consider the case of two images of a 3D scene taken from two cameras. The point in the left image is represented by the homogeneous vector $\mathbf{m} = (x, y, 1)^T$. Its corresponding point $\mathbf{m}' = (x', y', 1)^T$ in the right image is constrained to lie on the epipolar line l' derived from $\mathbf{m}$. This is known as the epipolar constraint, and algebraically it can be expressed as

$$\mathbf{m}'^T \mathbf{F} \mathbf{m} = 0 \qquad (1)$$

where $\mathbf{F}$ is a 3×3 fundamental matrix with rank 2. It incorporates information about the relative transformation and internal geometry of the camera.

The classic method to estimate epipolar geometry is Hartley's eight-point algorithm [10], which greatly improves the performance of the original work of Longut-Higgins [11] by applying a simple normalization to the image data. The method may be formulated in the following two steps:

(1) Least squares minimization. After data normalization, rewrite the epipolar constraint as a linear and homogenous equation in terms of the nine unknown coefficients in $\mathbf{F}$

$$\mathbf{Zf} = 0$$

where $\mathbf{f} = (F_{1,1}, F_{1,2}, F_{1,3}, F_{2,1}, F_{2,2}, F_{2,3}, F_{3,1}, F_{3,2}, F_{3,3})^T$ and

$$\mathbf{Z} = \begin{pmatrix} z_1 \\ \vdots \\ z_n \end{pmatrix} = \begin{pmatrix} x'_1 x_1 & x'_1 y_1 & x'_1 & y'_1 x_1 & y'_1 y_1 & y'_1 & x_1 & y_1 & 1 \\ \vdots & \vdots & \vdots & \vdots & \vdots & \vdots & \vdots & \vdots & \vdots \\ x'_n x_n & x'_n y_n & x'_n & y'_n x_n & y'_n y_n & y'_n & x_n & y_n & 1 \end{pmatrix}$$

Then a solution of $\mathbf{F}$ can be obtained from the vector $\mathbf{f}$ corresponding to the smallest singular value of $\mathbf{Z}$ in the least squares sense.

(2) Singularity enforcement. Replace $\mathbf{F} = \mathbf{V}_F \Lambda_F \mathbf{U}_F^T$ ($\Lambda_F = diag\{\sqrt{\lambda_1}, \sqrt{\lambda_2}, \sqrt{\lambda_3}\}$, λ_1, λ_2 and λ_3 are in decreasing order) with the nearest rank 2 matrix $\mathbf{F}^+ = \mathbf{V}_F \Lambda_F^+ \mathbf{U}_F^T$ ($\Lambda_F^+ = diag\{\sqrt{\lambda_1}, \sqrt{\lambda_2}, 0\}$).

Hartley's method delivers results comparable with those of some nonlinear methods, and is an good tool for initialization. Readers are referred to [10] for more details.

2.2 Heart Motion Analysis

The motion of the heart surface is a caused by a combination of cardiac and respiratory motion. Usually these two independent motions need to be separated by way of signal processing. In this paper, we avoid this problem using geometry estimation under an affine assumption, and analyze the heart motion directly from the image sequence.

Although the effect of respiration on the heart surface is nonlinear, it has been shown that an affine transformation can provide a good approximation to model the respiratory motion of the heart surface [12, 13]. This is especially true for an endoscope with a narrow field-of-view, which captures images covering only a small region of the heart surface. We therefore assume we can use the affine assumption in our method and consider respiration to be an extra affine transformation of the heart surface. We put this extra affine transformation into the fundamental matrix as a relative transformation between the camera and the heart surface. The result of this is that the movement of the heart surface can now be considered as being solely due to cardiac motion. Unless noted otherwise, the term "heart motion" refers to cardiac motion in the remainder of this paper.

The heart motion is a periodic (quasi-periodic) motion. For a 3D point on the heart surface, we can write $\mathbf{X}(t) = \mathbf{X}(t + kT)$, where T is the length of the heart cycle and $k = 1, 2, \cdots$. If a camera captures two images of the heart surface at times t and $t + kT$, the image projections of $\mathbf{X}$ can be denoted as

$$\mathbf{m}^t = \mathbf{P}^t \mathbf{X}(t), \qquad \mathbf{m}^{t+kT} = \mathbf{P}^{t+kT} \mathbf{X}(t + kT) = \mathbf{P}^{t+kT} \mathbf{X}(t) \qquad (2)$$

where $\mathbf{P}$ is the projective matrix, including intrinsic and extrinsic parameters.

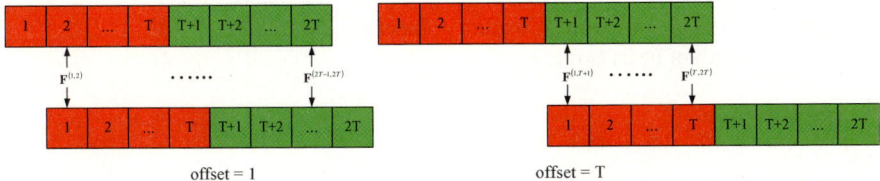

Fig. 1. Estimation of the heart cycle length based on geometric constraints. The image sequence moves from left to right with different offset and epipolar distances are computed between corresponding pairs.

Interestingly, we find that feature pair $(\mathbf{m}^t, \mathbf{m}^{t+kT})$ still satisfies the epipolar constraint, $(\mathbf{m}^{t+kT})^T \mathbf{F} \mathbf{m}^t = 0$, although they are taken at different time and using different projective matrices. But if the image points are not captured at the same position of the heart cycle, for example, at times t and $l \neq t + kT$, Eq. 1 will no longer hold for correspondence $(\mathbf{m}^t, \mathbf{m}^l)$ and this error can be evaluated by using an appropriate distance measure. The simplest measure is the algebraic distance, namely, the residual $r = (\mathbf{m}^l)^T \mathbf{F} \mathbf{m}^t$.

Unfortunately, r has no geometrical significance. Therefore in this paper we use the epipolar distance [10], which is the perpendicular distance of correspondence $(\mathbf{m}^t, \mathbf{m}^l)$ to the epipolar lines in frames t and l, defined as:

$$d_e = r \cdot \left(\frac{1}{(r_x^t)^2 + (r_y^t)^2} + \frac{1}{(r_x^l)^2 + (r_y^l)^2} \right)^{\frac{1}{2}} \quad (3)$$

where $r_x^t = F_{1,1} x^l + F_{2,1} y^l + F_{3,1}$, $r_y^t = F_{1,2} x^l + F_{2,2} y^l + F_{3,2}$, $r_x^l = F_{1,1} x^t + F_{1,2} y^t + F_{1,3}$ and $r_y^l = F_{2,1} x^t + F_{2,2} y^t + F_{2,3}$. It ensures that each image receives equal consideration.

Thus we can use the epipolar constraints to analyze the heart motion if a long enough image sequence is available, for example, with at least two or three heart cycles. As demonstrated in Fig. 1, the method is similar to self-correlation, but the criterion is based exactly on epipolar geometry. The image sequence moves from left to right with different *offset* frames, and for each offset, the fundamental matrix $\mathbf{F}^{(j-\mathit{offset}, j)}$ is computed between each frame pair $(j - \mathit{offset}, j)$ and the epipolar distance $d_e^{(j-\mathit{offset}, j)} = \frac{1}{n} \sum_{i=1}^{n} d_{ei}$ between this pair is calculated accordingly. Then the average epipolar distance of all these $m - 2 \cdot \mathit{offset}$ pairs of frames can be written as

$$d_e = \frac{1}{m - 2 \cdot \mathit{offset}} \sum_{j=\mathit{offset}+1}^{m-\mathit{offset}} d_e^{(j-\mathit{offset}, j)} \quad (4)$$

When $\mathit{offset} = kT$, the error d_e can reach a minimum value according to the geometric constraint. The first time a minimum appears, the offset should be equal to the length of the heart cycle T. An overview of the complete algorithm is given in Fig. 2.

Here we want to emphasize that there are several advantages using geometric constraint in heart motion analysis. Firstly, it can deal with the movement and also the change of internal geometry of the camera, since we do not rely directly on the feature

> **Input**: image sequence with n feature points from m frames
> **Output**: length of heart cycle T
>
> **Algorithm**:
> For $\textit{offset} = Min\_offset : Max\_offset$
>   For $j = \textit{offset} + 1 : m - \textit{offset}$
>   Estimate the fundamental matrix $\mathbf{F}^{(j-\textit{offset},j)}$ between frames $j-\textit{offset}$ and j
>   Compute the epipolar distance $d_e^{(j-\textit{offset},j)}$ using $\mathbf{F}^{(j-\textit{offset},j)}$ with Eq. (3)
>   End
>   Calculate the average epipolar distance with Eq. (4)
> End
> Find T, the first time a minimum average epipolar distance appears

Fig. 2. The algorithm for heart motion analysis based on geometric constraint

points' values in X, Y, or Z directions, which become meaningless if the camera parameters are changed. The fundamental matrix encapsulates both the intrinsic and extrinsic parameters, so we can concentrate on the heart cycle analysis using the geometry distance only. Secondly, the geometry estimation uses multiple image points and is based on a least squares minimization, so it is more robust to image noise compared with the traditional methods which use only one feature. Moreover, the geometric constraint helps us successfully separate the respiration from the heart motion under an affine assumption. The fundamental matrix encodes the respiration-induced motion as a relative movement of the camera, so the motion estimated is the heart motion itself without any respiration.

2.3 Sub-frame Accuracy

The accuracy of cycle length T we compute in Section 2.2 is limited to be an integer number of frames. In order to achieve sub-frame accuracy the following method is used.

Although heart tissue deforms nonlinearly, we can assume that the motion of a point from one frame to the next is approximately linear if the images are captured at a sufficiently high frame rate. As a result, sub-frame feature point $\mathbf{m}(t+\alpha)$ ($1 \geq \alpha \geq 0$) can be generated by using linear interpolation of image points either side of $\mathbf{m}(t+\alpha)$

$$\mathbf{m}(t+\alpha) = (1-\alpha)\mathbf{m}^t + \alpha\mathbf{m}^{t+1} \quad 1 \geq \alpha \geq 0 \tag{5}$$

Thus it is possible to estimate the offset for a range of values around the expected value, T, at an arbitrary resolution. Furthermore, we can use the Gaussian-Newton algorithm or other optimization techniques to obtain the optimal solution with sub-frame accuracy.

2.4 Experimental Design

In order to assess the performance of the proposed method, a beating heart phantom made of silicone rubber (The Chamberlain Group, Great Barrington, MA, USA) was employed to provide gold standard for evaluation. The phantom is continuously inflated and deflated using an air pump with an integrated controller. In order to create a beating heart model, it was scanned while beating at the rate of 55bpm with a Philips 64-slice CT scanner, producing 10 uniformly-spaced phases.

The first of these was manually segmented and converted into a tetrahedral mesh of 709 elements and 747 degrees of freedom. The Image Registration Toolkit [14] was then used to create a sequence of 3D tensor product cubic B-spline deformations, mapping the initial mesh onto each phase in turn.

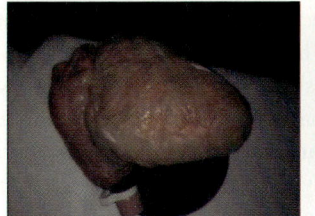 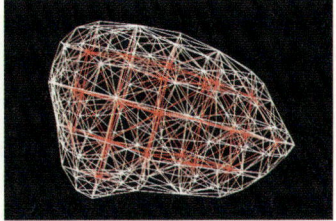

Fig. 3. Beating heart phantom and FEM mesh from CT data

To improve temporal stability of the FEM simulation 1D cubic B-splines were fitted through each node with respect to time, thus making the second order temporal derivatives continuous. Smoothness is also maintained across the coincident start and end of the cardiac cycle by arranging the basis functions. Fig. 3 shows the heart phantom and resulting mesh. Readers are referred to [15] for more details about the beating heart simulation.

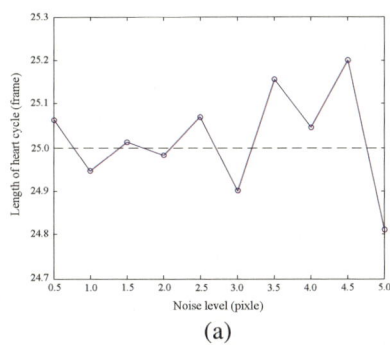 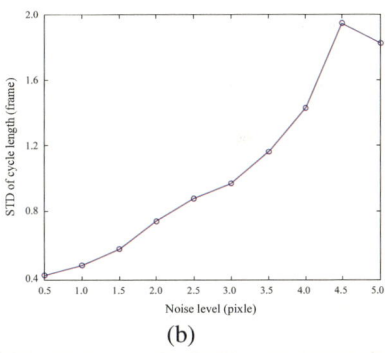

Fig. 4. Experimental results of synthetic data testing. (a) shows the estimated cycle length under different noise level (STD=0.5~5.0 pixels). (b) displays the standard deviation (STD) of estimated cycle length of 200 trials of each noise level.

3 Experimental Results

3.1 Synthetic Data

In synthetic data testing, 50 points were randomly selected from the beating heart model described in Section 2.4. For simplicity, we adjust the beating heart rate to

60bpm, that is, once per second. Then a moving camera was simulated with frame rate 25fps, and all these 3D points were projected to 50 image planes sequentially using the simulated camera, with different intrinsic and extrinsic (rotation and translation) parameters. So the ground truth for the length of heart cycle, T, is 25 frames per heart cycle.

Next, 10 different ranges of Gaussian noise were added to the image measurements, with a zero mean and standard deviation varying from 0.5 to 5.0 pixels. For each noise level, we ran 200 trials and the final results were the average of results from these 200 independent experiments. A graph of these results is shown is Fig. 4 (a). It can easily be noticed that the proposed method obtained an accurate heart cycle length over all the experiments, with error below 0.2 frame. In particular, when the noise reaches a high level ($\sigma = 4, 5$), the estimated results are still very close to the ground truth. Fig. 4 (b) illustrates the standard deviation of cycle length plotted against noise level. We can see that the standard deviation increases with noise, but errors are less than 2 frames. This strongly suggests that the proposed method can obtain an accurate result and is robust to image noise due to the use of multiple image features and data normalization for geometry estimation.

3.2 Phantom Model

The *da Vinci*™ robotic surgical system (Intuitive Surgical, Inc., Sunnyvale, CA, USA) was used to obtain images of the heart phantom. The heart phantom was beating with different rates, and the endoscopic camera was moving around the scene as well. The video endoscopic images were digitized at 25 frames per second (fps) using a frame grabber (LFG4 PCI64, Active Silicon, Uxbridge, U.K.). Therefore the ground truth for 55bpm testing was $60/55*25 = 27.27$ frames per heart cycle (fpc). 100 images were captured from the endoscope and the first and last frames are shown in Fig. 5 (a) and (b) respectively. A feature tracker based on optical flow was used to track 50 feature points over the image sequence. The proposed method was employed to calculate the length of heart cycle, and the estimated result was 27.37 frames per heart cycle, very close to the ground truth. The experiment was also repeated at higher frequency of 75bpm. In this situation, the ground truth was 20 frames per cycle. The experimental result was 20.18 frames per cycle, still very close to the ground truth.

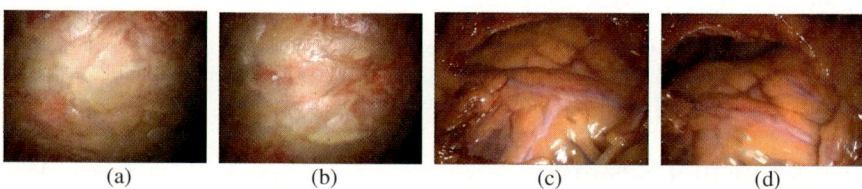

Fig. 5. Image sequences of heart phantom (a, b) and heart surface from TECAB surgery (c, d)

3.3 *In vivo* Data

Finally, the accuracy of the proposed method was evaluated using in vivo data. Our in vivo data set consisted of 50 images from a TECAB surgical procedure using the *da Vinci* system and the first and last frames are shown in Fig. 5 (c) and (d) respectively. These images were captured sequentially from the endoscope with a frame rate of 25fps and 10 feature points were manually detected and tracked from them. In order to provide a ground truth for evaluation, the electrocardiogram (ECG) signal was recorded as well during the beating heart surgery. In our experiment, the ECG reading was 76bmp and the computed cycle length was 19.57 frames per cycle, which is still close to the ground truth, i.e., $60/76*25 = 19.73$ fpc.

4 Discussion and Conclusions

This paper describes a novel technique for heart motion analysis using an image sequence from a moving camera. Epipolar geometry is employed to deal with the change of the camera parameters and to separate respiratory motion from heart motion under an affine assumption. Our approach has been evaluated using simulated data, a heart phantom and *in vivo* data from TECAB surgery. The results indicate the proposed method performs well in terms of both accuracy and robustness to noise, even when high-level noise is involved. Importantly our approach does not require any extra hardware, such as a high speed camera or a laser sensor, to assist the analysis.

Efforts in the near future will focus on further improvement of the robustness to image noise and outliers. Since the heart motion is estimated accurately using the proposed method, we can convert 4D dynamic surface reconstruction into 3D static scene reconstruction, and use the existing techniques i.e. [2] to solve it. Our long term goal is to automatically reconstruct the internal organ surfaces not only the beating heart surface, but also other organ surfaces with periodic motion, such as lung and liver) and register these with the preoperative data (CT or MRI).

Acknowledgments. The authors would like to thank Dr. Roberto Casula at St. Mary Hospital, London for his help in collecting the in vivo data. A special thanks also goes to Dr. Dean Barratt at CMIC, UCL for his helpful suggestions.

References

1. Szpala, S., Wierzbicki, M., Guiraudon, G., Peters, M.T.: Real-time fusion of endoscopic views with dynamic 3-D cardiac images a phantom study. IEEE Trans. Med. Imaging 24(9), 1207–1215 (2005)
2. Hu, M.X., Penney, G.P., Edwards, P.J., Figl, M., Hawkes, D.J.: 3D Reconstruction of Internal Organ Surfaces for Minimal Invasive Surgery. In: Ayache, N., Ourselin, S., Maeder, A. (eds.) MICCAI 2007, Part I. LNCS, vol. 4791, pp. 68–77. Springer, Heidelberg (2007)
3. Nakamura, Y., Kishi, K., Kawakami, H.: Heartbeat Synchronization for Robotic Cardiac Surgery. In: Proc. ICRA, pp. 2014–2019 (2001)

4. Thakral, A., Wallace, J., Tomlin, D., Seth, N., Thakor, N.V.: Surgical Motion Adaptive Robotic Technology (S.M.A.R.T): Taking the Motion out of Physiological Motion. In: Niessen, W.J., Viergever, M.A. (eds.) MICCAI 2001. LNCS, vol. 2208, pp. 317–325. Springer, Heidelberg (2001)
5. Gröger, M., Ortmaier, T., Sepp, W., Hirzinger, G.: Tracking local motion on the beating heart. In: Proc. SPIE Medical Imaging: Visualization, Image-Guided Procedures, and Display, vol. 4681, pp. 233–241 (2002)
6. Ortmaier, T., Groeger, M., Boehm, D.H., Falk, V., Hirzinger, G.: Motion Estimation in Beating Heart Surgery. IEEE Transactions on Biomedical Engineering 52, 1729–1740 (2005)
7. Ginhoux, R., Gangloff, J.A., de Mathelin, M.F., Soler, L., Arenas Sanchez, M.M., Marescaux, J.: Beating heart tracking in robotic surgery using 500 hz visual servoing, model predictive control and an adaptive observer. In: Proc. ICRA, pp. 274–279 (2004)
8. Ginhoux, R., Gangloff, J., de Mathelin, M., Soler, L., Sanchez, M.M.A., Marescaux, J.: Active Filtering of Physiological Motion in Robotized Surgery Using Predictive Control. IEEE Transactions on Robotics 21, 67–79 (2005)
9. Bader, T., Wiedemann, A., Roberts, K., Hanebeck, U.D.: Model-Based Motion Estimation of Elastic Surfaces for Minimally Invasive Cardiac Surgery. In: Proc. ICRA, pp. 2261–2266 (2007)
10. Hartley, R.I., Zisserman, A.: Multiple view geometry in computer vision. Cambridge University Press, Cambridge (2004)
11. Longuet-Higgins, H.C.: A computer algorithm for reconstructing a scene from two projections. Nature 293, 135 (1981)
12. Manke, D., Rosch, P., Nehrke, K., Bornert, P., Dossel, O.: Model evaluation and calibration for prospective respiratory motion correction in coronary MR angiography based on 3-D image registration. IEEE Trans. Med. Imaging 21, 1132–1141 (2002)
13. Shechter, G., Shechter, B., Resar, J.R., Beyar, R.: Prospective motion correction of X-ray images for coronary interventions. IEEE Trans. Med. Imaging 24, 441–450 (2005)
14. Image registration toolkit, http://www.doc.ic.ac.uk/~dr/software/
15. Pratt, P., Bello, F., Edwards, E., Rueckert, D.: Finite element simulation of the beating heart for image-guided robotic cardiac surgery. In: Proc. MICCAI workshop, Computational Biomechanics for Medicine, pp. 74–83 (2007)

On-the-Fly Motion-Compensated Cone-Beam CT Using an a Priori Motion Model

Simon Rit, Jochem Wolthaus, Marcel van Herk, and Jan-Jakob Sonke

The Netherlands Cancer Institute - Antoni
van Leeuwenhoek Hospital, Department of Radiation Oncology, The Netherlands
j.sonke@nki.nl

Abstract. Respiratory motion causes artifacts in slow-rotating cone-beam (CB) computed tomography (CT) images acquired for example for image guidance of radiotherapy. Respiration-correlated CBCT has been proposed to correct for the respiratory motion, but the use of a subset of the CB projections to reconstruct each frame of the 4D CBCT image limits their quality, thus requiring a longer acquisition time. Another solution is motion-compensated CBCT which consists of reconstructing a single 3D CBCT image at a reference position from all the CB projections by using an estimate of the respiratory motion in the reconstruction algorithm. In this paper, we propose a method for motion-compensated CBCT which allows to reconstruct the image on-the-fly, i.e. concurrent with acquisition. Before the CB acquisition, a model of the patient motion over the respiratory cycle is estimated from the planning 4D CT. The respiratory motion is then computed on-the-fly from this model using a respiratory signal extracted from the CB projections and incorporated into the motion-compensated CBCT reconstruction algorithm. The proposed method is evaluated on 26 CBCT scans of 3 patients acquired with two protocols used for static and respiration-correlated CBCT respectively. Our results show that this method provides CBCT images within a few seconds after the end of the acquisition where most of the motion artifacts have been removed.

1 Introduction

Recently, cone-beam (CB) computed tomography (CT) scanners have been integrated with linear accelerators to acquire 3D images of the patient during the fractions of the radiotherapy treatment. These CBCT images allow to correct for the tumor misalignments and, if necessary, to adapt the treatment plan. However, respiratory motion causes artifacts in the thoracic and upper abdominal regions, such as blur and streaks, which can disturb the extracted information.

A first solution to account for the respiratory motion is respiration-correlated CBCT imaging which consists in sorting the CB projections using a respiratory signal depending on their position in the respiratory cycle [1]. Each subset of CB projections is then used to reconstruct a 3D image (or frame) representing one phase of the respiratory cycle, thus obtaining a 4D image over the respiratory cycle. This approach has been successfully implemented clinically in our institution [2] but the use of only a subset of the CB projections to reconstruct each frame limits the image quality due to view-aliasing artifacts. These artifacts were reduced by slowing down the gantry rotation from 200°/min to 50°/min but this caused a longer acquisition time (4 min instead of 1 min) while view-aliasing was still present. Even longer acquisition times were not feasible in clinical practice.

Another solution is to compensate for the respiratory motion in the reconstruction. The non-rigid motion of the patient during the acquisition is estimated and used in the reconstruction algorithm to obtain a 3D CBCT image at a reference position using all the CB projections [3]. It has been shown on simulated data that this method can correct for the respiratory motion without view-aliasing artifacts [3], but the motion estimation on real CB projections is still a challenge. Several solutions have been proposed [4] but their computational cost has prevented the use of motion-compensated CBCT concurrent with acquisition.

In this paper, we propose a solution for on-the-fly motion-compensated CBCT reconstruction. Before acquisition, we estimate a model of the patient motion over the respiratory cycle from a 4D CT image acquired on a conventional scanner. The estimated motion model allows estimation of the respiratory motion from the CB projections on-the-fly, i.e. concurrent with acquisition, using a respiratory signal extracted from the CB projections. The estimated motion is then used in a motion-compensated CBCT reconstruction algorithm. The proposed method is evaluated on patient images and compared to non-corrected and respiration-correlated CBCT images.

2 Method

The complete method is summarized in Fig. 1. Each step is described in detail below.

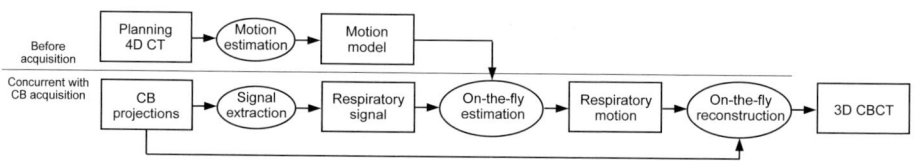

Fig. 1. Flow chart description of the method. Rectangles represent data and ellipses represent processes.

2.1 Motion Model of the Respiratory Cycle

A model of the patient motion over the respiratory cycle was built from the 4D CT image obtained for each patient on a multislice spiral CT scanner. This 4D CT image is acquired approximately 2 weeks prior to the the first treatment fraction and used for the treatment planning. A phase-based optical flow method

[5] adapted for thoracic images [6] was used to estimate the 3D deformation vector fields (DVF) from the end-exhale frame to the other frames of the planning 4D CT. We obtained thus a 4D motion model described by a 4D DVF which represents the piece-wise linear motion of each voxel over the respiratory cycle described by the planning 4D CT image. The average 3D DVF over the frames was subtracted from each frame of the 4D DVF to use the mean position as a reference.

2.2 On-the-Fly Extraction of the Respiratory Signal

The respiratory signal was extracted from the CB projections as implemented previously for on-the-fly respiration-correlated CBCT [2]. Each CB projection was processed to enhance the diaphragm with a derivative filter in the cranio-caudal direction and projected on the cranio-caudal axis in a 1D signal. The concatenation of these 1D signals for a few projections gives a 2D image from which the respiratory signal can be extracted with a linear correlation of adjacent columns.

2.3 On-the-Fly Motion Estimation

The on-the-fly motion estimation assumes that the motion over all the respiratory cycles during the acquisition of the CB projections is identical to the motion described by the planning 4D CT. This approximation is based on the observed stability of the shape of the tumor trajectory from fraction to fraction in a large set of patients [7]. A limited number of parameters remains then to be estimated.

First, each voxel of the CBCT image must be linked to a point of the planning CT. This was done by taking into account the rigid transformation from the coordinate system of the planning CT scanner to the one of the CBCT scanner. We thus assume that anatomical changes and patient setup errors do not significantly affect the motion estimation based on the smoothness of the vector fields in the lungs. This assumption was evaluated by comparing the motion-compensated CBCT images reconstructed with and without correcting for the setup error retrospectively measured with a rigid registration of the non-corrected CBCT image on the planning CT image.

Second, the respiratory displacement of each voxel must be known for each CB projection. This was computed from the motion model by interpolating a 3D DVF from the 4D DVF depending on the respiratory phase value.

2.4 On-the-Fly Reconstruction Algorithm

The reconstruction algorithm was similar to that proposed by [3], i.e. motion compensation based on the local application of the Feldkamp algorithm [8]. The only difference with the static filtered backprojection algorithm of Feldkamp *et al.* is that the backprojection is no longer performed along the straight acquisition lines corresponding to X-rays but along the curved lines corresponding to the acquisition lines warped from the acquisition position to the reference position with the estimated motion (Fig. 2). A high-speed version of the algorithm

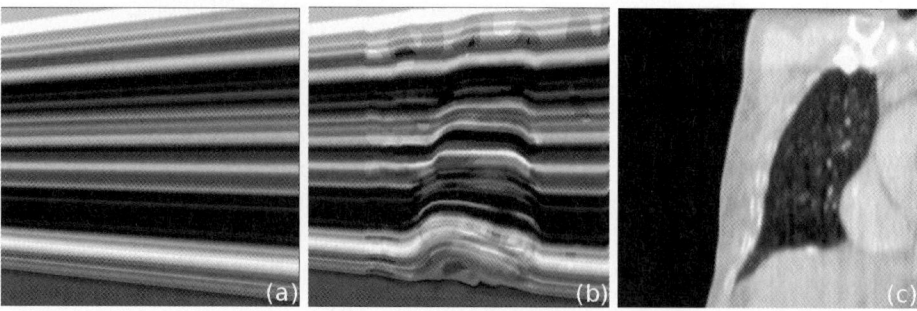

Fig. 2. Coronal slice of one backprojection acquired at end-inhale with the panel perpendicular to the left-right axis in (a) the static case and (b) the motion compensated case. (c) Corresponding slice of the motion-compensated CBCT image of the mean position.

was implemented by optimizing the computation and the memory management and by approximating the respiratory motion in the cranio-caudal direction with a piece-wise linear vector field.

3 Experiments

3.1 Datasets

Three patients were retrospectively selected based on the substantial motion of their lung tumor compared to its volume. For each patient, 3 sets of CB projections were acquired during 3 different fractions using the Elekta Synergy system (Elekta Oncology Systems Ltd., Crawley, West Sussex, UK). Two different gantry rotation speeds were used, a slow acquisition (200° in 4 min), currently used for respiration-correlated CBCT, and a fast acquisition (200° in 1 min), currently used for static CBCT. Table 1 summarizes for each patient the tumor characteristics and the number of scans. Besides the acquisition time, the acquisition and geometric parameters were similar for all acquisitions: X-ray tube: 120 kV, 40 ms and 16 mA; flat-panel: 5.5 fps, 41×41 cm^2, 512 × 512 pixels; source-to-isocenter distance: 100 cm and source-to-panel distance: 154 cm.

Table 1. Tumor characteristics of the 3 patients and number of scans acquired per protocol

	Gross tumor volume (cm^3)	Cranio-caudal tumor motion amplitude (cm)	Number of scans	
			4 min	1 min
Patient 1	6	1.1	3	6
Patient 2	10	2.5	3	6
Patient 3	31	1.9	5	3

3.2 Reconstructed CBCT Images

For each set of CB projections, four different CBCT images were reconstructed: the non-corrected 3D CBCT image (reconstructed as in the static case), the respiration-correlated 4D CBCT image and two motion-compensated 3D CBCT images, with and without a setup error correction for the motion estimation (Sec. 2.3). The 3D CBCT images were reconstructed at a 256^3 grid with 1-mm^3 voxel size and the 4D CBCT images were reconstructed in 10 equidistant phases at a 128^3 grid with 2-mm^3 voxel size.

3.3 Image Analysis

Reconstructed CBCT images were analyzed in two groups depending on the acquisition protocol used for the acquisition (4 min vs. 1 min). Two different criteria were used.

Image quality. The image quality was evaluated relative to the planning CT within a shaped region-of-interest (ROI) manually drawn on the mean position 3D CT to encompass the tumor. The mean position 3D CT was obtained from the planning 4D CT by averaging the frames after warping them to the mean position of each voxel with the estimated motion model. The resulting CT was rigidly registered on each reconstructed CBCT image (or each frame for the 4D CBCT images) using the correlation ratio in the ROI as a similarity measure. After registration, the correlation ratio in the ROI was used to evaluate quantitatively the image quality of reconstructed CBCT images compared to the planning CT. For a fair comparison, all 3D CBCT images were downsampled at a 128^3 grid before performing this evaluation.

Tumor position error. The ROI registration described above is currently used clinically with respiration-correlated 4D CBCT images to correct the position of the patient before the treatment by computing the time-weighted average of the registrations of the tumor in each frame [7]. We compared the position obtained with respiration-correlated 4D CBCT images (reference) with the position obtained with the non-corrected and motion-compensated 3D CBCT images by measuring the Euclidian distance of the misalignment processed by the ROI registration.

4 Results

Fig. 3 shows coronal slices of reconstructed CBCT images of a same patient with two different sets of CB projections, one with the 4 min protocol and the other with the 1 min protocol. For both protocols, the blur induced by the respiratory motion is clearly visible on non-corrected CBCT images around the tumor (center of the slice) and the diaphragm (bottom of the slice). This blur is substantially reduced on respiration-correlated CBCT images but the images are then degraded by view-aliasing artifacts, particularly with the 1 min protocol, as

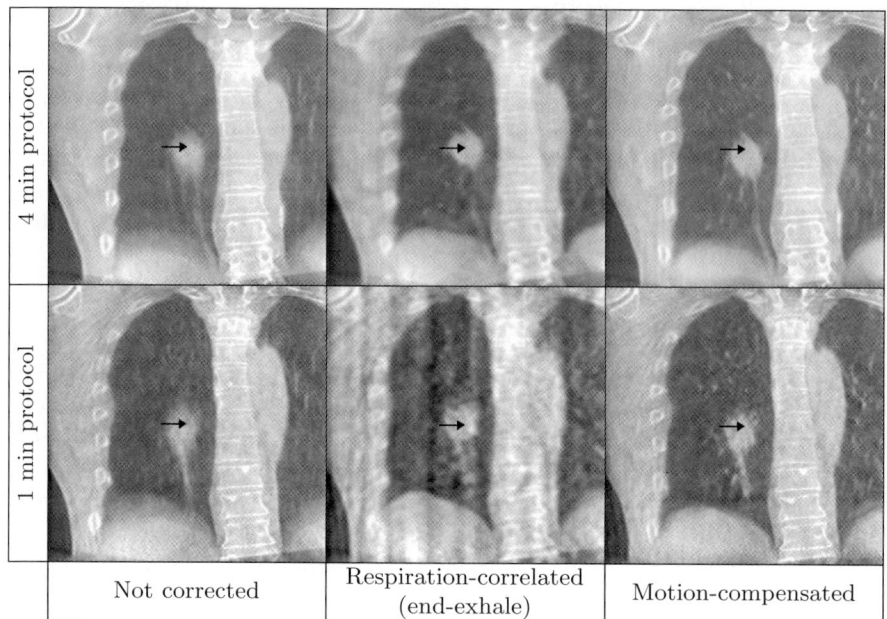

Fig. 3. Coronal slices of reconstructed CBCT images from sets of CB projections acquired with the two different protocols. The motion-compensated CBCT images have been reconstructed without taking into account the setup error. Arrows indicate the isocenter, i.e. the tumor location.

only around 10% of the CB projections are used to reconstruct each frame of the 4D CBCT. Finally, motion-compensated CBCT allows removal of most of the motion artifacts without degradation of the image quality with both protocols.

Fig. 4 depicts the quantitative results. In terms of image quality in the shaped ROI, respiration-correlated CBCT only improves the result with the 4 min acquisition protocol compared to non-corrected CBCT, whereas motion-compensated CBCT improves the image quality with both protocols. Motion-compensated CBCT images reconstructed with the 1 min protocol even have a quality comparable to respiration-correlated CBCT images reconstructed with the 4 min protocol. On average, the distance from the tumor position registered with the respiration-correlated CBCT image was higher with the non-corrected CBCT image (1.9 mm/1.3 mm with the 4 min/1 min protocol) than with the motion-compensated CBCT images (0.4 mm/0.6 mm with the 4 min/1 min protocol). No substantial difference was observed in the ROI between the motion-compensated CBCT images reconstructed with and without setup error correction for the motion estimation.

Computation times were estimated on a desktop computer (dual-core Pentium 4 3.2 GHz station with 3.5 GB RAM). The pre-acquisition part, i.e. the estimation of the motion vector fields of the motion model, took around 3 hours. The per-acquisition part, i.e. the on-the-fly motion estimation and image

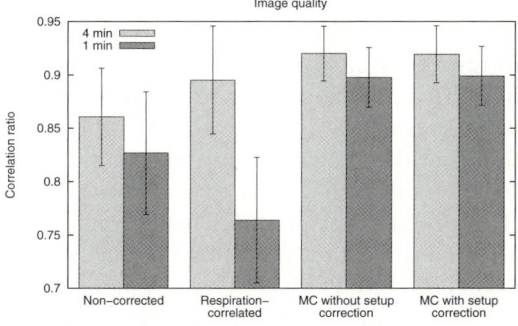 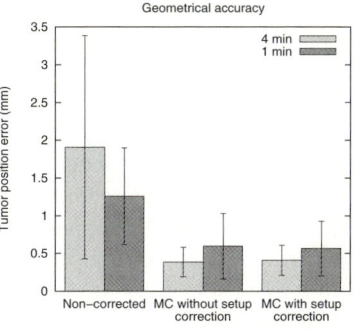

Fig. 4. Average of quantitative criteria over all 4 min and 1 min scans with plus or minus one standard deviation error bars. Left: image quality measured with the correlation ratio between the reconstructed CBCT images and the planning CT image in a shaped ROI encompassing the tumor. Right: tumor position accuracy measured with the respiration-correlated CBCT image as a reference.

reconstruction, took on average 230 s/67 s for the 4 min/1 min protocol (to process the 1360/370 CB projections), i.e. within the order of the acquisition time, such that on-the-fly implementation is possible.

5 Discussion and Conclusion

In this work, we proposed a motion-compensated CBCT method which is suitable for on-the-fly reconstruction, and evaluated it on several CB acquisitions acquired on 3 patients with two different protocols. To minimize the computational time during the acquisition, the patient motion was estimated based on a model computed from the planning 4D CT which was supposed to be still valid for all the respiratory cycles during the CB acquisition. We thus assumed that the respiratory cycle is stable both inter- and intra-fractions. Although this seems to be a strong approximation, the visual (Fig. 3) and quantitative (Fig. 4) results indicate that most of the respiratory artifacts are still corrected. This confirms previous observations of good inter-fraction motion stability measured on respiration-correlated CBCT images which also assumes no intra-fraction variability [7].

The comparison between the two CB acquisition protocols highlights the advantages of motion-compensated CBCT compared to respiration-correlated CBCT. Indeed, the image quality of respiration-correlated CBCT images acquired with a 1 min protocol is not acceptable for clinical applications due to the low number of CB projections per frame subset. The induced view-aliasing artifacts made us change the protocol to a 4 min acquisition. In comparison, the motion-compensated method produces CBCT images with the 1 min protocol where the respiratory motion artifacts are reduced without loss of image quality because all the CB projections are used to correct a single 3D CBCT image.

The proposed method can only be used on-the-fly, i.e. concurrent with the acquisition of the CB projections, if the patient setup error is neglected for the motion estimation because the setup error is usually measured from the reconstructed CBCT image. The quantitative comparison indicates no appreciable improvement when the setup error was taken into account (Fig. 4) which can be explained by the observed smoothness of the vector fields in the lungs. Combined with the fast reconstruction time, ignoring the setup error allows then to have the motion-compensated CBCT image available within a few seconds after the end of the acquisition, keeping thus an important advantage of our current implementation of static and respiration-correlated CBCT. Lower image quality should nevertheless be expected for tumors near the lung walls where the gradient of the vector fields is higher due to the so-called sliding tissue effect. The setup error could then be measured from the non-corrected image and a new reconstruction performed, in which case the time gained by using the 4 min protocol instead of the 1 min one would be partially lost but other advantages kept.

Future work will include validation on more patients as well as more elaborated motion estimation or reconstruction methods to improve the image quality off-line (outside the fractions). The degradation of the image quality due to a wrongly estimated respiratory motion will also be evaluated quantitatively on simulated data.

References

1. Sonke, J.J., Zijp, L., Remeijer, P., van Herk, M.: Respiratory correlated cone beam CT. Med. Phys. 32(4), 1176–1186 (2005)
2. van Herk, M., Zijp, L., Remeijer, P., Wolthaus, J., Sonke, J.J.: On-line 4D cone beam CT for daily correction of lung tumour position during hypofractionated radiotherapy. In: ICCR, Toronto, Canada (2007)
3. Li, T., Schreibmann, E., Yang, Y., Xing, L.: Motion correction for improved target localization with on-board cone-beam computed tomography. Phys. Med. Biol. 51(2), 253–267 (2006)
4. Li, T., Koong, A., Xing, L.: Enhanced 4D cone-beam CT with inter-phase motion model. Med. Phys. 34(9), 3688–3695 (2007)
5. Hemmendorff, M., Andersson, M., Kronander, T., Knutsson, H.: Phase-based multidimensional volume registration. IEEE Trans. Med. Imag. 21(12), 1536–1543 (2002)
6. Wolthaus, J., Sonke, J.J., van Herk, M., Zijp, L., Lebesque, J., Damen, E.: Motion estimation and compensating in 4D CT images using phase-based constraint models. In: ICCR, Toronto, Canada (2007)
7. Sonke, J.J., Lebesque, J., van Herk, M.: Variability of four-dimensional computed tomography patient models. Int. J. Radiat. Oncol. Biol. Phys. 70(2), 590–598 (2008)
8. Feldkamp, L., Davis, L., Kress, J.: Practical cone-beam algorithm. J. Opt. Soc. Am. A 1(6), 612–619 (1984)

A Statistical Motion Model Based on Biomechanical Simulations for Data Fusion during Image-Guided Prostate Interventions

Yipeng Hu[1], Dominic Morgan[1], Hashim Uddin Ahmed[2], Doug Pendsé[3,4], Mahua Sahu[3], Clare Allen[4], Mark Emberton[2], David Hawkes[1], and Dean Barratt[1]

[1] Centre for Medical Image Computing, University College London, London, UK
[2] Department of Urology, University College London, London, UK
[3] National Medical Laser Centre, University College London, London, UK
[4] Department of Radiology, University College Hospital, London, UK

Abstract. A method is described for generating a patient-specific, statistical motion model (SMM) of the prostate gland. Finite element analysis (FEA) is used to simulate the motion of the gland using an ultrasound-based 3D FE model over a range of plausible boundary conditions and soft-tissue properties. By applying principal component analysis to the displacements of the FE mesh node points inside the gland, the simulated deformations are then used as training data to construct the SMM. The SMM is used to both predict the displacement field over the whole gland and constrain a deformable surface registration algorithm, given only a small number of target points on the surface of the deformed gland. Using 3D transrectal ultrasound images of the prostates of five patients, acquired before and after imposing a physical deformation, to evaluate the accuracy of predicted landmark displacements, the mean target registration error was found to be less than 1.9mm.

Keywords: Transrectal ultrasound, minimally-invasive interventions, prostate, statistical shape modelling, biomechanical modelling.

1 Introduction

Transrectal ultrasound (TRUS) is used routinely to guide needle biopsy and therapeutic interventions for prostate cancer. However, TRUS images typically provide only very limited information on the spatial location of tumours. Therefore, the ability to fuse additional information on tumour location, derived from magnetic resonance (MR) imaging as well as needle and novel optical biopsy techniques, with TRUS images represents a major step towards improving the accuracy of image-guided interventions for prostate cancer. In particular, as the sensitivity and specificity of functional and structural MR imaging techniques for detecting and localising prostate cancer continue to improve, and new molecular imaging methods become available, these techniques potentially provide important information for targeting biopsy sampling and therapy delivery. Furthermore, as new minimally-invasive therapies, such as cryotherapy and high-intensity focused US (HIFU), gain popularity, there is an increasing clinical demand for technology that enables preoperative data to be used to deliver therapy at a specific location in order to spare adjacent tissue and minimise the risk of side effects.

Unfortunately, significant gland motion (including deformation) can occur between different image acquisitions due to forces exerted by the bladder and rectum, different patient positions, and the insertion of an endorectal US probe or MR coil [1]. Large changes in gland volume also commonly occur during and following interventions as a physiological response to needle insertion, ablative therapy, or both. In general, most conventional (geometrically constrained) image registration techniques perform poorly when significant organ motion is present due to physically implausible deformations being allowed. Consequently, there is a great deal of interest in motion modelling techniques to help constrain standard algorithms so that the output deformation fields are physically plausible. Statistical models have been reported for describing prostate deformation, which are based on training data drawn from a sample population of patient images [2]. However, establishing anatomical correspondence, both between and within patients, and analysing a sufficiently large training dataset to accurately estimate the variance in both shape and deformation, are challenging tasks. Furthermore, modelling methods based purely on the statistics of shape and deformation can be highly inaccurate when applied to an "atypical" gland that has a shape (or other properties) not represented adequately in the training population.

Some of the limitations highlighted above may be overcome by adopting physically based, biomechanical modeling techniques, such as finite element analysis (FEA), to predict motion given a 3D model of the prostate gland and surrounding tissue [3]-[5]. However, the accuracy of displacements predicted using this approach normally depends on the accuracy of boundary conditions (such as the position and orientation of the TRUS probe) and the values assigned to the elastic properties of soft tissues, which are known to vary considerably between patients: Chi et al., for example, report a registration error of up to 4.5mm due solely to a 30% uncertainty in material properties for a solid FE model of the prostate [5]. Furthermore, the computation time of FEA increases with the complexity of the model, which can make this method impractical in the interventional situation due to clinical time constraints, even when, for example, graphical processor units are employed.

In this paper, we adopt a combined biomechanical-statistical approach similar to that proposed to that by Mohamed et al. [6] in which a statistical deformation model is constructed from simulated deformations of a FE model of the prostate gland under different boundary conditions (TRUS probe position). However, we extend this approach to include material properties as variable parameters in the biomechanical simulations and validate the accuracy of a deformable registration algorithm, which uses information on gland deformation provided by the statistical model. This approach addresses the problem of uncertainty in material properties associated with direct FEA by using a statistical approach to capture variability in these parameters. Furthermore, since a SMM is inherently compact, it can be used to compute 3D solid models of the deformed prostate very rapidly, and is therefore well suited to intraoperative use. Alterovitz et al. [7] describe a method for estimating prostate deformation in 2D using FEA of a model based on MR images, which includes material properties and external forces as unknown parameters in the estimation algorithm. However, to the best of the Authors' knowledge, the present study is the first to report on the application and validation of full 3D FEA to estimate gland motion in a statistical framework without requiring accurate knowledge of material properties or the position of the TRUS probe and pelvic bone relative to the prostate.

2 Methods

A schematic overview of the registration scheme developed in this work is shown in Fig. 1. The steps involved can be summarised as follows:

a) Build a patient-specific 3D FE model based on a manually segmented 3D TRUS image (i.e., source image). In this work, the prostate gland was segmented using manual contouring, but a more automated method would be highly desirable.
b) Perform a large number of FEA simulations using a range of boundary conditions (specifically, the position of the TRUS probe/balloon and position and size of the pelvis relative to the prostate gland) and range of different material properties assigned to homogeneous regions of the FE model.
c) Apply principal component analysis (PCA) on the predicted displacement of FE mesh node points and build a SMM using the principal modes of variation in node displacement.
d) Identify a small number of surface points in planes corresponding to 6 slices through a 3D TRUS image of the deformed gland (i.e., the target image).
e) Register the deformable gland model to the target surface points by optimising the weights of the principal modes of variation of the SMM such that the distance between the target point set and the deformed model surface is minimised.

To enable rigorous validation without using implanted fiducial markers, in this study both the target and source TRUS images were acquired at the start of a procedure. However, it is intended that, in clinical practice, the source image would be acquired prior to a procedure, using either 3D TRUS or MR. Stages a–c are computationally intensive and would be performed before the intervention, whereas stages d and e would take place during an intervention (in realtime). Details of the experimental methods used in this study are provided in the following sections.

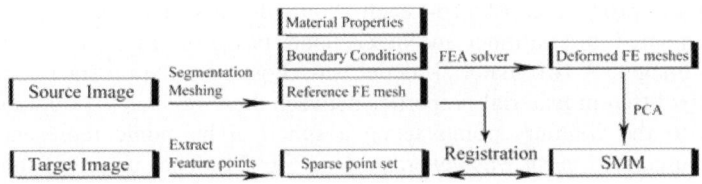

Fig. 1. Schematic overview of the method adopted. In this study, the source and target images were 3D TRUS images obtained before and after expanding the saline-filled balloon around the TRUS probe, respectively.

2.1 3D TRUS Volume Acquisition

Three-dimensional TRUS images of the prostate were acquired for 5 patients undergoing a template-guided biopsy, or HIFU or photodynamic therapy (PDT) for treatment of prostate cancer. All patients were recruited to clinical research studies, approved by the local research ethics committee at University College Hospital, and gave written consent to participate. In the case of biopsy and PDT, a set of parallel transverse B-mode US images was obtained using a B-K ProFocus scanner (B-K Medical, Berkshire, UK) and a mechanical stepper mechanism (Tayman Medical Inc., MO, USA) to translate the probe (B-K 8658T, 5-7.5MHz transducer) axially along the rectum. Images were captured at 2mm intervals and stored on the US scanner. In the case of HIFU therapy, 3D volumes were acquired automatically using a Sonablate® 500 system (Focus Surgery, Inc., Indiana, USA). Two volumes were acquired for each patient at the start of the procedure: one with the balloon at minimal expansion, and the other after expanding the balloon by injecting saline with a syringe in order to deform the prostate gland. Expanding the balloon in this way simulates the motion of the prostate gland that might typically occur due to the presence of a TRUS probe or an endorectal MR imaging coil. The first volume was chosen as the source image for building the SMM, whilst the second was used for accuracy evaluation.

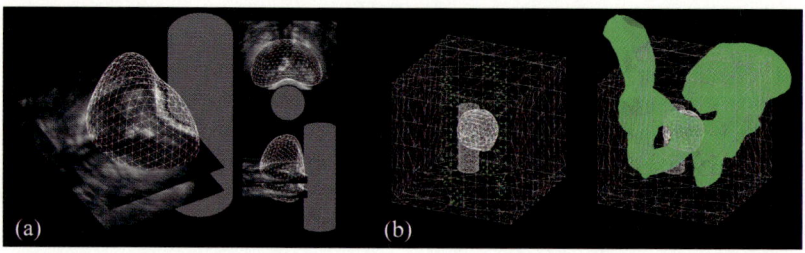

Fig. 2. (a) Three views of the triangulated surface mesh and cylinder representing the rectal balloon surface. (b) Illustration of the two methods used to constrain displacements away from the prostate: left – simple constraint (fixed node points are shown in green); right – realistic pelvis-shaped constraint (shown in green).

2.2 Finite Element Model Construction

In this study, the prostate was segmented from each 3D TRUS volume by manually contouring the prostate capsule on each acquired transverse slices. The gland was further segmented into an inner and outer gland, based on differences in echotexture on the US images. A two material model was chosen for the prostate because of the significantly different material properties between these regions [3]. A smooth surface was fitted to the contours points using a spherical harmonic representation from which a triangulated mesh was generated (see Fig. 2a). The surface of the balloon in contact with the rectum was modelled as a cylinder. The diameter and position of the cylinder was determined automatically by performing a least squares fit to points on the balloon surface, extracted from the TRUS images using Canny edge detection. The tissue surrounding the prostate was modelled as a homogeneous block with dimensions 20×20×20 cm^3. The surface meshes and the block structure were imported into the commercial FEA software ANSYS (ANSYS Europe Ltd., Oxfordshire, UK) using the solid modelling tool. The FE model was then constructed and meshed into 30-40,000 tetrahedral elements using trimmed parametric surfaces and Delaunay tessellation techniques provided by the software. Ten-node tetrahedral elements were used as these support non-linear geometries using unstructured meshes. Regions corresponding to the each part of the prostate gland, the rectal wall, and surrounding tissue were labelled separately. All tissues were assumed to behave as isotropic, linear elastic materials under loading, and node displacements were computed using the pre-conditions conjugate gradient iterative equation solver in ANSYS.

2.3 Boundary Conditions

FEA simulations of prostate motion were performed using the three different sets of boundary conditions are summarised in Table 1. These are explained as follows:

Table 1. Summary of boundary condition configurations used for FEA simulations

SMM	Balloon position	Bony constraints	Degrees of freedom
M1	Fixed	Fixed – Simple constraint	1
M2	Fixed	Variable pelvis position and size	5
M3	Variable	Variable pelvis position and size	8

Balloon/TRUS probe displacement: The expansion of the balloon was modelled by displacing the cylinder surface nodes radially to lie on the surface of an enlarged cylinder fitted to balloon surface points detected in the target (i.e., deformed) TRUS image. This step provided a fixed boundary condition for the FEA simulations, which could be easily and automatically performed during an intervention. However, as the assumption of no probe/patient motion may not always be valid, a random displacement in the range -5.0 to 5.0mm was added to each of the x, y and z co-ordinates of the cylinder to compare the performance of the resulting SMMs.

Bony constraints: Because only a very small part of the pelvic bone is visualised in TRUS images, it was not possible to accurately estimate its location relative to the prostate. Two methods for introducing bony constraints into the FE model were used, as shown in Fig. 2b. In the first, mesh nodes lying on four-strips around the gland were fixed. In the second, the nodes on the surface of a realistically-shaped model of the pelvic bone were fixed. The pelvis model was generated by a statistical shape model derived from CT images [8]. The initial size of the bone was set to the mean and the initial position was determined using the method described in [9]. In two of the series of biomechanical simulations the position and size of the pelvis were varied by adding a random (normally distributed) displacement of 0.0 ± 5.0mm (mean ± SD) to the x-, y-, and z-components of the pelvis position vector, and by varying a global scaling factor with a mean of 1.0 and a SD of 0.2.

2.4 Material Properties

Since it can been argued that the assumption of incompressibility (Poisson's ratio, $v = 0.5$) may not be appropriate for the prostate (and perhaps other soft-tissue) because of fluid gain and loss, and the presence of a collapsible urethra, both the Young's modulus (E) and the Poisson's ratio (v) assigned to different materials in the FE model were assumed to be unknown. Therefore, the relative values of these parameters were varied for the prostate compartments and surrounding tissue block in the FEA simulations. The values assigned to E and v for the inner and outer prostate gland and the surrounding tissue were sampled at 4 uniformly-spaced intervals over the ranges 10–200kPa and 0.01–0.49, respectively. The rectal wall in contact with the balloon was however assumed to be nearly incompressible as it is thin and already compressed, and was assigned the fixed values E=100kPa and v=0.49, which had the effect of reducing the number of degrees of freedom in the simulations to 6. Subsequently, 4^6=4096 simulations were performed for each of the 3 boundary condition configurations given in Table 1.

2.5 Statistical Motion Model

For each of M (=4096) simulated gland deformations, the 3D displacement of every node in the prostate gland mesh was calculated and combined to form a $3N\times 1$ vector, **x**, which describes the predicted displacement of the gland mesh nodes (N is the number of nodes). The principal modes of variation in **x** were then calculated using PCA. If $\mathbf{S}_0$ is a vector containing the co-ordinates of the node points of the initial model, the vector, **S**, containing the corresponding node positions of a deformed prostate is given by:

$$\mathbf{S} = \mathbf{S}_0 + \bar{\mathbf{x}} + \sum_{i=1}^{L} c_i \mathbf{e}_i, \quad 1 \leq L \leq M, \tag{1}$$

where $\bar{\mathbf{x}}$ is the mean displacement vector, $\mathbf{e}_i$ is the ith eigenvector of the covariance matrix, and c_i is a scalar weight. L was chosen so that the SMM covered >99% of variance in the training data and gave a model reconstruction error, ε, < 0.1mm, where

$$\varepsilon = \sqrt{\frac{1}{3N}\left(\sum_{i=1}^{M}c_i\mathbf{e}_i - \sum_{i=1}^{L}c_i\mathbf{e}_i\right)^T\left(\sum_{i=1}^{M}c_i\mathbf{e}_i - \sum_{i=1}^{L}c_i\mathbf{e}_i\right)}. \tag{2}$$

2.6 Model Registration

In practice, a full segmentation of the prostate surface in the target TRUS image is impractical during a surgical procedure because manual contouring remains the most reliable and accurate way of delineating the capsule. However, since the resulting SMM is very well constrained, only a sparse set of surface points is required to register the deformable prostate model. To simulate a simple and clinically feasible protocol for defining target points, the segmented target TRUS image was resliced in 3 sagittal and 3 transverse planes and 6 evenly-spaced points computed along the surface contours in each slice. Starting with the mean shape, the first L weights, $\{c_1, c_2, \ldots, c_L\}$, were optimised to minimise the distance between the target points and the deformed model surface in MATLAB using a nonlinear least-squares optimisation algorithm. Once registered, the positions of any point inside the deformed gland can be calculated by interpolating the node point positions. For the purposes of comparison with a rigid registration algorithm, the source (i.e., undeformed) surface was registered to the target points using the well-known ICP algorithm.

2.7 Accuracy Validation

A number of corresponding landmarks, including cysts, calcifications and the urethra, were identified manually in the source and target TRUS volumes. The landmarks in

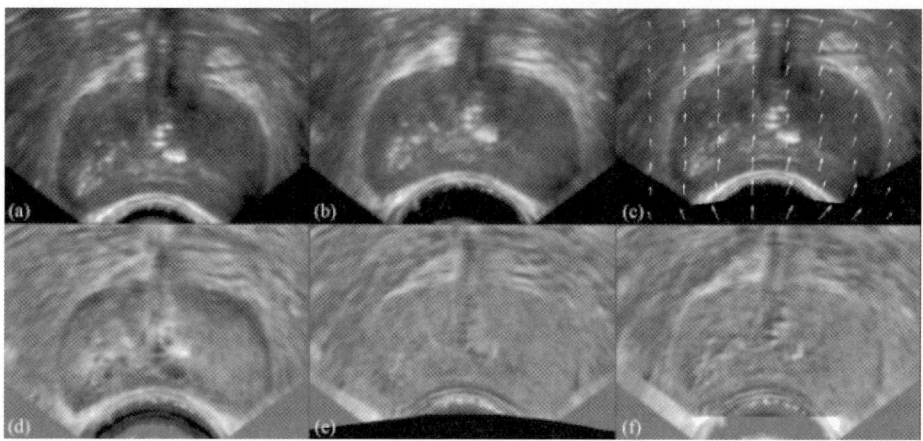

Fig. 3. Example transverse slices through 3D TRUS images (Case 1). From top left: (a) Source image (balloon minimally expanded); (b) Target image (balloon maximally expanded); (c) Source image after warping using the interpolated displacement field generated by registering the SMM (shown as white arrows); (d)-(f) Subtracted images: (d) target – source (b – a); (e) target – warped source (b – c); (f) target – source after rigid registration.

Table 2. Target registration errors calculated for anatomical landmarks (the boundary conditions used for the models M1, M2 and M3 are summarised in Table 1)

Case No.	No. Landmarks	Mean±SD TRE (mm)				
		Start	Rigid	M1	M2	M3
1 (Biopsy)	12	5.45 ± 1.16	3.32 ± 0.98	1.90 ± 0.54	1.83 ± 0.61	2.04 ± 0.61
2 (PDT)	7	4.32 ± 1.39	2.59 ± 0.50	1.45 ± 0.96	1.45 ± 0.92	2.06 ± 0.76
3 (HIFU)	8	5.03 ± 0.78	2.23 ± 1.28	1.77 ± 0.54	1.86 ± 0.52	2.05 ± 0.67
4 (Biopsy)	15	4.47 ± 1.02	2.63 ± 0.77	1.86 ± 0.52	1.80 ± 0.51	1.49 ± 0.68
5 (HIFU)	6	6.42 ± 1.48	3.73 ± 0.98	2.38 ± 0.86	2.32 ± 0.86	2.22 ± 0.76
All	48	5.03 ± 1.29	2.87 ± 1.01	1.86 ± 0.67	1.83 ± 0.67	1.89 ± 0.71

the source image were then propagated into the target image space using the displacement field produced by the SMM. For each pair of landmarks, a target registration error (TRE) was calculated, defined as the distance between the manually defined position and the propagated position of a landmark in the target image space.

3 Results

The landmark-based TREs are given in Table 2. Fig. 3 illustrates the difference between transverse TRUS slices after deformable versus rigid registration for Case 1. All registrations were completed within 10s on a PC with a 2.33GHz Intel® Core™ dual CPU processor and 3GB of RAM (between 7 and 11 principal modes were used for the SMMs). The average time taken to compute each SMM was approximately 50 hours. Inspection of the results in Table 2 reveals that the most accurate registrations were achieved using an SMM to constrain the deformation. Although a significant proportion of gland motion (~40%) is recovered using a rigid registration scheme, the

SMM-constrained deformable registration on average recovered approximately 60% of the motion, depending on the amount of deformation. An interesting observation is that including bony constraints and associated additional degrees of freedom in the SMM relating to the position of the pelvic bone made very little difference to the overall registration accuracy inside the gland.

4 Discussion

The approach in this study combines statistical shape modelling techniques with biomechanical simulations to generate a patient-specific, 3D deformable model that can be rapidly registered to a small number of surface points identified from TRUS slices. Since the model can be generated before a procedure and does not require accurate estimates of material properties, this method is clinically feasible, although further work is required to reduce the amount of pre-procedural computation and manual interaction, and to investigate the accuracy of generating an SMM from other imaging modalities, such as MR. In this case, the diameter and pose of the TRUS balloon are unknown *a priori* and therefore some additional degrees of freedom would be required (although good estimates could easily be obtained, particularly if a standardised protocol is adopted for probe insertion). The results of this study suggest that a complex FE model with accurate bony constraints derived from MR or CT data may be unnecessary when only the motion of the prostate is of interest. The use of TRUS data made it much easier to determine an accurate gold standard for landmark displacements compared with multimodal images, since identifying multiple corresponding intra-gland landmarks is difficult without using fiducial markers.

References

1. Byrne, T.E.: A review of prostate motion with considerations for the treatment of prostate cancer. Medical Dosimetry 30, 155–161 (2005)
2. Dam, E.B., et al.: Prostate shape modelling based on principal geodesic analysis bootstrapping. In: Barillot, C., Haynor, D.R., Hellier, P. (eds.) MICCAI 2004. LNCS, vol. 3217, pp. 1008–1016. Springer, Heidelberg (2004)
3. Bharatha, A., et al.: Evaluation of three-dimensional finite element-based deformable registration of pre-and intraoperative prostate imaging. Med. Phys. 28, 2551–2560 (2001)
4. Crouch, J.R., et al.: Automated finite element analysis for deformable registration of prostate images. IEEE Trans. on Med. Imag. 26, 1379–1390 (2007)
5. Chi, Y., et al.: A material sensitivity study on the accuracy of deformable organ registration using linear biomechanical models. Med. Phys. 33, 421–433 (2006)
6. Mohamed, A., et al.: A combined statistical and biomechanical model for estimation of intra-operative prostate deformation. In: Dohi, T., Kikinis, R. (eds.) MICCAI 2002. LNCS, vol. 2489, pp. 452–460. Springer, Heidelberg (2002)
7. Alterovitz, R., et al.: Registration of MR prostate images with biomechanical modeling and nonlinear parameter estimation. Med. Phys. 33, 446–454 (2006)
8. Thompson, et al.: Use of a CT statistical deformation model for multi-modal pelvic bone segmentation. In: Proc. SPIE Medical Imaging (2008)
9. Schallenkamp, J., et al.: Prostate position relative to pelvic bony anatomy based on intra-prostatic gold markers and electronic portal imaging. Int. J. Radiation Oncology Biol. Phys. 63, 800–811 (2005)

Spherical Demons: Fast Surface Registration

B.T. Thomas Yeo[1,*], Mert Sabuncu[1], Tom Vercauteren[2], Nicholas Ayache[3], Bruce Fischl[4,1], and Polina Golland[1]

[1] Computer Science and Artificial Intelligence Laboratory, MIT, USA
[2] Mauna Kea Technologies, Paris, France
[3] Asclepios Group, INRIA, France
[4] Athinoula A. Martinos Center for Biomedical Imaging, MGH/HMS, USA

Abstract. We present the fast Spherical Demons algorithm for registering two spherical images. By exploiting spherical vector spline interpolation theory, we show that a large class of regularizers for the modified demons objective function can be efficiently implemented on the sphere using convolution. Based on the one parameter subgroups of diffeomorphisms, the resulting registration is diffeomorphic and fast – registration of two cortical mesh models with more than 100k nodes takes less than 5 minutes, comparable to the fastest surface registration algorithms. Moreover, the accuracy of our method compares favorably to the popular FreeSurfer registration algorithm. We validate the technique in two different settings: (1) parcellation in a set of in-vivo cortical surfaces and (2) Brodmann area localization in ex-vivo cortical surfaces.

1 Introduction

Motivated by the spherical representation of the cerebral cortex, this paper deals with the problem of registering two spherical images. Cortical folding patterns are correlated with both cytoarchitectural [13] and functional regions [11]. In group studies of cortical structure and function, determining corresponding folds across subjects is therefore important. There has been much effort focused on registering cortical surfaces in 3D [9,10,14]. Since cortical areas – both structure and function – are arranged in a mosaic across the cortical surface, an alternative approach is to model the surface as a 2D closed manifold in 3D and to warp the resulting spherical coordinate system [11,18,20,21,23].

Unfortunately, many spherical warping algorithms are computationally expensive. One reason is the need for invertible deformations that preserve the topology of structural or functional regions across subjects. Previously demonstrated methods for cortical registration [11,18,23] rely on soft regularization constraints to encourage invertibility. They require computationally expensive steps of unfolding the mesh triangles or small optimization steps to achieve invertibility [11,23]. Elegant regularization penalties to guarantee invertibility exist [2,16] but make certain assumptions valid only in Euclidean spaces.

---

* Corresponding author: ythomas@csail.mit.edu

An alternative approach to achieve invertibility is to work in a Lie group of diffeomorphisms [3,4,9,15,22], the theory of which can be extended to manifolds [15]. The Large Deformable Diffeomorphic Metric Mapping (LDDMM) [4,9,15] is a popular framework under this paradigm that seeks diffeomorphisms parametrized by time-varying velocity fields. Because LDDMM optimizes over the entire path of the diffeomorphism, the resulting algorithm is slow.

In this paper, we take the approach, previously demonstrated in the Euclidean space [22], of restricting the deformation space to be a composition of diffeomorphisms, each of which is parameterized by a stationary velocity field. In each iteration, the algorithm greedily seeks the best diffeomorphism to be composed with the current transformation, resulting in much faster updates.

Another challenge in registration is the tradeoff between the image similarity measure and the regularization in the objective function. Since most regularizations favor smooth deformations, the gradient computation is complicated by the need to take into account the deformation in neighboring regions. For Euclidean images, the demons objective function [19,6,22] facilitates a fast two-step optimization where the second step handles the warp regularization via a single convolution with a smoothing filter.

Based on spherical vector spline interpolation theory [15] and other differential geometric tools, we show that the two-stage optimization procedure of the demons algorithm can be efficiently applied on the sphere. The problem is not trivial since tangent vectors at different points on the sphere are not comparable. We also emphasize that the extension of the demons algorithm to the sphere is *independent* of our choice of the space of admissible warps.

The Spherical Demons algorithm takes less than 5 minutes on a Xeon 3.2GHz processor, comparable to other non-linear cortical surface registration algorithms whose runtimes range from minutes [10,18] to more than an hour [11,23]. However, these fast algorithms [10,18] suffer from folding spherical triangles and intersecting triangles in 3D since only soft constraints are used.

Unlike [9,15], we do not assume the existence of corresponding landmarks. While landmark-free registration is harder, we demonstrate that our algorithm is accurate in both cortical parcellation and cyto-architectonic localization applications.

The contributions of this paper are multi-fold. First, we show that the demons algorithm can be efficiently applied on the sphere. Second, the use of a limited class of diffeomorphisms yields a speed gain of more than an order of magnitude compared with other landmark-free diffeomorphic spherical registration methods. Finally, we validate our algorithm by showing accuracy comparable to the popular FreeSurfer algorithm [11] on two data sets.

2 Background - Demons Algorithm

We choose to work with the modified demons objective function, essentially identical to [6,22], with a slightly different interpretation:

$$(s^*, c^*) = \underset{s,c}{\operatorname{argmin}} \|F - M \circ c\|^2 + \frac{1}{\sigma_x^2}\operatorname{dist}(s, c) + \frac{1}{\sigma_T^2}\operatorname{Reg}(s) \qquad (1)$$

where F is the fixed image, M is the moving image, c is the desired registration and s is a hidden transformation that acts as a prior on c. The fixed image F and warped moving image $M \circ c$ are treated as $N \times 1$ vectors. Typically, $\text{dist}(s, c) = \|s - c\|^2$, encouraging the resulting transformation c to be close to the hidden transformation s and $\text{Reg}(s) = \|\nabla s\|^2$, i.e., the regularization penalizes the gradient magnitude of the hidden transformation s. σ_x and σ_T provide a tradeoff among the different terms of the objective function.

This formulation facilitates a two-step optimization procedure that alternately optimizes the first two and last two terms of Eq. (1). Starting from an initial displacement field s^0, the demons algorithm iteratively seeks an update transformation to be composed with the current estimate.

Algorithm: Demons

Step 1. Given $s^{(t)}$, minimize the first two terms of Eq. (1)

$$u^{(t)} = \underset{u}{\arg\min} \, \|F - M \circ \{s^{(t)} \circ u\}\|^2 + \frac{1}{\sigma_x^2} \text{dist}(s^{(t)}, \{s^{(t)} \circ u\}) \tag{2}$$

where u is any admissible transformation. Compute $c^{(t)} = s^{(t)} \circ u^{(t)}$.

Step 2. Given $c^{(t)}$, minimize the last two terms of Eq. (1):

$$s^{(t+1)} = \underset{s}{\arg\min} \, \frac{1}{\sigma_x^2} \text{dist}(s, c^{(t)}) + \frac{1}{\sigma_T^2} \text{Reg}(s) \tag{3}$$

In the original demons algorithm [19], the space of admissible warps include all displacement fields: u, s and c are 3D displacement fields, and the composition operator $\circ$ corresponds to the addition of displacement fields. In the Diffeomorphic Demons algorithm [22], u is a diffeomorphism from $\mathbb{R}^3$ to $\mathbb{R}^3$ parameterized by a stationary velocity field v. Under certain smoothness conditions, a stationary velocity field v is related to a diffeomorphism through the exponential mapping $u = \exp(v)$. In this case, $\exp(v)$ is the solution at time 1 of the stationary ODE $\partial x(t)/\partial t = v(x(t))$, with $x(0) \in \mathbb{R}^3$. Deformation $\exp(v)(\cdot)$ maps point $x(0)$ to point $x(1)$.

The demons algorithm and its variants are fast because for certain forms of $\text{dist}(s, c)$ and $\text{Reg}(s)$, step 1 reduces to a non-linear least-squares problem that can be efficiently minimized via Gauss-Newton optimization and step 2 can be solved by a single convolution of the displacement field c with a smoothing filter.

3 Spherical Demons

In this section, we show that suitable choices of $\text{dist}(s, c)$ and $\text{Reg}(s)$ lead to efficient optimization on the sphere S^2. We work with updates u that are diffeomorphisms parameterized by a stationary velocity field v. We emphasize that unlike [22], v is tangent to the sphere and not an arbitrary 3D vector. It is also easy to extend our results to other transformations, e.g., spherical splines.

Choice of dist(s, c). Suppose the transformation c maps a point $x_n \in S^2$ to a point $c(x_n) \in S^2$. Let $T_{x_n} S^2$ be the tangent space at x_n. We define $\vec{c}_n \in T_{x_n} S^2$ to be the tangent vector at x_n, pointing along the great circle connecting x_n to $c(x_n)$, with length equal to the sine of the angle between x_n and $c(x_n)$. There is a 1-to-1 correspondence between $c(x_n)$ and $\vec{c}_n$, assuming the angle is less than $\pi/2$, which is reasonable even for relatively large deformations. On a unit sphere, $\vec{c}_n = -x_n \times (x_n \times c(x_n)) = -D_n^2 c(x_n)$, where D_n is the 3 × 3 skew-symmetric matrix representing the cross-product of x_n with another vector.

For a mesh of N vertices $\{x_n\}_{n=1}^N$, the set of transformed points $\{c(x_n)\}_{n=1}^N$ (or equivalently tangent vectors $\{\vec{c}_n\}_{n=1}^N$), together with a choice of an interpolation function, define the transformation c completely. Similarly, we can define s through $\{\vec{s}_n\}_{n=1}^N$. We emphasize that these tangent vector fields are just convenient representations of the transformations s and c and should not be confused with the velocity vector field v. We define $\text{dist}(s, c) = \sum_{n=1}^N \|\vec{s}_n - \vec{c}_n\|^2$, which is well-defined since both $\vec{c}_n$ and $\vec{s}_n$ belong to $T_{x_n} S^2$.

Choice of Reg(s). With a slight abuse of notation, we use s to denote both the transformation and its equivalent tangent vector field representation. We assume s belongs to the Hilbert space V of vector fields obtained by the closure of the space of smooth vector fields on S^2 via a choice of the so-called energetic norm denoted by $\|\cdot\|_V$ [15]. We define $\text{Reg}(s) = \|s\|_V$. With a proper choice of the energetic norm, a smaller value of $\|s\|_V$ corresponds to a smoother vector field. As we will see, the exact choice of the norm is unimportant for our purposes.

Step 1. With our choice of dist(s,c), Step 1 of the demons algorithm is a minimization with respect to the velocity field v defined by $\{\vec{v}_n \in T_{x_n} S^2\}_{n=1}^N$:

$$\{\vec{v}_n^{(t)}\} = \underset{\{\vec{v}_n\}}{\operatorname{argmin}} \|F - M \circ \{s^{(t)} \circ \exp(v)\}\|^2 + \frac{1}{\sigma_x^2} \sum_{n=1}^N \|\vec{s}_n^{(t)} + D_n^2 \{s^{(t)} \circ \exp(v)\}(x_n)\|^2 \quad (4)$$

$\vec{v}_n$ is a 3 × 1 tangent vector on the sphere. Let $\vec{e}_1, \vec{e}_2$ be 3 × 1 orthogonal basis vectors of the tangent space $T_{x_n} S^2$. We can write $\vec{v}_n = [\vec{e}_1 \vec{e}_2] \vec{v}'_n$ where $\vec{v}'_n$ is a 2 × 1 vector. We can thus optimize Eq. (4) with respect to $\{\vec{v}'_n\}$. The above non-linear least-squares form can be optimized efficiently with the Gauss-Newton method, which requires finding the gradient of both terms with respect to $\{\vec{v}'_n\}$ at $\{\vec{v}'_n = 0\}$ and solving a linearized least-squares problem. By switching back and forth between the tangent representation $\vec{v}'_n$ and embedding space representation $\vec{v}_n$, we construct an update rule *independent* of the choice of coordinate frames.

To see that, let $\overline{M}$ be a 3D image defined to be any smooth extension of $M \circ s^{(t)}$. For example, for all $x \in \mathbb{R}^3 \backslash 0$, $\overline{M}(x) = M \circ s^{(t)}(x/\|x\|)$. Similarly, we extend $s^{(t)}$ to $\overline{s}$. Let $\vec{m}_n^T = \nabla \overline{M}(x_n)$ be the 1x3 gradient of $\overline{M}$ at x_n and $B_n^T = \nabla \overline{s}(x_n)$ be the 3×3 gradient of $\overline{s}$. Since the differential of $\exp(v')$ at $v' = 0$ is the identity, the derivative of the entries corresponding to vertex n in both terms of Eq. (4) with respect to $\vec{v}'_k$ is 0 if $n \neq k$. With some algebra, we get:

$$\frac{\partial}{\partial \vec{v}'_n} \left[F(x_n) - M \circ \{s^{(t)} \circ \exp(\vec{v})\}(x_n) \right]_{\vec{v}=0} = -\vec{m}_n^T \left[\vec{e}_1 \vec{e}_1^T + \vec{e}_2 \vec{e}_2^T \right] \quad (5)$$

$$\frac{\partial}{\partial \vec{v}'_n} \left[\vec{s}_n^{(t)} + D_n^2 \{s^{(t)} \circ \exp(\vec{v})\}(x_n) \right]_{\vec{v}=0} = D_n^2 B_n^T \left[\vec{e}_1 \vec{e}_1^T + \vec{e}_2 \vec{e}_2^T \right] \quad (6)$$

The above equations involve the projection of the spatial gradients of $\overline{M}$ and $\overline{s}$ onto the tangent space $T_{x_n}S^2$ and are therefore independent of the choices of $\vec{e}_1, \vec{e}_2$ or the extension mechanism for $\overline{M}$ and $\overline{s}$. This leads to the following Gauss-Newton update for velocity vector $\vec{v}'_n$:

$$\vec{v}'^{(t)}_n = (F(x_n) - M \circ s^{(t)}(x_n)) \times$$

$$\times \left(\begin{bmatrix} \vec{e}_1^T \\ \vec{e}_2^T \end{bmatrix} \left[\vec{m}_n \vec{m}_n^T + \frac{1}{\sigma_x^2} B_n (D_n^2)^T D_n^2 B_n^T \right] [\vec{e}_1 \; \vec{e}_2] \right)^{-1} \begin{bmatrix} \vec{e}_1^T \\ \vec{e}_2^T \end{bmatrix} \vec{m}_n \quad (7)$$

Eq. (7) is used to compute $\vec{v}'^{(t)}_n$ for each vertex n independently and is therefore fast. We can then compute $\vec{v}^{(t)}_n = [\vec{e}_1 \; \vec{e}_2] \vec{v}'^{(t)}_n$ and use scaling and squaring to estimate $\exp(v^{(t)})$ [1], which is then composed with the current transformation estimate $s^{(t)}$ to form $c^{(t)} = s^{(t)} \circ \exp(v^{(t)})$. It is less obvious here, but the update is independent of the choice of basis vectors $\vec{e}_1, \vec{e}_2$ and extensions $\overline{s}^{(t)}$ and $\overline{M}_s$.

Step 2. The optimization in Step 2 of the demons algorithm

$$s^{(t+1)} = \underset{s}{\mathrm{argmin}} \; \frac{1}{\sigma_x^2} \sum_{n=1}^{N} \|\vec{s}_n - \vec{c}_n^{(t)}\|^2 + \frac{1}{\sigma_T^2} \|s\|_V \quad (8)$$

seeks a smooth vector field s that approximates the tangent vectors $\{\vec{c}_n^{(t)}\}_{n=1}^N$. The optimum $s^{(t+1)}$ is unique and is computed by solving a large system of linear equations [15]. We extend the results in [15], proving that the optimum vector field $s^{(t+1)}$ at x_n always has the form

$$\vec{s}_n^{(t+1)} = \sum_{i=1}^{N} \lambda(x_i, x_n) T(x_i, x_n) \vec{c}_i^{(t)} \quad (9)$$

where $T(x_i, x_n)\vec{c}_i$ is a linear transformation that parallel transports $\vec{c}_i$ along the great circle from $T_{x_i}S^2$ to $T_{x_n}S^2$ and $\lambda(x_i, x_n)$ is a non-negative scalar function that monotonically decreases as a function of the distance between x_i and x_n. We omit the proof due to space constraints.

In contrast to [15], Eq. (9) implies that we can avoid solving a large system of equations. The optimal tangent vector $\vec{s}_n^{(t+1)} \in T_{x_n}S^2$ is given by a linear combination of $\vec{c}_i^{(t)} \in T_{x_i}S^2$ parallel transported to $T_{x_n}S^2$, where the tangent vectors of closer points are given more weights via λ. One can interpret Eq. (9) as a spherical convolution of vector fields. This is the exact analogue of the convolution method of optimizing Step 2 in the demons algorithm [6,19,22] and is also similar to the convolution-based fast fluid registration in the Euclidean space [7].

The exact form of $\lambda(\cdot, \cdot)$ is determined by the choice of the energetic norm, the relative locations of all the mesh points and the constant σ_x^2/σ_T^2. In particular, increasing σ_x^2/σ_T^2 increases the "width" of λ. Rather than picking the energetic norm, we can simply choose a convenient λ. In practice, we replace the convolution operation with iterative smoothing: at each iteration, for each vertex x_n, tangent vectors of neighboring vertices are parallel transported to $T_{x_n}S^2$ and linearly combined in a weighted fashion with the current estimate of $\vec{s}_n$. Using more iterations of this process is equivalent to increasing the width of λ. Technically, the resulting λ might not correspond to any choice of the energetic norm. However, in practice, this does not appear to be a problem.

4 Experiments and Discussion

We use two sets of experiments to compare the accuracy of Spherical Demons and FreeSurfer [11]. The FreeSurfer registration algorithm uses the same similarity measure as Spherical Demons, but penalizes for metric and areal distortion. As mentioned earlier, its runtime is more than an hour while our runtime is less than 5 minutes.

Parcellation of In-Vivo Cortical Surfaces. We consider a set of 39 left and right cortical surface models extracted from in-vivo MRI. Each surface is spherically parameterized and represented as a spherical image with geometric features at each vertex (e.g., sulcal depth and curvature). Both hemispheres are manually parcellated by a neuroanatomist into 35 major sulci and gyri. We validate our algorithm in the context of automatic cortical parcellation.

We co-register all 39 spherical images of cortical geometry with Spherical Demons by iteratively building an atlas and registering the surfaces to the atlas. The atlas consists of the mean and variance of cortical geometry. One can easily modify the demons objective function (Eq. (1)) to use an atlas.

We then perform cross-validation parcellation 4 times, by leaving out subjects 1 to 10, training a classifier [8,12] using the remaining subjects, and using it to classify subjects 1 to 10. We repeat with subjects 11-20, 21-30 and 31-39.

We also perform registration and cross-validation with the FreeSurfer algorithm [11] using the same features and parcellation algorithm [8,12]. Once again, the atlas consists of the mean and variance of cortical geometry.

The average Dice measure (defined as the ratio of cortical surface area with correct labels to the total surface area averaged over the test set) on the left hemisphere is 88.9 for FreeSurfer and 89.6 for Spherical Demons. While the improvement is not big, the difference is statistically significant for a one-sided t-test with the Dice measure of each subject treated as an independent sample ($p = 2 \times 10^{-6}$). On the right hemisphere, FreeSurfer obtains a Dice of 88.8 and Spherical Demons achieves 89.1. Here, the improvement is smaller, but still statistically significant ($p = 0.01$).

Because the average Dice can be deceiving by suppressing small structures, we analyze the segmentation accuracy per structure. On the left (right) hemisphere, the segmentations of 16 (8) structures are statistically significantly improved by Spherical Demons with respect to FreeSurfer, while no structure got worse (False Discovery Rate = 0.05 [5]). Fig. 1 shows the percentage improvement of individual structures. Parcellation results suggest that our registration is at least as accurate as FreeSurfer.

Brodmann Areas Localization on Ex-vivo Cortical Surfaces. In this experiment, we evaluate the registration accuracy on ten human brains analyzed

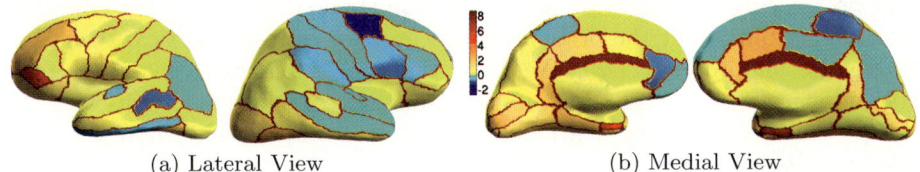

(a) Lateral View   (b) Medial View

Fig. 1. Percentage dice improvement over FreeSurfer. Yellow regions indicate structures scoring better than FreeSurfer. Blue regions correspond to decrease in accuracy. We note that no structure is statistically worse than FreeSurfer (see text).

Table 1. Average alignment errors of Brodmann areas in mm for the two registration methods. Lowest errors are shown in SD: Spherical Demons. FS: FreeSurfer.

	Left Hemisphere								Right Hemisphere							
	V1	BA4a	BA4p	BA2	V2	BA6	BA44	BA45	V1	BA4a	BA4p	BA2	V2	BA6	BA44	BA45
SD10	**3.1**	**3.3**	**3.3**	**5.4**	**3.7**	**6.4**	7.7	**6.4**	**3.2**	**3.4**	**2.8**	**5.4**	**3.5**	**6.4**	10.4	**8.6**
FS10	3.8	4.4	3.8	6.3	4.6	7.0	**7.4**	6.8	3.8	3.8	3.1	5.9	4.0	6.5	**11.5**	9.9

histologically postmortem [17]. The histological sections were aligned to postmortem MR with nonlinear warps to build a 3D volume. Eight manually labeled Brodmann areas from histology were sampled onto each hemispheric surface model and sampling errors were manually corrected [13]. Brodmann areas are cyto-architectonically defined regions closely related to cortical function.

It has been shown that nonlinear surface registration of cortical folds can significantly improve Brodmann area overlap across different subjects [13,24]. Registering the ex-vivo surfaces is more difficult than in-vivo surfaces because the reconstructed volumes are extremely noisy, resulting in noisy geometric features.

We co-register the ten surfaces to each other by iteratively building an atlas and registering the surfaces to the atlas. We compute the average distance between the boundaries of the Brodmann areas for each pair of registered subjects. For future reference, we call this experiment **SD10**. We repeat this process using FreeSurfer, referred to as **FS10** in the remainder of this section.

Table 1 presents the summary of the results. We see that SD10 outperforms FS10. We perform a permutation test to test for statistical significance. Compared with FS10, SD10 improves the alignment of 5 (2) Brodmann areas on the left (right) hemisphere (False Discovery Rate = 0.05 [5]) and no structure gets worse. These results suggest that the Spherical Demons algorithm is at least as accurate as FreeSurfer in aligning Brodmann areas. Another experiment (not shown) which involves registering the ex-vivo surfaces to an in-vivo atlas also results in comparable performance between Spherical Demons and FreeSurfer.

5 Conclusion

In this paper, we presented the fast Spherical Demons algorithm for registering spherical images. We showed that the characteristic two-step optimization of the

Demons algorithm can also be applied on the sphere. A clear future challenge is to take into account the original metric properties of the cortical surface in the registration process [11,20]. We tested the algorithm extensively on two data sets and show that the accuracy of the algorithm compares favorably with the widely used FreeSurfer registration algorithm [11], while offering more than one order of magnitude speedup.

Acknowledgments. We would like to thank Hartmut Mohlberg, Katrin Amunts and Karl Zilles for the histological dataset. Support for this research is provided in part by the NAMIC (NIH NIBIB NAMIC U54-EB005149), the NAC (NIT CRR NAC P41-RR13218), the mBIRN (NIH NCRR mBIRN U24-RR021382), the NIH NINDS R01-NS051826 grant, the NSF CAREER 0642971 grant, NCRR (P41-RR14075, R01 RR16594-01A1), the NIBIB (R01 EB001550, R01EB006758), the NINDS (R01 NS052585-01) and the MIND Institute. Additional support was provided by The Autism & Dyslexia Project funded by the Ellison Medical Foundation. B.T. Thomas Yeo is funded by the A*STAR, Singapore.

References

1. Arsigny, V., et al.: A Log-Euclidean Framework for Statistics on Diffeomorphisms. In: Larsen, R., Nielsen, M., Sporring, J. (eds.) MICCAI 2006. LNCS, vol. 4190, pp. 924–931. Springer, Heidelberg (2006)
2. Ashburner, J., Andersson, J., Friston, K.: High-dimensional Image Registration using Symmetric Priors. NeuroImage 9, 619–628 (1999)
3. Ashburner, J.: A Fast Diffeomorphic Image Registration Algorithm. NeuroImage 38, 95–113 (2007)
4. Beg, M., et al.: Computing Large Deformation Metric Mapping via Geodesic Flows of Diffeomorphisms. International Journal of Computer Vision 61(2), 139–157 (2005)
5. Benjamini, Y., Hochberg, Y.: Controlling the False Discovery Rate: A Practical and Powerful Approach to Mult. Testing. J. Roy. Stats. Soc. 57(1), 289–300 (1995)
6. Cachier, P.: Iconic Feature Based Non-rigid Registration: The PASHA Algorithm. CVIU 89(2-3), 272–298 (2003)
7. Bro-Nielsen, M., Gramkow, C.: Fast Fluid Registration of Medical Images Visualization in Biomedical Computing, 267–276 (1996)
8. Desikan, R., et al.: An automated labeling system for subdividing the human cerebral cortex on MRI scans into gyral based regions of interest. NeuroImage (2006)
9. Durrleman, S., et al.: Measuring Brain Variability via Sulcal Lines Registration: a Diffeomorphic Approach. In: Ayache, N., Ourselin, S., Maeder, A. (eds.) MICCAI 2007, Part I. LNCS, vol. 4791, pp. 675–682. Springer, Heidelberg (2007)
10. Eckstein, I., et al.: Generalized Surface Flows for Deformable Registration and Cortical Matching. In: Ayache, N., Ourselin, S., Maeder, A. (eds.) MICCAI 2007, Part I. LNCS, vol. 4791, pp. 692–700. Springer, Heidelberg (2007)
11. Fischl, B., et al.: High-resolution intersubject averaging and a coordinate system for the cortical surface. HBM 8(4), 272–284 (1999)
12. Fischl, B., et al.: Automatically Parcellating the Human cerebral Cortex. Cerebral Cortex 14, 11–22 (2004)

13. Fischl, B., et al.: Cortical Folding Patterns and Predicting Cytoarchictecture. Cerebral Cortex (2007)
14. Geng, X., et al.: Transitive Inverse-Consistent Manifold Registration. In: Christensen, G.E., Sonka, M. (eds.) IPMI 2005. LNCS, vol. 3565, pp. 468–479. Springer, Heidelberg (2005)
15. Glaunès, J., et al.: Landmark Matching via Large Deformation Diffeomorphisms on the Sphere. Journal of Mathematical Imaging and Vision 20, 179–200 (2004)
16. Nielsen, M., et al.: Brownian Warps: A Least Committed Prior for Non-rigid Registration. In: Dohi, T., Kikinis, R. (eds.) MICCAI 2002. LNCS, vol. 2489, pp. 557–564. Springer, Heidelberg (2002)
17. Schleicher, A., et al.: Observer independent method for microstructural parcellation of cerebral cortex: a quantitative approach to cytoarchitectonics. NeuroImage 9, 165–177 (1999)
18. Tosun, D., Prince, J.: Cortical Surface Alignment Using Geometry Driven Multispectral Optical Flow. In: Christensen, G.E., Sonka, M. (eds.) IPMI 2005. LNCS, vol. 3565, pp. 480–492. Springer, Heidelberg (2005)
19. Thirion, J.: Image Matching as a Diffusion Process: an Analogy with Maxwell's Demons. Medical Image Analysis 2(3), 243–260 (1998)
20. Thompson, P., et al.: Mathematical/Computational Challenges in Creating Deformable and Probabilistic Atlases of the Human Brain. HBM 9(2), 81–92 (2000)
21. Van Essen, D., et al.: Functional and structural mapping of human cerebral cortex: solutions are in the surfaces. PNAS 95(3), 788–795 (1996)
22. Vercauteren, T., et al.: Non-parameteric Diffeomorphic Image Registration with the Demons Algorithm. In: Ayache, N., Ourselin, S., Maeder, A. (eds.) MICCAI 2007, Part II. LNCS, vol. 4792, pp. 319–326. Springer, Heidelberg (2007)
23. Yeo, B.T.T., et al.: Effects of Registration Regularization and Atlas Sharpness on Segmentation Accuracy. In: Ayache, N., Ourselin, S., Maeder, A. (eds.) MICCAI 2007, Part I. LNCS, vol. 4791, pp. 683–691. Springer, Heidelberg (2007)
24. Yeo, B.T.T., et al.: What Data to Co-register for Computing Atlases. In: MMBIA, Proc. ICCV, pp. 1–8 (2007)

Symmetric Log-Domain Diffeomorphic Registration: A Demons-Based Approach

Tom Vercauteren[1], Xavier Pennec[2], Aymeric Perchant[1], and Nicholas Ayache[2]

[1] Mauna Kea Technologies, France
[2] Asclepios, INRIA Sophia-Antipolis, France

Abstract. Modern morphometric studies use non-linear image registration to compare anatomies and perform group analysis. Recently, log-Euclidean approaches have contributed to promote the use of such computational anatomy tools by permitting simple computations of statistics on a rather large class of invertible spatial transformations. In this work, we propose a non-linear registration algorithm perfectly fit for log-Euclidean statistics on diffeomorphisms. Our algorithm works completely in the log-domain, i.e. it uses a stationary velocity field. This implies that we guarantee the invertibility of the deformation and have access to the true inverse transformation. This also means that our output can be directly used for log-Euclidean statistics without relying on the heavy computation of the log of the spatial transformation. As it is often desirable, our algorithm is symmetric with respect to the order of the input images. Furthermore, we use an alternate optimization approach related to Thirion's demons algorithm to provide a fast non-linear registration algorithm. First results show that our algorithm outperforms both the demons algorithm and the recently proposed diffeomorphic demons algorithm in terms of accuracy of the transformation while remaining computationally efficient.

1 Introduction

Non-linear image registration has opened the way for computational characterization of morphological evolution and morphological variability. Most computational anatomy tools make use of registration results [1,2,3,4] but require that they satisfy some advanced properties such as invertibility and symmetry with respect to the order of the inputs. Image registration schemes can thus only be used if they meet the requirements of these tools. Large deformation diffeomorphic methods have initially been developed for this purpose. Transformations are determined by a time-varying ordinary differential equation (ODE) [5]. Following the seminal work on inverse consistency [6], the large deformations framework has also been extended to enforce the symmetry of the solution [3,7].

A widely acknowledged issue with the large deformation setting lies in its computational complexity and memory requirements. Recent work has strived towards bridging the gap between these rigorous mathematical tools and very efficient non-linear registration schemes such as Thirion's demons algorithm [8]. On one hand it has been proposed to constrain the large deformation setting by using transformations that satisfy the initial momentum conservation [9,10]. Similarly, in [1], the authors proposed to parameterize the diffeomorphisms with *stationary* velocity fields to allow easy computations of statistics on diffeomorphisms. This parameterization was used for registration in [11,12]. These algorithms are well-fit for further statistical processing [1,2,4]. On the other hand, in [13] the authors proposed an efficient diffeomorphic registration scheme based on the demons algorithm that encodes the optimization steps, but not the complete transformation, with such stationary velocity fields. Between these attempts, we believe that there is still a gap to be bridged. Second generation large deformation algorithms still need to solve rather large Euler-Lagrange equations at each iteration and the diffeomorphic demons cannot be directly used by the recent statistical tools we mentioned. Furthermore, the demons algorithm is not symmetric with respect to the order of the images to register.

In this work, we propose an image registration scheme that uses a demons-like alternate optimization approach for efficiency but represents the complete deformation as an exponential of a smooth velocity field. This approach will hereafter be referred to as log-domain one. Thanks to such representation, our results are symmetric and can be directly used for computational anatomy.

The remainder of this paper is organized as follows. Classical and diffeomorphic demons are presented in Section 2. Our log-domain approach is developed in Section 3 and evaluated in Section 4. Finally Section 5 concludes the paper.

2 Additive and Diffeomorphic Demons Algorithms

Non-linear image registration aims at finding a well-behaved spatial transformation $s(.)$ that best aligns two given images $I_0(.)$ and $I_1(.)$. Typically, a similarity criterion $\text{Sim}(I_0, I_1, s)$ is used to measure the resemblance of the aligned images while a regularization energy $\text{Reg}(s)$ estimates the likelihood of the transformation. *Non-parametric* methods need to find the displacement $s(p)$ of each point p in order to optimize the following energy functional:

$$E(s) = \frac{1}{\sigma_i^2} \text{Sim}(I_0, I_1, s) + \frac{1}{\sigma_T^2} \text{Reg}(s),$$

where σ_i accounts for the noise on the image intensity, and σ_T controls the amount of regularization we need. The desired properties of the final spatial transformation can be encoded within the regularization term or can be enforced by constraining the search space. Instead of looking for a solution in the complete space of non-parametric spatial transformations, it is for example possible to search only within a subspace of diffeomorphisms.

Additive Demons. Even if we use a simple transformation space and a classical regularization term, approaching the registration problem directly often leads to computationally expensive iterations that need the solution of an Euler-Lagrange equation. Contrastingly, Thirion's demons algorithm uses an efficient two-step procedure at each iteration [8]. It first looks for an unconstrained update step with an optical flow computation and then uses a simple Gaussian smoothing on the updated transformation. It has been shown in [14] that the demons algorithm could be cast to the minimization of a well-posed criterion by introducing a hidden variable c for point correspondences. The interest of this auxiliary variable is that it decouples the optimization into easily tractable sub-problems. Each iteration walks towards the optimum of the global energy

$$E(I_0, I_1, c, s) = \frac{1}{\sigma_i^2} \mathrm{Sim}\,(I_0, I_1, c) + \frac{1}{\sigma_x^2} \mathrm{dist}\,(s, c)^2 + \frac{1}{\sigma_T^2} \mathrm{Reg}\,(s), \qquad (1)$$

where σ_x accounts for a spatial uncertainty on the correspondences. We classically have $\mathrm{Sim}\,(I_0, I_1, c) = \|I_0 - I_1 \circ c\|^2$, $\mathrm{dist}\,(s, c) = \|c - s\|$ and $\mathrm{Reg}\,(s) = \|\nabla s\|^2$ but more advanced criteria can be used [14].

In the additive demons algorithm, the optimization is performed within the complete space of non-parametric transformation using additive updates of the form $s + u$. The optical flow procedure solves for the correspondence energy

$$E_{\mathrm{add}}^{\mathrm{corr}}(I_0, I_1, s, u) = \mathrm{Sim}\,(I_0, I_1, s + u) + \|u\|^2 \qquad (2)$$

with respect to u, while the Gaussian smoothing solves for the regularization. Different optimizers lead to different forces that have been justified in [15].

Diffeomorphic Demons. In [13], the authors proposed to adapt the demons algorithm to provide diffeomorphisms. The diffeomorphic demons algorithm uses Thirion's alternate optimization approach to maintain the computational efficiency but works in a space of diffeomorphisms to enforce the invertibility.

An efficient computational framework for diffeomorphisms was proposed in [1]. It uses a Lie group structure that defines an exponential mapping from the vector space of smooth stationary velocity fields to diffeomorphisms. The exponential $\exp(u)$ of a velocity field is given by the flow at time one of the stationary ODE: $\partial p(t)/\partial t = u(t)$. The nice property of this framework lies in the low computational requirement needed to compute the exponential.

At each iteration, the diffeomorphic demons takes advantage of this exponential mapping by looking for an update step u in the Lie algebra (the vector space of velocity fields) and then by mapping it in the space of diffeomorphisms through the exponential. The update step is thus of the form $s \circ \exp(u)$. The advantage of this approach is that it can compute u with an unconstrained optimizer that has the same form and complexity as the classical demons forces [13]. The diffeomorphic demons retains the simple Gaussian smoothing of Thirion's algorithm for its efficiency. With this approach the first step optimizes the modified correspondence energy

$$E_{\mathrm{diffeo}}^{\mathrm{corr}}(I_0, I_1, s, u) = \mathrm{Sim}\,(I_0, I_1, s \circ \exp(u)) + \|u\|^2. \qquad (3)$$

3 A Log-Domain Approach to Diffeomorphic Demons

The parameterization of diffeomorphic transformations through stationary velocity fields proposed in [1] provides a very efficient means of dealing with diffeomorphisms. In the diffeomorphic demons of [13], the exponential is used only to encode the adjustment made at each iteration to the current transformation. This leads to a computationally attractive scheme but lacks some of the characteristics of log-domain registration tools [11, 12] that encode the complete transformation with stationary velocity fields: namely the ability to compute the inverse of the transformation at a very low cost, the symmetry of the registration result and the adequacy of the representation for the statistical tools of [1, 2].

Our main contribution in this paper is to show that the diffeomorphic demons can be extended to represent the complete spatial transformation in the log domain. The main idea of the proposed algorithm is to represent the current transformation s as an exponential of a smooth velocity field v, i.e. $s = \exp(v)$, and use the diffeomorphic demons to efficiently compute a field u for an update of the form $s \circ \exp(u)$, i.e. $\exp(v) \circ \exp(u)$. With this idea, there are two questions that come to mind. First of all, given that we want to represent everything in the log-domain, we need to know whether for any v and u there exists a velocity field w such that $\exp(w) = \exp(v) \circ \exp(u)$. Then we need to design a regularization scheme that is consistent with the log-domain representation.

Baker-Campbell-Hausdorff Approximations. Our first goal is to find a smooth velocity field $Z(v, \varepsilon u)$ such that

$$\exp\left(Z(v, \varepsilon u)\right) \approx \exp(v) \circ \exp(\varepsilon u), \tag{4}$$

where ε is simply used to emphasize the fact that we look for an approximation valid for small εu (to encode the update) but arbitrary v (to encode the complete transformation). Since we deal with an infinite-dimensional space which has a Lie group structure but is not an actual Lie group, the question of the existence of such a velocity field is a tough mathematical one that needs further investigation. In practice though, it has been shown in [2] that the the Baker-Campbell-Hausdorff (BCH) formula which is valid for finite-dimensional spaces could be applied successfully on diffeomorphisms. By using the first terms of the BCH formula, the authors of [2] obtained an approximation that seems well-fit for the demanding application of brain atlas construction. In our setting, since only εu is assumed to be small, the first order approximation of $Z(v, \varepsilon u)$ is:

$$Z(v, \varepsilon u) = v + \varepsilon u + \frac{1}{2}[v, \varepsilon u] + \frac{1}{12}[v, [v, \varepsilon u]] + O(\|\varepsilon u\|^2), \tag{5}$$

where the Lie bracket $[v, u]$ provides a velocity field defined at each point p by[1]:

$$[v, u](p) = \text{Jac}(v)(p).u(p) - \text{Jac}(u)(p).v(p). \tag{6}$$

This first-order approximation provides a good candidate for our update rule but is still somewhat complex as it requires three Lie brackets. This might also lead to an unstable numerical scheme as the imbricated Lie bracket amounts to

---

[1] Most authors define the Lie bracket as the opposite of (6). Numerical simulations, and personal communication with M. Bossa, showed the relevance of this definition. Future research will aim at fully understanding the reason of this discrepancy.

using second-order derivatives. An *ad hoc* simplification can be made by simply considering the first terms of the BCH expansion. We chose to evaluate the quality of the following approximations: $Z_A(\boldsymbol{v}, \varepsilon\boldsymbol{u}) \triangleq \boldsymbol{v} + \varepsilon\boldsymbol{u}$, $Z_B(\boldsymbol{v}, \varepsilon\boldsymbol{u}) \triangleq \boldsymbol{v} + \varepsilon\boldsymbol{u} + \frac{1}{2}[\boldsymbol{v}, \varepsilon\boldsymbol{u}]$ and $Z_C(\boldsymbol{v}, \varepsilon\boldsymbol{u}) \triangleq \boldsymbol{v} + \varepsilon\boldsymbol{u} + \frac{1}{2}[\boldsymbol{v}, \varepsilon\boldsymbol{u}] + \frac{1}{12}[\boldsymbol{v}, [\boldsymbol{v}, \varepsilon\boldsymbol{u}]]$.

In order to test the validity of these approximations for our application we set up a small experiment to measure the error between $\exp(Z_X(\boldsymbol{v}, \varepsilon\boldsymbol{u}))$ and $\exp(\boldsymbol{v}) \circ \exp(\varepsilon\boldsymbol{u})$. We generate a random $\boldsymbol{v}$ at a given energy, a random $\boldsymbol{u}$ at a lower energy and measure $\|\exp(Z_X(\boldsymbol{v}, \varepsilon\boldsymbol{u})) - \exp(\boldsymbol{v}) \circ \exp(\varepsilon\boldsymbol{u})\|^2$. Due to space constraints, only the conclusions of these experiments can be presented here. The best results are as expected provided by Z_C with Z_B being only a few percents away from it. Z_A surprisingly still provide decent results but the error is however one order of magnitude away from the error resulting from Z_C.

Log-Domain Diffeomorphic Demons. The BCH approximations allow us to cast the update step $s \leftarrow s \circ \exp(\boldsymbol{u})$ used in the diffeomorphic demons into a log-domain update $\boldsymbol{v} \leftarrow Z_X(\boldsymbol{v}, \boldsymbol{u})$ provided that the current transformation s can be expressed as an exponential $s = \exp(\boldsymbol{v})$. It might however be unclear why one would resort to such a BCH approximation. It could indeed be possible to directly look for an update of the form $\boldsymbol{v} \leftarrow \boldsymbol{v} + \boldsymbol{u}$. The problem with this kind of approach used for example in [11] lies in its computational complexity. Since the exponential is not used around zero, the author cannot take advantage of the fact that $\partial \exp(\boldsymbol{u})/\partial \boldsymbol{u}|_{\boldsymbol{u}=0} = \text{Id}$. The non-trivial derivative introduces a coupling between the transformation and the update contrarily to our algorithm.

Finally, in order to be consistent with the log-domain representation but keep the simplicity of the demons algorithm, we chose to perform a Gaussian smoothing directly in the log-domain. Our framework can simply be linked to (1) by using $\text{dist}(s, c) = \|\log(s^{-1} \circ c)\|$ and $\text{Reg}(s) = \|\nabla \log(s)\|^2$.

Algorithm 1 (Log-Domain Demons)
- Choose a starting spatial transformation $s = \exp(\boldsymbol{v})$
- Iterate until convergence:
    - Given the current transformation $s = \exp(\boldsymbol{v})$, compute a correspondence update field $\boldsymbol{u}$ by minimizing $E_{\text{diffeo}}^{\text{corr}}(I_0, I_1, s, \boldsymbol{u})$ with respect to $\boldsymbol{u}$
    - For fluid-like regularization let $\boldsymbol{u} \leftarrow K_{\text{fluid}} \star \boldsymbol{u}$
    - Let $\boldsymbol{v} \leftarrow Z_X(\boldsymbol{v}, \boldsymbol{u})$, e.g. $\boldsymbol{v} \leftarrow \boldsymbol{v} + \boldsymbol{u} + \frac{1}{2}[\boldsymbol{v}, \boldsymbol{u}]$
    - For diffusion-like regularization let $\boldsymbol{v} \leftarrow K_{\text{diff}} \star \boldsymbol{v}$ ∎

Symmetric Extension. The inverse of a spatial transformation s parameterized in the log-domain $s = \exp(\boldsymbol{v})$, can be obtained at almost no cost by a backward computation $s^{-1} = \exp(-\boldsymbol{v})$. A symmetric registration framework can be obtained from the non-symmetric one by symmetrizing the global energy:

$$s_{opt} = \arg\min_{s} \left(E(I_0, I_1, s) + E(I_1, I_0, s^{-1}) \right), \tag{7}$$

where c has been omitted from (1) for clarity. Other approaches appear in [16].

Our second main contribution in this work is to provide an efficient scheme for solving this symmetrized system. We formulate it as a constrained optimization using two diffeomorphisms: $[s_{opt}, s_{opt}^{-1}] = \arg\min_{[s,t] \mid t = s^{-1}} E(I_0, I_1, s) +$

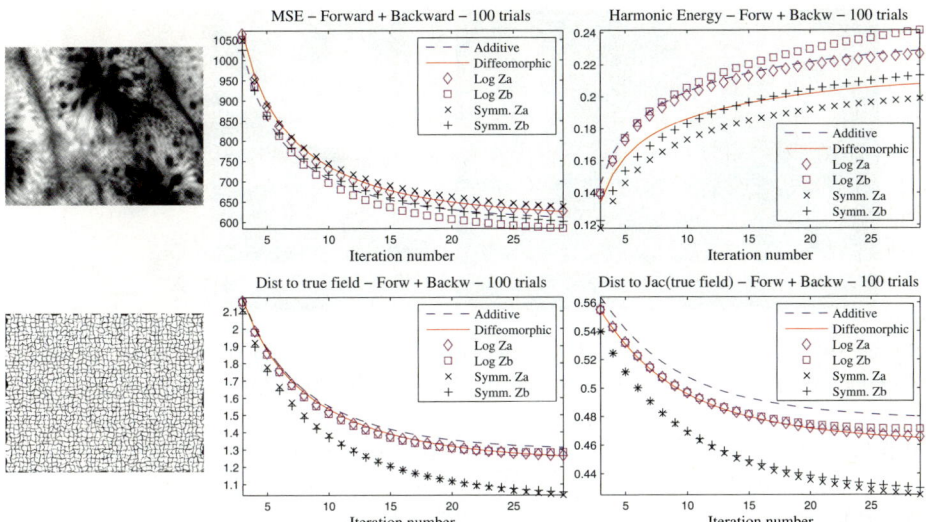

Fig. 1. Left column: Reference image, in vivo microscopy of normal colonic mucosa, courtesy of A. Meining, Klinikum rechts der Isar, Munich, and one example random warp. Other columns: Registration results on 100 random experiments. The log-domain diffeomorphic performs similarly to the diffeomorphic demons while our symmetric approach outperforms it. We see the small impact of the BCH expansion that we use.

$E(I_1, I_0, t)$. We propose to use an unconstrained optimization step on the pair $[s, t]$ and then to project the new transformations onto the space of symmetric transformations $\{[s, t] \,|\, t = s^{-1}\}$. By using a complete log-domain demons iteration starting from $s = \exp(v)$ to optimize the first term $E(F, M, \exp(\varsigma))$, we get $\varsigma = K_{\text{diff}} \star Z(v, K_{\text{fluid}} \star u^{\text{forw}})$, where u^{forw} is the demons force. Similarly, the second term $E(M, F, \exp(-\tau))$ is optimized with $\tau = -K_{\text{diff}} \star Z(-v, K_{\text{fluid}} \star u^{\text{back}})$, where u^{back} is the demons force for reversed inputs.

Thanks to the log-domain representation, we deal with a vector space and can design an easy projection operator that guarantees the symmetry of the results. We simply average, in the log-domain, the forward and backward iterations:

$$v \leftarrow \frac{1}{2} K_{\text{diff}} \star \left(Z(v, K_{\text{fluid}} \star u^{\text{forw}}) - Z(-v, K_{\text{fluid}} \star u^{\text{back}}) \right). \quad (8)$$

As an example, using Z_A provides $v \leftarrow K_{\text{diff}} \star \left(v + \frac{1}{2} K_{\text{fluid}} \star (u^{\text{forw}} - u^{\text{back}}) \right)$.

Algorithm 2 (Symmetric Iteration using Z_A)
- Compute the demons forces u^{forw} to minimize $E_{\text{diffeo}}^{\text{corr}}(I_0, I_1, \exp(v), u^{\text{forw}})$
- Compute the demons forces u^{back} to minimize $E_{\text{diffeo}}^{\text{corr}}(I_1, I_0, \exp(-v), u^{\text{back}})$
- For fluid-like regularization let $u \leftarrow \frac{1}{2} K_{\text{fluid}} \star (u^{\text{forw}} - u^{\text{back}})$
- For diffusion-like regularization let $v \leftarrow K_{\text{diff}} \star (v + u)$ else let $v \leftarrow v + u$ ∎

4 Experiments

The proposed algorithms were evaluated as follows. A reference image I_{ref} is deformed through a random diffeomorphism. Some random noise is added to

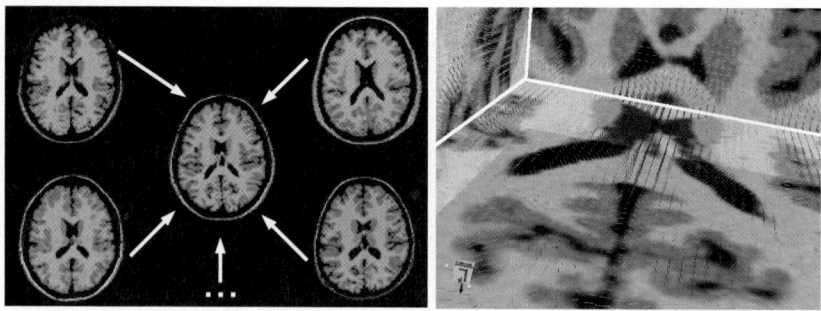

Fig. 2. 19 3D synthetic MRs of distinct anatomies were registered to an arbitrary reference. We show the principal direction of variability found by statistical analysis.

both the reference and warped image. The pair of images is registered first using $I_{\text{ref}} = I_0$ and then using $I_{\text{ref}} = I_1$. We compare the additive and diffeomorphic demons, the proposed log-domain demons with two different BCH expansions (using Z_A and Z_B), and the proposed symmetric log-domain demons again with two different BCH expansions. To make a fair comparison, each algorithm uses the same expression of the demons forces. Figure 1 shows the evolution of several criterion over the iterations. The choice of the BCH expansion does not significantly change the performance of our schemes. Hence we advocate the use of the simplest one (Z_A). Our log-domain schemes perform similarly to the diffeomorphic demons but allow an easy computation of the inverse and are well-fit for statistical analysis. Finally our symmetric extension outperforms the other algorithms in terms of distance to the ground truth transformation. The computational time is only twice the one of the diffeomorphic demons.

Finally Fig. 2 illustrates the adaptation of our algorithms for computational anatomy. A simple atlas is built from the 20 synthetic anatomies [17]. Of course more advanced techniques [1,2,3] should be used, but this proof of concept opens the way to neat future work. Thanks to our regularization by a simple smoothing, the integration of deformation statistics could be as simple as performing a non-stationary smoothing. Local covariance matrices could indeed be used to replace the norm used in the regularization by a Mahalanobis distance.

5 Conclusion

We proposed en efficient diffeomorphic algorithm that combines the efficiency of the demons algorithm and the desirable properties of modern large deformation algorithms such as invertibility with respect to the order of the inputs and memory efficient representations. Since we consider the spatial transformations as exponentials of smooth velocity fields, our results can directly be used by the recent statistical tools of [1,2]. We focused on a simple similarity criterion but our approach can easily be extended to other intensity relationships by borrowing ideas from [7,14,18]. The next step will be to integrate deformation statistics within the algorithm by locally adapting the regularization.

References

1. Arsigny, V., Commowick, O., Pennec, X., Ayache, N.: A Log-Euclidean framework for statistics on diffeomorphisms. In: Larsen, R., Nielsen, M., Sporring, J. (eds.) MICCAI 2006. LNCS, vol. 4190, pp. 924–931. Springer, Heidelberg (2006)
2. Bossa, M., Hernandez, M., Olmos, S.: Contributions to 3D diffeomorphic atlas estimation: Application to brain images. In: Ayache, N., Ourselin, S., Maeder, A. (eds.) MICCAI 2007, Part I. LNCS, vol. 4791, pp. 667–674. Springer, Heidelberg (2007)
3. Joshi, S., Davis, B., Jomier, M., Gerig, G.: Unbiased diffeomorphic atlas construction for computational anatomy. Neuroimage 23(S1), 151–160 (2004)
4. Vaillant, M., Miller, M.I., Younes, L., Trouvé, A.: Statistics on diffeomorphisms via tangent space representations. Neuroimage 23(S1), 161–169 (2004)
5. Beg, M.F., Miller, M.I., Trouvé, A., Younes, L.: Computing large deformation metric mappings via geodesic flows of diffeomorphisms. Int. J. Comput. Vis. 61(2), 139–157 (2005)
6. Christensen, G.E., Johnson, H.J.: Consistent image registration. IEEE Trans. Med. Imag. 20(7), 568–582 (2001)
7. Avants, B.B., Epstein, C.L., Grossman, M., Gee, J.C.: Symmetric diffeomorphic image registration with cross-correlation: Evaluating automated labeling of elderly and neurodegenerative brain. Med. Image Anal. 12(1), 26–41 (2008)
8. Thirion, J.P.: Image matching as a diffusion process: An analogy with Maxwell's demons. Med. Image Anal. 2(3), 243–260 (1998)
9. Marsland, S., McLachlan, R.I.: A Hamiltonian particle method for diffeomorphic image registration. In: Karssemeijer, N., Lelieveldt, B. (eds.) IPMI 2007. LNCS, vol. 4584, pp. 396–407. Springer, Heidelberg (2007)
10. Younes, L.: Jacobi fields in groups of diffeomorphisms and applications. Quart. Appl. Math. 65, 113–134 (2007)
11. Ashburner, J.: A fast diffeomorphic image registration algorithm. Neuroimage 38(1), 95–113 (2007)
12. Hernandez, M., Bossa, M.N., Olmos, S.: Registration of anatomical images using geodesic paths of diffeomorphisms parameterized with stationary vector fields. In: Proc. MMBIA Workshop of ICCV 2007, pp. 1–8 (2007)
13. Vercauteren, T., Pennec, X., Perchant, A., Ayache, N.: Non-parametric diffeomorphic image registration with the demons algorithm. In: Ayache, N., Ourselin, S., Maeder, A. (eds.) MICCAI 2007, Part I. LNCS, vol. 4791, pp. 319–326. Springer, Heidelberg (2007)
14. Cachier, P., Bardinet, E., Dormont, D., Pennec, X., Ayache, N.: Iconic feature based nonrigid registration: The PASHA algorithm. Comput. Vis. Image Underst. 89(2-3), 272–298 (2003)
15. Vercauteren, T., Pennec, X., Malis, E., Perchant, A., Ayache, N.: Insight into efficient image registration techniques and the demons algorithm. In: Karssemeijer, N., Lelieveldt, B. (eds.) IPMI 2007. LNCS, vol. 4584, pp. 495–506. Springer, Heidelberg (2007)
16. Tagare, H.D., Groisser, D., Skrinjar, O.: A geometric theory of symmetric registration. In: Proc. MMBIA Workshop of CVPR 2006, p. 73 (June 2006)
17. Aubert-Broche, B., Griffin, M., Pike, G.B., Evans, A.C., Collins, D.L.: Twenty new digital brain phantoms for creation of validation image data bases. IEEE Trans. Med. Imag. 25(11), 1410–1416 (2006)
18. Hermosillo, G., Chefd'Hotel, C., Faugeras, O.: Variational methods for multimodal image matching. Int. J. Comput. Vis. 50(3), 329–343 (2002)

EEG to MRI Registration Based on Global and Local Similarities of MRI Intensity Distributions

Žiga Špiclin[1], Arne Hans[2], Frank H. Duffy[2], Simon K. Warfield[2],
Boštjan Likar[1], and Franjo Pernuš[1]

[1] Faculty of Electrical Engineering, University of Ljubljana, Slovenia
{ziga.spiclin,bostjan.likar,franjo.pernus}@fe.uni-lj.si
[2] Department of Radiology, Children's Hospital Boston, USA
simon.warfield@childrens.harvard.edu

Abstract. In this paper, a novel method for EEG to MRI registration is proposed. Initial registration is achieved by extracting and matching symmetry planes of MRI and EEG data, followed by iterative registration based on minimizing a cost function. Comparison of the intensity distributions of the whole MR image and MRI voxels around a head surface point yields global similarities, while the comparison of intensity distributions of MRI voxels around corresponding EEG points, which reflects the head's sagittal symmetry, yields local similarities. Therefore, when the EEG points are registered to the MR image, maximal global and local similarities should be obtained. The cost function, incorporating global and local similarities, was the sum of Kullback-Leibler divergences between corresponding intensity distributions. The proposed method was evaluated on clinical MRI data with simulated EEG data, yielding mean registration error of 0.48 ± 0.33 mm, while with real EEG data an average root-mean-square point-to-surface error of 2.27 ± 0.02 mm was obtained.

1 Introduction

Correlating functional information with anatomical localization offers the ability to understand how the brain functions. For in vivo neurophysiological studies of the brain, for example to localize the epileptogenic foci, magnetic resonance imaging (MRI) is usually integrated with functional information like electroencephalography (EEG), magnetoencephalography (MEG) or transcranial magnetic stimulation (TMS). EEG techniques, especially, allow for high-resolution measurements of temporal and, if related to brain anatomy derived from MRI, also spatial dimensions of brain's electrical activity [1]. However, regarding the anatomical precision of clinically relevant locations of brain's electrical activity, accurate registration of MRI and EEG data is needed.

Retrospective registration of MRI and EEG, which is concerned with spatial localization of EEG electrodes in the MRI image, is usually solved by 1) extracting head surface from MR image, 2) acquiring EEG coordinates in physical space by some 3-D point localization technology and 3) using a surface-matching technique [2] to align the head surface and the localized 3-D coordinates of EEG electrodes. Previously published methods for EEG/MEG to MRI registration [3,4,5,6,7] or for TMS to MRI registration [8] typically utilize the three above-mentioned steps. However, using the head surface as the only feature of the information rich MRI data renders the registration process an ill-posed problem, especially due to the spherical symmetry of the head shape. Therefore, to get a well-behaved registration process, we propose to avoid segmentation of the head surface and choose to exploit the image intensities of the original MRI data.

In this paper, the main idea is to use MRI intensity information to drive the registration of MRI and EEG. Given a set of localized 3-D coordinates of EEG electrodes or EEG points that resemble the head's shape, we pursue to exploit the sagittal symmetry of the head by analyzing the topology of the EEG points, which yields the so-called *local similarities*. On the other hand, we also take account of the so-called *global similarities*, i.e. the similarities between the global intensity distribution and the intensity distribution of MRI voxels in the neighbourhood of each EEG point. By this approach a *cost function* is designed that yields a highly accurate and robust spatial registration of MRI and EEG.

2 Materials and Methods

In this section, a novel method for registration of MRI and EEG is presented. The outline of the proposed registration method is depicted in Fig. 1. Registration of the MRI and EEG input data is performed by: 1) computing the symmetry planes of MRI and EEG data and defining point-to-point correspondences of EEG points, 2) initial closed-form registration and 3) local iterative registration. In the following subsections, the MRI and EEG input data preprocessing and the initial and local EEG to MRI registrations are explained.

2.1 MRI and EEG Datasets

Three sets of MRI and EEG data were acquired for the present study. All patients were 8 to 10 years old volunteers, including normal controls and subjects born prematurely, enrolled in a separate ongoing study of the impact of premature birth on brain development. T1–weighted MR images were acquired by Siemens 3T Tim Trio MRI scanner using MPRAGE acquisition sequence with 18 cm FOV, 1.0 mm contiguous slice thickness, 256×256 sagittal slices covering the entire head, TR/TE=1410 ms/2.27 ms, TI=800 ms, flip angle=9 degrees, iPAT=2. Scan time was approximately 3 min 40 s. To acquire the EEG data, the EGI GES 250 system (www.egi.com) with HydroCel geodesic sensor net cap utilizing 128 EEG electrodes was used. The EEG sensor net cap was mounted on the patient's head and by using the EGI geodesic photogrammetry system, the 3-D coordinates of EEG electrodes were digitized in a few seconds.

2.2 MRI and EEG Data Preprocessing

Prior to registration, the input MRI and EEG data is preprocessed to get an initial registration of MRI and EEG and to derive the corresponding pairs of

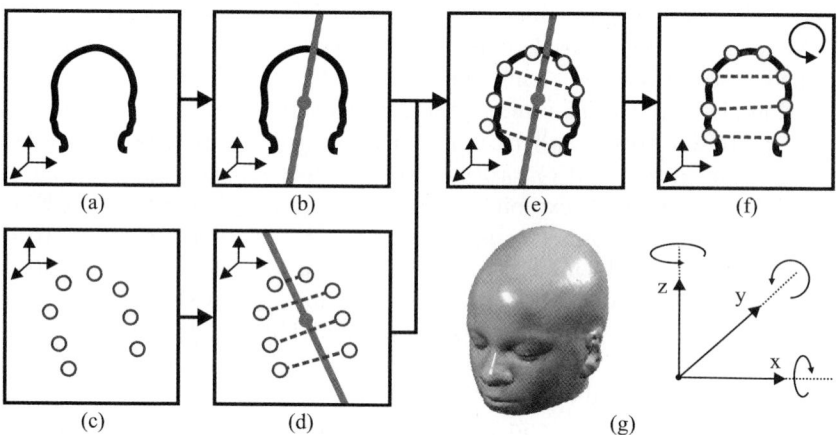

Fig. 1. Proposed method for registration of MRI and EEG: (a) input MR image and (b) the extracted mid-sagittal plane of the brain [9], (c) input EEG points and (d) the extracted symmetry plane and point-to-point correspondences of EEG points. An initial closed-form registration step (e) aligns the extracted symmetry planes of the MR image and the EEG points, followed by (f) local iterative registration procedure. The extracted head surface and corresponding MR image coordinate system (g).

EEG points that reflect the sagittal symmetry of the head. To obtain an initial registration of MRI and EEG, we propose to extract and match the symmetry planes of both the MRI and the EEG points. The center of gravity and the symmetry plane of the MR image, also called the mid-saggital plane (MSP), are computed by the method of Ardekani et al. [9].

The symmetry plane of EEG points (ESP) is computed from its 3-D geometrical moments [6], i.e. the center of gravity and the principal axes derived from the inertia matrix of EEG points. Parameters of the ESP are estimated by using the center of gravity of EEG points as the plane origin and the cross-product between two principal axes, corresponding to the smallest and the largest eigenvalue of the inertia matrix, as the plane normal. Such an estimation of the ESP is valid without loss of generality, since the fixed and physically constrained configuration of the EEG sensor net cap preserves the distribution of EEG points for different patients. As the distribution of EEG points resembles the head shape of the patient, the ESP, therefore, corresponds to the MSP derived from MRI.

Let the ESP plane $^{ESP}p(x,y,z) = 0$ divide the EEG points $V = \{V_i ; i = 1 \ldots N\}$ into subsets $\{V1, V2\}$:

$$V_i \in \begin{cases} V1 & \text{if } ^{ESP}p(V_i) \geq 0 \\ V2 & \text{otherwise} \end{cases} \qquad (1)$$

Using $\{V1, V2\}$ that contain n_1 and n_2 points ($n_1 + n_2 = N$), respectively, a maximum cardinality bipartite graph [10] is constructed according to the sorting criterion:

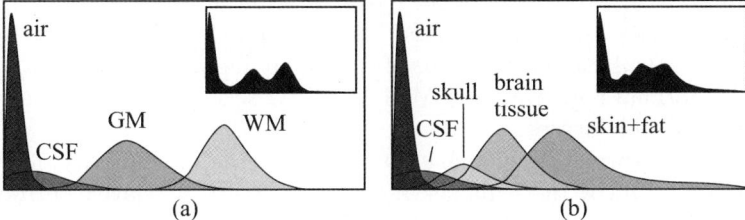

Fig. 2. Intensity distributions of (a) T1-weighted MR image and (b) local MRI voxels of a head surface point. Generally, modes of MR image intensity distribution correspond to *air*, cerebrospinal fluid (*CSF*), grey matter (*GM*) and white matter (*WM*), while modes of local intensity distribution correspond to *air, CSF, brain tissue, skin and fat*.

$$\{V1_{i*}, V2_{j*}\} = \underset{\substack{i=1...n_1 \\ j=1...n_2}}{\operatorname{argmin}} \|V1_i^\perp - V2_j^\perp\| \quad (2)$$

where points $V1_i^\perp$ and $V2_j^\perp$ correspond to $V1_i$ and $V2_j$, respectively, projected onto the ESP plane and $\|\cdot\|$ denotes the L_2−norm. In this way, the $N_p \leq N/2$ corresponding point pairs $\{V1_{i*}, V2_{j*}\}$ reflect the sagittal symmetry of the head.

2.3 Initial Closed-Form Registration

Initial registration of MRI and EEG is obtained by first aligning the centers of gravity of the EEG points and the MR image, followed by a rotation that aligns the normals of MSP and ESP. The initial registration results in a coarse alignment of MRI and EEG, but incorporates a π ambiguity around the z−axis and an undefined rotation around x−axis. The rotation ambiguities are resolved by minimizing, using a discrete angular step along the corresponding axes, the same *cost function* (4) that is used by the local iterative registration.

2.4 Local Iterative Registration

The initial registration is refined by the local iterative registration that uses a cost function based on the following two observations. First, the general shape of the T1-weighted MR image intensity distribution or global distribution (Fig. 2a) consists of four partially overlapping modes, corresponding to the air, cerebrospinal fluid (CSF), grey matter (GM) and white matter (WM). Second, a general local distribution, i.e. a distribution of intensities of MRI voxels around a head surface point (Fig. 2b), contains partially overlapping modes, corresponding to the air, CSF, skull, brain tissue, skin and fat. Computed from a large enough volume around a head surface point, the local intensity distribution is very similar to the global intensity distribution, because most of the image voxels correspond to the same anatomical structures (Fig. 2).

EEG points registered to the MRI should ideally lie on the head surface. Therefore, the local distributions corresponding to the registered EEG points should exhibit a high similarity to the global distribution. We call this similarity the global similarity. On the other hand, the local similarity is defined as the similarity between the local distributions of corresponding point pairs $\{V1_{i*}, V2_{j*}\}$ (Eq. 2). An optimal registration of MRI and EEG should yield maxima of both global and local similarities.

Instead of measuring the similarity, we measure the dissimilarity of two distributions p_1 and p_2 by the Kullback-Leibler divergence or relative entropy [11]:

$$KL(p_1\|p_2) = \sum_i p_{1i} \log \frac{p_{1i}}{p_{2i}} \quad (3)$$

Local intensity distributions are estimated by histograms, which are obtained by sampling a sphere of radius r with a step s along the $x-$, $y-$ and $z-$axes at locations of EEG points in the MRI image. Partial volume interpolation [12] is used to obtain the histograms of local intensity distributions, which results in a smooth cost function:

$$CF = \sum_{k=1}^{N} KL(p(V_k)\|p_g) + \frac{N}{N_p} \sum_{k=1}^{N_p} KL(p(V1_{i*(k)})\|p(V2_{j*(k)})) \quad (4)$$

with p_g being the global intensity distribution and $p(V_k)$ being the local intensity distribution computed at point V_k. In (4), the first sum measures the global dissimilarity, while the second sum measures the local dissimilarity. Finally, optimal parameters for rigid registration of MRI and EEG are found by iteratively minimizing the cost function (4) using Powell's multi-dimensional directional set method and Brent's one-dimensional optimization algorithm [13].

3 Experiments and Results

Cost function validation. Histograms of local intensity distributions were obtained from a spherically shaped volume with radius $r = 10$ mm and sampling step $s = 1$ mm. Histograms of both the local and global intensity distributions had 32 equally sized bins. Typical plots of the cost function (4) around the registered position of EEG points are shown in Fig. 3.

Registration results. Registration of MRI and EEG was evaluated on real data and by Monte Carlo simulations, as suggested by Singh et al. [14]. For this purpose, the head surface was extracted from MRI by interactive thresholding and manual correction (Fig. 1g). From the extracted head surface, 128 points were uniformly sampled to obtain the simulated EEG data. Transforming the simulated EEG points with a known rigid transformation and running the local iterative registration enabled the estimation of mean registration error (MRE), computed as a mean distance between the true and the registered positions of the simulated EEG points. By combined random translations and rotations of the simulated EEG, initial MREs were generated in the range of [0, 30] mm, with 10 misregistrations for each 1 mm MRE subinterval, yielding 300 starting

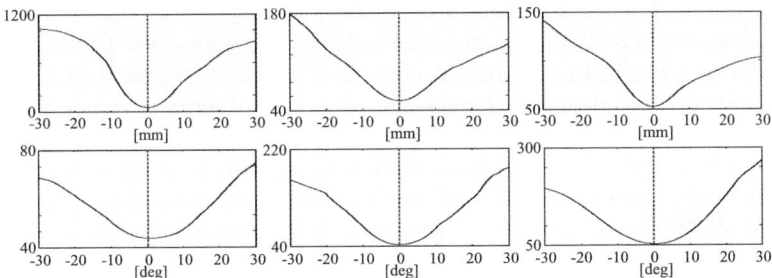

Fig. 3. Plot of the cost function (4) with respect to $x-$, $y-$ and $z-$ translations (*top*) and rotations (*bottom*) in the range of $[-30, 30]$ mm and $[-30, 30]$ degrees, respectively, from registered position of EEG points

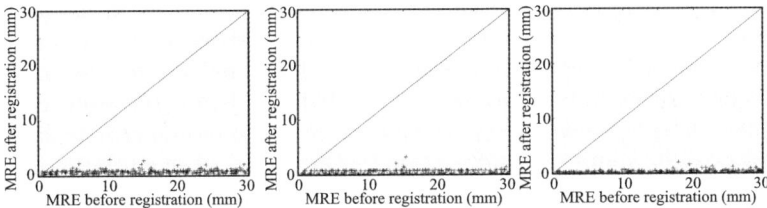

Fig. 4. Registration results with simulated EEG data for the three datasets, showing mean registration error (*MRE*) of simulated EEG points before and after registration. By random translation and rotation of the simulated EEG points, 300 initial MREs were generated in the range of $[0, 30]$ mm MRE, with 10 misregistrations for each 1 mm subinterval.

Table 1. Registration results of the simulations and the patient's studies from the proposed and the previously published methods

Method	Simulation	Patient's study
Schwartz el al. [3]	0.37 ± 0.15 mm	
Huppertz et al. [4]		3.39 ± 0.24 mm
Brinkmann et al. [5]		3.36 ± 0.91 mm
Kozinska el al. [6]	$0.73 - 1.22$ mm	1.55 ± 0.07 mm
Lamm et al. [7]	0.61 ± 0.26 mm	2.43 ± 0.22 mm
Noirhomme et al. [8]	0.17 ± 0.30 mm	1.17 ± 0.38 mm
Proposed method	0.48 ± 0.33 mm	2.27 ± 0.02 mm

positions. After the local iterative registration, the obtained average MREs were 0.77 ± 0.36, 0.39 ± 0.38 and 0.28 ± 0.24 mm for each of the three datasets. Fig. 4 shows Monte Carlo simulation results for the three datasets.

Using real EEG data, the initial closed-form registration was first executed. By a combined random translation and rotation in the range of $[-30, 30]$ mm and $[-30, 30]$ degrees, respectively, 300 displacements of the initially registered

EEG points were generated, followed by the local iterative registration. Root-mean-square error (RMS) was computed between the extracted head surface and the registered EEG data, yielding 2.41 ± 0.04, 2.26 ± 0.02 and 2.14 ± 0.01 mm for each of the three datasets. Computing the overall average RMS enabled us to compare our results to previously published results (Table 1).

4 Discussion

Accurate registration of MRI and EEG was obtained by employing MRI intensity information into the registration process. The proposed method initially aligned the MRI and EEG by extracting and matching the symmetry planes of MRI and EEG data. To refine the initial registration, the local iterative registration based on minimizing a cost function (4) was executed. The cost function was a sum of local and global similarities, expressed as the Kullback-Leibler divergences [11] between corresponding local and between local and global intensity distributions, respectively. Using only the global similarities as the cost function yielded successful registrations of MRI and EEG. However, employing local similarities improved the distinctivness of global minima for translation in $x-$ and rotation around $y-$ and $z-$axes, while unbiased global minima for the remaining parameters of rigid transformation were observed. Due to the smooth cost function (Fig. 3), the global minima was reached in 5–10 iterations, yielding an overall execution time < 2 minutes, acceptable for a routine clinical use.

Results with simulated EEG data gave an average MRE of 0.48 ± 0.33 mm, while the results on the real EEG data gave an average RMS of 2.27 ± 0.02 mm. It is important to emphasize that with the proposed method, the evaluation metrics (MRE, RMS) are independent of the optimizing cost function (4), contrary to the methods [3,4,5,6,7,8]. Nevertheless, as Table 1 indicates, the results obtained by the proposed method are comparable to the results in [3,4,5,6,7,8]. The methods [3,4,5,6,7,8] are exclusively based on the free-form surface matching techniques [2], that rely on proper segmentation of the head surface from MRI. According to Noirhomme et al. [8], registration errors due to segmentation of MRI can amount to as much as 1 mm in MRE and RMS. Due to the spherical symmetry of the head shape, more points than there are EEG electrodes are required by methods [3,4,5,6,7,8]. This problem has been solved by using either spline interpolation of EEG points [7], acquiring more than 1000 virtual EEG points [3,4,5,6] or applying a special point pattern during point acquisition [8], resulting in 200–800 virtual EEG points. Generally, the less points are used for the free-form surface matching, the poorer is the registration accuracy. Moreover, reducing the set of EEG points can lead to local minima in the distance measure, used in [3,4,5,6,7,8]. The proposed method, on the other hand, uses only the original 128 EEG points. By exploiting the MRI intensities it yielded accurate registration of MRI and EEG. Besides, because the cost function contained no local minima (Fig. 3), the proposed registration method had a large capturing range (> 30 mm, > 30 degrees).

Errors between the registered EEG points and corresponding true electrode coordinates in the MR image are not directly reflected by the RMS metric. In addition to registration inaccuracy, noise in the acquired EEG points and surface extraction errors contribute to the RMS. Thus, a ground truth for EEG to MRI registration, e.g. using MRI-visible markers attached to EEG electrodes, must be established to additionally validate the proposed, and any other, method.

To conclude, a fully automatic MRI intensity-driven method for registration of MRI and EEG was presented and evaluated on simulated and real EEG data. By incorporating MRI intensity information in the registration process, segmentation of MRI can be omitted without deteriorating the registration accuracy (Table 1). Moreover, using the framework of the proposed method (Fig. 1), other anatomical (CT) or functional (positron emission tomography and functional MRI) information can be correlated with modern point-based functional methods (EEG, MEG, TMS). In this way, the clinical neurophysiology would benefit from the ability of matching any tomographic data with the point-based functional methods [1], thus reducing cost and time of patient care.

Acknowledgements. This work has been supported by the Ministry of Higher Education, Science and Technology, Slovenia, under grants P2-0232, L2-7381, L2-9758, and J2-0716, in part by the NIH grants R01 RR021885, R01 GM074068 and R01 EB008015, and by a research grant from CIMIT.

References

1. Michel, C.M., Murray, M.M., Lantz, G., Gonzalez, S., Spinelli, L., de Peralta, R.G.: EEG source imaging. Clinical Neurophysiology 115(10), 2195–2222 (2004)
2. Audette, M.A., Ferrie, F.P., Peters, T.M.: An algorithmic overview of surface registration techniques for medical imaging. Medical Image Analysis 4(3), 201–217 (2000)
3. Schwartz, D., Lemoine, D., Poiseau, E., Barillot, C.: Registration of MEG/EEG data with 3D MRI: Methodology and precision issues. Brain Topography 9(2), 101–116 (1996)
4. Huppertz, H.J., Otte, M., Grimm, C., Kristeva-Feige, R., Mergner, T., Lucking, C.H.: Estimation of the accuracy of a surface matching technique for registration of EEG and MRI data. Electroencephalography and Clinical Neurophysiology 106(5), 409–415 (1998)
5. Brinkmann, B.H., O'Brien, T.J., Dresner, M.A., Lagerlund, T.D., Sharbrough, W., Robb, R.A.: Scalp-recorded EEG localization in MRI volume data. Brain Topography 10(4), 245–253 (1998)
6. Kozinska, D., Carducci, F., Nowinski, K.: Automatic alignment of EEG/MEG and MRI data sets. Clinical Neurophysiology 112(8), 1553–1561 (2001)
7. Lamm, C., Windischberger, C., Leodolter, U., Moser, E., Bauer, H.: Co-registration of EEG and MRI data using matching of spline interpolated and MRI-segmented reconstructions of the scalp surface. Brain Topography 14(2), 93–100 (2001)
8. Noirhomme, Q., Ferrant, M., Vandermeeren, Y., Olivier, E., Macq, B., Cuisenaire, O.: Registration and real-time visualization of transcranial magnetic stimulation with 3-D MR images. IEEE Transactions on Biomedical Engineering 51(11), 1994–2005 (2004)

9. Ardekani, B.A., Kershaw, J., Braun, M., Kanno, I.: Automatic detection of the midsagittal plane in 3-D brain images. IEEE Transactions on Medical Imaging 16(6), 947–952 (1997)
10. Kreyszig, E.: Advanced Engineering Mathematics, 9th edn. John Wiley and Sons, Hoboken (2006)
11. Kullback, S., Leibler, R.A.: On information and sufficiency. The Annals of Mathematical Statistics 22(1), 79–86 (1951)
12. Maes, F., Collignon, A., Vandermeulen, D., Marchal, G., Suetens, P.: Multimodality image registration by maximization of mutual information. IEEE Transactions on Medical Imaging 16(2), 187–198 (1997)
13. Press, W.H., Teukolsky, S.A., Vetterling, W.T., Flannery, B.P.: Numerical recipes in C: The art of scientific computing. Cambridge University Press, Cambridge (1992)
14. Singh, K.D., Holliday, I.E., Furlong, P.L., Harding, G.F.A.: Evaluation of MRI-MEG/EEG co-registration strategies using Monte Carlo simulation. Electroencephalography and Clinical Neurophysiology 102(2), 81–85 (1997)

Nonrigid Registration of Dynamic Renal MR Images Using a Saliency Based MRF Model

Dwarikanath Mahapatra and Ying Sun

Department of Electrical and Computer Engineering, National University of Singapore, 4 Engineering Drive 3, Singapore 117576, Singapore
{dmahapatra,elesuny}@nus.edu.sg

Abstract. Nonrigid registration of contrast-enhanced MR images is a difficult problem due to the change in pixel intensity caused by the wash-in and wash-out of the contrast agent. In this paper we propose a novel saliency based Markov Random Field approach for effective nonrigid registration of contrast enhanced images. Saliency information obtained from the neurobiology-based saliency model alongwith intensity information is used to quantify the degree of similarity between images in the pre- and post-contrast stages. Information from these two features is combined by using an exponential function of the saliency difference such that it assigns low values to small differences in saliency and at the same time ensures that saliency information does not bias the energy term. Rotationally-invariant edge information from edge-orientation histograms was used to complement the saliency information resulting in better registration results. Tests on real patient datasets show that our algorithm results in accurate registration. We also simulated elastic motion on images, and the deformation field recovered by our algorithm was nearly the inverse of the simulated field.

1 Introduction

Nonrigid image registration, also referred to as warping, is an essential step in medical image analysis. Over the years, a number of methods have been proposed to meet the challenges arising from registration of images where the object of interest has been elastically deformed. Some of the earliest methods include elastic models [1], fluid flow models [2,3] and an optical flow approach [4]. In [5] the registration problem has been solved using thin-plate splines where the images are deformed over a regular grid having numerous control points. The disadvantage of thin-plate splines is that they have a global region of support i.e., changing the position of one control point changes the entire deformation field. Rueckert et al. in [6] overcome this problem by using B-splines which have a local region of support. Rohde et al. in [7] introduce the adaptive bases algorithm which uses radial basis functions instead of traditional B-splines and allows for spatial adaptation of the displacement field in regions of misregistration only.

Recently, Markov random field (MRF) model has also been used to achieve nonrigid image registration. In an MRF formulation of the problem of nonrigid image registration, the solution is obtained as the maximum *a-posteriori* (MAP) configuration or equivalently, by minimizing the energy of the corresponding MRF. Roy and Govindu in [8], applied an MRF model for the optical flow problem by modeling the flow orientation and magnitude as separate fields. The $\alpha-\beta$ swap algorithm proposed by Boykov *et al* in [9] used graph cuts to find the minimum of an energy function in the case of 2D motion estimation. Shekhovtsov *et al.* in [10] have proposed an algorithm that uses blocks of pixels to effectively register non-rigid deformations in synthetic and real images and is computationally more tractable. Tang *et al.* in [11] use an MRF based model to elastically register brain images. In [12], to avoid the effects of contrast enhancement on the process of image registration, Zheng *et al.* propose an MRF framework to de-enhance dynamic contrast-enhanced MRI and then register them using the B-Spline based algorithm in [6].

In this paper, we propose a novel saliency based approach for the nonrigid registration of dynamic renal MR images that can effectively correct elastic deformations in the presence of contrast enhancement due to wash-in of the contrast agent. In our approach, nonrigid registration is achieved by integrating saliency and edge information alongwith pixel intensity into the MAP-MRF framework. Saliency information of the pre- and post-contrast stages combined with pixel intensity are used to quantify the degree of similarity between two regions in the presence of intensity changes. By the use of orientation histograms, edge information has been used to complement saliency information.

The rest of the paper is organized as follows. In Section 2, we describe the neurobiology-based saliency model and its advantage over an entropy-based saliency model. Section 3 describes our saliency based MRF model and its optimization. We present our results in Section 4 and conclude with Section 5.

2 Neurobiology-Based Saliency Model

Saliency is a concept which states that there are regions in a scene that are more "attractive" than their neighbors and hence draw attention. Fig. 1(a)-(c) show respectively the cropped image corresponding to the right kidney (of the patient) in one slice, the saliency map generated by an entropy-based approach [13], and by a neurobiology-based approach [14]. The saliency map shown in Fig. 1 (b) gives a lot of importance (in terms of saliency values) to less important regions surrounding the kidney. In contrast, the saliency map in Fig. 1 (c) shows distinct salient regions corresponding to the kidney. Therefore, we opt for the neurobiology-based saliency model described in [14] and use *luminance* and *edge* information to calculate the saliency.

Saliency Map for Pre- and Post-Contrast Enhanced Images: In dynamic contrast enhanced images, the intensity of certain areas in the image changes with time (see Fig. 1 (d) for a post-contrast image of the same kidney shown in Fig. 1 (a)). By increasing the intensity of an already salient region, the saliency map does not change. Saliency being a measure of how one region differs from its

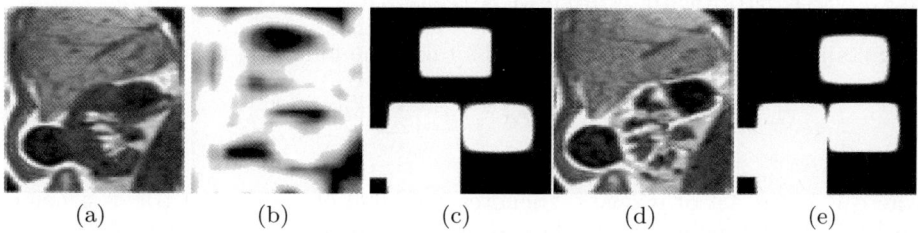

(a)   (b)   (c)   (d)   (e)

Fig. 1. (a) Kidney in one typical frame of pre-contrast stage; (b) saliency map generated by entropy-based method; (c) by neurobiological model; (d) kidney image in post-contrast stage; and (e) saliency map in post-contrast stage

immediate surroundings, is a relative quantity and is a good measure of establishing correspondence between regions in the pre- and post-contrast enhanced phases. From our experiments we observe that the saliency maps for the pre- and post- contrast stages are nearly identical, i.e., salient regions still remain salient after contrast enhancement. To demonstrate this, we display the saliency map of the kidney in the pre- and post-contrast stages in Fig. 1 (c) and (e), respectively. As shown, the two saliency maps are very close in spite of changes in image intensity due to the wash-in of the contrast agent. This suggests that the difference between saliency values of two corresponding regions is a good indicator of their similarity in the presence of contrast enhancement. Hence, it is desirable to facilitate the registration of dynamic renal MR images by exploiting the saliency information. For more details about the advantages of the neurobiology model over an entropy based approach refer [15].

3 Method

3.1 Overview of Our Algorithm

We model the displacement field of the elastic deformation as a Markov random field. MRF models use neighborhood relations between pixels of an image to model the interaction field. In registration of dynamic renal MR images where the kidney could have undergone elastic displacement, the correspondence between structure in two sets of images can be improved by including neighborhood information in the registration process. In our algorithm we use a combination of pixel intensity, saliency information and edge-orientation histograms to register dynamic contrast enhanced images. Integrating both saliency and edge information into the MRF framework ensures that the resulting matching is between pixels that are semantically as well as perceptually similar. Including saliency and intensity information from a neighborhood ensures smoothness of the deformation field. The displacements were denoted as discrete labels and the optimal labeling was determined by graph-cuts.

3.2 MRF Model for Nonrigid Registration

The standard energy function in MRFs takes the following form

$$E(x|\theta) = \sum_{s \in V} \theta_s(x_s) + \sum_{(s,t) \in N} \theta_{st}(x_s, x_t), \qquad (1)$$

where V is the set of pixels; x_s denotes the label of pixel $s \in V$; N is a neighborhood system defined on V. The term θ_s is a unary data penalty function and θ_{st} is a pairwise potential function that incorporates neighborhood information into the energy function.

We introduce an additional pairwise potential term θ_{edge}, and define our energy function as

$$E(x|\theta) = \sum_{s \in V} \theta_s(x_s) + \sum_{(s,t) \in N} \theta_{st}(x_s, x_t) + \sum_{(s,t) \in N} \theta_{edge}(x_s, x_t). \qquad (2)$$

In our experiments, the interaction potential is defined at the level of pixel-blocks and the neighborhood information is collected over a window comprising of blocks of pixels. Therefore s in equation (2) denotes blocks of pixels. We detail now each of the terms in equation (2).

A. Unary Data Term: $\theta_s(x_s)$

Let x_i^1 denote the pixel intensity in the floating image and x_i^2 the pixel intensity in the reference image. The data term is given by

$$\theta_s(x_s) = \sum_{i=1}^{m} w_i \times \left(x_i^1 - x_i^2\right)^2. \qquad (3)$$

It is the sum-of-squared differences of pixel intensities for each pixel block in the floating image and the reference image weighted by a function of the saliency difference between the constituent pixels. The weight w_i for the ith pixel in the pixel block is defined as

$$w_i = \frac{\exp\left(|sv_i^1 - sv_i^2|\right)}{1 + \exp\left(|sv_i^1 - sv_i^2|\right)} \qquad (4)$$

where sv_i^1 and sv_i^2 are the normalized saliency value of the corresponding pixel in the floating and reference image respectively. In equation (3), m is the total number of pixels in each block, i.e., $m = n \times n$, where n is the size of the square block.

B. Pairwise Interaction Term: $\theta_{st}(x_s, x_t)$

Recall that $\theta_{st}(x_s, x_t)$ is the interaction term between the block and its neighbors. Let $s + (x_s, x_t)$ be the block s shifted by (x_s, x_t). Therefore,

$$\theta_{st}(x_s, x_t) = \sum_j d\left(x_s, x_{s+(x_s, x_t)}\right), \qquad (5)$$

where $d\left(x_s, x_{s+(x_s,x_t)}\right) = \sum_{i=1}^{m} w_i \times |x_i^1 - x_i^2|$ is the dissimilarity measure between blocks s and $s + (x_s, x_t)$ and j denotes all neighboring blocks. In our formulation, we constrain the range of allowed displacements by imposing a large penalty for blocks with a displacement greater than 6 pixel units from the central block.

Here we explain the rationale behind the weight function w_i introduced in equation (3). The requirement for a weighting function was that it should assign low values to small difference in saliency and at the same time ensure that saliency information does not bias the energy term. To avoid dealing with very large numbers, a function is chosen so that its value lies between 0 and 1. Our choice of the weighting function was determined empirically and is not unique. In the scenario that the blocks of pixels being compared belong to the same region, the difference in their normalized saliency values is very small and the corresponding w_i is small. Also, the difference in intensity values is minimum for identical regions even in the face of intensity change due to wash-in of contrast agent. Thus the resultant product of the two terms is minimal.

When the two blocks in question are from different regions then the saliency values are different and a large difference results in a high value of w_i. This combined with the large intensity difference makes the terms $\theta_s(x_s)$ and $\theta_{st}(x_s, x_t)$ in equation (2) have a higher value. There is the possibility that we might have pixel blocks from regions having significantly different intensities but similar saliency values. In that case, the product of w_i and $|x_i^1 - x_i^2|$ takes a high value and the terms $\theta_s(x_s)$ and $\theta_{st}(x_s, x_t)$ are not minimal. In the normalized saliency map from the neurobiology based model, the salient regions are distinctly different from their neighbors. Thus, in a local neighborhood it is highly improbable to find pixels with identical or nearly identical values. In our experiments, the images have been registered for rigid transformations prior to nonrigid image matching. As a result, considering the amount of elastic motion a kidney could undergo, we constrain the range of allowed displacements for a pixel to ±6 pixel units in each direction. In such a setup, the scenario that pixel blocks being compared are from vastly different locations and have nearly identical saliency values does not arise.

C. Edge Potential Term: $\theta_{edge}(x_s, x_t)$

Elastic deformations in a kidney are like local rotations. As a potential term, $\theta_{edge}(x_s, x_t)$ is a rotation invariant metric that is used to match the edges of the object of interest, i.e., the kidney. We use edge-orientation histograms to define rotation invariant features [16] which are important for matching landmarks. The degree of dissimilarity between two sets of edges is determined by taking the histogram distance of the distribution of their orientations, as in equation (6). We observe that in the post-enhancement stage, the direction of edges at certain points is inverted due to increased intensity. In such a scenario, we ensured that gradient directions differing by π radians are grouped in identical bins.

$$\theta_{edge}(x_s, x_t) = \sum_{k=1}^{K} \left(h_k^1 - h_k^2\right)^2, \tag{6}$$

where h_k is the value in the kth bin of edge orientation histogram h, and K is the number of histogram bins. K was set to 5 in our experiments.

3.3 Optimization

The range of displacements was denoted as a series of discrete labels and the optimal labeling determined the displacement of each pixel block. Optimization of equation (2) was carried out using graph-cuts, [9], via a sequence of alpha-expansion (α-expansion) moves. Details of the method can be found in [9].

4 Experimental Results

4.1 Implementation

We tested our algorithm on 5 different datasets. The MR images of the kidney were of dimensions 256×256. There were 41 volumes acquired for each patient with each volume having 40 slices. The intensity values of the images and also that of the saliency map were normalized to lie in the range $[0, 1]$. All images were pre-registered for rigid transformations before implementing our algorithm. Non-overlapping pixel blocks of size 3×3 were used.

4.2 Results on Real Datasets

In registration of contrast-enhanced MR images, the difference image between the pre- and post-contrast stages after registration should show only the renal tissues (i.e, renal cortex) whose intensity is enhanced due to the contrast agent. We first evaluate the registration results by visual examination. Fig. 2 (a) shows the unregistered difference image between a reference pre-contrast image and the floating post-contrast image. We can see the significant error due to elastic deformation. Fig. 2 (b) shows the difference image after our registration algorithm has been applied to the floating image without using saliency (by setting $w_i=1$ in equations (3) and (5)) or edge information. Fig. 2 (c) shows the difference image when using saliency information alone. The registration results are not optimum with some regions improperly registered. Fig. 2 (d) shows the difference image after edge information along with saliency information has been used in our registration algorithm. This image clearly shows that in spite of large intensity differences due to the wash-in of the contrast agent, our MRF based method accomplishes registration very effectively.

4.3 Results of Simulated Deformation

In each dataset, pre-contrast images were elastically deformed using the free-form deformation (FFD) method in [6]. These deformed images were then registered to the original undeformed image using our MRF based algorithm. The difference images for a typical pre-contrast image are shown in Fig. 3 (a)-(b). Fig. 3 (a) shows the difference image before registration and Fig. 3 (b) shows

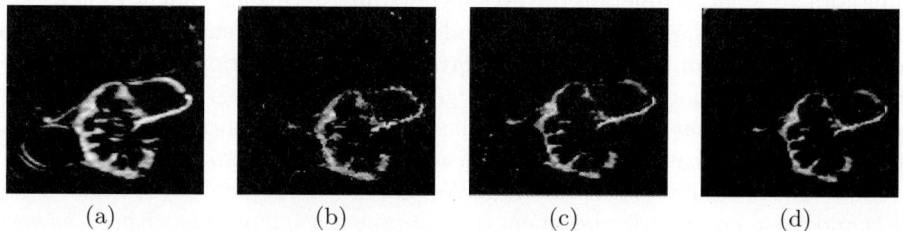

Fig. 2. Difference images: (a) before registration; after registration (b) using only intensity information; (c) saliency combined with intensity information; (d) using saliency and edge information together with intensity information

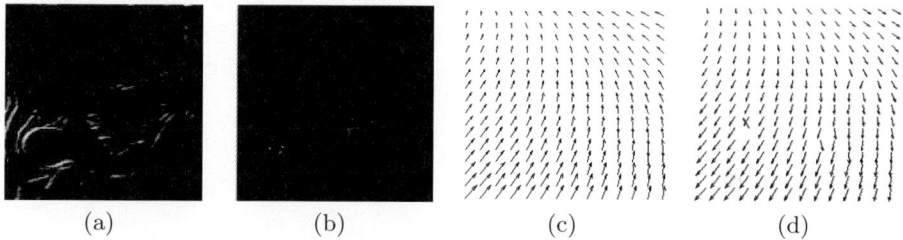

Fig. 3. Results of simulated elastic deformation (for pre-contrast stage): (a) difference image before registration; (b) difference image after registration; (c) simulated displacement field about the kidney region; and (d) recovered displacement field about the kidney region

the difference image after registration. From Fig. 3 (b) we conclude that our registration algorithm does well to recover the flow field. In Fig. 3 (c) we show the displacement field generated by applying the FFD algorithm and Fig. 3 (d) shows the displacement field recovered by our method. From the two images it is apparent that our algorithm could recover the simulated flow field with a considerable degree of accuracy. Similar results were obtained in our attempt to recover the flow field of a post-contrast image. The average error (Euclidean distance) between the actual deformation field and recovered flow field was found to be {0.0053, 0.0125, 0.0046, 0.0061, 0.0097} units for the datasets.

5 Conclusion

In this paper we have proposed a saliency based MRF model for registration of dynamic contrast enhanced images in the presence of intensity changes due to flow of contrast agent. To obtain the saliency information we used a neurobiology-based saliency model that works better than an entropy-based saliency model. Difference of saliency values from a normalized saliency map combined with intensity information was used to quantify the degree of similarity between two regions at different time intervals. Information from these two maps was fused using an exponential function of the saliency difference such that it assigns low values to small differences in saliency and at the same time ensures that saliency information does not bias the energy term. In the formulation of the cost function of the MRF model we used the edge-orientation histogram to incorporate rotationally-invariant edge information. Tests on 5 real patient datasets with different degrees of elastic deformation of the kidneys, demonstrate the effectiveness and accuracy of our method. We simulated elastic deformations using FFD and the recovered displacement field obtained using our algorithm was very close to the inverse of the simulated field.

Acknowledgements

The authors would like to thank Dr. Vivian Lee, Professor of Radiology, Physiology and Neuroscience, Vice-Dean for Science, Senior Vice-President and Chief Scientific Officer, New York University Medical Center, for providing the datasets. This work was supported by NUS grant R-263-000-470-112.

References

1. Bajcsy, R., Kovacic, S.: Multiresolution elastic matching. Computer Vision, Graphics, and Image Processing 46(1), 1–21 (1989)
2. Christensen, G., Miller, M.I., Vannier, M.: 3D brain mapping using a deformable anatomy. Phy. Med. Biol. 39, 609–618 (1994)
3. Bro-Nielsen, M., Gramkow, C.: Fast fluid registration of medical images. In: Höhne, K.H., Kikinis, R. (eds.) VBC 1996. LNCS, vol. 1131, pp. 267–276. Springer, Heidelberg (1996)
4. Thirion, J.P.: Image matching as a diffusion process: an analogy with maxwell's demons. Med. Image Anal. 2(3), 243–260 (1998)
5. Meyer, C., et al.: Demonstration of accuracy and clinical versatility of mutual information for automatic multimodality image fusion using affine and thin-plate spline warped geometric deformations. Medical Image Analysis 1(3), 195–206 (1997)
6. Rueckert, D., Sonoda, L.I., Hayes, C., Hill, D.L., Leach, M.O., Hawkes, D.J.: Non-rigid registration using free-form deformations: application to breast mr images. IEEE Trans. Med. Imaging 18(8), 712–721 (1999)
7. Rohde, G.K., Aldroubi, A., Dawant, B.M.: The adaptive bases algorithm for intensity based nonrigid image registration. IEEE Trans. Med. Imaging 22(11), 1470–1479 (2003)
8. Roy, S., Govindu, V.: Mrf solutions for probabilistic optical flow formulations. In: ICPR 2000: Proceedings of the International Conference on Pattern Recognition, p. 7053 (2000)
9. Boykov, Y., Veksler, O., Zabih, R.: Fast approximate energy minimization via graph cuts. IEEE Trans. Pattern Anal. Mach. Intell. 23(11), 1222–1239 (2001)
10. Shekhovtsov, A., Kovtun, I., Hlaváč, V.: Efficient mrf deformation model for non-rigid image matching. In: CVPR. IEEE Computer Society, Los Alamitos (2007)
11. Tang, T.W.H., Chung, A.C.S.: Non-rigid image registration using graph-cuts. In: Ayache, N., Ourselin, S., Maeder, A. (eds.) MICCAI 2007, Part I. LNCS, vol. 4791, pp. 916–924. Springer, Heidelberg (2007)

12. Zheng, Y., Yu, J., Kambhamettu, C., Englander, S., Schnall, M.D., Shen, D.: De-enhancing the dynamic contrast-enhanced breast mri for robust registration. In: Ayache, N., Ourselin, S., Maeder, A. (eds.) MICCAI 2007, Part I. LNCS, vol. 4791, pp. 933–941. Springer, Heidelberg (2007)
13. Kadir, T., Brady, M.: Saliency, scale and image description. International journal of Computer Vision 45(2), 85–105 (2001)
14. Itti, L., Koch, C.: A saliency-based search mechanism for overt and covert shifts of visual attention. Vision Research 40, 1489–1506 (2000)
15. Mahapatra, D., Sun, Y.: Registration of dynamic renal mr images using neurobiological model of saliency. In: Intl. Symp. Biomed. Imaging, pp. 1119–1122 (2008)
16. Lowe, D.G.: Distinctive image features from scale-invariant keypoints. Int. J. Comput. Vision 60(2), 91–110 (2004)

A Constrained Non-rigid Registration Algorithm for Use in Prostate Image-Guided Radiotherapy

W.H. Greene[1], S. Chelikani[2], K. Purushothaman[2], Z. Chen[3], J.P.S Knisely[3], L.H. Staib[1,2], X. Papademetris[1,2] and J. Duncan[1,2]

[1] Department of Biomedical Engineering,
[2] Department of Diagnostic Radiology
[3] Department of Therapeutic Radiology,
Yale University, New Haven, CT, USA
william.h.greene@yale.edu

Abstract. A constrained non-rigid registration (CNRR) algorithm for use in updating prostate external beam image-guided radiotherapy treatment plans is presented in this paper. The developed algorithm is based on a multi-resolution cubic B-spline FFD transformation and has been tested and verified using 3D CT images from 10 sets of real patient data acquired from 4 different patients on different treatment days. The registration can be constrained to any combination of the prostate, rectum, bladder, pelvis, left femur, and right femur. The CNRR was tested with 5 different combinations of constraints and each test significantly outperformed both rigid and non-rigid registration at aligning constrained bones and critical organs. The CNRR was then used to update the treatment plans to account for articulated, rigid bone motion and non-rigid organ deformation. Each updated treatment plan outperformed the original treatment plan by increasing radiation dosage to the prostate and lowering radiation dosage to the rectum and bladder.

1 Introduction

External-beam radiotherapy (EBRT) is one of the primary treatment modalities for prostate cancer [1]. Three-dimensional conformal radiotherapy (3DCRT) and intensity modulated radiotherapy (IMRT) have significantly increased the ability of EBRT to generate highly conformal radiation dose distributions for the prostate tumor volume with sharp dose falloff in the surrounding normal tissues. IMRT allows increased doses to be delivered to the prostate with acceptable acute and late toxicities for the nearby organs at risk, such as the rectum and bladder. However, when higher doses are to be delivered, precise and accurate targeting is essential because of unpredictable inter- and intra-fractional organ motions over the course of the daily treatments that often last more than seven weeks. Patient setup errors and internal organ motions must be taken into account in the treatment plan before dose-escalation trials are implemented in order to ensure accurate delivery of the planned dose to the prostate and to minimize the dose received by the rectum and bladder [2].

The latest advancement of Image-guided radiotherapy (IGRT) integrates an in-room cone-beam CT (CBCT) with radiotherapy linear accelerators for treatment day imaging. The CBCT images acquired on the treatment day enable the radiotherapist to rigidly adjust the position of the patient to best align the patient to the position used in the planning of the EBRT treatment. In addition to rigidly adjusting the position of the patient, a successful implementation of IGRT requires a robust non-rigid image registration and analysis technique to accurately align the patient anatomy on the treatment day to the patient anatomy on the planning day [3].

In this paper, we present a CNRR algorithm based on a multi-resolution cubic B-spline Free Form Deformation (FFD) transformation to capture the unpredictable articulated, rigid bone motion and internal organ deformation. The prostate, rectum, and bladder are used as non-rigid constraints and the pelvis, right femur, and left femur are used as rigid constraints. The constraint objects are independently registered prior to running the CNRR and the results are used in the CNRR to constrain the objects to their estimated position.

The transformation determined from the CNRR algorithm is used to update the planning day treatment plan to accurately account for bone and organ motion. An updated treatment plan that accurately accounts for bone and organ motion would allow for smaller planning margins and an escalated radiation dose, all while maintaining or lowering bladder and rectum toxicity levels [3][4].

2 Method

The CNRR algorithm consists of two steps. (**1**) Planning day organs {prostate, rectum, bladder} are independently registered to treatment day organs using a non-rigid transform. Planning day bones {pelvis, left femur, right femur} are independently registered to treatment day bones using a rigid transform. (**2**) The registration results are used to constrain the objects in the CNRR to their estimated transformations, generating $T_{0 \to d}$, the transformation from the planning day image I_0 to the treatment day image I_d.

The estimated transformation $T_{0 \to d}$ is used to update the planning day treatment plan P_0 to account for rigid bone motion and organ deformation, creating P_d, the updated treatment plan for treatment day d.

2.1 Independent Organ Registration

The segmented, binary prostate, rectum, and bladder images are independently registered using a non-rigid transform based on a multi-resolution cubic B-Spline FFD. A FFD based transform was chosen because a FFD is locally controllable due to the underlying mesh of control points which are used to manipulate the image [5].

A cubic B-spline FFD is defined by designating the image volume as $\Omega = \{(x, y, z) | 0 \leq x < X, 0 \leq y < Y, 0 \leq z < Z\}$. Φ denotes a $(l+3) \times (m+3) \times (n+3)$ mesh of control points $\phi_{i,j,k}$ with uniform spacing $\delta_x, \delta_y, \delta_z = \delta$. The parameter domain of the image is defined as $\Theta = \{(u,v,w) | 0 \le u \le l, 0 \le v \le m, 0 \le w \le n\}$. The FFD can then be written as a 3D tensor product of 1D cubic B-splines

$$T_{0 \to d}(x,y,z) = \sum_{i=0}^{3} \sum_{j=0}^{3} \sum_{k=0}^{3} B_i(u - \lfloor u \rfloor) B_j(v - \lfloor v \rfloor)$$
$$B_k(w - \lfloor w \rfloor) \phi_{(\lfloor u \rfloor + i)(\lfloor v \rfloor + j)(\lfloor w \rfloor + k)} \quad (1)$$

where $T_{0 \to d}$ maps the planning day image I_0 to the treatment day image I_d, and $u = \frac{x}{\delta_x}, v = \frac{y}{\delta_y}, w = \frac{z}{\delta_z}$. In addition, B_i represents the ith basis function of the cubic B-spline

$$B_0(u) = \frac{(1-u)^3}{6} \qquad B_2(u) = \frac{(-3u^3 + 3u^2 + 3u + 1)}{6}$$

$$B_1(u) = \frac{(3u^3 - 6u^2 + 4)}{6} \qquad B_3(u) = \frac{u^3}{6}.$$

The degree of non-rigid motion captured depends on the spacing of the control points in the mesh Φ. In order to create an algorithm with an adequate degree of non-rigid deformation, a hierarchical multi-resolution approach is implemented in which the control point resolution is increased in a coarse to fine fashion [6][7].

Let $\Phi^1, \Phi^2, \ldots, \Phi^N$ denote a hierarchy of control point meshes, each improving in resolution over the previous mesh. $T^1, T^2, \ldots, T^N$ are the transformations associated with each control point mesh. The composition of all transformations $\bar{T}(\Omega) = T^N \circ \cdots \circ T^2 \circ T^1(\Omega)$, is a map that defines the deformation of image volume Ω [6][7]. Thus, the transformation from the segmented planning day organ I_0^{obj} to the segmented treatment day organ I_d^{obj} is

$$\hat{T}_{0 \to d}^{obj}(x,y,z) = \hat{T}_{0 \to d}^{obj-N} \circ \cdots \circ \hat{T}_{0 \to d}^{obj-2} \circ \hat{T}_{0 \to d}^{obj-1}(x,y,z). \quad (2)$$

In order to determine each individual transformation $\hat{T}_{0 \to d}^{obj-n}$, we developed an objective function based on a sum of squared differences intensity matching term (C_{SSD}) and a transformation smoothing term (C_{smooth}).

The sum of squared differences intensity match function C_{SSD} is written as

$$C_{SSD}(T_{0 \to d}(\Phi)) = \frac{1}{N} \sum_{i=0}^{N} [I_d(i) - I_0(T_{0 \to d}(i, \Phi))]^2 \quad (3)$$

where i indexes over the voxels.

To ensure the transformation is smooth, each control point is restricted to move within a sphere of radius $r < R$, where $R \approx 0.4033 \times \delta$ [8][9][7]. The smoothing function is posed as

$$C_{smooth}(\Phi) = \sum_k f(\Phi_k) \quad (4)$$

where k indexes over the control points and

$$f(\Phi_k) = \begin{cases} 0 & \text{if } |\Phi_k| < 0.4033 \times \delta \\ |\Phi_k| & \text{otherwise} \end{cases}.$$

Each individual transformation $\hat{T}_{0 \to d}^{obj-n}$ in (2) is estimated by using a conjugate gradient optimizer to minimize the following objective function with respect to $T_{0 \to d}^{obj-n}$

$$\hat{T}_{0 \to d}^{obj-n} = \arg \min_{T_{0 \to d}^{obj-n}} \left[C_{SSD}(T_{0 \to d}^{obj-n}(\Phi^{obj-n})) + C_{smooth}(\Phi^{obj-n}) \right]. \quad (5)$$

The control point mesh Φ^{obj-n} is used as a constraint in the CNRR.

2.2 Independent Bone Registration

The segmented, binary pelvis, left femur and right femur images are independently registered using a rigid transformation to find the optimal $\hat{T}_{0 \to d}^{r, obj}$ which maps I_0^{obj} into I_d^{obj}

$$\hat{T}_{0 \to d}^{r,obj}(x,y,z) = \hat{T}_{0 \to d}^{r,obj-N} \circ \cdots \circ \hat{T}_{0 \to d}^{r,obj-2} \circ \hat{T}_{0 \to d}^{r,obj-1}(x,y,z). \quad (6)$$

To estimate each $\hat{T}_{0 \to d}^{r,obj-n}$, we minimize C_{SSD} with respect to $T_{0 \to d}^{r,obj-n}$ using a conjugate gradient optimizer

$$\hat{T}_{0 \to d}^{r,obj-n} = \arg \min_{T_{0 \to d}^{r,obj-n}} C_{SSD}(T_{0 \to d}^{obj-n}). \quad (7)$$

Each rigid transformation $\hat{T}_{0 \to d}^{r,obj-n}$ is applied to an associated control point mesh Φ^{obj-n}, which is used as a constraint in the CNRR.

2.3 Constrained Non-rigid Registration

The constrained non-rigid registration algorithm uses the same FFD transform developed in Sec. 2.1 to estimate the optimal $\hat{\bar{T}}_{0 \to d}$ which maps the planning day image I_0 into the treatment day image I_d.

$$\hat{\bar{T}}_{0 \to d}(x,y,z) = \hat{T}_{0 \to d}^N \circ \cdots \circ \hat{T}_{0 \to d}^2 \circ \hat{T}_{0 \to d}^1(x,y,z) \quad (8)$$

To estimate each $\hat{T}_{0 \to d}^n$, we developed a cost function based on C_{SSD}, C_{smooth}, and an object matching function (C_{object}).

The object matching function C_{object} aligns the organs and bones by forcing the control points that lie within the segmented objects to their position estimated by the individual object registration.

$$C_{object}(\Phi^n) = \sum_{obj} \sum_{k \in obj} \left[\Phi_k^n - \Phi_k^{n-obj} \right]^2 \quad (9)$$

where k indexes over the control points and obj indexes over any combination of constraint objects {prostate, rectum, bladder, pelvis, right femur, left femur} used in the registration.

Each $\hat{T}^n_{0 \to d}$ in (8) is estimated using a conjugate gradient optimizer to minimize the following objective function using weight α with respect to $T^n_{0 \to d}$

$$\hat{T}^n_{0 \to d} = \arg\min_{T^n_{0 \to d}} \left[C_{SSD}(T^n_{0 \to d}(\Phi^n)) + \alpha C_{object}(\Phi^n) + \alpha C_{smooth}(\Phi^n) \right]. \quad (10)$$

2.4 Updating and Assessing the Treatment Plan

The dose distributions in the tumor and organs at risk are analyzed by using the dose volume histogram (DVH), which plots the dose distribution throughout the organs (prostate, rectum, bladder). The prostate DVH can be reduced to a single metric known as the tumor control probability (TCP) and the normal tissue DVH can be reduced to the normal tissue complication probability (NTCP), which is calculated for both the rectum and bladder [10][11]. An optimal treatment plan maximizes the TCP while minimizing both rectal and bladder NTCP.

The treatment day TCP and NTCP values are calculated using the planning day treatment plan P_0 and treatment day image I_d and compared to the planning day values calculated using P_0 and I_0. If the treatment day NTCP for a healthy organ is greater than the planning day NTCP, then that organ is used as a constraint in the CNRR. The prostate is always used as a constraint. The transformation estimated from the CNRR result is used to warp P_0 into P_d, the updated treatment plan for day d.

3 Results

We used ten sets of real patient data acquired from four different patients. Two patients each had three treatment day CT images, and an additional two patients each had two treatment day CT images. Each of the four patients analyzed had an associated planning day 3DCRT treatment plan and CT image. The images and treatment plans were re-sliced to a clinically applicable spatial resolution of $4mm \times 4mm \times 4mm$. The prostate, rectum, and bladder were hand segmented by a qualified clinician. The pelvis, left femur, and right femur were segmented using *BioImage Suite* [12].

The CNRR was tested for robustness using 5 different constraint scenarios (Table 1); The weighting factor in (10) was set to infinity. The treatment plans were then updated by selecting registration constraints as described in Sec. 2.4. Registration and treatment plan results are presented below.

3.1 Registration Results

The CNRR algorithm was tested using 5 different constraint scenarios (Table 1) to determine how the constrained organs and bones affected the transformation of the unconstrained organs and bones. The control point spacing started at

Table 1. Registration Tests

Test	# Constraints	Objects Constrained
NRR	0	None – Non-Rigid Registration
CNRR-1	1	Prostate
CNRR-2	2	Bladder, Prostate
CNRR-3	3	Pelvis, L. Femur, R. Femur
CNRR-5	5	Pelvis, L. Femur, R. Femur, Bladder, Prostate
CNRR-6	6	Pelvis, L. Femur, R. Femur, Bladder, Rectum, Prostate

$\delta = 25mm$ and was refined to $\delta = 14mm$ over 10 iterations. For comparison, a non-rigid registration (NRR) and rigid registration (RR) were performed on all ten sets of real patient data. Object overlap was tracked at each iteration of the registration and was used as a metric to assess the quality of the registration and the improvement generated at each iteration.

The RR performed the poorest out of all the registrations algorithms, generating an identity transform for all ten sets of patient data. The RR results are not discussed further.

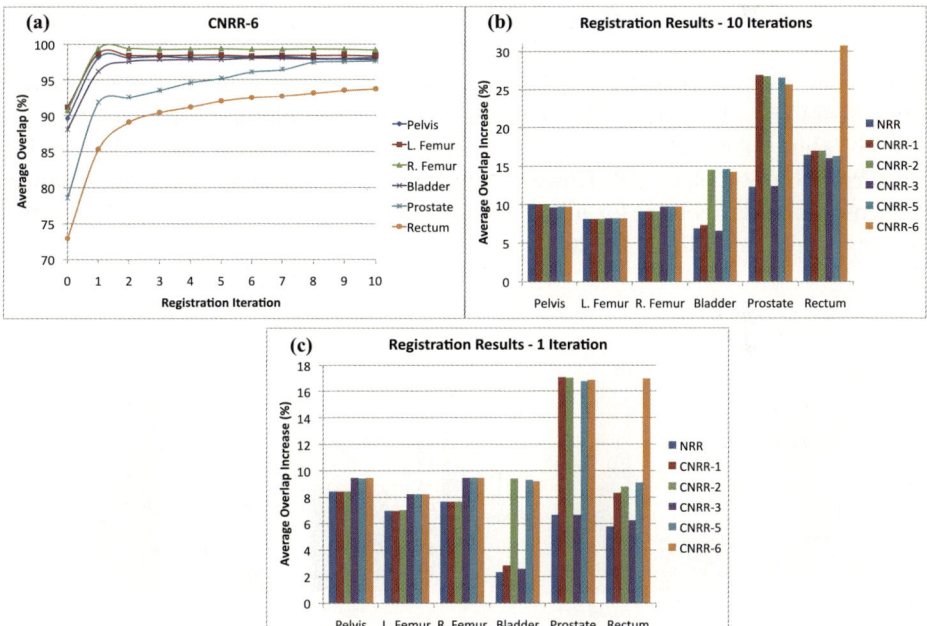

Fig. 1. Registration results presented are averaged over 10 sets of real patient data acquired from 4 different patients. (a) Average object overlap results at each iteration of CNRR-6, where iteration '0' represents the initial object overlap. (b) Average object overlap increase achieved after 10 iterations. Results are from NRR and 5 CNRR tests performed. (c) Average object overlap increase achieved after 1 iteration. Results are from NRR and 5 CNRR tests performed. For each object, more than 40% of the overlap increase acquired after 10 iterations was achieved in the first iteration.

The CNRR significantly outperformed the NRR at aligning constrained organs and bones. The overlap increase for each object after 10 iterations is presented in Fig. 1b. The best overlap results were generated when all 6 objects were used as constraints in CNRR-6 (Fig 1a). The most significant object overlap gains were made in the first registration iteration (Fig. 1c). The results indicate that constrained objects did not improve the overlap of unconstrained objects. All results presented in Fig. 1 are averaged over the ten sets of real patient data.

3.2 Treatment Plan Results

All four 3DCRT treatment plans were updated for each associated treatment day CT image. Due to set-up errors, inter- and intra-organ motion, treatment plan results varied from patient to patient and day to day. For this reason, results must be presented on an individual and daily basis.

As an example, normalized results from two treatment days for patient 2 are presented in Fig. 2. On both treatment days, the TCP and bladder NTCP were poorer than the planning values, so only the prostate and bladder were used as constraints. We tested three constraint scenarios, CNRR-1,2,5, with 10 iterations each. The best results occurred when both the prostate and bladder were held as constraints (CNRR-2). For both days, the TCP value did not decrease much from the planning TCP value due to the large planning margins used in 3DCRT that ensure the prostate receives the complete dose of radiation, so little correction was observed. However, updating the treatment plan significantly decreased bladder NTCP for all constraint scenarios tested. Including the bones as constraints in addition to the prostate and bladder (CNRR-5) did not further

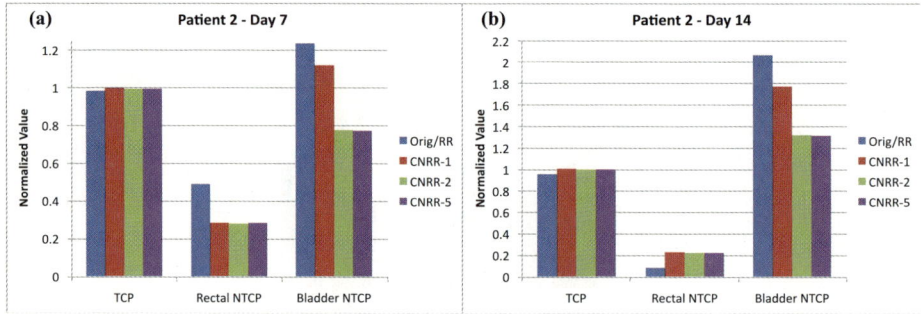

Fig. 2. TCP, NTCP Results for Patient 2 acquired from original and updated treatment plans. Results normalized by dividing treatment day value by planning day value. Original treatment plan was updated using RR, CNRR-1,2,5. For both days, CNRR-1,2,5 increased TCP and decreased bladder NTCP. CNRR-2,5 decreased bladder NTCP the most due to the bladder constraint. Bone constraints in CNRR-5 did not improve values when compared to CNRR-2. (a) Day 7 results. CNRR-1,2,5 improved rectal NTCP. (b) Day 14 results. Rectal NTCP was slightly increased in CNRR-1,2,5.

improve treatment plan results when compared to those with just the prostate and bladder (CNRR-2).

4 Discussion

For each patient and constraint combination tested, the CNRR proved to be highly robust and significantly improved the overlap for each constrained object and outperformed the results achieved from the RR and NRR.

Updating each treatment plan to account for prostate deformation and motion slightly improved the treatment day TCP for each patient. Although the treatment day TCP did not decrease much in each case due to the large planning margins used around the prostate in 3DCRT plans, nominal TCP improvements were achieved. Had IMRT plans, which provide more highly conformal and smaller dose planning margins, been used, significant improvements in the TCP would have been achieved.

Updating the treatment plans to improve the treatment day NTCP for normal organs significantly lowered the NTCP for these organs. When used to update the treatment plan, the CNRR transformation pulled the low radiation areas that were initially planned in the healthy organs back into the organs, improving the NTCP.

While the updated treatment plans may not be immediately realized without making corresponding modifications to the treatment beams, the updated plan will (**1**) serve as the new dose prescription for optimizing the fluence map of the treatment beams so that the updated plan can be physically delivered or (**2**) serve as a guide so that a closely matched realizable plan, selected from a library of pre-approved plans, can be used to deliver the updated dose distribution. While the first approach would be ideal, it is not clinically feasible due to time constraints. The latter approach, however, is time efficient and can be implemented clinically.

References

1. Potosky, A.L., Legler, J., Albertsen, P.C., Stanford, J.L., Gilliland, F.D., Hamilton, A.S., Eley, J.W., Stephenson, R.A., Harlan, L.C.: Health outcomes after prostatectomy or radiotherapy for prostate cancer: Results from the prostate cancer outcomes study. J. Nat. Cancer Inst. 92, 1582–1592 (2000)
2. Ghilezan, M., Yan, D., Liang, J., Jaffray, D., Wong, J., Martinez, A.: Online imageguided intensity-modulated radiotherapy for prostate cancer: How much improvement can we expect? A theoretical assessment of clinical benefits and potential dose escalation by improving precision and accuracy of radiation delivery. Int. J. Radiation Oncology Biol. Phys. 60(5), 1602–1610 (2004)
3. Dawson, L.A., Sharpe, M.B.: Image-guided radiotherapy: rationale, benefits, and limitations. Lancet. Oncol. 7, 848–858 (2006)
4. Klein, E.E., Drzymala, R.E., Purdy, J.A., Michalski, J.: Errors in radiation oncology: a study in pathways and dosimetric impact. J. Appl. Clin. Med. Phys. 62, 1517–1524 (2005)

5. Rogers, D.: An Introduction to NURBS: with Historical Perspective, 1st edn. Morgan Kaufmann Publishers, San Francisco (2001)
6. Rueckert, D., Sonoda, L., Denton, E., Rankin, S., Hayes, C., Leach, M.O., Hill, D., Hawkes, D.J.: Comparison and evaluation of rigid and non-rigid registration of breast MR images. In: SPIE, vol. 3661, pp. 78–88 (1999)
7. Greene, W.H., Chelikani, S., Papademetris, X., Knisely, J.P.S., Duncan, J.: A constrained non-rigid registration algorithm for application in prostate radiotherapy. In: ISBI, pp. 740–743 (April 2007)
8. Choi, Y., Lee, S.: Local injectivity conditions of 2D and 3D uniform cubic b-spline functions. In: Proc. of Pacific Graphics, pp. 302–311 (1999)
9. Rueckert, D., Aljabar, P., Heckemann, R., Hajnal, J.V., Hammers, A.: Diffeomorphic registration using b-splines. In: Larsen, R., Nielsen, M., Sporring, J. (eds.) MICCAI 2006. LNCS, vol. 4191, pp. 702–709. Springer, Heidelberg (2006)
10. Cozzi, L., Buffa, F.M., Fogliata, A.: Comparative analysis of dose volume histogram reduction algorithms for normal tissue complication probability calculations. Acta Oncologica. 39(2), 165–171 (2000)
11. Kutcher, G.J., Burman, C., Brewster, L., Goitein, M., Mohan, R.: Histogram reduction method for calculating complication probabilities for three-dimensional treatment planing evaluations. Int. J. Radiation Oncology Biol. Phys. (21), 137–146 (1991)
12. Papademetris, X., Jackowski, M., Rajeevan, N., Constable, R., Staib, L.: BioImage Suite: An integrated medical image analysis suite, Section of Bioimaging Sciences, Dept. of Diagnostic Radiology, Yale School of Medicine,
http://www.bioimagesuite.org

Identifying Regional Cardiac Abnormalities from Myocardial Strains Using Spatio-temporal Tensor Analysis

Zhen Qian[1], Qingshan Liu[1], Dimitris N. Metaxas[1], and Leon Axel[2]

[1] Center for Computational Biomedicine Imaging and Modeling (CBIM), Rutgers University, New Brunswick, NJ, USA
[2] Department of Radiology, New York University, New York, NY, USA

Abstract. Myocardial deformation is a critical indicator of many cardiac diseases and dysfunctions. The goal of this paper is to use myocardial deformation patterns to identify and localize regional abnormal cardiac function in human subjects. We have developed a novel tensor-based classification framework that better conserves the spatio-temporal structure of the myocardial deformation pattern than conventional vector-based algorithms. In addition, the tensor-based projection function keeps more of the information of the original feature space, so that abnormal tensors in the subspace can be back-projected to reveal the regional cardiac abnormality in a more physically meaningful way. We have tested our novel method on 41 human image sequences, and achieved a classification rate of 87.80%. The recovered regional abnormalities from our algorithm agree well with the patient's pathology and doctor's diagnosis and provide a promising avenue for regional cardiac function analysis.

1 Introduction

Myocardial deformation (or strain) is an important early indicator of many cardiac diseases and dysfunctions, such as ischemia and infarction. Recently, the technique of MRI tagging (tMRI) [1] has been extensively used in research and clinical applications to extract detailed information on myocardial deformation in vivo. This technique generates sets of equally spaced tagging lines or grids within the myocardium as temporary material markers, through spatial modulation of the magnetization. For deformation extraction from the images, many motion and strain estimation methods have been proposed for tMRI. In [2], deformed tags were tracked and interpolated using a spline method to obtain a dense displacement map, from which the 2D Lagrangian strain was calculated. In [3] the spatio-temporal continuity constraint was used to derive the myocardial displacement field. In [4], the myocardial velocity field and pathlines were calculated from the phase map using the HARP technique. Then the strain was obtained from the HARP phase *tracking* results. The left ventricle was divided into 8 sectors and regional myocardial strains were calculated, which demonstrated the inhomogeneous strain distribution in the ventricle. In [5,6,7], $3D + t$

strains were derived from 3D parametrical deformable models using either FEM or B-Spline tensor techniques.

Some of the aforementioned strain estimation methods [2,6,7] have been implemented to compare normal and pathological data. Their results show noticeable differences in the strain pattern of normal and abnormal hearts, which reveals the potential of using strain to identify pathology in cardiac function. However, limited research has been conducted to fulfill this potential in a quantitative manner. In [8], an exploratory normal contraction reference model has been set up, based on the principal component analysis (PCA) of tMRI scans from 8 healthy subjects using their spatio-temporal deformation. Abnormalities could be found by comparing with the reference model in the PCA subspace.

The goal of this paper is to use the spatio-temporally distributed myocardial strain pattern to identify and localize abnormal cardiac function in human subjects. The main difficulty behind this is the large strain variance among normal subjects, and the even larger variance in patients, which makes it difficult to define a normal or abnormal criterion. On the other hand, the spatio-temporally distributed myocardial strain is far more complicated to quantitatively interpret than the 1D ECG signal or the scalar ejection fraction. Pathology develops with complicated and systematic consequences. For example, a region of ischemia might cause the rest of the heart to contract more vigorously to compensate. In this case, the spatial or temporal pattern of the strain could be of more importance than strain value alone in detecting cardiac malfunctions.

In this paper, to solve these two difficulties, we formulate the detection of abnormality into a novel spatio-temporal tensor-based linear discriminant analysis (LDA) classification framework. In order to learn the classifier in a supervised fashion, we gathered a group of normal and patient tMRI sequences acquired in short axis (SA), and applied a non-tracking-based strain estimation method [9] to extract the radial strain, circumferential strain and tissue rotation angles to construct the training data. Then a tensor-based LDA classifier was employed, based on the Fisher criterion to find an optimal linear projection that maximizes the between-class, i.e., the normal and patient, scatter and minimizes the within-class scatter. Compared with the vector-based conventional LDA that projects the feature space onto a scalar, the advantage of using our spatio-temporal tensor-based LDA is that its dimension reduction is separately operated in the spatial and temporal domains, so that it conserves better the spatio-temporal structure and information of the training data. On the other hand, the advantage of using a linear classifier, rather than nonlinear approaches such as SVM, is that by using the pseudo-inverse matrix of the linear projection function, we are able to back-project the abnormality found in the subspace to the original feature space, so as to localize the regional cardiac abnormality in a more physically meaningful way. We have tested our novel classification algorithm on a clinical dataset of forty one tMRI sequences from normal and patient subjects, and have achieved a higher or comparable detection accuracy rate compared to conventional classification algorithms, such as PCA, LDA and SVM. The recovered regional abnormalities from our algorithm agree well with

2 Methodology

2.1 Strain Estimation and Data Preparation from tMRI

Non-tracking-based strain estimation. We adapt a non-tracking-based strain estimation method [9] to extract the motion information from the tMRI sequences. We assume that the myocardium is incompressible, and that it undergoes three possible deformations: stretching, compression, and local rotation. Instead of calculating the strain values in terms of the gradient of the displacement by tracking the tag pattern [2] or the embedded tag phase [4], this non-tracking based method directly analyzes the tag deformation gradient by locally applying a 2D Gabor filter and optimizing its parameters, i.e., the orientation ϕ and spacing S of a 2D Gabor's sinusoidal modulation in the spatial domain. This optimization procedure can be applied in each temporal frame independently, so that it can avoid the tracking step, which might be problematic when temporal resolution is relatively low and "tag-jump" can occur.

See Fig. 1 (a) for an illustration. The initial tag spacing $D_x = D_y = D$ and orientation ϕ_o are referred to as the initial state, so that the Lagrangian deformation gradient in the beating myocardium can be obtained by comparing the deformed tag spacing S and orientation change $\Delta\phi$ to the initial state. A 2D deformation gradient tensor $\mathbf{F}$ can be derived by:

$$\mathbf{F} = \begin{bmatrix} \frac{S_x \cos \Delta\phi_y}{D \sin \phi} & \frac{S_y \sin \Delta\phi_x}{D \sin \phi} \\ \frac{S_x \sin \Delta\phi_y}{D \sin \phi} & \frac{S_y \cos \Delta\phi_x}{D \sin \phi} \end{bmatrix} \quad (1)$$

where $\phi = \frac{\pi}{2} - \Delta\phi_x - \Delta\phi_y$. From $\mathbf{F}$, we can derive the Lagrangian finite strain tensor $\mathbf{E}$ and local rotation matrix $\mathbf{R}$ by:

$$\mathbf{E} = \frac{1}{2}(\mathbf{F}^T \cdot \mathbf{F} - \mathbf{I}) \quad (2)$$

$$\mathbf{R} = \mathbf{F}(\mathbf{F}^T \cdot \mathbf{F})^{-1/2} \quad (3)$$

where $\mathbf{I}$ is an identity matrix.

Rather than the 2D horizontal-vertical Lagrangian strain tensor in Equation 2, in myocardial deformation research, we are generally more interested in the radial and circumferential strains. Positive and negative radial strains indicate myocardial thickening and thinning, respectively, while myocardial stretching and shortening are represented by positive and negative circumferential strains, respectively. We define an angle θ about the centroid of the LV, and transform $\mathbf{E}$ into a radial-circumferential strain tensor $\dot{\mathbf{E}}$ with a rotation matrix $\mathbf{Q}(\theta)$, so that $\dot{\mathbf{E}} = \mathbf{Q}\mathbf{E}\mathbf{Q}^T$.

In Fig. 2, we show a visual comparison of our estimates of radial strain, circumferential strain and local rotation angle in a normal subject and a patient.

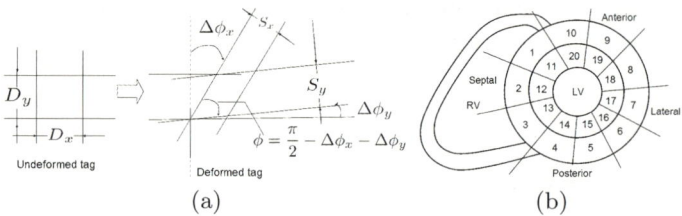

Fig. 1. (a): The illustration of **F** calculation. (b): The left ventricle is divided into 20 regions.

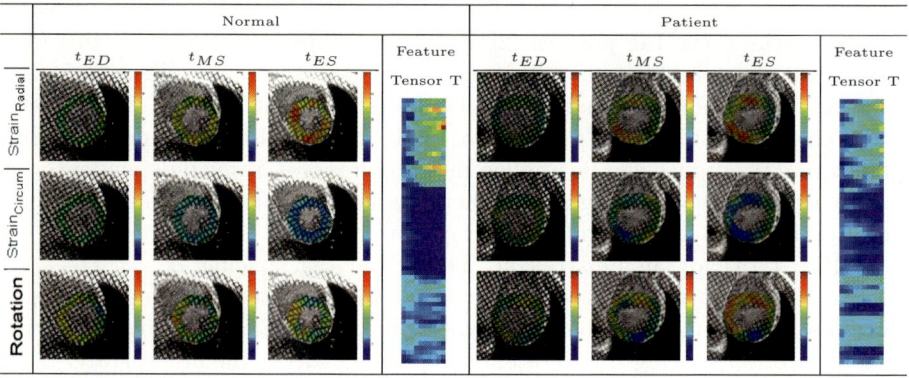

Fig. 2. Visual comparison of normal (left-hand-side) and patient's (right-hand-side) radial strain (first row), circumferential strain (second row) and rotation angle (third row) estimations at the time of ED, middle of systole (MS) and ES. For regional cardiac function analysis, we divide the left ventricle into 20 regions and interpolate the ED to ES deformation sequence into 10 frames, so as to form a 60×10-sized feature tensor **T**, which is illustrated as a pseudo-color bar.

Warm color stands for higher strain value or bigger rotation angle. It is interesting to see that the magnitudes of the strain or rotation angle value are not the only criteria that can be used to diagnose cardiac abnormality. Their spatial and temporal distributions seem potentially more important. Normal hearts seem to have smoothly distributed strains and rotation angle values. This suggests that the myocardial function should be assessed on a comprehensive basis, including the strain magnitude, the regional strain pattern, the regional tissue rotation pattern, and their temporal evolution.

Quantitative data preparation. For quantitative regional cardiac function analysis, we divide the left ventricle at a given base-apex level into two layers (endo- and epi-cardium) and ten sectors (septum is equally divided into 3 sectors and the rest of the heart is divided into 7). This results in 20 ordered regions in total, as can been seen in Fig. 1 (b). Within each region, we use the median value of the radial strain, the circumferential strain and the rotation angle to represent this region's deformation, so as to remove outliers and make the data preparation more robust. We denote them as $\mathbf{E}_R^i$, $\mathbf{E}_C^i$ and θ^i ($1 \leq i \leq 20$), respectively. Therefore, the myocardial deformation in a single time frame can be represented by a 60×1-sized vector $\mathbf{V} = (\mathbf{E}_R^1, ..., \mathbf{E}_R^{20}, \mathbf{E}_C^1, ...\mathbf{E}_C^{20}, \theta^1, ..., \theta^{20})^T$.

Due to the fading of the tags, myocardial deformation cannot be reliably extracted from frames after the end of systole (ES). Therefore, we only consider the image frames from end of diastole (ED) to ES. In addition, the heart beat rate varies in human subjects, and the absolute image frame rate varies between studies, so that the frame number from ED to ES ranges from 5 to 12 in our data. We implement a B-spline technique to interpolate them into 10 frames. Therefore, the myocardial motion of a tMRI time sequence can be represented by a 60×10-sized feature tensor $\mathbf{T} = [V_1, ..., V_{10}]$. As seen in Fig. 2, the feature tensor $\mathbf{T}$ exhibits noticeable differences between normal subjects and patients.

2.2 Spatio-temporal Tensor LDA

Learn the classifier. Suppose we have collected N samples (including normal and abnormal) for training purposes. We can train a typical two-class classifier to make the normal samples far away from the abnormal samples. LDA is a popular method to maximize the between-class scatter and minimize the within-class scatter, but it is a vector-based method. If we reshape the spatio-temporal tensor feature into a vector, it will collapse the spatio-temporal structure information, which is very important for identification. Additionally, the conventional LDA can only project the features into a scalar in the two-class case. In this paper, we propose to use spatio-temporal tensor LDA to deal with the above issues, as it can preserve the spatio-temporal information well, and it also has no limitation on dimensionality reduction.

Let $\mathbf{T}_i, i \in [1, 2, ..., N]$ be training tensor features with the labels of normal and abnormal. Similar to LDA, the spatio-temporal tensor-based LDA (ST-LDA) also employs the Fisher criterion that maximizes the between-class scatter and minimizes the within-class scatter, but it extends the vector-based norm into the Frobenius norm [10]. With the tensor features $\mathbf{T}_i \in \Re^{60 \times 10}$, the between-class scatter S_b and the within-class scatter S_w measured by the Frobenius norm are $S_b = \sum_{i=1}^{2} N_i \|M_i - M\|_F^2$ and $S_w = \sum_{i=1}^{2} \sum_{\mathbf{T}_j \in X_i} \|\mathbf{T}_j - M_i\|_F^2$, where N_i means the number of i-th class sample, M is the mean matrix of all the $\mathbf{T}_i$, M_i represents the mean matrix of the i-th class, and $\mathbf{T}_j \in X_i$ means that $\mathbf{T}_j$ belongs to the i-th class.

The goal is to find the optimal projection matrices $L \in \Re^{60 \times d_L}$ and $R \in \Re^{10 \times d_R}$ which maximize S_b and minimize S_w in the low dimensional subspace of $L \otimes R$, i.e., maximizing $S_b' = \sum_{i=1}^{2} N_i \|L^T(M_i - M)R\|_F^2$ and minimizing $S_w' = \sum_{i=1}^{2} \sum_{\mathbf{T}_j \in X_i} \|L^T(\mathbf{T}_j - M_i)R\|_F^2$ at the same time.

Because $\|X\|_F^2 = trace(XX^T)$, S_b' and S_w' can be written as $S_b' = trace(L^T D_b^R L)$ and $S_w' = trace(L^T D_w^R L)$ when R is given, where

$$D_b^R = \sum_{i=1}^{2} N_i(M_i - M)RR^T(M_i - M)^T \qquad (4)$$

$$D_w^R = \sum_{i=1}^{2} \sum_{\mathbf{T}_j \in X_i} (\mathbf{T}_j - M_i) R R^T (\mathbf{T}_j - M_i)^T \tag{5}$$

Then we can get the optimal projection L by maximizing $trace((L^T D_w^R L)^{-1}(L^T D_b^R L))$, i.e., computing the eigenvectors of $(D_w^R)^{-1} D_b^R$.

Similarly, if L is fixed, we can rewrite S_b' and S_w' as $S_b' = trace(R^T D_b^L R)$ and $S_w' = trace(R^T D_w^L R)$, because $trace(AB) = trace(BA)$, where

$$D_b^L = \sum_{i=1}^{2} N_i (M_i - M)^T L L^T (M_i - M) \tag{6}$$

$$D_w^L = \sum_{i=1}^{2} \sum_{\mathbf{T}_j \in X_i} (\mathbf{T}_j - M_i)^T L L^T (\mathbf{T}_j - M_i) \tag{7}$$

Then the optimal projection can be obtained by maximizing $trace((R^T D_w^L R)^{-1}(R^T D_b^L R))$, i.e., solving for the eigenvectors of $(D_w^L)^{-1} D_b^L$.

Thus, the final optimal solution can be computed by an iterative procedure, as shown in Table 1. It can be found that the ST-LDA algorithm not only avoids the eigen-decomposition in the 600-dimensional space, but also well preserves the geometric relations of row and column of $\mathbf{T}_i$. In addition, in the conventional LDA, the available dimension has the upper bound $C - 1$, which means it will project onto a scalar in our normal/abnormal two classes situation, while ST-LDA has no such constraint and is able to keep more information, which will be essential when we back-project the low dimensional subspace feature to the original feature space and look for the reasons for the classification.

For a new myocardial deformation pattern $\mathbf{T}_{test} \in \Re^{60 \times 10}$, its projection in the reduced dimensional subspace is: $Y_{test} = L^T \mathbf{T}_{test} R \in \Re^{d_L \times d_R}$. Classification is done in this subspace using a k-nearest neighbor scheme, where we empirically set $k = 3$.

Table 1. The ST-LDA algorithm

Input: $\mathbf{T}_1, \mathbf{T}_2, ..., \mathbf{T}_N$
Initialization: Set $R_0 = (I_{d_R}, 0)^T$, and compute the mean M_i of the i-th class for each class, and the global mean M.
Iteration: For $t = 1$ to t_{max}
　　1). For a given R_{t-1}, compute D_w^R and D_b^R using Equations 5 and 4, and get the optimal L_t by solving for the first d_L leading eigenvectors of $(D_w^R)^{-1} D_b^R$.
　　2). Based on L_t, compute D_w^L and D_b^L as in Equations 7 and 6, and get the optimal R_t by solving for the first d_R leading eigenvectors of $(D_w^L)^{-1} D_b^L$.
　　3). If $t > 1$, $\|L_t - L_{t-1}\| < \varepsilon$ and $\|R_t - R_{t-1}\| < \varepsilon$, break; else, continue.
End iteration.
Output: $L = L_{t_{max}}$ and $R = R_{t_{max}}$

Regional abnormality analysis. Identifying and localizing abnormal cardiac regions could be of more clinical value than just classifying a heart as normal or diseased. The intuition behind the ST-LDA algorithm is that the high dimensional feature tensor can be projected into a lower dimensional subspace that is optimal for classification. Therefore, the tensor distance between abnormal and normal features in the low dimensional subspace becomes a concise but accurate description of the abnormality. If we back-project this feature distance to the original space, we can recover the location of the pathology on the original spatio-temporal structure in a more physically meaningful way.

Because the linear projection functions L and R are not orthogonal matrices, the back-project operation needs to be done using their pseudo-inverse matrices L^+ and R^+. Suppose T_a is a feature tensor, and Y_a is its projection in the low dimensional subspace, which is classified as abnormal using the ST-LDA classifier. Then the feature distance in the original space can be derived by:

$$dT = (L^+)^T(Y_a - \bar{Y}_{normal})R^+ \tag{8}$$

Since $dT \in \Re^{60 \times 10}$ and we are more interested in recovering the spatial distribution of the cardiac function, we define an index of pathology $P_i, i = 1, 2, ..., 20$ that indicates each cardiac region's degree of functional abnormality. Note that P is a temporal and functional (including radial strain, circumferential strain and rotation angle) combination of the abnormal distances, therefore, it is no longer a descriptor of local strain or rotation angle, but rather a systematic indicator of the local cardiac function.

$$P_i = \sum_{t=1}^{10}(dT^2(i,t) + dT^2(20+i,t) + dT^2(40+i,t))^{\frac{1}{2}} \tag{9}$$

3 Experiments and Results

We acquired 41 time sequences of short-axis tagged MR images from 10 normal subjects and 12 patients. The patient's heart diseases varied from infarction or hypertrophy to general loss of myocardial function. The spatial positions of these SA images are confined to the mid-portion of the left ventricle, where the pathologies are usually prominent. In the ST-LDA classification algorithm, we empirically set the iteration number to 10, and the dimension of the subspace to 10×5, so that $L \in \Re^{60 \times 10}$ and $R \in \Re^{10 \times 5}$. To make comparisons with other conventional classification methods, we applied PCA, LDA and SVM algorithms to the same data set. Their parameters are also empirically set to be optimal.

The training and testing procedures are strictly done on a leave-one patient-out-basis, i.e., we leave one patient data for testing, and use the rest for training. In Table 2, we list the accuracy rate comparison of PCA, LDA, SVM and our proposed ST-LDA. We find that our novel algorithm outperforms PCA and LDA in accuracy, and has a similar accuracy rate with the nonlinear approach SVM. On the other hand, PCA and ST-LDA is able to recover the regional abnormality

Table 2. Comparison with other conventional classification algorithms

Classification Algorithm	PCA	LDA	SVM	ST-LDA
Classification Accuracy Rate	73.17%	85.37%	87.80%	87.80%

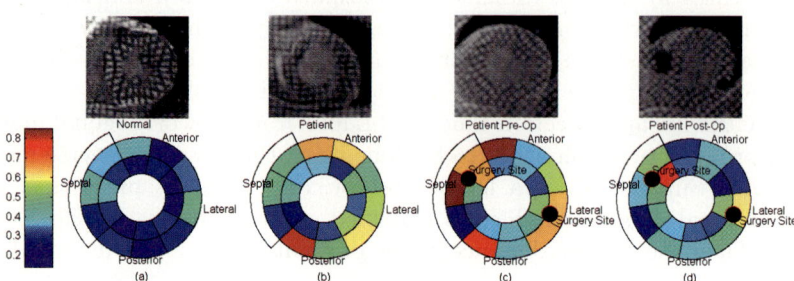

Fig. 3. Quantitative analysis of the regional abnormality from the back-projection. Warm color represents high P value, which means high degree of abnormality. The first row shows the sampling images at ES from 4 time sequences. The second row shows the analysis results. Column (a) is from a normal sequence. Column (b) is from an abnormal subject. (c) and (d) are from a patient before and after a surgery, respectively. The black dots show the surgery sites.

by back-projecting the subspace feature to the original feature space, while LDA and SVM cannot.

In Fig. 3, we show some representative results of the regional cardiac function analysis. The regional abnormality is represented by the index P, which is encoded in the pseudo color map. Column (a) is from a normal sequence. We can observe that the P index is low and smoothly distributed. Column (b) is from an abnormal subject. The warm color indicates possible abnormal regions, such as the 1 and 5 o'clock regions, which agree with doctor's diagnosis. The high abnormality at the 7 o'clock region very likely comes from the LV-RV connecting area, whose motion is affected by both ventricles and therefore sensitive to pathology. Columns (c) and (d) are from a patient before and after a surgery, respectively. This patient had insertion of a "Coapsys" device to reduce functional mitral regurgitation. We can observe that the doctor's diagnosis (indicated by the surgical sites, which appear as dark dots in the MR image, and depicted as black dots in the analysis results) coincides with the abnormal regions from our analysis results very well. Furthermore, the overall performance is more normal as depicted in the overall cooler color in (d), which shows the effectiveness of this surgery. However, the myocardium at the two surgical sites were impaired in the surgery, which is why the cardiac function is still (or even more) abnormal near the surgical sites in (d). Our regional cardiac function analysis results perfectly agree with the patient's pathologies before and after the operation.

4 Conclusion

In this paper, we have proposed a novel spatio-temporal tensor-based LDA classification framework to detect and localize regional cardiac abnormality. The advantage of our proposed method is that its dimension reduction is separately operated in the spatial and temporal domains, so that it conserves better the spatio-temporal structure and information of the training data. In addition, in order to analyze regional cardiac function, we back-project the abnormality distance found in the subspace to the original feature space, so as to localize the regional abnormality in a more physically meaningful way. Our experimental results show our ST-LDA approach achieves a higher classification rate than conventional linear approaches, and achieves comparable accuracy rate to non-linear methods, such as SVM. The recovered regional abnormalities agree with the doctor's diagnosis and patient's pathology very well.

References

1. Axel, L., Dougherty, L.: MR imaging of motion with spatial modulation of magnetization. Radiology 171, 841–845 (1989)
2. Axel, L., Chen, T., Manglik, T.: Dense myocardium deformation estimation for 2D tagged MRI. In: Frangi, A.F., Radeva, P.I., Santos, A., Hernandez, M. (eds.) FIMH 2005. LNCS, vol. 3504, pp. 446–456. Springer, Heidelberg (2005)
3. Clarysse, P., Basset, C., Khouas, L., Croisille, P., Friboulet, D., Odet, C., Magnin, I.E.: 2D spatial and temporal displacement and deformation field fitting from cardiac MR tagging. Medical Image Analysis 4, 253–268 (2000)
4. Osman, N.F., McVeigh, E.R., Prince, J.L.: Imaging heart motion using harmonic phase MRI. IEEE Trans. Med. Imaging 19(3), 186–202 (2000)
5. Park, J., Metaxas, D., Young, A., Axel, L.: Deformable models with parameter functions for cardiac motion analysis. IEEE Transactions on Medical Imaging 15(3), 278–289 (1996)
6. Hu, Z., Metaxas, D.N., Axel, L.: In-vivo strain and stress estimation of the left ventricle from MRI images. In: Dohi, T., Kikinis, R. (eds.) MICCAI 2002. LNCS, vol. 2488, pp. 706–713. Springer, Heidelberg (2002)
7. Declerck, J., Feldmar, J., Ayache, N.: Definition of a 4d continuous planispheric transformation for the tracking and the analysis of LV motion. Medical Image Analysis 2(2), 197–213 (1998)
8. Clarysse, P., Han, M., Croisille, P., Magnin, I.E.: Exploratory analysis of the spatio-temporal deformation of the myocardium during systole from tagged MRI. IEEE Trans. Biomed. Eng. 49, 1328–1339 (2002)
9. Qian, Z., Metaxas, D., Axel, L.: Non-tracking-based 2d strain estimation in tagged MRI. In: Proc. of the IEEE International Symposium on Biomedical Imaging (2007)
10. Ye, J.P., Janardan, R., Li, Q.: Two-dimensional linear discriminant analysis. In: Proc. of. Int. Conf. Neural Information Processing Systems (2004)

Volume Reconstruction by Inverse Interpolation: Application to Interleaved MR Motion Correction

Torsten Rohlfing, Martin H. Rademacher, and Adolf Pfefferbaum

Neuroscience Program, SRI International, Menlo Park, CA, USA
torsten@synapse.sri.com

Abstract. We introduce in this work a novel algorithm for volume reconstruction from data acquired on an irregular grid, e.g., from multiple co-registered images. The algorithm, which is based on an inverse interpolation formalism, is superior to other methods in particular when the input images have lower spatial resolution than the reconstructed image. Local intensity bounds are enforced by an L-BFGS-B optimizer, regularize the reconstruction problem, and preserve the intensity distribution of the input images. We demonstrate the usefulness of our method by applying it to retrospective motion correction in interleaved MR images.

1 Introduction

The fundamental problem addressed in this paper is the reconstruction of a volumetric image from data acquired on an irregular grid. This also includes data acquired on multiple regular grids, e.g., multiple images with general coordinate transformations between them. Such image reconstruction problems arise, for example, in freehand three-dimensional (3D) ultrasound acquisition [1] or in the reconstruction of high-resolution motion-corrected magnetic resonance (MR) images [4].

A common and straightforward volume reconstruction method, pursued for example by Moore et al. [2] in the construction of a cardiac MR atlas, is to interpolate the co-registered acquired images onto the target grid and average the interpolated images. This approach is limited, however, by the resolution of the input images (Fig. 1). It is, therefore, not satisfactory for reconstruction of high-resolution images from low-resolution images, as it is encountered in spatially interleaved image acquisitions. Such acquisitions are used in MR imaging to minimize crosstalk between neighboring slices without introducing slice gaps, and for covering large volumes when acquiring images with repetition times (TR) too short to allow data from all slices to be collected in a single pass. After acquisition of multiple interleaved passes, these are combined to form a high-resolution 3D image volume.

Movement of the subject is particularly a problem in the very young, the very old and in those suffering from neurodegenerative conditions. Motion artifacts within a pass are not recoverable post reconstruction, whereas motion across passes leads to misalignment of the images in the separate passes relative to each other. This, in turn, causes characteristic artifacts in the resulting image stacks (see Fig. 1 for an example), which makes them unsuitable for 3D image processing (e.g., registration, multi-spectral image segmentation). One application for the algorithm introduced in this paper is to

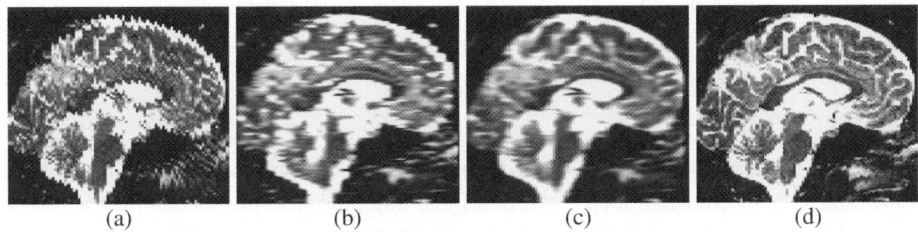

Fig. 1. Example of motion artifacts in a three-pass interleaved late-echo fast spin echo MR image (coronal slice orientation). The subject moved mostly between the first and second pass. (a) Characteristic artifacts are particularly evident in the sagittal view. (b) The pass images (here, pass #0) have 1/3 of the spatial resolution in between-slice direction (here, 6 mm instead of 2 mm). (c) The average of co-registered pass images (analogous to Ref. [2]) is blurry. (d) The image reconstructed using the proposed algorithm is crisp and free of between-pass motion artifacts.

reconstruct high-resolution, motion-corrected images from co-registered low-resolution passes with arbitrary rigid transformations between them.

2 Methods

The method for retrospective reconstruction of pass-to-pass motion artifact corrected images proposed in this paper comprises three distinct stages, which are described in detail below: 1) using image-to-image registration, the parameters of subject motion between the passes are estimated; 2) an initial reconstructed image is generated by volume injection of the co-registered pass images into the reconstructed image grid; 3) the final artifact corrected image is computed in an iterative image reconstruction stage, which represents the primary contribution of this paper. The reconstruction, which in effect serves to unblur the initial, volume-injected image, is based on an inverse interpolation formalism, which is solved using a gradient descent minimization of the mean squared difference (MSD) between the actually acquired pass images and those interpolated from the evolving artifact-corrected image.

2.1 Motion Estimation by Image Registration

The images acquired in the different passes are first combined into separate, contiguous 3D image stacks (rather than a single, interleaved high-resolution stack). To recover the motion between the passes, one of them (for example the first) is selected as the reference, and the images from the remaining passes are registered to the reference pass image using an established intensity-based 3D rigid registration algorithm [3], but using MSD as a more appropriate registration criterion in this application.

The transformation that relates the coordinate system of the n-th pass to the reference coordinate system is denoted as $\mathbf{T}_n$. Note that the we can restrict consideration to rigid coordinate transformations in this paper as dictated by the application, but this is not a limitation of the volume reconstruction method. Of course, estimating more complex nonrigid motion between low-resolution images is increasingly complicated and under-constrained, and registration errors will propagate to, and cause error in, the reconstruction stage.

2.2 Volume Injection

Image reconstruction from multiple co-registered views can be solved by push-forward interpolation and averaging [4]: Each pixel $\vec{y}$ is injected into the reconstructed image volume at all locations $\vec{x}$ within a radius d, weighted using a truncated Gaussian-shaped kernel,

$$G_{\vec{y},\sigma}(\vec{x}) \propto \begin{cases} \exp(-\frac{(\vec{x}-\vec{y})^2}{2\sigma^2}) & \text{if} ||\vec{x}-\vec{y}||_2 \leq d, \\ 0 & \text{otherwise.} \end{cases} \quad (1)$$

The accumulated intensities at each reconstructed pixel are subsequently normalized with the sum of all weights that contributed to them, so as to account for different numbers and distances of contributing pixels.

2.3 Volume Reconstruction by Inverse Interpolation

We now cast the actual image reconstruction of the high-resolution motion corrected 3D image stack from the co-registered passes as an inverse interpolation problem. Ignoring the spatial arrangement of its pixels, we can denote the (unknown) ground truth image as a vector of pixel values, $\vec{f} \in \mathbb{R}^M$, where M is the number of image pixels. The images from the separate passes are denoted $\vec{u}^{(n)} \in \mathbb{R}^{M_n}$ where n is the index of the pass, and M_n is the number of pixels acquired in the respective pass.

For the purpose of image reconstruction, the acquired pass images are modeled as if they were interpolated from $\vec{f}$. Each such interpolation can be written as a matrix-vector multiplication

$$\vec{u}^{(n)} = \mathbf{W}^{(n)} \vec{f}, \quad (2)$$

where $\mathbf{W}^{(n)} \in \mathbb{R}^{M_n \times M}$ is the matrix of interpolation coefficients for the n-th pass. The elements of each $\mathbf{W}^{(n)}$ essentially describe for each interpolated image pixel, which pixels in the original image contribute to it with what interpolation weight. The matrix entries are, therefore, determined by a) the spatial arrangements of the pixels in the images, b) the coordinate transformations between the images, and c) the interpolation kernel (e.g., linear, cubic, sinc).

The *inverse interpolation problem* is to find the image $\vec{f}$ that satisfies the system of equations defined by Eq. (2) over all n. Due to the size of the interpolation matrices, incomplete and inconsistent data, this system cannot be solved directly. Instead, we devised an iterative least-squares approach, for which we let $\vec{v}$ be some approximation of $\vec{f}$. Then the least-squares approximation error can be written as

$$E(\vec{v}) = \sum_n \left(\vec{u}^{(n)} - \mathbf{W}^{(n)} \vec{v} \right)^2 \quad (3)$$

and the true solution is approximated by solving the following minimization problem:

$$\vec{f} \approx \arg\min_{\vec{v}} E(\vec{v}). \quad (4)$$

The analytical gradient of E with respect to the elements of $\vec{v}$ (i.e., the pixel intensities in the evolving reconstructed image) is derived using elementary calculus as follows:

$$\frac{\partial}{\partial v_i} E(\vec{v}) = \sum_n \frac{\partial}{\partial v_i} \left(\vec{u}^{(n)} - \mathbf{W}^{(n)} \vec{v} \right)^2 = \sum_n \sum_j \frac{\partial}{\partial v_i} \left(u_j^{(n)} - \sum_k \mathbf{W}_{j,k}^{(n)} v_i \right)^2$$

$$= -2 \sum_n \sum_j \left[\mathbf{W}_{j,i}^{(n)} \left(u_j^{(n)} - \sum_k \mathbf{W}_{j,k}^{(n)} v_k \right) \right]. \quad (5)$$

Substituting into this equation for each pass n the error image, $\vec{e}^{(n)} = \vec{u}^{(n)} - \mathbf{W}^{(n)} \vec{v}$,

$$\frac{\partial}{\partial v_i} E(\vec{v}) = -2 \sum_n \sum_j \left[\mathbf{W}_{j,i}^{(n)} e_j^{(n)} \right]. \quad (6)$$

Note that E is non-negative, and zero if and only if the acquired pass images are identical to those interpolated in their spatial position from the reconstructed image, i.e., when $\vec{u}^{(n)} = \mathbf{W}^{(n)} \vec{v}$ for all n. Note also that if coordinate transformation $\mathbf{T}_n$ is the identity transformation, then for the common interpolation kernels the corresponding interpolation matrix $\mathbf{W}^{(n)}$ is the identity matrix. Therefore, if $\mathbf{T}_n \equiv \mathrm{Id}$ for all n (i.e., if there is no motion between the passes), then the acquired image itself is the global optimum of the reconstruction error functional in Eq. (3).

2.4 Implementation of the Inverse Interpolation

To compute the gradient of E, the inner sum in Eq. (6) must be evaluated for all j for which $\mathbf{W}_{j,i}^{(n)} \neq 0$, i.e., for all i, j, n such that the j-th pixel in the n-th interpolated pass image depends on the i-th pixel in the reconstructed image. The relationships between the pixels in reconstructed and interpolated images are schematically illustrated in Fig. 2. For forward interpolation, the interpolated image pixel is mapped into the reconstructed image via transformation $\mathbf{T}$ and its value determined from the neighboring reconstructed pixels.

The inverse interpolation determines the pixels in the interpolated image which depend on a given pixel in the reconstructed image. When the reconstructed pixel's interpolation neighborhood is mapped into the interpolated image via the inverse transformation, $\mathbf{T}^{-1}$, these are all interpolated image pixels that are located inside the mapped region. For affine (or rigid) transformations, an elegant and efficient way to compute the interpolated pixels inside the mapped neighborhood is via a volume intersection algorithm [5]. However, it is much easier (and almost as computationally efficient) to simply test for each pixel inside the bounding box (dashed rectangle in Fig. 2(b)) of the mapped region corners whether or not transformation $\mathbf{T}$ maps it into that region.

2.5 Local Intensity Thresholding

The acquired MR images represent a dense, approximately uniform sampling of the imaged object. Consequently, the intensity distribution in the original images should be

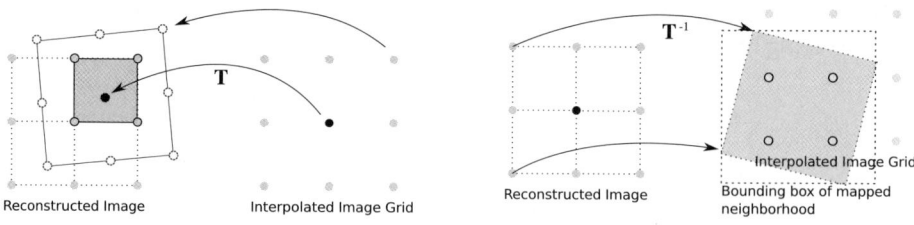

Fig. 2. Illustration of pixel relationships in forward (*left*) and inverse interpolation (*right*)

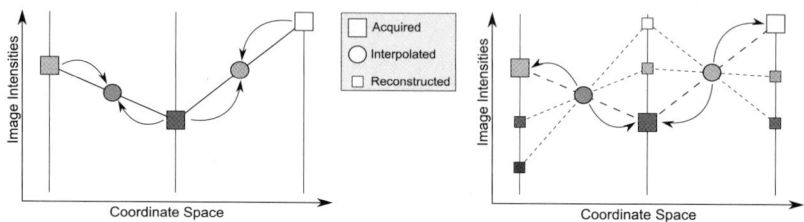

Fig. 3. Illustration of ill-posedness of inverse interpolation. *Left:* Given the acquired data (large squares), the forward problem of determining interpolated data (circles) between the grid positions is well-defined. *Right:* For the inverse problem to reconstruct the acquired data from the interpolated data, there is a continuum of solutions. Some examples of such solutions are represented here by smaller squares and dashed lines.

a good approximation of the "true" distribution for the given subject, and it is reasonable to expect that the reconstructed image should preserve this distribution. This is, however, not the case, largely due to the fact that inverse interpolation is an ill-posed problem for which there is no unique solution. This is schematically illustrated in Fig. 3. Meaningful boundary conditions are also not available in general, because at least one face of human MR image volumes is always a truncation surface.

A common remedy for this type of problem is to add a regularization term to the optimized cost function (here, the difference between interpolated and acquired pass images) that favors solutions which possess additional properties. For example, one could use the Kullback-Leibler (KL) divergence [6] between the acquired and the reconstructed image intensity distributions. Solutions would thus favor reconstructed images that have the same intensity distribution as the acquired images. However, we found such an approach difficult to implement due to the need to compute gradients of the KL divergence with respect to the reconstructed image intensities. It is also potentially too strict and may prevent effective optimization.

Instead, we apply a simple local thresholding scheme that makes use of the assumption that the intensity of any reconstructed pixel should be inside the range of pixel values in the original images that contribute to this pixel. In other words, the acquired intensity range in a reconstructed pixel's local neighborhood constrains the permissible intensities for that pixel. Our implementation enforces this constraint by hard truncation, rather than by soft penalty terms. This is more computationally efficient, completely avoids smoothing of the reconstructed image, and is easily enforced during the minimization of E using an L-BFGS-B optimizer [7].

3 Results

In the absence of a gold standard, we judge the reconstructed images by two criteria: 1) visual assessment of artifact reduction and definition of anatomical detail, and 2) preservation of acquired image intensity distribution. For visual assessment, Fig. 4 shows original and motion-corrected images from eight subjects. Inverse interpolation used cubic interpolation and local intensity thresholding. Note the visible increased crispness of the reconstructed images and the substantially reduced approximation error, E, after inverse interpolation compared with those after volume injection.

For one of the images in Fig. 4, the histogram plots in Fig. 5 show the intensity distributions of artifact-corrected images, reconstructed using three different interpolation kernels and with and without local thresholding. For comparison, the distribution of the original image data is also shown in each plot. For each combination, the final MSD

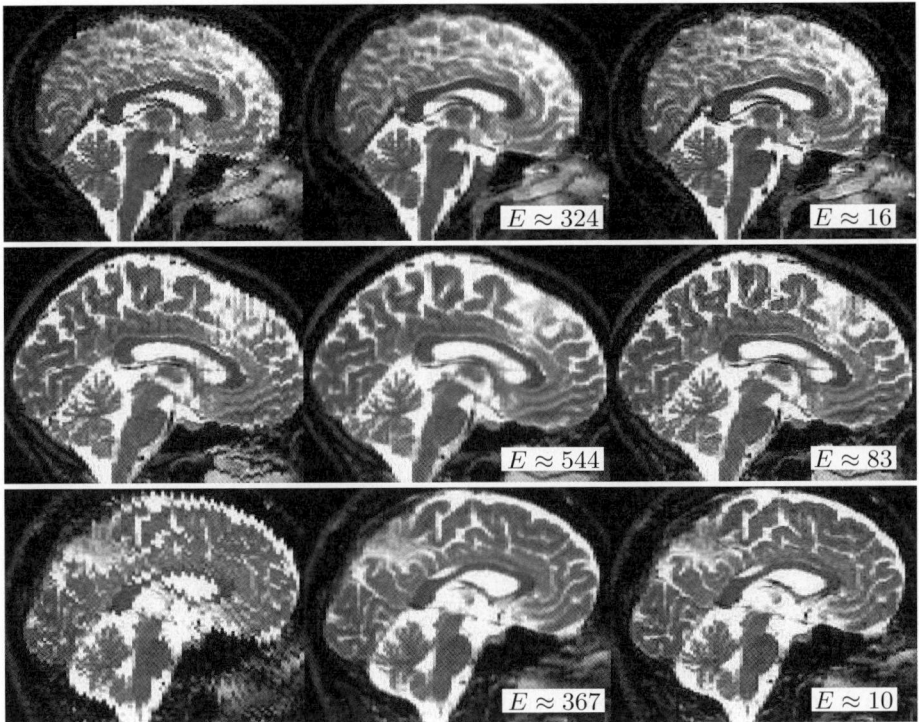

Fig. 4. Reconstructed motion-corrected images (volume injection and inverse interpolation) from three subjects. Image acquisition used a coronal fast spin echo sequence (94 slices 2 mm thick; TR/TE=11050/98 ms, matrix=256×192, FOV=240 mm), requiring three interleaved passes. For each reconstructed image, the approximation error, E, of the acquired images is provided.

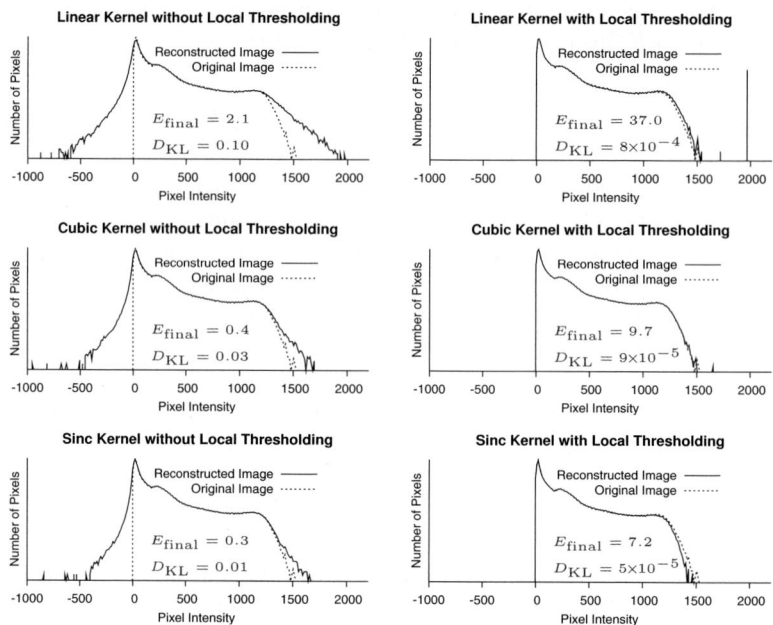

Fig. 5. Comparison of reconstructed vs. acquired image intensity distributions for different interpolation kernels, with and without local thresholding. Sinc interpolation used a cosine window with 3 samples window radius. All plots have logarithmic vertical axes. Note in particular the introduction of artificial high and low image intensities when local thresholding is not used. In each panel, E_{final} is the final MSD between interpolated and acquired pass images, and D_{KL} is the KL divergence between the original and reconstructed image intensity distributions.

Table 1. Computation times for evaluating the gradient $\frac{d}{d\vec{v}}E(\vec{v})$ and for a single evaluation of the approximation error (one forward interpolation). Times were measured on a dual-CPU Intel Xeon (E5345) server at 2.33 GHz clock speed. Sinc interpolation used a cosine window with 3 samples window radius. Optimization using the L-BFGS-B algorithm [7] typically converges in under 20 gradient search iterations.

	Computation Time: Single CPU (8 CPUs)		
	Linear	Cubic	Sinc
Gradient Computation	138 s (22 s)	354 s (55 s)	1964 s (262 s)
Error Computation	4 s (1 s)	9 s (2 s)	54 s (7 s)

between interpolated and acquired images, E_{final}, and the KL divergence, D_{KL}, between the original and the reconstructed image intensity distributions are also given.

The results in Fig. 5 are typical for all images to which we applied our algorithm. Higher-order interpolation improves the approximation, and to some extent it also reduces the frequency of artificial values outside the original image intensity range.

Local thresholding not only prevents values outside that range, which it is guaranteed to do by design, but also very effectively produces global intensity distributions that are virtually identical to the acquired image intensity distribution. This is remarkable because local thresholding does not explicitly enforce any global properties of the reconstructed image intensity distribution.

4 Conclusion

The algorithm introduced herein reconstructs high-resolution images from data acquired on an irregular grid, such as multiple co-registered lower resolution images. The coordinate transformations between the input images are arbitrary, i.e., the algorithm is not limited to in-plane transformations.

While this is by no means the only application of our method, we have demonstrated herein its usefulness for retrospective correction of between-pass motion in interleaved MR imaging. The qualitative (visual appearance) and quantitative (approximation error; preservation of intensity distribution) results in this paper suggest that a simple cubic kernel is effective, and it is also computationally efficient (Table 1). For comparison, we have demonstrated the superiority of our inverse interpolation reconstruction approach over interpolation-and-averaging schemes described in the literature [2]. It is also worth mentioning that our method can reconstruct image volumes from lower-dimensional acquired data (e.g., freehand ultrasound), which interpolation and averaging can not.

The advantage of our method over volume injection techniques [1,4] is more subtle, but still visually apparent (Fig. 4). Unlike volume injection, which requires tuning of injection kernel shape and truncation radius, our method is also data independent and parameter free. This is important because there may not be volume injection parameters that work equally well everywhere in the image, depending on the spatial arrangement of the acquired data.

Acknowledgments

This work was supported through Grants AA05965, AA12388, and AG17919. The authors thank Michael P. Hasak for many helpful comments and suggestions.

References

1. Prager, R.W., Gee, A., Berman, L.: Stradx: real-time acquisition and visualization of freehand three-dimensional ultrasound. Med. Image. Anal. 3(2), 129–140 (1999)
2. Moore, J., Drangova, M., Wierzbicki, M., Barron, J., Peters, T.: A high resolution dynamic heart model based on averaged MRI data. In: Ellis, R.E., Peters, T.M. (eds.) MICCAI 2003. LNCS, vol. 2878, pp. 549–555. Springer, Heidelberg (2003)
3. Studholme, C., Hill, D.L.G., Hawkes, D.J.: Automated three-dimensional registration of magnetic resonance and positron emission tomography brain images by multiresolution optimization of voxel similarity measures. Med. Phys. 24(1), 25–35 (1997)

4. Rousseau, F., Glenn, O., Iordanova, B., Rodriguez-Carranza, C., Vigneron, D., Barkovich, J., Studholme, C.: A novel approach to high resolution fetal brain MR imaging. In: Duncan, J.S., Gerig, G. (eds.) MICCAI 2005. LNCS, vol. 3749, pp. 548–555. Springer, Heidelberg (2005)
5. Rohlfing, T.: Incremental method for computing the intersection of discretely sampled m-dimensional images with n-dimensional boundaries. In: Medical Imaging: Image Processing, Proceedings of the SPIE, vol. 5032, pp. 1346–1354 (February 2003)
6. Kullback, S., Leibler, R.A.: On information and sufficiency. Ann. Math. Stat. 22, 79–86 (1951)
7. Byrd, R.H., Lu, P., Nocedal, J., Zhu, C.: A limited memory algorithm for bound constrained optimization. SIAM J. Sci. Comput. 16(5), 1190–1208 (1995)

A Hybrid System for the Semantic Annotation of Sulco-Gyral Anatomy in MRI Images

Ammar Mechouche[1], Xavier Morandi[1,2], Christine Golbreich[3,4], and Bernard Gibaud[1]

[1] Unit/Project VisAGeS U746, INSERM - INRIA - CNRS - Univ-Rennes 1, France
{Ammar.Mechouche,Bernard.Gibaud}@irisa.fr
http://www.irisa.fr/visages/
[2] University Hospital of Rennes, Department of Neurosurgery, France
Xavier.Morandi@chu-rennes.fr
[3] University of Versailles, Versailles
Christine.Golbreich@uvsq.fr
[4] LIRMM UMR 5506, Montpellier, France
http://www.lirmm.fr/tatoo/

Abstract. This paper presents an interactive system for the annotation of brain anatomical structures in Magnetic Resonance Images. The system is based on hybrid knowledge and techniques. First, it exploits both numerical knowledge from atlases and symbolic knowledge from a rule-extended ontology represented in OWL, the Web ontology language, and combines them with graphical data about cortical sulci, automatically extracted from the images. Second, the annotations of the parts of gyri and of sulci located in a region of interest are obtained with different reasoning techniques: Constraint Satisfaction Solving and Description Logics techniques. Preliminary experiments have been achieved on normal and also pathological data. The results obtained so far are very promising.

1 Introduction

Semantic annotation associates meaningful labels to images, in order to highlight their information content. Semantic annotation is becoming a major issue regarding wide scale sharing of information on the web and is of critical importance in biomedical research, notably for translational research aiming at facilitating the exploitation of experimental data across several disciplines and scales [1]. This is however a very challenging topic, due to the difficulty of defining consensual reference knowledge models, on the one hand, and to use them in image annotation tools, on the other hand. Such models, usually called ontologies, are often classified into two categories referred as lightweight and heavyweight ontologies, respectively [2]: 1) simple term lists, thesauri or taxonomies, 2) highly expressive knowledge models, according to which instances are created, involving complex assertions and constraints. Our primary application field is the preparation of surgical procedures in neurosurgery. Actually, the precise identification of gyri and sulci around the lesional area is of primary importance because they provide useful landmarks for the surgeon during surgery, especially in eloquent cortex [3]. The annotation of images, in our case anatomical MRI images, has two objectives: 1) to help to identify precisely the gyri and sulci around the lesion, and to provide the detailed annotation data relating anatomical conceptual entities to graphical primitives extracted from the images; 2) to use these metadata for cases retrieval in an images database. Our approach significantly differs from classical approaches of parcellation of cortex in MRI images [4,5,6,7]. Those are generally global (i.e. they analyze the whole cortex), have limited precision (i.e. they usually address gross anatomy), refer to simple term lists, are entirely automatic, mostly based on numerical priors (i.e. atlases), and primarily suited to normal anatomy. In contrast, our approach is local (i.e. focuses on a particular region in the image), may provide labels with high anatomical precision, can involve a human user participation, is based on symbolic prior knowledge (provided by a highly expressive ontology), and may be relevant to interpret pathological images as well as normal cases. The work presented here concerns a hybrid system designed according to the previous approach, i.e. a semantic approach, rather than morphometric or statistical. The knowledge supporting the labelling process consists of the mereo-topological relations between the different cortical features. This knowledge is described in an ontology of cortical gyri and sulci represented in OWL DL[1], according to the description logics (DL) paradigm [8]. The whole reasoning aims at producing instances of the ontology concerning the parts of sulci and of gyri involved in a set of graphical primitives extracted from the images (segments of cortical sulci, and parts of gyri called "patches"), that satisfy the axioms and constraints defined in the ontology. The very large number of possible combinations led us to adopt a hybrid approach, consisting in selecting a reasonable number of hypotheses for the labelling of patches, based on an atlas, and to select the valid combinations of such hypotheses, based on existing prior knowledge about the spatial arrangement of the gyri. This part constitutes a major extension of the method presented in [14]. Section 2 provides an overview of the method and further details of the system components; section 3 describes our first experiments with both normal and pathological data; section 4 discusses these preliminary results and highlights the capabilities and current limitations of the system.

2 Method

2.1 Definitions

Definition 1: A *segment* (figure 1) is a part of an external trace of a sulcus. The segments are organized in a graph describing the connections between them.

Definition 2: A *conventional separation* (figure 1) is a fictitious line added by the user in order to connect two segments separated by a gyrus.

---

[1] Ontology Web Language based on Description Logic formalism - http://www.w3.org/TR/owl-guide/

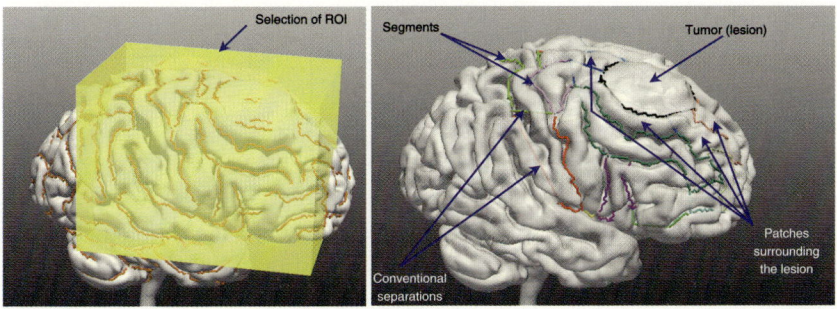

Fig. 1. ROI selection and Patches definition

Definition 3: A *patch* (figure 1) is a subset of the brain surface, corresponding to a part of a gyrus, and delimited by a set of continuous segments and conventional separations.

Definition 4: An *interpretation* consists of a set of labels associated with the patches and segments of a Region Of Interest (ROI); each patch and each segment has one label only.

Definition 5: A *consistent interpretation* is an interpretation, where each patch label and each segment label is consistent with our prior knowledge about the sulco-gyral anatomy and with the information supplied by the user.

2.2 System Overview

The overall labelling process involves three steps (figure 2): (1) the brain is segmented, the external traces of the sulci are extracted [9], the ROI is selected by the user, and the patches are defined (section 2.3); (2) patches identification: this is done by using Constraint Satisfaction Problem techniques (CSP) allowing to infer all the consistent interpretations for the patches with respect to prior knowledge about the spatial arrangement of the gyri (section 2.4). For that, the system uses a set of hypotheses (possible labels) derived from the matching of patch information with an atlas (SPAMs [10]); (3) sulci identification is done using the best interpretation computed for the patches and the logical definitions of the sulci in the ontology (section 2.5). The final annotations for the patches and the segments are generated in standard web languages to facilitate their exploitation by semantic web technologies. The paper focuses on (2) and (3).

2.3 Delimitation and Extraction of the Patches

The brain is automatically segmented from a T1-MRI scan and the graph of the external traces of the sulci is automatically extracted. Then, the user selects a ROI and the corresponding sub-graph is automatically extracted as shown on figure 1. Next, the user introduces a number of conventional separations, in order to produce a partition of the selected cortex area into a set of contiguous

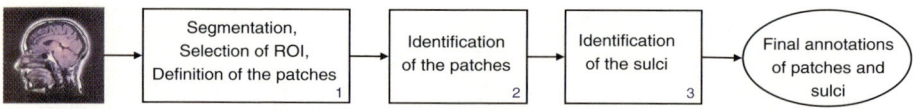

Fig. 2. General view of the labelling system

patches. Finally, the system computes the description of the topological relations and orientations between neighboring patches, and between the patches and the segments which form them. This description is represented in OWL ($file1$).

2.4 Identification of the Patches

Generation of Patches Labelling Hypotheses. The segments delimiting the patches within the ROI are realigned into the stereotaxic space (SPAMs space) thanks to the registration matrix produced during the segmentation process (figure 3). The position of each segment with respect to each SPAM is analyzed in order to determine whether it bounds this SPAM or not, and with which orientation. This analysis also provides a confidence index. All this information is represented in OWL ($file2$). The matching of information from $file1$ and $file2$ in the case of normal subjects is done by rules of the following form: $Bounds(x, y) \land SulcusPart(x) \land Patch(y) \land anteriorTo(x, y) \land Bounds(x, z) \land Gyrus(z) \land anteriorTo(x, z) \rightarrow partOf(y, z)$. This rule, for example, expresses that if we have a part of sulcus which bounds a given patch with an anterior orientation, and at the same time this part of sulcus bounds a given SPAM with the same orientation, then this patch is inferred to be part of the gyrus corresponding to this SPAM in the ontology. Six matching rules of this kind, corresponding to the six spatial orientations, are defined. Slightly different rules are used in pathological cases, taking into account only adjacency between the parts of sulci and the SPAMs, not orientations, because they might lead to erroneous decisions due to displacements related to the pathology. These rules assign to each patch a set of hypotheses. The correct label is assumed to belong to this set.

Determining the Consistent Interpretations Using a CSP Solver. A Constraint Satisfaction Problem (CSP) consists of a number of variables and a number of constraints. A variable is defined by its domain, i.e. the set of values that can be assigned to this variable. A constraint relates several variables and restricts the involved variables values to legal assignments. Constraint reasoning is the process of computing a solution to the given CSP, i.e. an assignment of values to the variables that satisfy all the given constraints on the variables [11]. In our case (figure 3-a), the patches represent the variables, the hypotheses computed for the patches represent the domains of the variables, and the spatial relations between the patches represent the constraints. The solutions of the CSP problem provide all possible interpretations for the patches with respect to our prior knowledge on the spatial arrangement of the gyri and parts of gyri. In order to find the best consistent interpretation for the patches among those computed by the CSP solver, the system

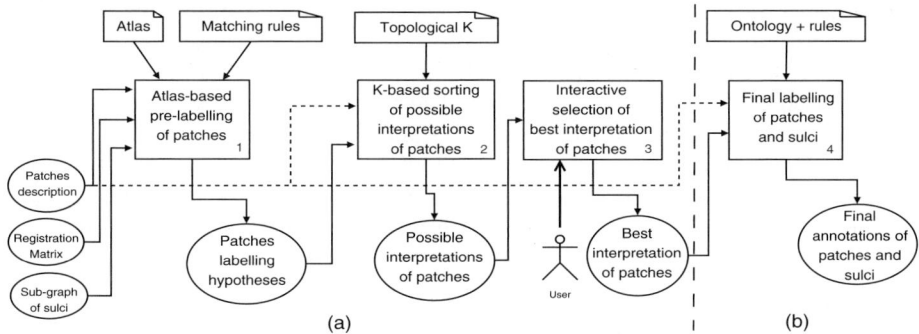

Fig. 3. The complete labelling process

allows interactions with the user. The latter is invited to select a preferred label for patches exhibiting different labels in different interpretations. Then the system eliminates those interpretations that are not consistent with the user information. The interactions are repeated until only one interpretation remains for the patches.

2.5 Identification of the Segments

To label the sulci segments the system uses the patches description, the best interpretation of the patches and the logical definitions of the sulci in the ontology (figure 3-b). The ontology contains the mereo-topological knowledge about the sulci and the gyri. To model the knowledge about the brain we have mainly used the Ono atlas [12], the Foundational Model of Anatomy (FMA[2]), and the expertise of a neuroanatomist. The concepts describing the sulci and gyri and their relations are defined in an ontology in OWL DL. An example of a concept definition of the ontology is the following: $RightCentralSulcusPart \equiv (\exists\ Bounds\ ((\exists\ hasEntity\ (\exists\ partOf\ RightPostCentralGyrus))\ \sqcap\ (\exists\ hasOrientation\ Anterior)))\ \sqcap\ (\exists\ Bounds\ ((\exists\ hasEntity\ (\exists\ partOf\ RightPreCentralGyrus))\ \sqcap\ (\exists\ hasOrientation\ Posterior)))\ \sqcap\ (\forall\ Bounds\ ((\exists\ hasEntity\ (\exists\ partOf\ RightPreCentralGyrus))\ \sqcup\ (\exists\ hasEntity\ (\exists\ partOf\ RightPostCentralGyrus))))$. This logical expression expresses that a part of the central sulcus of the right hemisphere bounds at least one part of the right postcentral gyrus with an anterior orientation and one part of the precentral gyrus with a posterior orientation, and only parts of such gyri. Our brain ontology contains for each hemisphere logical definitions of 49 gyri, 5 lobes, 3 operculum, 17 gyri parts, 44 sulci, 44 sulci parts (segments), and 31 relations. The ontology is enriched by some rules increasing its expressivity (see [14] for more details).

3 Results

3.1 Material

Preliminary experiments were made using T1-MRI images obtained with a 3T scanner (Philips Achieva) from three normal subjects and two patients

---

[2] http://sig.biostr.washington.edu/projects/fm/AboutFM.html

(pathological subjects). In the two pathological cases the lesion was located in the right frontal lobe. The brain segmentation and the extraction of the external traces of the sulci were done with Brainvisa[3] tools and Vistal[4] respectively. We have used 44 SPAMs corresponding to the gyri. The system is implemented in C++ and Java, the connection between C++ and Java programs is done thanks to JNI (Java Native Interface). The ontology is edited and created with the Protégé[5] software. The rules are edited and created with the SWRL[6] Plugin. The results were obtained with the Java Constraint Library[7], and the KAON2[8] reasoner.

3.2 Evaluation

The evaluation is done on a ROI defined by an expert neuroanatomist. It includes the superior frontal gyrus, the middle frontal gyrus, the inferior frontal gyrus, the precentral gyrus, the postcentral gyrus, the central sulcus, the superior precentral sulcus, the intermediate precentral sulcus, the inferior precentral sulcus, the superior frontal sulcus, and the inferior frontal sulcus regions. We compared the results provided by the system to the labels given by the expert considered as a gold-standard. The same procedure was applied to the five MRI datasets except for the matching rules, since orientations were not considered in case of pathological data. For each case, we report the type of the image (normal versus pathological), the number of patches extracted from the selected ROI, the number of consistent interpretations inferred for the patches, the number of user interactions needed to reach the best interpretation for the patches, the accuracy of patch labels (defined as the ratio of the accurately labelled patches over the total number of patches in ROI), and finally the accuracy for the sulci segments (defined as the ratio of the accurately labelled sulci segments over the total number of sulci segments in the ROI).

Table 1 reports the results for the five cases. We observe that the identification of the patches is complete after a reasonable number of interactions with the user (about 3). The sulci identification is quite accurate, although some segments are

Table 1. Results of the experiments

Brain MRI data	1	2	3	4	5
Normal (N) versus pathological (P)	N	N	N	P	P
Nb. of patches in ROI	16	18	16	17	15
Nb. of possible interpretations inferred for patches	7	6	6	4	3
Nb. of user interactions to best interpretation computing	3	3	3	2	2
Accuracy (patches)(%)	100	100	100	100	100
Accuracy (sulci segments)(%)	92.5	92.5	91	94.3	90.1

[3] http://brainvisa.info/index_f.html
[4] http://www.irisa.fr/vista/Themes/Logiciel/VIsTAL/VIsTAL.html
[5] http://protege.stanford.edu/
[6] http://www.w3.org/Submission/SWRL/
[7] http://liawww.epfl.ch/JCL/ (a CSP solver)
[8] http://kaon2.semanticweb.org/ (an inference engine for rule-extended ontologies)

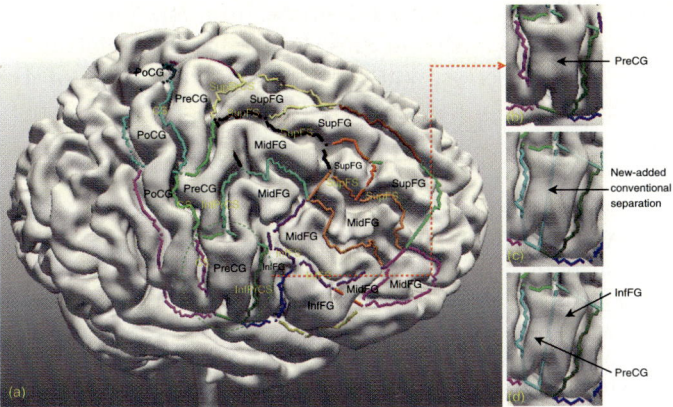

Fig. 4. (a) Inferred labels for the ROI and (b)(c)(d) influence of irrelevant conventional separations

not well classified due to the insufficient precision in the computation of the orientations between the patches and the segments. It is important to notice that the system performance is not decreased in pathological cases in spite of significant structures displacement according to the expert. An example of inferred annotations is reported figure 4-a. We observe on figure 4-(b,c,d) that if we add conventional separations where it is not necessary, then the system becomes less accurate. Regarding the time computing, the Atlas-based pre-labelling of the patches, the CSP reasoning, and the KAON2 reasoning take about 1 minute.

4 Conclusion

We have presented a hybrid system developed to semi-automatically label brain MRI images with semantic annotations and the first results obtained so far. The presented approach is novel with respect to several aspects: (1) the use of a CSP solver to select consistent interpretations of the gyri, (2) the easy generation of semantically-rich annotations of gyral/sulcal structures, (3) the use of explicit prior knowledge described in a formal ontology, (4) its representation in OWL, the Ontology Web Language, to facilitate knowledge sharing. Our first experiments using both normal and pathological data are very promising. We plan to still improve the system in the future with respect to several aspects. The definition of the conventional separations is defined manually in the current implementation, and could be automated. The use of atlases as a means to produce the initial hypotheses could be optimized, e.g. by using different types of numerical atlases, more adapted to the particular case under study. The orientations' computation could be improved, e.g. based on [13]. Finally, the ontology could be refined, in order to include more fine-grained gyri and sulci, and could be directly used to derive the orientations' definitions in the CSP problem. Moreover, the dependence of the system performance on initial processing steps (especially the definition of conventional separations) should be further investigated.

Acknowledgement. We thank **Louis Collins** from the Montreal Neurological Institute for providing us with the SPAMs database, **Christian Barillot** for his revision of the manuscript, and the **Regional Council of Brittany** for supporting this project.

References

1. Ruttenberg, A., Clark, T., Bug, W., Samwald, M., Bodenreider, O., Chen, H., Doherty, D., Forsberg, K., Gao, Y., Kashyap, V., Kinoshita, J., Luciano, J., Marshall, M., Ogbuji, C., Rees, J., Stephens, S., Wong, G., Wu, E., Zaccagnini, D., Hongsermeier, T., Neumann, E., Herman, I., Cheung, K.: Advancing translational research with the Semantic Web. BMC Bioinformatics 8(Suppl. 3), S2 (2007)
2. Corcho, O.: Ontology based document annotation: trends and open research problems. Int. Journal of metadata, semantics and ontologies 1(1), 47–57 (2006)
3. Jannin, P., Morandi, X., Fleig, O., Le Rumeur, E., Toulouse, P., Gibaud, B., Scarabin, J.: Integration of sulcal and functional information for multimodal neuronavigation. Journal of Neurosurgery 96(4), 713–723 (2002)
4. Tzourio-Mazoyer, N., Landeau, B., Papathanassiou, D., Crivello, F., Etard, O., Delcroix, N., Mazoyer, B., Joliot, M.: Automated anatomical labeling of activations in SPM using a macroscopic anatomical parcellation of the MNI MRI Single-Subject brain. Neuroimage 15(1), 273–289 (2002)
5. Cachia, A., Mangin, J., Rivière, D., Papadopoulos-Orfanos, D., Kherif, F., Bloch, I., Régis, J.A.: A generic framework for parcellation of the cortical surface into gyri using geodesic Voronoï diagrams. Medical Image Analysis 7(4), 403–416 (2003)
6. Fischl, B., van der Kouwe, A., Destrieux, C., Halgren, E., Ségonne, F., Salat, D., Busa, E., Seidman, L., Goldstein, J., Kennedy, D., Caviness, V., Makris, N., Rosen, B., Dale, A.: Automatically parcellating the human cerebral cortex. Cerebral Cortex 14, 11–22 (2004)
7. Clouchoux, C., Coulon, O., Anton, J., Mangin, J., Régis, J.: A new cortical surface parcellation model and its automatic implementation. In: Larsen, R., Nielsen, M., Sporring, J. (eds.) MICCAI 2006. LNCS, vol. 4191, pp. 193–200. Springer, Heidelberg (2006)
8. Franz, B., Diego, C., Deborah, L., Daniele, N., Peter, F.P.S.: The Description Logic Handbook: Theory, Implementation, and Applications. Cambridge University Press, Cambridge (2003)
9. Le Goualher, G., Barillot, C., Bizais, Y.: Modeling cortical sulci with active ribbons. IJPRAI 11(8), 1295–1315 (1997)
10. Collins, D.L., Zijdenbos, A.P., Baaré, W.F.C., Evans, A.C.: INSECT: Improved cortical structure segmentation. In: Kuba, A., Sámal, M., Todd-Pokropek, A. (eds.) IPMI 1999. LNCS, vol. 1613, pp. 210–223. Springer, Heidelberg (1999)
11. Krzysztof, A.: Principles of Constraint Programming (2003)
12. Ono, M., Kubik, S., Abernathey, C.: Atlas of the Cerebral Sulci (1990)
13. Yann, H., Aline, D.: Qualitative spatial relationships for image interpretation by using semantic graph. In: Escolano, F., Vento, M. (eds.) GbRPR 2007. LNCS, vol. 4538, pp. 240–250. Springer, Heidelberg (2007)
14. Mechouche, A., Golbreich, C., Gibaud, B.: Towards a hybrid system using an ontology enriched by rules for the semantic annotation of brain MRI images. In: Marchiori, M., Pan, J.Z., de Marie, C.S. (eds.) RR 2007. LNCS, vol. 4524, pp. 219–228. Springer, Heidelberg (2007)

Towards Multi-Directional OCT for Speckle Noise Reduction

L. Ramrath[1], G. Moreno[1], H. Mueller[2], T. Bonin[2], G. Huettmann[2], and A. Schweikard[1]

[1] Institute for Robotics and Cognitive Systems, University of Luebeck, Germany
ramrath@rob.uni-luebeck.de,
[2] Institute for Biomedical Optics, University of Luebeck, Germany

Abstract. Multi-directional optical coherence tomography (MD-OCT) applies and extends the concept of angular compounding for speckle noise reduction to the area of OCT imaging. OCT images are acquired from a wide range of angles of view. Averaging of the rotated images therefore requires compensation of the parallax which is achieved by simple image registration for image reconstruction. Test measurements of a sample structure in a low and highly scattering environment show that the method improves the signal-to-noise ratio by a factor of 4 and hence reduces speckle noise significantly. Experimental results also show that the proposed averaging increases the performance of common edge-detection algorithms.

1 Introduction

OCT is an evolving imaging technique with important contributions to several medical applications. Based on the principle of white light interferometry, it presents a high resolution non-invasive imaging technique in certain disciplines e.g. ophthalmology, dermatology, urology, and brain morphology [1]. The most severe problem in OCT imaging for diagnostic purposes is image corruption by speckle noise which complicates further analysis. A wealth of image-based speckle reduction filters have therefore been proposed [2]. All of these approaches, however, feature the disadvantage of altering structural information of the image. Another option of OCT image enhancement is spatial compounding by averaging multiple images by e.g. slightly displacing the sample [3]. These displacements eventually change the speckle patterns and a subsequent averaging process will improve image quality by approximately the square root of the number of averaged images. In this context, the concept of angular compounding by acquiring images from different angles has been proposed [4]. In previous studies, averaging of images was done without applying geometric image transformations. Thus, the effect of parallax was not compensated for which falsifies the averaged image. Also, in case of small displacements, speckle pattern might not really be independent and averaging is not suitable.

In this work, the concept of angular compounding is augmented by an automated parallax compensation applying image registration methods to construct

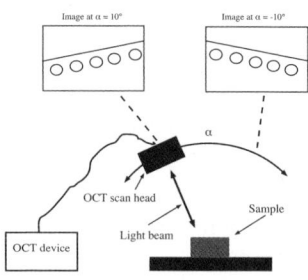 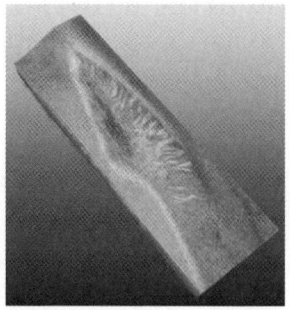

Fig. 1. The concept of multi-directional OCT

Fig. 2. Three-dimensional reconstruction of OCT B-scans of the rat brain showing the striatum with embedded white fibres

an averaged image. For that reason, an angular scanning method is proposed which is compatible with commercial OCT instruments. Applying the mentioned approach enhances structural image properties while reducing speckle noise contribution. An exemplary field of application include the neurosurgical scenario. Here, a robot-assisted microscope with an integrated OCT system is used to acquire multi-directional images automatically [5]. Such a system is able to provide the surgeon with information at microscale level leading to e.g. robust identification of residual tumor tissue or white matter fibres (see Fig. 2).

2 Method

2.1 Concept and Background of Multi-Directional OCT

The occurence of speckle noise is an inherent problem of OCT as it uses the coherence of backreflected light. An important characteristic of speckle is the statistical nature of the speckle pattern. If the scanning setup is not subject to any changes (e.g. movement, temperature), the speckle pattern is time-invariant. It is, however, spatially variant and scanning a sample from different directions will consequently yield a different speckle pattern. Speckle noise is usually modeled as a random multiplicative noise [1]. If f denotes the ideal image and g the speckled image, this assumption can be expressed as

$$g = fu, \tag{1}$$

where u is a signal-independent random variable. Applying the logarithmic operator to Eq. 1 transforms the multiplicative noise into a additive noise. In [6], the authors show that the additive noise component is approximately Gaussian distributed noise. This, in turn, motivates the use of a simple mean operator to estimate the structural component f. As the speckle pattern u is time-invariant averaging can be performed by taking B-scans from multiple direction. Averaging directional images thus reduces the Gaussian distributed noise but keep the structural information.

The idea of multi-directional OCT is visualized in Fig. 1. The OCT scanning head rotates along a circular path around the sample. For each directional B-scan, the angle of view $\Delta\alpha$ is known which will be of advantage in extracting structural information from speckled images. Images from different directions, however, can not be simply superimposed geometrically as the center of rotation of the scanning head, i.e. the distance to the probe, is not known exactly. Adequate averaging can therefore only be done if the effect of parallax is compensated.

2.2 Testbed Setup

To test the performance of the proposed approach, the following testbed scenario is chosen. Instead of rotating the OCT scanning head about the sample, the sample is rotated under the scanning head. The sample is attached to a micromanipulator stage comprising three cartesian stages and one rotary stage (see Fig. 3). The structural element of the sample consists of nylon wires which are chucked parallely with a distance of approximately 500μm. This element is placed into a sealed case which features a glas plate on top (see Fig. 4). Sealing is provided in order to put the sample into different media featuring different scattering properties. The mechanical setup is designed such that repetitive measurements of the same sample can be conducted although the scattering medium is changed. The scanning direction is adjusted to run across the wires such that B-scans image the circular cross-section of the wires. Fig. 5 shows a B-scan for an angle of $\alpha = -10°$ while Fig. 6 provides an image of the same sample at

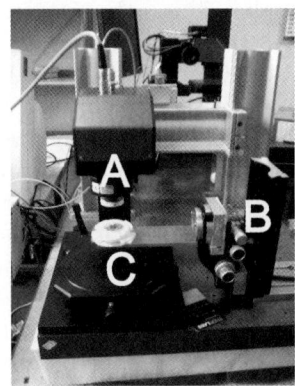

Fig. 3. Scanning setup for multi-directional OCT: [A] scanning head [B] micromanipulator stage for translational and rotational adjustments [C] sample

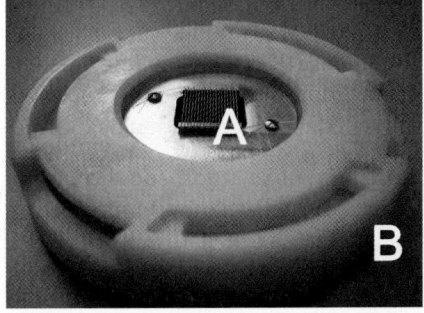

Fig. 4. Sample for multi-directional OCT: [A] nylon wires representing the structural element of the sample [B] sealing case

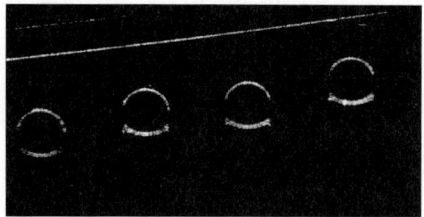 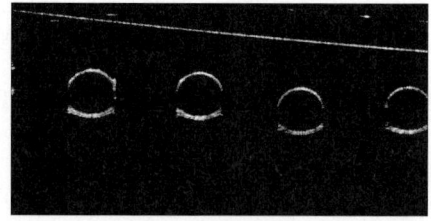

Fig. 5. B-scan showing the cross-sections of nylon wires in the aqueous environment at $\alpha = -10°$. The white line in the upper part corresponds to the sealing glas plate.

Fig. 6. B-scan showing the cross-sections of nylon wires in the aqueous environment at $\alpha = 10°$. The white line in the upper part corresponds to the sealing glas plate.

$\alpha = 10°$. Two imaging sequences with a stepsize of $\Delta\alpha = 1°$ are obtained, both having an angular range of $\alpha = [-10° \ldots 10°]$. For the first scenario, an aqueous environment was chosen which corresponds to a low scattering environment hereafter called water images. The second imaging sequence was done with the nylon wires embedded into a highly scattering milk suspension (10% milk, 90% water) which will be referred to as milk images.

2.3 Automated Registration Technique for Parallax Compensation

Imaging from different directions introduces the effect of parallax and establishes the need of an image correction for adequate averaging. This work proposes an automated registration method especially adapted to the described setup to provide the proof of concept of MD-OCT. This does, however, not limit the generality of the proposed approach as in other applications, other registration methods can be applied (see e.g. [7]).

As the sample geometry is not changed in the MD-OCT scenario, registration in the following is performed as a rigid registration consisting of translation and rotation [7]. The reference image is defined to be the zero degree image. As the angle of rotation of each image is known, the first step is to back-rotate all images to approximate the reference's angle. The back-rotation algorithm considers an arbitratry point outside the image as the center of rotation which does usually not correspond to the center of rotation of the scanning head. The back-rotated image therefore requires an additional alignement for correct averaging. Determination of the alignment parameters is based on a characteristic property of the obtained cross-sectional images. The single fibers from the sample appear to be circles with well-defined borders well suited for template matching. Analyzing the correlation with circular templates provides the coordinates of the circle centers. Additionally, a field of view is defined to delete the edges of the images that the whole set doesn't share. Knowing the location of the circles in the back-rotated and the reference image, the translational part of the registration is determined.

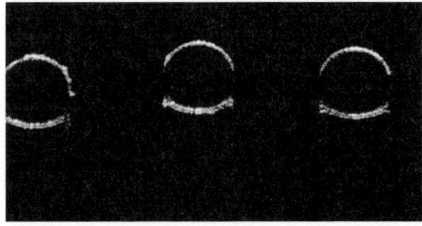 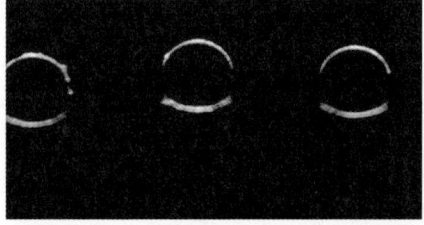

Fig. 7. B-scan showing the cross-sections of nylon wires in the aqueous environment at $\alpha = 0°$

Fig. 8. Averaged of 21 B-scan from different angles showing the cross-sections of nylon wires in the aqueous environment

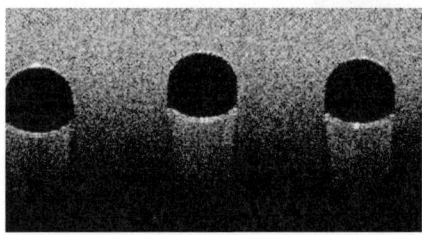 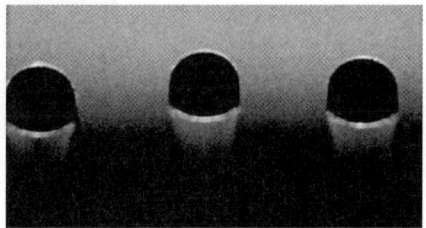

Fig. 9. B-scan showing the cross-sections of nylon wires in the milk suspension environment at $\alpha = 0°$

Fig. 10. Averaged of 21 B-scan from different angles showing the cross-sections of nylon wires in the milk suspension environment

3 Results

Fig. 7 shows a B-scan of the sample for $\alpha = 0°$. The average of all B-scans over an angular range $\alpha = [-10° \ldots 10°]$ after registration is visualized in Fig. 8. Analogous, results for the milk environment are given in Fig. 9 (showing a B-scan from a single angle of view) and Fig. 10 (showing the averaged results after registration). To evaluate the performance of the proposed approach, different measures were analyzed. First, the signal-to-noise ratio was evaluated for an increasing number of viewing directions. The SNR is evaluated as the ratio of the mean and the standard deviation. Fig. 11 shows the SNR course for an increasing number of B-scans acquired from different angular directions for the aqueous test scenario. For the milk trials, results are given in Fig. 12. It can be seen that the SNR improves by almost a factor of 4 for water and milk.

An additional performance evaluation is based on the capability of structure identification which is of great importance in medical image processing. In the following, identification refers to the detection of the circular borders in different scattering environments. Although no true OCT image of the sample in our test scenario is known, an approximation can be made by assuming the averaged water result as the ground truth. This assumption is supported by the low

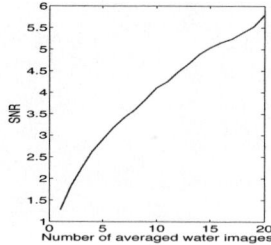
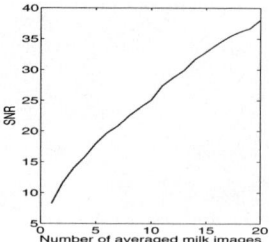

Fig. 11. SNR for an increasing number of averaged water images

Fig. 12. SNR for an increasing number of averaged milk images

Fig. 13. Edge detection with the Canny filter in averaged water image (ground truth)

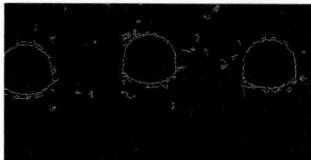
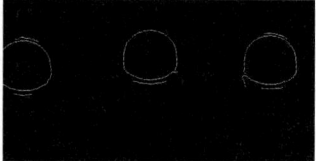

Fig. 14. Edge detection with the Canny filter in single view milk image

Fig. 15. Edge detection with the Canny filter in averaged milk image

scattering properties of water and the high SNR of the averaged B-scan (see Fig. 11). Equal geometrical settings of the measurement scenarios for both tests allow a direct comparison of structures identified in the ground truth (averaged water image) and images taken from the milk suspension testing. Edge detection is now performed by using the Canny operator. All following edge detection operations were performed with constant settings, no parameter adjustments have been made for different images. Fig.13 shows the edges detected in the average water image, Fig.14 the edges detected in $\alpha = 0°$ in milk suspension, and Fig. 15 the results of the edge detection on the averaged milk suspension. Clearly, the best edge detection is provided for the averaged water image. While edges in the single view milk images are irregular and non-existing edges are detected, the edge detection for the averaged milk images is much more similar to the averaged water one. To support these findings numerically, the correlation coefficient of the edge images of the averaged water B-scan and the averaged milk suspension images is given in Fig. 16. Additionally, the mean-square error of between the edge images of the milk enviroment and the averaged water image is plotted

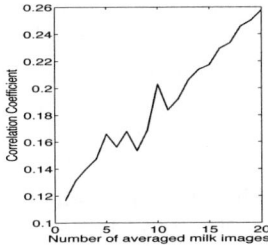
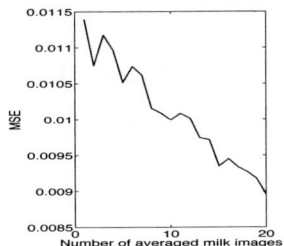

Fig. 16. Correlation performance for edge images with an increasing number of of averaged milk images and the averaged water (ground truth) image

Fig. 17. MSE performance for edge images with an increasing number of averaged milk images and the averaged water (ground truth) image

in Fig. 17. To compare the structure enhancement to existing approaches, edge detection performance on filtered images is analyzed. Filter performance of common filters as the median filter, the Frost filter, and the Perona-Malik filter are provided in Tab. 1.

4 Discussion

From visual inspection of the results shown in Fig. 8 and Fig. 10, it can be seen that the effect of speckle noise is clearly reduced while the structural elements, namely the wires, are enhanced. The reduction of speckle noise is also quantitatively supported by the course of the SNR which increases almost by the factor 4. This corresponds to theory which states that averaging improves the SNR by $\sqrt{n} = \sqrt{21} \approx 4.5$ where n is the number of images averaged. Note that the larger part of the improvement is achieved by averaging 10 images, while the remaining 10 images only provide a smaller improvement. As multi-directional imaging takes effort, e.g time consumption, the user has to decide which image quality serves his needs best. Note that Fig. 9 shows parallel structures (shadows) extending from the bottom of the nylon wires to the bottom of the image. In Fig. 10, these structures are tapered. This effect is related to the experimental setup where the probe is rotated rather than the sample. Shadows will therefore always appear in axial (scanning) direction. If the scanning head is rotated, the shadow direction will change from image to image thus reducing the tapering. Structure identification is also improved with the proposed technique. Simple edge dete-

Table 1. Mean square error between edge images and the averaged water (ground truth) image. Edge images were obtained by applying a simple edge detection after median filtering, Perona-Malik filtering, Frost filter filtering, and the proposed MD-OCT approach.

Median	Perona-Malik	Frost	MD-OCT
0.11	0.09	0.11	0.08

cion in averaged images taken from a highly scattering enviroment compares significantly better to edge detection in images in a low scattering environment. This is clearly validated by the increasing correlation coefficients (Fig. 16) and the decreasing MSE (Fig. 17). Compared to existing image filters for speckle noise reduction, the proposed approach performs better than existing filtering techniques (see Tab. 1). Performance of the MD-OCT approach is better than median and Frost filtering while only slightly better than Perona-Malik filtering. The good performance of the Perona-Malik filter in this case, however, might be related to the simple problem and is eventually worse for more complicated structures.

Although registration in the proposed approach is unique to the application, it provides a good proof of concept and indicates the generality of the approach. In clinical applications, especially for in vivo imaging, other methods of registration from a wealth of medical image registration methods can be taken [7]. The experimental testbed setup, however, has clear disadvantages since it is clearly unsuitable for use in-vivo and angular scanning is very slow. Future developments therefore concentrate on improving the hardware setup. An exemplary application includes a motorized OCT-equipped operating microscope for neurosurgery [5] which is able to perform automated angular scannings.

5 Conclusion

The concept of multi-directional OCT for speckle noise reduction and structure enhancement has been proposed. It is based on extending the idea of spatial compounding of multi-directional OCT images by a parallax compensation. Sample imaging of certain structures in a low and highly scattering environment show that the method significantly reduces speckle noise in OCT images and simplifies structure identification. The assets of the proposed approach present a valuable advantage for OCT-based medical imaging and subsequent diagnosis. In total, the findings motivate the design of (robot-assisted) OCT systems being able to acquire multi-directional images and thus enabling a system-based speckle noise reduction.

References

1. Bouma, B.E., Tearney, G.J.: Handbook of Optical Coherence Tomography. Marcel Dekker, Inc., New York (2002)
2. Brezinski, M.E.: Optical Coherence Tomography - Principles and Application. Academic Press, London (2006)
3. Schmitt, J.M., Xiang, S.H., Yung, K.M.: Speckle in optical coherence tomography. Journal of Biomedical Optics 4, 95–105 (1999)
4. Desjardins, A.E., Vakoc, B.J., Oh, W.Y., Motaghiannezam, S.M., Tearney, G.J., Bouma, B.E.: Angle-resolved optical coherence tomography with sequential angular selectivity for speckle reduction. Optics Express 15, 6200–6209 (2007)

5. Lankenau, E., Klinger, D., Winter, C., Malik, A., Mueller, H., Oelckers, S., Pau, H.-P., Just, T., Huettmann, G.: Combining Optical Coherence Tomography (OCT) with an Operating Microscope. Springer, Heidelberg (2007)
6. Arsenault, H.H., April, G.: Properties of speckle integrated with a finite aperture and logarithmically transformed. J. Opt. Soc. Am. 66, 1160–1163 (1976)
7. Modersitzki, J.: Numerical Methods for Image Registration. Numerical Mathematics and Scientific Computation, Oxford University Press Series (2004)

Automatic Tracking of Escherichia Coli Bacteria

Jun Xie[1], Shahid Khan[2,3], and Mubarak Shah[4]

[1] Janelia Farm Research Campus, HHMI, USA
xiej@janelia.hhmi.org
[2] Molecular Biology Consortium, Chicago, USA
[3] LUMS_SSE, Lahore, Pakistan
[4] Computer Vision Lab, University of Central Florida, USA

Abstract. In this paper, we present an automatic method for estimating the trajectories of Escherichia coli bacteria from *in vivo* phase-contrast microscopy videos. To address the low-contrast boundaries in cellular images, an adaptive kernel-based technique is applied to detect cells in sequence of frames. Then a novel matching gain measure is introduced to cope with the challenges such as dramatic changes of cells' appearance and serious overlapping and occlusion. For multiple cell tracking, an optimal matching strategy is proposed to improve the handling of cell collision and broken trajectories. The results of successful tracking of Escherichia coli from various phase-contrast sequences are reported and compared with manually-determined trajectories, as well as those obtained from existing tracking methods. The stability of the algorithm with different parameter values is also analyzed and discussed.

1 Introduction

The study of cell movement in response to chemical and environmental agents has been an important research area in the bio-medical and environmental science community for quite some time [1,2]. Biologists typically need manual or interactive computer-assisted tracking of cell motion to study chemotactic responses. Manual tracking becomes impractical for data sets where thousands of cells are involved. Automated tracking and analysis of the cells' motility thus becomes critical for time-resolved analysis of the underlying biological mechanisms.

The objective of this study is to track from microscopy videos the gram-negative organism *Escherichia coli bacteria* (E. coli), which can generally cause several intestinal and extra-intestinal infections such as urinary tract infections, meningitis, and peritonitis. Escherichia coli chemotaxis has been the system of choice for elucidation of the design principles of transmembrane and intracellular signal transduction. Automated tracking and motion analysis would significantly enhance the investigators' ability to study E. coli, improve data processing efficiency and remove operator bias.

Tracking typically consists of identifying unique objects in a complex environment where the background remains fairly constant and the target maintains a similar appearance. While numerous methods have been proposed for general object tracking [3], cellular videos pose many challenges to those existing techniques due to severe image noise and clutter, shape deformation, and high processing demand.

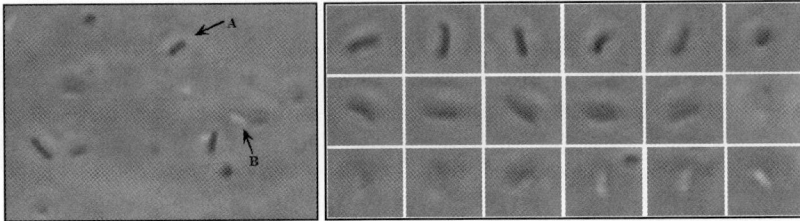

Fig. 1. (Left) A typical view of E. coli bacteria under a phase-contrast microscopy. The cell soma generally appears as a dark area surrounded with a white halo (A) when it is in the focal plane. Once it moves sufficiently out of focus, the contrast will be inverted and the same cell may appear as a white bulb (B). (Right) An sequence of E. coli bacteria.

Among the efforts devoted to cellular imaging, there is one class of methods that perform tracking using edge information [4,5]. Unfortunately, the close proximity of cells and occlusion in the *in vivo* microscopy videos make edge-based cell tracking difficult. A large number of adaptations are required for these methods to be successfully applied. Rather than segmenting the object precisely, some methods consider tracking as a problem of centroid relocation [1] to simplify the tracking task and avoid the requirement of boundary detection.

In order to track living E. coli from phase-contrast microscopy videos, we follow the idea of centroid tracking. Although there is no cell division in our case, serious collision and large overlapping pose more challenges to precise border detection. As shown in Fig. 1, the E. coli cells typically have a large range of motion patterns and the cell soma generally appears as a dark area surrounded with a white halo, but the contrast can be inverted and the cell appears white when it has moved sufficiently out of focus. Those facts make tracking based on the constancy in shape and intensity difficult. Padfield *et. al* [6] recently proposed to generate a dynamic model to describe the appearance change of nuclei over time for live cell tracking.

Another challenging issue in this specific tracking task is incomplete trajectories. Since individual E. coli bacteria can swim freely in 3D space, they may stray from the narrow focal plane and hence become temporarily lost, causing fragmentation of their trajectories. That is why we consider multi-cell tracking as a global optimal assignment problem.

2 Method

The proposed method starts with an object detection step which identifies the moving objects against the relative constant background. Then a global matching strategy is applied to estimate the cells' trajectories based on image appearance and motion patterns.

2.1 Cell Detection in Fuzzy Scene

In order to classify foreground and background, we apply our previous method [7] which is able to handle multiple objects with fuzzy edges. The method is based on

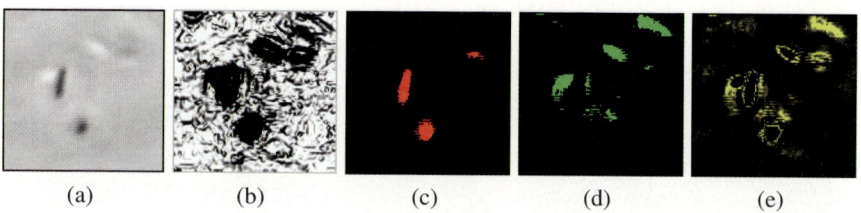

Fig. 2. An example of coli detection. (a) A patch from the original frame. (b) The homogeneity map computed using GVF measurement. (c) and (d) show the detected objects (without morphology operations). (e) The final entropy map.

the observation that the pixels with high class uncertainty accumulate mostly around object boundaries. We model the image as a mixture of Gaussians, and the optimal pixel classification is obtained by minimizing the loss function $L = L_{entropy} - \lambda L_{likelihood}$, where λ is a scale factor. $L_{likelihood} = \int_{\mathbf{x} \in \Omega_i} \log P(\mathbf{x})$ represents the likelihood and $L_{entropy}$ is the entropy term defined as:

$$L_{entropy} = \int_{\mathbf{x} \in \Omega_i} (1 - G(\mathbf{x}))U(\mathbf{x}) + (1 - U(\mathbf{x}))G(\mathbf{x}), \qquad (1)$$

where G is the normalized gradient vector flow (GVF) [8] serving as a measure of spatial information, and U is the normalized entropy describing the class uncertainty according to Shannon's theory. By minimizing the cost function, we can simultaneously optimize the parameters of the global model and the distribution of entropy for the detection process.

The optimization of those parameters can be achieved through the Quasi-Newton algorithm [9]. To improve the efficiency, we applied the EM method [10] at the initial stage to find the initial model parameters and the size of each object category. Figure 2 shows an example of the detection results. More details about this detection method can be found in [7]. After pixels are classified into different groups, the Connected Components Labeling technique [11] can be applied to generate connected regions (bulbs), and regions with sizes comparable with pre-selected thresholds are regarded as candidates.

2.2 Matching Gain for Candidate Selection

After detecting the candidates, an intuitive way to track the target, as applied in the Mean-Shift approach [12], is to compare the intensity similarity between the candidates and the targeted cells. Usually the intensity histogram will be employed to describe the intensity profile of each object.

In our context, where the appearance of the target changes very quickly (see Fig. 1 (Right) for an example), the single intensity similarity is not reliable enough to provide a robust measurement for the tracking. In addition, there are numerous cells moving in the field of view and interacting with each other so closely that it is difficult, even for human, to identify the correct tracks for those cells from one frame to the next. This is why we consider the global trajectory inference and promote the use of a graph based approach for optimal position estimation.

Multiple Cell Tracking: First, let's consider the simple case of multiple cells observed in two successive frames. Let c_i^p ($i = 1 \cdots l$) denote detected cells in the p-th frame and c_j^{p+1} ($j = 1 \cdots k$) represent those detected in the $(p+1)$-th frame. The task is to find the matching from $\{c_i^p\}$ to $\{c_j^{p+1}\}$. This context can be modeled with a complete bi-partite graph $G = (U, V, E)$ where $U = \{c_1^p, c_2^p ... c_l^p\}$, $V = \{c_1^{p+1}, c_2^{p+1} ... c_k^{p+1}\}$, and E represents the set of matching hypotheses between each pair of cells from frame p to $p + 1$. The correspondence problem can then be posed to find a matching of graph G, which is defined as a set of edges with no shared end-vertices. Assume there are pre-defined functions $\mathcal{W}$ associated with each of these edges. A minimum matching in a weighted graph is a matching with minimum weight among all matchings in the graph. Since any two detected cells may hypothetically match, the resulting bi-partite graph is complete. Given the weights defined by specific matching criteria, a unique matching $\widetilde{M}$ between the cells in two frames can be found as $\widetilde{M} = \arg\min_{M \in C} \sum \mathcal{W}(c_i^p, c_j^q)$, where C is the union of all the possible matching of G. There are several efficient algorithms (e.g., [13]) which can be used to find the minimum matching of a bipartite graph.

For multiple cells in multiple frames, it is a complete k-partite graph and this matching problem is NP-hard [14]. Fortunately, as demonstrated in [15], if the graph is an acyclic directed graph, a polynomial-time solution exists where the edges of the minimum matching of the split graph $\mathfrak{S}$ of an acyclic edge-weighted directed graph G correspond to the edges of minimum path cover of G. To model the multiple frame matching problem, we construct a weighted directed graph $G = (\{V_1, V_2, \cdots, V_k\}, E)$, where V_i represents the set of detected cells in frame F_i. Each edge $e = (c_i^p c_j^q)$ corresponds to a match hypothesis of coli c_i^p in frame F_i to coli c_j^q in frame F_j, and the weight w_e is defined as the matching cost, like in 2-frame cases.

If coli c_i^p has no correspondences in several consecutive frames and gets its forward matching $c_j^{p+\delta}$ in frame $F_{p+\delta}$ (due to occlusion or being out of focal plane), an edge $e = (c_i^p c_j^{p+\delta})$ can naturally handle broken trajectories and thus provide an overall coverage of the possible solutions. Since all the edges in graph G are in the temporal direction, it is guaranteed that G is acyclic. The only requirement for this graph is that the weight function must satisfy the inequality $\mathcal{W}(c_i^p, c_j^q) < \mathcal{W}(c_i^p, c_{i+1}^{p+1})\mathcal{W}(c_{j-1}^{q-1}, c_j^q)$ in order to penalize the choice of shorter trajectories when longer valid ones are present.

Matching Criteria: According to the discussion above, it is obvious that the weight function is critical for the correct matching of different cells across the long sequence. The weight of matching two cells c_i^p and c_j^q can be defined based on the cell appearances as follows:

$$\mathcal{W}_h(c_i^p, c_j^q) = \frac{1}{2} \sum_{b=1}^{B} \frac{[\mathbf{h}_i^p(b) - \mathbf{h}_j^q(b)]^2}{\mathbf{h}_i^p(b) + \mathbf{h}_j^q(b)}, \quad (2)$$

where $\mathbf{h}_i^t$ refers to the intensity histogram of the i-th cell in frame t and B indicates the total gray levels.

An alternative way is to define the gain function based on some assumption of the undergoing motion of the targeted cell, such as a constant direction or velocity. The prediction of the cell in a new frame is then estimated accordingly. Then the matching weight can be defined using motion measurements. A simple function for this is the nearest neighborhood criteria.

A matching function considering both direction and motion coherence has also been used in [16] for tracking feature points. The function is defined as follows:

$$\mathcal{W}(c_i^p, c_j^q) = \gamma \mathcal{W}_o + (1 - \gamma) \mathcal{W}_v, \tag{3}$$

where $\mathcal{W}_o = (\frac{1}{2} + \frac{\overrightarrow{c_i^p c_i^q} \cdot \overrightarrow{c_i^p c_j^q}}{2\|\overrightarrow{c_i^p c_i^q}\| \cdot \|\overrightarrow{c_i^p c_j^q}\|})$ is the orientation term, and $\mathcal{W}_v = \frac{2\sqrt{\|\overrightarrow{c_i^p c_i^q}\| \cdot \|\overrightarrow{c_i^p c_j^q}\|}}{\|\overrightarrow{c_i^p c_i^q}\| + \|\overrightarrow{c_i^p c_j^q}\|}$ represents the velocity term which prefers the match with less change in the magnitude of velocity.

Although those motion-based measures enforce the coherence of motion, they require initialization of correspondence obtained manually or by other criteria. Also, the motion coherence may not be sufficient in the presence of highly random motions as in our application. In addition, they are not suited to handle cells entering the field of view late.

Based on the observation that the significant changes of the coli's appearance are usually accompanied by the occurrence of contrast corruption, we define our matching gain function as following:

$$\mathcal{W}(c_i^p, c_j^q) = (1 - \omega_i^p) \mathcal{W}_h(c_i^p, c_j^q) + \omega_i^p (\mathcal{W}_d(c_i^p, c_j^q) + \mathcal{W}_o(c_i^p, c_j^q)), \tag{4}$$

where $\mathcal{W}_d(c_i^p, c_j^q) = (1 - \frac{\|\overrightarrow{c_i^p c_i^q} - \overrightarrow{c_i^p c_j^q}\|}{\sqrt{w_I^2 + h_I^2}})$ refers to the distance between the predicted and observed cells (w_I and h_I are the width and height of the frame, respectively). The term ω_i^p represents a scalar to balance the impact between the intensity and distance coherence. It is defined based on the contrast measurement of the targeted cell as follows:

$$\omega_i^p = \frac{\alpha}{2} \frac{(\bar{I}_i^p - \bar{I}_{\Omega_i})^2}{(\bar{I}_i^p + \bar{I}_{\Omega_i})}, \tag{5}$$

where α is a constant $0 \leq \alpha \leq 1$, $\bar{I}_i^p$ and $\bar{I}_{\Omega_i}$ refers to the average image intensity of region covered by c_i^p and its local window Ω_i, respectively.

The above matching gain function is a convex combination of the intensity measurement ($\mathcal{W}_h$) and motion gains ($\mathcal{W}_d$ and $\mathcal{W}_o$). They are adaptively combined based on the contrast of the tracked cell so that the intensity term will dominate the matching measurement when the target is clearly presented, while the motion clues will take over when the cell becomes blurry.

3 Experimental Results

In this section, we assess the proposed approach by comparing it with both popular tracking methods and manual tracking. Cultures for behavioral experiments were harvested at mid-exponential phase by centrifugation, washed three times, and re-suspended in a

Table 1. The Detection Validation and Tracking Performance on Each Sequence

Seq. No.	Res. (pixels)	Frames	Prec. (%)	Rec. (%)	MS	MSCE	MSAB	NEW
1	616 × 459	450	97.4	97.6	37.5	23.7	29.6	14.9
2	720 × 480	458	98.5	96.6	27.8	21.7	43.6	10.6
3	584 × 416	450	98.9	95.8	21.8	19.9	28.3	12.1
4	444 × 362	160	86.5	88.4	20.1	18.7	31.0	6.6
5	620 × 469	680	97.5	96.4	26.5	24.2	25.3	8.5
6	720 × 480	498	98.1	96.7	28.2	27.5	29.1	11.0
7	720 × 480	702	99.3	97.9	18.9	18.0	17.8	3.8
8	532 × 382	460	99.3	98.0	19.9	19.4	18.8	3.2
Avg.	620 × 441	482.2	96.94	95.93	25.09	21.64	27.93	8.83

potassium phosphate-EDTA motility buffer containing 5 mM lactate, as respiratory substrate, and 100 μM methionine to maintain vigorous swim-tumble bias. The sequences were imaged by a CCD camera mounted on a Nikon Optiphot microscope using a phase contrast objective (40x CF Fluor plan-apochromat, 0.85 numerical aperture) and zoom lens [17]. Due to variations in shutter time, light exposure, filtering and cell culture, the data sets vary among themselves in contrast, intensity and apparent proximity. Our trial data consists of eight sequences (Table 1), totaling nearly 3800 frames that contain numerous E. coli cells moving naturally in the three-dimensional space.

One advantage of our approach is that it does not require manual initialization. Starting from the first frame, the regions of interest are detected in each frame as discussed in Section 2.1. To evaluate the detection accuracy, as applied in [5], we compute the *precision* as the ratio of the number of detected cells to the total number of detected candidates, and the *recall* as the ratio of detected cells to the total number of cells actually in the frame. In order to obtain the ground-truth for validation, a tool has been developed for operators to identify the cell centroid in each of the frames. The computed precision and recall for each individual sequence are listed in Table 1.

After detection, the intensity profile for each candidate is computed and its contrast measurement is estimated within a local window, which is double the size of the candidate. To establish the initial correspondence, the first two frames are used to construct a bipartite graph, where the weights are computed using Eq. (4) with $\alpha = 1$. The following frames are then processed sequentially using a constant α which is selected empirically ($\alpha = 0.2$ in our experiment).

To improve the efficiency of the algorithm, we compute the correspondence within a spatial window. Given the initial correspondence, we extend the graph by computing the weights for the successive frame. The minimum path cover of the graph is then estimated, and this procedure is repeated until a specific number of frames have been included. The size of the sliding window k affects the computation complexity and the capability of the algorithm to handle occlusion and broken trajectory. In order to correct the mismatches in previous procedure, a backtracking can be performed by applying the same tracking method in the reverse time direction as applied in [18,19]. Figure 3 shows the cell tracking results on two trial sequences.

We compared the tracking performance of the proposed algorithm with that achieved by human operator. Also, several Mean Shift (MS) technique based algorithms are

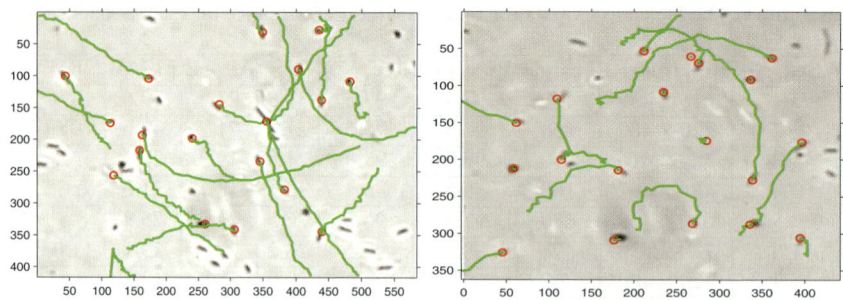

Fig. 3. Samples of estimated traces (red circles indicate start points)

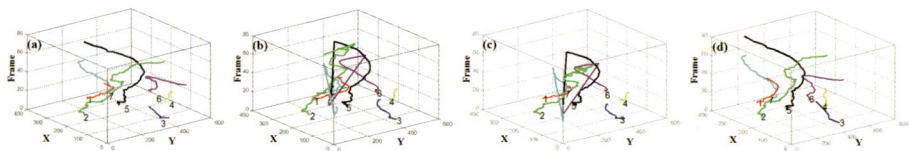

Fig. 4. Visualization of cell trajectories (in Sequence A) obtained using different methods: (a) Manual tracking, (b) Mean Shift, (c) MSCE, and (d) Our method. Each color curve shows a cell trajectory.

tested, including the classical Mean Shift [12], MS based on Contrast Enhancement (MSCE) [20], and MS using Adaptive Bandwidth (MSAB) [21]. For the proposed method, we assume there are three kernels for cell detection and the scale parameter λ was chosen as $1/N$ (N: the number of pixels in each frame). We also set $\alpha = 0.2$ and $k = 5$ for the test. For the classical Mean Shift algorithm, the histogram was generated using 64 levels and the model of the tracked cell was updated every 3 frames with a regression level of 0.3. Following the work in [20], we use the analysis resolution $\delta = 0.02$, outlier threshold $\tau = 0.01$ and distortion limit $\lambda = 5$ for the MSCE algorithm. As used in [21], we set the logarithmic coordinate base $b = 1$ and the scale level $s = 2$ in the MSAB method. The spatial-temporal plots in Fig. 4 demonstrate the three-dimensional views of several cells' traces obtained with different methods. As noted, the Mean-Shift based techniques, compared to the manual results (Fig. 4(a)), generated some incorrect jumps (line 5(black), 6(pink) and 7(cyan)) due to poor contrast of the frames and the interference from cells with similar intensity. In contrast, the proposed approach (Fig. 4(d)) solved those problems smoothly and provided a solid performance, which is comparable to manual results.

In order to evaluate the tracking performance quantitatively, we apply the following criteria to measure the accuracy of the tracking algorithms. For each automatic cell trajectory, we computed the average distance (in pixels) in each frame between the manually-marked locations and those computed by the algorithms. If the distance in one frame is smaller than a preselected threshold (for example, the half of the cell's size), the tracking result in this frame is considered to be correct and the frame is counted as a correct frame for the algorithm. Then the measure, called *frame-based error* [15], is

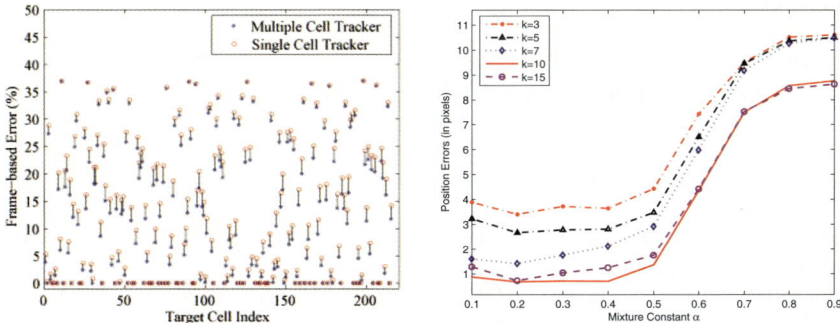

Fig. 5. (Left) The frame-based errors using the single-cell tracking method and multi-cell tracker. The horizontal axis represents the targeted cells. (Right) Tracking performance with respect to the mixture constant α: position errors (in pixels) for different size of sliding window k.

computed for the validation which is defined as $E_f = 1 - n_p/n_t$, where n_p is the number of correct frames generated by the tracker and n_t is the total number of frames the cell appears in the sequence.

The tracking errors of different tracking methods are illustrated in Table 1. In all the tested sequences, the proposed method has the best performance, with an average frame-based error of 8.83 ± 4.10%. Figure 5(Left) shows the difference between the tracking results using the single cell tracker and multi-cell tracker, which confirms that the optimal matching strategy is able to improve the overall tracking accuracy. In Fig. 5(Right) we demonstrate the average pixel-based tracking errors with different values of the mixture constant α and the size of temporal window. Notice that typically the value of constant α will affect the tracking accuracy, and the better results are achieved with low values. The plot also shows that the tracking errors can be generally reduced by increasing the size of the sliding window. However, since a large window will increase the computation complexity, there is a trade-off between the tracking accuracy and computation time. For our case, the tracking system typically takes 3.3s/frame with a Matlab implementation on a 2GHz PC.

4 Conclusion

This paper introduced a fully automated method for tracking Escherichia coli bacteria in phase-contrast microscopy videos. The proposed detection method has been successfully applied to detect cells in the low contrast frame images. To handle the ambiguity in cellular images, a global optimal matching strategy is also introduced to enable multi-cell tracking. We have demonstrated the utility of the proposed algorithm for tracking E. coli bacteria from classical phase-contrast microscopy videos. Coupled with additional parameters for measurement of morphology, we anticipate that this algorithm will find wide application in diagnosis of bacterial pathogens in clinics and in basic biomedical research on bacterial chemotaxis.

References

1. Debeir, O., VanHam, P., Kiss, R., Decaestecker, C.: Tracking of migrating cells under phase-contrast video microscopy with combined mean-shift processes. IEEE Trans. on Medical Imaging 24(6), 697–711 (2005)
2. Al-Kofahi, O., Radke, R., Goderie, S., Shen, Q., Temple, S., Roysam, B.: Automated cell lineage construction: a rapid method to analyze clonal development establis. Cell Cycle 5, 327–335 (2006)
3. Yilmaz, A., Javed, O., Shah, M.: Object tracking: A survey. ACM Journal of Computing Surveys 38(4), 13 (2006)
4. Mukherjee, D., Ray, N., Acton, S.: Level set analysis for leukocyte detection and tracking. IEEE Trans. on Image Processing 13(4), 562–572 (2004)
5. Li, K., Miller, E., Weiss, L., Campbell, P., Kanade, T.: Online tracking of migrating and proliferating cells imaged with phase-contrast microscopy. In: Proceedings of Intern. Works. on Comp. Vision and Pattern Recog., pp. 65–72 (June 2006)
6. Padfield, D., Rittscher, J., Thomas, N., Roysam, B.: Spatio-temporal cell cycle phase analysis using level sets and fast marching methods. In: Proc. of first Workshop on Microscopic Image Analysis with Applications in Biology, pp. 2–9 (2006)
7. Xie, J., Tsui, H.: Image segmentation based on maximum-likelihood estimation and optimum entropy-distribution (MLE-OED). Pattern Recognition Letter 25(10), 1133–1141 (2004)
8. Xu, C., Prince, J.L.: Snakes, shapes, and gradient vector flow. IEEE Trans. on Image Processing 7(3), 359–369 (1998)
9. Nocedal, J., Wright, S.J.: Numerical Optimization. Springer, Heidelberg (1999)
10. Empster, A.: Maximum likelihood from incomplete data via the em algorithm. J. Roy. Statist. Soc. 29, 1–38 (1997)
11. Rosenfeld, A., Kak, A.C.: Digital Picture Processing. Academic Press, London (1982)
12. Comaniciu, D., Ramesh, V., Meer, P.: Real-time tracking of non-rigid objects using mean-shift. In: Proc. of IEEE. Conf. Comp. Vision and Pattern Recog., vol. II, pp. 142–149 (June 2000)
13. Hopcroft, J., Karp, R.: An $n^{2.5}$ algorithm for maximum matchings in bipartite graphs. SIAM Journal on Computing 4(2), 225–230 (1979)
14. Garey, M.R., Johnson, D.S.: Computers and Intractability: A Guide to the Theory of NP-Completeness. W.H. Freeman, New York (January 1979)
15. Shafique, K., Shah, M.: A noniterative greedy algorithm for multiframe point correspondence. IEEE Trans. on Pattern Analysis and Machine Intelligence 27, 51–65 (2005)
16. Veenman, C., Reinders, M., Backer, E.: Resolving motion correspondence for densely moving points. IEEE Trans. on Pat. Anal. and Machine Intelligence 23(1), 54–72 (2001)
17. Wright, S., Walia, B., Parkinson, J., Khan, S.: Differential activation of escherichia coli chemoreceptors by blue-light stimuli. J. Bacteriol. 188, 3962–3971 (2006)
18. Deb, S., Yeddanapudi, M., Pattipati, K., Bar-Shalom, Y.: A generalized s-d assignment algorithm for multisensor-multitarget state estimation. IEEE Trans. Aerospace and Electronic Systems 33(2), 523–538 (1997)
19. Poore, A.: Multidimensional assignments and multitarget tracking. In: Proc. Partitioning Data Sets, pp. 169–196 (1995)
20. Grundland, M., Dodgson, N.A.: Automatic contrast enhancement by histogram warping. In: Proc. of Intern. Conf. Comp. Vision and Graphics, pp. 22–24 (September 2004)
21. Collins, R.: Mean-shift blob tracking through scale space. In: Proc. of IEEE. Conf. Comp. Vision and Pattern Recog., pp. 234–240 (June 2003)

Automatic Image Analysis of Histopathology Specimens Using Concave Vertex Graph

Lin Yang[1,3], Oncel Tuzel[2], Peter Meer[1], and David J. Foran[3]

[1] Dept. of Electrical and Computer Eng., Rutgers Univ., Piscataway, NJ, 08854, USA
[2] Dept. of Computer Science, Rutgers Univ., Piscataway, NJ, 08854, USA
[3] Center of Biomedical Imaging and Informatics, The Cancer Institute of New Jersey, UMDNJ-Robert Wood Johnson Medical School, Piscataway, NJ, 08854, USA

Abstract. Automatic image analysis of histopathology specimens would help the early detection of blood cancer. The first step for automatic image analysis is segmentation. However, touching cells bring the difficulty for traditional segmentation algorithms. In this paper, we propose a novel algorithm which can reliably handle touching cells segmentation. Robust estimation and color active contour models are used to delineate the outer boundary. Concave points on the boundary and inner edges are automatically detected. A concave vertex graph is constructed from these points and edges. By minimizing a cost function based on morphological characteristics, we recursively calculate the optimal path in the graph to separate the touching cells. The algorithm is computationally efficient and has been tested on two large clinical dataset which contain 207 images and 3898 images respectively. Our algorithm provides better results than other studies reported in the recent literature.

1 Introduction

As new therapies emerge for blood cancer screening, it becomes increasingly important to distinguish among subclasses of lymphocytes in advance. Processing the specimen using a reliable, image-based analysis system could reduce the cost and patient morbidity. In image-based analysis the first step is segmentation. However, the traditional methods usually fail to accurately segment touching cells in the digitized hematologic specimens. Touching cells are especially prominent in malignant cases. In Figure 1, we show representative morphologies for benign and five hematologic malignancies (hematoxylin-eosin staining): Chronic Lymphocytic Leukemia (CLL) [1], Mantle Cell Lymphoma, (MCL) [2], Follicular Center Cell Lymphoma (FCC) [3], Acute Myelocytic Leukemia (AML) and Acute Lymphocytic Leukemia (ALL) [2].

The watershed algorithm is the most commonly used method for performing touching object segmentation. However, it suffers from several major drawbacks.
– *Oversegmentation.* The algorithm is sensitive to noise and often produces many oversegmented small regions. Marker-based watershed [4] can partially remedy this issue, but it requires manual selection or accurate estimation of the markers.

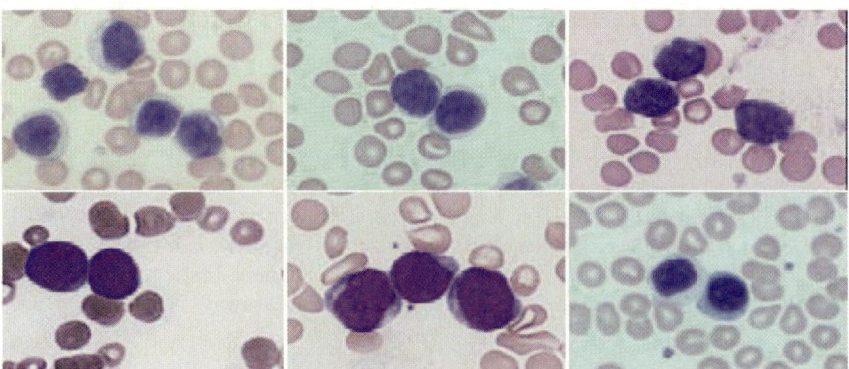

Fig. 1. Some representative morphologies of touching lymphocytes. In the first row, from left to right: CLL, MCL and FCC. In the second row, from left to right: ALL, AML and benign. The specimens were prepared at different hospitals and institutions therefore there exists large variations in staining.

- *Lack of shape prior.* It is generally difficult to include shape priors in the watershed transform. Although there are some efforts [5,6] proposed for specific cases, the general problem still exists.

In this paper, we propose a novel algorithm to separate touching cells. The algorithm starts from a deformable model which extracts the boundary contour of the touching cells. The concave vertex graph is constructed using the concave vertices on the contour and the edges detected in the region of touching cells. The segmentation is then treated as an optimal grouping of pixels, which can be solved by recursively searching optimal shortest path in the concave vertex graph.

2 Boundary Contour Extraction

The initial step of the algorithm is to extract the boundary contour of the touching cells. We first apply a L_2E robust estimation [7] to provide a rough estimation of the outer boundaries of the cells inside the region of interest (ROI). A robust gradient vector flow (GVF) snake [8] using Luv [9, Sec. 8.4] color gradients is further applied to extract the objects from the background. Since the deformable models are initialized using the results of robust estimation, the convergence speed is increased and the method can handle topological changes. In this paper, we focus our attention on the touching cases shown in Figure 2b, where the output contour represents the outer boundary of the touching cells.

3 Concave Points and Inner Edges Detection

In Figure 3, we show the construction of the concave vertex graph. The contour found by boundary contour extraction algorithm is shown in Figure 3a. We detect

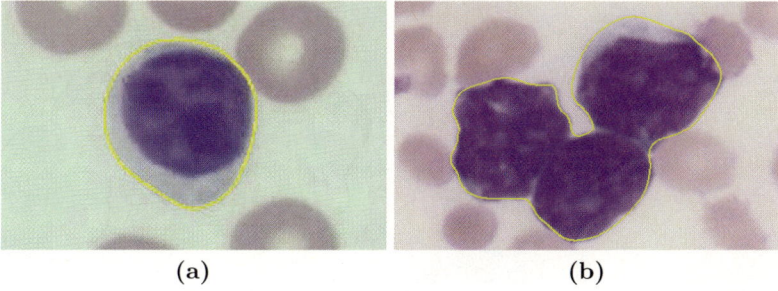

(a) **(b)**

Fig. 2. The segmentation result of robust color GVF snake. (a) The ROI contains only one cell. (b) The ROI contains the touching cells.

the high curvature points on the contour via [10](Figure 3b). At each point p on the contour a set of triangles are constructed. The points which satisfy

$$d_{\min} \leq |\boldsymbol{a}| \leq d_{\max} \qquad d_{\min} \leq |\boldsymbol{b}| \leq d_{\max} \qquad \alpha \leq \alpha_{\max} \qquad (1)$$

where $\alpha = \arccos \frac{|\boldsymbol{a}|^2 + |\boldsymbol{b}|^2 - |\boldsymbol{c}|^2}{2|\boldsymbol{a}||\boldsymbol{b}|}$, $d_{\min}, d_{\max} = 7, 9$ pixels and $\alpha_{\max} = 150°$ are kept. The candidates are further processed to suppress the local nonmaxima points. The final high curvature points correspond to both concave and convex points. We keep only the concave points, shown as red rectangles in Figure 3c. This can be calculated from the sign of the cross product $\boldsymbol{a} \otimes \boldsymbol{b}$, which has to be negative for concave points.

Canny edge detector is applied inside the cell region and straight line fitting is used to model the edges (Figure 3d). The separating curve combines a pair of convex vertices on the boundary and is enforced to pass through the inner edges.

4 Touching Cells Segmentation

The outer boundary of the touching cells is defined as C, and the region enclosed by C is $R(C)$. The concave points are the set V, e.g. $v1 - v5$ which are shown in Figure 3e. The inner edges are the set E, e.g. shown as white solid lines in Figure 3e and also illustrated by e_i in Figure 3f.

4.1 Concave Vertex Graph

In Figure 3f we construct the concave vertex graph G. Let W be the vertex set consisting of the end points of inner edges E, e.g. w_i and w_j in Figure 3f. The vertices of graph G are then equal to $V \cup W$.

The graph has two sets of edges E and F. The set E contains the inner edges found by the edge detection algorithm. The set F is constructed with *filling edges* by connecting the vertices in G which are not connected by inner edges, e.g. f_k in Figure 3f. The lengths of the inner edges are set to ϵ (10^{-16}), while the lengths of the *filling edges* in set F are given by the Euclidean distance between the two vertices of the edges.

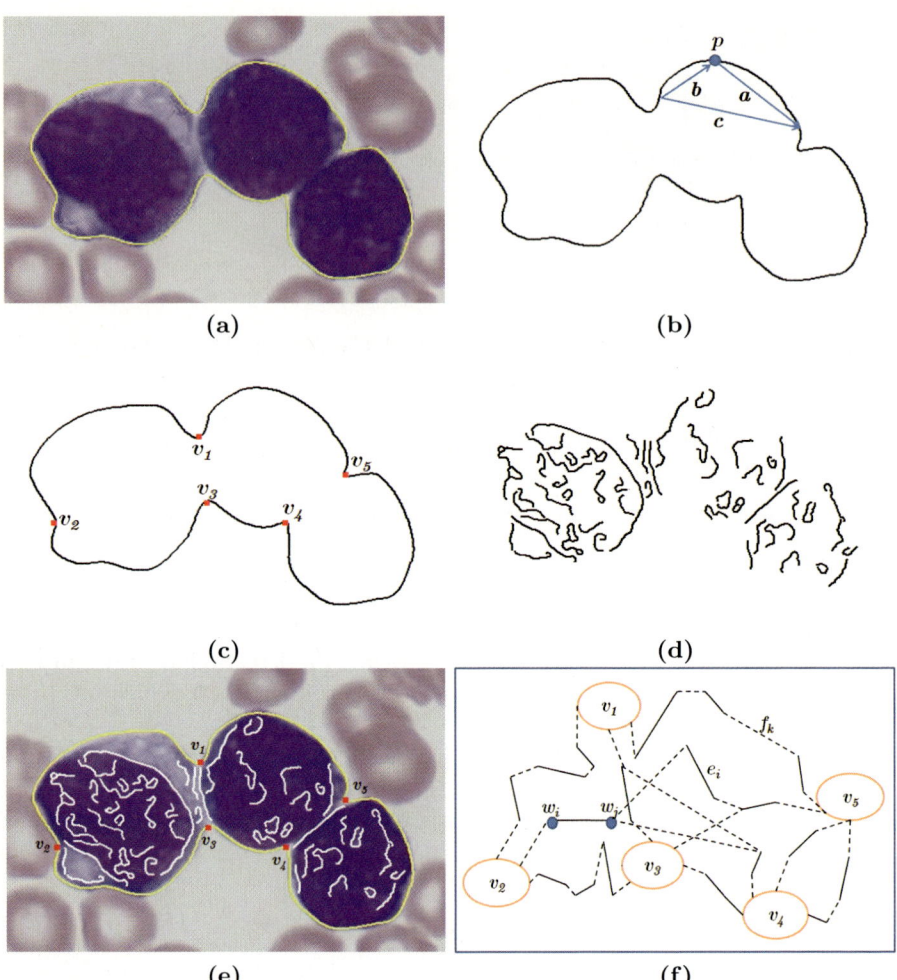

Fig. 3. Construction of the concave vertex graph. (a) The original image with the yellow boundary contour. (b) High curvature points detection. (c) Concave points detection. (d) Inner edges detection. (e) The outer boundary C, concave vertices V and inner edges E, superimposed on the original image. (f) The constructed concave vertex graph G. The filling edges are shown with dotted lines.

The Dijkstra algorithm is used to find the shortest path p_{ij} between v_i and v_j. The length of the p_{ij}, $\|p_{ij}\|$, is given by the total length of the *filling edges* f_k in p_{ij} because the length of real inner edges is set to be ϵ

$$\|p_{ij}\| = \sum_{f_k \in p_{ij}} length\,(f_k). \qquad (2)$$

In Figure 3f, as an example, we can see $\|p_{12}\| > \|p_{13}\|$ because p_{12} traverse longer *filling edges* than p_{13}. The defined path lengths enforce the segmentation

> **Input:** Given the region of interest (ROI) containing touching cells.
> - Extract the boundary contour C, detect the concave points V, the inner edges E in $R(C)$, construct the concave vertex graph G.
> - for each vertex $v(i) \in V$
>   • Find the path p_{ij} and calculate the length $\|p_{ij}\|$ using (2).
> - Initialize $mincost = +\infty$ and $Q = \varnothing$.
> - while (V is not empty)
>   • for each vertex $v(i) \in V$
>   * for each vertex $v(j \neq i) \in V$
>   · Apply the path p_{ij} to separate the graph G in to L and R.
>   · Calculate the cost c using (6) and save in Q.
>   • Sort Q and pick up the path p_{ij} with the lowest cost c.
>   • if ($c < 1.5 * mincost$)
>   * Record path p_{ij} and the region $R(C, p_{ij})$ with cost c in the $result$.
>   * The edges and zero degree vertices in the $R(C, p_{ij})$ are removed from G.
>   * Set $mincost = c$ and $Q = \varnothing$.
>   • else return $result$.

Alg. 1. The algorithm to separate touching cells using concave vertex graph

to follow inner edges since the trivial solution to directly connect two concave vertices using only *filling edges* in graph G would provide a longer path.

After the Dijkstra algorithm is applied, we find all the shortest pathes among concave vertices, p_{ij}, which are valid candidates to separate touching cells. The key idea of our algorithm is to treat the touching cells segmentation as recursively searching for the best path p_{ij} in G, which minimizes a cost function specifically designed to prefer cell-like object-cut.

4.2 Cost Function

We are looking for perceptually "good" segmentation of touching cells. For this purpose, we design the cost function to represent the clues that surgical pathologists use for judgement.

- The cells should be objects which are perceptually salient, since humans intend to separate such objects in an image. A good definition of saliency is proposed in [11] based on the Gestalt laws [12]. We apply the minimum of two saliency costs

$$c_s = \min\left(\frac{\|p_{ij}\|}{\sqrt{area_L(C, p_{ij})}}, \frac{\|p_{ij}\|}{\sqrt{area_R(C, p_{ij})}}\right) \quad (3)$$

where $\|p_{ij}\|$ is the length defined in (2), each path p_{ij} in G divides $R(C)$ into two regions L and R, and the min function in (3) selects the region with the smallest cost. The $area(C, p_{ij})$ denotes the area enclosed by C and path p_{ij}.
- The cells are objects which are close to elliptical shape and can be modeled by ellipse fitting using points on C and p_{ij}. The ratio between the long and

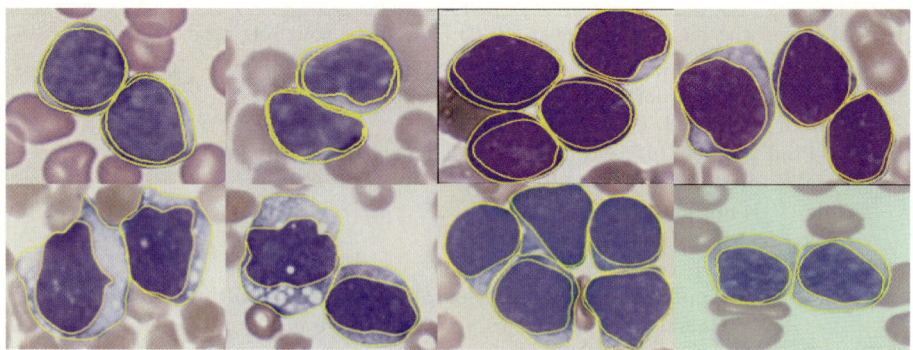

Fig. 4. The segmentation results using the concave vertex graph

short axes is recorded as tg. The segmented objects are expected to provide a ratio tg in the range $[tg_1, tg_2]$, in which case the $dist\,(tg, [tg_1, tg_2]) = 0$. Otherwise, we define $dist\,(tg, [tg_1, tg_2]) = \min\,(|tg - tg2|, |tg - tg1|)$.

$$c_g = \min\left(\frac{1}{1 + \exp\left(-dist\,(tg_L, [tg_1, tg_2])\right)}, \frac{1}{1 + \exp\left(-dist\,(tg_R, [tg_1, tg_2])\right)}\right) \quad (4)$$

where the L and R have the same definition as (3). The tg_1 and tg_2 represent the lower bound and upper bound of the long axes to short axes ratio.

- The cells are objects which have biologically reasonable areas. Following the definition above, we use ta_1 and ta_2 to represent the lower bound and upper bound of the cell area.

$$c_a = \min\left(\frac{1}{1 + \exp\left(-dist\,(ta_L, [ta_1, ta_2])\right)}, \frac{1}{1 + \exp\left(-dist\,(ta_R, [ta_1, ta_2])\right)}\right). \quad (5)$$

- The final cost c is the weighted sum

$$c = \lambda_1 c_s + \lambda_2 c_g + \lambda_3 c_a \qquad \sum_{i=1}^{3} \lambda_i = 1. \quad (6)$$

The optimal values of coefficients are selected as $\lambda_1 = 0.5, \lambda_2 = 0.3$ and $\lambda_3 = 0.2$, which are learned in an offline process using a training set and held constant throughout the experiments.

4.3 Algorithm

Using the concave vertex graph G and the cost function c, the method is described in Algorithm 1. It is recursively applied to separate touching cells until all the region $R(C)$ are allocated to the segmented cells. The algorithm only separates the cytoplasm of the touching cells. Since the colors of nuclei and cytoplasm are distinct, they can be easily separated. In order to provide smooth boundaries, we apply the quadratic splines to postprocess the boundaries of each segmented cell.

Table 1. Segmentation accuracy(%) using the concave vertex graph. The $accuracy_c$ and $accuracy_n$ represent the segmentation accuracy for cytoplasm and nuclei respectively.

	Benign	CLL	MCL	FCC	AML	ALL
$accuracy_c$ (%) of touching cells	90.1	90.8	86.4	86.9	86.3	85.2
$accuracy_n$ (%) of touching cells	92.3	91.2	88.1	88.7	87.5	87.9
$accuracy_c$ (%) of all cells	92.5	91.7	87.2	89.1	88.5	87.6
$accuracy_n$ (%) of all cells	95.8	92.8	90.1	91.0	88.9	89.2

Table 2. The segmentation accuracy(%) using the watershed algorithm and the concave vertex graph

	Mean	Variance	Median	Min	Max	80%
Watershed	74.3	9.8	75.1	65.4	82.7	72.9
Concave Vertex Graph	88.9	5.1	90.2	75.2	95.5	87.1

5 Experiments

The cell database consists of a mixed set of 86 hematopathology cases: 18 Mantle Cell Lymphoma (MCL), 20 Chronic Lymphocytic Leukemia (CLL), 9 Follicular Center Cell Lymphoma (FCC), 18 Acute Lymphocytic Leukemia (ALL), 19 Acute Myelocytic Leukemia (AML), and 19 benign cases. For each case, there are varying number of cell images from 10 to 90. In total there exists 3898 cell images in our complete database. All the cases were generated from the archives of City of Hope Hospital in California, University of Pennsylvania of School of Medicine, Spectrum Health System, Grand Rapids, MI and Robert Wood Johnson Medical School, University of Medicine & Density of New Jersey.

The imaging platform for the experiments consisted of an Intel-based workstation interfaced with a high-resolution Olympus DP70 camera equipped with 12-bit color depth on each color channel and 1.45 million pixel effective resolution. The system also includes a single 2/3 inch CCD digital camera, an Olympus AX70 microscope equipped with a Prior 6-way robotic stage, motorized objective turret and a magnification changer.

We compare the segmentation results with manually segmentation. Two sets of experiments are performed.

- The 207 touching cases of the histopathology cell image dataset.
- The complete database which contains 3898 histopathology cell images.

Figure 4 shows some segmentation results. In Table 1 we present the segmentation accuracies for the six different classes of lymphocytes in two set of experiments. We obtained an average accuracy 88.9% on the touching cells dataset and 90.1% on the complete database.

Only a limited number of recent literature addresses the issue of touching cells segmentation in histopathology images using hematoxylin staining in high resolution (60× in our case). The watershed algorithm [4] is widely accepted for touching object segmentation and successfully used in segmenting histopathology images [13]. We compared our method with watershed using the 207 touching cell image dataset and listed the results in Table 2. The 80% column in Table 2 represents the sorted 80% highest accuracy of all the results, and is commonly used by doctors to evaluate the usability of the system. The experiments demonstrate the superior performance of the presented approach.

6 Conclusion

In this paper, a novel segmentation algorithm has been proposed to address the challenges of touching cell segmentation in hematologic specimens. The results are validated using real clinical data containing six classes of hematologic blood cell images. We compare our algorithm with watershed and experimentally show the superior performance of the proposed algorithm.

For general pixel grouping problem using a normal graph, the optimization problem is NP-hard. Only certain cost function can be *approximately* solved using algorithm like normalized cut [14] in polynomial time. In our algorithm, the cost function is designed to meet the domain specific requirements. The concave vertex graph, which utilize the concave points of the outer contour, reduce the search space to the shortest pathes in the constructed graph G. Based on a MATLAB implementation, the algorithm can finish in less than 2 seconds for an 128×128 image.

References

1. Rozman, C., Montserrat, E.: Chronic lymphocytic leukemia. The New England Journal of Medicine 333(16), 1052–1057 (1995)
2. Cotran, R., Kumar, V., Collins, T., Robbins, S.: Pathologic basis of disease, 5th edn. W.B. Saunders Company, Philadelphia (1994)
3. Aisenberg, A.: Coherent view of non-Hodgkin's lymphoma. J. Clin. Oncol. 13, 2656–2675 (1995)
4. Moga, A.N., Gabbouj, M.: Parallel marker-based image segmentation with watershed transformation. Journal of Parallel and Distributed Computing 51(1), 27–45 (1998)
5. Grau, V., Mewes, A.U.J., Alcaniz, M., Kikinis, R., Warfield, S.K.: Improved watershed transform for medical image segmentation using prior information. ITMI 23(4), 447–458 (2004)
6. Nguyen, H.T., Ji, Q.: Improved watershed segmentation using water diffusion and local shape priors. CVPR 1, 985–992 (2006)
7. Scott, D.W.: Parametric statistical modeling by minimum integrated square error. Technometrics 43, 274–285 (2001)
8. Yang, L., Meer, P., Foran, D.: Unsupervised segmentation based on robust estimation and color active contour models. IEEE Trans. on Information Technology in Biomedicine 9, 475–486 (2005)
9. Wyszecki, G., Stiles, W.S.: Color Science: Concepts and Methods, Quantitative Data and Formulae, 2nd edn. Wiley, Chichester (1982)

10. Chetverikov, D., Szabó, Z.: A simple and efficient algorithm for detection of high curvature points in planar curves. In: The 23rd Workshop of the Austrian Pattern Recognition Group, pp. 175–184 (1999)
11. Stahl, J.S., Wang, S.: Convex grouping combining boundary and region information. ICCV 2, 946–953 (2005)
12. Elder, J.H., Goldberg, R.M.: Ecological statistics of Gestalt laws for the perceptual organization of contours. Journal of Vision 2(4), 324–353 (2002)
13. Adiga, P.S.U., Chaudhuri, B.B.: An efficient method based on watershed and rule-based merging for segmentation of 3D histo-pathological images. J. Pattern Recognition 34(7), 1449–1458 (2001)
14. Cai, W., Chung, A.C.: Multi-resolution vessel segmentation using normalized cuts in retinal images. In: Larsen, R., Nielsen, M., Sporring, J. (eds.) MICCAI 2006. LNCS, vol. 4191, pp. 928–936. Springer, Heidelberg (2006)

Analysis of Surfaces Using Constrained Regression Models

Sune Darkner[1,2], Mert R. Sabuncu[3], Polina Golland[3], Rasmus R. Paulsen[2], and Rasmus Larsen[1]

[1] Department of Informatics and Mathematical Modelling, Technical University of Denmark, Denmark
sda@imm.dtu.dk
[2] Oticon A/S, Denmark
[3] Computer Science and Artificial Intelligence Laboratory, MIT, USA

Abstract. We present a study of the relationship between the changes in the shape of the human ear due to jaw movement and acoustical feedback (AF) in hearing aids. In particular, we analyze the deformation field of the outer ear associated with the movement of the mandible (jaw bone) to understand its effect on AF and identify local regions that play a significant role. Our data contains ear impressions of 42 hearing aid users, in two different positions: open and closed mouth, and survey data including information about experienced discomfort due to AF. We use weighted support vector machines (WSVM) to investigate the separation between the presence and lack of AF and achieve classification accuracy of 80% based on the deformation field. To robustly localize the regions of the deformation field that significantly contribute to AF we employ logistic regression penalized with elastic net (EN). By visualizing the selected variables on the mean surface, we provide clinical interpretations of the results.

1 Introduction

One of the big challenges for hearing aid users is acoustical feedback (AF). When a customized hearing aid is produced, the ventilation size and gain are adjusted accordingly. However, when the ear changes shape due to movement of the mandible, false leaks and feedback can occur. Modern feedback cancellation algorithms exist, but they rely on the detection of feedback. The time lag between detection and cancellation causes a squeaking sound when a person talks or chews. Identifying and characterizing the main causes of AF can improve hearing aid designs to minimize AF risk. In this paper, we investigate the relationship between the deformation of the outer ear and AF. We are interested in localizing regions that play a significant role in this phenomenon. In our experiments, we work with surface scans of ear impressions from 42 subjects under two different conditions: open and closed mouth and questionnaire data that includes information about AF-related experience. The ear impressions are co-registered using a group-wise registration algorithm via a kernel-based nonlinear deformation model. We analyze the intra subject deformation fields using a classification method to illustrate the differences between the two groups: subjects who experience AF and subjects who do not. Using Weighted Support Vector Machines, we achieve 80% cross-validation accuracy on our data. Additionally, we employ logistic elastic net regression (logistic EN) to identify the surface points that consistently explain the difference between the two populations. Generalization performance and statistical significance of the fitted model are used to determine the parameters of the regression algorithm. We compute statistical significance based on a standard likelihood ratio test and the effective degrees of freedom for the model similar to [1]. The model is shown to be significant with $p < 0.001$ on the whole data set.

2 Prior Work

Previous studies investigated the deformation of the ear canal and concha using calipers[2], and deformable shape models [3,4]. Yet, the relationship between deformations of the ear and clinical observations have so far not been explored. In other medical contexts, such as neuroimaging, the relationship between image-derived features and clinical data has been extensively studied [5]. A popular method used to explore differences between two groups in a population is Support Vector Machines (SVM) [6]. The discriminative direction of an SVM can be used to illustrate the differences between classes [7]. However, an important challenge in such approaches, is the interpretation of discriminant features. Another problem commonly presented by medical data is its unbalanced nature: there are typically more negative samples than positive examples. To handle this, we use weighted SVMs [8]. Medical imaging provides further challenges: samples are high dimensional and few. Moreover, we expect that some of these dimensions exhibit significant correlations. Our goal is ideally to discover *all* these dimensions. Ridge regression [9] (or, in general Tikhonov ℓ_2 regularization [10]) takes this type of underlying structure into account. Additionally, we expect that only a small number of dimensions are related to the clinical outcome of interest. This prior knowledge can be formalized using a constraint on the ℓ_1 norm of the regression coefficients [11]. Elastic Net (EN) [12] combines these two approaches to achieve a sparse and correlated set of predictors. A Bayesian interpretation of this method yields an efficient implementation [12]. The method has been extended to fit the generalized linear model framework enabling various types of regressions through the canonical link functions including logistic regression. Analyzing multi-subject medical data requires spatial correspondence, usually determined via image registration. Motivated by group-wise registration methods [13], we use a co-registration formulation that simultaneously aligns all surfaces. We employ a kernel-based nonlinear deformation model [14][15] to achieve a dense, diffeomorphic correspondence within and across subjects.

3 Data

The data consists of 84 impressions from 42 hearing aid users. Two impressions were obtained from each individual in different positions. (i) Normal position, chosen as reference, (ii) mouth opened. A spacer was used to ensure consistency with respect to the angle of the mouth opening. The impressions were all acquired from the subjects' right ear. Each impression consists of ≈ 5500 points in 3D i.e. vertices, corresponding to a 16500 dimensional feature vector. In addition to the shape data, the subjects filled out a questionnaire, including questions regarding acoustical feedback (AF). All subjects that experienced frequent AF problems (once a week or more) were grouped together if the annoyance was related to ear deformation, i.e. jaw movement and facial expressions. The latter is included because it often involves jaw movement. Thus, we obtained two groups: subjects who experience AF and subjects who do not.

4 Methods

4.1 Co-registration and Preprocessing

The ear impressions were scanned to obtain surfaces, which were then manually preprocessed to remove artifacts. We represent each surface as a triangular mesh S, with vertices denoted by $x_S \in S \subset \mathbb{R}^3$. The registration framework is based on the method described in [16], which uses the difference between signed distance maps of the two surfaces S_1 and S_2 to compute a similarity metric. For computational efficiency, the distance is only computed on a narrow band $Q \subset \mathbb{R}^3$ that covers both surfaces, i.e., $Q \supset S_1, S_2$. The distance between S_1 and S_2 is then defined as:

$$f(S_1, S_2) = \frac{1}{\|Q\|} \sum_{x \in Q} (d_{S_1}(x) - d_{S_2}(x))^2, \quad (1)$$

where d_S denotes the signed distance map of the surface S and $\|Q\|$ denotes the volume of Q. The pairwise registration problem is formulated as the minimization of Eq. 1 and solved using Newton's method. We parameterize the deformations using a kernel-based approach [15] defined on a control grid in a coarse-to-fine fashion, from $2^3 - 40^3$ control points. The gradient of the objective function with respect to this parametrization can be easily computed. We extend this approach to a multi-subject setting by defining a mean surface $S_\mu = \frac{1}{N} \sum_i S_i$, where N is the number of subjects. The mean surface is updated at every iteration and a set of transformation parameters is computed for each subject based on its distance to the mean surface. To anchor the deformations, we constrain the average deformation across all subjects to be identity. In other words, the mean of the deformation parameters is zero.

4.2 Classification and Regression

Our goal is to analyze the deformation fields obtained from the co-registration step to show differences between subjects who experience Acoustical Feedback (AF) and subjects who do not. Ground truth labels were based on the questionnaire data, as described in Section 3. The localized nature of the deformation parametrization allows us to identify regions that influence AF. We use the popular SVM method with no kernel to classify the data based on the whole deformation field. Since our data contained 18 positive samples and 24 negative samples, we investigated weighted SVM (WSVM) [8]. In contrast with SVM where the penalty of misclassification is universal, WSVM sets a different penalty for each class and the the ratio between class penalties are inversely proportional to the class size ratio. In our experiments, this approach improves results by about 5% when compared with the uniform penalty on errors. Due to the challenges of interpreting the discriminant features, i.e., support vectors in the SVM experiment, we explored a logistic regression approach. Logistic regression models the probability P of a certain outcome, in our case subjects who experience AF and is estimated by the ratio of occurrences. This is accomplished through the canonical link $\log(\frac{p_i}{1-p_i})$, known as the log-odds or logit. Standard logistic regression can thus be formulated as:

$$\log\left(\frac{p_i}{1-p_i}\right) = \beta_0 + \boldsymbol{\beta}\mathbf{x_i}, \forall i \qquad (2)$$

where β_0 is the intercept, $\boldsymbol{\beta}$ is the regression coefficients of size 1× number of dimensions (16,500 in our case) and $\mathbf{x_i}$ is a column vector that represents an observation. Logistic elastic net extends standard logistic regression by penalizing the parameters $\boldsymbol{\beta}$ with the ℓ_1 and ℓ_2 penalty.

$$\log\left(\frac{p_i}{1-p_i}\right) = \beta_0 + \boldsymbol{\beta}\mathbf{x_i} + \epsilon_i, \quad \text{s.t.} \ \|\boldsymbol{\beta}\|^2 < \rho, |\boldsymbol{\beta}| < \xi \qquad (3)$$

for some $\rho, \xi > 0$ and for all i. The solution can be found via a MAP approach where the following prior on the parameters is used:

$$P_{\lambda,\alpha}(\boldsymbol{\beta}) = C(\lambda,\alpha)e^{-\lambda(\alpha\|\boldsymbol{\beta}\|^2 + (1-\alpha)\|\boldsymbol{\beta}\|)}, \qquad (4)$$

where λ is the hyper-parameter that determines the total amount of regularization, α determines the trade-off between the two penalty terms and C is the normalization. Logistic EN has the properties of ridge regression and yields sparse solutions thanks to the ℓ_1 constraint. Thus the model takes covariations into account while only consisting of a small subset of significant regression coefficients. This yields dimensionality reduction conditioned on the information in the data set.

5 Model Validation and Selection

We use cross-validation to select the hyper-parameters α and λ. Furthermore, by using the likelihood ratio test, we can ensure that the selected parameters yield statistically significant models, i.e., explain the data well. The likelihood ratio computes $\Lambda = \frac{L(\boldsymbol{\beta}|\mathbf{X})}{L(\beta_0|\mathbf{X})}$, where the numerator $L(\boldsymbol{\beta})$ is the log-likelihood of the fitted model, defined as:

$$L(\boldsymbol{\beta}|\mathbf{X}) = \sum_{i=1}^{N}\left[y_i\boldsymbol{\beta}^t\mathbf{x_i} - \log(1 + \exp(\boldsymbol{\beta}^t\mathbf{x_i}))\right], \qquad (5)$$

where $y_i \in \{0,1\}$ is the ground truth label, β_0 is included in $\boldsymbol{\beta}$ and $\mathbf{x_i}$ is the i'th observation in $\mathbf{X}$, the data to which the model is fitted. $L(\beta_0)$ is the null-hypothesis likelihood, computed with $\boldsymbol{\beta} = 0$. Note that $(-2\log \Lambda)$ is approximately χ^2 distributed with a parameter equal to the effective degrees of freedom of the model minus 1. Following [17], we can compute the effective degrees of freedom as $\sum_{j=1}^{P} \frac{\alpha_i}{\alpha_i + \lambda}$, where P is the number of dimensions and $\{\alpha_i\}$ are the eigenvalues of the data matrix $\mathbf{X}^T\mathbf{X}$.

6 Analysis

The analysis is divided into two parts, classification and regression. Performing classification demonstrates the difference between the two classes. To reveal how the deformation field relates to AF problem regression is performed. We fit a logistic regression model *to each variable i.e. vertex* independently and selects the significant models as determined by the likelihood test to identify *significant variables*. This approach does not take covariances into account since each variable is treated independently. We use logistic EN on all the data to perform variable selection while accounting for covariances. Logistic EN provides better and more robust localization, which yields interpretable results. Yet, SVM is typically superior with respect to classification accuracy.

6.1 Classification

To investigate if the data set size is sufficient for generalization, we use SVM to classify and perform cross validation (100 random trials) with an increasing number of samples included in the training set. The purpose is to investigate whether including further samples will improve the classification. The test error for each class vs. the number of samples included in the model is plotted in Fig. 1(c). From the figure it is clear that better results could be obtained with more data, however, the test error is around 22-25%, clearly showing separation in the data. Using WSVM reduces the error further to 20%. Fig. 2 illustrates the variable weights on a mean surface in four representative random trials. Comparing these four trials, one sees that even though the general patterns seem to be consistent, there is significant noise and the localization quality is not sufficient. Fig. 2(e)shows the frequency of each variable appearing in the top 20% quantile over all 100 trials. We notice that variables robustly (red regions) appearing in the top 20% quantile are sparse.

6.2 Regression

To get a base line, we perform a logistic regression of each parameter against the response variable. The significant variables are shown in Fig. 4(a), where red indicates a significant model. As can be seen significant variables cluster nicely. However, we expect significance in and around the canal as well, which is not present in this figure. This is due to the fact that each variable is treated

Analysis of Surfaces Using Constrained Regression Models 847

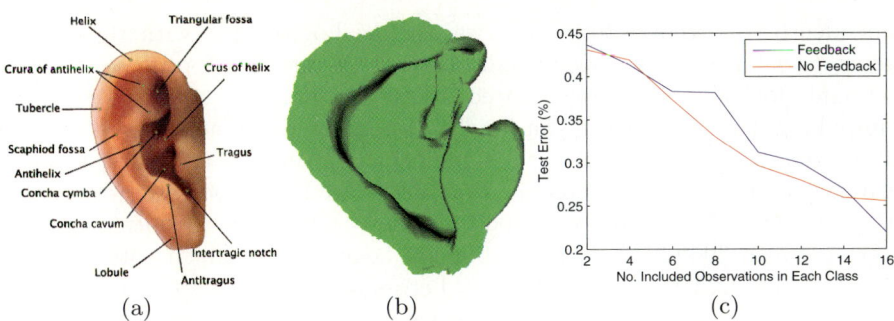

Fig. 1. (a) An anatomical atlas of the ear. (b) A typical ear impression. (c) Number of parameters for each class included in the model vs. the test error.

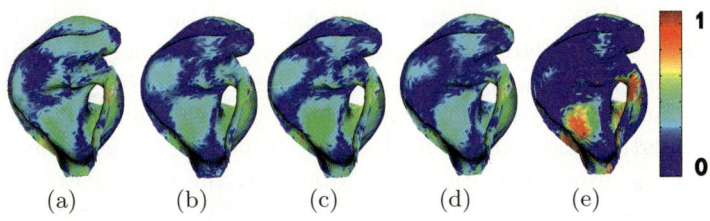

Fig. 2. The normalized coefficients from the SVM solution for 4 random cross validation iterations mapped to the mean surface.(e) the frequency of each vertex appearing in the to 20% quantile.

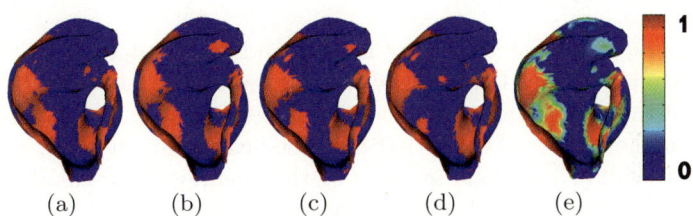

Fig. 3. The selected coefficients from the penalized logistic regression solution for 4 different cross validation iterations mapped to the mean surface. Red indicate a selected variable.3(e) Is the cross-validated probability of a variable being selected.

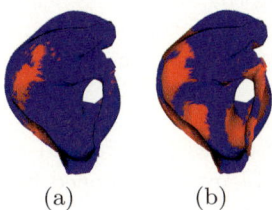

Fig. 4. (a) The significant logistic regression models on each variable mapped to the mean surface. (b) The selected variables of the full logistic EN regression model mapped to the mean surface. Red indicate a selected model/variable/vertex.

independently. To recover from this, we use the Logistic EN with the hyperparameters determined by cross validation and the likelihood ratio test. From the formula for effective degrees of freedom we can make an educated guess of the initial regularization parameter for the ℓ_2-penalty, which needs to be around 1000 for the model to be statistical significant. An interval around this value is searched to find a suitable combination where the likelihood ratio rejects the null hypothesis. This yields $\lambda = 1000$ and $\alpha = 0.997$. The resulting models contain between 2000-2500 variables but are heavily constrained with 2-3 free parameters. To validate the model, 10-fold cross validation is performed with an equal number of observations from each class used in training, which yields 73% accuracy for both classes. The regularization in the model increases test error to 5-10%. A representative selection of the resulting cross validation models can be seen in Fig. 3. We note that the models are consistent over different runs. Having estimated the regularization parameters we build a model on the full data set. The model is shown in Fig. 4(b). The estimated degrees of freedom for the model is 3.88, the model is significantly better than H_0 ($p < 0.001$). The resulting model is in very good correspondence with the individual models from the cross validation and includes far more of the surface in the model compared to the logistic regression in Fig. 4(a). Moreover, the logistic EN gives better and more consistent localization compared to the SVM, and the results are less noisy (Fig. 2 and Fig. 3). In addition the results are in good correspondence with clinical observations.

6.3 Clinical interpretation

The results are consistent with how hearing aids are situated in the ear. It is interesting that not only the entrance to the canal is important, but also the lower part of the outer ear, tragus and anti tragus (see Fig. 1(a)). The reason is that its often one or both of these that hold the hearing aid in place. The small In The Ear devices (ITE) are held in place by the opening of the canal and Tragus, where as Behind The Ear aids (BTE) are molded to the entire concha (most of the impression). Also the deformation, which we know occur deeper inside the canal seems to have little influence on the acoustical feedback. Only the bottom part of the inner canal seems to have a small influence, which corresponds to clinical observations made during normal practice. The results in Fig. 4(b) lead to the possibility of improving the fit with respect to feedback.

7 Conclusion

By using constrained logistic regression, we find parts of the ear canal surface that explain the feedback problems experienced by users. The regression model gives good localization and the outcome is easy to interpret. Furthermore, by using an extended framework for estimation of the free parameters in the model, a cross validation scheme based on significant models can be used. We show that the final model is significant ($p < 0.001$). In addition, we show that a classifier based on the WSVM can achieve a classification accuracy of 80% for both classes, with the possibility of improvement if more data were available.

References

1. Zou, H., Hastie, T., Tibshirani, R.: On the "degrees of freedom" of the lasso. Annals of Statistics 35(5), 2173–2192 (2007)
2. Oliviera, R., Hammer, B., Stillman, A., Holm, J., Jons, C., Margolis, R.: A look at ear canal changes with jaw motion. Ear and Hearing 13(6), 464–466 (1992)
3. Paulsen, R.R., Larsen, R., Laugesen, S., Nielsen, C., Ersbøll, B.K.: Building and testing a statistical shape model of the human ear canal. In: Dohi, T., Kikinis, R. (eds.) MICCAI 2002. LNCS, vol. 2489. Springer, Heidelberg (2002)
4. Darkner, S., Paulsen, R.R., Larsen, R.: Analysis of deformation of the human ear and canal caused by mandibular movement. In: Ayache, N., Ourselin, S., Maeder, A. (eds.) MICCAI 2007, Part II. LNCS, vol. 4792, pp. 801–808. Springer, Heidelberg (2007)
5. Sjoestrand, K., Cardenas, V.A., Larsen, R., Studholme, C.: A generalization of voxel-wise procedures for high-dimensional statistical inference using ridge regression. In: SPIE Medical Imaging (2008)
6. Boser, B., Guyon, I., Vapnik, V.: A training algorithm for optimal margin classifiers. In: Fifth Annual Workshop on Computational Learning Theory, pp. 144–152 (1992)
7. Golland, P.: Discriminative direction for kernel classifiers. In: NIPS, pp. 745–752 (2001)
8. Liu, S., Jia, C.Y., Ma, H.: A new weighted support vector machine with ga-based parameter selection, vol. 7, pp. 4351–4355 (2005)
9. Hoerl, A.E., Kennard, R.W.: Ridge regression: Biased estimation for nonorthogonal problems. Technometrics 12, 55–67 (1970)
10. Tikhonov, A.N.: Solutions of incorrectly formulated problems and the regularization method. Soviet Math. Dokl. 4, 1035–1038 (1963)
11. Tibshirani, R.: Regression shrinkage and selection via the lasso. J. R. Statist. Soc. B 58(1), 267–288 (1996)
12. Zou, H., Hastie, T.: Regularization and variable selection via the elastic net. J. R. Statist. Soc. B 67(part 2), 301–320 (2005)
13. Zöllei, L., Learned-Miller, E., Grimson, E., Wells, W.M.: Efficient population registration of 3d data. In: ICCV (2005)
14. Rueckert, D., Sonoda, L.I., Hayes, C., Hill, D.L.G., Leach, M.O., Hawkes, D.J.: Non-rigid registration using free-form deformations: Application to breast mr images. IEEE Transactions on Medical Imaging 18(8), 712–721 (1999)
15. Cootes, T., Twining, C., Taylor, C.: Diffeomorphic statistical shape models. In: Proc. British Machine Vision Conference, vol. 1, pp. 447–456 (2004)
16. Dakner, S., Vester-Christensen, M., Paulsen, R.R., Larsen, R.: Non-rigid surface registration of 2D manifolds in 3D euclidian space. In: SPIE Medical Imaging (2008)
17. Malthouse, E.C.: Shrinkage estimation and direct marketing scoring models 13(4), 10–23 (1999)

A Global Approach for Automatic Fibroscopic Video Mosaicing in Minimally Invasive Diagnosis

Selen Atasoy[1,3], David P. Noonan[2], Selim Benhimane[3],
Nassir Navab[3], and Guang-Zhong Yang[1,2]

[1] Department of Computing, Imperial College London
[2] Institute of Biomedical Engineering, Imperial College London
{catasoy,dnoonan,g.z.yang}@imperial.ac.uk
[3] Chair for Computer Aided Medical Procedures (CAMP), Technische Universität München
{atasoy,benhiman,navab}@cs.tum.edu

Abstract. Recent developments in bio-photonics have called for the need of bringing cellular and molecular imaging modalities to an in vivo – in situ setting to allow for real-time tissue characterization and functional assessment. Before such techniques can be used effectively in routine clinical environments, it is necessary to address the visualization requirement for linking point based optical biopsy to large area tissue visualization. This paper presents a novel approach for fibered endoscopic video mosaicing that permits wide region tissue visualization. A feature-based registration method is used to register the frames of the endoscopic video sequence by taking into account the characteristics of fibroscopic imaging such as non-linear lens distortion and high-frequency fiber optic facet pattern. The registration is combined with an efficient optimization scheme in order to align all input frames in a globally consistent way. An evaluation on phantom and *ex vivo* tissue images allowing free-hand camera motion is presented.

Keywords: Image mosaicing, visualization for diagnosis, fibered endoscopy.

1 Introduction

Fibered Endoscopic (fibroscope) systems are frequently used to visualize intra-luminal abnormalities ranging from benign polyps and lesions to carcinoma *in situ*, especially in constricted anatomical regions, where higher resolution tip-mounted camera systems are not suitable. The diagnosis of such abnormalities is generally based on initial visual inspection followed by necessary biopsy. Recent developments in bio-photonics have resulted in a major paradigm shift and clinical demand in bringing cellular and molecular imaging modalities to an *in vivo – in situ* setting to allow for real-time tissue characterization and functional assessment. Before such techniques can be used effectively in routine clinical environments, it is necessary to address the visualization requirement for linking point based optical biopsy to large area tissue visualization. The essence of this multi-scale integration problem is similar to video mosaicing.

In computer vision, image mosaicing is a well explored subject for stitching together sequential images with partial overlapping areas to create a seamless panoramic image with a widened field-of-view (FOV). The primary challenge is the registration of multiple partially overlapping images into a common coordinate system, or in other words, estimating the 3×3 homographic matrices mapping each frame to a chosen reference coordinate system. In theory, registration of image pairs which do not directly overlap can be performed by concatenation of pair-wise transformations of directly overlapping images. However, this can lead to the accumulation of small registration errors resulting in a large misalignment in the final mosaic [1, 2].

In medical imaging, mosaicing has been mainly used for retinal images [3-5]. For endoscopic images, Miranda-Luna *et al.* presented a method for the mosaicing of bladder endoscopic image sequences [6] using mutual information based image registration. In order to overcome the error accumulation, "back correction" with loop closing is proposed. Other applications include placenta image mosaicing [7], where global methods for improved alignment have been proposed. Vercauteren [8] presents a robust framework for endoscopic microconfocal image mosaicing. The method applies a tracking algorithm developed in the field of vision-based robot control for real-time applications [9]. The optimal global alignment of each image in the final mosaic is computed by defining the registration as an optimization problem on a Lie group. Unfortunately, the application of this technique is only possible for small inter-frame displacements.

The purpose of this paper is to present a novel endoscopic video mosaicing technique allowing free hand camera motion. To cater for potentially large inter-frame displacements, scale invariant feature transform (SIFT) and a descriptor-based matching is used [10]. A novel robust simultaneous approach for global alignment is proposed to overcome error accumulation. The method also takes into account non-linear lens distortions and high-frequency facet pattern introduced by the fibroscope. A mosaic validation with free hand camera motion is presented and results are evaluated with phantom and *ex vivo* tissue experiments.

2 Materials and Methods

2.1 Experiment Setup

In this paper, the fibroscopic video sequences are recorded using free-hand data acquisition by a laparoscopic test rig as shown in Fig. 1. The system features a flexible, coherent fibre image guide (Sumitomo IGN-05/10, 10,000 fibres, length 1.5 m, outer diameter 0.59mm) running down a rigid shaft in a configuration similar to a laparoscope. A graded index (GRIN) lens (Grintech GmbH) is cemented onto the end of the image guide (diameter 0.5mm, working distance 10mm, NA 0.5) to image an area of 35×35mm^2 at a working distance of 20mm onto the distal end of the image guide. The proximal end of the image guide is imaged onto a CCD camera (UEye, UI-2250-C/CM) using an achromatic ×10 microscope objective and 100mm focal length lens. The camera is pivoted around a point 174mm from its optical centre to simulate a laparoscope passing through a trocar port.

The camera motion introduced involves both rotation and translation of the camera centre. With such an arbitrary camera motion, correct mosaicing is only possible if the observed object is planar since the scene plane would introduce a homography

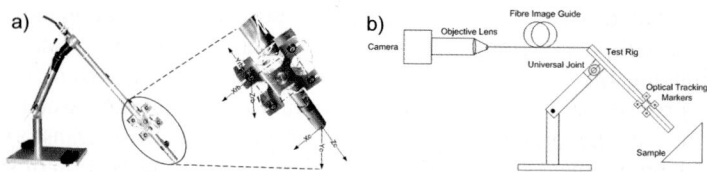

Fig. 1. (a) shows the fibroscope test-rig used to capture data. The optical tracking markers used to validate the results and the co-ordinate systems of the camera (x_c, y_c, z_c) and the rigid body defined by the markers, (x_{rb}, y_{rb}, z_{rb}) are also shown. (b) illustrates the schematic of the designed system.

between different views. The images captured by the fibroscope expose a small part of tissue surface. Therefore, the scene observed can be approximated as a planar surface patch. To correct for non-linear radial lens distortion before processing the images, camera calibration is performed to derive intrinsic parameters and radial distortion coefficients of the camera [11].

2.2 Feature Extraction

To achieve a fully automatic image mosaicing, a feature based approach is used. The detection of interest points in each frame is performed by extracting distinctive SIFT features [10]. The contribution of using SIFT features to create panaromic image mosaics is originally documented by Brown and Lowe [2]. SIFT features are detected at scale space extrema using a difference-of-Gaussian function leading to invariance in scale-change. At each feature location, an orientation is assigned based on local image gradients, which provides invariance to image rotation. The scale, location and orientation are represented by a distinctive descriptor vector and the use of image gradients and the normalization of the descriptor vector allows for the invariance to affine illumination changes. As no prior information about the anatomy of the tissue is present, a high-level feature extraction such as anatomical landmarks or vascular structures is not possible in the current experiment settings. Therefore, the reliability of the feature matching is crucial to the overall accuracy of the system.

It should be noted that the use of coherent fibre bundle can also introduce unwanted structural artifacts due to the boundary of individual fibre elements [6]. This is catered for in our method by avoiding small scale SIFT features. Only keypoints detected at a scale $\sigma^2 \geq t$ (with t being the scale threshold) are considered as interest points. Considering the frequency of the introduced fiber optic facet pattern we use $t = 2$ for our video sequences.

2.3 Feature Matching

After the extraction of SIFT keypoints, the match between them is established for each overlapping image pair. The matching process is performed by finding the nearest neighbor of each keypoint based on the Euclidean distance of the two descriptor vectors. In order to discard unreliable matches, a match is accepted only if the distance ratio of the first- and second-nearest neighbors is less then a prescribed threshold, where the threshold used determines the level of matching reliability. A value of

0.6 is used based on the statistics provided by Lowe [10]. Among all possible correspondences, the outliers are eliminated using a robust estimator. The homography between each overlapping image pair is estimated using Maximum Likelihood Sample Consensus (MLESAC) estimator [13] and only the feature matches that are consistent with this homography are used for global alignment.

MLESAC maximizes the likelihood $p(\varepsilon_H | H)$ of observing the error ε_H if H is the correct homography ($C_{\text{MLESAC}} = \arg\max_H [p(\varepsilon_H | H)]$). This leads to the minimization of the following function:

$$C_{\text{MLESAC}} = \arg\min_H \left[-\log\left(\left(\frac{1}{\sigma\sqrt{2\pi}}\exp\left(-\varepsilon_H^2/2\sigma^2\right)\right)p(\nu) + \left(\frac{1}{n}\right)(1 - p(\nu))\right) \right] \quad (1)$$

where ν is a mixing parameter controlling the relative importance of the probability distribution of the inliers and outliers, and n is a constant representing the uniform distribution of the outliers. Since MLESAC cannot yield a reliable homography using insufficient amount of point correspondences, we only use the homographies with a sufficient number of inliers. To consider only the image pairs with minimum 25 correspondences and a minimum inlier percentage of 80%, this number is chosen as 15.

2.4 Global Alignment

After the extraction and matching of feature points between overlapping image pairs, the homographies that map each frame to the reference frame are calculated by considering all overlapping images at the same time. An observed pair-wise homography $H_{i,j}$ between two directly overlapping frames I_i and I_j can be expressed as a combination of the global homographies $H_{i,j} = H_i^{-1} H_j$, where H_i and H_j map frames I_i and I_j to the reference frame, respectively. Let $F(i,j)$ be a set of feature matches between frame I_i and frame I_j and $P(i)$ be the set of frames directly overlapping frames with frame I_i. For each feature match $(p_m^i, p_n^j) \in F(i,j)$, where p_m^i denotes the position of m-th feature in frame I_i, we have an error vector $\varepsilon = p_m^i - (H_i^{-1} \cdot H_j) p_n^j$ caused by the image noise (or possibly by a mismatch). Note that ε is normalized and inhomogeneous coordinates are used. In this paper, we compute the global homographies successively for each frame by minimizing the reprojection error. To this end, two different alignment strategies are used. The first of these is *group-wise alignment*. With this method, the global homography H_i of a frame I_i is computed by considering all frames overlapping with frame I_i at the same time. This leads to minimization of the following objective function:

$$H_i^* = \arg\min_{H_i} \sum_{j \in P(i), (j<i)} \sum_{(p_m^i, p_n^j) \in F(i,j)} \omega(i,j) \cdot C(p_m^i - (H_i^{-1} \cdot H_j) p_n^j) \quad (2)$$

where C is the Huber cost function used to ensure the reprojection error is robust with σ being the expected image noise in pixels (In this paper we use $\sigma = 2$)

$$C(\mathbf{x}) = \begin{cases} |\mathbf{x}| & \text{for } |\mathbf{x}| < \sigma \\ 2\sigma|\mathbf{x}| - \sigma^2 & \text{otherwise.} \end{cases} \quad (3)$$

In Eq. (2), ω is a weight function assigning a quality weight to each pairwise homography depending on the number of feature matches between them, i.e. $\omega(i,j) = |F(i,j)| / |\sum_{k \in P(i)} F(i,k)|$. To minimize this non-linear least squares function, Levenberg-Marquardt minimization algorithm is used. Concerning the fact that the global homographies of two consecutive frames do not differ considerably, the parameters H_{i+1} of a new frame are initialized with the homography of the previous frame H_i. This alignment strategy is successfully performed in bundle-adjustment techniques, where for each new frame in a video sequence, the camera parameters and 3D feature positions are estimated jointly by minimizing the reprojection error over all features [2, 14].

A second strategy considered is *simultaneous alignment*. When using the groupwise alignment method, only the parameters of the current homography are updated by the minimization process. This means that the previously computed homographies are assumed to be optimal. However, with each new acquired frame new information is acquired, which can change the optimal solution for previous homographies. For this reason, we propose a new alignment strategy, where for each frame not only the parameters of the current homography, but also the parameters of all previously computed homographies, are updated. Note that the homographies of images which do not directly overlap with the new image are also updated as their optimal solution can depend on another updated homography. For each frame, the new objective function can therefore be minimized as:

$$[H_1^*, \ldots H_i^*] = \arg \min_{[H_1,\ldots,H_i]} \sum_{k=1}^{i} \sum_{j \in P(k),(j<k)} \sum_{(p_m^k, p_n^j) \in F(k,j)} \omega(k,j) \cdot C(p_m^k - (H_k^{-1} \cdot H_j) p_n^j) \quad (4)$$

At each step, all homographies are initialized with their optimal solutions from the previous step and the homography parameters of the newly introduced frame as the optimal homography of the previous frame.

2.5 Multi-band Blending

After warping each frame with the corresponding global homography, multi-band blending algorithm as described in [2] is used to create a seamless mosaic image. The use of this blending method is necessary because specular reflections and color shading due to the point light source of the laparoscopic camera and possible registration errors due to the parallax effect can lead to blurring of the final mosaic image if a simple average process is used. The idea of the multi-band blending is to partition the image in multiple frequency bands (3 bands in this study) to smooth out low frequencies while preserving the high frequencies. This leads to a seamless and smooth mosaic image with sharp high frequency details.

3 Experiment Results

To evaluate the practical value of the proposed technique, image sequences on a silicone soft tissue phantom and *ex vivo* kidney tissue are acquired using the experimental setup shown in Fig. 1. Fig. 2 illustrates the resulting mosaics for each video sequence created using the three alignment strategies; pair-wise homographies of consecutive frames, the group-wise and the simultaneous alignment strategies.

In the first experiment, 80 images of the phantom are captured while moving the camera in a closed loop. The use of pair-wise mosaicing leads to accumulation of the mis-registration error. A large misalignment between the two ends of the mosaic is evident in Fig 2-a(1) and Fig 2-b(1). Group-wise mosaicing provides improved alignment, although the error accumulation is still evident (Fig 2-a(2), Fig 2-a(3)). Simultaneous mosaicing leads to visually correct alignment in the final mosaic (Fig 2-a(3) and b(3)). In the second experiment, 80 images of *ex vivo* kidney tissue are acquired using a crescent-shaped camera motion. The pair-wise mosaicing results in misalignment of the line-like anatomical structures in the mosaic image as illustrated in Fig 2-c(1) and 2-d(1). The use of group-wise mosaicing improves the alignment of these structures (Fig 2-c(2), d(2)). Finally, a visually improved mosaic is achieved using the proposed simultaneous mosaicing technique (Fig 2-c(3), d(3)).

Due to the absence of real ground truth information, validation of image mosaicing is a difficult problem. Therefore, we track the camera motion using a NDI Optotrak Certus motion capture system (Northern Digital Inc, Canada) with four optical tracking markers attached to the shaft. These markers are defined as a rigid body with an

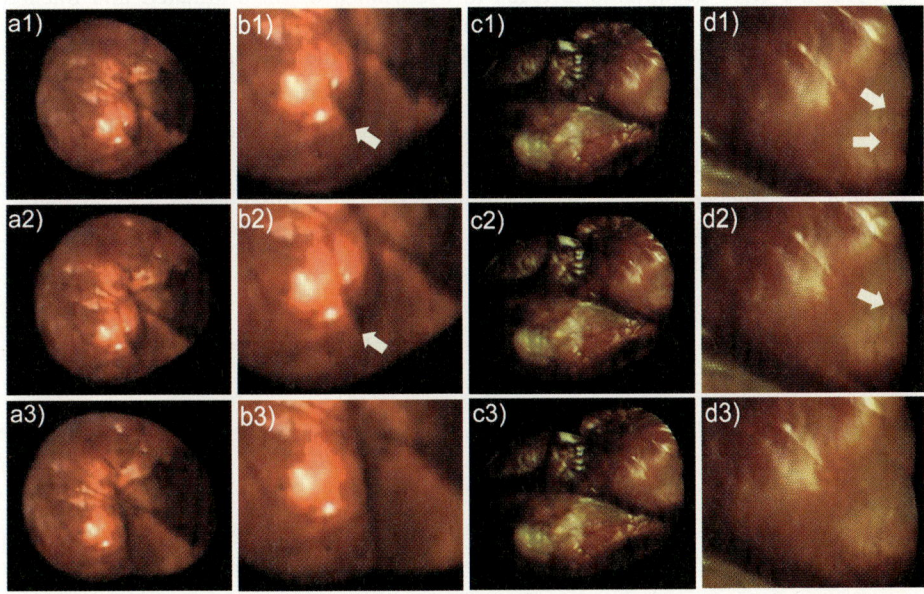

Fig. 2. A comparison of different image mosaicing results; (a1), (a2) and (a3) show using chained pair-wise homographies, group-wise alignment and simultaneous alignment, respectively; (b1), (b2) show the misalignment area in the first and second mosaic and (b3) shows the same area in the third mosaic; (c1), (c2) and (c3) show mosaics created using the three different strategies respectively. (d1), (d2) show the misalignment area in the first and second mosaic and (d3) shows the same area in the third mosaic.

origin located as shown in Fig. 1. A hand-eye calibration to compute the relative rotation and translation from the rigid body to the camera centre is then performed using the technique proposed by Tsai and Lens [12].

In an idealized situation and assuming that we observe a planar object, an image frame in the video sequence is related to the reference frame by a homography matrix $H = K(R + t \cdot n^T)K^{-1}$, where R and t are the relative rotations and translations of the camera centre with respect to first camera position respectively, n is the normal vector of the observed plane and d is the distance of the camera to the planar object. For each frame, we compute the relative rotation and translation of the camera with respect to the reference camera by decomposing the homographies as presented by Benhimane et al. [9]. Without knowing the distance and normal of the observed plane, the relative translations can only be estimated up to a scale factor. For each frame in the video sequence the tracked camera positions are compared to the estimated camera positions by decomposing the homographies which are computed using pair-wise, group-wise and simultaneous mosaicing. The results are illustrated Fig 3-(a) and Fig 3-(b). Changes in the scene depth can introduce small errors into the homographies due to the violation of the planarity assumption. This can be observed in the mismatch between the estimated and tracked camera paths after the 60. frame of the video sequence as shown in the marked region in Fig 3-(a) and Fig 3-(b). Furthermore, the error accumulation leads to a deviance of the estimated and tracked camera paths. It was observed that simultaneous mosaicing can best deal with this problem. This is illustrated in Fig 3-(c), which shows the normalized relative camera positions m_i computed as: $m_i = d_i / d_i^{gt} - \overline{d}_i / \overline{d}_i^{gt}$, where d_i and d_i^{gt} denote the estimated and tracked camera positions relative to the first camera, respectively and $\overline{d}_i$ and $\overline{d}_i^{gt}$ denote their mean values. This value is expected to be constant if the estimated and tracked camera paths correspond to each other up to a scale factor. Simultaneous mosaicing is shown to be more consistent with being similar to tracked camera path up to a scale factor.

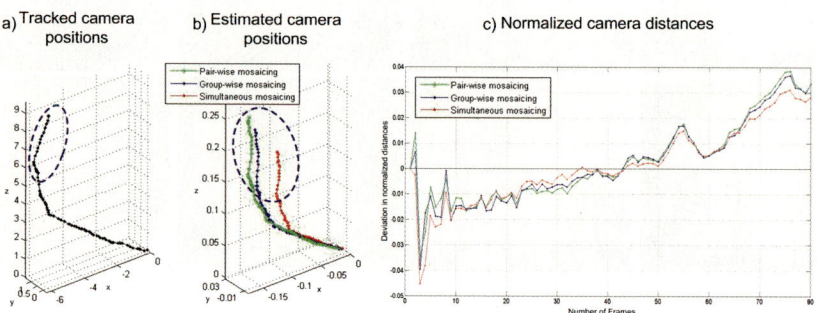

Fig. 3. (a) shows tracked camera positions and (b) shows camera positions estimated by decomposing the homographies computed by pair-wise, group-wise and simultaneous mosaicing methods. (c) shows the mean centered, ground truth normalized, relative camera positions to illustrate the proportionality of the tracked and estimated camera paths.

4 Conclusions

In this paper, we have presented a novel mosaicing technique for fibroscopic images. The proposed method takes into account particular properties introduced by the fibroscopic imaging such as lens distortions and fiber optic patterns. In order to overcome the error propagation in mosaicing, a new global alignment method is proposed. The accuracy of the presented method is demonstrated on *ex vivo* images of phantom and kidney tissue captured using free-hand camera motion. Future work will be to evaluate the accuracy of the proposed algorithm on *in vivo* studies and assess its potential clinical value.

Acknowledgments. The authors would like to thank Dan Elson, Danail Stoyanov and Adrian J. Chung for constructive discussions.

References

1. Shum, H.Y., Szeliski, R.: Panoramic Image Mosaics. Microsoft Research MSR-TR-97 23 (1997)
2. Brown, M., Lowe, D.G.: Automatic Panoramic Image Stitching using Invariant Features. International Journal of Computer Vision 74, 59–73 (2007)
3. Can, A., Stewart, C.V., Roysam, B., Tanenbaum, H.L.: A feature-based technique for joint, linear estimation of high-order image-to-mosaic transformations: mosaicing the curved human retina. IEEE Trans. on Pattern Analysis and Machine Intelligence 24, 412–419 (2002)
4. Choe, T.E., Cohen, I., Lee, M., Medioni, G.: Optimal Global Mosaic Generation from Retinal Images. International Conference on Pattern Recognition 03, 681–684 (2006)
5. Cattin, P.C., Bay, H., Van Gool, L., Szekely, G.: Retina Mosaicing Using Local Features. Medical Image Computing and Computer-Assisted Intervention. Springer, Heidelberg (2006)
6. Miranda-Luna, R., Daul, C., Blondel, W.C.P.M., Hernandez-Mier, Y., Wolf, D., Guillemin, F.: Mosaicing of Bladder Endoscopic Image Sequences: Distortion Calibration and Registration Algorithm. IEEE Trans. on Biomedical Engineering 55, 541–553 (2008)
7. Reeff, M., Gerhard, F., Cattin, P., Szekely, G.: Mosaicing of Endoscopic Placenta Images. GI Jahrestagung 93(1), 467–474 (2006)
8. Vercauteren, T.: Image Registration and Mosaicing for Dynami In Vivo Fibered Confocal Microscopy, PhD Thesis, Ecole des Mines de Paris (2008)
9. Benhimane, S., Malis, E.: Homography-based 2D Visual Tracking and Servoing. International Journal of Robotics Research 7, 661–676 (2007)
10. Lowe, D.G.: Distinctive Image Features from Scale-Invariant Keypoints. International Journal of Computer Vision 60, 91–110 (2004)
11. Zhang, Z.: A flexible new technique for camera calibration. IEEE Trans. on Pattern Analysis and Machine Intelligence 22(11), 1330–1334 (2000)
12. Tsai, R.Y., Lenz, R.K.: A new technique for fully autonomous and efficient 3D robotics hand-eye calibration. IEEE Trans. Robot Automat. 5(3), 345–358 (1989)
13. Torr, P.H.S., Zisserman, A.: MLESAC: a new robust estimator with application to estimating image geometry. Computer Vision and Image Understanding 78, 138–156 (2000)
14. Engels, C., Stewenius, H., Roysam, N.D.: Bundle Adjustment Rules. IEEE Trans. on Pattern Analysis and Machine Intelligence (PAMI) 24(3), 412–419 (2002)

Riemannian Framework for Estimating Symmetric Positive Definite 4th Order Diffusion Tensors

Aurobrata Ghosh[1], Maxime Descoteaux[2], and Rachid Deriche[1]

[1] Odyssee, INRIA Sophia Antipolis, France
Aurobrata.Ghosh@sophia.inria.fr
[2] NMR Lab, Neurospin, CEA Saclay, France

Abstract. DTI is an important tool to investigate the brain *in vivo* and non-invasively in spite of its shortcomings in regions of fiber-crossings. HARDI models such as QBI and Higher Order Tensors (HOT) were invented to overcome this shortcoming. HOTs, however, have not been explored extensively even though sophisticated estimation schemes were developed for DTI that guarantee positive diffusivity, such as the Riemannian framework. Positive diffusivity is an important constraint in diffusion MRI since it represents the physical phenomenon of molecular diffusion. It seems apt, to leverage the work done on DTI, to apply the positivity constraint to the HOT model. We, therefore, propose to extend the Riemannian framework from DTI to the space of 4th order diffusion tensors. We also review the existing methods for estimating 4th order diffusion tensors and compare all methods on synthetic, phantom and real datasets extensively to test for robustness and speed. Our contributions for extending the Riemannian framework from DTI to estimating 4th order diffusion tensors guarantees positive diffusivity, is robust, is fast, and can be used to discern multiple fiber directions.

1 Introduction

Diffusion Magnetic Resonance Imaging (dMRI) has proved to be an exquisite tool to investigate the anatomical connections of the human nervous system, *in vivo* and non-invasively. Diffusion Tensor Imaging (DTI) [1], was the first model proposed, and its value is only affirmed by its popularity till date. Its limitations are, however, well known in the regions that contain fiber-crossings. Recent High Angular Resolution Diffusion Imaging (HARDI) techniques have overcome that shortcoming with a plethora of new reconstruction schemes such as radial basis functions [2], Spherical Harmonics (SH) [3], Higher Order Tensors (HOT) [4] [5], etc. Notwithstanding its limitations, the DTI model has been extensively explored and sophisticated schemes for estimating it has been developed.

An important constraint in estimating DTI requires it to have a positive diffusivity profile, since it corresponds to the physical phenomenon of diffusion of water molecules. The sophisticated schemes for DTI rely on the native properties of the space of positive definite 2nd order diffusion tensors to guarantee the positive diffusivity profile. It seems appropriate, therefore, to explore HOT while leveraging the extensive framework already established for classical DTI. In this work, we propose a review and a comparison of the existing methods. We also propose an extension of the Riemannian framework [6][7] to the space of 4th order diffusion tensors. We compare our method to the other methods on synthetic, phantom and real data for robustness and speed.

The main contributions are directed towards extending the well established and tested Riemannian framework from DTI-2 to DTI-4. This provides a dMRI estimation method that guarantees positive diffusivity, is robust to noise, is computationally fast, and can also be used to discern multiple fiber directions.

2 Methods

To accommodate a multi-fiber distribution in a voxel, the Gaussian expression of the Stesjkal-Tanner equation was extended in [4], to incorporate a HOT of any order in the diffusivity function, generalizing it to $S = S_0 e^{-bD(\mathbf{g})}$ where $D(\mathbf{g}) = \sum_{j_1=1}^{3} \sum_{j_2=1}^{3} \cdots \sum_{j_k=1}^{3} D_{j_1 j_2 \ldots j_k} g_{j_1} g_{j_2} \cdots g_{j_k} = \mathbf{D}^k$. This generalization of DTI is sometimes referred to as GDTI-2. Another generalization along similar lines was done in [5], where the diffusivity function was written as $D(\mathbf{g}) = \mathbf{D}^2 + i\mathbf{D}^3 + \mathbf{D}^4 + i\mathbf{D}^5 + \ldots$, with $i = \sqrt{-1}$. This approach, sometimes referred to as GDTI-1, however, requires more complex aquisition and reconstruction techniques and therefore, we restrict ourselves to the GDTI-2 model. In GDTI-2 limiting k to 4 results in a 4th order diffusion tensor model. We now review the existing methods for estimating the 4th order diffusion tensor.

2.1 State of the Art

Least Squares (LS). The simplest approach to estimate the coefficients of a HOT, is to solve the over-determined linear least squares inverse problem, as suggested in [4]. This method is fast, is not limited to 4th order diffusion tensors but does not guarantee positive diffusivity, $D(\mathbf{g}) > 0 \ \forall \mathbf{g} \ st \ ||\mathbf{g}|| = 1$.

Ternary Quartic (TQ). In [8] the authors are the first to propose a method which guarantees positive diffusivity of the estimated 4th order diffusion tensor. They formulate the diffusivity function as a ternary quartic. Applying Hilbert's theorem on non-negative TQs, the diffusivity function is expressed as $D(\mathbf{g}) = (\mathbf{v}^T \mathbf{q}_1)^2 + (\mathbf{v}^T \mathbf{q}_2)^2 + (\mathbf{v}^T \mathbf{q}_3)^2 = \mathbf{v}^T \mathbf{Q} \mathbf{Q}^T \mathbf{v}$ where $\mathbf{Q}$ is estimated from the HARDI acquisitions, and the coefficients of the 4th order diffusion tensor – $\mathbb{A}$, are extracted from $\mathbf{Q}\mathbf{Q}^T$. Since $\mathbf{Q}$, however, can only determine $\mathbb{A}$ uniquely up to a rotation matrix, it is parameterized as $\mathbf{Q} = [\mathbf{B}, \mathbf{C}]^T = [\mathbf{TR}, \mathbf{C}]^T$ where $\mathbf{TR}$ is the qr-decomposition of $\mathbf{B}$ and $\mathbf{T}$ is taken to be $\mathbf{I}$ to reduce this indeterminacy. However, this method to reduce the number of parameters doesn't seem to have a physical explanation, and other methods may also exist. Also, this approach can only estimate positive semi-definite tensors due to its non-negative TQ formulation.

From Spherical Harmonics (SH). As proposed in [9], it is possible to compute the independent HOT coefficients from the even spherical harmonic coefficients of the same order. Since it is possible to use regularization to estimate the spherical harmonic coefficients, this provides another interesting method for estimating a HOT. This method is also extensible to any order, but again does not assure positive diffusivity.

2.2 Riemannian Approach (RM)

We now propose to extend the Riemannian framework from 2nd order diffusion tensors [6][7] to the space of 4th order tensors. First we consider 4th order tensors to be linear transformations $\mathbb{A} : Lin(V) \to Lin(V)$, where V is a vector space over $\mathbb{R}^n$ [10]. We can then define the double-dot-product $\mathbb{A} : \mathrm{D} = \mathbb{A}_{ijkl}\mathrm{D}_{kl}$ where D is a 2nd order tensor (T-2). Then we define the transpose $\langle \mathbb{A} : \mathrm{D} \mid \mathrm{C} \rangle = \langle \mathrm{D} \mid \mathbb{A}^t : \mathrm{C} \rangle$ using the inner-product $\langle . \mid . \rangle$ in the space of T-2s, and also define the inner-product in the space of 4th order tensors $\langle \mathbb{A} \mid \mathbb{B} \rangle = tr(\mathbb{A}^t\mathbb{B})$.

We then study the symmetries of 4th order tensors. As stated in [10] if a 4th order tensor has major and minor symmetries then it has 21 independent coefficients, in three dimensions, and has an eigen decomposition. If it satisfies total symmetry it has 15 independent coefficients. A proposition in [10] states that $\langle \mathbb{A}^s \mid \mathbb{B}^a \rangle = tr(\mathbb{A}^s\mathbb{B}^a) = 0$ where $\mathbb{B}^a$ is the remainder or anti-symmetric part that remains when the totally symmetric part $\mathbb{B}^s$ of a tensor is subtracted from itself $\mathbb{B}$ (see [10]).

When a 4th order tensor $\mathbb{A}$, in three dimensions, satisfies major and minor symmetries it can be mapped to a symmetric T-2 in 6 dimensions [11][10] (6x6) – A. And the double-dot-product $\mathbb{A} : \mathrm{D}$ can be rewritten as a matrix vector product $\mathbb{A} : \mathrm{D} = \mathrm{Ad}$, where $\mathrm{d} = [D_{11}, D_{22}, D_{33}, \sqrt{2}D_{12}, \sqrt{2}D_{13}, \sqrt{2}D_{23}]^T$. We can then rewrite the diffusivity function as $D(\mathbf{g}) = \mathrm{D}_i : \mathbb{A} : \mathrm{D}_i = tr(\mathbb{A}\mathbb{G}_i)$ where $\mathrm{D}_i = g_i \otimes g_i$ with $\otimes$ =outer-product and $\mathbb{G}_i = g_i \otimes g_i \otimes g_i \otimes g_i$ which is totally symmetric. Of course for computations we can use the equivalent matrix formulation $D(\mathbf{g}) = \mathrm{d}_i^t \mathrm{A} \mathrm{d}_i$.

We then proceed exactly as in [6] and estimate A in $S^+(6)$, the space of symmetric positive definite 6x6 matrices, by using the Riemannian metric defined in that space, with an M-estimator Ψ, minimizing the error energy function

$$E(\mathrm{A}) = \sum_{i=1}^{N} \Psi\left(-\frac{1}{b_i}\ln\left(\frac{S_i}{S_0}\right) + \mathrm{d}_i^t \mathrm{A} \mathrm{d}_i\right) \qquad (1)$$

as a non-linear gradient descent problem. Since A, is estimated in $S^+(6)$, the diffusivity function is guaranteed to be positive definite. We, however, realize that since A is estimated in $S^+(6)$, it has 21 independent coefficients, while a 4th order diffusion tensor is totally symmetric and has only 15 independent coefficients. This indeterminacy can be overcome by noticing that $\mathbb{G}$ is totally symmetric, therefore

$$D(\mathbf{g}) = tr(\mathbb{A}\mathbb{G}_i) = tr((\mathbb{A}^s + \mathbb{A}^a)\mathbb{G}_i) = tr(\mathbb{A}^s\mathbb{G}_i) \qquad (2)$$

where $\mathbb{A}^s$ contains the coefficients of the 4th order diffusion tensor and $\mathbb{A}^a$, the residue, contains the excess parameters. We can, therefore, apply the symmetry constraint of $||\mathbb{A}^a|| = 0$ by projecting $\mathbb{A}$ to its symmetric part $\mathbb{A}^s$.

3 Results

Here we present the details of the various datasets, explain our experiments and their motivations, and finally present the results.

Synthetic Data Experiment. We used a synthetic dataset to compare the robustness of the various methods under varying controlled conditions. The synthetic dataset to simulate fiber-crossings was generated using the multi-tensor model [9]. The synthetic diffusion weighted images S_i were generated from $S_i(b, g_i) = \sum_{k=1}^{n} p_k e^{-b g_i^T \mathbf{D_k} g_i} + \xi$, where b is the b-value, g_i is i-th gradient direction for $i \in \{1, N\}$, $n \in \{0, 1, 2, 3\}$ is the number of fibers and ξ is the Rician noise generated with a complex Gaussian noise with standard deviation of $1/\sigma$, producing an SNR of σ. The diffusion tensor profile used for a single fiber was diag($\mathbf{D_k}$) = [1390,355,355]x10^{-6}mm^2/s and for isotropic voxels was diag($\mathbf{D_k}$) = [700,700,700]x10^{-6}mm^2/s. Crossing voxels were composed of equal volume fractions ($p_k = 1/n$). This synthetic data generation is relatively standard and has the advantage of producing known ground truth ADC and ODF profiles as well as ground truth fiber orientations.

In our experiment to compare robustness, we varied the SNR from $\sigma = 2$ to $\sigma = 50$ to estimate the 4th order diffusion tensor using the different methods. Then we computed the mean and the standard deviation of the squared error between the estimated ADCs and the ground truth ADC. The results are plotted in Fig. 1. We repeated the experiment for $b = 1000 s/mm^2$ and for $b = 3000 s/mm^2$.

The Riemannian approach compares favourably to the exisiting methods. The TQ method, whose performance may seem surprising, perhaps needs a word of explanation. This was coded by us from [8], using the same guidelines and standards used for the rest of the methods. It seems to us, however, that it is highly sensitive to the optimization algorithm and to the initial conditions used, and we might not have the optimal implementation.

Estimation from Human Brain Data. In the next experiment we used a relatively large human brain dataset of 128 x 128 x 60 voxels for estimation. We used a mask to effectively work on 249352 voxels. This dataset was aquired on a 1.5T scanner at $b = 700 s/mm^2$ using 41 encoding directions, with voxel dimensions of 1.875mm x 1.875mm x 2mm[1].

In this experiment we checked the ADC profiles of the estimated tensors on a set of 81 gradient directions distributed evenly on a hemisphere, to examine the compliance of the estimation methods to the positive diffusivity constraint.

---

[1] The NMR database can be obtained by contacting Cyril Poupon directly by email, cyril.poupon@cea.fr.

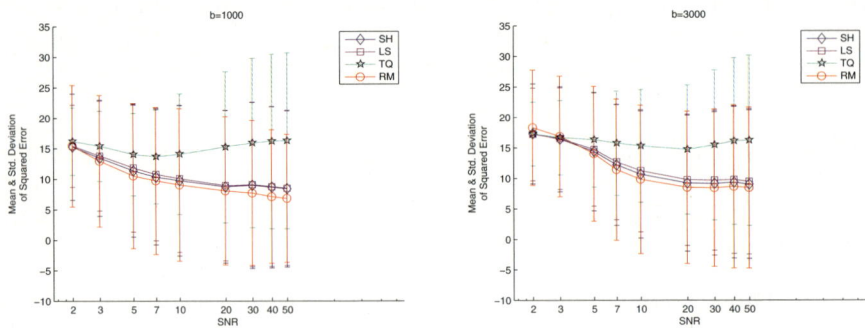

Fig. 1. Comparison of the DTI-4 estimation methods with varying SNR, computed for $b = 1000s/mm^2$ and for $b = 3000s/mm^2$. The SNR varies from $\sigma = 2$ to $\sigma = 50$. The Riemannian approach compares favourably to the exisiting methods.

Table 1. The estimated ADCs from 249352 tensors are checked for positive diffusivity on a set of 81 gradient directions distributed evenly on a hemisphere. The Riemannian and the TQ, are the only methods which guarantee a positive diffusivity profile.

(81 dirs)	LS	SH	TQ	RM
Positive	181757	249263	249352	249352
Negative	67595	89	0	0

Table 2. Time taken to estimate 249352 4th order diffusion tensors from a real dataset. The Riemannian method performs competitively when compared to the LS and SH methods, and still guarantees positive diffusion.

	LS	SH	TQ	RM
Time (sec)	7	28	22526 (6h 15min)	146 (2min 26s)

The results are presented in Table 1. The Riemannian and the TQ, are the only methods which guarantee a positive diffusivity profile.

In this experiment, we also timed the different methods, to compare their running times. It can be expected that as the estimation methods get more complex by trying to accomodate the positivity constraint, they also get computationally expensive. The motivation behind this experiment was to investigate the difference in performances of the simple estimation methods (LS, SH) and the more complex methods (TQ, RM). The results are presented in Table 2. The Riemannian method performs competitively when compared to the LS, and the SH methods, and it still guarantees positive diffusion (Table 1), making it a practical method to apply on large datasets.

Fiber Orientation on Biological Phantom Data. Next we worked on a biological phantom dataset to move beyond the ADC, and to compute the ensemble-average diffusion propagator (EAP) from the 4th order diffusion tensor.

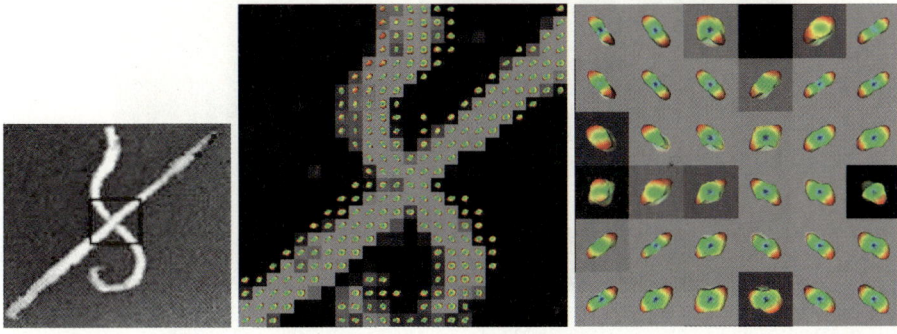

Fig. 2. The ensemble-average diffusion propagator (EAP) in every voxel on a biological phantom data. It is computed from the 4th order diffusion tensor which in turn has been estimated using the Riemannian method. The background is coloured using the GFA, while the glyphs are colour-encoded to indicate directional anisotropy. The image to the right zooms into the crossing section to provide a close up. T1 image to the left.

Since the peaks of the ADC do not necessarily correspond to the orientations of the underlying fiber bundles, it becomes necessary to compute the EAP to infer the correct directions. The EAP, $P(\mathbf{r})$, is given by the Fourier transform $P(\mathbf{r}) = \int E(\mathbf{q}) \exp\left(-2\pi i \mathbf{q}^T \mathbf{r}\right) d\mathbf{q}$, where $\mathbf{q}$ is the reciprocal displacement vector, $E(\mathbf{q})$ is the signal value associated with the vector $\mathbf{q}$ divided by the zero gradient signal, and $\mathbf{r}$ is the spin displacement vector. We computed the Fourier Transform numerically to estimate the EAP from the 4th order diffusion tensor.

The phantom contained exactly two fiber bundles, and this provided us with a framework to validate the estimated EAP. The biological phantom was created from two excised rat spinal cords embedded in 2% agar (see [12]). The acquisition was done on a 1.5T scanner using 90 encoding directions, with b = $3000 s/mm^2$, TR= 6.4 s, TE= 110 ms, 2.8 mm isotropic voxels and four signal averages per direction. The SNR of a single DW image in the spinal cord was estimated to be 5 and the corresponding averaged DW image had an SNR value of 10.

Fig 2, provides a qualitative result of the estimated EAP. In the figure each glyph represents an iso-surface of the corresponding EAP. We first estimated the 4th order diffusion tensors using the Riemannian method. Then we numerically computed the Fourier Transform to estimate the EAP. The background is coloured using the Generalised Fractional Anisotropy (GFA)[2], while the glyphs are colour-encoded to indicate directional anisotropy, with red representing high anisotropy and blue representing low values. The image to the right zooms into the crossing section to provide a close up. It can be seen that the EAP provides the correct orientation of the underlying fiber bundles.

Fiber Orientation on Human Brain Data. This dataset was aquired with 60 encoding gradient directions, a b-value of 1000 s/mm^2, twice-refocused spin-echo EPI sequence, TE = 100 ms, GRAPPA/2, 1.72 mm x 1.72 mm x 1.7 mm

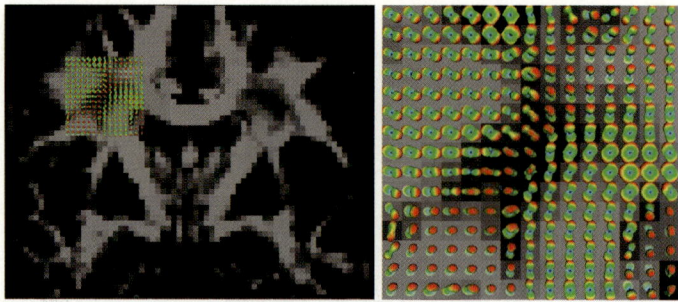

Fig. 3. We used the Riemannian method to estimate the 4th order diffusion tensors in a coronal slice, within a region of interest (ROI). From these we computed the ensemble-average diffusion propagator (EAP). In the ROI we see crossing fibers between the cortico spinal tract, superior longitudinal fibers (traversing the plane) and the corpus callosum (in the plane).

voxel resolution, with three repetitions, and corrected for subject motion. It was acquired on a whole-body 3T Trio scanner.

In this dataset we particularly looked at a Region of Interest (ROI) of a coronal slice, where complex fiber structures are known to exist in the white matter. The ROI contained fiber bundles from the cortico-spinal tract, superior longitudinal fibers (traversing the plane) and the corpus callosum (in the plane). We looked at this ROI to detect these different fiber bundles.

First we used the Riemannian method to estimate the 4th order diffusion tensors in every voxel, and then we computed the Fourier Transform to estimate the EAP.

4 Conclusion

Diffusion MRI is today the cutting edge tool to investigate the human brain anatomy. DTI was the first model proposed, and still remains today of immense value to both the clinician and the neuro-scientist. It has a major shortcoming in regions of fiber crossings, and therefore, other HARDI reconstruction techniques were invented to overcome this limitation. One among these is the HOT model, which has not been extensively researched.

We proposed to take this model further, since sophisticated esimation techniques have been established and well tested for DTI, which guarantee the compliance with the important constraint of positive diffusivity. To that goal we extended the Riemanian framework from DTI to the space of 4th order diffusion tensors. We also compared our Riemannian method to the existing methods on synthetic, phantom and real datasets. We tested all the methods for robustness, speed and also computed the diffusion propagator (EAP) to infer underlying fiber bundle orientations.

In the synthetic dataset tests, the Riemannian method performed well for varying sets of noisy data. This can be attributed to the fact that it inherently satisfies the positive difusivity constraint. This positive diffusivity was confirmed when the method was tested on large real datasets. A feather in the cap was also its computational speed on these large datasets. It performed very competitively when compared to simpler methods like the LS and the SH. Computing the EAP from the Riemannian method also proved to be successful. This was verified qualitatively on a controlled biological phantom, and we also tested the EAP on a real human brain dataset.

In short the performance of the Riemannian method proved to be favourable on all three accounts of robustness and positive diffusivity, computation-time and estimation of the EAP, on synthetic and real datasets. Its fast computational time made it valuable practically. We plan to explore the 4th order tensor model further for fiber-tracking, segmenting and registration in the future.

References

1. Basser, P., Mattiello, J., LeBihan, D.: Estimation of the effective self-diffusion tensor from the NMR spin echo. Journal of Magnetic Resonance B(103), 247–254 (1994)
2. Tuch, D.: Q-ball imaging. Magnetic Resonance in Medicine 52(6), 1358–1372 (2004)
3. Frank, L.: Characterization of anisotropy in high angular resolution diffusion-weighted MRI. Magnetic Resonance in Medicine 47(6), 1083–1099 (2002)
4. Ozarslan, E., Mareci, T.: Generalized diffusion tensor imaging and analytical relationships between diffusion tensor imaging and high angular resolution imaging. Magnetic Resonance in Medicine 50, 955–965 (2003)
5. Liu, C., Bammer, R., Moseley, M.E.: Generalized diffusion tensor imaging (gdti): A method for characterizing and imaging diffusion anisotropy caused by non-gaussian diffusion. Israel Journal of Chemistry 43, 145–154 (2003)
6. Lenglet, C., Rousson, M., Deriche, R., Faugeras, O.: Statistics on the manifold of multivariate normal distributions: Theory and application to diffusion tensor MRI processing. Journal of Mathematical Imaging and Vision 25(3), 423–444 (2006)
7. Arsigny, V., Fillard, P., Pennec, X., Ayache, N.: Log-Euclidean metrics for fast and simple calculus on diffusion tensors. Magnetic Resonance in Medicine 56(2), 411–421 (2006)
8. Barmpoutis, A., Jian, B., Vemuri, B.C.: Symmetric positive 4th order tensors & their estimation from diffusion weighted MRI. In: Karssemeijer, N., Lelieveldt, B. (eds.) IPMI 2007. LNCS, vol. 4584, pp. 308–319. Springer, Heidelberg (2007)
9. Descoteaux, M., Angelino, E., Fitzgibbons, S., Deriche, R.: Apparent diffusion coefficients from high angular resolution diffusion imaging: Estimation and applications. Magnetic Resonance in Medicine 56, 395–410 (2006)
10. Moakher, M.: The algebra and geometry of fourth-order tensors with application to diffusion MRI. In: Weickert, J., Hagen, H. (eds.) Perspectives Workshop: Visualization and Image Processing of Tensor Fields, vol. 04172 (2006)
11. Basser, P.J., Pajevic, S.: Spectral decomposition of a 4th-order covariance tensor: Applications to diffusion tensor MRI. Signal Processing 87, 220–236 (2007)
12. Savadjiev, P., Campbell, J.S.W., Pike, B.G., Siddiqi, K.: 3D curve inference for diffusion MRI regularization and fibre tractography. Medical Image Analysis 10, 799–813 (2006)

Non-uniform Gradient Prescription for Precise Angular Measurements Using DTI

Nathan Yanasak[1], Jerry D. Allison[1], Qun Zhao[2], Tom C.-C. Hu[1], and Krishnan Dhandapani[3]

[1] Department of Radiology, Medical College of Georgia, USA
[2] Department of Physics, University of Georgia, USA
[3] Deparment of Neurosurgery, Medical College of Georgia, USA
nyanasak@mcg.edu

Abstract. Diffusion Tensor Imaging (DTI) calculates a tensor for each voxel, representing the mean diffusive characteristics in volume-averaged tissue. Gradients that phase-encode spins according to the amount of their diffusion are usually applied uniformly over a sphere during a DTI procedure for minimal bias of tensor information. If prior knowledge of diffusion direction exists, the angular precision for determining the principle eigenvector of cylindrically-symmetric ("prolate") tensors can be improved by specifying gradients non-uniformly. Improvements in precision of 30-40% can be achieved using a restricted band of zenith angle values for gradient directions. Sensitivity to the *a priori* angular range of the principle eigenvector can be adjusted with the width of the band. Simulations and phantom data are in agreement; a preliminary validation is presented.

1 Introduction

The technique of diffusion tensor imaging (DTI) provides information about the anisotropy of diffusive water movement in tissue as well as the magnitude of diffusion. Clinical use of DTI has focused primarily on pathological changes as observed in the mean apparent diffusion coefficient (ADC) in a region of interest, or the fractional anisotropy (FA). Examples of this include the reduction of anisotropy from myelin destruction in sclerotic lesions [1], or the evolution of Wallerian degeneration following stroke [2].

Generally, no assumptions are made about the nature of tissue imaged with DTI. To measure tissue diffusivity precisely, gradients that create phase dispersion in proportion to diffusion along an axis are applied uniformly over a sphere [3]. However, information concerning anisotropy of a set of ADC measurements is not uniformly distributed among those gradient directions. If some prior knowledge of the tissue directionality is given (e.g., corticospinal tracts), gradients can be applied non-uniformly to improve DTI metrics, leading to pathological specificity [4]. For example, Peng, et al. [5] demonstrated an optimization scheme that specified gradient directions for maximum sensitivity to FA if the tissue had prolate diffusion characteristics, where the ADC measurements form a "peanut"-shaped spatial distribution. In general, other parameters such as b-value could also be varied non-uniformly during acquisition. Considering the use of multiple diffusion weightings in techniques such as in high angular resolution diffusion imaging (HARDI, [6]), this approach would be critical; parametric optimization methods used in previous studies (e.g., [5], [7]) would provide an efficient framework to search for solutions.

For tissues exhibiting diffusion predominantly along one direction (e.g., white matter tracts), DTI reveals the principle axis of diffusion within an image voxel. By "connecting" these principle axes together, Diffusion Tensor Tractography has been employed to reconstruct tissue structure orientation. Recent applications include characterization of tumor infiltration of white matter [8], coronary muscle fiber remapping in heart failure [9], and diseases and trauma of the spinal cord [10]. As with studies involving ADC or FA, improvement of angular precision in measuring principle diffusion directions could increase clinical specificity. For example, improved tracking could set quantitative limits on normal white matter tract deviation in the presence of tumors, in the case of tissues such as spinal cord or brain stem.

In this study, we demonstrate that a non-uniform set of gradient directions can lead to improved angular precision of the principle eigenvector for a prolate-like ADC distribution. Because of the azimuthal symmetry of a prolate distribution in spherical coordinates, gradient directions from a uniform distribution were compressed along the zenith angle to identify angles for optimal sensitivity to angular precision. It was anticipated that the optimal sensitivity would correspond to angular ranges, or "bands", that balance two characteristics: 1) curvature of the ADC distribution that changes quickly as a function of angle, and 2) distance away from the poles of the distribution, where signal attenuation may contribute more error proportionally to the ADC distribution. Using angular bands of different widths, the sensitivity of angular precision to uncertainty in the principle eigenvalue of the prolate distribution was characterized. Simulations were verified using phantom data, and improvement in angular precision was validated using human brain DTI images.

2 Method

2.1 Simulation

DTI data were simulated using Matlab (The Mathworks, Natwick, MA), and they were fit to a tensor to determine the angular dispersion of the principle eigenvalue for a set of noisy measurements. Water diffusivity was assumed to follow a prolate distribution with the following eigenvalues: λ=[2.4, 0.65, 0.65]$\times 10^{-3}$ mm^2/sec (FA=0.68). Beginning with gradient directions specified for a GE clinical scanner, new gradient directions for diffusion-weighting were determined by compressing the original directions into a limited range of zenith angles, assuming that the largest eigenvalue points along the $\hat{z}$-axis.

Given the prolate diffusion distribution and a non-diffusion-weighted signal intensity for water, diffusion-weighted intensities were calculated for each prescribed gradient direction. For each gradient direction, the diffusion-weighted intensity was duplicated into multiple samples and Fourier transformed. Gaussian noise was added to complex data before inverse Fourier transform, yielding multiple, unique samples of the prolate distribution as a proxy to multiple voxels within an ROI. Tensors were fit to each sample using a weighted least-squares method [11]. A dot product between the principle diffusion axis for each tensor and the prolate distribution axis was employed to find the angle between the two vectors (η), characterizing angular precision. Angular dispersion, σ_η, was defined as the angle at which 68% of the measurements were equal or smaller.

2.2 Phantom

A phantom with arrays of glass capillaries (20 μm i.d.) was used to verify simulation results. The phantom consisted of a 5×5×5 in.^{3} water-filled container, with a 1×1×0.3 in.^{3} region of capillary arrays. Characteristics of these arrays have been reported previously [12].

DTI images were acquired using a GE Excite HDx 3T MRI scanner (GE Medical Systems, Milwaukee, WI), with an eight-channel head coil. The following DW-EPI protocol was used: 3 slices; TR/TE=3000/80msec; 128×128 matrix; 16cm FOV; 4mm slice thickness; 1.5mm gap; ASSET factor=2; b=1000 mm^{-2}; 3 b=0 images. The image plane of the second slice was aligned in parallel with the capillary arrays, with the largest eigenvalue in the phantom parallel to the $\hat{y}$-axis. Gradient directions and number of directions were specified as per the simulation, switching the $\hat{z}$ and $\hat{y}$ coordinates for alignment of the long axis of the prolate. Capillary ROIs were chosen for each image series, resulting in $\approx$ 280-325 voxels. The SNR values of the b=0 images were $\approx$ 38 within the ROIs. Noise characteristics and number of sampled measurements in the simulations were chosen to match these values.

When comparing angular dispersion, Bartlett's test was used to verify a significant difference between one or more gradient direction schemes. Once a significant difference was found between multiple schemes, two-sample F-tests were used to identify significance of differences between pairs. Using a Bonferroni correction to account for multiple comparisons, α was lowered to 0.005. For $\sim$ 300 measurements per dispersion, values of F $\geq$ 1.34 were considered to be significant.

2.3 Validation

A previously-acquired clinical DTI scan was used for validation of the phantom and simulation results. The following DW-EPI protocol was used: 22 slices; TR/TE=6000/78msec; 128×128 matrix; 24cm FOV; 5mm slice thickness; 1.5mm gap; ASSET factor=2; 25 directions; b=1000 sec mm^{-2}; 2 b=0 images. Six small ROIs containing neural fibers from the corpus callosum were selected. Within each ROI, the angular dispersion of the principle eigenvector around their mean was less than $5°$. The ROIs, composed of 91 voxels total, were defined using an atlas to interpret the FA map [13].

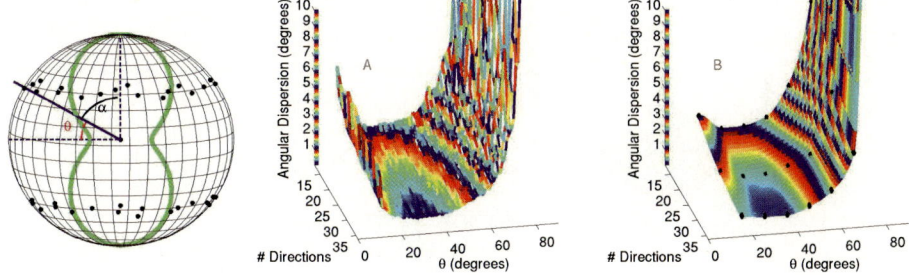

Fig. 1. Angular precision for measuring the eigenvector of principle diffusion for a prolate ADC distribution (green). The gradient directions, specified in a ring at elevation angle θ, are shown as black dots on a unit sphere. The zenith angle, α, is also shown. Panel A: simulated precision; Panel B: measured precision. One color cycle (e.g., red to red) = $1°$.

Using the mean principle eigenvector in each ROI determined from the 25-direction image series, two subsets of directions were chosen for recalculation of the tensor. The first subset, selected for higher angular precision, consisted of directions within a band of elevation angles $15° < \theta < 45°$. The elevation angle is given as the complementary angle to the zenith angle, α, in spherical coordinates (see Figure 1). The second subset, selected for ordinary angular precision, used a set of directions distributed evenly over the surface of a sphere. The number of directions in the second subset was the same as the first subset (10-12), allowing a direct comparison of the angular precision of the principle eigenvalue between both sets of directions. For each direction set, the angular difference of each principle eigenvector from the mean eigenvector was determined within each ROI, and the composite angular precision was determined using all of these differences. The significance of differences in the angular precision was characterized using a two-sample F-test ($F \geq 1.42$ corresponds to $p<0.05$ for 91 degrees of freedom). The choice of a smaller number of directions in the second subset, from the 25 directions distributed evenly over a sphere, resulted in a distribution that was approximately homogeneous. As a result, this procedure may be considered to be only a partial, preliminary validation.

3 Results

Simulations examined the sensitivity of angular precision to elevation angle, given a prolate distribution with the thin "waist" defined by $0°$ elevation. Gradient directions were compressed into a band of angles $10°$ wide, with a mean elevation angle of θ as shown in Figure 1. Panel A in Figure 1 shows the angular dispersion as a function of θ and the number of gradient directions. For the FA value in this simulation and for a DTI sequence having 36 gradient directions, the optimal elevation angle is $\theta=28.7°$, resulting in a dispersion of the measured principle eigenvector $\sigma_\eta=1.1°$. Phantom measurements, shown as black

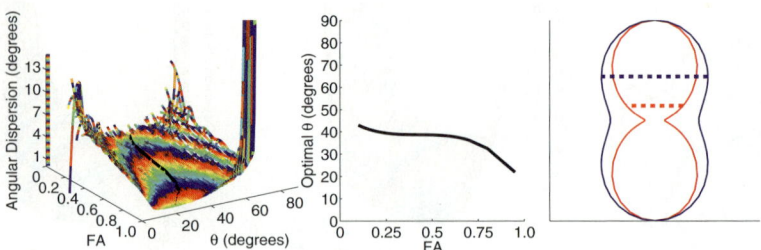

Fig. 2. Angular precision for measuring the eigenvector of principle diffusion for a prolate ADC distribution, as a function of prolate FA and elevation angle, $0° \leq \theta \leq 70°$. The optimal elevation angle is also shown in black, as a function of FA. One color cycle = $1°$. Right Panel: Dashed lines show the region of optimal θ, for ADC distributions with FA=0.5 (blue) and FA=0.9 (red).

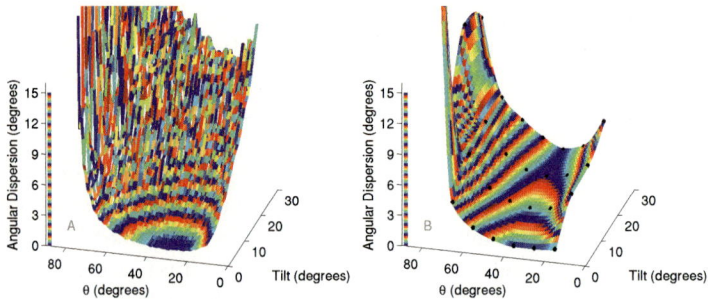

Fig. 3. Angular precision for measuring the eigenvector of principle diffusion for a prolate ADC distribution, with gradient directions specified in Figure 1. In this case, the principle eigenvector is tilted away from the poles of the sphere. Panel A: simulated precision; Panel B: measured precision. One color cycle = $1°$.

points on an interpolated surface in Panel B of Figure 1, qualitatively match with simulations. Data for a DTI sequence having 36 directions, acquired at $10°$ increments in the elevation angle, gives an optimal elevation angle of $\theta \approx 35°$, with an angular dispersion of $1.2°$.

The dependence of optimal elevation angle on FA is shown in Figure 2. The minimum angular dispersion for each value of FA is shown as a black line in the left and right panels, indicating the optimal elevation angle. Up to a value of FA=0.8 or so, the optimal elevation angle is fairly consistent at $\sim 30°$-$40°$. As shown in the right panel of Figure 2, the optimal angle corresponds to areas where the contours of the ADC distribution are changing rapidly, as expected.

Gradient specification within a thin angular band yields improved angular precision if the prolate direction is known. In practice, the direction is known coarsely, and the precision will depend on how far the prolate is tilted with respect to the band. Figure 3 compares angular precision from simulations (Panel A) and phantom data (Panel B) for a DTI sequence having 36 directions, as a function of θ and tilt of the prolate eigenvector. Once again, both data and simulation qualitatively compare favorably, with some difference in behavior at higher tilt angles. At an elevation angle of $35°$, simulated angular dispersion increases by $\Delta\sigma_\eta=11.5°$ as the prolate tilts from a zenith angle of $0°$ to $30°$. For measured data, the precision degrades by $\Delta\sigma_\eta=1.9°$. Simulations appear to deviate from measurements along the surface near the optimal angle in Figure 3, as the tilt angle increases. The origin of this difference is under investigation.

Figure 4 shows four different gradient prescriptions for comparison, using bands of different angular width to balance tilt effects. All bands were centered at an elevation angle of $30°$, where angular precision is near optimal. Simulations demonstrate that, as the band width increases, the immunity to tilt also increases while retaining low angular dispersion. At this FA value (0.68), a band width of $36°$ is the best compromise between minimal angular dispersion and tilting effects out to $30°$. Increasing the width continues to improve the immunity to tilt but decreases the angular precision (as in Figure 3). This trend is also present in phantom data, although angular dispersion increases more slowly as a function of tilt angle. Unlike the simulation, the widest band ($58°$) does not show a significant increase in mean dispersion for all tilt angles. Clearly, for a band somewhat thicker than $58°$, the gradient directions will approximate spherically-homogeneous sampling, and curve "D" in the right panel of Figure 4 will conform to the curve for the spherical distribution of gradient directions as per the simulations.

Bartlett's test identified significant differences between precision at all four measured tilt angles ($p<0.001$). Using two-sample F-tests corrected via Bonferroni for 10 different comparisons at each tilt angle, groups of precision values that were *not* significant to $p<0.005$ are indicated in Figure 4 within red circles. It should be noted that without the Bonferroni correction, precision for curves "C" and "D" at $10°$ tilt are significantly different from all others ($p<0.05$). Considering the multiple-comparison correction to be conservative, this suggests marginal significance for the phantom results at these tilt angle, although more precise measurements are required for confirmation.

The importance of the angular thickness of the band for scheme C in Figure 4 can be understood using the sensitivity of angular dispersion to elevation angle shown in Figure 1. In the angular range of the band ($\theta=15°-45°$), the distribution of angular dispersion is fairly flat, although the angular dispersion increases fairly quickly for larger and smaller elevation angles. By confining the band to this range, the "trough" in the angular dispersion surface is utilized, while tilt becomes less influential due to the band width.

Expectedly, the improvement of angular precision scales with SNR according to simulation. From Figure 4, use of scheme C results in an improvement in the precision $\sim$ 30-40% at maximum. Phantom data supports a similar improvement.

Figure 5 shows the angular distribution in an ROI of the principle eigenvectors for a human brain scan, for a homogeneous distribution of gradient directions and for gradients within an angular band ($\theta=15°-45°$). The angular precision values using these 10-12 gradient directions are $\sigma_\eta=6.5°$ and $3.8°$, respectively.

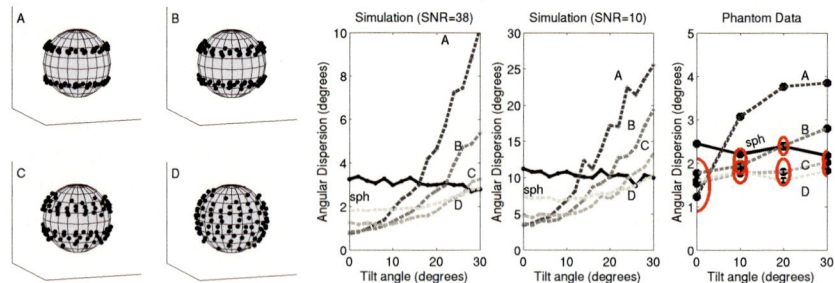

Fig. 4. Angular precision as a function of tilt angle, for four different gradient direction schemes. Note that the north and south hemispheres are mirrored. A: 10° thick ring; B: 18° thick band; C: 36° thick band; D: 58° thick band. The black line indicates the angular precision of a spherically-homogeneous set of gradient directions. Red circles indicate values of precision that are *insignificantly* different (p>0.005, Bonferroni-corrected).

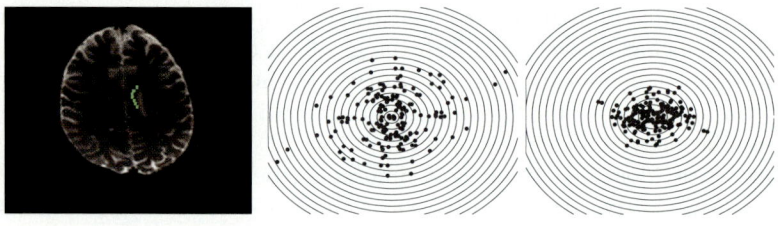

Fig. 5. Angular precision using data from the corpus callosum (green ROIs, left panel). Center panel: deviation of principle eigenvalues from 0°, for uniform distribution of gradient directions. Right panel: deviation of principle eigenvalues, for gradient directions within an angular band. Each ring represents 1°.

For comparison, the angular precision from analysis of the 25-direction scheme is 3.1°. The F-test verifies that the 10-12 gradient schemes are significantly different (F=2.84; p<0.001), indicating an improvement of $\Delta\sigma_\eta$=42% using the distribution within an angular band, and consistent with Figure 4. A slight significance between the 10-12 direction ring scheme and the 25-direction scheme is indicated (F=1.53; p=0.04). This observation affirms previous conclusions that increasing the numbers of gradient directions is generally better, although the gained improvement in precision is only 18%.

4 Discussion

If tissue geometry is prolate and the direction of the principle eigenvector is known to within ≤30°, we have shown that angular precision in determining the principle eigenvector can be optimized using a non-uniform gradient direction prescription. Most of the information describing the orientation of the prolate tissue is contained within a band of elevation angles $\theta \approx 15^\circ$-45° degrees. Simulations and phantom data show that the use of gradients within a band can give better precision than using the same number over a sphere. This improvement could be used to improve clinical specificity; additionally, the number of directions could be decreased from typical clinical protocols to achieve similar precision at a time savings. While elevation of the band determines the sensitivity of gradients to angular precision, band width provides some immunity to uncertainty in the tilt of the prolate to the scan plane. A band width of $\sim 30^\circ$-50° provides a reasonable amount of tilt immunity and angular precision for a large range of FA values, based on Figure 2. This preliminary study does not address whether the precision and accuracy of FA degrades while angular precision is optimized. FA accuracy could be improved by combining gradient bands with a small number of directions near the poles. Further validation of improvement in the angular precision in DTI using biological samples is warranted.

References

1. Filippi, M., et al.: Diffusion tensor magnetic resonance imaging in multiple sclerosis. Neurology 56, 304–311 (2001)
2. Gupta, R.K., et al.: Focal wallerian degeneration of the corpus callosum in large middle cerebral artery stroke: Serial diffusion tensor imaging. Journal of Magnetic Resonance Imaging 24, 549–555 (2006)
3. Papadakis, N.G., et al.: A comparative study of acquisition schemes for diffusion tensor imaging using MRI. Journal of Magnetic Resonance 137, 67–82 (1999)
4. Schmierer, K., et al.: Diffusion tensor imaging of post mortem multiple sclerosis brain. NeuroImage 35, 467–477 (2007)
5. Peng, H., Arfanakis, K.: Diffusion tensor encoding schemes optimized for white matter fibers with selected orientations. Magnetic Resonance Imaging 25, 147–153 (2007)
6. Frank, L.: Characterization of anisotropy in high angular resolution dw MRI. Magnetic Resonance in Medicine 47, 1083–1099 (2002)
7. Alexander, D.C.: Axon radius measurements in vivo from diffusion MRI: a feasibility study. In: Proceedings of the 11th ICCV, pp. 1–8 (2007)
8. Yu, C.S., et al.: Diffusion tensor tractography in patients with cerebral tumors: A helpful technique for neurosurgical planning and postoperative assessment. European Journal of Radiology 56, 197–204 (2005)
9. Helm, P.A., et al.: Evidence of structural remodeling in the dyssynchronous failing heart. Circulation Research 98, 125–132 (2006)
10. Vargas, M.I., et al.: Clinical applications of diffusion tensor tractography of the spinal cord. Neuroradiology 50, 25–29 (2008)
11. Salvador, R.G., et al.: Formal characterization and extension of the linearized diffusion tensor model. Human Brain Mapping 24, 144–155 (2005)
12. Yanasak, N., Allison, J.D.: Use of capillaries in the construction of an MRI phantom for assessment of diffusion tensor imaging: Demonstration of performance. Magnetic Resonance Imaging 24, 1349–1361 (2006)
13. Mori, S., Wakana, S., Nagae-Poetscher, L.M., Van Zijl, P.C.M.: MRI Atlas of Human White Matter. Elsevier, Amsterdam (2005)

Spatial Weighed Element Based FEM Incorporating a Priori Information on Bioluminescence Tomography*

Jin Shi[1,2], Jie Tian[1,2], Min Xu[1,2], and Wei Yang[1,2]

Medical Image Processing Group,
Institute of Automation Chinese Academy of Science
Graduate School of the Chinese Academy of Science
tian@ieee.org,
shijin@fingerpass.net.cn

Abstract. Bioluminescence tomography (BLT) is a promising imaging technique which may dynamically and real-timely detect the molecular and cellular activity at the whole-body level in small animal studies. In view of the ill-posedness of the BLT, it is hard to fully reconstruct source density. In addition, the uniqueness theorem on BLT indicates that it is important to employ a priori information for accurate source reconstruction. Hence, we adopt diffuse optical tomography (DOT) technique to provide optical parameters of main tissues as a priori information. Besides, we restrict the range of real source to a permissible region to raise the numerical stability and reduce the ill-posedness of BLT. Next, we forward Spatial Weighed Element based Finite Element Method and compare it's solutions with analytic formula and MOSE. Numerical simulation of homogeneous and heterogeneous phantom demonstrates the source location and density with prior information is better than that not using a priori information.

Keywords: bioluminescence tomography (BLT), diffuse optical tomography (DOT), spatial weighed element based FEM, a priori information.

1 Introduction

Currently, bioluminescence tomography (BLT) has become an important technique for studying living small animals, especially mice, on the cellular and molecular levels. BLT reconstructs near infrared light source distribution and density from transmission measurements detected on the surface of small animal. To perform BLT experiment, the mice's main organs are transfected with the reporter gene. This mechanism is currently often used in the real-time study of immune cell trafficking and of various genetic regulatory [1]. In bioluminescence tomography, luciferase enzymes are employed to real-timely in vivo monitor the already tagged cells in living animals. After luciferin is injected into a living

---

* This paper is supported by the Project for the National Key Basic Research and Development Program (973) under Grant No.2006CB705700.

animal, those cells in the organism which express the luciferase transgene emit photons of light. Photon propagation in the biological environment is subject to both scattering and absorption.

The biological environment is a turbid media that both scatters and absorbs photons. Because the biological environment does not emit photons and no external light source is needed for excitation, the signal-to-noise ratio (SNR) is high in BLT. Photon propagation in biological tissue is modeled as radiative transfer equation (RTE) [2]. However, RTE is computationally expensive in the practical medical imaging environment. Because the scattering is dominant over absorption in the living animal, diffusion approximation (DA) can provide a quite accurate description of the imaging model [3].

Based on diffusion approximation, the uniqueness theorem states that BLT reconstruction solution is not unique generally [4]. Because of the ill-posedness of BLT problem, we can get many solutions which meet the boundary measured data. In fact, because BLT is ill-posed, it is significant to evaluate background optical parameters as essential a priori information for later quantitative BLT reconstruction. At present, most BLT researchers read the optical properties of the main anatomical tissues from the references, which cannot be very accurate in practice due to individual variation. On the other hand, 3D BLT reconstruction is a high ill-posed inverse problem and it is difficult to fully reconstruct the source density information [5]. One reason is the inner unknown source density dimensions are far greater than the light flux dimensions which are detected on the surface.

In this paper, we use diffuse optical tomography (DOT) technique to provide accurate spatial distribution of optical properties. Here we use time-resolved optical absorption and scattering tomography (TOAST) code from University College London to reconstruct main organs respectly. With TOAST, we can get comparatively accurate absorption and scattering coefficients of main anatomical tissues. And we set up a source permissible region to reduce the dimensions and complexity of reconstruction. To reconstruct BLT light sources density, we propose Spatial Weighed Element based Finite Element Method (SWEFEM) to raise the accuracy of reconstructing source density based on steady-state diffusion equation. An optimization method of gradient projection with Armijo rule can iteratively solve this kind of least squares problem. The reconstructed results demonstrate the feasibility and potential of this method.

2 Algorithms

2.1 Formulation

The tissue of small animal is a kind of turbid media in which photons are absorbed and highly scattered. Transport theory can be used as an accurate mathematical description for propagation of photons in this environment [2]. However, RTE is difficult to deal with and computationally expensive. In practical tissues, the effect of photon scattering is far larger than that of photon absorption, so we can use diffusion approximation to describe the light transport process. In this context, the propagation of light can be described by the steady-state diffusion equation and Robin boundary condition [6,7] as followed:

$$-\nabla(D(x)\nabla\phi(x)) + \mu_a(x)\phi(x) = S(x)(x \in \Omega) \quad (1)$$

$$\phi(x) + 2A(x; n, n')D(x)(v(x)\nabla\phi(x)) = 0 (x \in \partial\Omega) \quad (2)$$

where Ω and $\partial\Omega$ are the tissue region and its boundary correspondingly; $\phi(x)$ represents the photon flux density distribution; S(x) denotes source energy density distribution; $D(x) = 1/[3(\mu_a(x) + (1-g)\mu_s(x))]$ is the diffusion coefficient; $\mu_a(x)$ is the absorption coefficient, while $\mu_s(x)$ is the scattering coefficient; and g is anisotropic parameter; v is the unit outer normal to $\partial\Omega$ at location x; n is the refractive index of Ω and n' is the refractive index of the external medium; $A = (1+R)/(1-R)$, in which R depends on the refraction properties of the medium and can be approximated by $R = -1.4399n-2+0.7099n-1+0.6681+0.0636n$ [8].

In bioluminescence tomography, the measured value is the outgoing flux density Q(x):

$$Q(x) = -D(x)(v\nabla\phi(x)) = \frac{1}{2A(x; n, n')}\phi(x)(x \in \partial\Omega) \quad (3)$$

Thus, BLT problem is defined to reconstruct inner source S(x) from Q(x) detected on the surface of small animal by Eqs. (1) - (3). The below weak solution of flux density $\phi(x)$ is described based on steady diffusion equation:

$$\int_\Omega (D(x)(\nabla\phi(x)) \cdot (\nabla\psi(x)) + \mu_a(x)\phi(x)\psi(x))dV$$
$$+ \int_{\partial\Omega} \frac{1}{2A(x; n, n')}\phi(x)\psi(x)dA = \int_\Omega S(x)\psi(x)dV, \forall \psi(x) \in H^1(\Omega) \quad (4)$$

where $\phi(x) \in H^1(\Omega)$ is the Sobolev space and $\psi(x)$ is a test function.

In this article, finite element method is employed to discretize the domain Ω into small and regular subdomains such that we can transfer an infinite dimensional problem into a finite dimensional problem. The selectable finite elements in three dimensional regions include tetrahedron, hexahedron and prism. Because of the flexible characteristic, tetrahedron is generally used as the finite element in the complicated and irregular biological environments. By the standard FEA [9,10], the left items of (4) can be written as $M \cdot \Phi$. The right items are treated as followed: take any tetrahedron i as example:

$$\int_i S(x)\psi(x)dV = [\psi_{i_1}\psi_{i_2}\psi_{i_3}\psi_{i_4}][w_{i_1} w_{i_2} w_{i_3} w_{i_4}]^T * S_i \quad (5)$$

where S_i represents ith reconstruction element; $\psi_{i_1}\psi_{i_2}\psi_{i_3}\psi_{i_4}$ are the nodal variables of the element; $w_{i_1} w_{i_2} w_{i_3} w_{i_4}$ are the basis function, which can describe the spatial location and shape of the tetrahedron and is very important in later reconstruction. And then we can get (6) and construct the linear relationship between the source energy density distribution and the photon flux density on the whole mesh.

$$M \cdot \Phi = F \cdot S \qquad (6)$$

By deleting internal flux density information and selecting source permissible region, we can construct the linear relationship between the unknown inner source and the photon flux density on the boundary.

$$M^{mod} \cdot \Phi^{bound} = F^{mod} \cdot S^{pr} \qquad (7)$$

where Φ^{bound} represents the vector of the photon flux density on the boundary and S^{pr} represents the vector of the unknown inner source. Hence, BLT problem can be transferred to an optimization problem.

$$\min_{S^{low} \leq S^{pr} \leq S^{up}} ||M^{mod} \cdot \Phi^{bound} - F^{mod} \cdot S^{pr}||_\wedge + \lambda \xi(S^{pr}) \qquad (8)$$

where S^{low} and S^{up} are the low and up bounds of the source density; $\wedge$ is the weight matrix, $||V||_\wedge = V^T \wedge V$; λ is the regularization parameter; ξ is the penalty function. Here, an optimization method of gradient projection with Armijo rule can iteratively solve (8) effectly [11].

2.2 Fusion of a Priori Information

In the complicated biological tissues, bioluminescence source emits photons. Photons are then highly scattered and absorbed by the tissues, which leads to the difficulty of source localization and quantification. Hence three-dimensional bioluminescence source reconstruction problem is highly ill-posed. Theoretically speaking, we can get the unique reconstruction solution in bioluminescence tomography only if we adopt some practical restricts and a priori information [4].

In this paper, we adopt a practical restrict to the range of real source, which is partitioned into a source permissible region and a source impermissible region to raise the numerical stability and efficiency and reduce the ill-posedness of BLT. In eq.6, the vector S represents the source distribution on the whole mesh. Then S is divided into two sub vectors: S^{pr} and S^{upr}, which represents the distribution in the source permissible region and that in source impermissible region. Obviously, S^{upr} is zero on assumption or experiment observation. By deleting internal density information, selecting source permissible region on the photon flux density and matrix transformation of M and F, we can construct the linear relationship between the unknown inner source and the photon flux density on the boundary, which is showed in eq.7.

It is very important to gain background optical parameters that can be used as essential a priori information for accurate BLT reconstruction. Up to now, most BLT groups in the world get the optical properties of the main anatomical tissues from the literature [6,7,12], which cannot be very accurate in practice because of the diversity of individuals. In this paper, before BLT reconstruction, we adopt Diffuse Optical Tomography (DOT) technique to reconstruct optical parameters as a priori information. Here we use time-resolved optical absorption and scattering tomography (TOAST) software code from University College London to reconstruct main organs respectly. TOAST has a forward solver to simulate light propagation in highly scattering media using finite element method (FEM) and an inverse solver to reconstruct the spatial distribution of optical coefficients using some kinds of optimization methods such as Newton-based and gradient-based algorithms. With TOAST, we can get comparatively accurate absorption and scattering coefficients of main anatomical tissues.

3 Experimental Results

3.1 Homogeneous Experiment

To validate the method that is proposed, two numerical experiments are performed. In the first one, we adopt one homogeneous phantom. As shown in Figure1, a uniform spherical ideal source is centered in the spherical tissue. The source radius is r mm and its power is s watt.

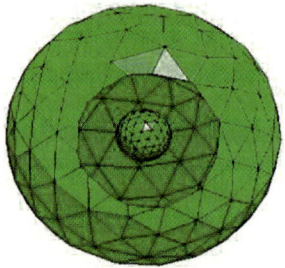

Fig. 1. finite element mesh of homogeneous phantom

We use TOAST software to reconstruct main organs. The reconstructed results of main mouse tissues are illustrated as Table1, which is the average of reconstructed values of the identical tissue. The reconstructions of lung tissue are showed in Fig.2. With TOAST, we can get comparatively accurate absorption and scattering coefficients of main anatomical tissues, which provide a priori information for later BLT reconstruction.

We compare forward solutions of SWEFEM, analytic formula and MOSE (http://www.mosetm.net/) as shown in Fig.3, in which the tissue radius ranges form 1mm to 10mm. The analytic formula is developed by Cong in Virginia Polytechnic Institute and State University [13]. MOSE is a forward model for bioluminescence light propagation based on Monte Carlo method [14]. MOSE simulates bioluminescent phenomena in the mouse imaging and predicts bioluminescent signals around the mouse. Seen from the chart, the SWEFEM forward solution meets with analytic solution and MOSE results very well.

In addition, we contrast SWEFEM reconstruction with DOT to that without DOT as shown in Fig.4. The background absorption coefficient $\mu_a = 0.12mm^{-1}$,

Table 1. Comparision of reconstructed and real optical parameters of main tissues

Material	Muscle	Lung	Heart	Bone	Liver
$real\_\mu_a$	0.01	0.35	0.2	0.002	0.035
$real\_\mu_s$	4	23	16	20	6
Rec_μ_a	0.01	0.35	0.2	0.002	0.035
Rec_μ_s	4	22.9	16	20	6

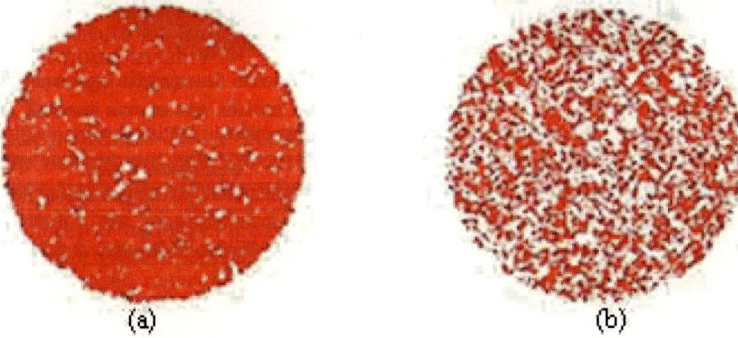

Fig. 2. A cross section of reconstruction in lung. (a) Absorption coefficient whose average value equals real value 0.35.(b)Scattering coefficient whose average value equals real value 23.

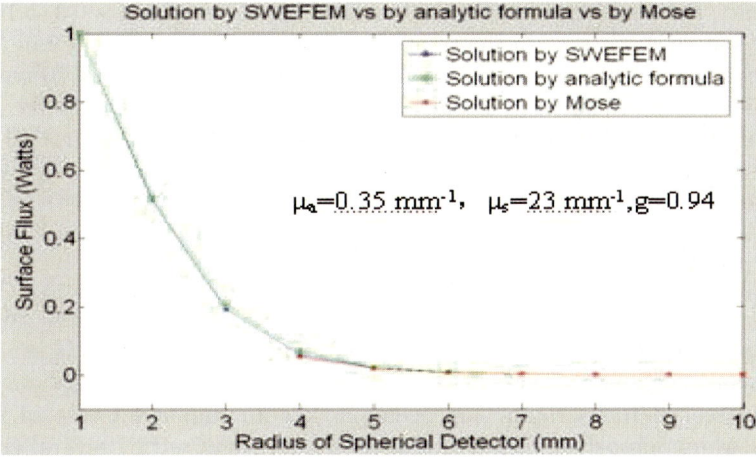

Fig. 3. The comparison of forward solutions of SWEFEM, analytic formula and MOSE

the scattering coefficient $\mu_s = 20mm^{-1}$, anisotropic parameter g=0.9. Without DOT, the optical coefficients have 40% errors and the maximal reconstruct density is about 0.09 $watts/mm^3$. While using DOT, the maximal reconstruct density is about 0.148 $watts/mm^3$ that equals the real density and the total

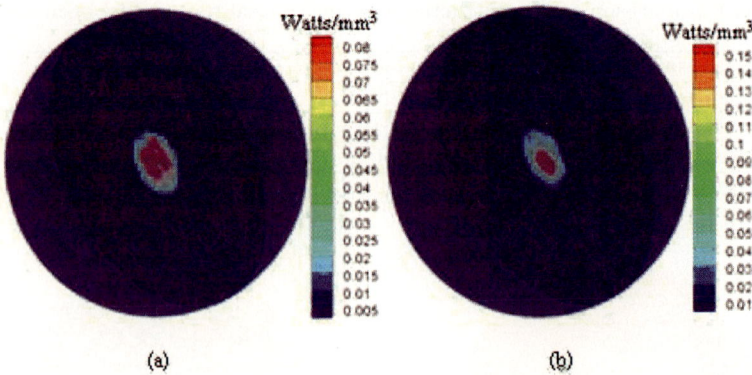

Fig. 4. A comparison of SWEFEM reconstruction with DOT and without DOT. (a) A cross section without DOT. (b) A cross section with DOT.

reconstruction energy amount to the initial total energy, which can approve the validation of SWEFEM.

3.2 Heterogeneous Experiment

In the second experiment, we adopt a heterogeneous cylindrical phantom [15], which is 30mm high and the radius is 10mm. It represents muscle. In the cylinder, there are four ellipsoid parts and one cylinder one to represent left lung, right lung, heart, bone and liver respectly. The location of right lung is (-3,-5,15). And the true source is centered in the right lung and the total power is 1 nano-Watts.

Optical parameters are reconstructed using the Diffuse Optical Tomography technique, which are listed in Table1. Similarly, we contrast relevant reconstruction using DOT with that not using it. Without DOT, the background optical coefficients have 50% errors and the maximal reconstructed density is nearly $0.077\ nano-watts/mm^3$. while with DOT, the maximal reconstructed density is about $0.22\ nano-watts/mm^3$ and approximately equals the real source density $0.238\ nano-watts/mm^3$.

4 Discussions

Bioluminescence tomography has been playing an important role in medical imaging. Many important results in this area are bought out by several groups in the world [5,7,12,16,17]. However, BLT is still faced with challenge, such as more accurate mathematical model, the improvement of the reconstruction algorithm, the deeper depth reconstruction of small animal, and so on.

In conclusion, we have forwarded a novel spatial weighed element based finite element method taking the optical parameters and source permissible region as a priori information which can accurately reconstruct source distribution and

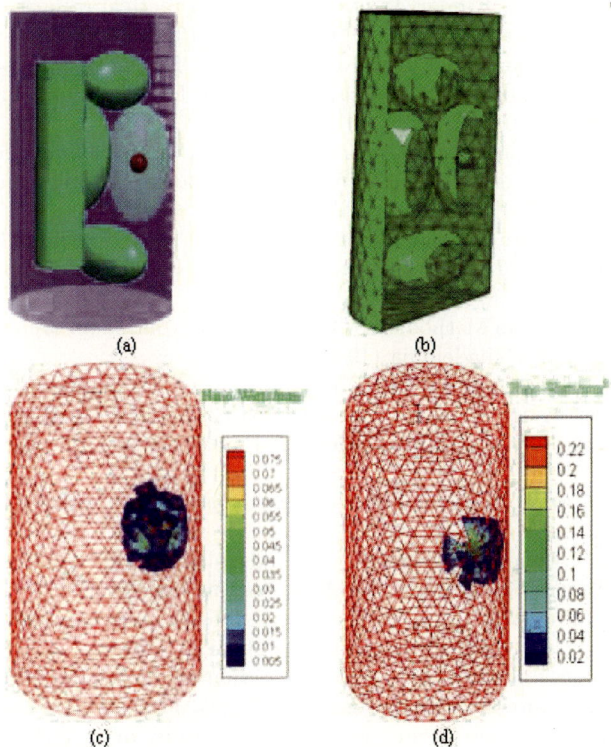

Fig. 5. Heterogeneous phantom. (a) A heterogeneous phantom with a real source in right lung region. (b) The discretized mesh of the phantom (c) Reconstructed result without DOT. (d) Reconstructed result without DOT.

density. And the feasibility and potential of this method is demonstrated. Next step, we will validate the method in real experiments using BLT experiment system and further results will be reported later.

References

1. Contag, C., Bachmann, M.: Advances in Bioluminescence imaging of gene expression. Annu. Rev. Biomed. Eng. 4, 235–260 (2002)
2. Klose, A.D., Ntziachristos, V., Hielscher, A.: The inverse source problem based on the radiative transfer equation in optical molecular imaging. Comput. Phys. 202, 323–345 (2005)
3. Arridge, S.R., Schweiger, M., Hiraoka, M., Delpy, D.: A finite element approach for modeling photon transport in tissue. Med. Phys. 20, 299–309 (1993)
4. Wang, G., Li, Y., Jiang, M.: Uniqueness theorems in bioluminescence tomography. Med. Phys. 31, 2289–2299 (2004)
5. Dehghani, H., Davis, S., Jiang, S.D., Pogue, B., Paulsen, K., Patterson, M.: Spectrally resolved bioluminescence optical tomography. Optics Letters 31, 365–367 (2005)

6. Cong, W., Wang, G., Kumar, D., Liu, Y., et al.: Practical reconstruction method for bioluminescence tomography. Optics Express 13(18), 6756–6771 (2005)
7. Chaudhari, A.J., Darvas, F., Bading, J.R., Moats, R.A., et al.: Hyperspectral and multispectral bioluminescence optical tomography for small animal imaging. Phys. Med. Biol. 50, 5421–5441 (2005)
8. Schweiger, M., Arridge, S.R., Hiraoka, M., Delpy, D.T.: The finite element method for the propagation of light in scattering media: Boundary and source conditions. Med. Phys. 22, 1779–1792 (1995)
9. Schwarz, H.R.: Finite element methods. Academic Press, London (1988)
10. Rao, S.S.: The finite element method in engineering. Butterworth-Heinemann, Boston (1999)
11. Kelley, C.T.: Iterative Methods for Optimization. Frontiers in Applied Mathematics, vol. 18. SIAM, Philadelphia (1999)
12. Alexandrakis, G., Rannou, F.R., Chatziioannou, A.F.: Tomographic bioluminescence imaging by use of a combined optical-PET (OPET) system: a computer simulation feasibility study. Phys. Med. Biol. 50, 4225–4241 (2005)
13. Cong, W.X., Wang, L.H., Wang, G.: Formulation of photon diffusion from spherical bioluminescent sources in an infinite homogeneous medium. Biomed. Eng. Online 4, 12 (2004)
14. Li, H., Tian, J., et al.: Development of a molecular optical simulation enviroment. Journal of Pattern Recognition and Artificial Intelligence (2006)
15. Lv, Y., Tian, J., et al.: A multilevel adaptive finite element algorithm for bioluminescence tomography. Optics Express 14, 8211–8223 (2006)
16. Jiang, M., Zhou, T., et al.: Image reconstruction for bioluminescence tomography from partial measurement. Optics Express 15(18), 11095–11116 (2007)
17. Kuo, C., Rice, B., et al.: Bioluminescent tomography for in vivo localization and quantification of luminescent sources from a multiple-view imaging system. Molecular Imaging 4, 370 (2005)

Geometric Deformable Model Driven by CoCRFs: Application to Optical Coherence Tomography

Gabriel Tsechpenakis[1], Brandon Lujan[2], Oscar Martinez[1], Giovanni Gregori[2], and Philip J. Rosenfeld[2]

[1] Dept. of Electrical and Computer Engineering, University of Miami
gavriil@miami.edu, o.martinez4@umiami.edu
[2] Bascom Palmer Eye Institute, Miller School of Medicine, University of Miami
{BLujan,GGregori,prosenfeld}@med.miami.edu

Abstract. We present a geometric deformable model driven by dynamically updated probability fields. The shape is defined with the signed distance function, and the internal (smoothness) energy consists of a C^1 continuity constraint, a shape prior, and a term that forces the zero-level of the shape distance function towards a connected form. The image probability fields are estimated by our collaborative Conditional Random Field (CoCRF), which is updated during the evolution in an active learning manner: it infers class posteriors in pixels or regions with feature ambiguities by assessing the joint appearance of neighboring sites and using the classification confidence. We apply our method to Optical Coherence Tomography fundus images for the segmentation of geographic atrophies in dry age-related macular degeneration of the human eye.

1 Introduction

A challenging problem in computer and medical vision is to segment regions with boundary insufficiencies, i.e., missing edges and/or lack of texture contrast between regions of interest (ROIs) and background. In this paper we focus on two general categories of segmentation methods, namely the deformable models and the learning-based classification approaches.

Deformable models are divided into two main categories. The first class is the *parametric* or *explicit* deformable models [11,2,15,23], or active contours, which use parametric curves to represent the model shape. Edge-based parametric models use edges as image features, which usually makes them sensitive to noise, while region-based methods use region information to drive the curve [20,24,8]. A limitation of the latter methods is that they do not update the region statistics during the model evolution, and therefore local feature variations are difficult to be captured. Region updating is proposed in [3], where active contours with particle filtering is used for vascular segmentation.

Another class of deformable models is the *geometric* or *implicit* models [16,17,14], which use the level-set based shape representation, transforming the curves into higher dimensional scalar functions. In [16], the optimal function is the one that best fits the image data, it is piecewise smooth and presents discontinuities across the boundaries of different regions. In [17], a variational framework is proposed, integrating boundary and region-based information in PDEs that are implemented using a level-set approach. These methods assume piecewise or Gaussian intensity distributions within each partitioned image region, which limits their ability to capture intensity inhomogeneities and complex intensity distributions. In [7], the Metamorphs was introduced, which updates a kernel-based approximation of the model interior texture during the evolution. The model dynamics are defined parametrically using Free Form Deformations, which sometimes is a limiting factor for capturing region details. Also, merging different curves on the image plane is formulated as detection of collision of different models, and therefore merging is not a property inherently defined in the model representation.

Learning-based region classification is also among the most popular approaches to medical image segmentation, with representative example the Markov Random Fields (MRFs) [6]. To obtain better probability smoothing, Conditional Random Fields (CRFs) were introduced in computer vision [13]. Although CRFs were first used to label sequential data, extensions of them are used for image segmentation [12,5,22]. The main advantage of CRFs is that they handle the known label bias problem [13], avoiding the conditional independence assumption among the features of neighboring sites. In [12] the Discriminative Random Fields (DRFs) are presented, which allow for computationally efficient MAP inference. Also, in [5], CRFs are used in different spatial scales to capture the dependencies between image regions of multiple sizes. A potential limitation of CRFs is that they do not provide robustness to unobserved or partially observed features, which is a common problem in most discriminative models.

Integrating deformable models with MAP inference methods is a recently introduced framework for propagating deformable models in a probabilistic manner, by formulating the *traditional* energy minimization as a MAP estimation problem. In the survey of [15], methods that use probabilistic formulations are described. In the work of [8] the integration of probabilistic active contours with MRFs in a graphical framework is proposed to overcome the limitations of edge-based probabilistic active contours. In [6], a framework that tightly couples 3D MRFs with deformable models is proposed for the 3D segmentation of medical images. Finally, to exploit the superiority of CRFs compared to common first-order MRFs, a coupling framework is proposed in [22], where a CRF and an implicit deformable model are integrated in a simple graphical model.

In this paper we present a probabilistic geometric deformable model that is driven by a *collaborative* CRF. The model evolution is solved as a joint MAP estimation problem for the model position and the image label field. In section 2, we define the model's shape and its internal energy, which consists of a C^1 continuity constraint, a shape prior, and a term that forces the zero-level of the shape distance function towards a connected form. The latter can be seen as a term that forces different closed curves on the image plane to merge, and therefore our model inherently carries the property of merging regions. During the evolution, described in 2.1, the model interior statistics are dynamically updated, and the new distributions are used in our CRF in an active learning manner. In section 3 we describe our *collaborative* CRF, which infers class posteriors in pixels and regions with feature ambiguities by assessing the joint appearance of neighboring sites and using classification confidence. In 4 we show our results on the segmentation of geographic atrophies in dry age-related macular degeneration of the human eye, from Optical Coherence Tomography (OCT) fundus images. Finally, in 5 we give our conclusions.

2 Deformable Model

The model boundary $\mathcal{M}$ defines two regions in the image domain Ω, namely the region $\mathcal{R}_\mathcal{M}$ enclosed by the model $\mathcal{M}$ and the background $\Omega \backslash \mathcal{R}_\mathcal{M}$. The model shape $\Phi_\mathcal{M}$ is represented implicitly by its distance transform, as in [7,22]. The internal energy of the model consists of three individual terms, namely the smoothness constraint E_{smooth}, the distance from the target shape E_{shape}, and a partitioning energy E_{part},

$$E_{int}(\Phi_\mathcal{M}) = E_{smooth}(\Phi_\mathcal{M}) + E_{part}(\Phi_\mathcal{M}) + E_{shape}(\Phi_\mathcal{M}) \quad (1)$$

The smoothness term is defined as,

$$E_{smooth}(\Phi_\mathcal{M}) = \varepsilon_1 \mathcal{A}(\mathcal{R}_\mathcal{M}) + \varepsilon_2 \int\int_{\partial \mathcal{R}_\mathcal{M}} \|\nabla \Phi_\mathcal{M}(\mathbf{x})\| d\mathbf{x} \quad (2)$$

where ε_1 and ε_2 are weighting constants, $\partial \mathcal{R}_\mathcal{M}$ denotes a narrow band around the model boundary, and $\mathcal{A}(\mathcal{R}_\mathcal{M})$ denotes the area of the model interior. The minimization of this energy forces the model to the position with the minimum area enclosed and the maximum first-order smoothness along the model boundary; $\nabla \Phi_\mathcal{M}$ is defined $\forall \mathbf{x} \in \Omega$, and is used similarly as in the Mumford-Shah formulation [16].

The partitioning energy forces the regions $\Phi_\mathcal{M} \geq 0$ towards a connected form. It can be also seen as a term that minimizes the entropy of a set of particles, where the particles are assumed to be the connected components of $\Phi_\mathcal{M} \geq 0$, or equivalently the connected regions of $\mathcal{H}(\Phi_\mathcal{M})$. Let $\{\varphi_\mathcal{M}^{(i)}\}_{i=1}^{N} \subseteq \mathcal{H}(\Phi_\mathcal{M})$ be the set of N connected regions, and $e_{part}(\varphi_\mathcal{M}^{(i)})$ be the energy of each connected region $\varphi_\mathcal{M}^{(i)}$. We define this energy in terms of the distances between $\varphi_\mathcal{M}^{(i)}$ and the rest of the connected regions in the set $\mathcal{H}(\Phi_\mathcal{M})$,

$$e_{part}(\varphi_\mathcal{M}^{(i)}) = \sum_{j=1, j \neq i}^{N} \tilde{d}(\varphi_\mathcal{M}^{(j)}, \varphi_\mathcal{M}^{(i)}), \quad \tilde{d}(\varphi_\mathcal{M}^{(j)}, \varphi_\mathcal{M}^{(i)}) = \min_{\mathbf{x} \in \varphi_\mathcal{M}^{(j)}} \|\varphi_\mathcal{M}^{(i)} - \mathbf{x}\| \quad (3)$$

Then, the partitioning energy of the model is expressed as,

$$E_{part}(\Phi_\mathcal{M}) = \frac{1}{2} \sum_{i=1}^{N} e_{part}(\varphi_\mathcal{M}^{(i)}), \quad (4)$$

The minimization of this energy forces the model towards the minimum distances between the connected components of $\mathcal{H}(\Phi_\mathcal{M})$, i.e., forces different regions (curves) on the image plane to merge.

Finally, we define the shape energy term in a similar way as in [18,1], in terms of the distance between the model $\Phi_\mathcal{M}$ and the target shape $\Phi_{shape}(\mathbf{x})$: $\|\Phi_\mathcal{M} \mathcal{H}(\Phi_\mathcal{M}) - \Phi_{shape} \mathcal{H}(\Phi_{shape})\|$, where we include in the calculations only the regions of the model and target shape.

2.1 The Model Evolution

We formulate the deformable model evolution as a joint MAP estimation problem for the model position and the image label field,

$$\langle \Phi_{\mathcal{M}}^*, \mathcal{L}^* \rangle = \arg \max_{(\Phi_{\mathcal{M}}, \mathcal{L})} P(\Phi_{\mathcal{M}}, \mathcal{L}|F), \qquad (5)$$

where $\mathcal{L}$ is the sites' (pixels or image patches) labels, i.e., $\mathcal{L} = \{-1, 1\}$, where -1 and 1 denote *background* and *model interior* respectively, and F is the observations set, i.e., the intensity distributions. For the posterior probability $P(\Phi_{\mathcal{M}}, \mathcal{L}|F)$, we adopt the decomposition of [22],

$$P(\Phi_{\mathcal{M}}, \mathcal{L}|F) \propto P(\Phi_{\mathcal{M}}) \cdot P(F) \cdot P(\mathcal{L}|\Phi_{\mathcal{M}}) \cdot P(\mathcal{L}|F), \qquad (6)$$

where $P(\Phi_{\mathcal{M}})$ is the model prior, $P(\mathcal{L}|F)$ represents the pixel/region classification in a discriminative manner, and $P(\mathcal{L}|\Phi_{\mathcal{M}})$ is a likelihood term that introduces uncertainty between the classification and the deformable model position. The data prior $P(F)$ is calculated using the nonparametric intensity distribution of the model interior in every instance of the evolution process.

The model prior $P(\Phi_{\mathcal{M}})$ corresponds to the energy of eq. (1), and is defined in terms of the gibbs functional,

$$P(\Phi_{\mathcal{M}}) = (1/Z_{int}) \exp\{-E_{int}(\Phi_{\mathcal{M}})\}, \qquad (7)$$

where the individual terms of $E_{int}(\Phi_{\mathcal{M}})$ are calculated using the definitions we described above; Z_{int} is a normalization constant. The maximization of this prior forces the model towards a position with the minimum enclosed area and maximum smoothness along the boundary, with the smallest distance to the target shape, and the minimum *entropy* as defined in eqs. (3)-(4).

We define the likelihood $P(\mathcal{L}|\Phi_{\mathcal{M}})$ as the softmax function,

$$P(l_i|\Phi_{\mathcal{M}}) = \frac{1}{1 + \exp\{-\Phi_{\mathcal{M}}(\mathbf{x}_i)\}}, \qquad (8)$$

where $l_i = \{-1, 1\}$ is the label of the i-th pixel or region $\mathbf{x}_i$. This term indicates that the probability of a site belonging to the model interior rapidly increases as $\Phi_{\mathcal{M}}(\mathbf{x}) > 0$ increases, and converges to zero as $\Phi_{\mathcal{M}}(\mathbf{x}) < 0$ decreases; also $P(l_i|\Phi_{\mathcal{M}}) = 0.5$ $\forall \mathbf{x}_i \in \Omega : \Phi_{\mathcal{M}}(\mathbf{x}_i) = 0$. Also, if $\mathbf{x}_i$ is a region, we consider its center to estimate this probability.

The remaining term $P(\mathcal{L}|F)$ in eq. (6) is calculated using our CRF framework described below.

3 The Collaborative CRF

We use a Conditional Random Field (CRF) formulation to calculate the probability field $P(\mathcal{L}|F)$ that drives the deformable model evolution, according to eqs. (5) and (6). We implement interactions that enforce similar class labels (*model interior* or *background*) between all sites containing similar intensity distributions; these interactions are driven by the classification confidence to assist weakly labeled sites. To improve classification in cases of region ambiguities, we also use correlative information between neighboring sites, by estimating their joint intensity distributions.

Let $F = \{f_i\}_{i \in S}$, where f_i is the intensity distribution from a site i, and S is the set of all sites. Also, let $\mathcal{L} = \{l_i\}_{i \in S}$ be the set of corresponding labels for all sites in S, with $l_i = \{-1, 1\}$ (background, ROI). If N_i denotes the spatial neighborhood of each site i, we can then say that conditioned on the discrete observations F, the distribution over the labels $p(\mathcal{L}|F)$ can be written as a first order CRF of the form,
$$p(\mathcal{L}|F) = \frac{1}{z} \exp\left\{ \sum_{i \in S} \mathbf{A}(l_i, f_i) + \sum_{i \in S} \sum_{j \in N_i} \left[\mathbf{I}(l_i, l_j, f_i, f_j, K_i, K_j) + \mathbf{C}(l_i, l_j, f_{ij}) \right] \right\}, \quad (9)$$

where z is a normalization constant.

The unary *association potential* $\mathbf{A}(y_i, x_i)$ is estimated using a discriminative classifier (Support Vector Machine) to directly calculate the class posterior as mapping between the distribution f_i and the class l_i [12],
$$\mathbf{A}(l_i, f_i) = \log P(l_i|f_i), \quad (10)$$

The *interaction potential* $\mathbf{I}(l_i, l_j, f_i, f_j, K_i, K_j)$ compares the intensity distributions f_i and f_j and enhances classification by forcing smoothness between the neighboring l_i and l_j,
$$\mathbf{I}(l_i, l_j, f_i, f_j, K_i, K_j) = \frac{1}{z_{int}} \exp\left\{ \frac{\delta(l_i - l_j)}{\sigma^2} \right\} \beta(f_i, f_j) \gamma(K_i, K_j) \quad (11)$$

where z_{int} is a normalizing constant, $\delta(l_i - l_j) = 0$ if $l_i \neq l_j$, and $\delta(l_i - l_j) = 1$ if $l_i = l_j$, σ^2 controls the smoothing, and $\beta(f_i, f_j)$ measures the distance between i and j in the feature space; here we use the Bhattachayya distance for measuring the distributions similarity. We modulate the role of the interaction potential by the relative classification confidence $\gamma(K_i, K_j)$ of the sites i and j; K_i and K_j are the corresponding confidences representing how strong the discriminative classification of each site is. As a measure of confidence we use the distance from the classification boundary, although more efficient measures can be found in the literature [10]. To measure the relative confidence between two neighboring sites, we use the pairwise softmax function,
$$\gamma(K_i, K_j) = \frac{1}{1 + \exp\{\alpha(K_i - K_j)\}}, \quad \alpha > 0, \quad (12)$$

where K_i and K_j are the classification confidence values for the sites i and j respectively, and α is a constant regulating the confidence similarity. The value of $\gamma(K_i, K_j)$ is only dependent on the relative value of K_i with respect to K_j: $K_i \gg K_j \Leftrightarrow \gamma \to 0$ and $K_i \ll K_j \Leftrightarrow \gamma \to 1$. This weighing function allows the interaction in eq. (11) between i and j only if site j is more confidently classified than site i. This guarantees that interaction will generally *flow* from sites labeled with relative confidence to sites labeled with relative uncertainty.

The *correlative potential* $\mathbf{C}(l_i, l_j, f_{ij})$ is used to improve classification in instances of region ambiguities by evaluating neighboring sites that could be portraying a single region,

$$\mathbf{C}(l_i, l_j, f_{ij}) = \log P(l_i = l_j | f_{ij}), \tag{13}$$

where f_{ij} is the joint intensity distribution of the sites i and j. To consider the joint appearance of two sites, we evaluate whether they are complimentary to each other with respect to their classification confidence: f_i and f_j are complimentary if $\{j \in N_i : K_i, K_j \leq K_{ij}\}$, where K_{ij} is the classification confidence for the joint distribution f_{ij}. In other words the classifier treats neighboring sites as possible regions of the same class that have erroneously been segmented apart, and decides whether or not they belong to the same class. Note that here, as confidence measurement we use the same classification probabilities (using the distance from the decision boundaries [19]); currently we are working towards generalizing this confidence-driven approach using the *belief* and *plausibility* terms from the Dempster-Shafer evidence theory.

4 Segmentation of Geographic Atrophy in the Retina

Age-related Macular Degeneration (AMD) has become the most common cause of severe irreversible vision loss in developed countries. In patients with advanced dry AMD, most of the severe vision loss results from atrophy of the retinal pigment epithelium (RPE). Confluent areas of RPE atrophy are clinically referred to as **geographic atrophy (GA)**, which can cause legal blindness if it affects the central macula. GA is currently present in 3.5% of all people 75 years and older in the United States [21], and this number is expected to double by 2020 [4]. There is currently no effective treatment for GA and there is only a rudimentary understanding of its pathophysiology. Furthermore, its visibility by standard photography depends on the degree of pigmentation present in the surrounding intact RPE. A new imaging modality, **Spectral Domain Optical Coherence Tomography (SDOCT)**, demarcates areas of GA precisely even when it cannot be identified by photography. It utilizes the principles of reflectometry and interferometry to obtain structural information from the retina and layers under the retina at different depths along each axial scan (A-scan). One commercially available model, the Cirrus HD OCT (Carl Zeiss Meditec, Dublin, CA) images a $6mm \times 6mm \times 2mm$ volume of the central macula at a rate of $27,000$ A-scans/sec. It utilizes a broadband superluminescent diode with a wavelength centered at $840nm$. This provides an axial resolution of $5\mu m$ and a lateral resolution of $20\mu m$. SDOCT can be reconstructed to generate an *enface* SDOCT image, allowing for precise topographic localization of GA [9].

We used our method to automatically segment GA from *en face* SDOCT images. In both examples we present here, we used a circle as target shape. **Fig. 1** illustrates our results using a set of A-scans, where the brighter region is the GA: the three images were obtained using the intensity values (a) in a predefined depth across the A-scans, (b) of all depths from each scan (with averaging), and (c) a specific depth range from each scan (bounded by the so-called *anatomic countour*); the latter is the fundus image used for patient evaluation. We illustrate these three cases to show the performance of our approach on the same data and under different rates of region ambiguities. In Fig. 1(d) and (e) we illustrate the model evolution on the image of Fig. 1(c), using one

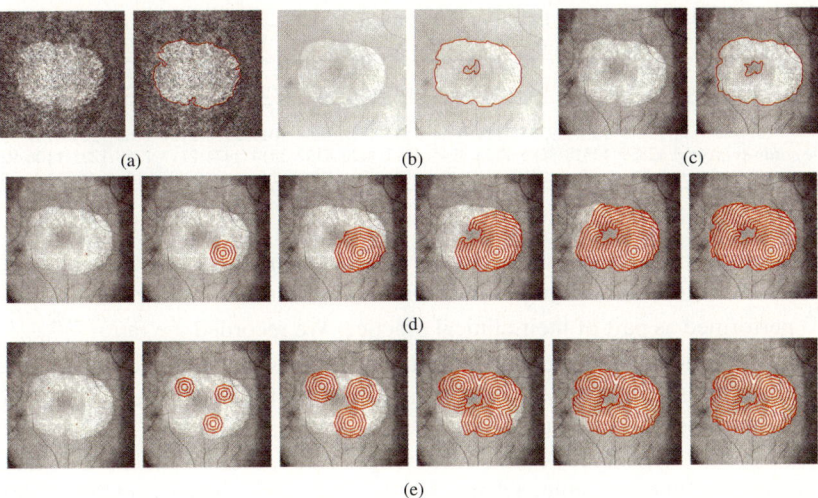

Fig. 1. GA segmentation in SDOCT fundus images: (a)-(c) images obtained using intensities from different depths across the A-scans; (d)-(e): model evolution using one and three markers for the model initialization. The model boundaries are shown in red.

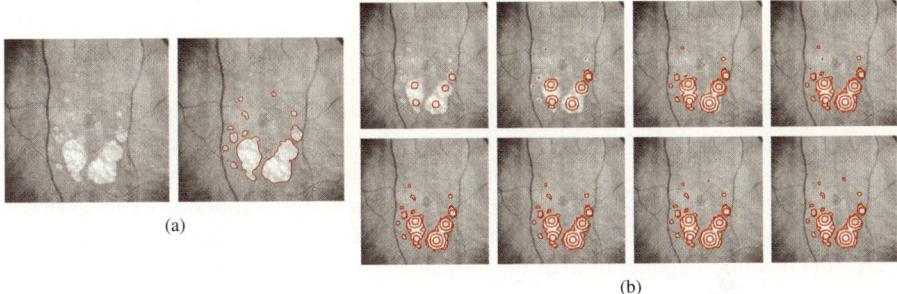

Fig. 2. GA segmentation: our dynamically updated CoCRF detects new GA regions during the model evolution. The model boundaries are shown in red.

and three markers for initialization respectively. The image resolution is 200×200 pixels, and in our CoCRF we used 5×5 patches as sites. **Fig. 2** illustrates another example of GA segmentation: (a) the original image (left) and the segmentation result (right); (b) the model evolution using five markers for initialization. During the evolution, new regions are detected by our CoCRF, due to the dynamic updating of the model interior statistics, and the confidence-driven classification. In this case, the CoCRF probability field overcomes the effect of the partitioning energy term of eqs. (3)-(4), which forces the zero-level of the model distance function towards a connected form. In this example we used pixels as sites in our CoCRF.

For the numerical validation of our method's performance, we used 15 subjects (A-scan sets), from which we manually selected a depth value and a depth range (inside the anatomic contour) to produce the fundus images similar to Fig. 1(a), (c). We

Table 1. Segmentation results for the fifteen subjects (see text). Image size $= 200 \times 200$ pixels.

Subject	#1	#2	#3	#4	#5	#6	#7	#8	#9	#10	#11	#12	#13	#14	#15
Ground-truth	12871	10347	9305	7127	4955	4553	4432	4201	3019	2978	2121	1763	1229	1109	931
True positives (pixels)	12839	10318	9285	7113	4945	4542	4420	4192	3014	2974	2117	1758	1225	1106	928
False positives (pixels)	23	32	21	11	13	12	16	9	14	6	8	12	7	11	8

compared our segmentation results with the detailed manual segmentation that two experts from Bascom Palmer Eye Institute (*www.bpei.med.miami.edu*, University of Miami) performed as part of their clinical practice. We recorded the ratio $\frac{\mathcal{A}(\mathcal{R}_m \cap \mathcal{R}_a)}{\mathcal{A}(\mathcal{R}_m)}$, where $\mathcal{R}_m$, $\mathcal{R}_a$ denote the manually and automatically estimated regions, and $\mathcal{A}(\cdot)$ denotes the area. The ratio variations for the three kinds of fundus images were: (i) single A-scan depth: $98.6 - 99.3\%$, (ii) entire A-scan depth range: $98.9 - 99.7\%$, and (iii) anatomic contour-determined A-scan depth range: $99.7 - 99.8\%$. Table 1 illustrates the validation results for the examined data set, where the fundus images are 200×200 pixels: the false positives (background regions that were detected as GA) are mainly due to small brighter background regions outside the main (bigger) GA segments. Currently we are using our method in clinical trials for further validation.

5 Conclusions

We presented a deformable model integrated with discriminative learning-based classification, with the model interior statistics being dynamically updated and used in an active learning manner. For the classification, we used a new CRF-based collaborative framework (CoCRF), which infers class posteriors in regions with intensity ambiguities, by using the joint appearance and the classification confidence of neighboring sites. We demonstrated our results on the segmentation of geographic atrophies in dry age-related macular degeneration of the human eye, from SDOCT fundus images.

References

1. Chan, T., Zhu, W.: Level Set Based Shape Prior Segmentation. In: CVPR (2005)
2. Cohen, L.D., Cohen, I.: Finite-element Methods for Active Contour Models and Balloons for 2-D and 3-D Images. IEEE PAMI 15, 1131–1147 (1993)
3. Florin, C., Williams, J., Paragios, N.: Globally Optimal Active Contours, Sequential Monte Carlo and On-line Learning for Vessel Segmentation. In: ECCV (2006)
4. Friedman, D.S., O'Colmain, B.J., Muñoz, B., Tomany, S.C., McCarty, C., de Jong, P.T., Nemesure, B., Mitchell, P., Kempen, J.: Prevalence of age-related macular degeneration in the United States. Arch. Ophthalmol. 122(4), 564–572 (2004)
5. He, X., Zemel, R., Carreira-Perpinan, M.: Multiscale Conditional Random Fields for Image Labeling. In: CVPR (2004)
6. Huang, R., Pavlovic, V., Metaxas, D.: A Tightly Coupled Region-Shape Framework for 3D Medical Image Segmentation. In: ISBI (2006)
7. Huang, X., Metaxas, D., Chen, T.: Metamorphs: Deformable Shape and Texture Models. In: CVPR (2004)

8. Huang, R., Pavlovic, V., Metaxas, D.: A Graphical Model Framework for Coupling MRFs and Deformable Models. In: CVPR (2004)
9. Jiao, S., Knighton, R., Huang, X., Gregori, G., Puliafito, C.: Simultaneous acquisition of sectional and fundus ophthalmic images with spectral-domain optical coherence tomography. Optics Express 13(2), 444–452 (2005)
10. Kapoor, A., Grauman, K., Urtasun, R., Darrell, T.: Active Learning with Gaussian Processes for Object Categorization. In: ICCV (2007)
11. Kass, M., Witkin, A., Terzopoulos, D.: Snakes: Active contour models. Int'l. Journal of Computer Vision 1, 321–331 (1987)
12. Kumar, S., Hebert, M.: Discriminative Fields for Modeling Spatial Dependencies in Natural Images. Advances in Neural Information Processing Systems (2004)
13. Lafferty, J., McCallum, A., Pereira, F.: Conditional Random Fields: Probabilistic Models for Segmenting and Labeling Sequence Data. In: ICML (2001)
14. Malladi, R., Sethian, J., Vemuri, B.: Shape Modeling with Front Propagation: A Level Set Approach. IEEE PAMI 17(2), 158–175 (1995)
15. McInerney, T., Terzopoulos, D.: Deformable Models in Medical Image Analysis: A Survey. Medical Image Analysis 1(2) (1996)
16. Mumford, D., Shah, J.: Optimal Approximations by Piecewise Smooth Functions and Associated Variational Problems. Communications on Pure and Applied Mathematics 42(5), 577–685 (1989)
17. Paragios, N., Deriche, R.: Geodesic Active Regions and Level Set Methods for Supervised Texture Segmentation. Int'l Journal of Computer Vision 46(3), 223–247 (2002)
18. Paragios, N., Rousson, M., Ramesh, V.: Matching Distance Functions: A Shape-to-Area Variational Approach for Global-to-Local Registration. In: Heyden, A., Sparr, G., Nielsen, M., Johansen, P. (eds.) ECCV 2002. LNCS, vol. 2351, pp. 775–789. Springer, Heidelberg (2002)
19. Platt, J.C.: Probabilistic outputs for support vector machines and comparisons to regularized likelihood methods. In: Advances in Large Margin Classifiers, pp. 61–74. MIT Press, Cambridge (1999)
20. Ronfard, R.: Region-based strategies for active contour models. Int'l Journal of Computer Vision 13(2), 229–251 (1994)
21. Smith, W., Assink, J., Klein, R., Mitchell, P., Klaver, C.C., Klein, B.E., Hofman, A., Jensen, S., Wang, J.J., de Jong, P.T.: Risk factors for age-related macular degeneration: Pooled findings from three continents. Ophthalmology 108(4), 697–704 (2001)
22. Tsechpenakis, G., Metaxas, D.: CRF-driven Implicit Deformable Model. In: CVPR (2007)
23. Xu, C., Prince, J.L.: Snakes, Shapes and Gradient Vector Flow. IEEE Trans. on Image Processing 7(3), 359–369 (1998)
24. Zhu, S., Yuille, A.: Region Competition: Unifying snakes, region growing, and Bayes/MDL for multi-band image segmentation. IEEE PAMI 18(9), 884–900 (1996)

Contractile Analysis with Kriging Based on MR Myocardial Velocity Imaging

Su-Lin Lee, Andrew Huntbatch, and Guang-Zhong Yang

Royal Society/Wolfson Foundation MIC Laboratory,
Imperial College London, United Kingdom
{su-lin.lee,a.huntbatch,g.z.yang}@imperial.ac.uk

Abstract. Diagnosis and treatment of coronary artery disease requires a full understanding of the intrinsic contractile mechanics of the heart. MR myocardial velocity imaging is a promising technique for revealing intramural cardiac motion but its ability to depict 3D strain tensor distribution is constrained by anisotropic voxel coverage of velocity imaging due to limited imaging slices and the achievable SNR in patient studies. This paper introduces a novel Kriging estimator for simultaneously improving the tracking and dense inter-slice estimation of the myocardial velocity data. A harmonic embedding technique is employed to determine point correspondence between left ventricle models between subjects, allowing for a statistical shape model to be reconstructed. The use of different semivariograms is investigated for optimal deformation reconstruction. Results from *in vivo* data demonstrate a marked improvement in tracking myocardial deformation, thus enhancing the potential clinical value of MR myocardial velocity imaging.

1 Introduction

Coronary artery disease has been the focus of much research due to its considerable morbidity and poor prognosis. The interpretation and prediction of changes induced require a full understanding of the underlying mechanics of coronary flow and myocardial contraction. While visualization of global changes in contractile patterns is possible, examination of local changes in the myocardium requires a more sensitive and quantitative technique. In recent years, Cardiovascular Magnetic Resonance (CMR) has emerged as a versatile technique for non-invasive assessment of intramural motion of the myocardium and has taken a key role in diagnosing myocardial contractile abnormalities.

Historically, the most popular CMR technique for measuring myocardial deformation is MR tagging [1]. More recently, the use of motion tracking with Harmonic Phase (HARP), displacement encoding (DENSE), and myocardial velocity mapping has received increased attention. For myocardial velocity mapping, recent work on pulse sequence design has significantly improved its sensitivity, SNR, and resilience to blood flow artifacts. Detailed, reliable myocardial contractility information is obtained that can be directly used for myocardial modeling. One of the drawbacks of myocardial velocity mapping is that its direct visualization is less intuitive than strain/strain rate information as revealed by myocardial tagging, due to the superimposition of global, as well as local myocardial motion. Reliable integration of myocardial velocity information requires physical based 3D modeling combined with correct noise estimation of the velocity data.

Thus far, research into 3D modeling of intramural cardiac motion using velocity imaging has been limited. Current modeling techniques require extensive *a priori* data, many of which are difficult to obtain on a per subject basis - for example, material properties and fiber orientation. Bergvall *et al.* [2] used Fourier tracking to examine myocardial deformation. Motion was calculated using an iterative scheme involving regularization to remove the effects of noise. The method was extended by considering data certainty and regularity of the model to improve performance [3]. Masood *et al.* [4] introduced the *virtual tagging* framework to derive strain distribution from myocardial velocity data. In virtual tagging, an artificial tag pattern is superimposed onto the velocity data and the subsequent deformation is observed. If the deformation of the virtual tags is correct, the estimated velocity distribution should be identical to the directly measured CMR velocity data in a least-mean-squares sense. Under this framework, *a priori* information is not required and hence the technique is suitable for subject specific modeling. More recently, the method has been extended by introducing a prediction framework based on kernel-partial least squares regression to predict the distortion of a fine mesh from that of a coarse one [5]. Results from training sets based on a leave-one-out analysis were shown to be promising but the technique would be more effective with training sets from multiple subjects. For this reason, the left ventricles of the subjects must be aligned and mesh correspondence must be found. With correspondence achieved, a model can be built from the resulting training set; such a model could be used for segmentation or as input to the described prediction framework.

Recent work on myocardial velocity data has revealed problems due to anisotropic voxel coverage caused by limited imaging slices and the achievable SNR in patient studies. The purpose of this paper is to introduce a novel Kriging estimator for simultaneously improving the tracking and dense inter-slice estimation of the myocardial velocity data. Kriging is a geostatistical technique to interpolate the value of a random field and it has been used in 3D medical imaging for isosurface generation and tensor estimation and registration [6, 7]. In this paper, we incorporate the Kriging estimator into the virtual tagging framework with surface harmonic embedding such that improved tracking with material correspondence can be achieved. Detailed validation is performed on *in vivo* MR velocity data sets from five normal subjects.

2 Methods

2.1 Virtual Tagging and the Kriging Estimator

The concept of virtual tagging was introduced for myocardial contractility analysis for improved strain visualization to avoid the explicit use of tissue properties that are not readily available *in vivo*. A 3D grid is overlaid onto the velocity image slices and is manipulated based on the surrounding velocity vectors. The cost function E to be minimized is

$$E = \sum_i |\Delta \vec{v}_i|^2 \Delta t^2 + \alpha \sum_i |\xi_i - 1| S_i \,. \tag{1}$$

Δv is the difference between the estimated and measured velocity vectors, Δt is the difference in time between two consecutive timeframes, α is a weighting function, ξ is the change in volume of each element, and S is the surface area of the element. In this paper, we incorporate the *ordinary Kriging estimator* into the framework to improve the tracking of the myocardial velocity vectors across the cardiac cycle. Kriging is used to interpolate the estimated velocity value at each pixel based on the surrounding mesh nodal values.

Kriging estimation is a modified linear regression technique and is based on the spatial distribution of the samples. The interpolated value is calculated using a neighborhood of the N closest points surrounding the chosen location. The basic Kriging equation is

$$\hat{Z}(p) = \sum_{i=1}^{N} w_i Z_i (p_i) \,. \tag{2}$$

where $\hat{Z}(p)$ is the estimated value at point p, $Z_i(p_i)$ are the known regionalized variables at known points p_i, and w_i are the weights. Kriging is considered the best linear unbiased estimator due to the following two conditions:

$$\begin{aligned} \mathrm{E}\left(\hat{Z} - Z\right) &= 0 \\ \mathrm{E}\left(\hat{Z} - Z\right)^2 &\text{ is minimum} \end{aligned} \tag{3}$$

The system is solved for by using a Laplacian Multiplier λ to obtain this system of equations:

$$\begin{aligned} \sum_j w_i g(h_{ij}) + \lambda &= g(h_{ip}) \quad (i = 1, \ldots, N) \\ \sum_j w_j &= 1 \end{aligned} \tag{4}$$

Weights w for each point are calculated based on a variogram, half of the variance of the difference between two variables, describing the degree of spatial dependence of the spatial field. A variogram is the expected squared increment of the values between two locations, making it suitable for interpolation. In some applications, a semivariogram (half the variogram) is chosen by fitting a model to empirical data but many now utilize a model semivariogram $g(h)$.

To our knowledge, the choice of model semivariogram has not been studied in medical image applications. In this paper, we compare three model semivariograms to be used within the virtual tagging framework: the exponential semivariogram,

$$g(h) = c \left(1 - \exp\left(\frac{-3h}{a}\right)\right) \tag{5}$$

the Gaussian semivariogram,

$$g(h) = c\left[1 - \exp\left(\frac{-3h^2}{a^2}\right)\right] \quad (6)$$

and the spherical semivariogram.

$$g(h) = \begin{cases} c \cdot \left[1.5\left(\frac{h}{a}\right) - 0.5\left(\frac{h}{a}\right)^3\right] & \text{if } h \leq a \\ c & \text{otherwise} \end{cases} \quad (7)$$

where h is the distance between the samples of interest, c is the sill, *i.e.*, the limit of the variogram tending to infinity distances, and a is the range, a distance in which the difference of the variogram from the sill is negligible. While the sill requires an accurate value, the range value can be dispersed.

2.2 Data Acquisition

For *in vivo* validation of the proposed method, five normal subjects were scanned using a gradient-echo phase-contrast protocol (TR = 53ms, TE = 7.1ms, in-plane pixel resolution = 1.17×1.17mm, FOV = 30×30cm, VENC = -15 to +15 cm/s), obtaining a total of 12 to 14 short axis velocity mapping images of the heart with 10-18 timeframes spanning the cardiac cycle on a 1.5T Siemens Sonata MR scanner. The images were restored using a rigid body motion correction and a Total Variational (TV) restoration technique [8, 9]. In the sequence, a specially designed black-blood RF pulse is applied every other time frame followed by the imaging pulse and a k-space viewsharing scheme is incorporated to reduce the total scan time needed, hence allowing for one reference image and three orthogonally encoded velocity images to be acquired. Free-breathing data acquisition is possible through the use of diaphragmatic navigator echoes and this ensures geometrical and functional consistency of the 3D cine myocardial velocity data.

2.3 Volumetric Left Ventricle Model

The left ventricles are first semi-automatically segmented from the reference MR images. Epi- and endocardial surfaces are generated from the slice contours and a volumetric model is built by connecting these surfaces together. However, the points defining these volumes do not correspond across subjects.

To establish correspondence between the two volume models, surface harmonic embedding was applied [10]. With this technique, the epi- and endocardial surfaces are first harmonically mapped to a hollow half sphere. A template of points is then overlaid on the normalised space, providing each surface, regardless of size or subject, with the same number of points defining it. Correspondence is established across two or more subjects through the use of the Minimum Description Length (MDL) criterion. The points are manipulated such that the MDL cost function is minimised, indicating that the model is compact and is unlikely to have spurious modes of variation when Principal Components Analysis (PCA) is applied. After optimisation is complete, the resultant surfaces are reconnected to reform the volumetric mesh.

Correspondence is only found between the left ventricles at the first timeframe of each subject. The application of virtual tagging ensures that these points are tracked across time and therefore, correspondence will remain.

3 Results

In Figure 1, the difference made by the incorporation of the Kriging estimator is visually presented. The use of the Kriging estimator gives a smoother output, especially with the strains, but still tracks the correct movement of the left ventricle. The differences in the virtual tagging due to the use of different semivariograms are shown in Table 1. While all the errors are at a sub-pixel level, use of the Gaussian and spherical semivariograms currently causes slower convergence of the virtual tagging program.

In Figure 2, the strain results are shown from one subject across the cardiac cycle. The results are as expected with the strains following the expected movement in all components. The heart has complex motion that can be broken down into three components – longitudinal, circumferential, and radial. Longitudinally, the heart shortens and lengthens; radially, the heart wall thickens and thins; and circumferentially, there is twisting, leading to contraction and expansion. Component strains are also examined in the left ventricle at each region of the standard AHA 17 segment model [11] in Figure 2. Longitudinal, radial, and circumferential strains are all displayed – in particular, the longitudinal strains are much improved over many existing techniques.

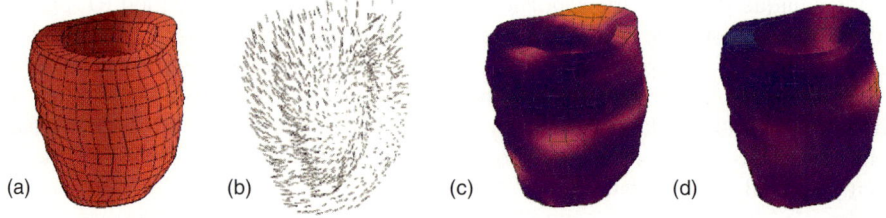

Fig. 1. An example of strain analysis results based on MR phase contrast velocity mapping with and without Kriging. (a) The input shape to the virtual tagging framework, (b) the sampled velocity field showing the noise that can affect the deformation, (c) the deformation found without Kriging, with radial strain overlaid, and (d) the deformation recovered with Kriging.

Table 1. Mean position errors from one subject across three time frames comparing exponential, spherical, and Gaussian model semivariograms

	Semivariogram		
TF	Exponential	Gaussian	Spherical
1	0.154	0.109	0.120
2	0.292	0.228	0.202
3	0.166	0.192	0.120

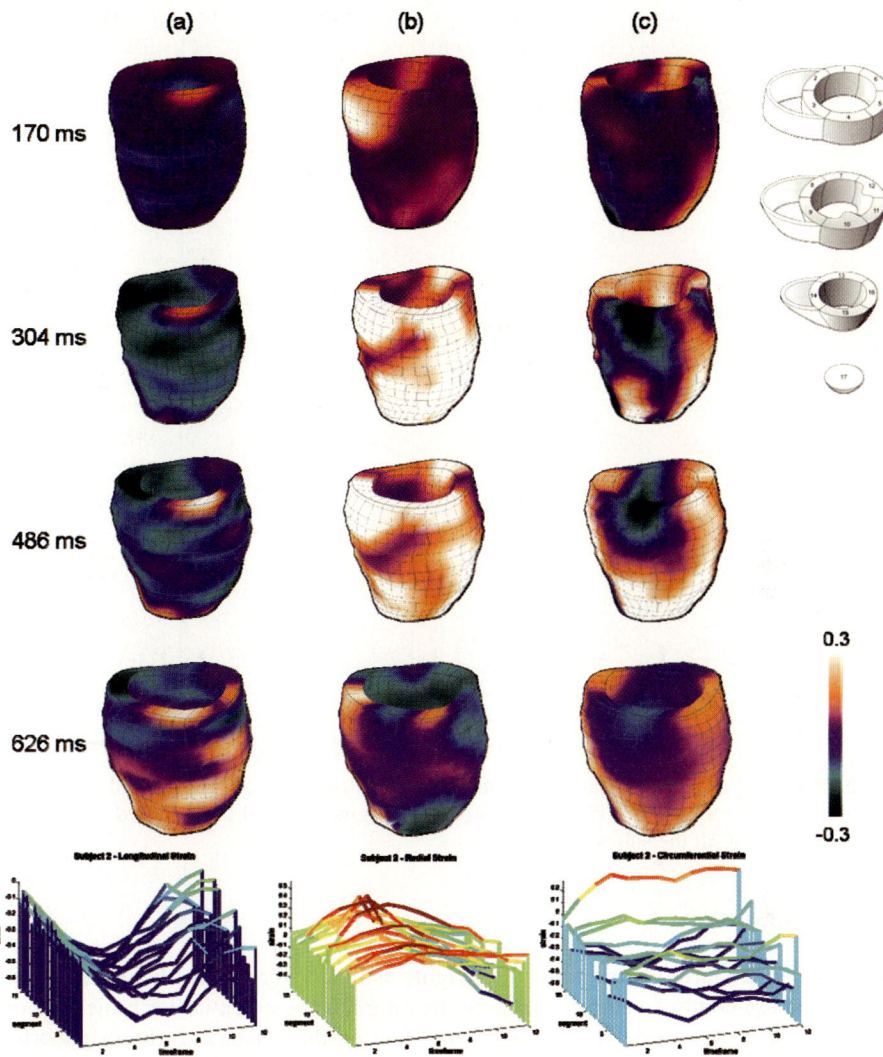

Fig. 2. Strain results from one of the subjects studied – (a) longitudinal, (b) radial, and (c) circumferential strain distribution after Kriging. The seventeen segment model of the left ventricle and the component strains at each of the segment regions are shown to the right and below.

While both the longitudinal strains and radial strains strongly correlate with previous investigations, with the left ventricle clearing showing longitudinal shortening and radial contraction, the circumferential strains are less strong. In Figure 3, the mean values of each strain components are shown for each of the left ventricle segments (except Segment 17 - the apical segment).

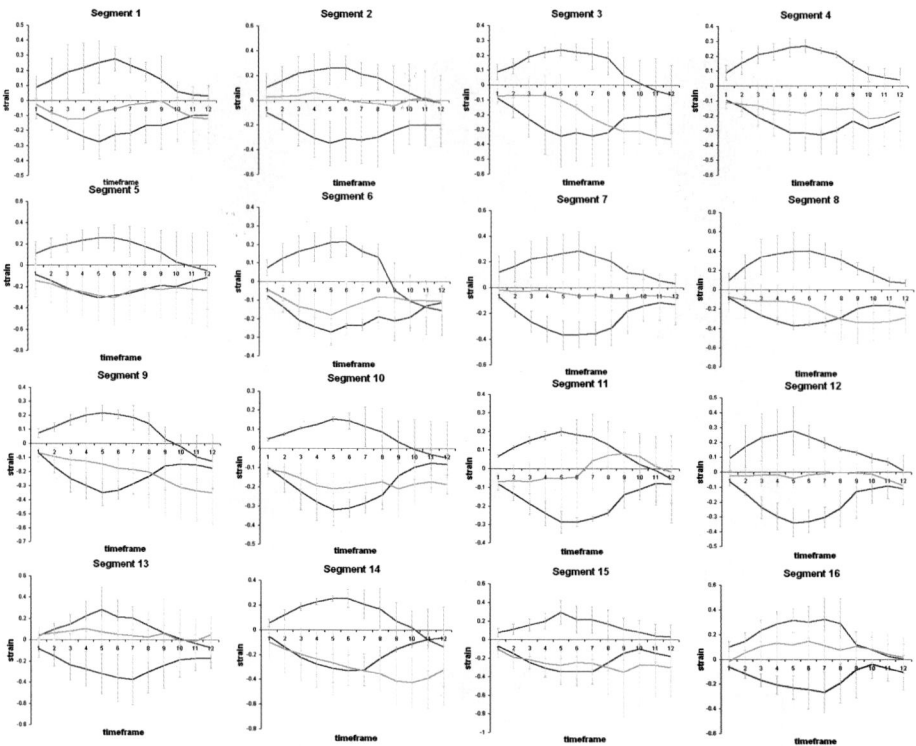

Fig. 3. Mean and standard deviations of the longitudinal (blue), radial (pink), and circumferential (green) strains for each of the segments (except Segment 17) of the standard AHA 17 segment model across all the subjects studied

4 Conclusions

In this paper, we have incorporated the Kriging estimator for myocardial strain analysis based on phase contrast velocity mapping. Kriging has the potential for projecting optimal interpolation estimates and is only dependent on the distance to the neighborhood samples. We have shown that the final result is relatively immune to the choice of semivariogram, but the convergence of the algorithm can be affected by different semivariograms. The proposed technique has provided promising results in the tracking of the left ventricle throughout the cardiac cycle with MR velocity images. When combined with the virtual tagging framework, the method allows accurate material correspondence, and thus can serve as a valuable tool for detailed myocardial strain analysis.

Acknowledgements

The authors wish to thank the team at the Royal Brompton Hospital, London, UK, for their assistance in image acquisition and Robert Merrifield for his assistance with images.

References

1. Axel, L., Dougherty, L.: MR Imaging of Motion with Spatial Modulation of Magnetization. Radiology 171, 841–845 (1989)
2. Bergvall, E., Cain, P., Arheden, H., Sparr, G.: A Fast and Highly Automated Approach to Myocardial Motion Analysis Using Phase Contrast Magnetic Resonance Imaging. Journal of Magnetic Resonance Imaging 23, 652–661 (2006)
3. Bergvall, E., Hedstrom, E., Arheden, H., Sparr, G.: Model Based Cardiac Motion Tracking Using Velocity Encoded Magnetic Resonance Imaging. In: Ersbøll, B.K., Pedersen, K.S. (eds.) SCIA 2007. LNCS, vol. 4522, pp. 82–91. Springer, Heidelberg (2007)
4. Masood, S., Gao, J., Yang, G.-Z.: Virtual Tagging: Numerical Considerations and Phantom Validation. IEEE Transactions on Medical Imaging 21, 1123–1131 (2002)
5. Lee, S.-L., Wu, Q., Huntbatch, A., Yang, G.Z.: Predictive K-PLSR Myocardial Contractility Modeling with Phase Contrast MR Velocity Mapping. In: Ayache, N., Ourselin, S., Maeder, A. (eds.) MICCAI 2007, Part II. LNCS, vol. 4792, pp. 866–873. Springer, Heidelberg (2007)
6. Parrott, R.W., Stytz, M.R., Amburn, P., Robinson, D.: Towards Statistically Optimal Interpolation for 3-D Medical Imaging. IEEE Engineering in Medicine and Biology 12, 49–59 (1993)
7. Ruiz-Alzola, J., Westin, C.-F., Warfield, S.K., Alberola, C., Maier, S., Kikinis, R.: Nonrigid Registration of 3D Tensor Medical Data. Medical Image Analysis 6, 143–161 (2002)
8. Ng, Y.-H.P., Yang, G.-Z.: Vector-valued image restoration with applications to magnetic resonance velocity imaging. Journal of WSCG 11 (2003)
9. Ng, Y.-H., Carmo, B., Yang, G.-Z.: Flow Field Abstraction and Vortex Detection for MR Velocity Mapping. In: Ellis, R.E., Peters, T.M. (eds.) MICCAI 2003. LNCS, vol. 2878, pp. 424–431. Springer, Heidelberg (2003)
10. Horkaew, P., Yang, G.-Z.: Construction of 3D Dynamic Statistical Deformable Models for Complex Topological Shapes. In: Barillot, C., Haynor, D.R., Hellier, P. (eds.) MICCAI 2004. LNCS, vol. 3216, pp. 217–224. Springer, Heidelberg (2004)
11. Cerqueira, M.D., Weissman, N.J., Dilsizian, V., Jacobs, A.K., Kaul, S., Laskey, W.K., et al.: Standardized Myocardial Segmentation and Nomenclature for Tomographic Imaging of the Heart. Circulation 105, 539–542 (2002)

Averaging Centerlines: Mean Shift on Paths

Theo van Walsum[1], Michiel Schaap[1], Coert T. Metz[1],
Alina G. van der Giessen[2], and Wiro J. Niessen[1]

[1] Biomedical Imaging Group Rotterdam
Departments of Radiology and Medical Informatics
[2] Hemodynamics Laboratory
Department of Biomedical Engineering
Erasmus MC – University Medical Center Rotterdam
t.vanwalsum,michiel.schaap,c.metz,
a.g.vandergiessen,w.niessen@erasmusmc.nl

Abstract. Generation of a reference standard from multiple manually annotated datasets is a non-trivial problem. This paper discusses the weighted averaging of 3D open curves, which we used to generate a reference standard for vessel tracking data. We show how weighted averaging can be implemented by applying the Mean Shift algorithm to paths, and discuss the details of our implementation. Our approach can handle cases where the observer centerlines take different branches in a natural way. The method has been evaluated on synthetic data, and has been used to generate reference centerlines for evaluation of vessel tracking algorithms.

1 Introduction

It is commonly understood that thorough evaluation of methodologies and algorithms is essential for progress in the field of medical imaging. Such evaluations require a set of test data, a reference standard (we prefer to use this phrase if there is no ground truth available), and a set of measures to quantify the results for evaluation.

The authors are involved in the coronary artery tracking challenge (http://cat08.bigr.nl), and therefore these issues were to be addressed in this context. As no ground truth central lumen lines are available for our clinical datasets, three observers manually annotated the central lumen lines: from a fixed starting position, the centerline of the main vessel should be annotated as distal as possible. However, the observers did not always take the same decision at bifurcations and also the handling of vessel pathology such as stenoses or regions with non-circular lumen cross sections was not always consistent. In our efforts to come to a reference standard from a set of three manually drawn centerlines we therefore soon came to the conclusion that plain averaging does not work. The most important requirement of the averaging process is that it should give reference centerlines that are nearly always inside the vessel lumen, i.e. the reference centerline should follow the "majority votes" centerline. The main contribution of this paper is a method to "average" these centerlines into a reference standard.

Many publications have appeared that implement a way to compare open curves. If correspondence between centerlines is known, and bifurcations are not a problem, then approaches to estimate the mean of a set of curves can be applied [1]. To the best of our knowledge, no work has been published that addresses how to generate a reference centerline from several manually annotated lines, if there is no explicit correspondence between the lines.

Warfield et al. [2] address the related issue of generating a ground truth segmentation and propose a method called STAPLE. They use a Maximum Likelihood Expectation Maximization algorithm to estimate the performance parameters of the observers (and possibly software algorithms) given a set of segmentations, with the reference standard segmentation modelled as hidden data. This approach is appealing, as it not only determines a reference standard from multiple segmentations, but also addresses the issue of sensitivity and specificity of the observers and automated approaches.

More recently, Jomier et al. [3] showed how STAPLE could be used for evaluating centerlines in vessel segmentation. They propose to voxelize the open curves, dilate them and then apply STAPLE to the resulting segmentations, which yields a probability map of the ground truth segmentation. Their work is most related to ours.

The remainder of the paper is organized as follows. In Sect. 2 and 3, we describe our method and the implementation, in Sect. 4 our experiments are described, followed by Results and Discussion in Sect. 5 and 6 and Conclusions in Sect. 7.

2 Averaging Via Mean Shift

We propose to perform a weighted averaging to determine the reference centerline, where the weights depend on the distance from the reference. This suggests that averaging can be performed via the Mean Shift algorithm [4,5], which is an algorithm that iteratively shifts a data point along the gradient of a density that is determined by a set of data points and kernel functions, until the gradient vanishes, and the point has arrived at a mode (maximum) of the density.

More formally, the Mean Shift algorithm with Gaussian kernels G_σ and for a set of m datapoints can be described by the following iterative procedure (see e.g. Carreira-Perpinan [5]):

$$\mathbf{x}^{\tau+1} = \sum_{m=1}^{M} \frac{G_\sigma(|\mathbf{x}^\tau - \mu_\mathbf{m}|)}{\sum_{m'=1}^{M} G_\sigma(|\mathbf{x}^\tau - \mu_{\mathbf{m'}}|)} \mu_\mathbf{m} \;, \tag{1}$$

where μ_m represents the mth data point. After convergence of the algorithm, the mean shifted position x is the weighted average of the data points, where the weights are determined by the distance to the weighted average and the kernel function used.

This Mean Shift algorithm is a well-known algorithm, that has, among others, been used to find the modes of clusters in feature space analysis in image processing [4]. We adapt Eq. 1 for our application to paths (we will use path instead of centerline to underline that our method is applicable to any open 3D curve) in the following way.

Let $p_i(t)$ with $0 \leq i < m$ (m number of paths) and $t \in [0, 1]$ be the path annotated by the ith observer and parametrized by parameter t, and $r_i(t)$, $t \in [0, 1]$ be the mean shifted path to be determined. Furthermore, let $s_i(t)$ be a bijection from $[0, 1]$ to $[0, 1]$ that defines the correspondence between r_i and p_i, i.e. $r_i(t)$ corresponds to $p_i \circ s_i(t)$. Thus s_i relates positions along r_i to positions along p_i that will be used in the Mean Shift algorithm. The mean shift r_i of path p_i is then given by the following equation:

$$r_i^{\tau+1} = \sum_j \frac{G_\sigma(|r_i^\tau - p_j \circ s_j|)}{\sum_k G_\sigma(|r_i^\tau - p_k \circ s_k|)} p_j \circ s_j , \qquad (2)$$

where the corresondence function s_i may change after each iteration, and $r_i^0 = p_i$. This equations states that each point along r_i is shifted to the weighted average of the corresponding points on all paths p_j.

We apply this adapted Mean Shift algorithm to each of the manually drawn paths, using the manually annotated paths as data points. This results in a set of mean shifted paths, of which some will coincide for some part (following the same mode), and some may diverge at certain locations. To obtain the final reference path, the largest common part of the shifted paths is determined in a post processing step. Implementation details are discussed in the next section.

3 Implementation

3.1 Correspondence

Equation 2 contains correspondence functions s_i, which relate points from the path being shifted to the observer paths and also vice versa, as s_i is a bijection. Point correspondence must be known, as it determines which points of the paths p_i are involved in the mean shift of a position on r_i.

In our implementation, we use a discretized version S_i of the correspondence function s_i. Equidistant resampling of the input paths is performed before determining the correspondence. Next, the correspondence is determined by finding the minimum of the sum of the Euclidean lengths of all point-point connections that are connecting two paths over all valid correspondences.

Let O be a path, represented by an ordered set of n points $\{o_i\}$, $i \in [1, n]$, and let Q be a second path, represented of an ordered set of m points $\{q_j\}$, $j \in [1, m]$. We define a correspondence C for paths O and Q as the ordered set of connections $\{c_k\}$, $k \in [1, n+m-1]$ where c_k is a tuple $[i, j]$ that represents a connection from o_i to q_j, and we define a valid correspondence as a correspondence satisfying the following conditions:

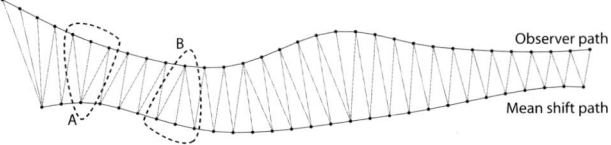

Fig. 1. Correspondence between two lines, as determined by the Dijkstra algorithm. A and B show regions where one point on one path corresponds to multiple points on the other path.

- The first connection c_1 connects the start points: $c_1 = [1, 1]$.
- The last connection c_{n+m-1} connects the end points: $c_{n+m-1} = [n, m]$.
- If connection c_k ($k < n + m - 1$) equals $[i, j]$ then connection c_{k+1} equals either $[i+1, j]$ or $[i, j+1]$.

These conditions guarantee that each point of O is connected to at least one point of Q and vice versa. Note that this is not a bijection, as multiple points on O may be connected to Q, and vice versa. A Dijkstra graph search algorithm [6] on a Cartesian grid with connection lengths as edge costs is used to determine the global minimum Euclidean length correspondence. See Fig. 1 for an example.

3.2 Mean Shift on Paths

Equation 2 shows how to determine the reference path given the positions and weighting factors, by taking the weighted average over all points involved. The correspondence as defined in Sect. 3.1 is not a real bijection, see Fig. 1: a point on the mean shifted path may be connected to several points on an observer path (case A), and vice versa (case B). To account for multiple observer points connected to one point on the mean shifted path (A), the weights are normalized with a factor of $\frac{1}{n_j}$, where n_j is the number of nodes on the observer path that is connected to a point of the mean shifted path. This means that the total weight of a path is not affected by the number of points connected to a point on the mean shifted path. In case one point on the observer path is connected to several points on the mean shifted path (B), that point is used in the mean shifts for each of the points of the mean shifted path it is connected to.

Equation 2 is thus implemented in our discretized Mean Shift algorithm as follows, with R_i, P_i and S_i the discretized versions of respectively the mean shifted path r_i, the observer path p_i and the correspondence s_i:

$$R_i^{\tau+1} = \sum_j \sum_l^{n_j} \frac{\frac{1}{n_j} G_\sigma\left(|R_i^\tau - P_j \circ S_{j,l}|\right)}{\sum_k \sum_{l'}^{n_k} \frac{1}{n_k} G_\sigma\left(|R_k^\tau - P_k \circ S_{k,l'}|\right)} P_i \circ S_{j,l} \ , \qquad (3)$$

where n_j is the number of connections of path j to the position of R_i that is being evaluated, and $S_{j,l}$ corresponds to the lth connection from the position on R_i to P_i and $\frac{1}{n_j}$ is the weighting factor for point multiplicity. This equation is evaluated for each of the points along R_i. The correspondence S_i is redetermined after each mean shift iteration, i.e. after a shift of all points on R_i.

3.3 Post Processing

The implementation of the Mean Shift algorithm on paths returns three shifted paths: each observer path is shifted to a mode of all input paths. In a subsequent post processing step, these paths are merged into one resulting path, representing the "major mode" of the paths. We perform this clustering task in a straightforward way. The local distance between each tuple of mean shifted paths is determined via correspondences established as described in Sect. 3.1. After thresholding this distance, the length of the common part that two paths share can be determined. The tuple with maximum common path length is subsequently chosen, and the average of the two paths of this tuple over the part of the paths that they share is determined.

4 Experiments

The method described in the previous section has been implemented and evaluated. Evaluation was done visually on synthetic test cases, to inspect the behaviour of the algorithms in case of paths ending at different positions, single bifurcations and double bifurcations. In these experiments, the bandwidth σ was set to 2 mm (the path length was around 80 mm, initial sampling distance as shown in the images was 1 mm). The effect of varying the bandwidth was also evaluated, with σ varying from 1 mm to 16 mm, where σ was doubled in each next experiment. These bandwidth experiments are shown together with a plain averaged path, i.e. a path that would be obtained if we would average without weighting factors. This averaging is performed by iteratively averaging tuples of observer paths over all connections that have been determined by the same Dijkstra algorithm, i.e. the plain average path is determined by iterating the following over all i: $p_i^{\tau+1} = \frac{1}{2} \left(p_i^{\tau} + p_{i+1}^{\tau} \right)$ where τ is the iteration number, and $i+1$ wraps at 3 in our case. This iterative approach converges to the average of the three paths.

The method was also used to generate the reference standards from manually annotated centerlines for evaluation of vessel tracking algorithms. Currently, four coronaries have been annotated in 24 coronary CTA datasets by three observers. The method has been tested on all 96 triplets of paths, and the reference paths generated in this way have been checked visually by displaying them in Curved Multiplanar Reformatted images and locally orthogonal views (oriented with the tangential of the centerline), together with interobserver variations. The observer centerlines contained centerlines that take different branches at bifurcations or that ended prematurely and also centerlines that have local deviations. For the mean shift of the centerlines of these coronary arteries we used a σ of 2 mm, which is approximately the average radius of the coronary vessels that we are tracking in this application. This implies that paths running apart much more than 2 mm will not converge to the same mode, which is exactly what we want. The mean shifted paths were determined at a sampling distance of 0.2 mm, and the input observer paths were resampled to a sampling distance of 0.03 mm.

5 Results

Results of the method for the experiments with synthetic data are shown in Fig. 2a–h. In all cases, the reference path is not much affected by a path that chooses another vessel, although a small bump is sometimes noticeable, the size of which depends on the bandwidth of the algorithm. Also paths that end less distal than others do not affect the reference path.

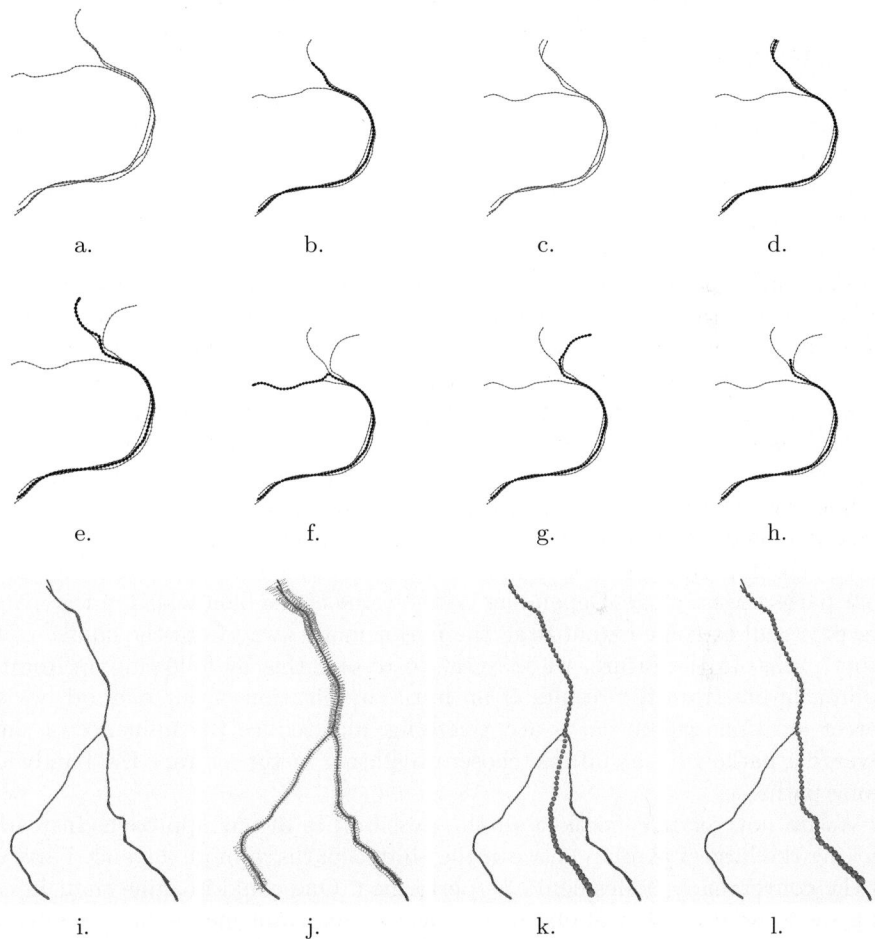

Fig. 2. Examples of the Mean Shift algorithm: a–h to 2D synthetic data, i–l to the 3D paths data. a) three paths, where not all paths run to the distal end; b) mean shift result of a; c) bifurcation in observer paths; d) mean shift result of c; e), f) and g) mean shift result for each of the three observer paths separately; h) final result after clustering the paths; i) centerlines; j) vessels; k) average path; l) mean shift path.

The effect of varying σ on the final reference path is small if changes in σ are small. When σ is large enough, all vessels will be averaged, even if they follow different branches, and the resulting path will be outside all vessels. A slight bump can be observed at the bifurcations with low values for σ, as the bifurcating path initially is near enough to also contribute to the major mode.

All the CTA reference paths have been visually inspected, and all could be used directly for the evaluation of tracking algorithms, none of them needed additional manual editing. Examples are shown in the bottom row of Fig. 2.

6 Discussion

We have shown how the Mean Shift algorithm can be used to determine a weighted average of three manually annotated open curves. Correspondence between two curves was determined by the set of connections with minimal total Euclidean length. Our application involves averaging of three 3D (spatial) curves, and the algorithms discussed have been developed for this specific case. Both the spatial dimensionality and the number of input curves, however, are not essential to the algorithm: our approach can easily be applied to curves in higher- or lower-dimensional space, and also on sets of more than three curves.

The choice of a kernel and bandwidth determines the final result of the algorithm. We chose our bandwidth according to the expected variance of the data: all paths should be in the same vessel, and thus the bandwidth was similar to the vessel radius. We choose the Gaussian kernels because of their assumed better behaviour. The infinite support of the Gaussian kernel, which makes them computationally expensive in other cases [4], is not an issue in our case.

The resulting paths in our implementation may have slight bumps or kinks near paths that diverge. Depending on the value of the bandwidth σ, the diverging path will to some extent drag the major mode away from the course of the other paths. In the future, we may try to resolve this by following an iterative approach: based on the results of an initial application of our method, we can detect locations where paths are diverging, and reduce the influence of single diverging paths with a suitable chosen weighting factor, or vary the bandwidth along paths.

We do not yet fully exploit all the possibilities of our approach. Instead of picking the largest overlap between the shifted paths, a more advanced analysis of the convergence modes could be performed. One could imagine that, in case of a substantial number of observers, several important modes can be detected, even consisting of varying sets of observer paths, all of which should be part of the final reference. In the future, we intend to investigate this issue.

The work most closely related to ours is the STAPLE approach of Jomier et al. [3]. Our approach differs from theirs in several aspects. First, the STAPLE approach requires a voxelization of the input centerlines, whereas our approach is subvoxel accurate. Second, the STAPLE approach yields an explicit probability map that can be used for evaluation, whereas our approach gives a reference centerline, that can be used to derive quantitative measures on the position of other centerlines. The probability map could be used to derive a reference path, but this is not trivial, and it is not discussed in the work of Jomier et al. Third, the STAPLE approach gives a sensitivity and specificity value for the complete curve, whereas we use a weighting factor that varies along the curve. The advantage of the latter approach is that in proximal regions, where all curves track the same vessel, all curves are incorporated in calculating the average with approximately the same weights, even if one of the curves would track another part incorrect, e.g. by tracking the wrong branch at a distal bifurcation, and that weights are decreased locally in case of local errors.

In the future, we want to extend the approach to sets of more than three vessels. Also, we want to investigate how the analysis of the resulting modes can contribute to a better definition of the reference standard. Furthermore, a similar approach could be pursued to determine reference standards for other types of data.

7 Conclusion

We have shown how the Mean Shift algorithm can be used to determine the average centerline from a set of centerlines annotated by observers. The method can handle bifurcating centerlines and centerlines that stop at different distances along the vessel in a natural way. The technique has been applied successfully to 96 manually annotated coronary artery centerlines, and will be used in the evaluation of vessel tracking algorithms.

Acknowledgment

This work was sponsored by the Dutch Foundation for Scientific Research, NWO, STW.

References

1. Rice, J.A., Silverman, B.W.: Estimating the Mean and Covariance Structure Non-parametrically when the Data are Curves. Journal of the Royal Statistical Society. Series B (Methodological) 53(1), 233–243 (1991)
2. Warfield, S.K., Zou, K.H., Wells, W.M.: Simultaneous truth and performance level estimation (STAPLE): an algorithm for the validation of image segmentation. IEEE Transactions on Medical Imaging 23(7), 903–921 (2004)
3. Jomier, J., LeDigarcher, V., Aylward, S.R.: Comparison of vessel segmentations using staple. In: Duncan, J.S., Gerig, G. (eds.) MICCAI 2005. LNCS, vol. 3749, pp. 523–530. Springer, Heidelberg (2005)
4. Comaniciu, D., Meer, P.: Mean Shift: A robust approach toward feature space analysis. IEEE Transactions on Pattern Analysis and Machine Intelligence 24(5), 603–619 (2002)
5. Carreira-Perpiñán, M.: Gaussian Mean-Shift is an EM algorithm. IEEE Transactions on Pattern Analysis and Machine Intelligence 29(5), 767–776 (2007)
6. Dijkstra, E.W.: A note on two problems in connexion with graphs. Numerische Mathematik 1, 269–271 (1959)

On Classifying Disease-Induced Patterns in the Brain Using Diffusion Tensor Images

Peng Wang[1,2] and Ragini Verma[1]

[1] Section of Biomedical Image Analysis, Department of Radiology, University of Pennsylvania, Philadelphia PA, 19104*
[2] Department of Integrated Data Systems, Siemens Corporate Research, Princeton NJ, 08540

Abstract. Diffusion tensor imaging (DTI) provides rich information about brain tissue structure especially in the white matter, which is known to be affected in several diseases like schizophrenia. Identifying patterns of brain changes induced by pathology is therefore crucial to clinical studies. However, the high dimensionality and complex structure of DTI make it difficult to apply conventional linear statistical and pattern classification methods to identify such patterns. In this paper, we present a novel framework that uses a combination of DTI-based anisotropy and geometry features to effectively identify brain regions with pathology-induced abnormality, and to classify brains into the diseased and healthy groups. Our method first directly estimates the underlying overlap between the patient and control groups, based on a semi-parametric Bayes error estimation method. By ranking voxels based on these estimation results, the method identifies abnormal brain regions from which features are extracted through Kernel Principal Component Analysis (KPCA) for subsequent classification. Application of the method to a dataset of controls and patients with schizophrenia, demonstrates promising accuracy of this framework in identifying brain patterns to separate two groups, and hence aiding in prognosis and treatment.

1 Introduction

Diffusion tensor imaging (DTI) [1] characterizes brain tissue structure based on underlying water diffusivity, providing effective and unique characterization of the white matter. It has therefore been extensively used for studying pathology of diseases, such as schizophrenia, where the white matter is known to have been affected [2]. In clinical research, it is important to analyze group differences between patients and controls, by identifying brain abnormality patterns induced by pathology, to provide insight into the progression of the disease. There are usually two types of analysis: voxel-based analysis, which identifies regions of difference between the two groups based on statistics per voxel in the brain or region-of-interest (ROI) [3], and pattern classification that uses the whole brain to classify the patients and controls. Although much research has been done on DTI visualization, segmentation, registration [4,5,6], and group difference analysis for clinical discovery [2], little work has been done in classifying brain patterns using DTI data [7]. In this paper, we present a framework for combining the two types of

---

* This work was done in Section of Biomedical Image Analysis, University of Pennsylvania.

analysis on DTI data, by first identifying abnormal regions at a voxel level, and then incorporating them into a pattern classification framework to differentiate diseased from healthy brains.

The tensorial structure of a 3×3 positive-definite symmetric matrix at each voxel, combined with the high dimensionality of the brain data, make classification of such data challenging. Most of current voxel-based methods apply conventional linear statistical methods, such as t-test and Fisher discriminant analysis (FDA), to single scalar measures of anisotropy and/or diffusivity computed from tensors [2,7]. However, such single scalar measurements do not fully used the rich information in diffusion tensors. FDA usually assumes single Gaussian distribution for each class, and may fail on high dimensional complex DTI data, especially when only limited samples are available in most clinical studies. In [7], a shaving procedure, which iteratively discards small weights in FDA, has been applied to a single scalar measure of anisotropy to select a certain percentage of voxels for classifying brains induced by schizophrenia. The method provides a cross-validation accuracy only between 65% and 75% when using a single type of scalar features. Nonlinear classifiers, such as Support Vector Machine (SVM), have been used to effectively classify structural MRI data [8], but it has not been applied to a combination of DTI features, and its performance is linked with the choice of features different from DTI data.

In this paper, we present a novel framework for DTI-based brain pattern analysis. Our method can identify brain regions where disease induces abnormality of brain tissue, and can combine information from multiple measures extracted from tensors to classify diseased and healthy brains. The framework includes three major parts: ranking voxels based on their discriminant capability, selecting voxels and regions from which features are extracted for pattern analysis, and classifying brains based on the extracted features. First, rooted in the pattern classification theory, our method estimates the underlying overlap between different groups using a semi-parametric Bayes error estimation. Unlike the linear discriminant analysis or t-test, this method does not assume global Gaussian distribution for each class, but only considers data distribution to be locally smooth, thus being able to handle the complex structure in DTI data. Also multiple measures of anisotropy and diffusivity that are extracted from diffusion tensors are incorporated into the Bayes error estimation. Second, individual voxels are ranked according to their estimated Bayes error, and are then grouped into local regions to identify brain patterns induced by disease. Finally, multiple scalar measures are combined through Kernel Principal Component Analysis (KPCA) in local regions, and are input to nonlinear classifiers for region-based group classification. The presented methods are validated on real data sets, and experimental results demonstrate encouraging classification results.

2 Methods

We present in this section a framework of identifying brain patterns induced by diseases with the use of DTI data. In this paper, scalar values are represented by regular lower case letters, while bold lower case letters, such as **x**, and **y**, represent vectors. Capital bold letters, such as **V**, represent sets of vectors. In feature selection and classification, all the DT images are from two classes $C_i \in \{-1, 1\}$, which represent two groups: healthy controls (positive class) and patients with disease (negative class).

2.1 Scalar Features of Diffusion Tensors

In diffusion tensor images, a diffusion tensor at a voxel is a 3×3 positive-definite symmetric matrix D, which can be represented by its eigen-decomposition as $D = \lambda_1 \mathbf{g}_1 \mathbf{g}_1^T + \lambda_2 \mathbf{g}_2 \mathbf{g}_2^T + \lambda_3 \mathbf{g}_3 \mathbf{g}_3^T$, where $\lambda_1 \geq \lambda_2 \geq \lambda_3$ and $\mathbf{g}_1, \mathbf{g}_2, \mathbf{g}_3$ are the eigenvalues and eigenvectors of D respectively. Multiple measures, called "scalar features" in the paper, can be extracted from tensor data. For classification, we focus on two types of features, i.e., anisotropy and geometry based scalar features. We choose Fractional Anisotropy (FA) to characterize the anisotropy of diffusion tensor. The geometry based features characterizes different aspects of tensors in terms of anisotropy and diffusivity: linearity ($C_l = \frac{\lambda_1 - \lambda_2}{\lambda_1}$), planarity ($C_p = \frac{\lambda_2 - \lambda_3}{\lambda_1}$) and sphericity ($C_s = \frac{\lambda_3}{\lambda_1}$). Such scalar features provide different information about brain structures, and their combination is expected to provide comprehensive information of the underlying tissue structure. In this paper, we demonstrate that the combination of multiple scalar features can provide better discriminative accuracy than using single features. Since $C_l + C_p + C_s = 1$, our method uses only two of them, i.e, C_l, C_p, as well as FA.

2.2 Bayes Error Estimation for DTI Feature Selection

A common difficulty in classification of DT images is that they are high dimensional, but there are only a limited number of samples available in any disease-specific classification problem. Therefore for the purposes of analysis, it is important to select a subset of voxels in the brain, which comprehensively represents the underlying abnormality induced by disease. This is equivalent to a typical feature selection task in machine learning [9]. In DTI classification, we re-formalize the feature selection as selecting a subset of voxels, such that the scalar features, including possible combinations of FA, C_l and C_p, in these voxels can well discriminate brains with pathology from healthy brains. Although numerous methods have been proposed to rank and select features [9], identifying a "better choice" is still problem-dependent and hence challenging, in most scenarios. Due to the high dimensionality of medical images, it has been shown that the feature ranking based on the discriminant criteria, followed by classifier-dependent feature selection, is a realistic solution to classification of medical images [8]. However, there is little work in this regard in DT images.

In our framework, we adopt a fundamental method of ranking voxels by estimating their corresponding Bayes error. By its definition, the Bayes error is the minimal error rate that a probabilistic classifier can achieve when applying the Bayes rule [10]. Our method directly estimates Bayes error at each voxel, based on the k-NN and Parzen window method [11,10]. Unlike linear statistical methods that usually assume global Gaussian distributions, this method only assumes the local smoothness in kernel density estimation, therefor it can naturally handle non-Gaussian data. Also this method is able to combine multiple scalar features for voxel selection.

In the Parzen window kernel density estimation, the likelihood probability of **x** for class C_i is given as Eqn. (1):

$$P(\mathbf{x}|C_i) = \frac{1}{nh^d} \sum_{\mathbf{y} \in C_i} K(\frac{\mathbf{y}-\mathbf{x}}{h}) \quad (1)$$

In Eqn. (1), **x** and **y** are feature vectors, which are combinations of scalar features extracted at a voxel from different brains. **y** corresponds to a DT image of the class C_i. n is the total number of samples, d is the feature dimensionality, K is the kernel function, and h is the kernel window size. In our framework, we adopt the widely used Gaussian kernel. Since the $K(\mathbf{y}-\mathbf{x})$ is small when **y** is far from **x**, we only use the data in a k-nearest neighborhood in the kernel density estimation to reduce computational complexity. From the Bayes rule, the posterior probability of class C_i given **x** is

$$P(C_i|\mathbf{x}) \propto P(C_i) \sum_{\mathbf{y} \in C_i, \mathbf{y} \in NN_\mathbf{x}} K(\frac{\mathbf{y}-\mathbf{x}}{h}) \quad (2)$$

where NN_x is a k-nearest neighborhood of **x**. Two parameters in the Gaussian kernel function, i.e., the covariance matrix and kernel size h, can be optimally estimated from training samples assuming local smoothness [12]. According to its definition, the Bayes error rate P_e can be estimated as Eqn. (3):

$$P_e = \sum (1 - \max_i \{(C_i|\mathbf{x})\}) P(\mathbf{x}) \quad (3)$$

Our method estimates error rate P_e at each individual voxel in the brain. The range of P_e is between 0 to 0.5, where 0 means perfect separability and 0.5 means total overlap between classes at a voxel level. The voxels with small error rates are more discriminative of different patterns.

2.3 Region Selection, Feature Extraction, and Classification

For each voxel **v** in the 3D brain image, the Bayes error rate $P_e(\mathbf{v})$ is estimated based on Eqns. (2) and (3), to represent its discriminative capability for pattern classification. To select a subset of voxels for pattern classification, only those voxels with error rate less than a threshold P_{th} are preserved. The selected voxels sets are denoted as $\mathbf{V}^s = \{\mathbf{v}|P_e(\mathbf{v}) < P_{th}\}$. Usually brain tissue changes occur in regions instead of at single voxels; therefore, the selected voxels are further grouped into local regions by connected component analysis. Small local regions are removed to eliminate noisy regions caused by registration error. As a result of region selection, we obtain a set of disjointed local regions, with each local region containing a subset of connected voxels in the brain.

Features are then extracted from the selected regions to characterize brain patterns. Our method first extracts Kernel Principal Component Analysis (KPCA) features from each of the local regions, to remove the nonlinear correlation among scalar features and reduce feature dimensionality. All the local features are then combined into a pattern feature vector $\mathbf{f} = \{\mathbf{f}_1, ..., \mathbf{f}_i, ...\}$ where $\mathbf{f}_i$ is the KPCA feature extracted at i-th local region. The feature vector **f** represents the global brain pattern of a DT image, and is ready to be used for pattern recognition.

For each testing DT image, extracted pattern features **f** are used to predict its class label (healthy/patient). The classification can validate whether selected regions reflect the underlying differences between the healthy and patient groups, and can also provide numerical outputs indicating the degree of class membership, and thereby can assist in disease diagnoses. We adopt a probabilistic k-NN classifier, which follows the same principle of k-NN/Parzen window based kernel density estimation as described in Section 2.2. For a DT image **x** for testing, its posterior probability of belonging to class C_i is estimated as $P(C_i|\mathbf{x}) \propto P(C_i) \sum_{\mathbf{y} \in C_i, \mathbf{y} \in NN_\mathbf{x}} K(\frac{|\mathbf{f_y}-\mathbf{f_x}|}{\sigma'})$, where $\mathbf{f_x}$ and $\mathbf{f_y}$ are pattern features extracted from the testing image **x** and training images **y**, and σ' is the kernel parameter. The predicted class is the one with the maximal posterior probability, i.e., $\hat{C} = \arg_{C_i} \max P(C_i|\mathbf{x})$. In our experiments shown in Section 3, the k-NN classifier has outperformed the commonly used Support Vector Machine (SVM) [13].

3 Experiments

In this study, we apply our method to real datasets. The data set consists of 36 healthy controls (17 male and 19 female) and 34 patients (21 male and 13 female) diagnosed with schizophrenia. The males and females are analyzed separately as the progression of the schizophrenia is known to be different in the genders [14]. All the DTI data has been acquired on a Siemens 3T scanner, at the dimensions of $128 \times 128 \times 40$, with voxel resolution of $1.72 \times 1.72 \times 3.0$ mm. For each subject, DTI images were registered to a common template space using a deformable registration method [6]. Scalar features of FA, C_l and C_p are computed for these normalized images. In the following experiments, abnormal brain regions that can distinguish patients from controls are first identified, and then validated through pattern classification experiments.

3.1 Identifying Abnormal Brain Regions

In the first experiment, we identify brain regions where abnormal tissue changes occur. For each voxel in the brain, the Bayes error is estimated using combinations of scalar features, and then local regions are selected by ranking and filtering voxels, as described in Section 2.3. Since DTI mainly characterizes the white matter, the method is applied to voxels where FA is greater than 0.10 (a loose threshold to mainly discard the CSF). Due to limited space, only the results of female participants with the use of combinations of FA, C_l and C_p are displayed in Figure 1. Figure 1 (a) shows color maps of estimated Bayes error, overlayed on FA maps of a heathy control. For visual effect, the red color shows regions with smaller estimated error rate, meaning higher group separation between patients and healthy people, and blue color represents regions with lower group separation. Figure 1 (b), (c), (d) show identified abnormal regions. Such regions are obtained by setting threshold $P_{th} = 0.40$, which represents a significant group difference at the voxel level. The affected regions are mainly located in the corpus callosum, corona radiata, corticospinal tract, and cingulum bundle. These regions have been confirmed to be affected in schizophrenia by other researchers [2] using completely different methods.

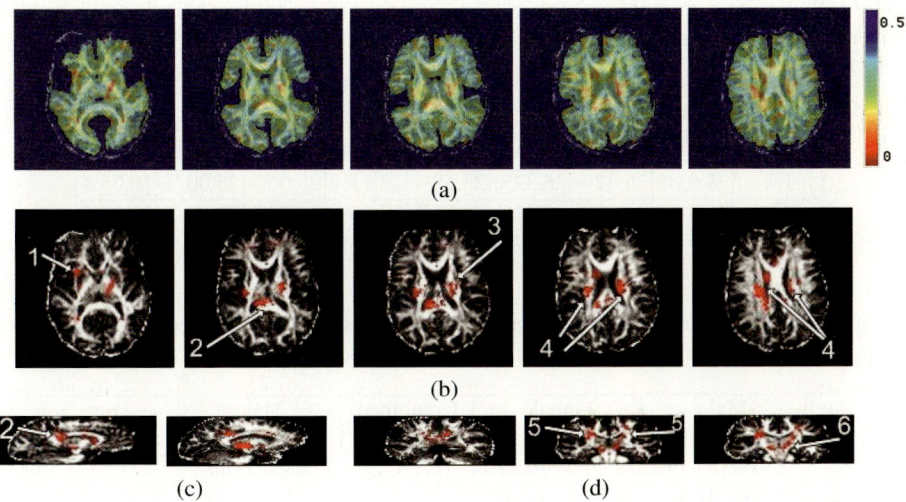

Fig. 1. Bayes error estimation and identified abnormal brain regions in female participants by using combinations of FA, C_l and C_p. (a): map of estimated Bayes error overlayed on FA maps of a healthy control at the axial view. The red color shows smaller estimated error rate, i.e., more discriminative regions; (b) (c) (d): some identified regions (P_{th} = 0.40) at the axial, sagittal and coronal views respectively. Some of those regions lie in: (1) external capsule; (2) corpus callosum; (3) internal capsule; (4) cingulum bundle; (5) corona radiata; (6) corticospinal tract.

3.2 Validation of Classification

The identified regions indicate possible existence of disease-induced abnormal tissue changes in the brain. To evaluate how such regions can be used to distinguish between brain patterns of patients and healthy controls, cross-validation experiments [10] are performed. *We first validate that our framework provides better accuracy than a commonly used correlation based feature selection method, through experiments on single features, and then we demonstrate that combinations of multiple features can further improve classification accuracy.* In the cross-validation, only the training set will be used for the feature selection and classifier training. The Bayes error estimation based feature selection is compared with a commonly used feature selection method based on linear correlation coefficients, applied to both SVM and k-NN classifiers. In the correlation based feature selection, the linear correlation coefficient γ between a scalar feature variable x and class label c is calculated as $\gamma = \frac{\sum_j (x_j - \bar{x})(c_j - \bar{c})}{\sqrt{\sum_j (x_j - \bar{x})}\sqrt{\sum_j (c_j - \bar{c})}}$ [9]. Such correlation indicates the dependence between features and class label, and is optimal when each class is a single Gaussian distribution. Following the procedure of feature extraction described in Section 2.3, extracted features are then input to two types of classifiers, i.e., SVM and k-NN, for the prediction of class label. In all of the experiments, classifier parameters are optimized automatically through cross-validation within training samples only. Such parameters include the kernel type and kernel size in SVM, and the size of nearest neighborhood and the kernel size in k-NN. The threshold P_{th} is empirically set to select a certain number of voxels, e.g. between 600 to 1000 voxels. When more

Table 1. Recognition error of leave-one-out (LOO) cross-validations using single scalar features. Lower error indicates better performance.

Features	Male				Female			
	Correlation		Bayes Error		Correlation		Bayes Error	
	SVM	k-NN	SVM	k-NN	SVM	k-NN	SVM	k-NN
FA	28.95%	26.32%	26.32%	**23.68%**	28.13%	25.00%	25.00 %	**18.75%**
C_l	36.84%	31.58%	31.21%	28.95%	37.50%	33.75%	25.00 %	21.88%
C_p	39.47%	34.21%	39.47%	36.84%	31.25%	31.25%	28.13 %	28.13%

Table 2. Recognition error of 10-fold cross-validations using single and combined scalar features. Lower error indicates better performance.

Single features	Male		Female		Combined features	Male		Female	
	SVM	k-NN	SVM	k-NN		SVM	k-NN	SVM	k-NN
FA	32.11%	25.79%	28.75 %	26.87%	(FA, C_p)	23.68%	**19.68%**	33.75%	28.13%
C_l	32.61%	31.58%	29.69 %	25.00%	(C_l, C_p)	27.11%	21.84%	24.37%	**17.81%**
C_p	40.79%	37.87%	34.06%	30.63%	(FA, C_l, C_p)	27.89%	22.37%	25.62 %	19.06%

voxels are added, the classification accuracy starts decreasing due to more noise and limited number of samples. The comparison of leave-one-out (LOO) cross-validation accuracy using single scalar features are summarized in Table 1. Results show that our method outperforms the correlation based method, for both SVM and k-NN classifiers. Among the three scalar features, FA and C_l provide better accuracy than C_p. Furthermore, for both feature selection methods, the k-NN classifier provides a slightly better accuracy than commonly used SVM.

We further validate that the DTI pattern classification accuracy can be significantly improved with the use of combined features. Since only limited number of samples are available, for a robust evaluation of our method, we adopt multiple times of 10-fold cross-validations. The final ROC is obtained from the outputs from multiple times cross-validation. Compared to a single cross-validation, such multiple cross-validations provide a more robust evaluation that is less sensitive to parameter tuning, especially when the data number is limited. Comparisons between pattern recognition using single and combined scalar features based on 10 times 10-fold cross-validation are summarized in Table 2, where the 10-fold cross-validation accuracy is slightly worse than the leave-one-out cross-validation. From the table, it can be observed that combining different scalar features significantly improves the pattern classification accuracy. For example, when combining FA and C_p features, the cross-validation recognition error of male participants is decreased to 19.68% from 25.79% of using FA features. Other combinations, such FA+ C_p, also improves the recognition accuracy. For female participants, the combination of FA and C_p greatly improves the recognition accuracy, i.e, recognition error decreased from around 25.00% to 17.81%. Furthermore, from all the experiments, the k-NN classifier consistently outperforms the SVM classifier. ROC curves corresponding to different combinations of scalar features, displayed in Figure 2, further confirm the advantages of combining scalar features.

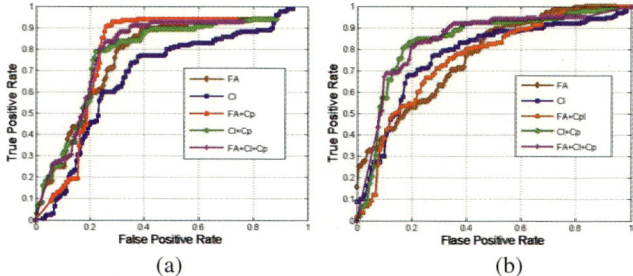

Fig. 2. Comparison of ROCs from 10-fold cross-validations using different combination of scalar features. (a) ROCs of male participants; (b) ROCs of female participants.

We notice that, although in general, combinations of different scalar features improve the recognition accuracy, the optimal combinations that achieve the best accuracy are different for female and male sets. Hence the regions that are involved in the classification are also different for the two genders. This supports the clinical observation that the progression of schizophrenia is different in men and women [14]. Also, our experiments show that the combinations of the planar index C_p, which can be seen as a measure of diffusivity, with other features of anisotropy can significantly improve the recognition accuracy, although C_p on its own cannot effectively distinguish patients from healthy people. This demonstrates that C_p carries complimentary information to the other two features (FA and C_l) which characterize the anisotropy. The results confirm the benefits of combining multiple tensor features by our method. Furthermore, the combination of all the features does not necessarily provide the best accuracy. This is probably caused by insufficient samples in estimating pattern overlap when the feature dimensionality increases.

4 Conclusion

We have presented a novel method of identifying regions in the brain affected by disease, based on the pattern classification of DTI data. The method is able to detect non-linear group differences between patients and controls, and can be used to distinguish disease-affected brains from healthy controls, and potentially aid in disease diagnosis. We show that the combination of multiple scalar features from tensors characterizing the anisotropy and the shape can improve the classification accuracy due to the complementary nature of physical properties that the features characterize. Our future work will focus on generalizing the framework to other medical image group classifications such as in aging and to multi-modality data.

Acknowledgement

This work is supported by NIH grants R01-MH-079938 and 1R01MH73174-01. The authors would like to thank the Brain Behavior Laboratory, University of Pennsylvania, for providing us the data.

References

1. Basser, P.J., Mattiello, J., LeBihan, D.: MR diffusion tensor spectroscopy and imaging. Biophysical Journal 66, 259–267 (1994)
2. Kubicki, M., McCarley, R.W., Westin, C.F., Park, H.J., Maier, S., Kikinis, R., Shenton, M.E., Jolesz, F.A.: A review of diffusion tensor imaging studies in schizophrenia. Journal of Psychiatric Research 41, 15–30 (2007)
3. Ashburner, J., Fristonn, K.J.: Voxel-based morphometry: The methods. NeuroImage 11, 805–821 (2000)
4. Westin, C.F., Maier, S.E., Mamata, H., Nabavi, A., Jolesz, F.A., Kikinis, R.: Processing and visualization of diffusion tensor MRI. Med. Image Anal. 6(2), 93–108 (2002)
5. Lenglet, C., Rousson, M., Deriche, R.: DTI segmentation by statistical surface evolution. IEEE Trans. Med. Img. 25(6), 685–700 (2006)
6. Xu, D., Mori, S., Shen, D., van Zijl, P.C.M., Davatzikos, C.: Spatial normalization of diffusion tensor fields. Magnetic Resonance in Medicine 50, 175–182 (2003)
7. Caan, M., Vermeer, K., van Vliet, L., Majoie, C., Peters, B., den Heeten, G., Vos, F.: Shaving diffusion tensor images in discriminant analysis: a study into schizophrenia. Med. Image Anal. 10, 841–850 (2006)
8. Fan, Y., Shen, D., Gur, R.C., Gur, R.E., Davatzikos, C.: COMPARE: Classification of morphological patterns using adaptive regional elements. TMI 26, 93–105 (2007)
9. Guyon, I., Elisseeff, A.: An introduction to variable and feature selection. Journal of Machine Learning Research 3, 1157–1182 (2003)
10. Duda, R., Hart, P., Stork, D.: Pattern Classification, 2nd edn. John Wiley Sons, Chichester (2000)
11. Fukunaga, K., Hummels, D.M.: Bayes error estimation using Parzen and k-NN procedures. IEEE Trans. Pattern Anal. Mach. Intell. 9(5), 634–643 (1987)
12. Silverman, B.: Density Estimation for Statistics and Data Analysis. Chapman & Hall / CRC (1986)
13. Cortes, C., Vapnik, V.: Support-vector networks. Machine Learning 20(3), 4
14. Nopoulos, P., Flaum, M., Andreasen, N.C.: Sex differences in brain morphology in schizophrenia. Am. J. Psychiatry 154, 1648–1654 (1997)

Findings in Schizophrenia by Tract-Oriented DT-MRI Analysis

Mahnaz Maddah[1], Marek Kubicki[2,3], William M. Wells[3], Carl-Fredrik Westin[3], Martha E. Shenton[2,3], and W. Eric L. Grimson[1]

[1] Computer Science and Artificial Intelligence Laboratory, Massachusetts Institute of Technology, Cambridge, MA, USA
mmaddah@mit.edu
[2] Psychiatry Neuroimaging Laboratory, Brigham and Women's Hospital, Harvard Medical School, Boston, MA, USA
[3] Surgical Planning Laboratory, Brigham and Women's Hospital, Harvard Medical School, Boston, MA, USA

Abstract. This paper presents a tract-oriented analysis of diffusion tensor (DT) images of the human brain. We demonstrate that unlike the commonly used ROI-based methods for population studies, our technique is sensitive to the local variation of diffusivity parameters along the fiber tracts. We show the strength of the proposed approach in identifying the differences in schizophrenic data compared to controls. Statistically significant drops in fractional anisotropy are observed along the genu and bilaterally in the splenium, as well as an increase in principal eigenvalue in uncinate fasciculus. This is the first tract-oriented clinical study in which an anatomical atlas is used to guide the algorithm.

1 Introduction

Schizophrenia is one of the major disabling brain disorders. It has been hypothesized that oligodendroglial dysfunction and subsequent myelin abnormalities contribute to the schizophrenic syndrome [1]. Diffusion tensor MRI has been employed by several groups in the past to investigate myelin integrity in patients with schizophrenia. Reduced diffusion anisotropy has been reported in prefrontal cortex [2], cingulum [3], uncinate fasciculus [4,5], corpus callosum [6,7], and arcuate facsiculus [4]. However, other studies find no significant difference in some of the above structures [3,8,9]. We believe that the inconsistency in experimental results is in part due to the difference in specifying the regions over which the anisotropy is measured. Clinical studies in the past are mostly either based on averaging the quantitative parameters over expert-specified regions of interest (ROIs) or used a voxel-by-voxel comparison. The former is sensitive to the accuracy of specifying the ROI, while the latter are susceptible to registration errors. Most recently, a tract-specific analysis has been proposed to more accurately define the measurement regions [10]. Jones *et. al* perform tractography to obtain the pathways of each fiber tract and then report a single number by averaging the parameter of interest along all pathways that belong to a given tract. However, local variation of the quantitative parameters is not captured in their analysis.

In this work, we propose a tract-oriented analysis in which parameters of interest are studied along the arc length of the tract. This allows us to study local variations that are missed in an ROI-based analysis or in the study performed in [10]. We apply the proposed procedure on a population of 18 patients with chronic schizophrenia and 19 normal subjects, analyze several fiber bundles that have been indicated in schizophrenia research, and demonstrate the sensitivity of our approach to identifying the group differences in diffusivity measures such as fractional anisotropy (FA) and mean diffusivity (MD).

2 Method

In this study, the probabilistic tract-oriented quantitative analysis described in [11] is extended to incorporate an anatomical atlas of fiber tracts. We use an atlas of fiber tracts [12], which is composed of a set of labeled ROIs, each corresponding to an anatomically-known bundle of fiber tracts in human brain. These ROIs are used to seed the tractography and to guide the clustering algorithm as detailed in this section. We add prototype curves to the atlas to represent the shape of the trajectories in each tract. This is a one-time process done by an expert by manual selection of trajectories that are representative of the shape of the tracts. These prototype curves are also used as the initial cluster centers in the clustering algorithm.

Fractional anisotropy maps calculated from DT-MRI data are first mapped into a common coordinate system using a congealing registration [13] and then into the atlas (MNI) space using an affine registration [14]. As opposed to a series of pair-wise subject-template registrations, this approach prevents the introduction of bias in the population study.

Atlas-specified regions corresponding to each fiber tract are mapped to the coordinate system of each case using the affine transformation obtained from registration. We then apply a dilation operation on those regions to ensure that they contain the fiber tract of interest. These regions are used to seed a streamline tractography [15] that produces fiber trajectories by following the principal eigenvector of the tensor at each voxel. We terminate the trajectory propagation when an FA value less than 0.15 is reached. The quantitative parameters of interest, such as fractional anisotropy and the diffusivity eigenvalues, are collected at each point on the trajectories and stored for further quantitative analysis.

Trajectories obtained from the tractography algorithm on each case are all mapped into the common MNI space and then clustered using our expectation-maximization (EM) algorithm first proposed in [11]. We employ the atlas-specified ROIs as the spatial prior information while the prototype trajectories of the atlas are used as the initial cluster centers for initializing the EM iteration. A gamma mixture model is used to describe the distribution of the distance between the trajectories and 3D cluster centers as detailed in [11]. This distance includes both the Euclidean distance and the shape difference between the trajectories and cluster

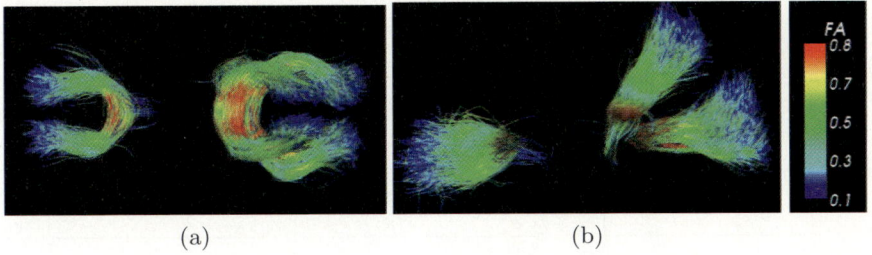

Fig. 1. (a) Axial and (b) saggital view of the clustered trajectories from genu and splenium parts of the corpus collasum. Trajectories from all cases are registered into the atlas space, clustered, and colored with the local fractional anisotropy.

centers and is obtained by establishing the point-by-point correspondences between them. Atlas-specified membership prior for each trajectory is determined by mapping the trajectory to the atlas ROI and counting the number of overlapping points. The membership likelihood from the mixture model is then combined with the atlas prior in a Bayesian framework to determine the membership probability. The output of the clustering algorithm is the probabilistic assignment of the trajectories to each cluster, a set of cluster centers, and the point correspondence between the trajectories and the cluster centers. Outliers are identified as those trajectories that receive small membership likelihood from all clusters, and they are removed from further processing.

Tract-oriented quantitative analysis is performed by calculating the weighted averages of the parameters of interest along the arc length of the cluster centers. By doing so, trajectories with low membership probability contribute less to the quantitative analysis. Such analysis can be performed on a case-by-case basis or on all cases that belong to a group. Analysis of variance (ANOVA) and permutation test with 1000 iterations are used for statistical group analysis. The correction for multiple comparison is not made.

3 Experiments and Results

For this experiment, we used DTI images acquired on a 3 Tesla GE system using an echo planar imaging (EPI) DTI sequence. We used a double echo option to reduce eddy-current related distortions, and an 8-Channel coil that allows us to perform parallel imaging using ASSET (Array Spatial Sensitivity Encoding Techniques, GE) with a SENSE-factor (speed-up) of 2 to reduce the impact of EPI spatial distortions. Eighty-five axial slices parallel to the AC-PC line covering the whole brain were acquired, with the following parameters: 51 directions with $b = 900$, 8 baseline scans with $b = 0$, TR = 17000 ms, TE = 78 ms, FOV = 24 cm, 144×144 encoding steps, and 1.7 mm slice thickness.

As mentioned above, at least some of the schizophrenia symptoms are hypothesized to be related to the disruptions of the interhemisphere connectivity, which makes study of corpus collasum of great interest. To analyze corpus

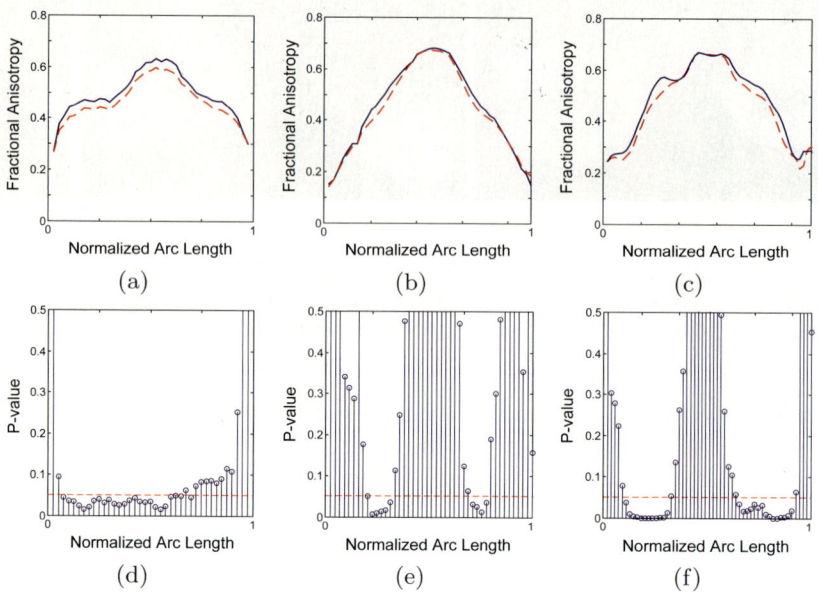

Fig. 2. The variation of FA along the arc length, from left to right of the brain, for genu (a), upper splenium (b) and lower splenium (c) for healthy (solid lines) and diseased (dashed lines) subjects and the corresponding p-values. Significant difference is observed on the left side of the genu and lateral portion of the splenium.

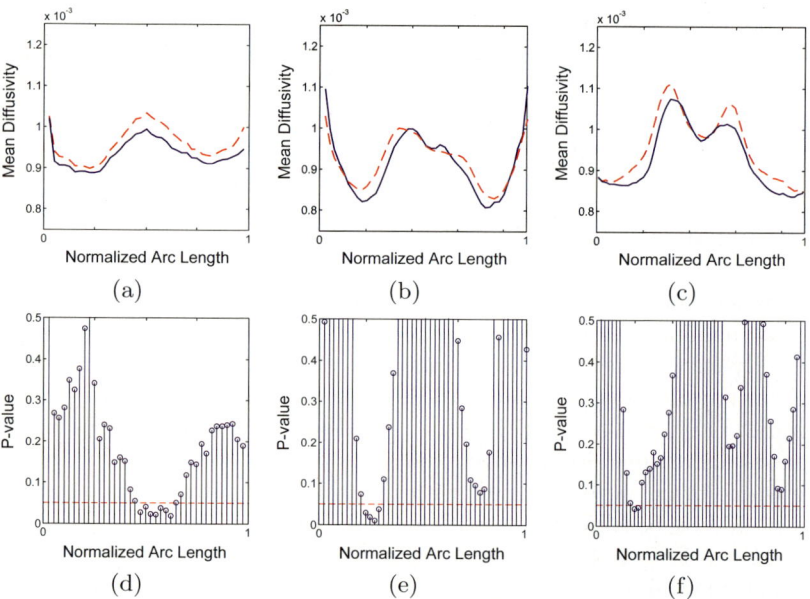

Fig. 3. Similar to Fig. 2 but for mean diffusivity along the tract

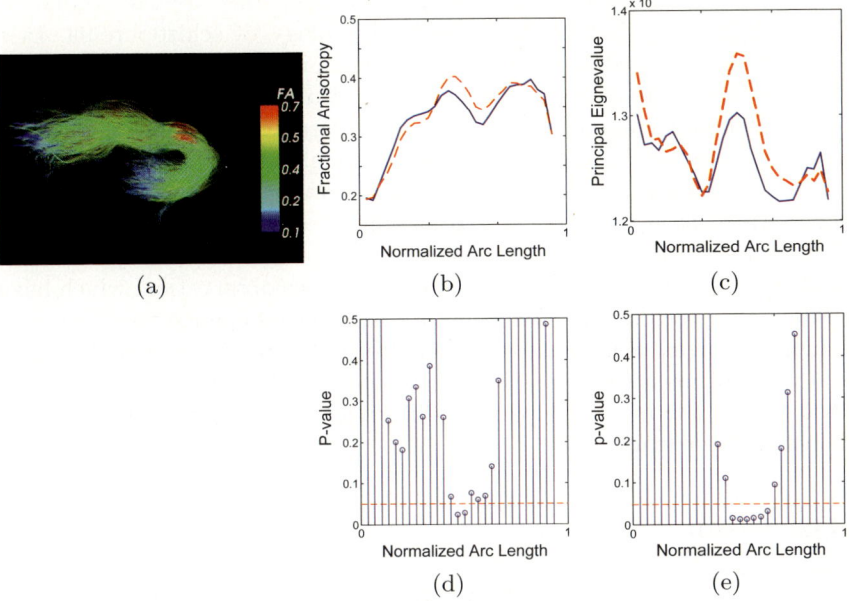

Fig. 4. (a) Sagittal view of the clustered trajectories from left uncinate fasciculus (UF). Trajectories from all subjects are mapped into the atlas space, clustered, and colored with the local FA. Variation of fractional anisotropy (b) and the major diffusivity eigenvalue (c) along the tract arc length for left UF in healthy (solid lines) and diseased (dashed lines) subjects and the corresponding p-values (d) and (e).

callosum in schizophrenia, we analyzed DTI data from 19 control subjects, and 18 chronic schizophrenics, matched on age, gender and parental socioeconomic status. Figure 1 shows the clustered trajectories from genu and splenium of the corpus collasum, colored based on the local fractional anisotropy. Our method allows us to divide the splenium into its upper and lower parts (tracts interconnecting parietal and occipital lobes respectively), as they pose different shapes. Figure 2 compares the fractional anisotropy in genu and upper and lower splenium for healthy and schizophrenic subjects. Significant FA reduction is observed in genu, which confirms earlier reports of similar observations [16]. Moreover, our analysis clearly indicates that FA reduction is primarily in left part of the genu which is consistent with a few detailed voxel-based studies [16].

We also observed significant reduction of the fractional anisotropy in splenium, especially in its lower part. As can be seen in Fig. 2, the FA reduction is seen bilaterally, in the middle of each side. To our knowledge, only one voxelwise analysis [7] was sensitive enough to observe such a bilateral FA reduction in splenium. Similar analysis is performed for mean diffusivity and the results are given in Fig. 3. Increased mean diffusivity is only significant in small portions of the genu (in the middle) and the splenium (in the left).

Besides corpus callosum, fronto-temporal connections are the second most frequently indicated fiber tracts in pathophysiology of schizophrenia. In this work, we thus examined the uncinate fasciculus, which is the most prominent of all white matter fiber tracts connecting the frontal and temporal lobes, and which has been implicated in schizophrenia in several publications [4]. Figure 4(a) depicts the trajectories from left uncinate fasciculus from all subjects mapped into the atlas space and colored with the local fractional anisotropy. As shown in Fig. 4, increase in FA and MD is significant only for a small part at the middle of this structure. However, significant increase in the major diffusivity eigenvalue, i.e. parallel to the tract, is observed. This observation, which has not been reported in the past, indicates that FA alone is not enough for DTI analysis. Although the origins of increased parallel diffusivity are unknown and it opposes general views of axonal damage, it should be noted that such an increase is not impossible. In fact, increased parallel diffusivity has been reported previously for displaced fiber tracts [17].

4 Discussion

As shown in the previous section, our tract-oriented method is able to reveal the local variations of the diffusion parameters. This approach is thus very sensitive compared to ROI-based methods, as the differences might be lost when parameters (such as FA) over the entire tract are being averaged and compared between groups. Although voxel-based methods are potentially able to show the local variations, the results are very sensitive to registration errors. Abnormalities within the genu of the corpus callosum are localized in the midsagittal region, thus appear in the portion of the tract where the fibers of the tract run all alone, which suggests disruptions in tracts interconnecting frontal lobes. On the other hand, changes observed in schizophrenia group in the parasagittal, but not midsagittal portion of the splenium of the corpus callosum are suggestive of factors other than disruption of corpus collasum integrity, such as interfering and crossing fibers.

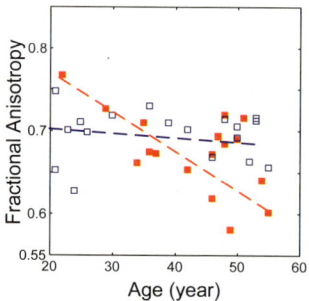

Fig. 5. Age-dependence of the fractional anisotropy in mid-saggital point of the lower splenium for healthy (open squares) and schizophrenic (closed squares) subjects

We would like to stress that a comprehensive DTI analysis requires examination of both anisotropy measures, such as FA, and the diffusivity magnitude, e.g. MD, or equivalently the parallel and radial diffusivity eigenvalues [18]. The diffusivity perpendicular to the fiber tract reflects changes in axonal membrane, myelin, or extracellular space [19], whereas membrane disintegration and gliosis may create diffusion barriers in the direction of the fiber tract and reduce the parallel diffusivity [19]. Axonal damage may also result in reduced diffusivity perpendicular to the fiber tract [19]. The analysis performed on the uncinate fasciculus clearly demonstrates the fact that fractional anisotropy alone is not sufficient to study white matter integrity.

Another important issue, which is essential in group analysis and was discussed in previous schizophrenia studies [10], is the age and/or disease-dependence of the diffusion parameters. To illustrate this point, in Fig. 5 we have plotted the age-dependence of the fractional anisotropy in the mid-saggital point of the lower splenium. While healthy subjects exhibit small age-dependence in our age range, considerable reduction of FA is observed in schizophrenic cases upon aging.

5 Conclusion

A tract-oriented quantitative analysis of genu, splenium, and left uncinate fasciculus in schizophrenia was presented. The method is able to reveal the local variations of the fiber integrity, which are lost when the quantitative parameters are averaged over the entire fiber tract in ROI-based methods. Significant reduction in fractional anisotropy in the left part of the genu and bilaterally in the middle of each side of the splenium was observed. While FA analysis shows no significant change in uncinate fasciculus, significant increase in the parallel diffusivity was observed in this structure. Although the origins of this increase are unknown, this finding emphasizes the fact that FA alone is not enough for quantitative analysis. Finally, it was shown that age-dependence of the diffusivity parameters is an important factor when performing group analysis.

References

1. Davis, K., Stewart, D., Friedman, J., Buchsbaum, M., Harvey, P., Hof, P., Buxbaum, J., Haroutunian, V.: White matter changes in schizophrenia: Evidence for myelin-related dysfunction. Arch. Gen. Psychiatry 60, 443–456 (2003)
2. Buchsbaum, M., Friedman, J., Buchsbaum, B., Chu, K., Hazlett, E., Newmark, R., Schneiderman, J., Torosjan, Y., Tang, C., Hof, P., Stewart, D., Davis, K., Gorman, J.: Diffusion tensor imaging in schizophrenia. Biological Psychiatry 60, 1181–1187 (2006)
3. Sun, Z., Wang, F., Cui, L., Breeze, J., Du, X., Wang, X., Cong, Z., Zhang, H., Li, B., Hong, N., Zhang, D.: Abnormal anterior cingulum in patients with schizophrenia: a diffusion tensor imaging study. Neuroreport 14, 1933–1936 (2003)
4. Burns, J., Job, D., Bastin, M., Whalley, H., Macgillivray, T., Johnstone, E., Lawrie, S.: Structural disconnectivity in schizophrenia: a diffusion tensor magnetic resonance imaging study. Br. J. Psychiatry 182, 439–443 (2003)

5. Kubicki, M., Westin, C.F., Maier, S., Mamata, H., Frumin, M., Ernst-Hirshefeld, H., Kikinis, R., Jolesz, F., McCarley, R., Shenton, M.: Cingulate fasciculus integrity disruption in schizophrenia: a magnetic resonance diffusion tensor imaging study. Biological Phychiatry 54, 1171–1180 (2003)
6. Agartz, I., Andersson, J., Skare, S.: Abnormal white matter in schizophrenia: a diffusion tensor imaging study. Neuroreport 12, 2251–2254 (2001)
7. Ardekani, B., Nierenberg, J., Hoptman, M., Javitt, D.: MRI study of white matter diffusion anisotropy in schizophrenia. Neuroreport 14, 2025–2029 (2003)
8. Steel, R., Bastin, M., McConnell, S., Marshall, I., Cunningham-Owens, D., Lawrie, S., Johnstone, E., Best, J.: Diffusion tensor imaging (DTI) and proton magnetic resonance spectroscopy (1H MRS) in schizophrenic subjects and controls. Psych. Res.: Neuroimage 106, 161–170 (2001)
9. Foong, J., Symms, M., Barker, G., Maier, M., Miller, D.: MRI study of white matter diffusion anisotropy in schizophrenia. Neuroreport 13, 333–336 (2002)
10. Jones, D., Catani, M., Pierpaoli, C., Reeves, S., Shergill, S., O'Sullivan, M., Golesworthy, P., McGuire, P., Horsfield, M., Simmons, A., Williams, S., Howard, R.: Age effects on diffusion tensor magnetic resonance imaging tractography measures of frontal cortex connections in schizophrenia. Human Brain Mapping 27, 230–238 (2006)
11. Grimson, W.E.L., Warfield, S.K., Wells, I.W.M., Westin, C.-F., Maddah, M.: Probabilistic Clustering and Quantitative Analysis of White Matter Fiber Tracts. In: Karssemeijer, N., Lelieveldt, B. (eds.) IPMI 2007. LNCS, vol. 4584, pp. 372–383. Springer, Heidelberg (2007)
12. Wakana, S., Jiang, H., Nagae-Poetscher, L.M., van Zijl, P.C.M., Mori, S.: Fiber tract-based atlas of human white matter anatomy. Radiology 230, 77–87 (2004)
13. Zöllei, L., Learned-Miller, E., Grimson, E., Wells, W.: Efficient population registration of 3D data. In: Workshop on Computer Vision for Biomedical Image Applications: Current Techniques and Future Trends (2005)
14. Wells, W., Viola, P., Atsumi, H., Nakajima, S., Kikinis, R.: Multi-modal volume registration by maximization of mutual information. Medical Image Analysis 1, 35–51 (1996)
15. Basser, P., Pajevic, S., Pierpaoli, C., Duda, J., Aldroubi, A.: In vivo fiber tractography using DT-MRI data. Magn. Reson. Med. 44, 625–632 (2000)
16. Park, H.J., Westin, C.F., Kubicki, M., Maier, S.E., Niznikiewicz, M., Baer, A., Frumin, M., Kikinis, R., Jolesz, F.A., McCarley, R.W., Shenton, M.E.: White matter hemisphere asymmetries in healthy subjects and in schizophrenia: A diffusion tensor MRI study. NeuroImage 24, 213–223 (2004)
17. Schonberg, T., Pianka, P., Hendler, T., Assaf, Y.: Characterization of displaced white matter tracts using DTI and fMRI. In: Proc. ISMRM, p. 468 (2005)
18. Hasan, K.: Diffusion tensor eigenvalues or both mean diffusivity and fractional anisotropy are required in quantitative clinical diffusion tensor MR reports: Fractional anisotropy alone is not sufficient. Radiology 239, 611–613 (2006)
19. Pierpaoli, C., Basser, P.: Toward a quantitative assessment of diffusion anisotropy. Magn. Reson. Med. 36, 893–906 (1996)

Task-Specific Functional Brain Geometry from Model Maps

Georg Langs[1,2], Dimitris Samaras[1,3], Nikos Paragios[1,2], Jean Honorio[3],
Nelly Alia-Klein[4], Dardo Tomasi[4], Nora D. Volkow[4], and Rita Z. Goldstein[4]

[1] Laboratoire de Mathématiques Appliquées aux Systèmes,
Ecole Centrale de Paris, France
georg.langs@ecp.fr, nikos.paragios@ecp.fr*
[2] Equipe GALEN, INRIA Saclay, Île-de-France, France
[3] Image Analysis Laboratory, Stony Brook University, USA
samaras@cs.sunysb.edu, jhonorio@cs.sunysb.edu
[4] Medical Department, Brookhaven National Laboratory, USA
rgoldstein@bnl.gov
[5] National Institute on Drug Abuse - National Institutes of Health, USA

Abstract. In this paper we propose *model maps* to derive and represent the intrinsic functional geometry of a brain from functional magnetic resonance imaging (fMRI) data for a specific task. Model maps represent the coherence of behavior of individual fMRI-measurements for a set of observations, or a time sequence. The maps establish a relation between individual positions in the brain by encoding the blood oxygen level dependent (BOLD) signal over a time period in a Markov chain. They represent this relation by mapping spatial positions to a new metric space, the *model map*. In this map the Euclidean distance between two points relates to the joint modeling behavior of their signals and thus the co-dependencies of the corresponding signals. The map reflects the functional as opposed to the anatomical geometry of the brain. It provides a quantitative tool to explore and study global and local patterns of resource allocation in the brain. To demonstrate the merit of this representation, we report quantitative experimental results on 29 fMRI time sequences, each with sub-sequences corresponding to 4 different conditions for two groups of individuals. We demonstrate that drug abusers exhibit lower differentiation in brain interactivity between baseline and reward related tasks, which could not be quantified until now.

1 Introduction

Despite the tremendous progress in studying the brain, little is known about its function and flexibility for specific activities. One way to understand these

---
* This work has been partially supported by the Region Île-de-France; by NIDA 1 R01 DA020949-01; by grants from the National Institute on Drug Abuse (RZG: 1R01DA023579 and R21DA02062); Laboratory Directed Research and Development from U.S. Department of Energy (OBER; to RZG: LRDR #07-055), National Institute on Alcohol Abuse and Alcoholism (NDV: AA/ODO9481-04), and General Clinical Research Center (5-MO1-RR-10710).

processes is through a statistical analysis of functional brain imaging datasets. Neural activity can be captured by functional magnetic resonance imaging (fMRI). It takes advantage of the hemodynamics response caused by active nerve cells that consume oxygen. The resulting fMRI signal is different depending on the level of oxygenation, and can be detected by using blood-oxygen-level dependent (BOLD) contrast.

Recently the extraction of information from fMRI was approached by various methodologies: In [1] the correlation of the BOLD signal *between* individuals while watching a movie was utilized to search for regions relevant for memory. Inter-subject synchronization was also studied in [2]. In [3] the strength of fMRI signals and its change for certain activities, and preconditions was assessed, in order to differentiate between drug addicts and control subjects. In [4], and [5] fluctuations within the brain were connected with the variability in subsequent fMRI observations. Even-though these works refer to the interdependency of brain regions, a comprehensive method to capture and represent this functional brain structure, and its dynamics, is still missing.

In this paper we address the question of synchronization within the brain. That is, we search for brain regions that exhibit highly coherent behavior as a strong indication of cooperation during an activity. We expect the BOLD signals corresponding to these regions to be observations stemming from a single source - the cooperative work caused by a certain condition. We propose a method to capture and represent these relationships in a transparent manner. It allows for data exploration, and for quantitative measurements of relationships between different regions of the brain, which are dynamic and task-specific. We call the set of these relationships the *functional geometry*. In addition to knowledge about functional regions [6] it offers information about their subtle mutual interaction patterns. The distance between the signals is derived from the joint model description length [7] of groups of signals, describing their joint modeling behavior [8]. In contrast to standard correlation, it can capture more complex or hidden relations, that go beyond mere synchronization. The method can be applied to other modalities like EEG/ERP or PET.

We use diffusion maps [9] to retrieve and encode the functional geometry. A diffusion map is a space constructed by the eigenfunctions of a Markov matrix. The Euclidean distance within this space offers a geometry that can capture complex relations between nodes in a Markov chain, and is related to spectral segmentation approaches [10]. In [11] diffusion maps were used to perform dimensionality reduction by parameterizing entire brain states, to represent relations between brains. In [12] they were used to segment activated regions. A related line of work addresses correlation analysis with regard to seed points, [13], while in [14] the brain is partitioned, and representative BOLD signals are searched for by a correlation and expectation maximization approach. The method presented in this paper tackles a different question: instead of differentiating between activated and non-activated voxels in the fMRI volume, or between subjects, we ask for a continuous functional relation between brain regions. We do not classify brain regions, but quantify their - often subtle - relations continuously.

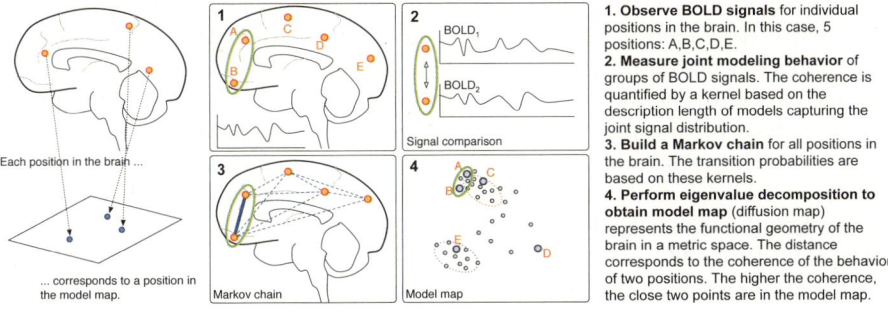

Fig. 1. Generating a model map generation from fMRI data

We propose to use *model maps* to explore the functional geometry of a brain for a certain task or time period. Each spatial position in the brain is mapped to a position in the map that is governed by the functional coherence of the corresponding observed BOLD signals in the brain (Fig. 1). The model map is built by calculating a Markov chain with nodes representing the positions in the brain, and transition probabilities defined by the description lengths [7] of models, that encode the joint density of the signals. The resulting model map captures joint modeling behavior of signals acquired at different positions, and reflects this functional geometry. It has several interesting properties: functional relations are translated to Euclidean distance, therefore groups of voxels, that have a high probability to stem from the same model, form clusters in the map. The density for positions in the map provides information about how *connected* a point is to any other region in the brain. High density indicates high coherence with many other signals, while low density indicates relatively independent behavior. These properties are essential for data exploration of complex fMRI sequences. Instead of a parcellation of the brain, they present the entire functional geometry including subtle dependencies. The unique position of points in the map makes a comparison between subjects, and between time-points for the same subject possible. These properties have considerable diagnostic value (as reported in the experiments), and we believe that they are an important tool, to explore and assess the changing distribution patterns of individual brain activities, that are not captured by the BOLD signal strength at individual positions. We evaluate the method on a challenging data set, that exhibits subtle cognitive changes regarding reward processing. Experiments show that the method is able to capture subtle differences, and interactions for different tasks.

2 Model Maps to Find Geometry in Functional Brain Data

We aim at a representation that maps measurements to positions in a space, so that low distance between two points indicates high compactness for a model that encodes both of them, or high temporal coherence of their signals. We derive model maps from a set of signals $\{\mathbf{x}_1, \ldots, \mathbf{x}_m\}$, where $\mathbf{x}_i \in \mathbb{R}^n$. The signals are mapped to a new manifold $\{\boldsymbol{\Psi}_i, \ldots, \boldsymbol{\Psi}_m\}$ in the model map, where the Euclidean distance relates to a similarity between signals. In our case, each $\mathbf{x}_i$ is the BOLD signal observed at one position in the brain for n time points. In this section we will first discuss how to define a similarity function, that captures relations between BOLD signals based on a multivariate Gaussian model. Then we will describe how to construct a Markov chain, and the corresponding model map with new positions $\boldsymbol{\Psi}_i$ for each signal $\mathbf{x}_i$. Finally we will explain how to perform measurements in the model map. The approach is closely related to *shape maps*, introduced in [8].

2.1 Comparing Signals: Compactness of a Gaussian Model

To establish a relation between a group of signals $\{\mathbf{x}_1, \ldots, \mathbf{x}_l\}$ we find the principal axes of the joint distribution, and approximate it by a multivariate Gaussian distribution with Gaussians along the principal axes. For each dimension of the eigenspace used to encode the data we can apply Shannons theorem [15] to the according one-dimensional distribution. That is we can estimate the description length or complexity of a model, that encodes the data. The description length comprises the cost L of communicating a model $\mathcal{M}$ itself (the parameters of the Gaussians) and the data D (i.e. BOLD signals) encoded with the model: $L(D, \mathcal{M}) = L(\mathcal{M}) + L(D|\mathcal{M})$. An extensive derivation of the description length calculation for Gaussian models is given in [16]. The description length reflects the complexity of the representation, and thus the plausibility of data stemming from a certain model. The method can be applied to models other than Gaussian straight-forwardly, and an optimal choice is subject of current research.

2.2 A Markov Chain That Describes Dependencies

Given a set of n examples, each consisting of BOLD signal observations for m points, we derive a metric on the set of points, that reflects their joint modeling behavior. The construction of such a diffusion map is explained in detail in [9]. The Markov chain consists of m nodes X which correspond to the individual signals $\mathbf{x}_i$, and pair-wise relations $d(i,j)$. We define $d_k(i,j)$ for two signals and *kernel size* k based on the minimum description length of models encompassing the two signals i and j and $k-2$ others: $d_k : \{1, 2, \ldots, n\}^2 \to \mathbb{R}$: $d_k(i,j) = \min_{\mathcal{M}}(\mathcal{L}(\mathcal{M})|i, j \subseteq \mathcal{M}$ and $\#\mathcal{M} = k)$, where the model $\mathcal{M}$ with cardinality $\#\mathcal{M} := \#\{h_1, \ldots, h_k\} = k$ represents k signals. $\mathcal{L}(\mathcal{M})$ denotes the description length $\mathcal{L}(\mathbf{x}_{\{h_1, \ldots, h_k\}})$ as defined in Sec. 2.1, and $i, j \subseteq \mathcal{M} :\Leftrightarrow i, j \in \{h_1, \ldots, h_k\}$ for $\mathcal{M}$. That is, $d(i,j)$ is the minimum of the description lengths of all models representing i and j, and arbitrary $k-2$ other entries of the observations. Note that for $k > 2$, $d_k(i,j)$ not only depends on the behavior of the two signals i and j but on the behavior of a larger sub set that is most *affine* to the two, i.e., that can be described by the least complex model. With increasing k only larger coherent sub-sets will benefit in terms of the distance in the model map, allowing for a multi-resolution approach. d_k is non-negative, and symmetric, and the nodes X and edges weighted according to d_k between the nodes build a symmetric graph (X, d_k). In practice we can estimate d_k by randomly choosing sub-sets of the data, calculating the according value $d_k(i, j)$ for all pairs in the sub-set and keeping the minimum of all samples for (i, j). Using this set of pairwise relations, one can proceed to form a Markov chain that encompasses the notion of compactness in the entire set of fMRI signals.

From this, the normalized graph Laplacian construction [17] generates a reversible Markov chain, resulting in a diffusion operator P and its powers P^t. P is the Markov matrix with the entries $p(i, j)$, which are the transition probabilities in the Markov chain. P^t allows to propagate information through the Markov chain. The probability of the transition from any point i to another point j in t timesteps is given by the according kernel $p_t(i, j)$. By increasing t we can analyze the data at multiple *scales* i.e., propagate the relations between pairs of nodes. This operator P defines the geometry on the set of signals we are looking for, which can be mapped to an Euclidean geometry by an eigenvalue decomposition of P. Corresponding to P^t we can define a family of *diffusion distances* parameterized by t on the set of fMRI signals:

$$D_t(i,j) = \sum_{l=1,\ldots,m} \frac{(p_t(i,l) - p_t(j,l))^2}{\pi(l)} \quad \text{where} \quad \pi(i) = \frac{d(i)}{\sum_j d(j)} \qquad (1)$$

is the probability of i in the unique stationary distribution (the uniqueness is fulfilled if the graph is connected). D_t is an L^2 distance and captures the connectivity in the Markov chain, summing over all possible paths from i to j. The distance D_t is low if there is a large number of paths of length t with high transition probabilities between the nodes i and j.

2.3 Constructing Model Maps of Functional Data

We now construct the space the encodes the functional relations of all fMRI signals from this chain. An eigenvalue decomposition of the operator P results in a sequence of eigen values $\lambda_1, \lambda_2 \ldots$ and corresponding eigen functions $\Psi_1, \Psi_2, \ldots$ that fullfill $P\Psi_i = \lambda_i \Psi_i$. In [9] the authors explain how a *diffusion map*, the space spanned by the eigenfunctions of a Markov chain relates to the geometry determined by a diffusion distance D_t. We use this to create a metric space, a *model map* $\Psi_t : X \to \mathbb{R}^w$, that embeds the nodes (fMRI signals) $i = 1, \ldots, m$ which are represented in the Markov chain into a Euclidean space where the diffusion distance in Eq. 1 corresponds to the euclidean distance in the eigen space:

$$\Psi_t(i) \triangleq \begin{pmatrix} \lambda_1^t \Psi_1(i) \\ \vdots \\ \lambda_w^t \Psi_w(i) \end{pmatrix}, \text{ and } \|\Psi_t(i) - \Psi_t(j)\| = D_t(i,j). \qquad (2)$$

Thereby the *functional* relations between fMRI signals are translated into spatial distances in the model map. The local density in the map corresponds to

Table 1. Relative increase of model map density from baseline. Left: entire brain, right: right orbitofrontal cortex. Right: corresponding plots for the absolute values.

	Full		ROFC	
	Abuser	Control	Abuser	Control
BL	0	0	0	0
C0	0.68	0.94	0.63	0.77
C1	0.70	1.04	0.68	1.14
C45	0.74	0.77	0.82	0.91

the amount of other signals, that are closely related. We can perform standard density estimation, clustering, or the definition of neighborhoods in this space. Closest neighbors indicate high coherence, and the scatter of specific brain regions in the map indicates the level of co-dependency of their sets of signals. Such a process captures the relations between the fMRI signals during the observation time.

3 Experiments

Data and set-up: We conducted experiments with previously acquired fMRI data from 29 individuals, 16 of which were cocaine abusers (group A), and 13 were control subjects (group B) provided by the authors of [3]. The MRI scans were acquired by a 4-T whole body MRI scanner (Varian), and BOLD responses were measured for 91 time points. The dataset focused on the way different subjects process monetary rewards. The overall neuropsychological experiment design included six blocks each consisting of three monetary reward conditions: 0 cent, 1 cent and 45 cents. This results in 3 baseline conditions (BL) without stimulus and the stimulus conditions ($Co0/1/45$). To assess if the model maps provide quantitative diagnostically relevant information, we assess their ability to differentiate between the subject groups, and between tasks. We measure the model map density for each point. We evaluate the mean density for the entire map, and the densities for the map positions corresponding to anatomical regions, e.g. the orbitofrontal cortex. We performed three comparisons: 1. We expect functionally connected regions within the brain to be in close proximity in the model map. Thus the density should increase if a specific task is performed, and we compared the model map density for $Co0$, $Co1$, and $Co45$ with $BL1$. 2. For the drug abusers the relative increase of interaction between $BL1$ and $Co0$, $Co1$, and $Co45$ is expected to be lower, thus we compared the relative increase of density for the two subject groups. 3. We observed the model map scatter for the cortical region of *orbitofrontal cortex*, *lateral prefrontal cortex*, and *anterior cingulate cortex*, regions previously found to be important in the

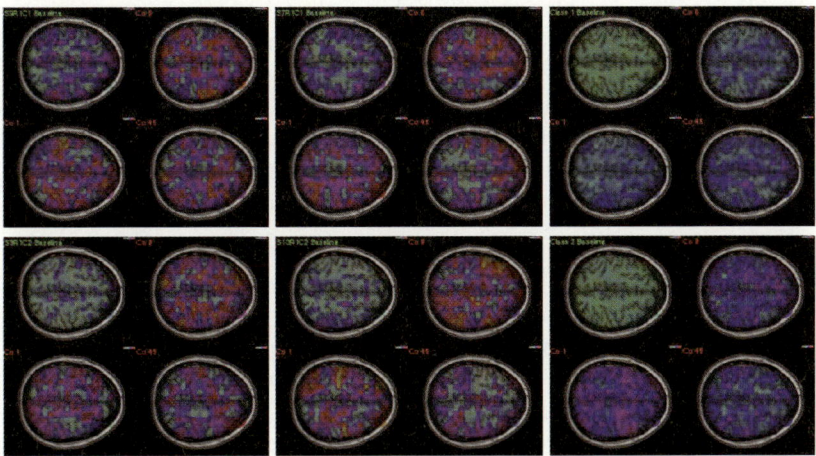

Fig. 2. Functional integration within the brain: the model map density values were projected back to the spatial coordinate system. Top row: two series for drug abusers, and median values, bottom row: two series for controls, and median values. For each subject baseline, and the three conditions are depicted. The differences between baseline (top left in each panel) and reward conditions are less pronounced for the drug abusers.

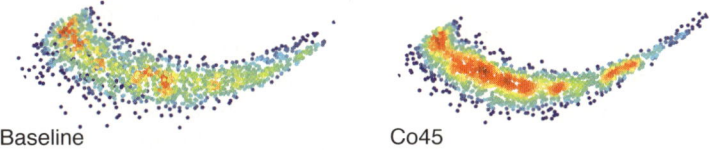

Fig. 3. Two model maps for one subject: one corresponding to baseline, one to Co45

context of reward processing [3]. Scatter indicates the level of integration of the activity in this region. We also report qualitative results for the model maps, to demonstrate the visual information they provide for data exploration, and visualize the model map density - the connectivity - in the spatial brain space.

Results: In Tab. 1 the increase in model map density relative to BL is reported, and plots for the absolute values for both drug abusers, and control subjects are depicted. For all subjects, the density values for Co0/1/45 are significantly higher than for BL ($p=0.05$). The relative increase is more pronounced for control subjects. An interesting observation is that the scatter of the points in the model map that correspond to the cortical regions is significantly lower for group A, compared to group B during BL ($p=0.034$). This indicates that these regions behave in a more coherent manner during baseline for drug abusers. In Fig. 2 the model map density is visualized on corresponding structural (T1) data. The top row shows two examples, and the median values for group A, while the bottom row shows the same for group B. The more pronounced increase of connectivity for group B is visible in this example. The median images show a similar trend for the entire population. However, since these results exhibited a certain level of heterogeneousity more research is needed to understand their implications. In Fig. 3 the model maps are shown for conditions BL, and Co45. The color encodes the local density in the map. The rather sparse structure with scattered local density maxima of the BL map changes to a dense map for Co45. This corresponds to increased interactions between brain regions.

4 Conclusion

We propose a method to capture, and to represent the functional geometry of brains in model maps. The representation is built by quantifying the joint modeling behavior of individual BOLD signals over time for all positions in the brain. The model map represents the functional relations between brain positions. In addition to mere signal strength, the distance in the map can indicate subtle co-dependencies between regions, while the density represents the functional connectivity to the rest of the brain. Experimental results demonstrate that the method extracts clinically relevant information, and can be used for data exploration, since in contrast to seed-point based approaches, it is built in an unsupervised manner, and encodes the structure of the entire brain in a single map. We expect this method to be relevant when searching for differentiating regions in the brain for the detection of certain changes over time. The functional connectivity can be used to establish functional trajectories. Promising directions both from the practical as well as theoretical point of view are to introduce dependencies that go beyond pair-wise interactions between the nodes and to relax the multi-variate Gaussian assumption. The proposed method could have an impact on understanding the relationships of measurements from heterogeneous domains (functional, anatomical), which is one of the challenges in the field of biological and biomedical analysis.

References

1. Hasson, U., Furman, O., Clark, D., Dudai, Y., Davachi, L.: Enhanced intersubject correlations during movie viewing correlate with successful episodic encoding. Neuron 57(3), 452–462 (2008)
2. Hasson, U., Nir, Y., Levy, I., Fuhrmann, G., Malach, R.: Intersubject synchronization of cortical activity during natural vision. Science 303(5664), 1634–1640 (2004)
3. Goldstein, R.Z., Alia-Klein, N., Tomasi, D., Zhang, L., Cottone, L.A., Maloney, T., Telang, F., Caparelli, E.C., Chang, L., Ernst, T., Samaras, D., Squires, N.K., Volkow, N.D.: Is decreased prefrontal cortical sensitivity to monetary reward associated with impaired motivation and self-control in cocaine addiction? Am. J. Psychiatry 164(1), 43–51 (2007)
4. Fox, M.D., Snyder, A.Z., Vincent, J.L., Raichle, M.E.: Intrinsic fluctuations within cortical systems account for intertrial variability in human behavior. Neuron 56(1), 171–184 (2007)

5. Fox, M.D., Raichle, M.E.: Spontaneous fluctuations in brain activity observed with functional magnetic resonance imaging. Nat. Rev. Neurosci. 8(9), 700–711 (2007)
6. Brett, M., Johnsrude, I.S., Owen, A.M.: The problem of functional localization in the human brain. Nat. Rev. Neurosci. 3(3), 243–249 (2002)
7. Rissanen, J.: Modeling by shortest data description. Automatica 14, 465–471 (1978)
8. Langs, G., Paragios, N.: Modeling the structure of multivariate manifolds: Shape maps. In: Proc. of CVPR 2008 (2008)
9. Coifman, R.R., Lafon, S.: Diffusion maps. Appl. Comp. Harm. An. 21, 5–30 (2006)
10. Yan, J., Pollefeys, M.: A general framework for motion segmentation: Independent, articulated, rigid, non-rigid, degenerate and non-degenerate. In: Leonardis, A., Bischof, H., Pinz, A. (eds.) ECCV 2006. LNCS, vol. 3954, pp. 94–106. Springer, Heidelberg (2006)
11. Meyer, F.: Learning and predicting brain dynamics from fMRI: a spectral approach. In: Wavelet XII conference, Proceedings of SPIE, vol. 6701(2007)
12. Shen, X., Meyer, F.: Analysis of Event-Related fMRI Data Using Diffusion Maps. Inf. Process Med. Imaging 19, 652–663 (2005)
13. Wang, Y., Xia, J.: Functional interactivity in fMRI using multiple seeds' correlation analyses – novel methods and comparisons. In: Karssemeijer, N., Lelieveldt, B. (eds.) IPMI 2007. LNCS, vol. 4584, pp. 147–159. Springer, Heidelberg (2007)
14. Golland, P., Golland, Y., Malach, R.: Detection of spatial activation patterns as unsupervised segmentation of fMRI data. Med. Image Comput. Comput. Assist. Interv. Int. Conf. Med. Image Comput. Comput. Assist. Interv. 10(Pt 1), 110–118 (2007)
15. Shannon, C.: A mathematical theory of communication. Bell Systems Technical Journal 27, 379–423 (1948)
16. Davies, R.H., Twining, C., Cootes, T.F., Waterton, J.C., Taylor, C.J.: A minimum description length approach to statistical shape modeling. IEEE TMI 21(5), 525–537 (2002)
17. Chung, F.R.: Spectral Graph Theory. American Mathematical Society (1997)

Texture Classification in Lung CT Using Local Binary Patterns

Lauge Sørensen[1], Saher B. Shaker[2], and Marleen de Bruijne[1,3]

[1] Department of Computer Science, University of Copenhagen, Denmark,
{lauges,marleen}@diku.dk
[2] Department of Cardiology and Respiratory Medicine, Hvidovre University Hospital, Copenhagen, Denmark
[3] Biomedical Imaging Group Rotterdam, Erasmus MC, The Netherlands

Abstract. In this paper we propose to use local binary patterns (LBP) as features in a classification framework for classifying different texture patterns in lung computed tomography. Image intensity is included by means of the joint LBP and intensity histogram, and classification is performed using the k nearest neighbor classifier with histogram similarity as distance measure.

The proposed method is evaluated on a set of 168 regions of interest comprising normal tissue and different emphysema patterns, and compared to a filter bank based on Gaussian derivatives. The joint LBP and intensity histogram, achieving a classification accuracy of 95.2%, shows superior performance to using the common approach of taking moments of the filter response histograms as features, and slightly better performance than using the full filter response histograms instead. Classification results are better than some of those previously reported in the literature.

1 Introduction

Chronic obstructive pulmonary disease (COPD) is a major cause of death and a growing health problem worldwide. In the United States it is the fourth leading cause of morbidity and mortality and it is estimated to be ranked the fifth most burdening disease worldwide by 2020 [1]. COPD is a chronic lung disease characterized by limitation of airflow in the airway and it comprises two components: Chronic bronchitis, which is an inflammation of the small airways, and emphysema, which is characterized by gradual loss of lung tissue.

The primary diagnostic tools for COPD are the lung function tests (LFT). However, LFT has a low sensitivity and is not capable of detecting early stages of COPD. Another diagnostic tool that is gaining more and more attention is computed tomography (CT) imaging. CT is a sensitive method for diagnosing emphysema and both visual and quantitative CT are closely correlated with the pathological extent of emphysema [2]. This makes CT suitable for both early detection and study of COPD as well as to monitor effect of different treatments.

We focus on the assessment of emphysema, which is thought to be the main cause of shortness of breath and disability in COPD. In CT emphysema lesions,

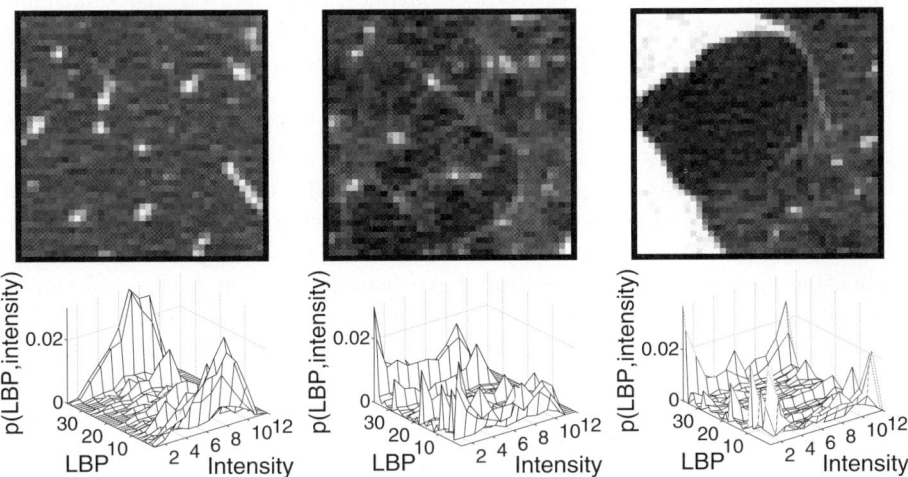

Fig. 1. Example ROIs and corresponding joint LBP and intensity histograms. **Top row:** 41 × 41 pixel ROIs showing examples of the appearance of the three classes used in the experiments. **Top Left:** Normal tissue. **Top middle:** Centrilobular emphysema **Top right:** Paraseptal emphysema. **Bottom row:** Joint histogram between LBP ($R = 1$ and $P = 8$) and intensity in the center pixel corresponding to the example ROIs in the top row.

or bullae, are visible as areas of abnormally low attenuation values, close to that of air. Different objective parameters for quantification of emphysema can be derived from the histogram of CT attenuation values, and the most common one is the relative area of emphysema [3]. Usually emphysema is classified into three subtypes and we will adopt the naming and definitions from Webb et al. [4]. These subtypes are: Centrilobular emphysema (CLE) defined as multiple, small, spotty lucencies, that may have thin walls, paraseptal emphysema (PSE) defined as multiple, lucencies in a single layer along the pleura, commonly with thin walls visible, and panlobular emphysema (PLE) defined as a lucent lung with small pulmonary vessels. The middle and right column of the top row of Figure 1 show examples of CLE and PSE respectively. Common for the quantitative methods based on the attenuation histogram are that they ignore the possibly valuable information inherent in the emphysema disease patterns, such as subtype, shape, and size distribution. This was exemplified in a recent clinical study that reported discrepancies between disease pattern based visual scoring and relative area of emphysema for assessing the craniocaudal distribution of emphysema in the three subtypes [5].

One way to objectively analyze the properties of the disease patterns is to use texture analysis [6]. This can be turned into a quantitative measure by performing pixel classification of each pixel in the lung based on textural appearance in a local region around the pixels. Several publications exist on classifying emphysema and other disease patterns in lung CT images using texture features.

[7,8,9] uses measures on co-occurrence matrices, measures on run-length matrices, moments of the attenuation or intensity histogram, and in some cases fractal dimension as features. Sluimer et al. [10] used a filter bank of Gaussians and Gaussian derivatives.

In this paper we propose to use local binary patterns (LBP), formulated by Ojala et al. [11], as texture features in a pattern classification system for discriminating between normal tissue (NT), CLE, and PSE. Using LBP it is possible to unify structural and statistical information by histograms of microstructures, and LBP are simple to compute. LBP have shown promising results in various applications in computer vision, and have been applied in other problems in medical imaging, for example resulting in a reduction of the number of false positives in mammographic mass detection [12]. To our knowledge LBP have not been applied to lung texture classification before. LBP is by design invariant to intensity, thus we also propose to include the intensity distribution. Previous work on lung texture classification has used moments of the intensity histogram as features [7,8,9,10]. We propose to instead use the full intensity histogram, together with LBP, by means of the joint LBP and intensity histogram, and to use it in a k nearest neighbor (kNN) classifier with histograms similarity as distance measure. The proposed method is compared to that of a filter bank based on Gaussian derivatives.

2 Methods

In the following the classification system is described. Section 2.1 describes the LBP features we use for characterizing the lung texture, Section 2.2 presents an alternative group of features used for comparison purposes, and Section 2.3 describes the classification framework.

2.1 Local Binary Patterns

The features that we use are based on the local binary patterns (LBP) proposed by Ojala et al. [11]. In general, LBP measures the local structure at a given pixel using P samples on a circle of radius R around the pixel and summarizes this information with a unique code for each local structure or pattern. The operator is highly non-linear and detects microstructures in the image at different resolutions governed by the parameter R, for example spots, edges, corners, etc., exemplified in the right part of Figure 2. The basic steps for calculating the LBP code in a pixel position in a given image are illustrated in the left part of Figure 2. Applying the LBP operator to an image results in a LBP code image. Based on this an LBP histogram is formed. Note that no quantization is needed and that the LBP codes are directly accumulated into a histogram. The LBP histogram combines structural and statistical approaches, LBP detects microstructures in the image, and the histogram captures the distribution of these microstructures. We use the rotation invariant formulation of LBP which is accomplished as illustrated in Figure 2 (c), see [11] for more details.

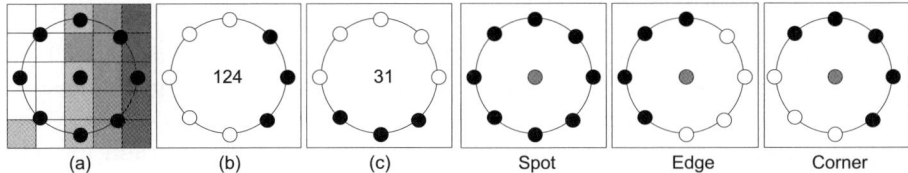

Fig. 2. Illustration of LBP. **Left:** The basic steps in computing the LBP code for a given pixel position: (a) the operator is centered on the given pixel and P equidistant samples are taken on the circle of radius R around the center; (b) the obtained samples are turned into 0's and 1's by applying a sign function with the center pixel value as threshold. By choosing a fixed sample position on the circle as the leading bit, the samples can be turned into a binary number. Thus each pattern has an associated unique binary number; (c) rotation invariance is achieved by bitwise shifting the binary pattern clock-wise until the lowest binary number is found. **Right:** Some of the microstructures that LBP are measuring.

LBP are invariant to any monotonic gray-scale transformation of the image. This is however not a desired property when dealing with CT images, where values are measurements of a physical property of the tissue displayed. [11] describes how to include contrast into LBP by making a joint histogram between the LBP and the variance of the intensities in the LBP samples. In a similar fashion we include the distribution of the intensities in the center pixels, by forming the joint histogram between the LBP and the intensities in the center pixels. This results in a histogram containing information about how the LBP varies at different intensity ranges, which we expect to be valuable information. The bottom row of Figure 1 contain examples of joint LBP and intensity histograms computed from the ROIs shown in the top row.

2.2 A Filter Bank Based on the Gaussian Function and Its Derivatives

For comparison we introduce a second group of features, which are based on the Gaussian function $G(\mathbf{x}; \sigma)$ and combinations of derivatives of the Gaussian function. By varying the standard deviation σ of the function in a discrete manner we obtain a whole bank of filters that can be applied to the images. Using a filter bank of various derivatives of the Gaussian function for lung texture classification was proposed by Sluimer et al. [10], where the Gaussian function itself was also included to make the filter bank sensitive to offsets in absolute intensity. The filters that we use are similar to those used in [10], except that the filters we use are all rotation invariant. The filter bank comprise the following filters: $G(\mathbf{x}; \sigma)$; the Laplacian of the Gaussian $\nabla^2 G(\mathbf{x}; \sigma)$; the gradient magnitude $|\nabla G(\mathbf{x}; \sigma)|_2$; the Gaussian curvature $K(\mathbf{x}; \sigma) = \partial^2 G(\mathbf{x}, \sigma)/\partial x^2 + \partial^2 G(\mathbf{x}, \sigma)/\partial y^2 - 2\partial^2 G(\mathbf{x}, \sigma)/\partial xy$.

2.3 Classification Framework

Classification is done using the kNN classifier [13]. When using the filter bank features, of Section 2.2, feature selection is applied using the sequential forward selection algorithm [13] for deciding which filters at which scales to use. When using the LBP features, of Section 2.1, several combinations of radii for multiresolution analysis are evaluated.

In [7,8,9,10] intensity and filter response distributions were represented by up to four moments of the histogram. This way a more compact representation is obtained at the expense of information loss. We use the full histogram instead and apply histogram similarity as distance measure in the kNN classifier. The histograms of the intensities and the filter responses are constructed using non-linear binning, where the binning is found by employing two rules on the total distribution of the ROIs in the training set: The distribution of the total distribution should be uniform and the number of bins is $\lfloor \sqrt[3]{N} \rfloor$, where N is the number of pixels in the ROI. Histogram intersection is used as the similarity measure between histogram H and histogram K

$$L_{hist}(H, K) = 1 - \sum_{b=1}^{B} \min(H_b, K_b), \quad (1)$$

where H_b denotes bin b of histogram H, B is the number of histogram bins and the histograms are assumed normalized to sum to one. Other histogram similarity measures could be used, for example the G statistic [11] or the earth movers distance [14]. In the case of measuring combined histogram similarity of N different histograms, we sum the individual histogram similarities computed using (1)

$$L_N = \sum_{n=1}^{N} L_{hist}(H^n, K^n). \quad (2)$$

3 Experiments and Results

The data used for the experiments is collected from a set of thin-slice CT images of the thorax. CT was performed using GE equipment (LightSpeed QX/i; GE Medical Systems, Milwaukee, WI, USA) with four detector rows, using the following parameters: 1.25-mm collimation, tube voltage 140 kV and tube current 200 milliampere (mA). The slices were reconstructed using a high spatial resolution (bone) algorithm. A population of 25 individuals, 8 healthy non-smokers, 4 smokers without COPD, and 13 smokers diagnosed with moderate or severe COPD according to LFT [1] were scanned in the upper, middle, and lower lung, resulting in a total of 75 CT slices. Visual assessment of the leading pattern, either NT, CLE, PSE, or PLE, in each of these slices was done individually by an experienced chest radiologist and a CT experienced pulmonologist. In 47% of the slices there was disagreement and in the slices where both human observers agreed on an emphysematous leading pattern, there was disagreement on the

Table 1. Left: Evaluation of the six different lung texture classification approaches. **Right:** Confusion matrices for the six approaches, in which the rows define the true class and the columns the estimated class. The top left matrix is for FB1, the top middle FB2, etc.

Approach	Accuracy (%)	p		NT	CLE	PSE	NT	CLE	PSE	NT	CLE	PSE
FB1	61.3	≈ 0	NT	17	27	15	55	0	4	41	8	10
FB2	94.0	0.724	CLE	19	31	0	2	48	0	6	42	2
LBP1	79.2	≈ 0	PSE	4	0	55	4	0	55	3	6	50
INT	87.5	0.004	NT	51	3	5	56	1	2	55	0	4
LBP2	92.3	0.228	CLE	2	48	0	1	49	0	1	49	0
LBP3	95.2	-	PSE	8	3	48	8	1	50	2	1	56

emphysema class in 40% of the cases. Consensus readings were obtained in all cases of disagreement. 168 non-overlapping ROIs were annotated in the slices representing the three classes: NT (59 observations from non-smokers), CLE (50 observations), and PSE (59 observations). The NT ROIs were annotated in the non-smokers and the CLE and PSE ROIs were annotated in the two smokers patient classes, within the area(s) of the leading pattern. PLE was excluded due to underrepresentation in the data set (only 2 out of 20 individuals diagnosed with COPD).

Six different approaches are evaluated and compared:

- A filter bank with the first four moments of filter responses, standardized to unit variance, as features. In this approach we use Euclidean distances in a feature space in the kNN classifier (FB1).
- A filter bank with histograms of filter responses, combined using (2), as features (FB2).
- Basic rotation invariant LBP histograms (LBP1).
- Intensity histograms (INT).
- LBP histograms and intensity histograms, combined using (2) (LBP2).
- Joint LBP and intensity histograms (LBP3).

The six different approaches are each evaluated using leave-one-out on patient level, thus in each trial all ROIs from one patient are held out and used for testing. The remaining ROIs are split into a training set and validation set using a 50%/50% split on patient level on each class, such that all ROIs from half the patients of each class are put in the training set and the rest in the validation set. Using the training set and validation set the model is trained, meaning that the optimal setting for the parameters listed in the next paragraph are selected. Subsequently, the held out ROIs are classified with the selected parameter setting using all the samples in the training set and validation set in the kNN.

The following parameter values are considered during training. In the Gaussian based filter bank the following scales are used for all filters $\sigma = [0.5, 1, 2, 4, 8]$ pixels. In the LBP the following radii are used $R = [1, 2]$ pixels with corresponding number of samples $P = [8, 16]$. Single radii as well as a combination of the two are tried during training. Combining operators results in a multiresolution analysis, and the combination is done using (2). Common parameters for all six approaches are: ROI size $= [31 \times 31, 41 \times 41, 51 \times 51]$ pixels and number of neighbors in the kNN classifier $k = [1, 2, \ldots, 10]$ neighbors.

The performance of the six approaches is summarized in Table 1 left, where the best performance (95.2% classification accuracy) is achieved by LBP3. The table also includes p-values found using McNemar's test [15], comparing our proposed approach, LBP3, against the other approaches. Further, confusion matrices are shown in Table 1 right.

4 Discussion and Conclusion

LBP3 performs best achieving a classification accuracy of 95.2%, however, it is not significantly different ($p = 0.72$) from the second best approach, FB2 which achieves an accuracy of 94.0%. There is an indication that there is a gain in modeling the joint LBP and intensity histogram instead of using the individual LBP and intensity histogram together, which is evident from the fact that LBP2 has a lower performance (92.3%), but this difference is not significant ($p = 0.23$). We expect that a larger data set would make the importance of joint modeling more evident, but LBP2 may remain a viable, computationally cheaper, alternative. LBP alone achieves a decent performance (79.2%) but including intensity information improves the performance considerably as expected; LBP3 is significantly better than LBP1 ($p \approx 0$). That the intensity information is important is also evident from the fact that INT achieves better performance than LBP1. In this setting, moments of the histogram clearly provide a too simple representation of the full distribution; the performance of FB1 is the lowest of all (61.3%). This is an interesting finding that should be investigated further, since most previous work on texture classification in lung CT uses moments, for example [7,8,9,10].

Comparing our results to some of the previous work, the performance of LBP3 is actually very good. [8] reports an overall sensitivity of 60.3% and an overall specificity of 86.7%, where for LBP3 the sensitivity is 97.3% and the specificity is 93.2% (when comparing NT versus CLE and PSE). [10] reports a classification accuracy of 76% when using a kNN classifier, whereas the classification accuracy of LBP3 is 95.2%. Off course the results are not directly comparable, due to differences in the data, the choice of classes, etc., but this comparison at least gives an indication of the usefulness of our proposed approach.

The relatively high level of disagreement between the two human expert observers on determining the leading pattern, illustrates the importance and usefulness of developing objective methods for characterizing emphysema patterns. These methods should be based on consensus readings of as many experts as possible, or be unsupervised.

In this paper we focus on evaluating a new proposed approach based on LBP for texture classification in lung CT. In future work, we will evaluate the performance of this classification system for emphysema quantification. Another issue that would be interesting to investigate is to use the combination of LBP and filter responses, for example the filters described in Section 2.2. LBP3 and FB2 achieve almost the same overall performance, but do not classify exactly the same ROIs correctly as indicated by the confusion matrices. Perhaps a combination of these features may further reduce classification errors.

To conclude, we have proposed to use local binary patterns combined with intensity for classification of texture in lung CT, achieving a classification accuracy of 95.2% on a three-class problem comprising normal tissue, centrilobular emphysema, and paraseptal emphysema.

Acknowledgements. This work is partly funded by the Danish Council for Strategic Research (NABIIT), the Netherlands Organisation for Scientific Research (NWO), and AstraZeneca, Lund, Sweden.

References

1. Rabe, et al.: Global strategy for the diagnosis, management, and prevention of chronic obstructive pulmonary disease: GOLD executive summary. Am. J. Respir. Crit. Care. Med. 176(6), 532–555 (2007)
2. Shaker, et al.: Identification of patients with chronic obstructive pulmonary disease (COPD) by measurement of plasma biomarkers. The Clinical Respiratory Journal 2(1), 17–25 (2008)
3. Müller, et al.: density mask, an objective method to quantitate emphysema using computed tomography. Chest 94(4), 782–787 (1988)
4. Webb, et al.: High-Resolution CT of the Lung, 3rd edn. Lippincott Williams & Wilkins (2001)
5. Stavngaard, et al.: Quantitative assessment of regional emphysema distribution in patients with chronic obstructive pulmonary disease (COPD). Acta Radiol. 47(9), 914–921 (2006)
6. Tuceryan, M., Jain, A.K.: Texture analysis. In: The Handbook of Pattern Recognition and Computer Vision, 2nd edn., pp. 207–248. World Scientific Publishing, Singapore (1998)
7. Uppaluri, et al.: Quantification of pulmonary emphysema from lung computed tomography images. Am. J. Respir. Crit. Care. Med. 156(1), 248–254 (1997)
8. Chabat, et al.: Obstructive lung diseases: texture classification for differentiation at CT. Radiology 228(3), 871–877 (2003)
9. Xu, et al.: MDCT-based 3-D texture classification of emphysema and early smoking related lung pathologies. IEEE Trans. Med. Imaging 25(4), 464–475 (2006)
10. Sluimer, et al.: Computer-aided diagnosis in high resolution CT of the lungs. Med. Phys. 30(12), 3081–3090 (2003)
11. Ojala, et al.: Multiresolution gray-scale and rotation invariant texture classification with local binary patterns. IEEE Trans. Pattern Anal. Mach. Intell. 24(7), 971–987 (2002)
12. Oliver, et al.: False positive reduction in mammographic mass detection using local binary patterns. MICCAI 10(Pt. 1), 286–293 (2007)
13. Jain, et al.: Statistical pattern recognition: a review. IEEE Trans. Pattern Anal. Mach. Intell. 22(1), 4–37 (2000)
14. Rubner, et al.: A metric for distributions with applications to image databases. In: Sixth International Conference on Computer Vision, 1998, January 4-7, pp. 59–66 (1998)
15. Dietterich, T.G.: Approximate statistical test for comparing supervised classification learning algorithms. Neural Computation 10(7), 1895–1923 (1998)

A Symmetry-Based Method for the Determination of Vertebral Rotation in 3D

Tomaž Vrtovec, Franjo Pernuš, and Boštjan Likar

University of Ljubljana, Faculty of Electrical Engineering, Slovenia
{tomaz.vrtovec, franjo.pernus, bostjan.likar}@fe.uni-lj.si

Abstract. In the past, a number of methods were proposed for quantitative assessment of vertebral rotation from three-dimensional (3D) images. However, these methods were based on manual identification of distinctive anatomical landmarks, required manual determination of cross-sections from 3D images, and measured only axial vertebral rotation instead of the rotation in 3D. In this paper, we propose an automated method for quantitative assessment of vertebral rotation in 3D that is based on finding the planes of vertebral symmetry by matching image intensity gradients on both sides of each plane. The method was evaluated on 28 images of normal and pathological vertebrae, obtained by computed tomography (CT) and magnetic resonance (MR). For each vertebra, final angle displacements of 200 initial angle displacements, uniformly distributed within 30° from manually obtained reference angles, were obtained. The results show that by the proposed method, vertebral rotation can be successfully estimated in 3D with an average accuracy of 1.0° and precision of 0.5°.

1 Introduction

Vertebral rotation is important for the understanding of normal and pathological spine conditions. In the past, many methods for quantitative assessment of vertebral rotation were developed for two-dimensional (2D) X-ray images, while the measurements in three dimensions (3D) became possible with the development of 3D imaging techniques. Earlier methods were based on identifying a number of distinctive anatomical landmarks on vertebrae in both computed tomography (CT) and magnetic resonance (MR) axial cross-sections [1,2,3,4]. Recently, methods based on image analysis techniques have been proposed for measuring vertebral rotation in 3D. Rogers et al. proposed a method that measured the axial vertebral rotation between two axial MR [5] or CT [6] cross-sections by maximizing the correlation of intensities inside manually defined circular areas. Oblique CT cross-sections were used by Adam and Askin [7], who determined the axial vertebral rotation with the line that bisected the manually defined area around the vertebral body, so that the correlation of thresholded intensities in the bisected regions was maximal. Kouwenhoven et al. measured vertebral rotation in manually selected axial cross-sections from CT [8] and MR [9] images of normal spines. The rotation was defined with the line passing through the center of the vertebral canal and the center of the anterior half of the vertebral body, both obtained by an automatic region growing segmentation technique. These methods required manual initialization of parameters, which may lead to errors because:

1. Manual identification of distinctive anatomical landmarks is difficult due to variable vertebral anatomical structure (e.g. pathological cases) and variable image quality (e.g. low image resolution).
2. Manual determination of oblique (reformatted) cross-sections consists of determining one or two rotation angles and requires a relatively difficult navigation through 3D images.
3. The vertebrae are in general rotated in 3D, i.e. in sagittal, coronal and axial planes. In case of significant sagittal and/or coronal rotation, errors are induced in the measurement of axial rotation in 2D cross-sections.

To avoid these problems, we propose an automated method for quantitative assessment of vertebral rotation in 3D. The method is based on finding the planes of vertebral symmetry by matching image intensity gradients on both sides of each plane. The method can be applied to images of normal and pathological vertebrae, acquired either by CT or MR.

2 Method

2.1 Vertebral Rotation and Anatomical Correspondence in 3D

The rotation of a vertebra in a 3D image can be represented by the angles of rotation of the coordinate system V of the vertebra around the axes of the coordinate system I of the 3D image:

$$\boldsymbol{\omega} = (\omega_x, \omega_y, \omega_z). \qquad (1)$$

The axes of the image (global) coordinate system I and vertebral (local) coordinate system V can be represented by the Cartesian unit vectors $\{e_{Ix}, e_{Iy}, e_{Iz}\}$ and $\{e_{Vx}, e_{Vy}, e_{Vz}\}$, respectively. The angles ω_x, ω_y and ω_z then represent the rotation of the vertebral coordinate system V around vectors e_{Ix} (pitch), e_{Iy} (roll) and e_{Iz} (yaw), respectively.

If the origin of V is located at the vertebral body center and V is rotationally aligned with the vertebra in I, anatomically corresponding (symmetrical) parts of the vertebra can be observed within volumes of interest (VOIs) along positive/negative directions of each axis e_{Vj}, $j = x, y, z$, of V (Fig. 1a). This means that the vertebra is symmetrical in left/right ($\pm e_{Vx}$) directions, and that the vertebral body is symmetrical in anterior/posterior ($\pm e_{Vy}$) and upward/downward ($\pm e_{Vz}$) directions. Because the observed correspondences decrease with increasing rotation between V and I, the angles $\boldsymbol{\omega}$ of vertebral rotation can be obtained by evaluating these anatomical correspondences of vertebral structures. It is important to note that the origin of V is located at the vertebral body center and not at the vertebral anatomical center of rotation, which was reported to be in

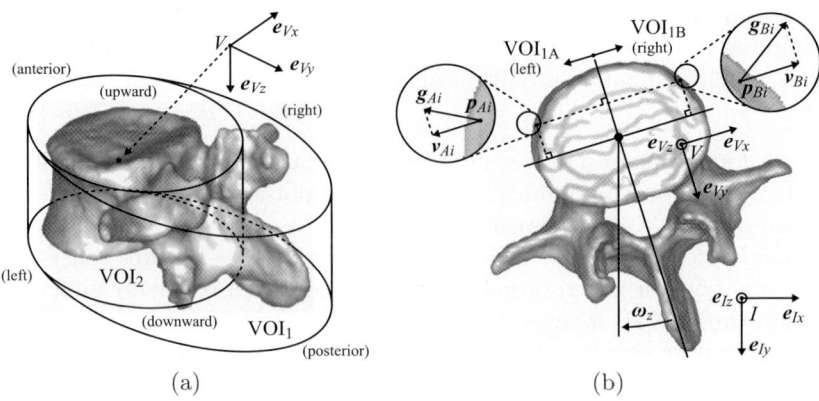

Fig. 1. (a) The vertebral coordinate system V and the observed volumes of interest (VOI$_1$ contains the whole vertebra, VOI$_2$ contains only the vertebral body). (b) Example of anatomical correspondence in left/right directions (S_x), shown for a symmetrical pair of points $\boldsymbol{p}_{Ai}$ and $\boldsymbol{p}_{Bi}$ inside VOI$_1$.

the mid-sagittal plane at the anterior wall of the vertebral canal [5] or at the center of the vertebral canal [8]. However, the rotation angles do not depend on the location of the origin of V, but on the axes of V, i.e. on the vectors $\boldsymbol{e}_{Vj}$, $j = x, y, z$, that have to be rotationally aligned with the vertebra in I.

2.2 Determination of Vertebral Rotation in 3D

The angles $\boldsymbol{\omega}$ of vertebral rotation can be determined by finding the planes of vertebral symmetry that define maximal anatomical correspondences. For each axis $\boldsymbol{e}_{Vj}$, $j = x, y, z$, we propose to measure the correspondences of two halves of a VOI (VOI$_A$ and VOI$_B$, Fig. 1b) by:

$$S_j(\text{VOI}) = \frac{\sum_{i=1}^{N} |\boldsymbol{v}_{Ai}| \cdot |\boldsymbol{v}_{Bi}| \cdot f}{\sum_{i=1}^{N} |\boldsymbol{v}_{Ai}| \cdot \sum_{i=1}^{N} |\boldsymbol{v}_{Bi}|} ; \quad f = \begin{cases} 1; & \boldsymbol{v}_{Ai} \cdot \boldsymbol{v}_{Bi} < 0 \\ 0; & \text{otherwise} \end{cases}, \quad (2)$$

where f is the weighting function, and $\boldsymbol{v}_{Ai} = proj_{\boldsymbol{e}_{Vj}} \boldsymbol{g}_{Ai}$ and $\boldsymbol{v}_{Bi} = proj_{\boldsymbol{e}_{Vj}} \boldsymbol{g}_{Bi}$ are the projections of the intensity gradient vectors $\boldsymbol{g}_{Ai} = grad\, I(\boldsymbol{p}_{Ai})$ and $\boldsymbol{g}_{Bi} = grad\, I(\boldsymbol{p}_{Bi})$ in the coordinate system I to the unit vector $\boldsymbol{e}_{Vj}$, $j = x, y, z$, of the coordinate system V at symmetrical pair of points $\boldsymbol{p}_{Ai}$ and $\boldsymbol{p}_{Bi}$, respectively. A total of N pairs of symmetrical points exist inside each VOI. By projecting the gradient vectors to the axis $\boldsymbol{e}_{Vj}$, $j = x, y, z$, and by applying the weighting function f, we retain the gradient components $\boldsymbol{v}_{Ai}$ and $\boldsymbol{v}_{Bi}$ that are relevant for defining the vertebral symmetry in the direction of the axis $\boldsymbol{e}_{Vj}$.

It is expected that the anatomical structures in VOI halves will correspond maximally when V is rotationally aligned with the vertebra in I. Therefore, the

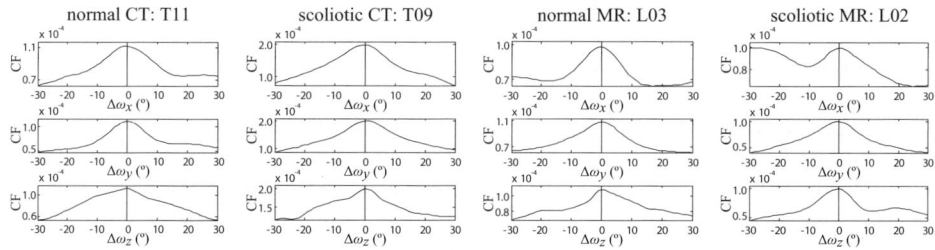

Fig. 2. Behavior of the criterion function CF for different vertebrae, obtained by independently varying the angles $\boldsymbol{\omega} = (\omega_x, \omega_y, \omega_z)$ for $-30° \div 30°$ from the reference angles $\boldsymbol{\omega}_R$

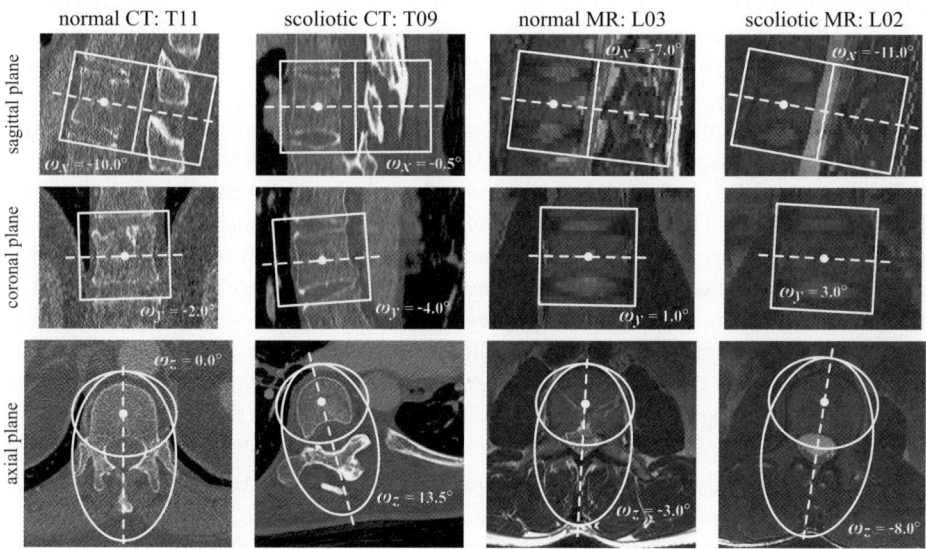

Fig. 3. Examples of the determination of reference angles $\boldsymbol{\omega}_R$ and the initialization of VOIs in 3D, shown for different vertebrae

rotation of the coordinate system V, i.e. the angles $\boldsymbol{\omega}$ of vertebral rotation, can be found by maximizing the following criterion function:

$$CF = S_x(\text{VOI}_1) + S_y(\text{VOI}_2) + S_z(\text{VOI}_2) \ . \qquad (3)$$

Figure 2 illustrates the behavior of the criterion function CF, obtained by independently varying the angles ω_x, ω_y and ω_z from reference angle values. The large capture ranges and distinctive maxima of CF indicate that the proposed criterion function is feasible for the estimation of vertebral rotation angles.

3 Experiments and Results

3.1 Data and Experiments

The anatomical structure of an arbitrary vertebra may significantly differ from the "normal" structure. This usually occurs in spinal diseases (e.g. scoliosis, hyper-kyphosis/lordosis) due to pathological vertebral growth. Besides, the rotation of an arbitrary vertebra in the 3D image depends on the orientation of image acquisition planes and on the position of the patient in scanner. To analyze the performance of the proposed method with respect to different vertebral shapes, we used 20 vertebrae from images of normal spines (CT: 10, voxel size $0.7 \times 0.7 \times 1.0 \, \text{mm}^3$; MR: 10, voxel size $0.4 \times 0.4 \times 3.0 \, \text{mm}^3$) and 8 vertebrae from images of scoliotic spines (CT: 4, voxel size $0.6 \times 0.6 \times 1.0 \, \text{mm}^3$, strong right thoracolumbar curve; MR: 4, voxel size $0.4 \times 0.4 \times 3.0 \, \text{mm}^3$, mild left lumbar curve). The scoliotic vertebrae were located around the apex of the deformity (usually most rotated and different from the normal shape). For each vertebra, reference rotation angles ω_R were determined by manually defining the vertebral body center and by aligning the VOIs with the vertebra in the sagittal, coronal and axial cross-sections. The size of the VOIs were based on vertebral morphometric data, so that VOI_1 and VOI_2 contained the whole vertebra and the vertebral body, respectively (Figs. 1a, 3). Before computing the intensity gradient vectors ($grad\,I$) in 3D, the images were blurred with a Gaussian filter ($\sigma = 3 \, \text{mm}$). For each vertebra, the origin of the vertebral coordinate system V was initialized in the manually defined vertebral body center. To study the influence of different vertebral orientations, we initialized the orientation of the vertebral coordinate system V in angles that were for $\Delta\omega$ displaced from the obtained reference angles ω_R, thus simulating an arbitrary initialization of the orientation of the vertebral coordinate system V. For each vertebra, 200 initial displacements were applied that were uniformly distributed within $|\Delta\omega| = \left(\Delta\omega_x^2 + \Delta\omega_y^2 + \Delta\omega_z^2\right)^{1/2} = 30°$, resulting in a total of 5600 displacements for all vertebrae. For each initial angle displacement, the angles ω were found by maximizing the criterion function (Eq. 3) with the Powell's optimization method.

3.2 Results

The results of the experiments are presented in Table 1. A single assessment of the rotation angles was considered successful if it resulted in an angle displacement less than $|\Delta\omega| = 2°$ (i.e. $2.0°$ for one or $1.1°$ for each angle) from the reference angles ω_R. The results show that for most vertebrae, the success rate was equal or close to 100% if the initial angle displacement was below $10°$ (i.e. $10°$ for one or $5.8°$ for each angle). For successful experiments, the average angle displacement was $\overline{|\Delta\omega|} = 0.95°$ ($\overline{|\Delta\omega_x|} = 0.58°$, $\overline{|\Delta\omega_y|} = 0.53°$, $\overline{|\Delta\omega_z|} = 0.53°$) and the average standard deviation was $|\sigma_{\Delta\omega}| = 0.47°$ ($\sigma_{\Delta\omega_x} = 0.28°$, $\sigma_{\Delta\omega_y} = 0.26°$, $\sigma_{\Delta\omega_z} = 0.26°$), which represent the accuracy and the precision of the method, respectively.

Table 1. Median of 200 final angle displacements and success rates for three initial displacement ranges

Vertebra image (level)		Median angle displacement (°)				Success rate ($|\Delta\omega| < 2°$) (%)		
		$\Delta\omega_x$	$\Delta\omega_y$	$\Delta\omega_z$	$|\Delta\omega|$	0°÷10°	10°÷20°	20°÷30°
CT normal	T07	−1.0	1.1	−0.9	1.7	70	64	46
	T08	−0.7	−0.2	0.1	0.8	100	100	98
	T09	−0.3	−0.3	−1.3	1.5	94	93	80
	T10	−0.5	−0.1	−1.3	1.5	86	73	71
	T11	**0.3**	**0.1**	**0.0**	**0.4**	**100**	**100**	**93**
	T12	−0.2	0.2	−0.4	0.5	100	100	90
	L01	**0.5**	**−1.5**	**−0.6**	**1.8**	**86**	**88**	**61**
	L02	0.9	−0.6	−0.5	1.2	100	97	72
	L03	1.2	0.3	0.5	1.3	98	97	67
	L04	0.0	0.0	0.2	0.4	86	85	55
CT scoliotic	T07	−0.1	−0.8	−1.3	1.5	98	76	54
	T08	−1.3	−0.7	−0.4	1.8	84	61	30
	T09	**−0.5**	**0.2**	**0.4**	**0.7**	**98**	**100**	**93**
	T10	**0.2**	**2.3**	**0.1**	**2.4**	**20**	**16**	**13**
MR normal	T07	0.0	−0.3	0.5	0.6	89	94	54
	T08	**−1.8**	**−0.4**	**0.4**	**2.2**	**52**	**36**	**28**
	T09	−1.2	−0.2	0.5	1.4	100	81	55
	T10	0.5	0.9	−0.3	1.2	100	94	80
	T11	0.2	−0.2	0.0	0.3	98	100	67
	T12	1.5	0.6	0.2	1.6	100	100	77
	L01	1.0	−0.2	−0.2	1.1	98	97	71
	L02	−0.5	−0.8	−0.2	1.0	100	100	83
	L03	**−0.1**	**0.1**	**0.1**	**0.3**	**100**	**99**	**57**
	L04	−0.2	−0.1	0.5	0.6	100	82	65
MR scoliotic	L01	0.2	0.5	−0.1	1.0	94	60	29
	L02	**0.1**	**−0.6**	**−0.5**	**0.8**	**100**	**73**	**52**
	L03	**0.1**	**−0.4**	**1.3**	**1.5**	**100**	**82**	**36**
	L04	−0.2	−0.7	−0.1	1.2	98	93	59

Figure 4 shows the scatter diagrams of the initial and final angle displacements for vertebrae that performed best and worst inside each group of normal CT, scoliotic CT, normal MR and scoliotic MR vertebrae (shown in bold in Tab. 1). It can be observed that the final displacements tend to converge to a value that is not equal to 0°, which means that the final angles were not equal to the reference angles. These constant displacements represent systematic errors, and when they were above 2°, the experiments were not considered successful. However, these systematic errors may originate in the reference angles ω_R, which were determined manually and may therefore not represent the "true" vertebral rotation. For example, although poor success rates are reported for the T10 scoliotic CT vertebra (Tab. 1), the scatter diagram (Fig. 4) shows that the angles always converged to approximately the same angle displacements with the median of 2.4°. This systematic error was mostly caused by the angle ω_y, which resulted in approximately −11°, while the reference angle was −9° ($\Delta\omega_y = 2.3°$). After examining this case in detail, we concluded that the reference angle ω_y could not be reliably defined manually due to the strong scoliotic nature of the vertebral anatomical structure, i.e. relatively strong shear of the vertebral body.

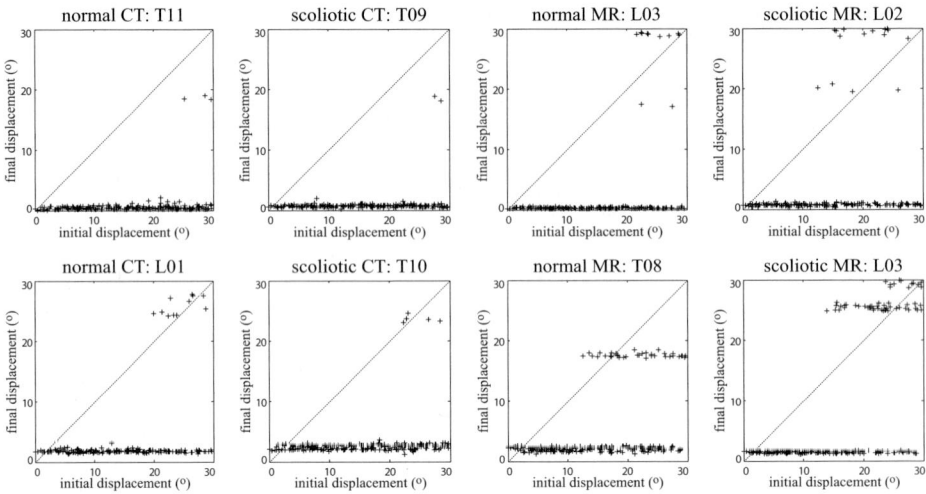

Fig. 4. Scatter diagrams of 200 initial and final angle displacements, shown for different vertebrae

4 Discussion and Conclusion

We proposed an automated method for quantitative assessment of vertebral rotation in 3D. The relation between the image and vertebral coordinate systems was obtained by matching image intensity gradients that, when the vertebral coordinate system is aligned with the vertebra, define the symmetry of the vertebral anatomical structure. The method proved to be applicable to normal and pathological vertebrae, obtained from CT or MR images.

The results of axial vertebral rotation (i.e. angle ω_z) are comparable to other methods that were based on image analysis techniques. Measurement errors of 0.2° were reported for the method of Rogers et al. [5,6]. Adam and Askin [7] claimed their method to be relatively insensitive to image thresholding, however, they reported that different intensity thresholds caused a 2.8° difference in rotation. Kouwenhoven et al. [8,9] reported the standard deviation of their method to be around 1°. By applying the proposed method, we achieved around 0.5° accuracy and 0.3° precision for the axial vertebral rotation. For the measurements of vertebral rotation in 3D, the accuracy and precision of the proposed method were around 1.0° and 0.5°, respectively.

The manual determination of reference rotation angles, required to assess the accuracy of any method, is usually based on the orientation of vertebral body and spinous process, shape of vertebral canal and other vertebral anatomical features. However, such features do not always represent a good anchor, as the anatomical structures are not always perfectly symmetrical and oriented in the same direction across the whole vertebra, resulting in different reference angles for different reference features. The reference angles have to be therefore considered with caution, as they may not represent the "true" rotation of the vertebra. The proposed method, on the other hand, estimates the vertebral rotation by finding the maximal possible symmetry of the entire vertebra. To conclude, the benefits of the method are at least the following:

1. The vertebral rotation can be defined with high accuracy and precision in 3D, i.e. all three angles of rotation ω_x, ω_y and ω_z around the three coordinate system axes are obtained. Errors due to projection of the vertebra onto a 2D plane are therefore eliminated.
2. The method may be used to determine the "true" ("gold standard") vertebral rotation, as the symmetry of the entire vertebral anatomical structure may represent an objective reference feature.

The symmetry of the vertebral anatomical structure may also be used to determine the reference center of rotation of the vertebral coordinate system. We are currently developing a method for robust determination of vertebral body centers in CT and MR images, which may allow an accurate determination of vertebral rotation and position in 3D.

Acknowledgements

This work has been supported by the Ministry of Higher Education, Science and Technology, Slovenia, under grants P2-0232, L2-7381, L2-9758, and J2-0716. The authors would like to thank the Image Sciences Institute, Utrecht, The Netherlands, and the Commonwealth Scientific and Industrial Research Organisation (CSIRO), Australia, for providing the CT and MR images used in this study.

References

1. Aaro, S., Dahlborn, M.: Estimation of vertebral rotation and the spinal and rib cage deformity in scoliosis by computer-tomography. Spine 6(5), 460–467 (1981)
2. Ho, E., Upadhyay, S., Chan, F., Hsu, L., Leong, J.: New methods of measuring vertebral rotation from computed tomographic scans: An intraobserver and interobserver study on girls with scoliosis. Spine 18(9), 1173–1177 (1993)
3. Krismer, M., Sterzinger, W., Christian, H., Frischhut, B., Bauer, R.: Axial rotation measurement of scoliotic vertebrae by means of computed tomography scans. Spine 21(5), 576–581 (1996)
4. Göçen, S., Havitçioglu, H., Alici, E.: A new method to measure vertebral rotation from CT scans. European Spine Journal 8(4), 261–265 (1999)
5. Rogers, B., Haughton, V., Arfanakis, K., Meyerand, E.: Application of image registration to measurement of intervertebral rotation in the lumbar spine. Magnetic Resonance in Medicine 48(6), 1072–1075 (2002)
6. Rogers, B., Wiese, S., Blankenbaker, D., Meyerand, E., Haughton, V.: Accuracy of an automated method to measure rotations of vertebrae from computerized tomography data. Spine 30(6), 694–696 (2005)

7. Adam, C., Askin, G.: Automatic measurement of vertebral rotation in idiopathic scoliosis. Spine 31(3), 80–83 (2006)
8. Kouwenhoven, J.W., Vincken, K., Bartels, L., Castelein, R.: Analysis of preexistent vertebral rotation in the normal spine. Spine 31(13), 1467–1472 (2006)
9. Kouwenhoven, J.W.M., Bartels, L., Vincken, K., Viergever, M., Verbout, A., Delhaas, T., Castelein, R.: The relation between organ anatomy and pre-existent vertebral rotation in the normal spine: Magnetic resonance imaging study in humans with situs inversus totalis. Spine 32(10), 1123–1128 (2007)

Spatio-temporal Speckle Reduction in Ultrasound Sequences

Noura Azzabou[1,*] and Nikos Paragios[1,2]

[1] Laboratoire MAS Ecole Centrale de Paris, France
[2] GALEN Group, INRIA Saclay, Ile-de-France, France
n.azzabou@institut-myologie.org, nikos.paragios@ecp.fr

Abstract. In this paper we will be concerned with speckle removal in ultrasound images. To this end, we introduce a new spatio-temporal denoising method based on a variational formulation. The regularization relies on a non parametric image model that describes the observed image structure and express inter-dependencies between pixels in space and time. Furthermore, we introduce a new data term adapted to the Rayleigh distribution of the speckle. The interaction between pixels is determined through the definition of new measure of similarity between them to better reflect image content. To compute this similarity measure, we take into consideration the spatial aspect as well as the temporal one. Experiments were carried on both synthetic and real data and the results show the potential of our method.

1 Introduction

Ultrasound imaging is a popular non invasive and low cost technique to observe the dynamical behavior of organs. The produced images inherit a multiplicative component that is the speckle. This signal may contain information useful to medical experts [1]. Nevertheless, for some applications like segmentation or registration the speckle affects the quality of images and complicates the diagnosis task. Therefore, speckle removal could be a tool to obtain better images while preserving details. In the literature, numerous methods for speckle suppression were proposed. Some of them transform the multiplicative noise problem into an additive one by considering the logarithm of the image and assume that the noise is Gaussian [2]. The limitation of such a method lies in the fact that the logarithm function reduces the contrast in the image and makes the task of denoising more complex. The anisotropic diffusion [3] relies on the gradient information which is not robust when dealing with high noise levels. We want to point out also that these methods, consider only fixed images and not sequences. The temporal aspect was addressed in [4] using temporal averaging. This technique is efficient tool of speckle removal but due to motion, fine details can be blurred unless an appropriate weight definition is done. Techniques that aim to perform signal correction through motion correction were also investigated [5]. Analysis

---

* The first author is affiliated now to AIM -CEA NMR Laboratory Institue of Myology.

in the transform domain like wavelet was also considered toward speckle reduction [6,7], but the transform selection is crucial for the performance of these methods.

In this paper, we will address the speckle removal problem in ultrasound images. Inspired from total variation techniques, our approach entails a functional minimization process. Such a functional is composed of two terms : the regularization term that is able to encode complex image structure and the data term that encodes the speckle model. In addition to the image structure, the regularization term is designed to take into consideration the temporal aspect. In this context, the interactions between pixels are determined by weights that reflect the similarity in the temporal and the spatial domain with implicit constraints imposing motion consistency. As far as fidelity to data term is considered, its formulation is based on the speckle model which is assumed to be a Rayleigh distribution. The paper is organized as follows, section 2 is devoted to the presentation of the method, we present in section 3 the definition of weights (or interaction between pixels), next we will focus on the experimental validation of our approach in section 4, and finally we conclude the paper in section 5.

2 Problem Statement

Let us consider two image sequences U and I defined on $T \times \Omega$ where T is the length of the sequence and Ω refers to a frame spatial domain. These two sequences are related according to $I = U * n$ with n being a multiplicative noise sequence that follows a Rayleigh distribution [1] defined as : $r(n) = \frac{n}{\sigma_n^2} \exp(-\frac{n^2}{2\sigma_n^2})$
In order to recover the noise free sequence U we have to minimize a cost function that insures smoothness, preserves boundaries, while imposing a fidelity constraint, to the observed sequence. To define the fidelity to data term, we will consider the link between the Maximum a Posteriori (MAP) estimation framework and the total variation formulation. The MAP estimator aims to minimize an energy composed of two terms : the image model that is the regularization term and the noise model that corresponds to the fidelity to data term. In the discrete case and for a frame U_t the observed noise likelihood is equivalent to the data term that can be expressed as

$$E_{data}(U_t) = -log(P(I_t|U_t)) = -log(P(n_t))$$

Under the assumption that (i) the noise observations are independent (ii) identically distributed, and (iii) U and I have non zero intensity for each pixel in the sequence, then we can write:

$$E_{data}(U_t) = -\log\left(\prod_{i=1}^{|\Omega|} r(n_t(i))\right) = \sum_{i=1}^{|\Omega|}\left[-\log\left(\frac{I_t(i)}{\sigma_n^2 U_t(i)}\right) + \frac{I_t^2(i)}{2\sigma_n^2 U_t^2(i)}\right]$$

Note that the assumption of independence between the noise observations is too simple for the speckle because it is correlated. However such an assumption yields a simpler energy and a computationally efficient formulation. Now, if we consider the substitute the continuous formulation of the data term to the discrete one, we obtain

$$E_{data}(U_t) = \int_\Omega \left[\log(U_t(\mathbf{x})) + \frac{I_t^2(\mathbf{x})}{2\sigma_n^2 U_t^2(\mathbf{x})} + Cte \right] d\mathbf{x} \quad (1)$$

Now, if we consider the function $f(x) = \log(x) + \frac{1}{2\sigma_n^2} \frac{I_t^2(\mathbf{x})}{x^2}$, it can be easily shown that the second derivative of f is positive for $x \leq \frac{\sqrt{6} I_t(\mathbf{x})}{2\sigma_n^2}$. This function is convex on the interval $]0, 255]$ if $\frac{\sqrt{6} I_t(\mathbf{x})}{2\sigma_n^2} > 255$ for any intensity value $I_t(\mathbf{x})$. In other words, if $\left(\sigma_n^2 \leq \frac{\sqrt{6} \times \mathrm{Inf}(I_t)}{2 \times 255}\right)$ then the designed function f is convex. In practice it is verified when $(\sigma_n \leq 0.1)$ which is equivalent to small noise amount. Hence for small value of σ_n, the data term E_{data} is a convex function.

Regarding the regularization, we selected the model introduced in [8] that is a generalized linear interpolation model where each pixel is expressed as a weighted mean of the remaining pixels of the sequence. Such a model involves a data driven image model were the interaction between pixels is defined according to the similarity between them in order to preserve image content. For this application, we will consider the extension of this formulation to ultrasound sequences to account for the time dimension and to perform a temporal filtering as well as a spatial one. In this case E_{reg} is defined as

$$E_{reg}(U) = \iint_{T \times \Omega} \left(\frac{\iint_{T \times \Omega} w(\mathbf{x}, t, \mathbf{y}, t_1) U_{t_1}(\mathbf{y}) d\mathbf{y} dt_1}{\iint_{T \times \Omega} w(\mathbf{x}, t, \mathbf{y}, t_1) d\mathbf{y} dt_1} - U_t(\mathbf{x}) \right)^2 d\mathbf{x} dt \quad (2)$$

where $w(\mathbf{x}, t, \mathbf{y}, t_1)$ is a similarity measure between two pixels $\mathbf{x}$ and $\mathbf{y}$ observed on the frame t and t_1. Finally, we define the global cost function that is minimized to estimate the restored image as

$$E(u) = E_{reg}(U) + \lambda \int_0^T E_{data}(U_t) dt \quad (3)$$

where λ is a trade-off parameter between the regularization and the fidelity to data term. The estimation of the noise free ultrasound sequence is obtained through minimizing the cost function given in equation (3). The minimization is done through a gradient descent scheme. Starting from the noisy observation $U^0 = I$, the restored image is obtained at the convergence of the sequence U_t^k

$$U_t^{k+1}(\mathbf{x}) = U_t^k(\mathbf{x}) - dt \left[\frac{\partial E_{reg}}{\partial U_t(\mathbf{x})} + \lambda \left(\frac{1}{U_t(\mathbf{x})} - \frac{1}{\sigma_n^2} \frac{I_t(\mathbf{x})}{U_t(\mathbf{x})^3} \right) \right] \quad (4)$$

In order to decrease the computation cost we will restrict the interaction between pixels to a local neighborhood domain and not the whole image. Therefore, we note : $\Pi_\mathbf{x}$ the spatial neighborhood centered on a pixel $\mathbf{x}$ and T_w the size of the temporal window (the number of frames that interact directly with a given frame). In this case, the derivative of the regularization term is equal to

$$\frac{\partial E_{reg}}{\partial U_t(\mathbf{x})} = 2\left(U_t(\mathbf{x}) - \int_{\Pi_\mathbf{x}} \int_{t-T_w}^{t+T_w} \frac{w(\mathbf{x},t,\mathbf{y},t_1)}{Z(\mathbf{x},t)} U_{t_1}(\mathbf{y})d\mathbf{y}dt_1\right)$$
$$+2\int_{\Pi_\mathbf{x}} \int_{t-T_w}^{t+T_w} \left(U_{t_1}(\mathbf{z}) - \int_{\Pi_\mathbf{z}} \int_{t_1-T_w}^{t_1+T_w} \frac{w(\mathbf{z},t_1,\mathbf{y},t_2)}{Z(\mathbf{z},t_1)} U_{t_2}(\mathbf{y})d\mathbf{y}dt_2\right) \frac{w(\mathbf{z},t_1,\mathbf{x},t)}{Z(\mathbf{z},t_1)} d\mathbf{z}dt_1 \quad (5)$$

with $Z(\mathbf{x},t) = \int_{\Pi_\mathbf{x}} \int_{t-T_w}^{t+T_w} w(\mathbf{x},t,\mathbf{y},t_1)d\mathbf{y}dt_1$ the normalization coefficient. Note that such a derivative formulation assumes that the weights are independent from the image U which is a valid assumption because weights are calculated in the beginning of the process on the noisy observations.

3 Weights Computation

In our algorithm we combine spatial and temporal filtering. Therefore, a robust weight definition is crucial to avoid details blurring due to motion. More explicitly, with a good definition of weights there is no need to estimate the motion of the organ. In this work, we will suggest a suitable definition of the weights in the case of multiplicative Rayleigh noise and we will consider a distance based on the spatial information as well as the temporal one. To this end, we use patch based similarity which is more robust to noise than the similarity between intensities at a pixel level. We recall that this measure relies on the assumption that an image is stationary (at least at local scale), and redundant which means that a given patch has several copies in the entire ultrasound sequence. Let us characterize a pixel $\mathbf{x}$ at the frame U_t by the set of neighboring pixels in the same frame. Let us consider now the L^2 distance between two patches of size $(2p+1) \times (2p+1)$ centered on $\mathbf{x}$ and $\mathbf{y}$ in two different frames U_{t_1} and U_{t_2} in the sequence.

$$d_s(\mathbf{x},t_1,\mathbf{y},t_2) = \sum_{\mathbf{z}\in[-p,p]^2} (I_{t_1}(\mathbf{x}+\mathbf{z}) - I_{t_2}(\mathbf{y}+\mathbf{z}))^2$$
$$= \sum_{\mathbf{z}\in[-p,p]^2} (U_{t_1}(\mathbf{x}+\mathbf{z})n_{t_1}(\mathbf{x}+\mathbf{z}) - U_{t_2}(\mathbf{y}+\mathbf{z})n_{t_2}(\mathbf{y}+\mathbf{z}))^2$$

In case the observed patches are derived from the same speckle free patch, we can write:

$$d_s(\mathbf{x},t_1,\mathbf{y},t_2) = \sum_{\mathbf{z}\in[-p,p]^2} U_{t_1}^2(\mathbf{x}+\mathbf{z})(n_{t_1}(\mathbf{x}+\mathbf{z}) - n_{t_2}(\mathbf{y}+\mathbf{z}))^2$$

This equation shows that contrarily to additive noise, the L^2 distance is not only dependent on noise distribution but also on the image intensity. To overcome this dependence one can compute

$$d_s(\mathbf{x},t_1,\mathbf{y},t_2) = \sum_{\mathbf{z}\in[-p,p]^2} \frac{(I_{t_1}(\mathbf{x}+\mathbf{z}) - I_{t_2}(\mathbf{y}+\mathbf{z}))^2}{U_{t_1}^2(\mathbf{x}+\mathbf{z})}$$

To determine the distance $d_s(\mathbf{x}, t_1, \mathbf{y}, t_2)$, one needs an estimation of $U_{t_1}(\mathbf{x})$. A simple way to do that is to compute the average of I_{t_1} over the patch around $\mathbf{x}$. Furthermore, in order to obtain a symmetric distance with respect to t_1 and t_2 we will consider $U_{t_1}^2 = U_{t_1} * U_{t_2}$. Thus, we obtain the following distance definition

$$d_s(\mathbf{x}, t_1, \mathbf{y}, t_2) = \sum_{\mathbf{z} \in [-p,p]^2} \frac{(I_{t_1}(\mathbf{x}+\mathbf{z}) - I_{t_2}(\mathbf{y}+\mathbf{z}))^2}{\tilde{U}_{t_1}(\mathbf{x}+\mathbf{z})\tilde{U}_{t_2}(\mathbf{y}+\mathbf{z})} \quad \tilde{U}_{t_1}(\mathbf{x}) = \sum_{\mathbf{z} \in [-p,p]^2} \frac{I_{t_1}(\mathbf{x}+\mathbf{z})}{(2p+1)^2}$$

Now if we consider the temporal aspect of the sequence, two similar pixels that belong to the same structure have similar displacement vectors. Thus, in addition to the distance between patches, the variation of pixel intensity over time should be taken into account. To this end, we consider temporal windows of size $(2t_c+1)$ and similarly to the spatial distance, we define

$$d_t(\mathbf{x}, \mathbf{y}, t_1, t_2) = \sum_{k=-t_c}^{t_c} \frac{[I_{t_1+k}(\mathbf{x}) - I_{t_2+k}(\mathbf{y})]^2}{\tilde{U}_{t_1+k}(\mathbf{x})\tilde{U}_{t_2+k}(\mathbf{y})} \quad (6)$$

Finally we define the similarity measure between $\mathbf{x}$ and $\mathbf{y}$ belonging to two different frames as a decreasing function of the distances $d_s(\mathbf{x}, \mathbf{y}, t_1, t_2)$ and $d_t(\mathbf{x}, \mathbf{y}, t_1, t_2)$. A possible weight definition is

$$w(\mathbf{x}, t_1, \mathbf{y}, t_2) = \exp\left(-\frac{d_s(\mathbf{x}, t_1, \mathbf{y}, t_2)}{2h_s^2}\right) \exp\left(-\frac{d_t(\mathbf{x}, t_1, \mathbf{y}, t_2)}{2h_t^2}\right) \quad (7)$$

h_s and h_t are parameters that have an impact on the selection degree of pixels that interact together. They have an influence on the smoothness of the final result. To summarize, the proposed weights are designed to take into account the noise properties, mainly the fact that it is multiplicative. With such definition, we restrict interactions between pixels only to similar ones in order to preserve details in each frame. We take also into account motion consistency by computing similarity measure on temporal windows.

4 Experimental Results

To assess the performance of the proposed method we used both synthetic and real data. In the first experiment, we used synthetic images with artificial speckle. The speckle is simulated by low pass filtering a complex Gaussian random field and computing its magnitude [2]. We compared our algorithm to the anisotropic diffusion algorithm [3] and a wavelet based technique [7]using the Matlab implementation provided by the authors. Regarding anisotropic diffusion the parameter is the number of iteration. For the wavelet based algorithm the parameter are the thresholding coefficient and the neighborhood size were local energy was computed. For the first method we tuned the iteration number to obtain the better possible results (PSNR and visually). The optimal parameters range of the second method was provided by the author in their paper but we slightly

Table 1. PSNR values for denoised image corrupted by Speckle

	Sythetic1 [7]			Synthetic2		
σ_n	1	0.5	0.25	1	0.5	0.25
Corrupted image	22.20	27.93	33.95	20.44	26.47	32.62
OurMethod	29.16	37.32	38.01	33.88	38.89	43.53
SRAD[3]	24.88	33.09	40.95	31.55	38.36	46.15
wav [7]	29.14	35.48	41.69	31.06	35.85	39.75

modified them to improve their performance with respect our data. Regarding our algorithm we considered 11×11 window size for Π_x while $\lambda = 0.05$. For weight computation the parameters setting is: $h_s = \frac{\sigma_n}{5}$ and a 3×3 patch size. We did not consider the temporal aspect for this experiment because the synthetic data are single images and not sequences. For an evaluation we considered the PSNR $\left[PSNR = 10log_{10}\frac{255^2}{MSE}\right]$ of the reconstructed images $\hat{U}$ that is a function of the mean square error with respect to the ground truth image noted $\left[MSE = \sum_{t=0}^{T}\sum_{\mathbf{x}\in\Omega}(U_t(\mathbf{x}) - \hat{U}_t(\mathbf{x}))^2\right]$.

In table (1) we reported the PSNR value for the different methods and with different noise variance. This results show that our method achieve high performance when the noise variance is important. Such a behavior is justified by the fact that we consider large spatial neighborhood (Π_x) for filtering which reduces considerably the variance inside each region. The anisotropic diffusion algorithm (SRAD)[3] is more local and its numerical scheme is based on interactions between pixels at local scale when compared to our algorithm. Besides, the gradient information is not reliable in case of high level noise. The approach presented in [7] and the choice of the parameter of threshold used in this algorithm to compute the noise free wavelet coefficients is critical to insure the balance between edge preserving and noise suppression. In figure [Fig.(1)] one can see the restoration results for the synthetic image using the different methods and different variance. The method based on the wavelet transform provides images with sharp contours but the noise remains in homogeneous regions. The anisotropic diffusion results in blurry edges while smoothing the homogeneous areas. Our algorithm reaches an optimal balance where the obtained images are completely smoothed inside each region while the edges being sharp. As we stated before we consider large neighborhood size to remove the speckle, while encoding the image structure in our weight definition to preserve image discontinuities and details. This figure shows that our method preserves the image discontinuities and contrast between regions better than the two other algorithms. As far as real data are concerned we considered an ultrasound sequence of the left ventricle on which we applied our speckle removal algorithm. The parameters used for this experiment are: a 7×7 window size for Π_x, $\lambda = 0.5$ and $T_w = 5$. The weight computation was performed using 3×3 patch size, a temporal window for comparison of size $t_c = 2$ and $h_s = h_t = 0.05$. In figure [Fig.(2)] we reported the restoration result on one frame of an ultrasound sequence. To evaluate the quality of restoration, we extracted the boundaries of the ventricle, using a level set based technique. The contours obtained using our method are smooth and

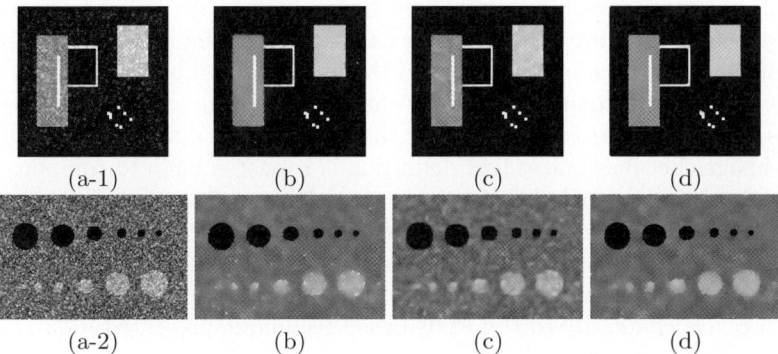

Fig. 1. (a-1) Image (Sythetic1) corrupted by the speckle $\sigma_n = 0.5$ (a-2) Image (Sythetic2) corrupted by the speckle $\sigma_n = 1$ (b) Result using the anisotropic diffusion [3] (c) Result using the wavelet based technique [7] (d) Result using our algorithm

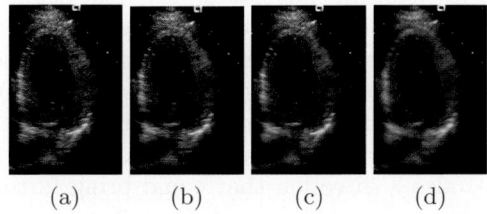

Fig. 2. Results of restoration on real ultrasound frames. (a) Observed image (b) Result using algorithm [7] (c) Anisotropic diffusion [3] (d) Results of our algorithm.

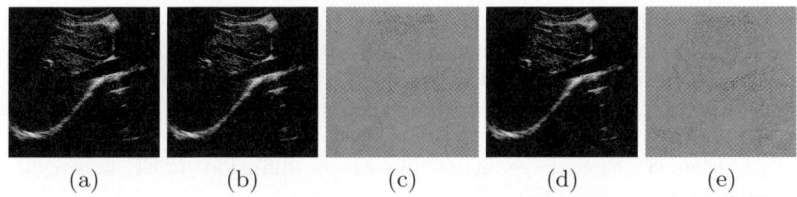

Fig. 3. Results of filtering real ultrasound frames (a) Observed image (b) Result of our algorithm without temporal component ($T_w = 0$) (frame by frame filtering) (c) Residual obtained with our algorithm without temporal component ($T_w = 0$) (frame by frame filtering)(d) Result of our algorithm using temporal filtering ($T_w = 2$) (e) Residual obtained with our algorithm using temporal filtering ($T_w = 2$)

the structure being present in the image were preserved. The contour extracted in the frame restored using our approach is similar to the one associated to the anisotropic diffusion, but this method yields piecewise smooth images. Regarding the wavelet based technique, it produces image with sharp details but the contours are not smooth. To evaluate the impact of the time component we compared the algorithm performance by processing the whole sequence using

$T_w = 2$ and by processing it frame by frame ($T_w = 0$). and the obtained results are shown in figure [Fig.(3)]. One can see that using a temporal window is more efficient for speckle reduction and this is illustrated by the residual images [Fig.(3-c),Fig.(3-e)](difference between the filtered image and the observed one). Besides, we notice that considering the time component doesn't introduce a blur on the images because our weight definition is robust enough to compensate the effect of motion. To conclude we can say that the experimental results show that our method can deal with correlated speckle even though we make the assumption of independence between pixels. We have to point out that the proposed speckle removal approach is flexible with the selection of the scale of interaction between pixels contrarily to the PDE based technique presented in [3].

5 Discussion

In this paper we proposed a new regularization technique for ultrasound sequences. The regularization term was based on weight definition adapted to the Speckle to impose some consistency with the observed structure in the image. We introduced also a data term that is coherent with the speckle distribution A future direction to improve our work will be considering anisotropic neighborhood shapes as well as variable size ones. This will ensure a better interaction between pixels lying on the same structure. Considering the fact that speckle is a correlated signal is also a direction that could bring further improvement to the method.

References

1. Wagner, R., Smith, S., Sandrik, J.M., Lopez, H.: Statistics of speckle in ultrasound b-scans. IEEE Trans. on Sonics and Ultrasonics 30(3), 156–163 (1983)
2. Achim, A., Bezerianos, A., Tsakalides, P.: Novel bayesian multiscale method for speckle removal in medical ultrasound images. IEEE trans. on Medical Imaging 20, 772–783 (2001)
3. Yu, Y., Acton, S.: Speckle reducing anisotropic diffusion. IEEE trans. on Image Processing 11(11), 1260–1270 (2002)
4. Abbott, J.G., Thurstone, F.L.: Acoustic speckle: Theory and experimental analysis. Ultrason. Imag. 1, 303–324 (1979)
5. Markosien, L.: A motion-compensated filter for ultrasound image sequences. Technical report, Providence, RI, USA (1996)
6. Angelini, E., Laine, A., Takuma, S., Holmos, J., Homma, S.: Lv volume quantification via spatiotemporal analysis of real-time 3-D echocardiography. IEEE trans. on Medical Imaging 20(6), 457–469 (2001)
7. Pizurica, A., Philips, W., Lemahieu, I., Acheroy, M.: A versatile wavelet domain noise filtration technique for medical imaging. IEEE trans. on Medical Imaging 22(3), 323–331 (2003)
8. Azzabou, N., Paragios, N., Guichard, F., Cao, F.: Variable bandwidth image denoising using image-based noise models. In: CVPR, pp. 1–7 (2007)

Surface-Based Structural Group Analysis of fMRI Data

Grégory Operto[1], Cédric Clouchoux[1], Rémy Bulot[1], Jean-Luc Anton[2], and Olivier Coulon[1]

[1] Laboratoire LSIS, UMR CNRS 6168, Marseille, France
gregory.operto@univmed.fr
[2] Centre d'IRM fonctionnelle de Marseille, Marseille, France

Abstract. As structural and surface-based analyses gain interest for activation detection, morphometry and intersubject matching purposes, this paper proposes a method to perform structural group analyses directly on the cortical surface. Scale-space blobs are extracted from surface-based functional maps and matched across subjects. The process aims at identifying activations within a population despite the various effects due to variability. Results of the method are presented with simulated activations and with data from a somatotopy protocol.

1 Introduction

Group analysis in fMRI aims at building descriptions of unicity and diversity across a pool of subjects of a same cognitive experiment. When the pool is sufficiently big, results may then be generalized to a population. Still, matching these subjects together strongly suffers from the intersubject variability that exists at different levels : anatomical, physiological, functional [1]. The usual procedure consists in normalizing every scanned subject to a common anatomical space. Hence, any location in that space is supposed to correspond to the same region in the brain of each subject. Since responses to a same protocol show variability from one subject to another, decisions concerning a group-scale effect are taken upon the hypothesis that the signals across subjects are normally distributed. This forms the general basis of any voxel-based activation detection technique. This general, historical and widely spread volume-based approach consider the voxels of the whole brain, including those in the white matter, whereas the main sources of the functional signal are located in the cortical ribbon. In this context, surface-based analysis schemes especially gain interest [2,3,4] as they focus on the main location of the cerebral activity. On the other hand, the framework of structural approaches [5,6] allows to match objects from one subject to another instead of voxels, a level at which variability is better addressed. In this paper, the proposed method aims at performing analyses of functional data across a group of subjects, in both a surface-based and a structural way (as opposed to the iconic voxel-based fashion). This approach gains sensitivity against volume-based approaches, first by restricting the analysis to the cortex and by focusing on objects rather than voxels. The method is inspired by the volume-based structural group analysis presented in [5]. After adapting its general algorithms to surfaces, such as building surface-based scale-space primal sketches, the intersubject anatomical matching is addressed via a 2D coordinate system defined on the cortical surface [2]. In this context, this work attempts to gather the advantages of two approaches, structural and surface-based, in order to overcome the intersubject variability as much as possible. This paper details in section 2 the method from the representation of data to the detection itself. Section 3 presents results on synthetic and real data. Discussion is then presented in section 4.

2 Surface-Based Structural Group Analysis

2.1 Data Preparation

For each subject, a triangulated mesh of the inner cortical surface (G/W interface) is first extracted from their anatomical volume using the Brainvisa package [7]. The advantages of using this surface reside in its geometry and its spherical topology. Functional volumes are coregistered with the anatomy, e.g. using SPM2 package [8]. Surface-based representations of functional data are then created using a volume-to-surface projection technique proposed in [9] and t-maps are built by an incremental statistical method [10]. Cortical localization and intersubject matching are performed via a surface-based coordinate system built on each cortical surface [2]. This pipeline finally allows to build individual surface-based statistical maps, used as inputs for the structural representation process described below.

2.2 Structural Representation of Data

The structural approach in fMRI data analysis is advocated by different works [5,6] for theoretical, computational and representation purposes. The voxels are only the acquisition space and have never had any anatomical meaning, other than the simple localization provided by spatial normalization. Moreover, the big amounts of information contained in raw 3D volumes lead to high computation costs, and not necessarily higher sensitivity. The main idea of the structural approach is to deal with representations of data closer to the objects under study than voxels. Some existing works choose to build a scale-space primal sketch of the activity, considering that objects of interest are found at multiple scales [11,12]. This multiscale approach is advocated for instance by [5,13]. Some others focus on supra-threshold regions [14], or activity peaks [1]. Subsequent objects are hence characterized by different, numerical or geometrical, features.

One part of the work presented here consisted in adapting the volume-based scale-space primal-sketch construction algorithm to a topologically and geometrically different domain such as a triangulated surface. Linear scale-space representations of the surface-based functional maps are obtained by smoothing along the meshes by solving the heat-equation, leading to a diffusion process which progressively removes details as in figure 1. In order to solve the heat equation on a triangular mesh, the laplacian is computed using a finite element approximation [15].

The method then defines a hierarchical description of the structure of each statictical map on the cortical surface. Different characteristics can be embedded with the scale-space blobs, from their lifetime across scales to geometrical or intensity-based measurements. We chose to attach the product between the blob's lifetime and the t-test value of the blob's maximum on the original functional map, hence describing both the intensity of the blobs and their saliency with respect with surrounding structures [5,13]. This has been shown to be an appropriate measurement for activation detection purpose [5].

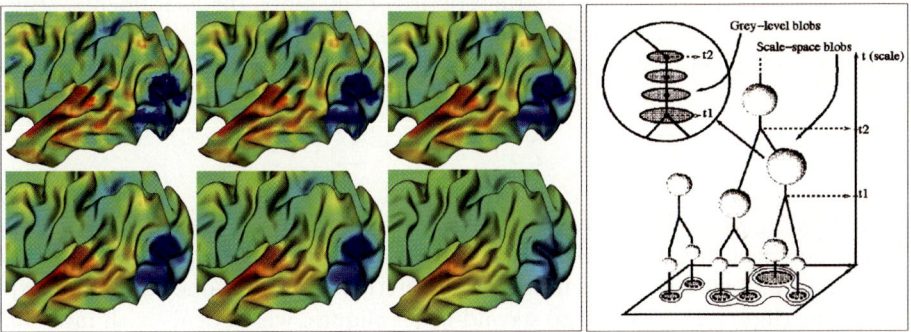

Fig. 1. (left) Example of scales from a scale-space of a surface-based statistical t-map (right) Symbolic representation of a scale-space primal sketch

2.3 Structural Analysis on the Cortical Surface

Let n_s be the number of subjects responding to a certain cognitive task. We build for each one a surface-based t-map, describing the relevance for each node to have been activated by the task. n_s primal sketches are created from these t-maps, with n_{bi} the number of scale-space blobs extracted from t-map $i, i \in \{1, ..., n_s\}$. By matching the primal sketches, the structural analysis aims at assigning a specific label to each of the $N = \sum_{i \in [1,...,n_s]} n_{bi}$ scale-space blobs, depending on the blob probability to represent an actual activation. As far as the matching can be achieved, corresponding activation clusters get assigned the same positive label across subjects and null label is given to blobs of non-interest (noise). This association relies on a model defined using the same set of rules as in [5], i.e. :

1. A blob representing an activation is likely to have high measurements;
2. Two blobs representing the same activation must be linked in the graph and have the same non-null label;
3. Two blobs representing the same activation (same non-null label) are likely to have spatial supports close to each other;
4. An activation is represented only once for each subject, ie, a positive label must have only one occurrence per primal sketch.

Group analysis is performed on a graph embedding primal sketches of all subjects and built as follow : graph nodes are blobs and edges are set between two blobs if those two blobs a) belong to two different subjects and b) are close enough in the common space defined by the surface-based coordinate system defined in [2] (namely, inter-blob distance must be below 20 mm).

As presented in [5], a blob is identified as an activation if its associated measurements are sufficiently high in the map and if it is repeated often enough across subjects. The label field is modeled as a Markov random field (MRF), whose optimal realization can be achieved in a Bayesian framework by maximizing the posterior probability $P(X|Y)$, with X the label field on the primal sketch graph and Y the data. In other terms, maximization of this probability drives to the optimal labeling given the characteristics of the blobs (measurements, scale) and the similarities observed between subjects. It is shown [5] to be equivalent to the minimization of an energy function $U(X|Y)$ defined as follow :

$$U(X|Y) = \sum_{s=1}^{N} V(y_s|x_s) + \sum_{c \in C} V_c(X|c)$$

where $V(y_s|x_s)$ is a data-driven potential function (rule 1) and $V_c(X|c)$ a contextual potential function calculated from every contextual clique $c \in C$ of the graph (rule 2, 3 and 4). Chosen potential functions are the same as in [5] except for the one (figure 2) attached to second-order cliques, which deals with intersubject similarities. Similarity between two blobs is computed using an intersubject

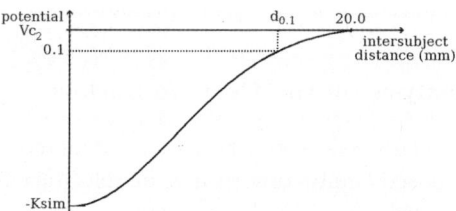

Fig. 2. The second-order inter-primal-sketches clique potential function

distance function $f(b_1, b_2)$. If b_1 and b_2 belong to different subjects and have the same non-null label, the potential V_{c_2} then equals :

$$V_{c_2} = -K_{sim} \cdot \frac{e^{-f(b_1,b_2)^2}}{2 \cdot \left(\frac{d_{0.1}}{\sqrt{2 \cdot log(10.0)}}\right)^2}$$

Otherwise (different or null labels), $V_{c_2} = 0$. The similarity function $f(b_1, b_2)$ is computed using the surface-based referential attached to each cortical mesh as a common referential. Given two blobs b_1 and b_2, $f(b_1, b_2)$ returns the length of the shortest geodesic path between the two blobs' maxima in the common referential. $d_{0.1}$ is a user-defined distance at which the potential V_{c_2} equals 0.1.

Once all potential functions are defined, the total energy function is defined. To minimize it, we use a stochastic algorithm, the Gibbs sampler with annealing [16]. After minimization, the process returns a set of positive labels, each one representing an activation and having an occurrence in a number of primal sketches. We therefore know the occurrence, or the non-occurrence, of each activation for any subject. These occurrences can then be mapped on the individual anatomy of the subject for localization considerations.

3 Experiments

3.1 Experiments on Simulated Data

The whole pipeline was applied to simulated activation maps on a spherical mesh. Gaussian background noise was first distributed all over the surface, then a set of 4 simulated activation clusters were added to the background. Since the experiment is run on a common spherical mesh, the similarity issue has no more anatomical meaning compared to as on real meshes. Still, the profile of the map was meant to recall the one of a typical functional t-map and some amount of variability was simulated in terms of activation intensity and location as illustrated on figure 3 : from the original location, a different node is randomly selected in a neighborhood as a new activation focus for each map. The neighborhood is taken as 10.0 mm-wide, equal to the typical intersubject variability magnitude δ_τ in [6]. Primal sketches are built for each of the 10 maps and minimization is run on the resulting graph and label field. Non-null labels are presented in figure 3. A set of 4 non-null distinct labels were attributed, each of them identifying the same specific simulated activation focus across all the maps. Blobs are represented as small spheres for visualization purposes.

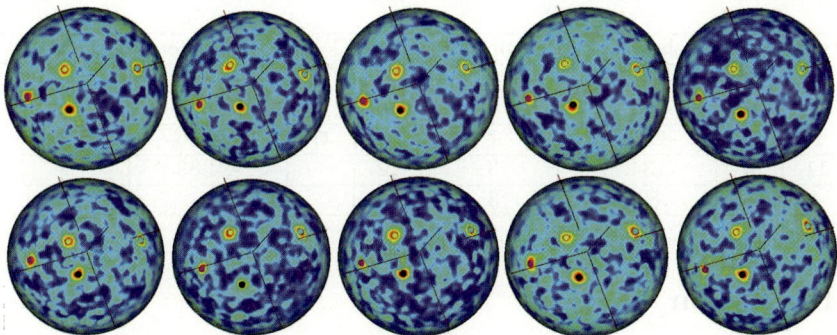

Fig. 3. Labeling after minimization on simulated activation maps and spherical atlas

3.2 Experiments on Real Data

We ran the activation detection pipeline on 8 subjects issued from a somatotopy experiment. Surface-based maps were computed for a simple (foot movement-rest) contrast and primal sketches were extracted from these. Minimization was performed on the primal sketches graph. Resultingly, there were 9 non-null labels generated. One of them is repeated across the 8 subjects, two of them exist in 7 subjects and one can be found in 6 subjects. The most frequently occurring labels are gathered at the top of the central sulcus, or on the medial face of the hemisphere, located either in the primary sensorimotor areas (M1-S1) or in the supplementary motor area (SMA), as the results one would expect from a neuroscientific point of view. One label appears near the insular cortex in 2 subjects. Figure 4 shows non-null labels for 4 subjects, together with individual statistical t-maps thresholded at $p < 0.05$ (corrected for multiple comparisons). Table 1 details the numbers of occurrences and the energies associated to these labels.

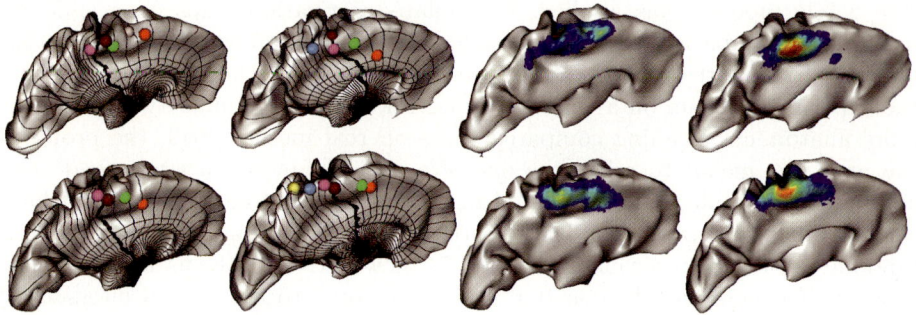

Fig. 4. Resulting activations from a right-motor contrast for 4 subjects. (left) labeled after minimization (right) thresholded individual statistical t-maps ($p < 0.05$ corrected).

Table 1. Energies and numbers of occurences of non-null generated labels

Label	Color	Global energy	Occurences	Label	Color	Global energy	Occurences
3	●	-586.82	8	7	●	-81.11	7
5	●	-368.92	6	10	○	-42.91	2
9	●	-236.56	7	8	○	-25.66	2
11	●	-134.71	3	12		-24.83	2
4		-89.75	3				

4 Discussion

The minimization aims at finding the label configuration which leads to fit with the initial model. Results on simulated data show that non-null labels were attributed to areas on the sphere showing relative high intensity and good matching across the simulated maps. Specifically, all clusters were properly labelled, with no false positive. On real data, results show that non-null labels appear in variable numbers of subjects, which correlates with the variability effects recognized by other works e.g. [5,1,6]. Overall, the label with the lowest energy (table 1) is the one existing in most subjects and identifies the primary motor activation. Then, the labels with the second lowest energies stand for somatosensory activations on one hand, and supplementary motor activations on the other. This complies precisely with our model and with the neuroscientific results expected for such study. Figure 4 compares the activations to thresholded individual statistical maps and shows that several components may exist under a single suprathreshold cluster, which is a specific valuable feature of structural approaches.

In order to assess similarities between subjects, a surface-based coordinate system is used as a common referential to all subjects. However, these coordinates cannot be used as is to compute distances. This illustrates the need for a common reference spatial support, i.e. a cortical surface atlas. Without such an atlas, our method chooses one subject as a reference used to calculate interblobs distances. Nevertheless, this subject presents specific anatomical features, which are not necessarily representative neither at a global nor at the group scale. This inevitably introduces a bias in the calculated distances [17]. The choice of a statistically representative and non-biased atlas is directly related to the performance in overcoming intersubject anatomical variability and therefore a crucial point in order to realize our measures on the cortical surface. By these considerations, structural group analysis using surface-based intersubject distances constitute a new approach, significantly different compared to voxel/node-based statistical methods.

5 Conclusion and Further Work

This paper presents a method which connects two distinct analysis frameworks, structural and surface-based. The method was applied to a set of simulated data and functional data from a somatotopy experiment. The results showed efficiency of the chosen model in retrieving simulated activations and detecting activations associated to a simple motor task. The paper underlines the importance of a common space to make comparisons between subjects. Future research will concern the creation of a cortical surface reference atlas and therefore the implementation of an anatomically meaningful intersubject distance.

References

1. Thirion, B., Flandin, G., Pinel, P., Roche, A., Ciuciu, P., Poline, J.B.: Dealing with the shortcomings of spatial normalization: Multi-subject parcellation of fMRI datasets. Human Brain Mapping 27(8), 678–693 (2005)
2. Clouchoux, C., Coulon, O., Riviere, D., Cachia, A., Mangin, J.F., Régis, J.: Anatomically constrained surface parameterization for cortical localization. In: Duncan, J.S., Gerig, G. (eds.) MICCAI 2005. LNCS, vol. 3750, pp. 344–351. Springer, Heidelberg (2005)
3. Andrade, A., Kherif, F., Mangin, J., Worsley, K., Paradis, A., Simon, O., Dehaene, S., Bihan, D.L., Poline, J.: Detection of fmri activation using cortical surface mapping. Human Brain Mapping 12, 79–93 (2001)

4. Van Essen, D.C., Drury, H.A.: Structural and functional analyses of human cerebral cortex using a surface-based atlas. J. Neurosci. 17(18), 7079–7102 (1997)
5. Coulon, O., Mangin, J.F., Poline, J.B., Zilbovicius, M., Roumenov, D., Samson, Y., Frouin, V., Bloch, I.: Structural group analysis of functional activation maps. NeuroImage 11(6), 767–782 (2001)
6. Thirion, B., Pinel, P., Tucholka, A., Roche, A., Ciuciu, P., Mangin, J.F., Poline, J.B.: Structural analysis of fmri data revisited: Improving the sensitivity and reliability of fmri group studies. IEEE Transactions on Medical Imaging 26(9), 1256–1269 (2007)
7. http://brainvisa.info
8. Ashburner, J., Friston, K.: Voxel-based morphometry: the methods. Neuroimage 11, 805–821 (2000)
9. Operto, G., Bulot, R., Anton, J.L., Coulon, O.: Projection of fmri data onto the cortical surface using anatomically-informed convolution kernels. Neuroimage 39(1), 127–135 (2007)
10. Roche, A., Lahaye, P.J., Poline, J.B.: Incremental activation detection in fMRI series using kalman filtering. In: IEEE International Symposium on Biomedical Imaging, pp. 376–379 (2004)
11. Worsley, K., Marrett, S., Neelin, P., Evans, A.: Searching scale space for activation in PET images. Human Brain Mapping 4, 74–90 (1996)
12. Poline, J.B., Mazoyer, B.: Analysis of individual brain activation maps using hierarchical description and multiscale detection. IEEE Transactions on Medical Imaging 13(4), 702–710 (1994)
13. Lindeberg, T., Lidberg, P., Roland, P.: Analysis of brain activation patterns using a 3-D scale-space primal sketch. Human Brain Mapping 7, 166–194 (1999)
14. Simon, O., Kherif, F., Flandin, G., Poline, J.B., Riviere, D., Mangin, J.F., Bihan, D.L., Dehaene, S.: Automatized clustering and functional geometry of human parietofrontal networks for language, space, and number. Neuroimage 23(3), 1192–1202 (2004)
15. Chung, M.K., Taylor, J.: Diffusion smoothing on brain surface via finite element method. In: IEEE International Symposium on Biomedical Imaging, vol. 1, pp. 432–435 (2004)
16. Geman, S., Geman, D.: Stochastic relaxation, gibbs distribution, and the bayesian restoration of images. IEEE Trans. on Pattern Anal. Machine Intell. 6, 721–741 (1984)
17. Devlin, J., Poldrack, R.: In praise of tedious anatomy. Neuroimage 37(4), 1033–1041 (2007)

Dynamic Cardiac Mapping on Patient-Specific Cardiac Models

Kevin Wilson[1,3], Gerard Guiraudon[1,2], Doug Jones[1,2,4], Cristian A. Linte[1,3], Chris Wedlake[1], John Moore[1], and Terry M. Peters[1,3,5]

[1] Imaging Research Laboratories, Robarts Research Institute,
[2] Canadian Surgical Technology and Advanced Robotics (CSTAR),
[3] Biomedical Engineering Graduate Program, University of Western Ontario,
[4] Department of Medicine, University of Western Ontario,
[5] Department of Medical Biophysics, University of Western Ontario,
London, Ontario, Canada
kevin.wilson@vanderbilt.edu, tpeters@imaging.robarts.ca

Abstract. Minimally invasive techniques for electrophysiological cardiac data mapping and catheter ablation therapy have been driven through advancements in computer-aided technologies, including magnetic tracking systems, and virtual and augmented-reality environments. The objective of this work is to extend current cardiac mapping techniques to collect and display data in the temporal domain, while mapping on patient-specific cardiac models. This paper details novel approaches to collecting spatially tracked cardiac electrograms, registering the data with a patient-specific cardiac model, and interpreting the data directly on the model surface, with the goal of giving a more comprehensive cardiac mapping system in comparison to current systems. To validate the system, laboratory studies were conducted to assess the accuracy of navigating to both physical and virtual landmarks. Subsequent to the laboratory studies, an in-vivo porcine experiment was conducted to assess the systems overall ability to collect spatial tracked electrophysiological data, and map directly onto a cardiac model. The results from these experiments show the new dynamic cardiac mapping system was able to maintain high accuracy of locating physical and virtual landmarks, while creating a dynamic cardiac map displayed on a dynamic cardiac surface model.

1 Introduction

Minimally invasive cardiac therapy, driven through computer-aided intervention, has made a large contribution to the advancement in the field of cardiac mapping and catheter ablation therapy. Dedicated systems such as the CARTO^{TM} XP Navigation System (Biosense-Webster), EnSite® System (St. Jude Medical), and more recently the combination of the CARTO RMT electroanatomical mapping system with the Stereotaxis Niobe magnetic steering technology, provide physicians with the tools necessary to record, display, and analyze the electrical activation patterns of the heart.

The motivation behind cardiac mapping systems for both clinical and research related use are to create a detailed description of the electrical activation of the heart to study the mechanisms of arrhythmias, and in some cases assist in a curative procedure such as catheter ablation therapy. In practice, atrial fibrillation (AF) is the most common type of cardiac arrhythmia affecting over 2.5 million North Americans, and due to an aging population is becoming more prevalent [1]. However, researchers are still investigating the sources of AF. As reported by Efimov and Fedorov [2] theories are being investigated whether AF is caused by single or multiple sources, the electrical circuits are focused or reentrant, and whether AF is purely and myogenic disease or whether there are neurological causes.

A key tool in this analysis is a cardiac map, which gives spatial representation to cardiac electrophysiological (EP) data by tracking the tip of the electrode catheter in real-time, while recording cardiac electrograms (CEGs). The tracked location data are reconstructed into a three dimensional model and the CEG data is interpolated across the structure so information such as activation time, signal amplitude, as well as abnormal patterns can be studied on the volumetric atrial/ventricle and epicardial/endocardial surfaces.

Until recently cardiac mapping systems were limited to maps displayed on reconstructed heart geometry created through the sampled locations collected from the tracked catheter. This limited the usefulness of the map to the ability of the physician to orient the data with its corresponding anatomical locations. Now, the CARTO^{TM} Merge and EnSite® Verismo modules provide tools for importing pre-operative patient data, segmenting heart geometry to create virtual models, and overlaying the models on the reconstructed cardiac map. This provides valuable information to the physician by allowing them to more easily associate the collected EP data with known anatomical locations.

The purpose of this work is to extend the current approaches in cardiac mapping to create a system that more accurately represents the collected information, allows physicians additional tools to interpret the data, and provides a more robust cardiac surgery platform to deliver therapy. We propose to do this by describing and evaluating a dynamic cardiac mapping system, using patient-specific cardiac models. This system extends the collection, analysis, and display of the spatially tracked CEGs into the temporal domain, while providing the ability for the data to be displayed directly on a patient-specific model created from pre-operative cardiac images. In addition, the cardiac mapping system is to be included in the our virtual-reality based cardiac surgery and therapy environment that supports integrated modular components [3,4], to provide a more robust platform for delivering cardiac care.

2   Method

The hardware components of our dynamic cardiac mapping system consist of a 3.0 GHz Pentium 4 computer workstation that serves as the central core. The workstation processes data from an Aurora magnetic tracking system (MTS) (Northern Digital Inc., Waterloo, Canada). The MTS sensors are rigidly attached to a standard electrode catheter for the purpose of tracking the location and orientation of the tip of the catheter. The electrode is connected to an analog-to-digital converter (ADC) (Data Translation, Marlboro, USA) for input to the workstation that also records the patient's digitized ECG signal. The workstation is based on running the Atamai Viewer software package, which is responsible for processing all the data. The Atamai Viewer cardiac surgery planning and therapy environment supports integrated module components including image viewing, volume rendering, ultrasound overlay, surgical tracking, as well as the dynamic EP cardiac mapping environment described in this work.

2.1 Pre-operative and Configuration

A dynamic structural cardiac scan (CT or MR) of the patient is taken in a pre-operative stage of the cardiac mapping procedure. This image is segmented to create a patient-specific dynamic cardiac model that will be used in our system as the geometric structure for displaying the cardiac map. The most simplistic approach to the segmentation is manually outlining the region(s) of interest in each image, and combining each outline to create a polygonal surface. More advanced software methods and programs for segmentation exist, examples in the cardiac mapping field are CARTO^{TM} Merge and EnSite® Verismo. For our system, we have used the method described by Wierzbicki et al. [5], which uses non-linear registration techniques to propagate a segmented surface from one cardiac phase to another in order to generate a dynamic cardiac model. The cardiac model is imported into the Atamai Viewer and the display is synchronized to the patient's heart rhythm using the ECG signal. Throughout the entire procedure the synchronization between the patient's heart pace and the model pace is constantly updated.

Following the synchronization of the display, a two-step procedure is completed to characterize the electrode catheter and the MTS. This step is necessary to transform the locations reported by the MTS relative to the field generator to locations relative to anatomical space. The first procedure is to find the transformation for the location of the sensor in respect to the catheter tip, and is achieved through a pivot calibration algorithm that finds a transformation to minimize the RMS distance between the sensor's location and a pivot point while posing the tracked catheter in different positions, keeping the tip on the pivot point. The second transformation is found to transform points from the MTS coordinate system to the cardiac model's coordinate system. Initially, this transformation is found through a landmark-based registration, to orient the coordinate systems and approximately align the cardiac model with the patient's heart. After the initial transformation is achieved, a fully automatic temporal based point registration as described previously [6], refines the alignment of the physical and virtual environments.

Once the patient-specific cardiac model is created, and the spatial locations reported by the MTS are transformed to represent known physical locations, the dynamic cardiac mapping system is prepared to collect data and create the cardiac map.

2.2 Data Collection

For each sampled location the system collects a dynamic set of spatial coordinates reported by the MTS, representing the locations at which the CEG is sampled. Associated with these locations are the CEG samples from the electrode catheter, which the system records through the ADC.

To sample a location the physician holds the catheter against the moving cardiac chamber wall, presses the acquisition button, and holds the catheter at the same location on the beating heart until the system indicates the acquisition is complete. From a systems point-of-view, once the acquisition is fired the system waits for the next R-wave trigger from the ECG signal, and begins to sample spatial locations and the CEG signal for an entire cardiac cycle. Temporal alignment occurs after data collection, as the timing of each device is derived from a single system clock, and the timestamps associated with each signal.

The data are stored within the system and are available to the physician to analyze in both time and frequency domains. In addition, to viewing the data in association with the patient-specific cardiac model, the data are grouped into separate point-cloud sets. The imported dynamic cardiac model has a finite number of surfaces that each represents a different phase of the cardiac model (10 surfaces). Through the time course of the collected data the values of the spatial coordinate and the CEG are extracted at each of these phases and inserted into a corresponding point cloud. The result of this procedure is 10 separate point cloud datasets where the location of each point is the physical location of the CEG along with the recorded value. Throughout the cardiac mapping procedure, additional locations are sampled over the myocardium and the point clouds become denser, leading to a more accurate cardiac map.

2.3 Surface Reconstruction and Interpolation

Once four or more locations have been collected the data may be constructed into a dynamic surface model. Similar to current cardiac mapping systems, this system allows users to reconstruct cardiac anatomy based on collected spatial locations. The points within a point cloud are connected using a Delaunay triangulation, and the resulting mesh is input into a geometry filter that extracts tetrahedral facets on the outer surface of the mesh, representing the geometry of the cardiac chamber. Data values from the CEG at each collected location are linearly interpreted onto the surface, and users are able the view the cardiac data as a color coded map, represented as either peak voltage or relative activation time.

The final step in the creation of a dynamic cardiac map is to interpolate the values from the raw data onto the patient-specific cardiac model. In the pre-operative stage the model was created from a dynamic CT or MR image, and registration between the physical and virtual environment was achieved with an automatic temporal based algorithm. Since the raw data and model are in the same coordinate system we can choose a radius of interpolation, Ri, which determines the distance around each raw data point that will receive an interpolated CEG value on the cardiac map. Once the areas to be interpolated are determined, the closest point on the patient-specific cardiac model to each point on the reconstructed raw dynamic cardiac map is calculated and assigned a value, completing the creation of the dynamic patient-specific cardiac model.

3 Experiments

Three separate experimental protocols were set up to evaluate the overall effectiveness of the dynamic cardiac mapping system. The experiments assessed the accuracy of locating a physical landmark, the accuracy of locating a landmark in image space, and the creation of a dynamic cardiac map in an in-vivo porcine experiment.

3.1 Physical Accuracy and Image Space Accuracy Experiments

Methodology. For the accuracy experiments we employed a realistic beating heart phantom (The Chamberlain Group, Great Barrington, MA, www.thecgroup.com) as the cardiac model. Five CT visible fiducial markers were fixed to the surface of the phantom, and a dynamic 10-phase CT image volume was acquired. These data were then used to create a dynamic cardiac surface model.

In both the physical and image space accuracy studies a dynamic experiment was conducted to represent our cardiac mapping environment, and a static experiment was performed to mimic current cardiac mapping system technology.

To measure physical and image space accuracy in the static environment, one phase of the cardiac model was imported into the system, and configured as described in the pre-operative stage above. To simulate a cardiac mapping procedure using the current technology, 20 locations were sampled around the epicardium of the phantom and an iterative closest point (ICP) registration was performed [7]. Seven users were asked to select the five fiducial markers using a tracked catheter while directly looking at the phantom for the physical accuracy study, and while looking only at the computer display (virtual environment) for the image space accuracy study. Each user repeated the physical study three times and the virtual study twice. The values were then compared with the ground truth, positions identified directly on the CT image.

Next, the cardiac mapping system was configured for dynamic mapping by importing all 10 phases of the cardiac model. The system was configured and 20 locations were sampled around the epicardium, however in this experiment the temporal based registration methods were used to align the coordinate systems of real space with image space. The same users were asked to repeat the same procedure as in the static environment. There were two key differences in this experiment; the system acquires multiple coordinates at each sampled location (corresponding to the movement of the cardiac wall throughout each phase), and in the virtual environment the users follow a dynamic target on the screen.

Results. The following errors are important in the evaluation of the systems. The fiducial localization error (FLE), measured as a RMS distance error, is defined by the NDI Aurora MTS system specifications as 0.9mm for translation and 0.8° for orientation. The target registration error (TRE) of the catheter tip was 1.54mm measured using the pivot calibration algorithm. These errors have a direct effect on the overall accuracy of the system.

The targeting accuracy was reported as the RMS distance from the recorded coordinates of the above experiments with the ground truth location of the given fiducial. Table 1 summarizes these errors for the dynamic and static mapping systems for each the physical and image space accuracies. Furthermore, a quantile-to-quantile (q-q) plot was created for each result set, comparing the quantiles of the error distribution against a normal distribution, with a linear result confirming a normal distribution of the errors.

Table 1. Accuracy measurements of the cardiac mapping system

Experiment	System	RMS Error
Physical Space Accuracy	Static	3.7 mm
	Dynamic	3.9 mm
Image Space Accuracy	Static	3.7 mm
	Dynamic	3.7 mm

Student's t-test analysis demonstrated no significant difference between the two cases in each experiment, and a one-way ANOVA test showed no significant differences between the performances of the various volunteers.

The results demonstrate that we are able to extend the current technology into a dynamic environment while maintaining the accuracy of locating landmarks. In context of catheter ablation therapy, these maintained accuracies are within our goal of 4mm, in order to create a fully connected isolation ring around an AF focal region using a standard 8mm ablation catheter in a clinical environment.

3.2 In-Vivo Porcine Experiment

Methodology. We evaluated this system clinically in an in-vivo porcine study. To create a gold standard comparison, a custom-made 63-electrode plaque (electrodes spaced at 4mm) was sutured on to the right atrium (RA) of a pig. The recordings from the electrode were input to a Prucka CardioLab EP System (GE Healthcare). Through this system, a 2D isochronal map of activation time can be created. Once the plaque was in place a quadripolar electrode was sutured on the RA superior to the plaque, and was used to pace the pig's heart at a rate of 1.9Hz.

The in-vivo experiment was conducted on the porcine heart exposed via a mini-thoracotomy as part of a separate porcine electrophysiology study. A CT-derived porcine dynamic heart model was imported in the Atamai Viewer software package, within which two dynamic cardiac maps were created. The first was a six-point dynamic isochronal cardiac activation map generated while

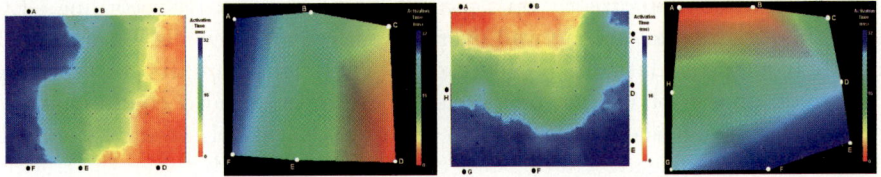

Fig. 1. Cardiac maps of the RA of a pig heart. From left to right: 63-point 2D isochronal map during pacing (Prucka System), 6-point 3D isochronal map during pacing (Dynamic System), 63-point 2D isochronal map during sinus rhythm (Prucka System), 8-point 3D isochronal map during sinus rhythm (Dynamic System).

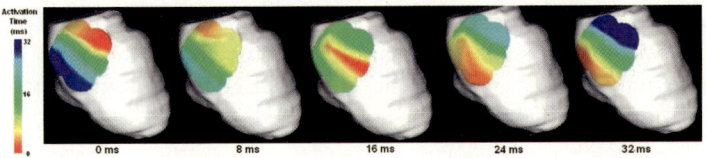

Fig. 2. Dynamic series of 6-point isochronal cardiac activation maps interpolated on a cardiac surface model created during pacing of the heart

pacing the heart, by sampling at each corner and one on either side at the middle of the plaque. The second was an eight-point map was created during sinus rhythm from sampling around the plaque (each corner and the middle of each edge).

Results. Figure 1 shows the cardiac maps created for each system during paced and sinus rhythm of the heart. On each pair of maps (paced/sinus for each system) the sampled location was marked to indicate overlapping portions of the map. All images are color coded, indicating reference activation time (red) to activation 32 ms later (blue).

From these images it can be seen that the activation patterns from the dynamic mapping system match well with those from the Prucka system. In the paced recording the activation is starting from the lower-right corner, where the quadripolar electrode was placed, and proceeding across the plaque area from right to left. During sinus rhythm the pacing initiates in the top-middle-left of the plaque area, where the sinoatrial (SA) node is closely located, and proceeds across the RA toward the bottom of the plaque area. These results demonstrate the system's ability to record CEG data in conjunction with their spatial location and reconstruct a meaningful dynamic cardiac map on a pre-operative CT model (Figure 2).

4 Conclusion

In this work we have introduced methods to extend the current cardiac mapping technologies to collect dynamic cardiac electrophysiology data and display the generated cardiac map directly on a patient-specific model. By recording CEGs and the motion of the cardiac wall over the entire cardiac cycle we are able to temporally align the data and create discrete point cloud datasets corresponding to different phases of the cardiac cycle. These datasets also correspond to a dynamic cardiac surface model that has been pre-operatively created from a 4D CT or MR image. The system registers coordinate systems between the tracking system and the imaging space, allowing users the ability to interpret the data onto the patient-specific model.

We have shown the ability to extend current cardiac mapping techniques to the dynamic patient-specific system without losing accuracy of locating physical landmarks or the ability to navigate using a dynamic virtual environment. In the in-vivo study we demonstrated that the system is able to collect and temporally align data to reproduce cardiac maps created using a commercial EP system. However, the system extends the usability of current technologies by allowing physicians to more freely analyze the entire CEG in context to the patient's anatomy throughout different phases of the cardiac cycle.

References

1. Go, A.S., Hylek, E.M., Phillips, K.A., Chang, Y., Henault, L.E., Selby, J.V., Singer, D.E.: Prevalence of diagnosed atrial fibrillation in adults: national implications for rhythm management and stroke prevention: the AnTicoagulation and Risk Factors in Atrial Fibrillation (ATRIA) Study. JAMA 285(18), 2370–2375 (2001)
2. Efimov, I.R., Fedorov, V.V.: Chessboard of atrial fibrillation: reentry or focus? Single or multiple source(s)? Neurogenic or myogenic? American Journal of Phyiology - Heart and Circulatory Physiology 289, H977–H979 (2005)
3. Moore, J., Guiraudon, G., Jones, D., Hill, N., Wiles, A., Bainbridge, D., Wedlake, C., Peters, T.: 2D ultrasound augmented by virtual tools for guidance of interventional procedures. Health Technology and Informatics 125, 322–327 (2007)
4. Linte, C.A., Wiles, A.D., Moore, J., Wedlake, C., Peters, T.M.: Virtual reality-enhanced ultrasound guidance for atrial ablation: In vitro epicardial study. In: Metaxas, D., et al. (eds.) MICCAI 2008, Part II. LNCS, vol. 5242, pp. 644–651. Springer, Heidelberg (2008)
5. Wierzbicki, M., Drangova, M., Guiraudon, G., Peters, T.: Validation of dynamic heart models obtained using non-linear registration for virtual reality training, planning, and guidance of minimally invasive cardiac surgeries. Medical Image Analysis 8(3), 387–401 (2004)
6. Wilson, K., Guiraudon, G., Jones, D., Peters, T.M.: 4D shape registration for dynamic electrophysiological cardiac mapping. In: Larsen, R., Nielsen, M., Sporring, J. (eds.) MICCAI 2006. LNCS, vol. 4191, pp. 520–527. Springer, Heidelberg (2006)
7. Besl, P.J., McKay, N.D.: A method for registration of 3-D shapes. IEEE Transactions on Pattern Analysis and Machine Intelligence 14(2), 239–256 (1992)

Detection of DTI White Matter Abnormalities in Multiple Sclerosis Patients

Olivier Commowick[1], Pierre Fillard[2], Olivier Clatz[2], and Simon K. Warfield[1]

[1] Computational Radiology Laboratory, Department of Radiology,
Children's Hospital, 300 Longwood Avenue, Boston, MA, 02115, USA
Olivier.Commowick@childrens.harvard.edu
[2] INRIA Sophia Antipolis - Asclepios Team, 2004 Rte des Lucioles BP 93
06902 Sophia Antipolis Cedex, France

Abstract. The emergence of new modalities such as Diffusion Tensor Imaging (DTI) is of great interest for the characterization and the temporal study of Multiple Sclerosis (MS). DTI indeed gives information on water diffusion within tissues and could therefore reveal alterations in white matter fibers before being visible in conventional MRI. However, recent studies generally rely on scalar measures derived from the tensors such as FA or MD instead of using the full tensor itself. Therefore, a certain amount of information is left unused.

In this article, we present a framework to study the benefits of using the whole diffusion tensor information to detect statistically significant differences between each individual MS patient and a database of control subjects. This framework, based on the comparison of the MS patient DTI and a mean DTI atlas built from the control subjects, allows us to look for differences both in normally appearing white matter but also in and around the lesions of each patient. We present a study on a database of 11 MS patients, showing the ability of the DTI to detect not only significant differences on the lesions but also in regions around them, enabling an early detection of an extension of the MS disease.

1 Introduction

Multiple sclerosis (MS) causes a demyelination of the white matter fibers. The origin and evolution of this disease are still not well understood, and numerous studies have been conducted to evaluate its evolution and its influence on neighboring brain structures. To this end, several methods have been proposed, mainly using conventional MR modalities like T1, FLAIR or T2 images to delineate lesions as in [1]. This task is challenging and crucial, as having access to the lesion load over time, coupled with measurements such as local brain atrophy, can bring a lot of information on the characterization of the disease.

The emergence of new modalities, and in particular diffusion tensor imaging (DTI) [2], is of great interest in MS. DTI gives information about water diffusion within tissues, and could therefore reveal alterations in normal appearing white matter fibers before being visible in conventional MRI. For this purpose,

Filippi *et al.* [3] evaluated the differences in fractional anisotropy (FA) between MS patients and controls on normal appearing white matter regions. While this type of studies tend to show that diffusion MRI could be beneficial to detect more accurately MS lesions, they generally rely on scalar measures derived from the tensor such as FA or mean diffusivity, instead of using the full tensor itself. A certain amount of information is thus lost in the processing of this data. In parallel, other studies have shown the interest of using the whole tensor information. For example, [4] showed that it was possible to compare diffusion tensors of two populations using Log-Euclidean (LE) metrics [5], and that the comparison was more sensitive, i.e. could reveal more differences, than considering only a scalar parameter such as the FA.

In this work, we propose a framework that relies on the whole diffusion tensor information to detect statistically significant differences between MS patients and controls. Recent work proposed methods for the detection of group differences between two tensor populations such as [4] on diffusion tensors, or [6] on Jacobian tensors derived from deformation fields. However, in our context, these methods are not directly applicable as lesions are not spatially consistent. Consequently, it is necessary to compare each patient individually with the group of control subjects. This approach also raises the question of the construction of an unbiased reference frame from the controls.

To address those problems, we propose a framework to compute an unbiased atlas of diffusion tensors from a database of controls. Based on this atlas, we show how to compute statistical differences between a patient and the atlas using a z-score derived from the whole tensor.

This framework was evaluated on a database of 11 MS patients and 31 normal controls, showing significant differences between each individual patient and the controls in regions identified as lesions on the T1 and FLAIR images. Interestingly, our results shows that DTI can remain sensitive inside a thick ribbon surrounding the lesions, suggesting that DTI could be more sensitive than conventional MRI to detect MS lesions.

2 Materials and Methods

2.1 Construction of a Diffusion Tensor Atlas of Controls

In order to compare the DTI of normal controls with the patient DTI, we need to bring all the DTI into the same reference frame. Using any subject as a reference would introduce a bias due to the specific anatomy of this reference image. Therefore, we chose to build a geometrically unbiased atlas from the dataset of controls extending the work of [7], and use this atlas as the reference for the rest of the study.

Our algorithm basically iterates over two steps until convergence (in our application the average image was built in 6 iterations). In a first step, all images I_k are non linearly registered onto an initial (randomly chosen) reference image R, using a block-matching based non linear registration method presented in [8]. These registrations produce the deformation fields T_k. A mean image M is built from all registered images by averaging them. In a second step, the deformation fields T_k are averaged to get a mean transformation $\overline{T}$, which inverse is applied to M. This new mean image is then used as the new reference image for the next iteration, i.e. $R = M \circ \overline{T}^{-1}$. Notice that we used the Log-Euclidean framework for diffeomorphisms [9] when averaging deformation fields to ensure the invertibility of $\overline{T}$. Transformations are calculated based on T1 images and then applied on DTIs, the main reason being that DTI registration is still not a mature research topic.

When warping diffusion tensor images, special attention must be paid to the reorientation of tensors. Indeed, tensors are supposed to remain aligned with underlying tissues under any transform. We chose the finite strain reorientation strategy proposed in [10] to reorient the tensors with respect to the Jacobian of the deformation. Note that the principal direction of diffusion preserving method [11] could be used as well. Tensors are resampled and averaged using Log-Euclidean metrics as they provide a fast way to extend any interpolation method to tensors while preserving the positive-definite constraint, and without suffering from the swelling effect as this is the case of the Euclidean calculus.

In summary, a set of transformations T_k is obtained for each T1 image I_k along with a mean T1 image $\bar{I}$. Each T_k is applied to its corresponding DTI. The DTI atlas is finally generated by averaging these images.

2.2 Evaluation of Statistical Differences between Atlas and Patient

In statistics, differences between a test data and a population are estimated through the Mahalanobis distance, also abusively called z-score in this article by analogy to the univariate z-test. This distance requires to know the covariance matrix of the population (of tensors in our case). We propose to detail its computation in a first step, and show in a second step how to extract a p-value from it to test for significance.

Covariance Matrix and z-Score. The covariance matrix is computed as follows. Tensor logarithms are turned into vectors by keeping only the 6 independent coefficients and multiplying off-diagonal elements by $\sqrt{2}$, so that the L_2 norm of tensors is compatible with the L_2 norm of vectors. We call this operation the Vec mapping. Then, the covariance matrix C of this 6-dimensional vector is calculated. Finally, the Mahalanobis distance between a tested tensor $\tilde{D}$ and the ensemble mean/covariance matrix of the atlas is given by:

$$z(\tilde{D}) = \left(\tilde{D}_{Log} - \bar{D}_{Log}\right)^T C^{-1} \left(\tilde{D}_{Log} - \bar{D}_{Log}\right)$$

where $\tilde{D}_{Log}$ and $\bar{D}_{Log}$ are the Vec mappings of the tensor logarithms, i.e. $\tilde{D}_{Log} = Vec\left(\log(\tilde{D})\right)$.

Computing the p-Value Associated to the z-Score. In our case, the null hypothesis is that the diffusion tensor being tested belongs to the normal population. As in the scalar case, the p-value is given by $P(X > I_c(z))$, where $I_c(z)$ is defined as the points x where $r \equiv (x - \bar{D}_{Log})^\top C^{-1}(x - \bar{D}_{Log}) = z^2$. In our specific context, the probability density function to be integrated is a 6D multivariate Gaussian, leading to the following formulation:

$$V(z) = 1 - P(X < I_c(z)) = 1 - \int_{r<z^2} G_{\bar{D}_{Log},C}(x) dx \qquad (1)$$

where G is a multivariate Gaussian of mean $\bar{D}_{Log}$ and covariance matrix C. It can be shown that this integration is equivalent to the integration of a multivariate Gaussian of mean 0 and covariance Id for values of x such as $x^\top x < z^2$. Using this simplification and a change of coordinates to spherical coordinates, we obtain the following expression for the p-value:

$$V(z) = e^{-\frac{z^2}{2}} \left(1 + \frac{z^2}{2} + \frac{z^4}{8}\right) \qquad (2)$$

Following the usual practice in voxel-based morphometry, average p-values are computed over spatially coherent regions of interest R (for instance MS lesions). To this end, we have chosen to compute first a mean z-score over the voxels i in region R and use it to compute the p-value, i.e. $\bar{V}_R = V(\frac{1}{N} \sum_{i \in R} z(\tilde{D}_i))$.

3 Results

3.1 Image Databases

Data. For this study, we used a dataset of 31 controls and 11 patients diagnosed with MS. For each control, a T1 image and a DTI were acquired. T1 images have a resolution of $256 \times 256 \times 176$ and a voxel size of $1 \times 1 \times 1$ mm^3. DTI images were acquired with 12 gradients and have a resolution of $256 \times 256 \times 60$ and a voxel size of $1 \times 1 \times 2.5$ mm^3.

For each patient, a T1 image (resolution $124 \times 256 \times 256$, voxel size $1.3 \times 1 \times 1$ mm^3) and a DTI (12 gradients, resolution $256 \times 256 \times 60$, voxel size $1 \times 1 \times 2.5$ mm^3) were also available, as well as T2 and FLAIR images.

Pre-Processing. For each control and each patient, the image sequence (DTI, FLAIR, T2) was rigidly registered onto the T1 image. For the DTI, the B0 image was rigidly registered on the T1 image, and the obtained transform was applied to the diffusion gradients. To correct for acquisition distortion in DTI, we applied a non rigid registration procedure between the B0 of the DTI acquisition and the T1 image using the B-Splines method of [12] with few control points ($5 \times 5 \times 5$). B0 to T1 registration results were visually validated by a radiologist. T1 and FLAIR images were finally used to manually delineate the MS lesions on each patient.

For each MS patient, non linear registration of the T1 image onto the atlas was done. Patient to atlas registration consists in two steps. First, a global affine transformation was computed between the T1 images. Then, non linear registration was performed to locally align the anatomies of the atlas and the patient. As intensities in voxels with lesions are different from those of the atlas,

Detection of DTI White Matter Abnormalities in Multiple Sclerosis Patients 979

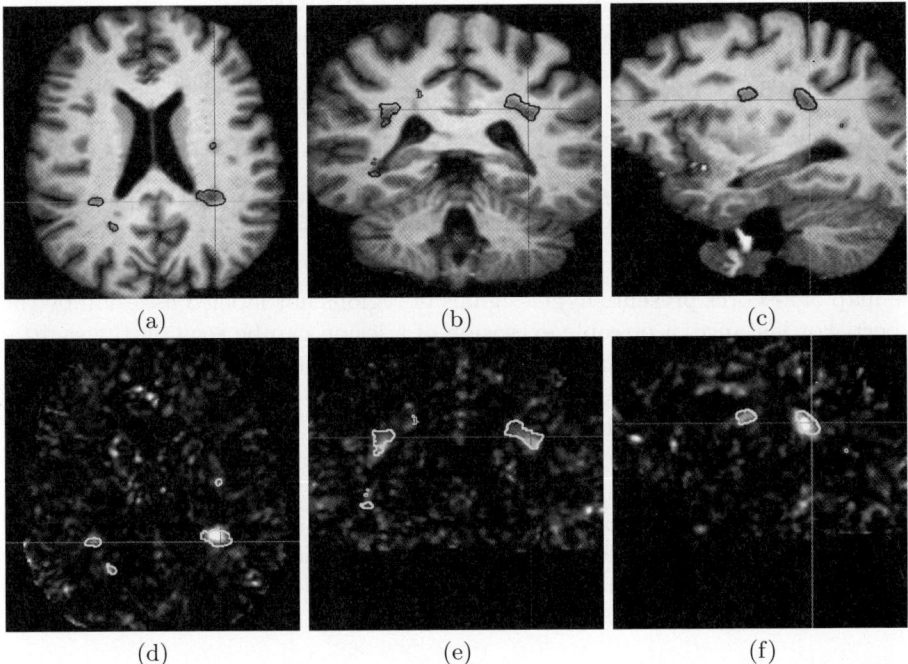

Fig. 1. Voxel-wise z-scores for a given MS patient. Illustration of the z-score maps obtained for a patient (images (d), (e), (f)) compared to the corresponding anatomy (axial (a),(d), coronal (b),(e) and sagittal slices (c),(f)). The contours correspond to the manual delineations of the MS lesions.

the transformation was interpolated inside a dilated mask of the patient's lesions following a method similar to [13]. Thus, abnormalities in lesions signal did not interfere during the registration process. The final transformations were then applied to the patient DTI as presented in Sec. 2.1. Finally, voxel-wise z-score and p-value calculation were done to obtain a map of statistical differences. Results are presented in the next section.

3.2 Diffusion Tensor Differences in MS Lesions

The initial evaluation consisted in looking at differences between patients and controls in the lesion regions. We present in Fig. 1 the maps of z-scores, with the manual delineations of the lesions superimposed, for one patient of the database.

This figure shows that MRI regions with visible lesions have the highest z-scores. This indicates that the diffusion tensor is affected by MS and that lesions are highly likely to be significantly different with respect to an atlas of controls. We can also see on this figure (particularly on the sagittal slice) that, for some lesions, the manual delineation does not correspond exactly to the high z-score values. This is mainly caused by local errors in manual delineation, as shown in the sagittal view of Fig. 1 (c) at the position of the axes. More interestingly,

Table 1. Quantitative evaluation results on the MS lesions. Mean p-values obtained on regions corresponding to the MS lesions for each patient.

Patient #	p-value	Patient #	p-value	Patient #	p-value
1	2.1×10^{-18}	5	4.2×10^{-7}	9	8.7×10^{-4}
2	7.9×10^{-5}	6	7.5×10^{-5}	10	6.8×10^{-4}
3	0.045	7	3.4×10^{-4}	11	4.2×10^{-7}
4	4.9×10^{-4}	8	1.8×10^{-7}		

the map of z-scores presents hyper-signals in regions not labeled as lesion by the expert. For instance, a possible extension of a lesion can be seen on the sagittal slice. There are indeed high z-score values around the large lesion on the right of this view that are not seen in the T1 image.

To verify and quantify the DTI signal difference between the patients and the control subjects, we computed the mean tensor-based p-value inside the manually delineated lesions. Results are presented in Table 1.

All p-values are below the critical value of 0.05, therefore rejecting for all patients the null hypothesis: tensors in lesions are not likely to belong to the normal variability represented by the atlas of controls. Interestingly, patient 3 is closer to 0.05 than the other patients.

3.3 Evaluation of Tensor Differences Around Lesions

The previous section has shown the existence of significant tensor-based differences between patients and controls inside the lesions. To go beyond this sensitivity analysis, we looked at surrounding regions to check whether regions around the lesions exhibit large z-score values.

These ring-like regions around the lesions were obtained by subtracting the binary mask of the manually segmented lesions to its dilation. P-values were then computed withing those regions surrounding the lesions. These results are presented in Table 2.

Results show, for 7 patients out of 11, a p-value that is below the threshold of 0.05. Remaining p-values are also very low (the maximum value being 0.101). This may suggest that some patients exhibit an extension of the lesions that is not visible in conventional MRI, but is detectable in DTI using higher order statistical analysis. These results tend to prove that DTI may effectively be used

Table 2. Quantitative evaluation results on regions around the MS lesions. Mean p-values obtained on regions around the MS lesions for each patient (see text).

Patient #	p-value	Patient #	p-value	Patient #	p-value
1	8.1×10^{-7}	5	0.009	9	1.9×10^{-3}
2	0.059	6	1.8×10^{-3}	10	0.028
3	0.101	7	0.079	11	0.019
4	0.066	8	0.016		

as a complementary diagnostic imaging modality to study and understand the evolution of MS.

4 Conclusion

We have presented in this article a new framework for the detection of significant differences between DTI of patients and normal controls. This framework was applied to the study of multiple sclerosis and highlighted the great interest of DTI measurements made on the whole tensor for a better understanding and characterization of the disease. Results indeed indicated, qualitatively and quantitatively, that diffusion tensors were not only significantly different inside the lesion regions, but also for some patients in regions around the lesions. This suggests the existence of an extension of the disease invisible in conventional MRI, but revealed by DTI.

This comparison framework is however dependent on the choice of the registration method to build and register the statistical atlas. This choice may indeed bias the p-values results. The comparison of different registration methods will therefore be interesting to quantify this dependency. This evaluation will also include the use of registration methods taking into account the specificities of the DTI such as [14], allowing to register more precisely regions such as the white matter, which has a uniform intensity in conventional MRI.

Another way to cope with this bias and possible preprocessing errors is the study of robust analysis methods, including more information on the local neighborhood of the tensors. An interesting solution could be the use of the STAPLE method [15] on each of the tensors components, allowing to compute at the same time a robust mean tensor image and error parameters of the patient tensors.

This work also opens wide and important perspectives for the understanding of multiple sclerosis. One of them will be the temporal study of the evolution of the lesions and the comparison of the invisible extents found through DTI with the real evolution of the disease. This will allow us to see if these extents effectively evolve into lesions or if they are more related to a local edema. This framework will also be used for the evaluation of the influence of the disease on normal appearing white matter regions such as the corticospinal tracts.

In the future, we would also like to perform a quantitative comparison of all available imaging modalities to independently detect and quantify the lesion volume in the brain. Finally, as an extension to the present work, it will be interesting to propose a multi modal statistical framework to compute statistics on multivariate data (i.e. DTI, FLAIR, T1, T2) of higher dimensions. Indeed, this statistical study will also allow to do a sensitivity analysis of the contribution of each modality in the final detection performance.

Acknowledgments

This investigation was supported in part by a research grant from CIMIT, grant RG 3478A2/2 from the NMSS, and by NIH grants R03 CA126466, R01 RR021885, R01 GM074068 and R01 EB008015.

References

1. Ge, Y.: Multiple sclerosis: The role of MR imaging. American Journal of Neuroradiology 27, 1165–1176 (2006)
2. Basser, P., Mattiello, J., Bihan, D.L.: MR diffusion tensor spectroscopy and imaging. Biophysical Journal 66, 259–267 (1994)
3. Filippi, M., Cercignani, M., Inglese, M., Comi, M.H.G.: Diffusion tensor magnetic resonance imaging in multiple sclerosis. Neurology 56, 304–311 (2001)
4. Whitcher, B., Wisco, J.J., Hadjikhani, N., Tuch, D.S.: Statistical group comparison of diffusion tensors via multivariate hypothesis testing. Magnetic Resonance in Medicine (57), 1065–1074 (2007)
5. Arsigny, V., Fillard, P., Pennec, X., Ayache, N.: Log-Euclidean metrics for fast and simple calculus on diffusion tensors. Magnetic Resonance in Medicine 56(2), 411–421 (2006)
6. Lepore, N., Brun, C.A., Chiang, M.C., Chou, Y.Y., Lopez, O.L., Aizenstein, H.J., Toga, A.W., Becker, J.T., Thompson, P.M.: Multivariate statistics of the jacobian matrices in tensor based morphometry and their application to HIV/AIDS. In: Larsen, R., Nielsen, M., Sporring, J. (eds.) MICCAI 2006. LNCS, vol. 4190, pp. 191–198. Springer, Heidelberg (2006)
7. Guimond, A., Meunier, J., Thirion, J.P.: Average brain models: A convergence study. Computer Vision and Image Understanding 77(2), 192–210 (2000)
8. Commowick, O., Malandain, G.: Evaluation of atlas construction strategies in the context of radiotherapy planning. In: Proc. of the SA2PM Workshop, Copenhagen. Held in conjunction with MICCAI 2006 (October 2006)
9. Arsigny, V., Commowick, O., Pennec, X., Ayache, N.: A Log-Euclidean framework for statistics on diffeomorphisms. In: Larsen, R., Nielsen, M., Sporring, J. (eds.) MICCAI 2006. LNCS, vol. 4190, pp. 924–931. Springer, Heidelberg (2006)
10. Ruiz-Alzola, J., Westin, C.F., Warfield, S.K., Alberola, C., Maier, S., Kikinis, R.: Nonrigid registration of 3D tensor medical data. MedIA 6(2), 143–161 (2002)
11. Alexander, D., Pierpaoli, C., Basser, P., Gee, J.: Spatial transformations of diffusion tensor magnetic resonance images. IEE TMI 20(11), 1131–1139 (2001)
12. Rueckert, D., Sonoda, L.L., Hayes, C., Hill, D.L.G., Leach, M.O., Hawkes, D.J.: Nonrigid registration using free-form deformations: Application to breast MR images. IEEE Transactions on Medical Imaging 18(8), 712–721 (1999)
13. Stefanescu, R., Commowick, O., Malandain, G., Bondiau, P.Y., Ayache, N., Pennec, X.: Non-rigid atlas to subject registration with pathologies for conformal brain radiotherapy. In: Barillot, C., Haynor, D.R., Hellier, P. (eds.) MICCAI 2004. LNCS, vol. 3216, pp. 704–711. Springer, Heidelberg (2004)
14. Goodlett, C., Davis, B., Jean, R., Gilmore, J.H., Gerig, G.: Improved correspondence for DTI population studies via unbiased atlas building. In: Larsen, R., Nielsen, M., Sporring, J. (eds.) MICCAI 2006. LNCS, vol. 4191, pp. 260–267. Springer, Heidelberg (2006)
15. Warfield, S.K., Zou, K.H., Wells, W.M.: Validation of image segmentation by estimating rater bias and variance. In: Larsen, R., Nielsen, M., Sporring, J. (eds.) MICCAI 2006. LNCS, vol. 4191, pp. 839–847. Springer, Heidelberg (2006)

Automatic Mitral Valve Inflow Measurements from Doppler Echocardiography

JinHyeong Park[1], S. Kevin Zhou[1], John Jackson[2], and Dorin Comaniciu[1]

[1] Integrated Data Systems, Siemens Corporate Research, Inc., Princeton, NJ, USA
{jin-hyeong.park,shaohua.zhou,dorin.comaniciu}@siemens.com
[2] Ultrasound Division, Siemens Medical Solution, Mountain View, CA, USA
jacksonjohn@siemens.com

Abstract. Doppler echocardiography is widely used for functional assessment of heart valves such as mitral valve. In current clinical work flow, to extract Doppler measurements, the envelopes of acquired Doppler spectra are manually traced. We propose a robust algorithm for automatically tracing the envelopes of mitral valve inflow Doppler spectra, which exhibit a large amount of variations in envelope shape and image appearance due to various disease conditions, patient/sonographer/instrument differences, etc. The algorithm is learning-based and capable of fully automatic detection and segmentation of the mitral inflow structures. Experiments show that the algorithm, running within one second, yields comparable performance to experts.

1 Introduction

Doppler echocardiography is widely used in clinical practices to assess the heart valve functionality as it records the blood velocity [1][2]. The current work flow of Doppler analysis requires manual tracing the envelopes of acquired Doppler spectra, based on which clinically relevant measurements are computed. The manual tracing is a main bottle-neck of the work flow. In the paper, we aim to propose an automatic algorithm for tracing the envelopes of the Doppler spectra belonging to mitral valve inflow (MI) only.

The MI patterns and measurements have been studied extensively as indices of left ventricular diastolic function [2]. Fig. 1 displays a few sample images of MI spectra with the expert envelopes overlaid to illustrate the challenges we confront. The MI pattern, occurring in the ventricular diastole phase, typically consists of an "early" wave (E-wave) and an "atrial" wave (A-wave). For normal hearts, the E- and A-waves do not overlap each other and the E-wave is higher than the A-wave. But for disease hearts, the following can occur: the E- and A-waves sometimes overlap depending on heart diseases; the E-wave is lower than or of the same height as the A-wave; only the E-wave is present with no A-wave. The above factors contribute significant variation in the envelope shape. In terms of image appearance, the variation is large too due to signal aliasing, difference in imaging setting, etc.

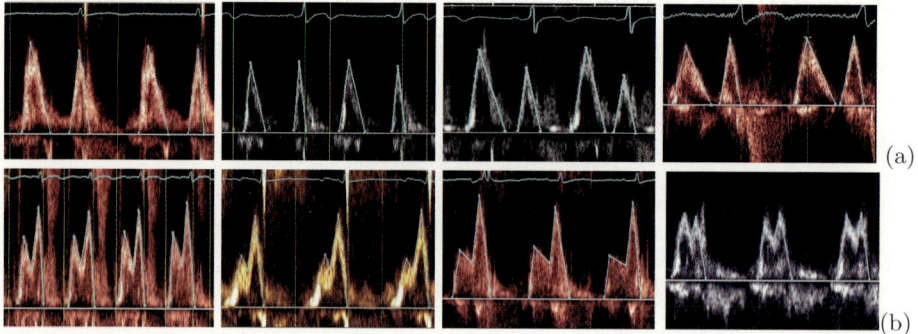

Fig. 1. Examples of MI Doppler spectra. (a) Isolated triangles. (b) Overlapping triangles.

There are a few previous approaches that address the automatic tracing of Doppler spectra envelopes. In [3][4], image processing/filtering techniques such as low-pass filtering, thresholding and edge detection are used. They, however, do not guarantee robustness in the presence of severe images artifacts. Recently a learning-based method, the so-called *PHD* framework [5], was proposed for detection and segmentation of deformable anatomic structures in medical images. This method was successfully applied for automatically tracing the envelopes of three Doppler flow types including MI. In [5], a triangle representation was used to model the MI envelope. This representation has inherent difficulty when dealing with severely overlapping E- and A-waves, rendering the missing triangle roots, which are often seen in the spectra of diseased hearts.

We propose a robust algorithm for automatically tracing the envelopes of mitral valve inflow Doppler spectra. The proposed algorithm builds upon the techniques used in the *PHD* framework [5]. However, unlike [5], it explicitly handles the overlapping E- and A-waves by separate detection and segmentation of non-overlapping E/A-wave and overlapping E/A-waves. The non-overlapping case is formulated as a problem of single triangle detection/segmentation, which means that the E- and A-waves are treated as the same object with a triangle shape. For the overlapping case, we detect and segment a pair of overlapping E- and A-waves. In addition, we introduce several novel components: direct shape inference from image appearance for the overlapping structures, shape score computation based on image gradient, information fusion for robust decision making, etc.

2 Automatic Computation of MI Measurements

To achieve automatic detection and segmentation of target deformable objects, the proposed algorithm first employs a series of detectors to anchor the location of the objects and then utilizes the shape information to segment the deformable object. Fig. 2 gives the schematic overview of the algorithm.

A single triangle object represents an isolated E-wave or A-wave, and a double triangle object represents a pair of overlapping E- and A-waves. A single triangle

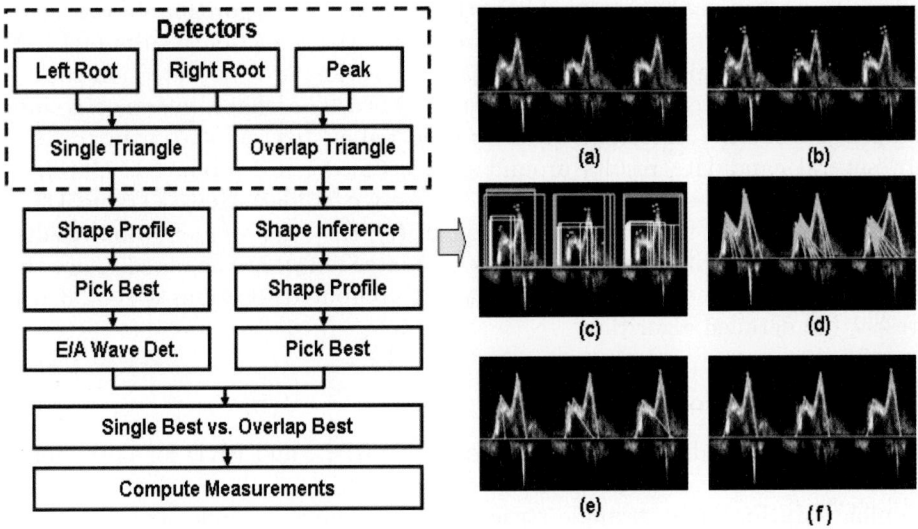

Fig. 2. Algorithm overview. (a) input image, (b) results of 1st layer detectors, (c) results of 2nd layer detectors, (d) results of shape inference, (e) Best candidates of single triangle and overlapped triangles, and (f) Final segmentation results.

model consists of three points: a left root, a right root and a peak; a double triangle model has five points: a left root, a right root, a left peak, a right peak, and an intersection point. Base on the observation that both single and double triangle objects share left root, right root, and peak(s), we train three part detectors: left root detector (LRD), right root detector (RRD), and peak detector (PKD). Note that the double triangle object has two peaks but we pool them together during training. We also train two global box detectors: a single triangle detector (STD) and a double triangle detector (DTD). These detectors are organized in a hierarchical manner to efficiently prune the search space down to a set of most promising candidates for both single triangle and double triangle objects. Each candidate is associated with a posterior detection probability $P_D(\Theta|I)$, where Θ is object parameter and the I denotes the image input. Refer to Section 2.1 and [5] for more detail about how they are organized and collaborated.

Once a candidate box for a single triangle is identified, the triangle shape is fully specified. But, this is not the case for a double triangle candidate box as the intersection point of the two overlapping triangles is unknown. We therefore insert a shape inference model for the double triangle object. For each shape candidate, either specified or inferred, the shape profile model is invoked to score it with a posterior probability $P_S(\Phi|I)$, where Φ is the shape model. Section 2.2 addresses how to compute $P_S(\Phi|I)$.

Based on the probabilities $P_D(\Theta|I)$ and $P_S(\Phi|I)$, the algorithm selects the best candidates from the single triangle candidate pool and the best double triangle candidate. Then we compare them to determine the final result.

Fig. 2(a-f) depicts the results of important steps in the algorithm. In Fig. 2(b), yellow dots, red dots, and green dots represent the detection results of LRD, RRD and PKD respectively. In (c), the white boxes are the detection results of STD and the green boxes are those of DTD. The shape inference results computed from the detection boxes are plotted in (d). As shown in (c) and (d), several candidate results around each structure are produced. In (e), it shows the results the algorithm selects the best candidates for STD and DTD independently from their candidate pool. In (f), the final segmentation results, obtained by comparing the better best candidates in (e), are depicted. Once the segmentation is done, measurements can be computed. Sections 2.1 - 2.3 will present the detailed algorithm.

2.1 The Detection Probability

As earlier mentioned, we train one set of LRD, RRD, and PKD for both single triangle and double triangle structures. For box detector, we collect separate training data for single triangle structures and double triangle structures and train the STD and DTD. We treat the detection problem as a two-class classification problem (positive vs. negative) and follow the probabilistic boosting network implementation [6] for testing efficiency. Each detection carries a detection probability. For example, the LRD outputs the posterior probability of being the left root object O_{LR} given an input image I and a hypothesized location θ_{LR}, which is denoted by $P(O_{LR}|I,\theta_{LR})$.

All the above detectors are organized into a two-layer hierarchy. The first layer consists of LRD, RRD, and PKD, which outputs independent candidates of the left root, right root, and peak. Note that in [5], there are no LRD, RRD trained for the MI type. Using LRD and RRD, we significantly speed up the processing time as they are simple and with light computation yet effectively prune the search space.

The second layer consists of STD and DTD. The STD further verifies if a particular combination of a left root, a right root and a peak point from the candidates form a valid E-wave or A-wave. If the combination passes the STD, the two root points and the peak point form a trace of a triangle envelope and no further segmentation process is needed. On the other hand, the DTD verifies if a combination of a left root, a right root and two peak points that lie in between the left and right roots forms a valid pattern. Even if the pattern is valid, however, we only have four points with the intersection point of E-wave deceleration line and the A-wave acceleration line missing. We need to estimate its location, which will be discussed in the next section.

A target object O parameterized by Θ consists of M parts $O = \{O_1, O_2, ..., O_M\}$ with part O_i parameterized by θ_i. In our case, we define two target objects: (i) a single triangle object with a left root (LR), a right root (RR) and a peak point (PK), i.e., $O_{ST} = \{O_{LR}, O_{RR}, O_{PK}\}$ and $\Theta_{ST} = \{\theta_{LR}, \theta_{RR}, \theta_{PK}\}$, and (ii) a double triangle object with a LR, a RR, an E-wave peak point (EPK), and an A-wave peak point (APK), i.e., $O_{DT} = \{O_{LR}, O_{RR}, O_{EPK}, O_{APK}\}$ and $\Theta_{DT} = \{\theta_{LR}, \theta_{RR}, \theta_{EPK}, \theta_{APK}\}$.

The *PHD* framework assumes conditional independence among the parts and the global structure. For the single triangle object, it evaluates the object detection probability as

$$P_D(\Theta_{ST}|I) \equiv \prod_{a \in A} P(O_a|I, \theta_a) \, P(O_{ST}|I, \Theta_{ST}), \tag{1}$$

where $A = \{LR, RR, PK\}$. A similar detection probability $P_D(\Theta_{DT}|I)$ can be define for the double triangle object. The conditional independence assumption brings computational advantage: If one of the classifiers fails, the overall detection fails.

2.2 The Shape Probability

For the double triangle structure, we need to estimate the missing intersection point of E-wave deceleration line and the A-wave acceleration line. To this end, we employed the shape inference algorithm proposed in [7].

Given training images and their corresponding shapes, we attempt to learns a nonparametric regression function that gives a mapping from an image to its shape. The training of shape inference model conducts a feature selection process. Each image is represented by an over-complete set of features. The training data are first clustered in the shape space into several clusters. The algorithm then selects a small set of features from the huge feature pool based on a forward feature framework by maximizing the Fisher separation criterion of the clusters. After training, a training image I_j, whose shape is Φ_j, is represented by a feature vector f_j. Given a query image I, we first compute its corresponding feature vector f, then invoke the nonparametric regression function to infer the shape s:

$$\Phi = \frac{\sum_j \Phi_j \, k(f_j, f)}{\sum_j k(f_j, f)}, \tag{2}$$

where k is a kernel function.

To define the shape probability $P(\Phi|I)$, we use the image evidence along the shape. Suppose that the trace of the envelope has N discrete points, $\{s_i = (x_i, y_i)\}_{i=1}^N$, distributed with equal distance along the trace. For each point s_i, we compute a shape profile score ψ_i based on the intensity gradients along the trace of the envelope. Let line l_i be perpendicular to the tangent of a point s_i. We denote points on the line l_i by $\{s_{ij} = (x_{ij}, y_{ij})\}_{j=i-\Delta}^{i+\Delta}$, where $\Delta > 0$ and $s_i = s_{ii}$, and assume that $\{s_{ij} = (x_{ij}, y_{ij})\}_{j=i-1}^{i-\Delta}$ corresponds to the outside of the contour and $\{s_{ij} = (x_{ij}, y_{ij})\}_{j=i+1}^{i+\Delta}$ the inside. Then, i^{th} shape profile score is defined as follow:

$$\psi_i = \sum_{j=i}^{i+\Delta} I(s_{ij}) - \sum_{i-\Delta}^{j=i} I(s_{ij}), \tag{3}$$

where $I(s_{ij})$ represents a pixel intensity at the location of s_{ij}. The shape probability, $P_S(\Phi|I)$ is then defined using a Sigmoid function:

$$P_S(\Phi|I) \equiv [1 + \exp(-\gamma \sum_i \psi_i)]^{-1}, \tag{4}$$

where $\gamma > 0$ is a pre-specified constant.

By integrating both the detection posterior probability $P_D(\Theta|I)$ and shape posterior probability $P_S(\Phi|I)$, we select the best candidates of single triangle and double triangle per each heart cycle among a cluster of detection results. Again we assume that the detectors and shape profiles are independent of each other, which is reasonable because they are two heterogeneous models, we obtain the fused probability as

$$P(\Theta, \Phi|I) = P_D(\Theta|I)P_S(\Phi|I), \qquad (5)$$

Finally we select the best candidates that locally maximizes the fused probability.

2.3 Measurement Computation

For the single triangle model, after selecting one best candidates from the cloud of candidates around a structure, we need to determine whether it is E-wave or A-wave in order to compute the necessary measurements. We rely on the given End of Systole (ES) and End of Diastole (ED) lines: the E-wave appears first and the A-wave follows in the diastole period.

For final decision to take the best solution from the single triangle model or that from the double triangle model, we only rely on the shape probability because the detection probabilities from the two models are heterogeneous.

Four MI measurements [1][2] are computed: E-Wave Peak Velocity (EPV), E-Wave deceleration time (EDT), A-Wave Peak Velocity (APV), and A-Wave duration (ADU). Fig. 3 illustrate the measuring process.

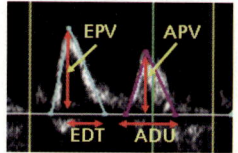
(a) Separated E/A-wave

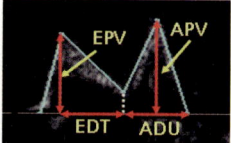
(b) Partially overlapped E/A-wave

Fig. 3. Four measurements: E-Wave Peak Velocity (EPV), E-Wave deceleration time (EDT), A-Wave Peak Velocity (APV), and A-Wave duration (ADU)

3 Experimental Results

We collected 255 Dicom files as training data and 43 Dicom files as test data, which have several cardiac cycles (3.8 cycles/file). The training data were annotated by a sonographer, and the test data were annotated by two sonographers. To best of our knowledge, this is the largest study so far in the literature. In [5], 153 images were used for training and 46 for testing. Also, it faced significant difficulty in dealing with severely overlapping E/A-waves.

For each cardiac cycle, we computed the consensus ground truth (GT) measurements by averaging the measurements individually computed using the annotations by the two experts. The GT measurements are compared with those

Table 1. comparison of correlation coefficient (CC), structure overlap ratio (OR), and delta Peak Velocity (PV) using test data set

	Correlation Coefficient				OR	$|dPV|$ (cm/s)
	EPV	EDT	APV	ADU		
Algorithm vs. Expert Ave.	0.987	0.821	0.986	0.481	85.2%	4.27
Expert 1 vs. Expert 2	0.985	0.903	0.973	0.767	85.8%	3.82

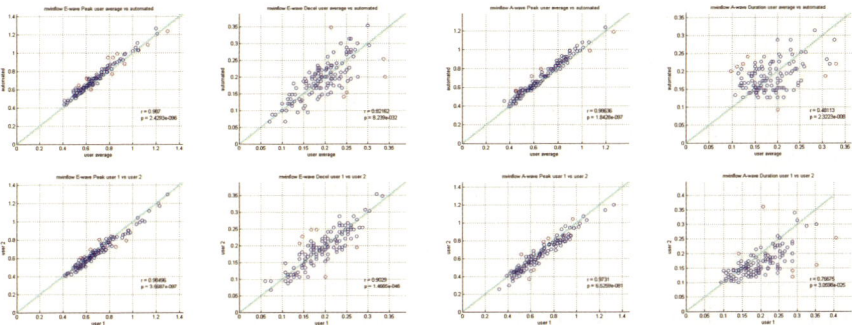

Fig. 4. Scatter plots of the four measurements. The 1st row: the algorithm vs. the average of the experts. The 2nd row: expert 1 vs. expert 2. The columns from left to right: EPV, EDT, APV and ADU.

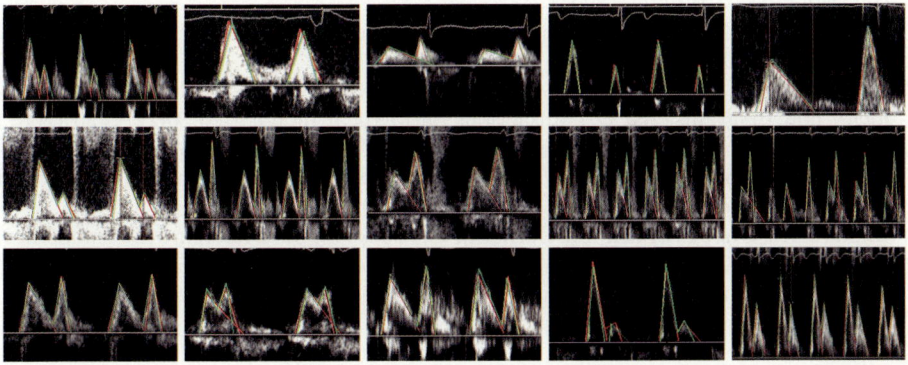

Fig. 5. Segmentation results

computed by our algorithm. We used correlation coefficient (CC) as a comparison metric. The CC between the two experts is also computed. Table 1 shows the comparison of CC between our algorithm vs. GT and that between the two experts, and Fig. 4 displays the scatter plot of the measurement results.

As shown in Table 1 and Fig. 4, our algorithm performs favorably for EPV and APV measurements when compared to the inter-expert variation. The automatic performance of EDT and ADU needs some improvement to match the expert level. To gauge the detection accuracy, we also measure the standard area overlapping ratio (OR), i.e., $OR = 2 * area(A \cup B)/(area(A) + area(B))$ and the absolute peak velocity difference ($|dPV|$). Again, the automatic algorithm yields results with the inter-user variability. The algorithm, implemented on a 2GHZ PC with 2GB RAM, runs very fast: it takes less than one second to process one image.

Fig. 5 presents the automatic tracing results on various images. In Fig. 5, the red line represents ground truth annotated by an expert and the green line corresponds automatic tracing computed by the proposed algorithm.

4 Conclusion

We have proposed a robust algorithm for automatic Doppler measurement of MI pattern in spite of significant variations in shape and appearance. To handle severely overlapping of E-wave and A-wave, the algorithm has trained two global structure detectors, one for non-overlapping structures and the other for overlapping structures. We have also proposed to use shape profile to compute shape probability, and implemented a novel framework to combine the detection results and the shape score. The experimental results show that the algorithm performs very comparable to experts while running within one second.

References

1. Feigenbaum, H., Armstrong, W., Ryan, T.: Feigebaum's Echocardiography. Lippincott Williams & Wilkins (2005)
2. Goldberg, B., McGahan, J.: Atlas of Ultrasound Measurements. Mosby Elsevier, Amsterdam (2006)
3. Tschirren, J., Lauer, R., Sonka, M.: Automated analysis of doppler ultrasound velocity flow diagrams. IEEE Transactions on Medical Imaging 20, 1422–1425 (2001)
4. Greenspan, H., Shechner, O., Scheinowitz, M., Feinberg, M.: Doppler echocardiography flow-velocity image analysis for patients with atrial fibrillation. Ultrasound in Medicine and Biology 31(8), 1031–1040 (2005)
5. Zhou, S.K., Guo, F., Park, J., Carneiro, G., Jackson, J., Brendel, M., Simopoulos, J., Otsuki, J., Comaniciu, D.: A probabilistic, hierarchical, and discriminant (phd) framework for rapid and accurate detection of deformable anatomic structure. In: Proc. of ICCV (2007)
6. Zhang, J., Zhou, S., Comaniciu, D.: Joint real-time object detection and pose estimation using probabilistic boosting network. In: Proc. of CVPR (2007)
7. Georgescu, B., Zhou, X.S., Comaniciu, D., Gupta, A.: Database-guided segmentation of anatomical structures with complex appearance. In: Proc. of CVPR, pp. 429–436 (2005)

Motion Robust Magnetic Susceptibility and Field Inhomogeneity Estimation Using Regularized Image Restoration Techniques for fMRI

Desmond Teck Beng Yeo[1,2], Jeffrey A. Fessler[1,2], and Boklye Kim[1]

[1] Department of Radiology, University of Michigan Medical School, MI 48109, USA
{tbyeo,fessler,boklyek}@umich.edu
[2] Department of Electrical Engineering and Computer Science, University of Michigan, MI 48109, USA

Abstract. In functional MRI, head motion may cause dynamic nonlinear field-inhomogeneity changes, especially with large out-of-plane rotations. This may lead to dynamic geometric distortion or blurring in the time series, which may reduce activation detection accuracy. The use of image registration to estimate dynamic field inhomogeneity maps from a static field map is not sufficient in the presence of such rotations. This paper introduces a retrospective approach to estimate magnetic susceptibility induced field maps of an object in motion, given a static susceptibility induced field map and the associated object motion parameters. It estimates a susceptibility map from a static field map using regularized image restoration techniques, and applies rigid body motion to the former. The dynamic field map is then computed using susceptibility voxel convolution. The method addresses field map changes due to out-of-plane rotations during time series acquisition and does not involve real time field map acquisitions.

Keywords: field inhomogeneity; susceptibility; geometric distortion; field map.

1 Introduction

In functional MRI (fMRI), time series images are acquired with high speed pulse sequences that are typically adversely affected by magnetic field-inhomogeneities. As a result, these images may be geometrically distorted or blurred, depending on the pulse sequence used. A static field-inhomogeneity map may be measured before or after a fMRI session to correct for such distortions [1,2], but it does not account for magnetic field changes due to head motion *during* the time series acquisition. To address this, several prospective dynamic field mapping techniques have been proposed [3,4]. However, they require pulse sequence modifications or high computational cost. Our work focuses on regularized image restoration methods to approximate dynamic field maps retrospectively without pulse sequence modifications.

A previous retrospective approach to approximate a dynamic field map applies rigid body transformations to an observed static field map [5], which may be sufficient only in the absence of significant out-of-plane rotations. In the presence of such rotations, that method may not be suitable since field-inhomogeneities may change nonlinearly [6]. Our approach is to retrospectively estimate the object's magnetic susceptibility (χ) map from an observed high-resolution susceptibility induced static field map using regularized image restoration principles. To compute the dynamic field maps, we apply rigid body motion to the χ-map estimate, and apply 3D susceptibility voxel convolution (SVC) [7] to the resultant spatially translated/ rotated χ-map. SVC is a deterministic, physics-based discrete convolution model for computing susceptibility induced field-inhomogeneity given a 3D χ-map. Our main contributions include: (i) recognizing and formulating the inverse SVC problem for dynamic field map estimation, and, (ii) the implementation of a penalized least squares approach to solve the inverse problem. Another way to approximate the object's χ-map is to segment a CT volume [6] into air, bone and soft tissue, and apply literature susceptibility values to different voxels. However, this may introduce segmentation errors and the use of incorrect susceptibility values. Our approach alleviates the burden of ensuring good accuracy in both the segmentation process, and the susceptibility values used. The approach is demonstrated with realistically simulated noisy 3D field maps of a spherical air pocket in water.

2 Theory

2.1 Susceptibility Voxel Convolution for Field Map Computation

Previous work [8] has shown that given an object with K independent closed compartments of constant χ values, a Lorentz-corrected boundary element approach to computing the z-component of the χ-induced magnetic field map, $\mathbf{B}_p(\mathbf{r})$, yields

$$\mathbf{B}_p(\mathbf{r}) \approx \frac{\chi(\mathbf{r})}{3}\mathbf{B}_0 + \frac{\hat{\mathbf{z}}}{4\pi}\sum_{k=1}^{K}(\chi_k^+ - \chi_k^-)\oint_{S_k}\frac{z-z'}{|\mathbf{r}-\mathbf{r}'|^3}\mathbf{B}_0 \cdot d\mathbf{S}' \text{ (Tesla)}, \quad (1)$$

where $\hat{\mathbf{z}}$ is a unit vector parallel to $\mathbf{B}_0$, χ_k^+ and χ_k^- denote the susceptibilities outside and inside the kth compartment, respectively, S_k is the kth surface, $\mathbf{r}'$ is a surface point, $d\mathbf{S}'$ is perpendicular to the surface at $\mathbf{r}'$. In the presence of out-of-plane rotations, the orientation of the surfaces with $\mathbf{B}_0$, i.e., $\mathbf{B}_0 \cdot d\mathbf{S}'$, changes, thus resulting in nonlinear field map changes.

Susceptibility voxel convolution (SVC) [7] applies Eq. 1 directly to voxels of an object. Each voxel is defined as a closed six-sided compartment of uniform susceptibility. The dot product, $\mathbf{B}_0 \cdot d\mathbf{S}'$, is non-zero only for the top and bottom surfaces of a voxel. Only the upper surface is used since the superposition principle allows each surface to be used only once in computing $\mathbf{B}_p(\mathbf{x})$. The values of χ_k^- and χ_k^+ are obtained from the kth voxel, and the voxel above it in the z direction, respectively. The χ-induced field equation now becomes

$$\mathbf{B}_p(\mathbf{r}) \approx \mathbf{B}_0\left[\frac{\chi(\mathbf{r})}{3} + \frac{1}{4\pi}\sum_{k=1}^{K}(\chi_k^+ - \chi_k^-)\int_{y_k-l_y/2}^{y_k+l_y/2}\int_{x_k-l_x/2}^{x_k+l_x/2}\frac{(z_k+l_z/2-z)}{|\mathbf{r}-\mathbf{r}'|^3}dx'dy'\right], \quad (2)$$

where (x_k, y_k, z_k) is the center of voxel k, and l_x, l_y, l_z are the x, y, and z lengths of a voxel. After discretisation in $\mathbf{r}$, Eq. 2 becomes a 3D discrete convolution in space domain. The convolution kernel can be written as

$$K(x-x_k, y-y_k, z-z_k) =$$
$$(z_k + l_z/2 - z) \int_{y_k-l_y/2}^{y_k+l_y/2} \int_{x_k-l_x/2}^{x_k+l_x/2} \left[(x'-x)^2 + (y'-y)^2 + (z_k+l_z/2-z)^2\right]^{-3/2} dx'dy', \quad (3)$$

and the SVC impulse response is

$$d(h,i,j) = \frac{\delta(l-l')\delta(m-m')\delta(n-n')}{3} + \frac{[K(h,i,j-1) - K(h,i,j)]}{4\pi}, \quad (4)$$

where (l,m,n) denotes the voxel where $\mathbf{B}_p$ is to be calculated, and (l',m',n') denotes voxels in the field of view. The discrete convolution of Eq. 2 becomes

$$\mathbf{B}_p(l,m,n) = \mathbf{B}_0 \sum_{l',m',n' \in \text{FOV}} \chi(l',m',n') d(l-l', m-m', n-n'), \quad (5)$$

which can be computed with

$$\mathbf{B}_p = \mathbf{B}_0 \chi *** d = \mathbf{B}_0 \mathfrak{J}_{3D}^{-1}\left(\mathfrak{J}_{3D}(\chi)\mathfrak{J}_{3D}(d)\right), \quad (6)$$

where *** denotes 3D convolution, and $\mathfrak{J}_{3D}$ denotes 3D Fourier transform. The discrete convolution can also be written in matrix-vector notation as

$$\mathbf{B}_p = \mathbf{D}\chi, \quad (7)$$

where $\mathbf{D}$ denotes the SVC "system" matrix and χ is the column-stacked χ-map vector. The χ-induced field map in Hz is $\Delta\omega_p = \gamma \mathbf{B}_p$, where γ is the gyromagnetic ratio of hydrogen.

2.2 Dynamic Field Map Estimation with Penalized Weighted Least Squares Estimation of Magnetic Susceptibility Map – A 3D Image Restoration Approach

A static field map, $\Delta\omega_{\text{static}}$, is typically approximated by taking the phase difference of a pair of gradient-echo images acquired at two different echo times [9], and may be composed of susceptibility and non-susceptibility induced field inhomogeneity sources. The two complex-valued images may be denoted by

$$I_j^{\text{TE1}} = f_j + \varepsilon_j^{\text{TE1}}, \quad (8)$$

$$I_j^{\text{TE2}} = f_j e^{-i\Delta\omega_{\text{static},j}\Delta\text{TE}} + \varepsilon_j^{\text{TE2}}, \quad (9)$$

where f is the complex transverse magnetization of the object, j is the voxel number, ΔTE is the echo time difference, and ε is independent identically distributed MR Gaussian noise. The echo time difference is typically small to prevent phase wrapping. In previous work [10], the maximum likelihood estimator for $\Delta\omega_{\text{static}}$ was shown to be

$$\Delta\hat{\omega}_{\text{static}} = \arg\min_{\Delta\omega_{\text{static}}} \sum_j \left|I_j^{\text{TE2}} I_j^{\text{TE1}}\right|\left[1 - \cos(\angle I_j^{\text{TE2}} - \angle I_j^{\text{TE1}} - \Delta\omega_{\text{static},j}\Delta\text{TE})\right]. \quad (10)$$

Ignoring phase wrapping, and decomposing $\Delta\omega_{\text{static},j}$ into susceptibility and system induced parts, i.e., $\Delta\omega_{\text{static},j} = \gamma[\mathbf{D}\boldsymbol{\chi}]_j + \Delta\omega_{\text{sys},j}$, and since a minimum exists when the cosine term in Eq. 10 is equal to one, the maximum likelihood estimator for χ is

$$\hat{\chi}_j = \frac{1}{\gamma}\left[\mathbf{D}^{-1}\left[\frac{\angle\mathbf{I}^{TE2} - \angle\mathbf{I}^{TE1}}{\Delta TE} - \Delta\omega_{\text{sys}}\right]\right]_j. \quad (11)$$

For simplicity, we assume that $\Delta\omega_{\text{sys}}$ is negligible, or can be measured empirically. Since the SVC frequency response has very small values at some frequencies, the inverse SVC problem is ill-posed, and thus 3D smoothness regularization is desirable when solving for χ. We propose to use a quadratic penalized weighted least squares (QPWLS) image restoration approach to estimate χ by minimizing the cost function

$$\Psi(\chi) = \frac{1}{2}\|\mathbf{g} - \gamma\mathbf{D}\boldsymbol{\chi}\|_{\mathbf{W}}^2 + \beta\|\mathbf{C}\boldsymbol{\chi}\|^2, \quad (12)$$

where $\mathbf{g}$ is the observed static field map ($\angle\mathbf{I}^{TE2} - \angle\mathbf{I}^{TE1}$)/$\Delta TE$, $\mathbf{W}$ is a weighting matrix that assigns higher weights to voxels where MR image intensity, i.e., $|I_j^{TE2}I_j^{TE1}|$, is higher, β is a regularization parameter that determines the amount of smoothing, and $\mathbf{C}$ is a first order finite-differencing matrix. We minimize the cost function using the conjugate gradient algorithm. Any available motion estimates for each slice or volume in the fMRI time series can then be used to rotate or translate the χ-map estimate. Since the SVC impulse response is linear shift invariant and depends only on the voxel size and orientation with respect to $\mathbf{B}_0$, it remains unchanged when a χ-map undergoes rigid body transformation. Thus, the same SVC matrix used in estimating the χ-map can be used to compute the dynamic field map after the desired motion has been applied.

The proposed QPWLS method was compared to three other methods of approximating the dynamic field map from an observed field map: thresholded inverse filtering [11], Wiener filtering [11], and direct rotation of the observed field map to the tilted positions [5]. The thresholded inverse filter ignores noise statistics and amplifies noise in frequency bands where the SVC frequency response has small values. To mitigate the latter, while preserving as much spatial information as possible, the threshold parameter needs to be chosen carefully, usually in an empirical manner. The Wiener filter assumes that χ and the additive field map noise are stationary processes, and assumes that their power spectra may be estimated accurately, which is often not true in the χ estimation problem.

3 Methods

3.1 Data Simulation

To measure the algorithms' performances, we generated 91 pairs of ground truth χ-maps of a simulated, off-centered spherical air pocket (χ_{air}=0.04 ppm [7]) in water (χ_{water}=-9.05ppm [7]) that was rotated counterclockwise about the x-axis by angles from 0° to 180°, in increments of 2°. The dataset with 0° rotation was defined to be in the *non-tilted* position. In addition, an observed field map in the 0° position was generated. Each 256×256×256 dataset had a voxel size of 1mm×1mm×1mm.

A SVC impulse response was formed (Eq. 4) and applied to all the ground truth χ-maps (Eq. 6) with B_0=1.5 T. The resultant ground truth field maps were then cropped to 128×128×128 voxel volumes. To form the weighting matrix **W** in Eq. 12, we simulated an image intensity map, **f**, with zeros in the air pocket region (no MR signal), and 100 in the water region. With the *non-tilted* ground truth field map ($\Delta\omega_{static}$), an arbitrary value for ΔTE (short enough to avoid phase wrapping), and **f**, we used Eqs. 8 and 9 to generate two independent, complex Gaussian images, each with a SNR of 100.0. An observed non-tilted field map, **g**, shown in Fig. 1(a), was then computed as described in the Theory section.

3.2 Experiments

The main goal of this work is to accurately estimate rotated χ-maps and field maps given (i) an originally observed non-tilted susceptibility induced field map, and, (ii) the respective rotation angles about the *x*-axis. We compared the field map estimation accuracy of our proposed method with those of thresholded inverse filtering, Wiener filtering and direct rotation of the original observed field map to tilted positions.

The first part of the experiment involved the estimation of the original, *non-tilted* χ-map using the various methods. We applied the SVC matrix to these χ-map estimates to compute field map estimates from which a few slices are shown in the top row of Fig. 1. Root mean-square-error (RMSE) values were then computed with reference to the 3D ground truth non-tilted field map, $\Delta\omega_{static}$. In the second part of the experiment, the χ-map estimates from the first part were all rotated about the *x*-axis by the same range of values used to create the 91 pairs of ground truth maps, i.e., 0° to 180° in increments of 2°. The SVC matrix was again applied to these rotated χ-map estimates to compute the dynamic field map estimates. RMSE values were then computed with reference to the 3D ground truth tilted field maps. The second row in Fig. 1 shows a few field map slices of the object rotated by 45°, and the field map RMSE values for all positions and methods were plotted in Fig. 2.

The QPWLS implementation was built upon previous work [12], and 50 iterations of the algorithm were performed for each dataset with β=0.7. The initial guess for the conjugate gradient algorithm was a volume filled with zeros. For the thresholded inverse filter, a threshold value of 10 (0.2 % of the maximum absolute value of the inverse of the SVC frequency response) was used. A flat χ power spectrum was used for the Wiener filter to contrast its higher dependence on object prior information with that of the spatial smoothness prior in the proposed method. All algorithms were implemented in MATLAB (The Mathworks Inc., Natick, MA, USA) and C++, and executed on Intel Pentium 4 Xeon 3.0GHz CPUs.

4 Results

The RMSE values over entire 3D field map estimates for all rotated positions using the various field map estimation methods are shown in Fig. 2. Comparing all the methods, it was observed that the QPWLS method had the lowest (best performing) RMSE values, and RMSE variability, across all rotated positions.

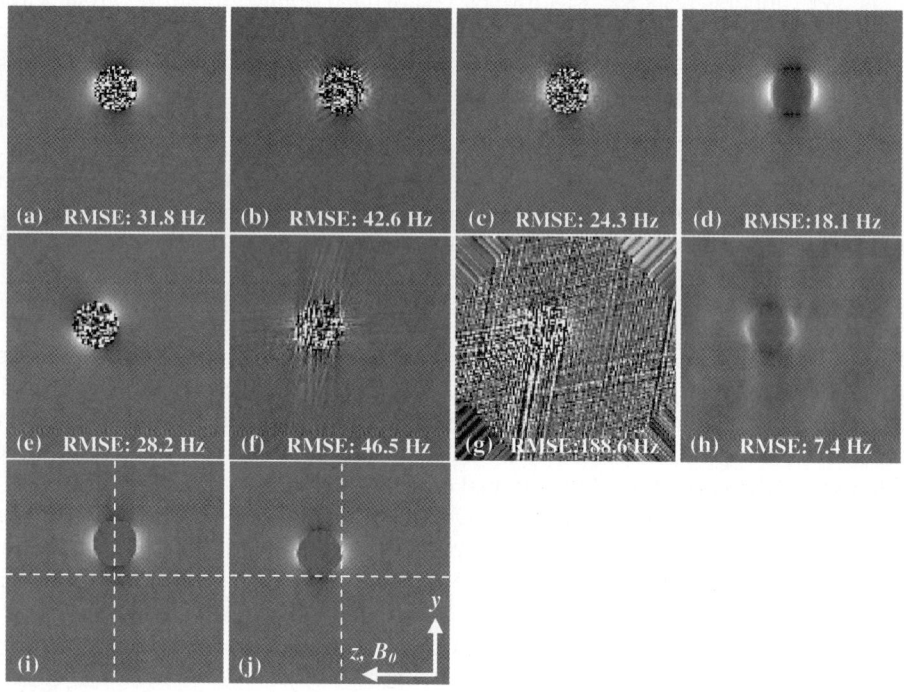

Fig. 1. (Top row) Non-tilted field map slice (y-z plane) from (a) *originally* observed field map, (b) thresholded inverse filter estimate, (c) Wiener filter estimate with flat object power spectrum, (d) QPWLS estimate with β=0.7. (Second row) 45° rotated field map slice from (e) rotation of *original* observed field map, (f) application of SVC on rotated estimate of χ from thresholded inverse filter, (g) application of SVC on rotated estimate of χ from Wiener filter, (h) application of SVC on rotated estimate of χ from QPWLS. (Bottom row) Ground truth field maps for (i) non-tilted, and (j) 45° tilted positions. Display scale: -200 to 450 Hz.

Fig. 1 shows the field map estimates' slices at the same spatial location in the y-z plane when the object was in the 0° and 45° rotated positions, i.e., same slice position from two rotation angles in Fig. 2. The x-axis points into the plane of the page. It was observed that the field map estimates in the spherical air region were invariably noisy for the inverse filter and Wiener filter in Figs. 1(b), 1(f), and Figs. 1(c), 1(g), respectively. The noise in this region was greatly reduced in the QPWLS estimates in Figs. 1(d) and 1(h) because the weighting matrix suppressed the data fidelity requirement in the air region, which allows for smoother χ-map estimates in this region. Since there were less abrupt susceptibility changes in the regularized χ-map estimates, the resultant field inhomogeneity estimate in the air region was small and smooth. For an EPI pulse sequence with a typical phase encode pixel bandwidth of about 20 Hz, the QPWLS RMSE values (<20 Hz) in Fig. 2 represent errors of less than one pixel shift. In contrast, the RMSE values for the other methods (>20 Hz) translate to errors of more than one pixel shift, which may reduce the accuracy of geometric distortion algorithms that depend on field maps. The SVC field map computation time was 1.5

secs for a 128×128×128 voxel χ-map. The computation times for χ-map estimation using the thresholded inverse filter, Wiener filter and QPWLS method were 4.1 secs, 5.8 secs, and 5.6 secs (one iteration), respectively.

5 Discussion and Conclusions

The proposed method estimates dynamic susceptibility induced field maps from an observed static susceptibility induced field map, while accounting for the proper MR noise model. It does not require segmentation or pulse sequence modifications, and may yield higher resolution dynamic field maps that address nonlinear changes due to out-of-plane rotations. Fig. 2 shows quantitatively that the QPWLS RMSE values were the lowest (best performing) among all the other methods. Figs. 1(d) and 1(h) show qualitatively that the field map estimates were close to the ground truths. For our spherical air pocket in water, nonlinear field map changes would typically be worst at the 90° position, hence the peak in Fig. 2 for the method that simply rotates the observed field map. In contrast, the low QPWLS RMSE variability across rotation angles in Fig. 2 suggests that the method performs reasonably well regardless of rotation angles. Further improvements may be possible upon optimizing the choice for the regularization parameter, coupled with the implementation of regularization functions that utilize prior spatial information specific to a brain's χ-map. A potential limitation of the proposed method may arise because $\Delta\omega_{sys}$ was ignored in Eq. 11. In future work, we will investigate methods to reliably measure non-χ induced field inhomogeneities, characterize their effects on the various approaches in this work, and validate the proposed method with real data.

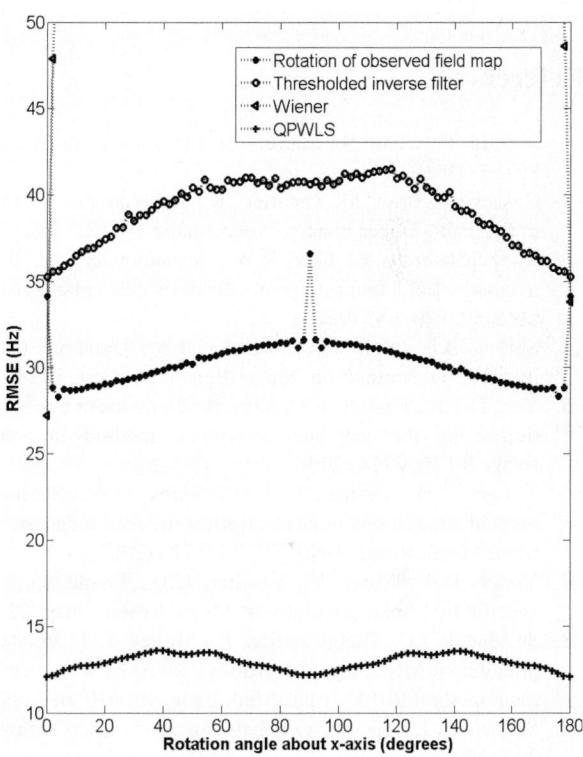

Fig. 2. Dynamic field map RMSE values versus rotation angles for different estimation methods when object was rotated about the x-axis from 0° to 180°. The Wiener filter results were truncated due to large RMSEs.

A novel regularized image restoration approach to estimate field maps of a moving object was proposed and shown, with simulated data, to be more effective than non-regularized methods or simple transformations of an observed field map. In fMRI, this may potentially improve dynamic field map estimates and hence, geometric distortion correction accuracy.

Acknowledgements

This work was supported in part by the National Institute of Health grants 1P01 CA87634 and 8R01 EB00309.

References

1. Jezzard, P., Clare, S.: Sources of distortion in functional MRI data. Hum. Brain Mapp. 8, 80–85 (1999)
2. Cusack, R., Brett, M., Osswald, K.: An evaluation of the use of magnetic field maps to undistort echo-planar images. Neuroimage 18, 127–142 (2003)
3. Roopchansingh, V., Cox, R.W., Jesmanowicz, A., Ward, B.D., Hyde, J.S.: Single-shot magnetic field mapping embedded in echo-planar time-course imaging. Magn. Reson. Med. 50, 839–843 (2003)
4. Sutton, B.P., Noll, D.C., Fessler, J.A.: Dynamic field map estimation using a spiral-in/spiral-out acquisition. Magn. Reson. Med. 51, 1194–1204 (2004)
5. Yeo, D.T.B., Fessler, J.A., Kim, B.: Concurrent correction of geometric distortion and motion using the map-slice-to-volume method in echo-planar imaging. Magn. Reson. Imag. 26, 703–714 (2008)
6. Truong, T.K., Clymer, B.D., Chakeres, D.W., Schmalbrock, P.: Three-dimensional numerical simulations of susceptibility-induced magnetic field inhomogeneities in the human head. Magn. Reson. Imag. 20, 759–770 (2002)
7. Yoder, D.A., Zhao, Y., Paschal, C.B., Fitzpatrick, J.M.: MRI simulator with object-specific field map calculations. Magn. Reson. Imag. 22, 315–328 (2004)
8. de Munck, J.C., Bhagwandien, R., Muller, S.H., Verster, F.C., Van Herk, M.B.: The computation of MR image distortions caused by tissue susceptibility using the boundary element method. IEEE Trans. Med. Imag. 15, 620–627 (1996)
9. Schneider, E., Glover, G.: Rapid in vivo proton shimming. Magn. Reson. Med. 47, 335–347 (1991)
10. Fessler, J.A., Yeo, D., Noll, D.C.: Regularized fieldmap estimation in MRI. In: Proc. IEEE Intl. Symp. Biomed. Imag., pp. 706–709 (2006)
11. Lim, J.S.: Two-dimensional signal and image processing. Prentice Hall, New Jersey (1990)
12. Fessler, J.A.: Image reconstruction toolbox (2007), http://www.eecs.umich.edu/~fessler

Cortical Surface Thickness as a Classifier: Boosting for Autism Classification*

Vikas Singh[1], Lopamudra Mukherjee[2], and Moo K. Chung[1]

[1] Biostatistics and Medical Informatics, University of Wisconsin-Madison,
vsingh@biostat.wisc.edu, mkchung@wisc.edu
[2] Computer Science & Engineering, State University of New York at Buffalo
lm37@cse.buffalo.edu

Abstract. We study the problem of classifying an autistic group from controls using structural *image data alone*, a task that requires a clinical interview with a psychologist. Because of the highly convoluted brain surface topology, feature extraction poses the first obstacle. A clinically relevant measure called the cortical thickness has shown promise but yields a rather challenging learning problem – where the dimensionality of the distribution is extremely large and the training set is small. By observing that each point on the brain cortical surface may be treated as a "hypothesis", we propose a new algorithm for LPBoosting (with truncated neighborhoods) for this problem. In addition to learning a high quality classifier, our model incorporates topological priors into the classification framework directly – that two neighboring points on the cortical surface (hypothesis pairs) must have similar discriminative qualities. As a result, we obtain not just a label $\{+1, -1\}$ for test items, but also an indication of the "discriminative regions" on the cortical surface. We discuss the formulation and present interesting experimental results.

1 Introduction

Learning in biomedical imaging employs training samples provided in the form of image data, with given class labels. We must learn a classifier to assign the correct "label" (positive or negative) to an unseen (test) image. The label may be a pathology (presence or absence of a disease), such as in computer assisted diagnosis. The label may also be a *clinical population group*: for instance, in this paper, our goal is to classify an autistic group from controls – a task that requires an extensive clinical interview with an experienced psychologist [1]. But can we achieve the same objective based on *structural imaging data alone* – efficiently and reliably?

In order to answer the above question, the first difficulty relates to the choice of the features to extract from the images for learning and classification. Feature and shape descriptors (e.g., medial axis, SIFT) that work well across a variety of applications in classical computer vision yield a less than satisfactory performance (in classification) when applied to highly convoluted brain surfaces (their variations are useful in volume

---

* The first author was supported in part by funds from Dept. of Biostatistics and Medical Informatics, UW-Madison and UW Institute for Clinical and Translational Research (ICTR).

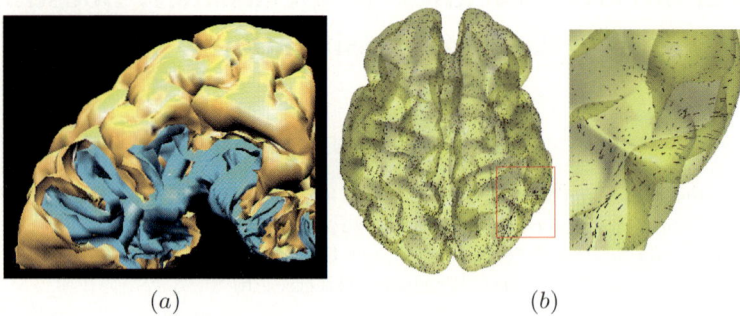

(a) (b)

Fig. 1. (a) Cortical thickness illustration: the outer cortical surface (in yellow) and the inner cortical surface (in blue). The distance between the two surfaces is the cortical thickness. (b) Subsampled surface displacement vector field showing the displacement for one surface (first control subject) to match the other surface (second control subject), as an illustration. The red rectangle region is enlarged to show the displacement vector field (black arrows). Note that the segmentation and cortical thickness calculation were performed in native space.

registrations, however). Among alternatives explored in literature, a promising option is cortical thickness – this measures the distance between the *outer cortical surface* (the interface between gray matter and cerebrospinal fluid), and the *inner cortical surface* (the interface between gray and white matter), see Fig. 1(a). Some neuroanatomical studies [2,3] have reported using this measure for discriminating a clinical population from controls. In cortical thickness based discrimination [3], the image volume is first segmented into tissue types, a mesh representation of the cortical surface (CS) is derived (by triangulation), and the thickness values are calculated at mesh vertex points (in the native space). Then, the standard procedure is to feed such values into a two-sample T statistic at each mesh vertex. However, to account for correlated T statistics at neighboring mesh vertices, we must solve the *multiple comparison problem* [4]: unfortunately, computing the P-value for multiple comparisons is quite challenging. Secondly, such hypothesis driven approaches must satisfy distributional assumptions (e.g., the normality assumption on the cortical thickness values) which may not hold in practice[1], making such approaches error-prone and subsequent quantitative analysis problematic. Since the problem at hand is a classification problem, let us briefly explore the applicability of the powerful support vector machine framework. Given that cortical thickness has a reasonable clinical interpretation, we may consider using it as the measure of choice. Therefore, if a CS (of a single subject) is represented as a mesh with ~ 40000 points, the vectorial representation (say, x) of the cortical thickness lives in $\Re^{40000}$. However, the sizes of datasets in brain imaging literature are typically small (< 100) due to difficulty of recruiting volunteers and cost issues. Therefore, with a finite (and small) training sample $n < 100$, the high-dimensional feature space ($d \gg 100$) where the classifier is calculated is *almost empty* [5]. Hence, as noted in [6], in such cases SVM-based

---

[1] The support of the normal distribution is $-\infty$ and ∞ but cortical thickness values are bounded in $[0\ mm, 6\ mm]$. Also, thickness values are defined on a mesh-vertex and cannot possibly be smooth and differentiable. It may also not be bell-shaped.

classifiers may perform well on training data but will generalize to test data poorly. While some authors have used SVM based methods for classification using brain image data [7], a pre-processing step (typically, a brute force dimensionality reduction using PCA) is used. This seems reasonable for simple shapes (e.g., hippocampus shape data used in [7]) but is too simplistic and immensely lossy for cortical thickness data, and more sophisticated classification tasks.

In this paper, we propose a novel approach for this classification problem. By viewing each set of point-wise correspondences in the training set as a "weak classifier", the training phase seeks to find their best weighted combination, given the correct labels for the training samples. Because the weak classifiers are inherently "spatial", we can exploit this relationship as *priors* within the LPboost framework [8] – which enables us to learn with a small dataset. The paper makes the following contributions: (1) In contrast to the statistical approaches, we do not need to test for the null hypothesis, we also do not compute P-values. Hence, we totally bypass the multiple comparisons problem; (2) In addition to $\sim 90\%$ accuracy, our model yields the goodness of each mesh point as a classifier. This has a physical interpretation – these are the discriminative points between autistic subjects and controls; (3) Because weak classifier pairs are related due to the CS mesh topology, we may derive the discriminative characteristics of "regions" by solving a modified model of LPBoost; (4) The model proposes an algorithm for classifying an autistic group from controls *using image data alone*.

2 Background

First, the raw MRI images must be processed to extract information for use in subsequent steps. We perform an intensity non-uniformity correction before tissue segmentation into three classes: cerebrospinal fluid (CSF), gray matter and white matter (segmentation was performed in native space). We then use a topology preserving deformable surface algorithm [9] to obtain the outer and inner cortical meshes. The details of tissue segmentation and the mesh construction are given in [9]. From the triangular mesh representation of the CS (vertices and triangles) and the spherical

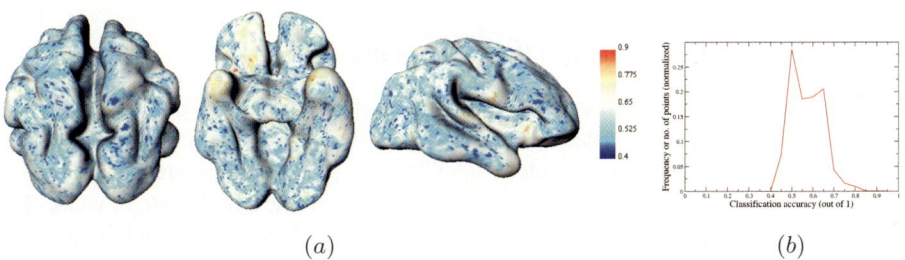

Fig. 2. (a) Unsupervised clustering on coordinates (correspondence sets) and classification accuracy (see color bar) of individual CS mesh points. (b) A histogram of accuracy. Note that given the clustering for each S_i (correspondence set), we know the color assignment (i.e., accuracy) for the cortical surface point i by comparing with ground-truth.

mapping, we may directly obtain the spherical harmonic representation (SPHARM) [3] of cortical thickness g and cortical surface coordinates $\mathbf{p}$ (specific details can be found in [10,3]). Briefly, SPHARM for surface coordinates is calculated as $\mathbf{p}(\theta, \varphi) = \sum_{l=0}^{k} \sum_{m=-l}^{l} \mathbf{p}_{lm} Y_{lm}(\theta, \varphi)$, where Y_{lm} is the spherical harmonic of degree l and order m, and θ, φ are the Euler angles that parameterize the CS. The Fourier coefficient vectors $\mathbf{p}_{lm}$ are estimated iteratively (low to high degree). The SPHARM representation for cortical thickness is $g(\theta, \varphi) = \sum_{l=0}^{k} \sum_{m=-l}^{l} g_{lm} Y_{lm}(\theta, \varphi)$. Here, we use degree $k = 42$ for the representation. In all, we have 1849 coefficients characterizing the cortical thickness. The surface coordinates $\mathbf{p}$ are represented similarly with 3×1849 coefficients. We may calculate the cortical thickness value at each point on the CS. Nonlinear surface correspondence (registration) may also be established using the spherical harmonic correspondence, see [10]. Fig. 1(b) shows the displacement vector field for warping one subject's CS on to another subject's CS, as an illustration. In §3, we turn our attention back to the classification problem.

3 Main Ideas

A useful observation in approaching our classification problem is the following. Because registration has been performed, we may pick a point i on a CS (and obtain the cortical thickness value), retrieve the correspondences for this point in the other $N - 1$ cortical surfaces (with their cortical thickness values), the N thickness values define a *correspondence set*, S_i. We may analyze clusters in this set: by performing a maximum margin clustering (identifying two consecutive points in a sorted set with maximum separation) on this set with two classes. Based on this clustering on S_i, CSs in our dataset belong to one of two classes. A classification at this stage assigns a "+1" or "−1" label based on cluster membership of a single point on the CS. Fig. 2(a) shows the classification accuracy of each point i on the average CS. Figure 2(b) shows a histogram of the corresponding values. The classification accuracy is in $[44\%, 92.5\%]$. Not all points on the CS are good class discriminators but a subset (1.8%) of points perform well and have an accuracy of $> 80\%$. The key lies in selecting the subset automatically. Note that we calculate the accuracy by comparing the CS classification to ground-truth data.

3.1 Supervised Classification on the Coordinates

With the large variation in classification accuracy of individual CS points, using individual correspondence set clustering for classification does not seem to be a good idea. However, notice that we may consider each CS point (i.e., correspondence set) to be a "weak classifier" (or hypothesis), then, our goal is to combine a multitude of weak classifiers to obtain a discriminative classifier using training. A powerful machine learning method called "boosting" offers this capability.

Boosting was proposed in [11,12] and has since found applications in many areas including biomedical imaging [13]. A popular boosting algorithm is AdaBoost [14]. Adaboost adds weak classifiers to the ensemble in an iterative fashion, by adjusting the *weight* of the classifier, and the training samples w.r.t. classification accuracy (on the training set). The vector of learnt weights of the unrelated classifiers may then be used with a new CS to determine class membership ($+1$ or -1). As the reader may have realized, a peculiar characteristic of the problem at hand is that the weak hypotheses are strongly correlated in a four or eight neighborhood sense. For example, two adjacent points on a CS surface (which correspond to two hypothesis) must be expected to have a similar discriminative power. Unfortunately, the solution from AdaBoost may not meet this requirement. Hence, calculated hypothesis weights (via boosting) have little physical interpretation in terms of the cortical surfaces. To address this difficulty, we will look at an alternate model for boosting proposed recently called LPBoost [8]. We will then analyze how it can be modified to include additional meta-information from our problem (e.g., point neighborhoods) in a natural manner.

Classifier Boosting using LPBoost. The method of LPBoost relies on applying the power of linear programming to boosting. Each weak classifier (divides the data set into $+1$ and -1. Rather than adding a new classifier (a combination of given weak classifiers) iteratively at each step, LPboost assumes all weak hypotheses are available. The labels generated by the weak classifiers are considered to be a new feature space, where the goal is to learn a function that minimizes the misclassification error and maximizes the maximum margin of separation. The model is given as [8]:

$$(\text{LPBoost}) \min \sum_{j=1}^{n} a_j + C \sum_{i=1}^{m} \xi_i$$

$$\text{s.t.} \sum_{j=1}^{n} y_i H_{ij} a_j + \xi_i \geq 1, \quad \forall i \in \{1, \cdots, m\}, \tag{1}$$

where $a_j \geq 0$. In (1), $\mathbf{y} \in \Re^m$ denotes class-membership for training set items whose entries take values $\{+1, -1\}$. H_{ij} tabulates the response of the j-th hypothesis on the i-th item and $a \in \Re^n_+$ weighs the hypotheses. Like in SVMs, we must allow for a small margin of error (appropriately penalized) to minimize the effects of a few outliers – this gives the so-called "slack" as ξ and C is a regularizer. For better generalization, we penalize the 1-norm of a in the objective which also suppresses redundant features [6].

Boosting with Neighborhoods (truncated smoothness penalty). The previous model of LPBoost does not provide a way to incorporate additional relational information between classifiers. While this may suffice for other applications, in our case, the classifier corresponds to a mesh point and is spatially related to other classifiers. We may model the given cortical surface triangulation as a graph $\mathcal{G} = (\mathcal{V}, \mathcal{E})$. The points on the CS constitute $\mathcal{V}$ and adjacent points p_i, p_j on the CS mesh are neighbors in $\mathcal{G}$: $v_i, v_j \in \mathcal{V}$ have an edge $e_{ij} \in \mathcal{E}$, $\sim$ denotes neighborhood. Since the cortical thickness (and accuracy of classification) cannot change abruptly across neighboring mesh points, the weights assigned to the classifiers i.e., a entries for neighbors should also be smoothly varying. We propose a model with the following objective function to incorporate such neighborhood information with the same constraints as (1).

$$(\text{LPBoost-N}) \quad \min \sum_{j=1}^{n} a_j + C \sum_{i=1}^{m} \xi_i + \sum_{v_j \sim v_{j'}} \gamma \|a_j - a_{j'}\| \tag{2}$$

where a_j is non-negative. We impose smoothness over the weights assigned to CS points, by penalizing the variation between weights assigned to neighbors v_j and $v_{j'}$, regularized by a parameter, γ. There is no penalty if v_j and $v_{j'}$ take the same weight. To address the difficulty with the 1-norm in the second term, we can introduce an additional variable, $t_{jj'}$. It can be easily verified that the following is an equivalent model

$$\text{(LPBoost-N')} \min \sum_{j=1}^{n} a_j + C \sum_{i=1}^{m} \xi_i + \sum_{v_j \sim v_{j'}} \underbrace{\gamma'}_{\rho_{ij}\gamma} t_{jj'}$$

$$\text{s.t.} \sum_{j=1}^{n} y_i H_{ij} a_j + \xi_i \geq 1 \quad \forall i \in \{1, \cdots, m\},$$

$$a_j - a_{j'} \leq t_{jj'}, \; a_{j'} - a_j \leq t_{jj'} \quad \forall e_{jj'} \in \mathcal{E},$$

$$a_j \geq 0 \quad \forall j \in \{1, \cdots, n\}. \tag{3}$$

A note on the third term, $\gamma' t_{jj'}$, in the objective in (3) is in order. Observe that in (2), if γ is constant in $\gamma \|a_j - a_{j'}\|$, we impose a smoothness penalty for all neighbors as a function of $\|a_j - a_{j'}\|$. This encourages the identification of smooth discriminative regions, but the term unnecessarily penalizes (j, j') pairs that lie on either side of the "regions" (analogous to edge pixels on the boundary of foreground/background in image segmentation). Ideally, a_j and $a_{j'}$ should *not* be similar, and the difference should not be penalized. To address this problem, we use a *truncated cost model* [15]: by imposing a smoothness penalty only if (j, j') had similar classification accuracy *on the training set*. This can be modeled using ρ_{ij} which is 1 if (j, j') had similar accuracy (within a threshold, t) and $\rho_{ij} = 0$ otherwise. Therefore, in the third term in (3), $\gamma' = \rho_{ij}\gamma$. To wrap up, the model in (3) is linear, and the requirement on a is only of non-negativity. So, (3) can be solved optimally in polytime.

4 Experimental Results

The experimental evaluation of the algorithm was designed to investigate the suitability of the framework in context of the following issues from §1: (1) Can we learn a classifier from training image data to reliably classify autism group and controls? If yes, what kind of accuracy can we hope for? (2) In addition to a binary class assignment, can we determine the *discriminative regions* that help us classify? This would be very useful information – the existence of such areas convey that the structural basis of autism is localized in brain regions, we may be able to better understand the structural connection to the functional deficit in autistic subjects. So, instead of trying to investigate every part of the brain, we may limit our investigation to these discriminative areas, possibly using more traditional hypothesis driven statistical inference.

Acquisition and Processing. We acquired three Tesla T_1-weighted MR brain image scans for 11 controls and 16 high functioning autistic subjects (27 subjects in all), see [1] for details. The autistic subjects were diagnosed by a certified psychologist, this was used as the "truth" classification, **y**. The standard image processing steps from §2 were performed, and the weak hypotheses were generated for boosting. Boosting using our model in (3) was performed on the cortical thickness vectors using k-fold cross validation procedure ($k = 9$), and the mean of the results analyzed. Since cross validation experiments can be repeated $n!$ times (for n items), which grows rapidly, we randomly permuted the data set and repeated the experiments 10 times and report on the mean for each case.

A large number of CS points have poor discriminative characteristics. Ideally, the boosting algorithm should ignore all such points, the weighted combination should include only the discriminative weak classifiers. However, when the number of hypotheses is large (with a relatively smaller training set), occasionally a few not-so-good hypotheses are assigned non-zero weights. Inclusion of such hypotheses reduces the generalization behavior of the boosted classifier. This can be partly mitigated in practice by moderately pruning the set of hypotheses and boosting only the better classifiers, i.e., classifiers that have lower training error for a particular training set. We performed this pruning step for classifiers by only including hypothesis with error (on training data) below a user specified threshold (15% − 45%).

The model in (3) has at most $27 + H + N$ variables and $27 + 2N$ constraints, where H is the maximum number of hypotheses (40392) and N is the number of neighbors ($< 6H$). Solving the model to obtain a solution using CPLEX took $\sim 20s$. To prune the set of hypothesis, we repeated each of the above experiments for hypotheses with 15%−45% training error. Each experiment was repeated for LPBoost without neighborhoods (1) and LPBoost-N′ with truncated neighborhoods (3). The regularizer, C, was set to 100. In all cases, we report on misclassification errors on the test data sets.

Fig. 3 compares the misclassification errors for LPBoost and LPBoost-N′ (truncated neighborhoods). We see that LPBoost-N′ outperforms LPBoost in all cases, with a mean error of $\sim$ 10% in cases where the maximum error in the included hypotheses is 25%. Also, analyzing misclassification error as a function of increasing the number of hypotheses considered (increasing training error) shows that the errors are relatively high when the size of the hypothesis set is very small. It improves as the size increases and plateaus between 25%−40%, with a slight deterioration as the set includes more hypotheses with very high error. In summary, by combining the discriminative power of cortical thickness at many CS points, we can classify the autism group from controls with $\sim$ 90% accuracy.

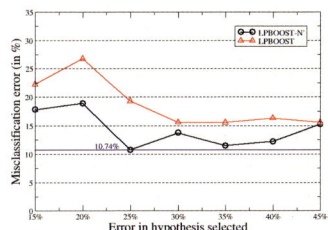

Fig. 3. Misclassification error for boosting on coordinates for LPBoost and LPBoost-N′

The entries of the weight vector, a, returned by our model are non-zero for a small subset of hypotheses, this gives a way of determining discriminative weak classifiers from a large set. Because of the spatial contiguity requirement in (3), we get contiguous discriminative regions on the cortical surface (see Fig. 4, regions in red). By incrementally including more hypotheses to boost (15% to 35%), most regions identified for fewer hypotheses exhibit an expansion, see Fig. 4 (left to right). It is also very encouraging to see that if we compare Fig. 4 with Fig. 2(a), the regions in Fig. 4 are a subset of the "good" regions in Fig. 2(a) (notice that since Fig. 2(a) corresponds to all 27 CS, it may serve as ground truth). It is expected that all high accuracy CS points in Fig. 2(a) are not selected by boosting because the model selects *only* a minimal subset of hypotheses needed to yield an accurate classifier. If desired, we may determine *all* discriminative regions by

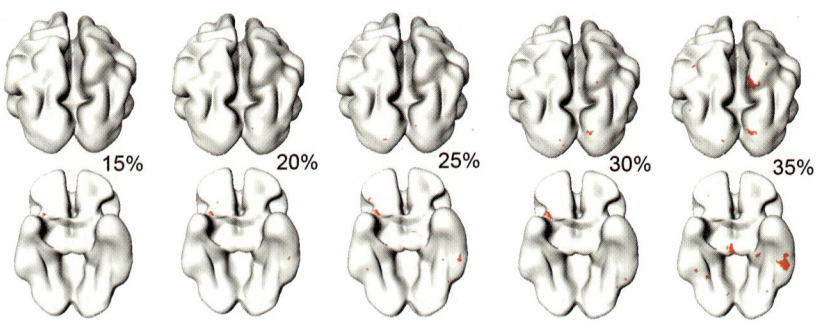

Fig. 4. The discriminating regions selected by the model (non-zero weights in a in (3)) in red corresponding to increasing set of hypotheses selected

repeatedly running the algorithm on a reduced set of hypotheses (by removing the regions already selected), we omit these results due to limited space.

5 Conclusions

We present a LPboosting based algorithm for classifying autistic subjects from controls based on cortical thickness. The model incorporates spatial priors – as a result we obtain discriminating regions on the cortical surface in addition to high classification accuracy ($\sim 90\%$) on test items. As future work, it will be interesting to see if improvements are possible by incorporating additional clinically relevant features (apart from cortical thickness) in the model. Given that in brain imaging, we often encounter datasets in high dimensions but with few data items, classifiers that learn from a wide spectrum of information may generalize better, and are desirable for robust classification systems.

References

1. Dalton, K.M., Nacewicz, B.M., Johnstone, T., Schaefer, H.S., Gernsbacher, M.A., Goldsmith, H.H., Alexander, A.L., Davidson, R.J.: Gaze fixation and the neural circuitry of face processing in autism. Nature Neuroscience 8, 519–526 (2005)
2. Kabani, N., Le Goualher, G., MacDonald, D., Evans, A.C.: Measurement of cortical thickness using an automated 3-d algorithm: a validation study. NeuroImage 13(2), 375–380 (2001)
3. Chung, M.K., Dalton, K.M., Shen, L., Evans, A.C., Davidson, R.J.: Weighted fourier representation and its application to quantifying the amount of gray matter. IEEE Trans. Med. Imaging 26, 566–581 (2007)
4. Worsley, K.J., Marrett, S., Neelin, P., Vandal, A.C., Friston, K.J., Evans, A.C.: A unified statistical approach for determining significant signals in images of cerebral activation. Human Brain Mapping 4, 58–73 (1996)
5. Hertz, J., Krogh, A., Palmer, R.G.: Introduction to the Theory of Neural Computation. Addison-Wesley, Reading (1991)
6. Bradley, P.S., Mangasarian, O.L.: Feature selection via concave minimization and support vector machines. In: International Conf. on Machine Learning, pp. 82–90 (1998)

7. Shen, L., Ford, J., Makedon, F., Saykin, A.: Surface-based approach for classification of 3d neuroanatomical structures. Intelligent Data Anal. 8, 519–542 (2004)
8. Demiriz, A., Bennett, K.P., Shawe-Taylor, J.: Linear programming boosting via column generation. Machine Learning 46(1-3), 225–254 (2002)
9. MacDonald, J.D., Kabani, N., Avis, D., Evans, A.C.: Automated 3-D extraction of inner and outer surfaces of cerebral cortex from MRI. NeuroImage 12, 340–356 (2000)
10. Chung, M.K., Hartley, R., Dalton, K.M., Davidson, R.J.: Encoding cortical surface by spherical harmonics. In: Statistica Sinica, Special Issue on Statistical Challenges and Advances in Brain Science (in press, 2008)
11. Schapire, R.E.: The strength of weak learnability. Machine Learning 5, 197–227 (1990)
12. Freund, Y.: Boosting a weak learning algorithm by majority. In: Proc. of Computational Learning Theory (1990)
13. Tu, Z., Zheng, S., Yuille, A.L., Reiss, A.L., Dutton, R.A., Lee, A.D., Galaburda, A.M., Dinov, I., Thompson, P., Toga, A.W.: Automated extraction of the cortical sulci based on a supervised learning approach. IEEE Trans. Med. Imaging 26(4), 541–552 (2007)
14. Freund, Y., Schapire, R.E.: A decision-theoretic generalization of on-line learning and an application to boosting. In: Conf. on Computational Learning Theory, pp. 23–37 (1995)
15. Gupta, A., Tardos, E.: Constant factor approximation algorithms for a class of classification problems. In: ACM Symposium on Theory of Computing, pp. 652–658 (2000)

Surface-Based Vector Analysis Using Heat Equation Interpolation: A New Approach to Quantify Local Hippocampal Volume Changes

Hosung Kim, Pierre Besson, Olivier Colliot, Andrea Bernasconi, and Neda Bernasconi

Department of Neurology and Brain Imaging Center, McGill University, Montreal Neurological Institute and Hospital, Montreal, Quebec, Canada

Abstract. Analysis of surface-based displacement vectors using spherical harmonic description (SPHARM) localizes shape changes accurately. However, it does not allow differentiating volume variations from shifting and/or bending. We propose a new approach to quantify local volume changes by computing the surface-based Jacobian determinant. This measurement is computed on the displacement vector fields estimated by a heat equation interpolation on the displacement vectors produced by SPHARM. Data simulation showed that the surface-based Jacobian determinant enables accurate quantification of local volume changes without interference of shifting/bending. In patients with temporal lobe epilepsy and left hippocampal atrophy, SPHARM detected widespread inward deformation related to atrophy in the hippocampal head and body, and showed areas of mirrored inward/outward deformations mostly at the level of the hippocampal tail. In these areas, the surface-based Jacobian determinant showed atrophy. Our method facilitates the interpretation of SPHARM because it allows decomposing volume changes and shifting/bending. Furthermore, it provides a better delineation of the extent of hippocampal atrophy.

Keywords: brain morphometry, shape analysis, Jacobian analysis, heat equation, hippocampus.

1 Introduction

Surface shape models are objective methods to assess morphometric changes not evident in the measurement of the total volume. These methods have been successfully applied to quantify hippocampal shape in a variety of neurological and psychiatric disorders including epilepsy [1], Alzheimer's disease [2] and schizophrenia [3]. Among surface-based shape analysis methods, medial surface and axis models have been used to assess local variations in thickness [3]. These approaches produce symmetrical measurements on two facing surfaces. Alternatively, vertex-wise analyses of displacement vectors using surface registration techniques [1, 2] or the spherical harmonics description (SPHARM) [3, 4] localize asymmetrically shape changes. The signed surface normal component of the displacement vector is generally used to describe inward/outward deformations, which have been interpreted as the result of local volume changes [1]. However, this metric also captures positional differences between a given object and a template. Thus, it does not allow differentiating local volume variations from mirrored inward/outward deformations.

Deformation-based morphometry (DBM) enables the quantification of local volume changes without the interference of shifting/bending effects [5, 6]. This technique produces 3D displacement vector fields between two non-linearly registered volume data. The Jacobian determinant map is computed on the vector fields and allows assessing local volume changes. DBM has been used to assess brain development [5] and atrophy in Alzheimer's disease [7].

The heat equation is a partial differential equation which describes the propagation process of heat over time [8]. Solving this equation from preset values on the boundary of a closed volume generates scalar fields within this volume. Therefore, this approach can be used to perform an isotropic and homogeneous interpolation.

Here, we propose an extension of SPHARM based on a heat equation interpolation method to estimate displacement vector fields inside a surface boundary. The vertex-wise Jacobian determinant computed on the displacement vector fields will enable assessment of local volume changes without interference of shifting/bending.

2 Methods

Our method includes three main steps. First, using spherical harmonics description and point distribution models [4], we compute vertex-wise displacement vectors on a surface. Secondly, we interpolate the displacement vector fields within the surface boundary using the heat equation [8]. Finally, we compute the surface-based Jacobian determinant from the displacement vector fields to quantify local volume changes. We evaluate this method using simulation shapes and human hippocampi.

2.1 Spherical Harmonics Description and Point Distribution Model

Simulated objects/anatomical labels undergo a minimal smoothing operation. They are then converted to surface meshes for which a spherical parameterization (SPHARM) is computed using an area-preserving, distortion-minimizing mapping. Based on a uniform icosahedron-subdivision of the SPHARM, we obtain a point distribution model (PDM). SPHARM-PDM surfaces of each individual are rigidly aligned to a template constructed across subjects with respect to the centroid and the longitudinal axis of the 1st order ellipsoid. Vertex-wise displacement vectors are calculated between each individual and the template. The surface normal component of this vector is analyzed to assess inner/outer deformations.

2.2 Heat Equation

The heat equation is a partial differential equation which describes the propagation process of heat in a given region over time [8]. For a function of three spatial variables x, y, z and a time variable t, the heat equation is:

$$\frac{\partial u}{\partial t} = k\left(\frac{\partial^2 u}{\partial x^2} + \frac{\partial^2 u}{\partial y^2} + \frac{\partial^2 u}{\partial z^2}\right) = k\Delta u \qquad (1)$$

where k is a constant called conductivity and Δ is the Laplacian operator. From fixed scalar values on a boundary, this equation allows diffusing fields by minimizing the sum of gradient changes so that smooth fields are obtained at the equilibrium status. Using Laplacian operator, this equation can be applied to 3 orthogonal vector components (x,y,z) without co-varying variables. Therefore, solving this equation with vectors on the surface S of a closed volume as a boundary condition diffuses smooth vector fields within the volume. We used the displacement vectors $\mathbf{u}_S$ obtained in **2.1** as boundary condition. If a displacement vector at position (x,y,z) in the volume domain is $\mathbf{u} = (u_x, u_y, u_z)$, its variation at time t can be defined as:

$$\frac{\partial \mathbf{u}}{\partial t} = \left(\frac{\partial u_x}{\partial t}, \frac{\partial u_y}{\partial t}, \frac{\partial u_z}{\partial t}\right) = (k\Delta u_x, k\Delta u_y, k\Delta u_z) \qquad (2)$$

Finally, the displacement vector fields in the volume inside S are estimated by solving equation (2) until reaching convergence ($\partial \mathbf{u}/\partial t \rightarrow 0$).

2.3 Implementation on Discrete Space

Let $\Omega = \{(x,y,z) \mid x=0, 1, \ldots, l;\ y=0, 1, \ldots, m;\ z=0, 1, \ldots, n\}$ be a discrete domain in 3D space. Consider a set of surface vertices $S = \{\mathbf{s}_1, \mathbf{s}_2, \ldots, \mathbf{s}_M\}$, on which the control lattice Ω is overlaid (Figure 1-a). Then, let $\mathbf{u}_S = \{\mathbf{u}_{S1}, \mathbf{u}_{S2}, \ldots \mathbf{u}_{SM}\}$ be displacement vectors on S calculated at the previous SPHARM-PDM stage. In 3D, we consider a surface point $\mathbf{s}_i$ located within a unit-size cube enclosed by its adjacent 8 points on Ω. To compute the heat equation on Ω with the boundary condition $\mathbf{u}_s(t) = \mathbf{u}_s$, $\mathbf{u}_{si}$ should be interpolated on domain Ω. Let $\mathbf{x}=(x,y,z)$ be one of these 8 points and $d(\mathbf{x}, \mathbf{s}_i)$ be the Euclidean distance between $\mathbf{x}$ and $\mathbf{s}_i$. Point $\mathbf{x}$ can be adjacent to one or more surface points (e.g., $\mathbf{s}_{i-1}$, $\mathbf{s}_{i+1}$ in Figure 1-b). We consider a general interpolation method at $\mathbf{x}$. Let $N_{s,\mathbf{x}}$ be the number of surface points adjacent to $\mathbf{x}$ and $A_{d,N}$ be the average of distances between $\mathbf{x}$ and the adjacent surface points $s = \{\mathbf{s}_i, \mathbf{s}_{i+1}, \ldots, \mathbf{s}_{i+N-1}\}$. Then, we can compute $\mathbf{u}_\mathbf{x}$ by iterative search from $\mathbf{s}_i$ to $\mathbf{s}_{i+N-1}$. When considering $\mathbf{s}_i$, $\mathbf{u}_\mathbf{x}$ is determined as:

$$\mathbf{u}_\mathbf{x}(t) = \mathbf{u}_{S_i},\ A_{d,1} = d(\mathbf{x}, \mathbf{s}_i) \qquad (3)$$

When $N_{s,\mathbf{x}}=N$, $\mathbf{u}_\mathbf{x}$ is updated from the N-1th computation ($\tilde{\mathbf{u}}_\mathbf{x}$, $A_{d,N-1}$) at $\mathbf{s}_{i+N-2}$ as:

$$\mathbf{u}_\mathbf{x} = \frac{\mathbf{u}_{S_{i+N-1}} \cdot A_{d,N-1} + \tilde{\mathbf{u}}_\mathbf{x} \cdot d(\mathbf{x}, \mathbf{s}_{i+N-1})}{A_{d,N-1} + d(\mathbf{x}, \mathbf{s}_{i+N-1})}, \qquad (4)$$

$$A_{d,N-1} = \frac{A_{d,N-2} \cdot (N-2) + d(\mathbf{x}, \mathbf{s}_{i+N-2})}{N-1}$$

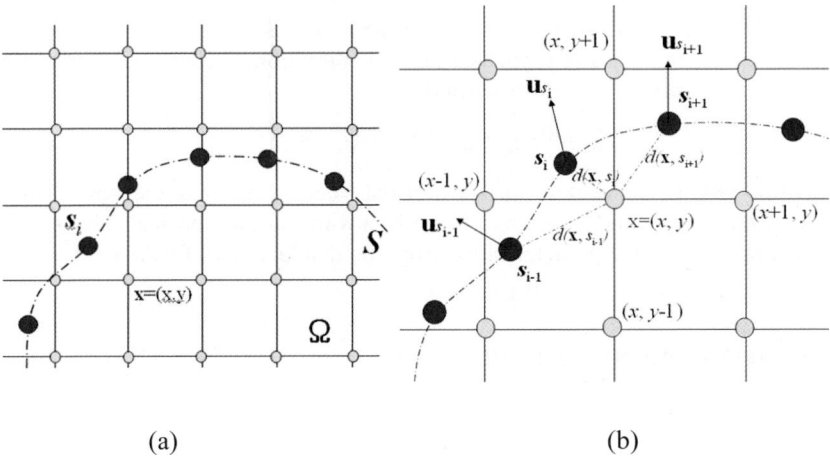

Fig. 1. (a) Schematic 2D representation of surface vertices overlaid on a discrete and rectangular control lattice Ω. (b) a vector $\mathbf{u}_x$, as a boundary condition, is interpolated from displacement vectors on surface vertices ($\mathbf{u}_{Si-1}$, $\mathbf{u}_{Si}$, $\mathbf{u}_{Si+1}$) adjacent to x.

Under the boundary condition determined in (4), the heat equation on the discrete domain Ω is defined as:

$$\mathbf{u}_x(t) - \mathbf{u}_x(t-1) = k\,\Delta \mathbf{u}_x(t-1) \tag{5}$$

$$= \frac{1}{6}(\mathbf{u}(x-1,y,z,t-1) + \mathbf{u}(x+1,y,z,t-1) +$$

$$\mathbf{u}(x,y-1,z,t-1) + \mathbf{u}(x,y+1,z,t-1) +$$

$$\mathbf{u}(x,y,z-1,t-1) + \mathbf{u}(x,y,z+1,t-1) - 6\mathbf{u}(x,y,z,t-1))$$

$\mathbf{u}_x(t)$ is updated by adding $\mathbf{u}_x(t-1)$ in (5).

The final displacement vector fields on Ω are determined when:

$$\sum_{\Omega} \|\mathbf{u}_x(t) - \mathbf{u}_x(t-1)\| < \alpha \tag{6}$$

In (6), the optimization threshold α was chosen to be 0.001.

2.4 Assessment of Local Volume Changes

Local volume changes are quantified by the Jacobian determinant J_S [5] on surface points S, being defined as:

$$J_S = \det(I + \nabla \mathbf{u}_S) = 1 + tr(\nabla \mathbf{u}_S) + \det_2(\nabla \mathbf{u}_S) + \det(\nabla \mathbf{u}_S) \tag{7}$$

where tr is the trace operator, $det_2(\nabla \mathbf{u}_S)$ is the sum of 2x2 principal minors of $\nabla \mathbf{u}$.

For the vector fields produced by an isotropic diffusion, which assumes no shear deformation, the higher order terms approach zero. Therefore, we can approximate $J \approx tr(\nabla \mathbf{u}_S)$ when 1 is subtracted. This Jacobian explains growth or shrinkage of a unit-size cube through each of the 3 orthogonal axes. For surface-based analysis, we are only interested in assessing surface-normal directional changes. Therefore, the Jacobian at a surface point s_i is simplified as:

$$J_{si} = \nabla \mathbf{u}_{si} \cdot \mathbf{n}_{si} = (\mathbf{u}_{si} - \mathbf{u}_{\hat{s}i}) \cdot \mathbf{n}_{si} \tag{8}$$

In equation (8), $\mathbf{n}$ is the unit surface normal vector and $\hat{s}_i$ is the point where the distance from s_i is 1 and its direction is the inward surface normal. Using tri-linear interpolation, $\mathbf{u}_{si}$ and $\mathbf{u}_{\hat{s}i}$ are determined from the displacement fields on Ω.

3 Experiments and Results

3.1 Simulation Data

We created a rounded cylindrical volume with a resolution of $0.25 \times 0.25 \times 0.25$ mm^3 (Figure 2-a) and applied the following deformations: bending (Figure 2-b, row 1), local shifting (Figure 2-b, row 2) and simultaneous local shrinking (0.5 mm) and shifting (2.0 cm) in z-axis (Figure 2-b, row 3). To compare the deformed object to the original, we first extracted SPHARM-PDM surfaces and calculated the displacement vectors. Then, at each vertex, we computed a signed surface-normal component of the displacement vector (SNV) and a surface-based Jacobian determinant (SJD). 3D mapping of the SNV showed *mirrored* inward/outward deformations on the two facing surfaces reflecting bending and shifting (Figure 2-d row 1, 2). However, in the case of simultaneous local shrinking and shifting, SNV did not allow differentiating shrinkage from shifting because of a stronger effect of shifting (Figure 2-d, row 3). Contrary to SNV, the SJD was not influenced by bending and shifting (Figure 2-e, row 1, 2) and accurately localized the shrinkage (Figure 2-e, row 3).

To investigate the influence of the heat equation interpolation kernel size in detecting volume changes, we measured SJD with respect to different grid sizes of the 3D domain Ω ranging from $0.125 \times 0.125 \times 0.125$ mm^3 to $4.0 \times 4.0 \times 4.0$ mm^3. For this experiment, SJD was computed from the displacement vectors between the reference object and its variant deformed by simultaneous local shifting and shrinkage. We defined the ROI as the vertices on which we modeled the shrinkage. Then, for each grid size, we measured the mean SJD in the ROI and a modified standard error (MSE) over the entire object. MSE was defined as:

$$MSE = \sum_{ROI} |SJD - (-0.5)| / n_{ROI} + \sum_{\overline{ROI}} |SJD| / n_{\overline{ROI}} \tag{9}$$

In equation (9), n_{ROI} is the number of vertices in the *ROI* and $\overline{ROI}$ defines the vertices outside the ROI. Mean SJD in the ROI showed that the target volume shrinkage was detected with a grid size ranging from $0.25 \times 0.25 \times 0.25$ (mean SJD: 0.53) to $0.5 \times 0.5 \times 0.5$ mm^3 (mean SJD: 0.49) (Figure 3-a). The MSE demonstrated that the minimum error is obtained at the grid size of $0.5 \times 0.5 \times 0.5$ mm^3 (Figure 3-b).

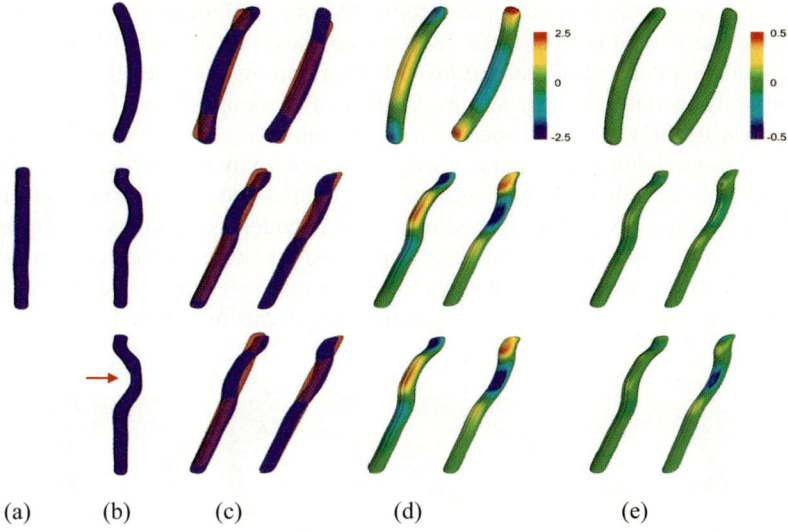

Fig. 2. Simulation. **(a)** Reference object. **(b)** Three deformed variants of the reference object: bending (top), local shifting (middle), simultaneous local shifting and shrinkage (bottom). The red arrow indicates the region where the local shrinking was applied. **(c)** Deformed objects (solid blue) aligned to the reference (transparent red). **(d)** Signed surface-normal components of the displacement vectors measured between the deformed objects and the reference (color scale in mm, -/+ signs indicate inward/outward deformation) **(e)** Surface-based Jacobian determinant maps (color scale in mm^3, -/+ signs indicate volume loss/growth).

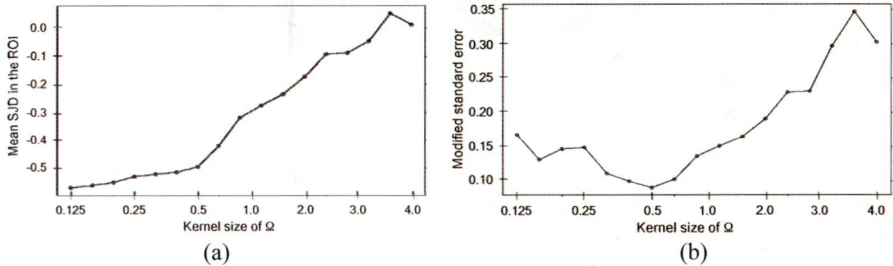

Fig. 3. Influence of the kernel size of the heat equation interpolation on the detection of 0.5mm shrinkage. Graph of mean SJD in the ROI (a) and modified standard error over the entire object (b) across blurring kernels.

3.2 Shape Analysis of the Hippocampus in Temporal Lobe Epilepsy

Temporal lobe epilepsy (TLE) is associated with hippocampal sclerosis, a pathology consisting of various degrees of neuronal loss throughout the hippocampus. The most conspicuous MRI feature of hippocampal sclerosis is atrophy.

We selected from our database 22 medically intractable TLE patients (11 males; mean age: 37 ± 11) with a left-sided seizure focus and 33 age- and sex-matched healthy controls. Based on a 2SD cutoff from the mean volume of healthy controls, all patients had unilateral hippocampal atrophy. Group differences were assessed by vertex-wise t-tests with correction for multiple comparisons using FDR.

In patients, SNV detected areas of inward deformations at the level of hippocampal head and body ipsilateral to the seizure focus, and areas of *mirrored* inward/outward deformations in the tail due to local shifting (Figure 4-a). There were also areas of subtle focal inward deformation at the level of the contralateral hippocampal body.

SJD analysis revealed areas of atrophy that overlapped with inward deformation regions seen on the SNV map. In addition, SJD revealed volume loss at the level of hippocampal tail where SNV had detected *mirrored* inward/outward deformation. The extent of ipsi- and contralateral atrophy in the SJD maps was more widespread than in SNV. Representative examples are shown in four patients in Figure 4.

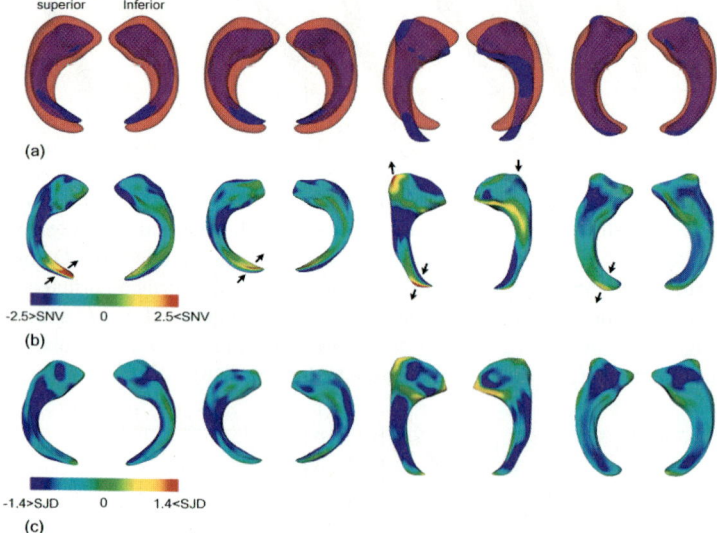

Fig. 4. Analysis of the left hippocampus in left TLE. **(a)** Four hippocampi (superior and inferior views) of TLE patients aligned to a template built from 33 control subjects. The template is shown in transparent red. The patients' hippocampi are in solid blue (purple shows areas of overlap with the template). **(b)** Signed surface-normal component maps of the displacement vectors (SNV; color scale in mm, -/+ signs indicate inward/outward deformation). Paired black arrows indicate the region where a local shifting/bending is detected. These changes at the level of the hippocampal tail are clearly visible in (a). **(c)** Surface-based Jacobian determinant maps (SJD; color scale in mm^3, -/+ signs indicate volume loss/growth).

4 Discussion and Conclusion

Medial surface and axis models allow assessing local volume changes [3]. However, these thickness-based approaches are limited to the detection of *symmetric* alterations [3]. Diseased-related morphological changes, nevertheless, may result in asymmetrical deformations. While SPHARM-PDM accurately localizes *asymmetrical* morphological changes it does not yield insights in the nature of the difference, i.e., whether it is due to shrinkage or a shifting/bending process.

We propose a new approach to differentiate these processes by computing the Jacobian determinant on the deformation field estimated from the displacement vectors produced by SPHARM. This is done by solving the heat equation using vertex-wise displacement vectors as a boundary condition. Our method enables the detection of local *asymmetrical* volume changes independent of shifting and bending, thus complementing SPHARM and providing new insights to the interpretation of morphological processes associated with neurological disorders.

Our experiments suggest that the heat equation interpolation kernel size should be equal or smaller than the expected volume changes, even though a too small kernel would decrease accuracy.

In a previous surface-based displacement analysis in TLE, the nature of posterior hippocampal deformations could not be interpreted [1]. In our study combining traditional SPHARM-PDM and surface-based Jacobian determinant, we were able to differentiate atrophy from displacement. In addition, surface-based Jacobian determinant allowed detecting atrophy where SPHARM showed mirrored changes.

In the current study, we adopted a template-dependent method to analyze the surface normal component of displacement vectors. Recently Styner et al. [4] developed a template free method to assess positioning changes. However, this method does not assess the direction of changes. Since our aim was to provide a biological meaningful interpretation of local volume changes, we favored a template-dependent approach. By creating a template made of a large number of hippocampal surfaces any bias related to shape was minimized.

References

1. Hogan, R.E., et al.: MRI-based high-dimensional hippocampal mapping in mesial temporal lobe epilepsy. Brain 127, 1731–1740 (2004)
2. Csernansky, J.G., et al.: Early DAT is distinguished from aging by high-dimensional mapping of the hippocampus. Neurology 55, 1636–1643 (2000)
3. Styner, M., et al.: Boundary and medial shape analysis of the hippocampus in schizophrenia. Medical Image Analysis 8, 197–203 (2004)
4. Styner, M., et al.: Statistical Shape Analysis of Brain Structures using SPHARM-PDM. In: MICCAI 2006 Opensource workshop (2006)
5. Chung, M.K., et al.: A unified statistical approach to deformation-based morphometry. NeuroImage 14, 595–606 (2001)
6. Ashburner, J., Friston, K.J.: Voxel-based morphometry: the methods. NeuroImage 11, 805–821 (2000)
7. Janke, A.L., et al.: 4D deformation modeling of cortical disease progression in Alzheimer's dementia. Magnetic Resonance in Medicine 46, 661–666 (2001)
8. Douglas Jr., J., Rachford Jr., H.H.: On the numerical solution of heat conduction problems in two and three space variables. Trans. Amer. Math. Soc. 82, 421–439 (1956)

Discovering Structure in the Space of Activation Profiles in fMRI

Danial Lashkari[1], Ed Vul[2], Nancy Kanwisher[2], and Polina Golland[1]

[1] Computer Science and Artificial Intelligence Laboratory, MIT, USA
[2] Brain and Cognitive Science Department, MIT, USA

Abstract. We present a method for discovering patterns of activation observed through fMRI in experiments with multiple stimuli/tasks. We introduce an explicit parameterization for the profiles of activation and represent fMRI time courses as such profiles using linear regression estimates. Working in the space of activation profiles, we design a mixture model that finds the major activation patterns along with their localization maps and derive an algorithm for fitting the model to the fMRI data. The method enables functional group analysis independent of spatial correspondence among subjects. We validate this model in the context of category selectivity in the visual cortex, demonstrating good agreement with prior findings based on hypothesis-driven methods.

1 Introduction

In contrast to early fMRI studies that commonly used a simple task-versus-fixation setup to localize functional areas of interest, modern fMRI experiments aim to explore and understand brain activations induced by an increasing number of tasks or stimuli. In this paper, we introduce a representation for fMRI activations that naturally lends itself to exploratory analysis of the space of observed activation patterns. We demonstrate a method for such analysis in individual subjects and in a population, using visual fMRI experiments to validate our approach.

Our motivation comes from fMRI studies of category selectivity in visual cortex (high level vision) where subjects are presented with several categories of visual stimuli. Using hypothesis-driven localization methods [1], investigators discovered regions with specific category selectivity which consistently appear in most subjects. For instance, the well-known fusiform face area (FFA) is associated with higher response to faces when compared to other visual stimuli. In addition, the parahippocampal place area (PPA), and extrastriate body area (EBA) exhibit high selectivity for places, and body parts, respectively [2].

While hypothesis-driven methods provide a convenient tool for testing highly specific hypotheses about activations, they usually consider and compare only two experimental conditions (categories) at a time. Spatial consistency of the localization maps across subjects serves as evidence for the validity of the corresponding hypothesis. With the increasing number of conditions or tasks, it becomes more challenging with these methods to search the entire set of possible activations, for instance, all hypothetical areas activated by more than one condition. Moreover, this approach leaves out the question of what constitutes a good hypothesis. This is in stark contrast with the goals of a fMRI experiment aiming to model visual processing in the brain by finding structure in the space of activations due to visual stimuli.

An alternative approach is to employ exploratory, unsupervised learning methods, which can be broadly grouped into two classes. The first class of methods works on the raw time courses and uses clustering [3,4,5] or Independent Component Analysis [6,7] to estimate a decomposition of the data into a set of distinct time courses of interest and their localization maps. However, this framework offers no clear mechanism for characterizing the relationship between the multitude of experimental conditions and the noisy representative time courses identified in such analysis. The second group of exploratory methods uses the information from the experimental setup to define a measure of similarity between voxels, effectively projecting the original high-dimensional time courses onto a low dimensional feature space, followed by clustering in the new space [3,8,9].

Here, we present an exploratory method that aims to identify patterns of activation (e.g., patterns of category selectivity in high level vision) in complex experimental setups. We introduce an *activation profile*, a low-dimensional representation that directly reflects the effects of experimental conditions. Working in the space of activation profiles, we employ mixture modeling to find the strongest patterns of activation present in the data. Rather than relying on spatial consistency to establish the validity of the detected activation pattern, we employ *functional* consistency across subjects to evaluate the robustness, and therefore relevance, of the detected profiles. Thus, we obtain a fully functional characterization of the data.

We emphasize that our goal is to find patterns of activation in complex experimental setups, unlike previous feature-based clustering methods [8,9] that mainly focused on identifying the "active" voxels in simple experiments. In the case of high level vision, our results agree with the findings in the field that were established as a result of numerous hypothesis-driven fMRI studies.

2 Methods

We present our method in three steps. First, we introduce the space of activation profiles, our representation of fMRI data. Then, we describe our mixture model which finds the prototypical activation profiles and their corresponding localization maps. Finally, we discuss our approach to group analysis.

2.1 Space of Activation Profiles for Category Selectivity

We define an activation profile to be a vector whose components describe selectivity to different categories. Given a set of raw fMRI time courses, we apply a General Linear Model (GLM) analysis [1] at each voxel and form a vector containing the estimated regression coefficients of the experiment stimuli. The norm

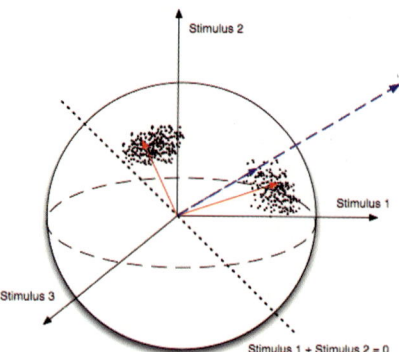

Fig. 1. An artificial population of voxels illustrating the space of activation profiles. The experiment presents three stimuli and evokes two distinct profiles. The blue, dashed line shows an original vector of regression coefficients. A hypothesis test comparing the first and second stimuli projects the vector of regression coefficients onto the dotted line; the significance is a function of the projection coefficient. The red vectors are the cluster mean profiles.

of these vectors is mainly a byproduct of irrelevant variables such as distance from major vessels or, the overall magnitude of response to the type of stimuli used in the experiment. Moreover, it is widely accepted that only relative values of responses are important in characterizing selectivity to different stimuli. To reflect these two properties in our representation, we choose to normalize the activation profiles to be unit length vectors. This removes the effect of the magnitude of activation while preserving the relative strength of activation across categories. With D categories of visual stimuli present in the experiment, our space of activation profiles is a unit sphere S^{D-1} in a D-dimensional space. A unit vector in this space represents a specific form of category selectivity. For instance, a profile completely parallel to a single dimension represents perfect selectivity to the corresponding category.

When represented in the space of activation profiles, an fMRI data set becomes a population of vectors on a unit sphere. Naturally, the interesting patterns of selectivity in this population correspond to the directions with highest concentration of data points around them (Fig. 1). It is easy to see that finding these patterns can be thought of as clustering the activation profiles and estimating the corresponding cluster means as described in the next section.

2.2 Estimating Patterns of Category Selectivity

Let $\{\mathbf{y}_v\}_{v=1}^V$ be a set of activation profiles of V brain voxels on a S^{D-1} sphere. We devise a mixture model based on correlation as the natural measure of similarity for unit vectors. We assume the vectors are i.i.d. samples from a mixture distribution

$$p(\mathbf{y}; \{q_k, \mathbf{m}_k\}_{k=1}^{K}, \mu) = \sum_{k=1}^{K} q_k f(\mathbf{y}; \mathbf{m}_k, \mu). \tag{1}$$

where $\{q_k\}_{k=1}^{K}$ denotes the weights of K model components and $f(\mathbf{y}; \mathbf{m}, \mu)$ is a distribution defined on a unit sphere. We choose the simplest such distribution, *von Mises-Fisher distribution* [10]

$$f(\mathbf{y}; \mathbf{m}, \mu) = C_D(\mu) e^{\mu \langle \mathbf{m}, \mathbf{y} \rangle}, \qquad C_D(\mu) = \frac{\mu^{D/2-1}}{(2\pi)^{D/2} I_{D/2-1}(\mu)} \tag{2}$$

where $\langle \cdot, \cdot \rangle$ denotes the inner product of two vectors and the normalizing constant $C_D(\mu)$ is defined in terms of the γ-th order modified Bessel function of the first kind I_γ. This distribution is an exponential function of the correlation between voxel activation vector $\mathbf{y}$ and the cluster activation profile $\mathbf{m}$. The *concentration parameter* μ controls the concentration of the distribution around the mean direction $\mathbf{m}$. In general, mixture components can have distinct concentration parameters but in this work, we use the same parameter for all the clusters to ensure a more robust estimation.

We use the EM algorithm [12] to solve the corresponding maximum likelihood estimation. We define $p^{(t)}(k|\mathbf{y}_v)$ to be the posterior probability that voxel v is associated with the mixture component k at step t. Through a bit of algebra, we the update rules:

E-step: $$p^{(t)}(k|\mathbf{y}_v) \propto e^{\mu^{(t)} \langle \mathbf{m}_k^{(t)}, \mathbf{y}_v \rangle}, \tag{3}$$

M-step: $$q_k^{(t+1)} = \frac{1}{V} \sum_{v=1}^{V} p^{(t)}(k|\mathbf{y}_v), \qquad \mathbf{m}_k^{(t+1)} \propto \sum_{v=1}^{V} \mathbf{y}_v p^{(t)}(k|\mathbf{y}_v), \tag{4}$$

$$\frac{I_{D/2}(\mu^{(t+1)})}{I_{D/2-1}(\mu^{(t+1)})} = \frac{1}{V} \sum_{l=1}^{K} \sum_{v=1}^{V} p^{(t)}(k|\mathbf{y}_v) \langle \mathbf{m}_k^{(t)}, \mathbf{y}_v \rangle, \tag{5}$$

where $q_k^{(t)}$, $\mathbf{m}_k^{(t)}$, and $\mu^{(t+1)}$ are the parameter estimates at step t. We normalize vectors $\mathbf{m}_k^{(t)}$ in each step to unit length. The nonlinear equation (5) for the estimation of $\mu^{(t+1)}$ can be solved with a simple zero-finding algorithm. We note that this model was independently developed previously in the context of clustering text data [11].

Using the above algorithm, we find K representative activation profiles $\mathbf{m}_k$ and a set of soft assignments $p(k|\mathbf{y}_v)$. The assignments define localization maps of different activation profiles.

2.3 Group Analysis of the Activation Profiles

Since we aim to discover activation patterns that robustly appear in brain activations, it is reasonable then to assume that the space of activation profiles is shared across subjects.

We denote a voxel in an experiment with S subjects by $\mathbf{y}_v^s$, where $s \in \{1, \cdots, S\}$ is the subject label and v is the voxel index as before. If the set of vectors $\mathbf{m}_k$ truly descbribes all noteworthy activation profiles of the brain, each voxel $\mathbf{y}_v^s$ could be thought of as an independent sample from the same distribution (1). Thus, we can combine the data from several subjects to form the *group data*, i.e., $\{\{\mathbf{y}_v^s\}_{v=1}^{V_s}\}_{s=1}^{S}$, to perform our analysis across subjects. Applying the same algorithm on the group data, the resulting $\{p(k|\mathbf{y}_{v,s})\}_{v=1}^{V_s}$ defines the localization map of activation profile k in subject s. We note that no spatial registration of subjects is required for this step.

3 Experimental Results

We demonstrate our method on the data from a block design fMRI experiment on 9 subjects using five categories of images: bodies, faces, objects, scenes, and scrambled images. Each block lasts 16 seconds and contains 20 images from one catcgory with an interval of fixation separating it from other blocks. Each run contains two blocks of each category; blocks of the same category do not share images. We perform motion-correction, spike detection, intensity normalization, and Gaussian smoothing with a kernel of 3-mm width using the standard package *FreeSurfer*. We apply General Linear Model [1] to estimate 5 regression coefficients for the stimulus categories and form a 5-dimensional vector for each voxel. To discard the voxels not activated by any of the visual categories, we run a t-test comparing the response of each voxel to fixation, keeping only the voxels which show significance with $p \leq 10^{-4}$. The resulting data is a set of 5-dimensional vectors corresponding to the voxels that demonstrate significant response to at least one category of presented images.

3.1 Activation Profiles

Since our main goal is to discover important patterns of activation, we first examine the resulting cluster profiles. Fig. 2 (Left) shows the selectivity profiles for the clusters found in the data from one of the subjects found for $K = 8$. The largest cluster corresponds to the visually responsive voxels that do not show differential response to the variety of categories presented in this experiment. Such a cluster appears in all our results from single-subject and group data sets. The smaller clusters exhibit the selectivity patterns expected based on the previous studies. According to the rough definition commonly used in the field, the response of a selective region to its category is at least two times stronger than that of any other category. We find such selective clusters for bodies (clusters 2, 5, and 6,) scenes (clusters 3 and 7,) and faces (clusters 4 and 8,) corresponding to the EBA, PPA, and FFA, respectively. These profiles only differ in their strengths of selectivity. The interesting aspect of this result is that *we do not find clusters corresponding to the types of category selectivity not observed before*. For instance, no scrambled-image-selective region or double-category selectivity is observed.

Using the data from all 9 subjects, we run a group data analysis. Fig. 2 (Right) shows the resulting group profiles. The group profiles are very similar to the ones found in the single subject data, supporting our assumption that

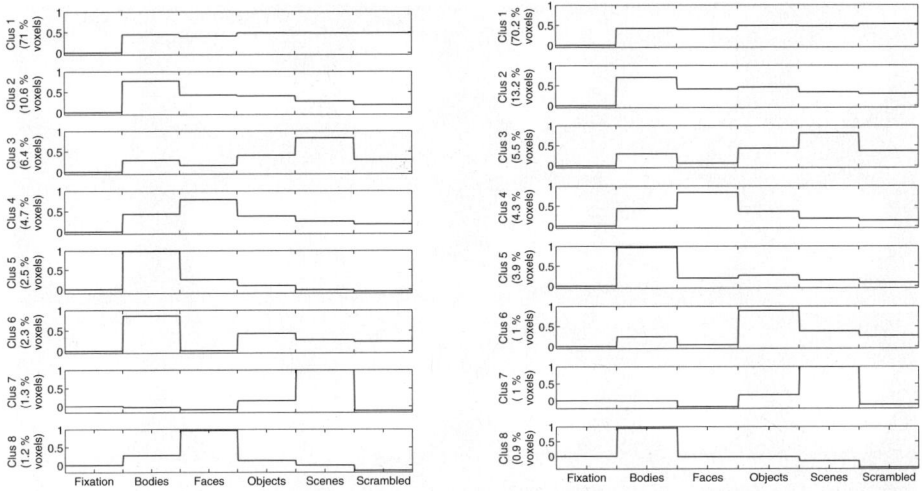

Fig. 2. Cluster profiles for (Left) a single subject and (Right) group data for 9 subjects. The clusters are ordered based on their estimated weight in the model.

the space of activations is shared across subjects. However, we also expect to see some differences due to factors such as subject variablitity and noise. Group data yields more robust estimates of the cluster profiles by providing more samples per cluster.

3.2 Spatial Maps

We examine the spatial maps our algorithm associates with cluster profiles by comparing them with the standard maps of FFA, PPA, and EBA. To find these standard maps, we apply t-tests comparing each voxel's response for faces, scenes, and bodies, to its response for objects, and threshold the resulting significance maps at $p = 10^{-4}$. From our algorithm's results, we accept any profile whose component for one of the three categories of interest is at least 1.5 times all other components. The cluster assignments found in our method represent probabilities over cluster labels. Here, we assign each voxel to its corresponding MAP cluster label to find a binary map. Fig. 3 shows the standard map of face selective region (FFA) for the same subject in Fig. 2 (Left). It also shows the voxels assigned by our method to clusters 4 and 8 in Fig. 2 (Left). These clusters are face-selective according to the above definition. Although the two maps are derived with very different assumptions, they clearly agree.

We quantify the agreement between these binary, spatial maps by measuring their uncentered correlation. For example, the correlation between the two maps presented in Fig. 3 is 0.29. We also form the map associated with the largest cluster as another case for comparison and call it the non-selective profile. Table 1 shows the resulting correlation values averaged across all subjects for $K = 7, 8$, and 9.

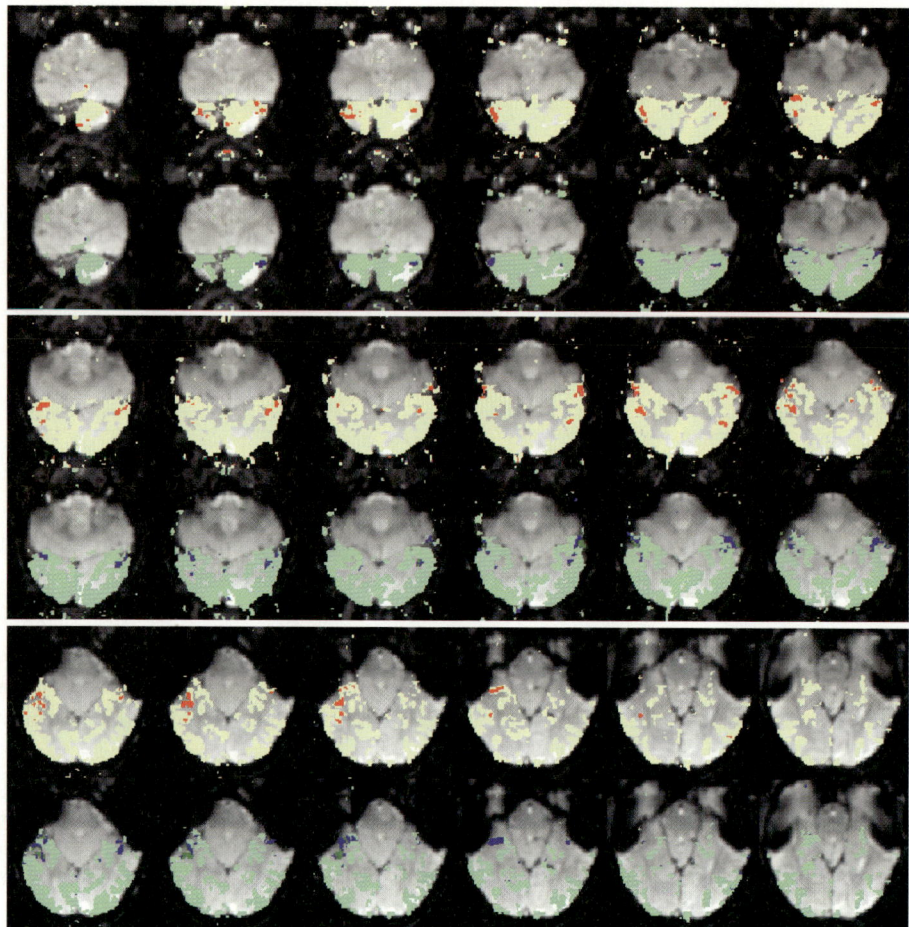

Fig. 3. Spatial maps of the face selective regions found by the statistical test (red) and the mixture model (dark blue). The same slices from the two maps are presented in alternating rows. The mask of visually responsive voxels is shown in different colors (yellow for the hypothesis test, and light green for ours) in the backgound of the two maps to help the visual comparison.

We first note that the correlation between the functionally related regions is significantly higher than the other ones. Moreover, the spatial correlation is insensitive to the number of clusters. In genereal, we observed that increasing the number of clusers results only in the split of some clusters, and does not significantly alter the pattern of the discovered profiles. In the table, we also present the spatial correlations obtained from subject-specific activation profiles. The correlation values are quite similar to the group analysis, which suggests that by forming the group data, we have not lost the accuracy of our method in identifying the functional areas in individual subjects. Moreover, we have

Table 1. Correlation between the spatial maps constructed with our method and those from the t-test. Values are averaged across all 9 subjects in the experiment.

Group $K=7$	FFA	PPA	EBA	Group $K=8$	FFA	PPA	EBA
Face Profile	0.37 ± 0.09	0.00	0.04 ± 0.03	Face Profile	0.37 ± 0.10	0.00	0.04 ± 0.03
Scene Profile	0	0.31 ± 0.14	0.00 ± 0.01	Scene Profile	0	0.31 ± 0.14	0.00 ± 0.01
Body Profile	0.04 ± 0.03	0.00	0.51 ± 0.07	Body Profile	0.05 ± 0.04	0.00	0.47 ± 0.08
Non-sel. Profile	0.05 ± 0.04	0.06 ± 0.04	0.04 ± 0.04	Non-sel. Profile	0.05 ± 0.04	0.06 ± 0.04	0.02 ± 0.03
Group $K=9$	**FFA**	**PPA**	**EBA**	**Indiv. $K=8$**	**FFA**	**PPA**	**EBA**
Face Profile	0.36 ± 0.10	0.00	0.04 ± 0.03	Face Profile	0.31 ± 0.13	0.00	0.02 ± 0.02
Scene Profile	0	0.31 ± 0.14	0.00 ± 0.01	Scene Profile	0	0.30 ± 0.13	0.00
Body Profile	0.03 ± 0.03	0.00	0.48 ± 0.08	Body Profile	0.03 ± 0.04	0.00	0.49 ± 0.09
Non-sel. Profile	0.05 ± 0.04	0.06 ± 0.04	0.02 ± 0.03	Non-sel. Profile	0.04 ± 0.04	0.06 ± 0.04	0.02 ± 0.01

established correspondence among these functionally defined areas, as all of them are now associated with the same profile of activation in the group data.

We emphasize that from our perspective, the statistical significance maps are not the ground truth but rather a competing hypothesis for explaining the data. In fact, the neuroscientific definition of the selective regions only includes a subset of the standard map, identified by the experts based on prior knowledge of the approximate locations. Therefore, we do not seek a perfect agreement between the spatial maps.

4 Conclusion

We presented a mixture-model algorithm which finds the profiles of fMRI activation due to different experimental condition. It enables group analysis without spatial co-registration of subjects. Our algorithm promises benefits in discovering new category selective regions in high level vision and other problems with complex experimental setup. Representing the fMRI data in the space of activation profiles makes it possible to define the consistency of a discovered profile aross subjects as an alternative for the traditionally used registration-based spatial consistency. We are currently working on methods for investigating cross-subject consistency in this space.

Acknowledgements. This research was supported in part by NIH grants NIBIB NAMIC U54-EB005149, and NCRR NAC P41-RR13218, and by the NSF CAREER grant 0642971.

References

1. Friston, K.J., et al.: Statistical parametric maps in functional imaging: a general linear approach. Hum. Brain Mapp. 2, 189–210 (1995)
2. Kanwisher, N.G.: The ventral visual object pathway in humans: evidence from fMRI. In: Chalupa, L., Werner, J. (eds.) The Visual Neurosciences. MIT Press, Cambridge (2003)

3. Goutte, C., et al.: On clustering fMRI time series. NeuroImage 9, 298–310 (1999)
4. Baumgartner, R., et al.: Fuzzy clustering of gradient-echo functional MRI in the human visual cortex. J. Magnetic Resonance Imaging 7(6), 1094–1108 (1997)
5. Golland, P., et al.: Detection of spatial activation patterns as unsupervised segmentation of fMRI data. In: Ayache, N., Ourselin, S., Maeder, A. (eds.) MICCAI 2007, Part I. LNCS, vol. 4791, pp. 110–118. Springer, Heidelberg (2007)
6. McKeown, J.M., et al.: Analysis of fMRI data by blind separation into independent spatial components. Hum. Brain Mapp. 10, 160–178 (2000)
7. Beckmann, C.F., Smith, S.M.: Tensorial extensions of independent component analysis for group fMRI data analysis. NeuroImage 25(1), 294–311 (2005)
8. Goutte, C., et al.: Feature-space clustering for fMRI meta-analysis. Hum. Brain Mapp. 13, 165–183 (2001)
9. Thirion, B., Faugeras, O.: Feature detection in fMRI data: the information bottleneck approach. In: Ellis, R.E., Peters, T.M. (eds.) MICCAI 2003. LNCS, vol. 2879, pp. 83–91. Springer, Heidelberg (2003)
10. Mardia, K.V.: Statistics of directional data. J. R. Statist. Soc. Series B 37, 349–393 (1975)
11. Banerjee, A., et al.: Clustering on the unit hypersphere using von Mises-Fisher distribution. J. Mach. Learn. Res. 6, 1345–1382 (2005)
12. Dempster, A., et al.: Maximum likelihood from incomplete data via the EM algorithm. J. R. Statist. Soc. Series B 39, 1–38 (1977)

Left Ventricle Tracking Using Overlap Priors

Ismail Ben Ayed[1], Yingli Lu[1], Shuo Li[1], and Ian Ross[2]

GE Healthcare, London, ON, Canada
London Health Sciences Centre, London, ON, Canada

Abstract. This study investigates *overlap priors* for tracking the Left Ventricle (LV) endo- and epicardium boundaries in cardiac Magnetic Resonance (MR) sequences. It consists of evolving two curves following the Euler-Lagrange minimization of two functionals each containing an original overlap prior constraint. The latter measures the conformity of the overlap between the *nonparametric* (kernel-based) intensity distributions within the three target regions–LV cavity, myocardium and background–to a prior learned from a given segmentation of the first frame. The *Bhattacharyya* coefficient is used as an overlap measure. Different from existing intensity-driven constraints, the overlap priors do not assume *implicitly* that the overlap between the distributions within different regions has to be minimal. Although neither shape priors nor curve coupling were used, quantitative evaluation showed that the results correlate well with independent manual segmentations and the method compares favorably with other recent methods. The overlap priors lead to a LV tracking which is more versatile than existing methods because the solution is not bounded to the shape/intensity characteristics of a training set. We also demonstrate experimentally that the used overlap measures are approximately constant over a cardiac sequence.

1 Introduction

Tracking the Left Ventricle (LV) endo- and epicardium boundaries in cardiac Magnetic Resonance (MR) sequences plays an essential role in diagnosing cardiovascular diseases. It consists of segmenting each frame into three regions: LV cavity, myocardium and background. Manual tracing is time-consuming. Therefore, an automatic tracking is desired. Although several techniques have addressed this task [2]–[7], [9]–[11], accurate LV tracking is still acknowledged as a difficult problem because of the overlap between the intensity distributions within the cardiac regions (cf. the typical example in Fig. 1), the lack of edge information and the intensity/shape variability from one patient to another [10].

As discussed by Freedman et al. in [15], most of existing methods in medical image segmentation compute a pixelwise correspondence between the current image (or frame) and model distributions of shape and appearance (or intensity). Model distributions are generally learned from a training set and embedded in the segmentation via two standard frameworks: variational level-sets [1] (such as [2]–[7]) and active appearance/shape models [8] (such as [9]–[11]).

In the level-set framework [2]–[7], the problem is commonly stated as the minimization of a functional containing two constraints: a shape prior constraint and an intensity-driven constraint based on the Maximum Likelihood (ML) principle. The latter maximizes the conditional probability of pixel intensity given the assumed model distribution within each region. Unfortunately, a ML intensity-driven constraint is sensitive to inaccuracies in estimating model distributions [12]. More importantly, it can not incorporate information about the *overlap* between the intensity distributions within different regions. Based on the evaluation of a pixelwise correspondence between the image and the models, ML intensity-driven constraints assume *implicitly* that the overlap between the distributions within different regions has to be *minimal*. The pixelwise information is misleading in the case of the LV due to the "significant" (cf. the typical example in Fig. 1) overlap between the distributions within the cardiac regions. Consequently, the use of geometric priors (such as shape) in conjunction with ML intensity-driven constraints was inevitable to obtain satisfying results [5], [6]. Similar to variational level-set approaches, active appearance/shape models compute a pixelwise correspondence between the image and the models [15]. As we will show in the experiments (section 3), embedding global information about the overlap between the intensity distributions within the segmentation regions is important. In the current study, we devise overlap priors for LV tracking.

The current study is most related to recent variational segmentation/tracking methods [12]–[14] using *similarity/dissimilarity* measures between intensity distributions. Using the Bhattacharyya coefficient as an overlap measure, we propose to track the endo- and epicardium boundaries in a cardiac MR sequence by evolving two active curves following the Euler-Lagrange minimization of two functionals each containing an original *overlap prior*. The latter measures the conformity of the overlap between the *nonparametric* (kernel-based) intensity distributions within the three target regions–LV cavity, myocardium and background–to a prior learned from a given segmentation of the first frame.

The overlap priors lead to a method which has several advantages over existing ones: (1) shape priors are not needed to obtain satisfying LV tracking because the overlap priors prevent the endo- and epicardium boundaries from spilling, respectively, into the cavity and the background; (2) no assumption is made as to the *parametric* distributions of intensity/shape data; (3) *explicit* curve coupling [7], [3] is not required because the proposed functionals and two-step minimization yield an *implicit* coupling. Those advantages lead to a LV tracking which is more versatile than existing ones because the solution is not bounded to the shape/intensity properties learned from a finite training set.

2 Formulation

Let $\mathcal{I}$ be a MR cardiac sequence containing N frames[1], $I^n : \Omega \subset \mathbb{R}^2 \to \mathbb{R}^+$, $n \in [1..N]$. The purpose of this study is to automatically detect the endocardium (yellow contour in Fig. 1.a) and the epicardium (green contour in Fig. 1.a) of the

---
[1] The number of frames N is typically equal to 20 or 25.

heart for each $n \in [2..N]$. We formulate the problem as the evolution of two closed planar parametric curves, $\boldsymbol{\Gamma}^n_{in}(s), \boldsymbol{\Gamma}^n_{out}(s) : [0, 1] \to \Omega$, toward, respectively, the endo- and epicardium. The curve evolution equations are sought following the minimization of two original functionals based on the notion of *overlap* between the intensity distributions within three target regions: (1) the heart cavity C^n corresponding to the interior of curve $\boldsymbol{\Gamma}^n_{in}$: $C^n = \mathbf{R}_{\boldsymbol{\Gamma}^n_{in}}$, (2) the myocardium M^n corresponding to the region between $\boldsymbol{\Gamma}^n_{in}$ and $\boldsymbol{\Gamma}^n_{out}$: $M^n = \mathbf{R}^c_{\boldsymbol{\Gamma}^n_{in}} \cap \mathbf{R}_{\boldsymbol{\Gamma}^n_{out}}$ and (3) the background B^n corresponding to the region outside $\boldsymbol{\Gamma}^n_{out}$: $B^n = \mathbf{R}^c_{\boldsymbol{\Gamma}^n_{out}}$.

The proposed functionals: For each $\mathbf{R} \in \{C^n, M^n, B^n, n = 1..N\}$, define $P_{\mathbf{R},I}$ as the nonparametric (kernel-based) estimate of intensity distribution within region $\mathbf{R}$ in frame $I \in \{I^n, n = 1..N\}$

$$\forall z \in \mathbb{R}^+, \; P_{\mathbf{R},I}(z) = \frac{\int_{\mathbf{R}} K(z - I(x))dx}{a_{\mathbf{R}}} \quad (1)$$

where $a_{\mathbf{R}}$ is the area of region $\mathbf{R}$: $a_{\mathbf{R}} = \int_{\mathbf{R}} d\mathbf{x}$. Typical choices of K are the Dirac function and the Gaussian kernel [12]. Let $\mathcal{B}(f/g)$ be the Bhattacharyya coefficient[2] measuring the amount of overlap between two statistical samples f and g [12]

$$\mathcal{B}(f/g) = \sum_{z \in \mathbb{R}^+} \sqrt{f(z)g(z)} \quad (2)$$

We assume that a segmentation of the first frame I^1, i.e., a partition $\{C^1, M^1, B^1\}$, is given. Consider

$$\mathbf{B}^n_{in} = \mathcal{B}(P_{C^n, I^n}/P_{M^1, I^1}); \; \mathbf{B}^n_{out} = \mathcal{B}(P_{M^n, I^n}/P_{B^1, I^1}) \;\; \forall n \in [1..N] \quad (3)$$

$\mathbf{B}^n_{in}$ measures the overlap between the intensity distributions within the LV cavity and the myocardium in I^n. $\mathbf{B}^n_{out}$ measures the overlap between the intensity distributions within the myocardium and the background in I^n. As we will demonstrate *experimentally* in section 3, $\mathbf{B}^n_{in}$ and $\mathbf{B}^n_{out}$ are *approximately constant* over a cardiac sequence. Consequently, measures $\mathbf{B}^1_{in}$ and $\mathbf{B}^1_{out}$ estimated from a given segmentation of the first frame in sequence $\mathcal{I}$ can be used as *overlap priors* to constrain the tracking in frames $I^2..I^N$. We adopt a two-step curve evolution for each $n \in [2..N]$. First, we evolve the endocardium boundary, $\boldsymbol{\Gamma}^n_{in}$, following the minimization of

$$\mathcal{F}^n_{in} = \underbrace{\alpha(\mathbf{B}^n_{in} - \mathbf{B}^1_{in})^2}_{\text{Overlap cavity/myocardium}} + \underbrace{\beta(\mu^n_{in} - \mu^1_{in})^2}_{\text{Cavity mean}} + \underbrace{\lambda \oint_{\boldsymbol{\Gamma}^n_{in}} (g_n + c)ds}_{\text{Endocardium boundary}} \quad (4)$$

where μ^n_{in} is the estimate of intensity mean within C^n_{in} for $n \in [1..N]$: $\mu^n_{in} = \frac{\int_{C^n} I^n d\mathbf{x}}{a_{C^n}}$, $g_n = \frac{1}{1+\|\nabla I^n\|^2}$ is an edge indicator function which biases the curve toward high gradient of intensity and c is a constant to enforce curve smoothness.

---

[2] Note that the values of $\mathcal{B}$ are always in $[0, 1]$, where 0 indicates that there is no overlap, and 1 indicates a perfect match.

α, β and λ are positive real constants to balance the contribution of each term. Second, we fix the obtained $\boldsymbol{\Gamma}_{in}^n$ and minimize the following functional with respect to the epicardium boundary, i.e., $\boldsymbol{\Gamma}_{out}$

$$\mathcal{F}_{out}^n = \underbrace{\alpha(\mathbf{B}_{out}^n - \mathbf{B}_{out}^1)^2}_{Overlap\ myocardium/background} + \underbrace{\beta(\mu_{out}^n - \mu_{out}^1)^2}_{Myocardium\ mean} + \underbrace{\lambda \oint_{\boldsymbol{\Gamma}_{out}^n} (g_n + c)ds}_{Epicardium\ boundary} \quad (5)$$

where μ_{out}^n is the estimate of intensity mean within M_{in}^n for $n \in [1..N]$: $\mu_{out}^n = \frac{\int_{M^n} I^n d\mathbf{x}}{a_{M^n}}$. In section 3, we will validate experimentally the usefulness of the proposed overlap terms: for ten different datasets, we will confirm with manual segmentations that $(\mathbf{B}_{in}^n - \mathbf{B}_{in}^1)^2$ and $(\mathbf{B}_{out}^n - \mathbf{B}_{out}^1)^2$ are approximately equal to zero (refer to table 2).

Curve evolution minimization equations: Curve evolutions are obtained by the Euler-Lagrange descent equations. We embed each curve $\boldsymbol{\Gamma} \in \{\boldsymbol{\Gamma}_{in}^n, \boldsymbol{\Gamma}_{out}^n\}$ in a one-parameter family of curves: $\boldsymbol{\Gamma}(s,t) : [0,1] \times \mathbf{R}^+ \to \Omega$, and solve the partial differential equations: $\frac{\partial \boldsymbol{\Gamma}_{in}^n(s,t)}{\partial t} = -\frac{\partial \mathcal{F}_{in}}{\partial \boldsymbol{\Gamma}_{in}^n}$, $\frac{\partial \boldsymbol{\Gamma}_{out}^n(s,t)}{\partial t} = -\frac{\partial \mathcal{F}_{out}}{\partial \boldsymbol{\Gamma}_{out}^n}$. After some algebraic manipulations, we obtain the final curve evolution equations

$$\frac{\partial \boldsymbol{\Gamma}_{in}^n}{\partial t} = \{\frac{\alpha(\mathbf{B}_{in}^n - \mathbf{B}_{in}^1)}{a_{C^n}}(\mathbf{B}_{in}^n - \sqrt{\frac{P_{M^1,I^1}}{P_{C^n,I^n}}}) + \frac{2\beta(\mu_{in}^n - \mu_{in}^1)}{a_{C^n}}(\mu_{in}^n - I^n)$$
$$+ \lambda[\nabla g_n . \boldsymbol{n}_{in}^n - (g_n + c)\kappa_{in}^n]\}\boldsymbol{n}_{in}^n$$
$$\frac{\partial \boldsymbol{\Gamma}_{out}^n}{\partial t} = \{\frac{(\mathbf{B}_{out}^n - \mathbf{B}_{out}^1)}{a_{M^n}}(\mathbf{B}_{out}^n - \sqrt{\frac{P_{B^1,I^1}}{P_{M^n,I^n}}}) + \frac{2\beta(\mu_{out}^n - \mu_{out}^1)}{a_{M^n}}(\mu_{out}^n - I^n)$$
$$+ \lambda[\nabla g_n . \boldsymbol{n}_{out}^n - (g_n + c)\kappa_{out}^n]\}\boldsymbol{n}_{out}^n \quad (6)$$

where $\boldsymbol{n}_{in}^n$ and $\boldsymbol{n}_{out}^n$ are the outward unit normals to, respectively, $\boldsymbol{\Gamma}_{in}^n$ and $\boldsymbol{\Gamma}_{out}^n$. κ_{in}^n and κ_{out}^n are the mean curvature functions of, respectively, $\boldsymbol{\Gamma}_{in}^n$ and $\boldsymbol{\Gamma}_{out}^n$. Partition (C^n, M^n, B^n) of frame I^n is obtained from $\boldsymbol{\Gamma}_{in}^n$ and $\boldsymbol{\Gamma}_{out}^n$ at convergence i.e., when $t \to \infty$. The level-set framework [1] is used to implement the evolution equations in (6). The level-set implementation has well-known advantages over explicit curve discretization and can be effected by stable numerical schemes.

3 Experiments

In the following, we first give a typical example which demonstrates clearly the advantage of using overlap constraints over the commonly used ML constraints. Then, we describe a statistical performance evaluation of the method by comparisons with manual segmentations and other variational methods [2], [3]. We also evaluate the statistics of the proposed overlap priors/measures over

Left Ventricle Tracking Using Overlap Priors   1029

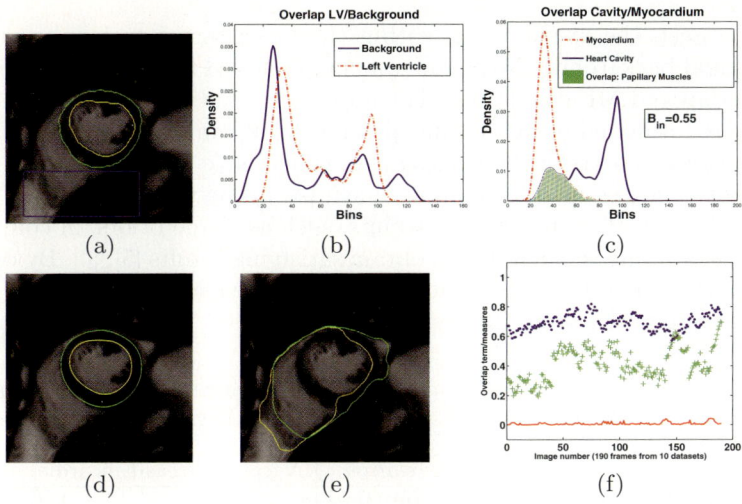

Fig. 1. Advantage of overlap constraints: (a) manual segmentation by a radiologist–yellow curve: endocardium, green curve: epicardium; (b) overlap between the distributions within the LV and the nearby background (region inside the blue curve in a); overlap between the distributions within the cavity and the myocardium; (d) segmentations obtained *with and overlap constraint*, i.e., with our method; (e) segmentations obtained *with a ML constraint*. **Both constraints were used without shape priors**. (f) The proposed overlap priors/measures versus the frame number (190 frames) in 10 manually segmented datasets: $\mathbf{B}_{out}^n$ (blue points); $\mathbf{B}_{in}^n$ (green markers); $(\mathbf{B}_{out}^n - \mathbf{B}_{out}^1)^2 + (\mathbf{B}_{in}^n - \mathbf{B}_{in}^1)^2$ (continuous red line).

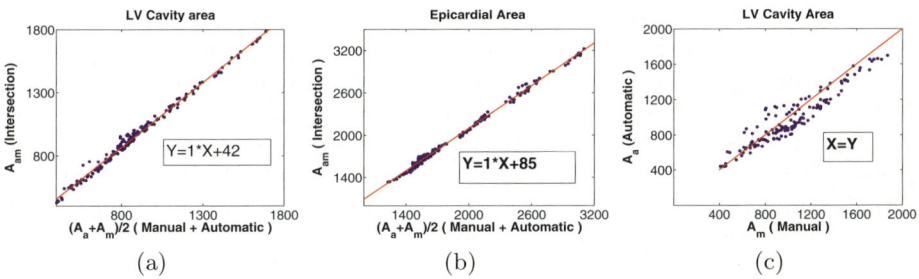

Fig. 2. Comparisons of manual and automatic segmentations in 190 images from 10 datasets. $\mathbf{A}_{am}$ versus $\frac{\mathbf{A}_a + \mathbf{A}_m}{2}$: (a) cavity area ($DM = \mathbf{0.92} \pm 0.03$); (b) epicardial area ($DM = \mathbf{0.94} \pm 0.01$). (c) Automatic versus manual LV cavity areas.

several datasets. Finally, we give a representative sample of the results for visual inspection.

(1) Overlap constraint vs. ML intensity-driven constraint: Figure 1 (a) shows a typical example of a MR mid-cavity frame. It depicts the expected segmentations of the LV cavity (region inside the yellow curve) and the epicardial region (region inside the green curve). Figs. 1 b and c illustrate the significant overlap between the distributions within the three target regions: cavity, myocardium and background. No shape priors were added for a fair comparison between overlap and ML constraints. For both constraints, model distributions of regions were estimated from the same pesegmented frame. *With a ML intensity-driven constraint*, parts of the background, which have intensity profiles similar to the cavity and the myocardium, are included inside the final curves (refer to Fig. 1.e). The use of geometric constraints, such as shape priors, in conjunction with ML constraints is inevitable to obtain satisfying results [5], [6]. By contrast, *using an overlap constraint* delineates accurately the cavity and the LV (refer to Fig. 1 d), thereby removing the need of shape priors.

Table 1. Comparisons of manual and automatic segmentations: *Dice metrics* and *correlation coefficients*. The higher the *Dice metric*, the better the segmentation.

Dice metrics	Mean	Std	*Correlation*	LV cavity areas	Epicardial areas
This method	0.93	0.02	**This method**	0.94	0.96
Method in [2]	0.81	0.16	**Method in [3]**	0.89	0.87

Table 2. Statistics of the overlap priors/measures (expressed as mean ± std) over ten datasets. The overlap priors are *approximately* equal to zero.

$\mathbf{B}_{out}^n$	$\mathbf{B}_{in}^n$	$(\mathbf{B}_{out}^n - \mathbf{B}_{out}^1)^2, (n>1)$	$(\mathbf{B}_{in}^n - \mathbf{B}_{in}^1)^2, (n>1)$
0.69 ± 0.05	0.42 ± 0.17	$1.9(10^{-3}) \pm 2.4(10^{-3})$	$6.5(10^{-3}) \pm 8.5(10^{-3})$

(2) Statistical performance evaluation: The performance of the proposed variational technique was evaluated by comparisons with independent manual segmentations approved by an experienced cardiologist. We applied the method to 2D mid-cavity MR sequences obtained from 10 patients, i.e., 10 different datasets: 190 frames were automatically segmented. *The free parameters were unchanged for all the datasets*: $\alpha = 1000, \beta = 10, \lambda = 0.1, c = 10$. Curve initializations and estimation of $B_{in}^1, B_{out}^1, \mu_{in}^1$, and μ_{out}^1 were obtained from a user-provided segmentation of the first frame in each sequence. Two clinically important measures were evaluated for performance appraisal: *LV cavity area* and *LV epicardial area*. Area measurements are expressed as the number of pixels within the region. We first used the *Dice Metric (DM)* to measure the *similarity* between manual and automatic segmentations. Let $\mathbf{A_a}$, $\mathbf{A_m}$ and $\mathbf{A_{am}}$ be the areas of, respectively, the automatically detected region, the corresponding hand-labeled region and the intersection between them. *DM* is given by $\frac{2\mathbf{A_{am}}}{\mathbf{A_a}+\mathbf{A_m}}$ [2][3]. Our algorithm yielded a *DM* equal to 0.93 ± 0.02 for all the data (*DM* is expressed as mean ± standard deviation). We obtained *DM* equal to 0.92 ± 0.03 for the LV cavity areas and *DM* equal to 0.94 ± 0.01 for the epicardial areas. Linear regression was also used to assess the differences between $\mathbf{A_{am}}$ and $\frac{\mathbf{A_a}+\mathbf{A_m}}{2}$

---

[3] *DM* is always in [0, 1]. *DM* equal to 1 indicates a perfect match between manual and automatic segmentation.

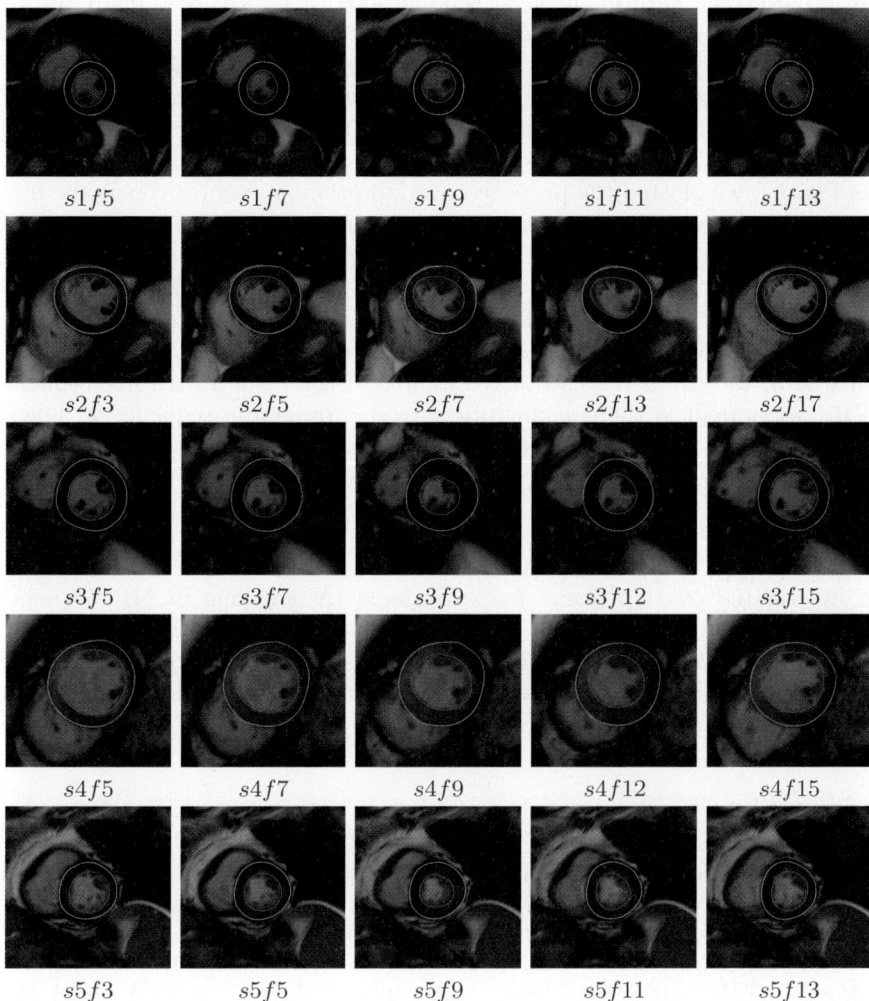

Fig. 3. Results for five MR sequences. Each row depicts the results for one sequence. $\alpha = 1000, \beta = 10, \lambda = 0.1, c = 10$. Γ_{in}^n: **red curve**, Γ_{out}^n: **green curve**.

(refer to Figs. 2 a and b). The smaller these differences, the higher the similarities between manual and automatic segmentations. The LV cavity and epicardial regression lines did not differ significantly from the identity line. We also report good correlation coefficients between manual and automatic endo- and epicardial areas (refer to table 1). To assess the differences between manual and automatic LV cavity areas, we give the linear regression plot in Fig. 2 c, displayed with the identity line.

To bear comparisons with other recent variational approaches to LV tracking, we give in table 1 the Dice metrics and correlation coefficients reported, respectively, in [2] and [3]. Our method leads to a significant improvement in accuracy over the variational level set methods in [2], [3]. Although the proposed functional does not embed shape knowledge, it compares very well with existing methods [2]-[7] which, in most cases, use shape priors. Different from ML intensity-driven constraints, the proposed overlap constraints measure the similarities between the intensity distributions within the cardiac regions, thereby removing the need of shape constraints.

In Fig. 1.f, we plotted the proposed overlap priors/measures versus the frame number (190 frames) using manual segmentations from 10 datasets. As reported in table 2, the overlap priors in Eqs. (4) and (5) are approximately equal to zero (refer to the continuous line in Fig. 1.f). This validates the usefulness of such priors for the LV tracking. It is also interesting to notice that overlap measures B_{in}^n and B_{out}^n do not vary much over different patients (refer to Fig. 1.f).

In Fig. 3, we give a representative sample of the results with five sequences ($s1$–$s5$). $sxfy$ depicts the tracking obtained for frame y in sequence x. The red and green curves represent, respectively, $\mathbf{\Gamma}_{in}^n$ and $\mathbf{\Gamma}_{out}^n$ at convergence.

4 Conclusion

We investigated overlap priors for variational LV tracking in MR sequences. Quantitative evaluation showed the advantages of overlap priors over existing intensity-driven constraints. Although neither shape priors nor curve coupling were used, the results correlated well with manual segmentations and the method compared favorably with other methods.

References

1. Cremers, D., Rousson, M., Deriche, R.: A Review of Statistical Approaches to Level Set Segmentation: Integrating Color, Texture, Motion and Shape. International Journal of Computer Vision 62, 249–265 (2007)
2. Lynch, M., Ghita, O., Whelan, P.F.: Segmentation of the Left Ventricle of the Heart in 3-D+t MRI Data Using an Optimized Nonrigid Temporal Model. IEEE Transactions on Medical Imaging 27(2), 195–203 (2008)
3. Lynch, M., Ghita, O., Whelan, P.F.: Left-ventricle myocardium segmentation using a coupled level-set with a priori knowledge. Computerized Medical Imaging and Graphics 30, 255–262 (2006)
4. Jolly, M.-P.: Automatic Segmentation of the Left Ventricle in Cardiac MR and CT Images. International Journal of Computer Vision 70(2), 151–163 (2006)
5. Kohlberger, T., Cremers, D., Rousson, M., Ramaraj, R., Funka-Lea, G.: 4D Shape Priors for a Level Set Segmentation of the Left Myocardium in SPECT Sequences. In: Larsen, R., Nielsen, M., Sporring, J. (eds.) MICCAI 2006. LNCS, vol. 4190, pp. 92–100. Springer, Heidelberg (2006)
6. Sun, W., Çetin, M., Chan, R., Reddy, V., Holmvang, G., Chandar, V., Willsky, A.: Segmenting and Tracking the Left Ventricle by Learning the Dynamics in Cardiac Images. Information Processing in Medical Imaging, 553–565 (2005)
7. Paragios, N.: A Variational Approach for the Segmentation of the Left Ventricle in Cardiac Image Analysis. IJCV 50(3), 345–362 (2002)

8. Cootes, T., Edwards, G., Taylor, C.: Active Appearance Models. IEEE Transactions on Pattern Analysis and Machine Intelligence 23(6), 681–685 (2001)
9. Andreopoulos, A., Tsotsos, J.K.: Efficient and Generalizable Statistical Models of Shape and Appearance for Analysis of Cardiac MRI. Medical Image Analysis (in press)
10. Zambal, S., Hladůvka, J., Bühler, K.: Improving Segmentation of the Left Ventricle Using a Two-Component Statistical Model. In: Larsen, R., Nielsen, M., Sporring, J. (eds.) MICCAI 2006. LNCS, vol. 4190, pp. 151–158. Springer, Heidelberg (2006)
11. Mitchell, S.C., Lelieveldt, B.P.F., van der Geest, R.J., Bosch, H.G., Reiber, J.H.C., Sonka, M.: Multistage Hybrid Active Appearance Model Matching: Segmentation of Left and Right Ventricles in Cardiac MR Images. IEEE Transactions on Medical Imaging 20(5), 415–423 (2001)
12. Michailovich, O.V., Rathi, Y., Tannenbaum, A.: Image Segmentation Using Active Contours Driven by the Bhattacharyya Gradient Flow. IEEE Transactions on Image Processing 16(11), 2787–2801 (2007)
13. Zhang, T., Freedman, D.: Improving performance of distribution tracking through background mismatch. IEEE Transactions on Pattern Analysis and Machine Intelligence 27(2), 282–287 (2005)
14. Ben Ayed, I., Li, S., Ross, I.: Tracking Distributions with an Overlap Prior. In: IEEE Computer Society Conference on Computer Vision and Pattern Recognition (CVPR 2008), Anchorage, Alaska (2008)
15. Freedman, D., Radke, R.J., Zhang, T., Jeong, Y., Lovelock, D.M., Chen, G.T.Y.: Model-Based Segmentation of Medical Imagery by Matching Distributions. IEEE Transactions on Medical Imaging 24(3), 281–292 (2005)

Mean q-Ball Strings Obtained by Constrained Procrustes Analysis with Point Sliding

Irina Kezele[1,2], Cyril Poupon[1,2], Muriel Perrin[3], Yann Cointepas[1,2], Vincent El Kouby[1,2], Fabrice Poupon[1,2], and Jean-François Mangin[1,2]

[1] NeuroSpin, CEA, Gif-sur-Yvette, France
[2] IFR49, France
[3] GE Healthcare, Buc, France

Abstract. The idea underpinning the work we present herein is to design robust and objective tools for brain white matter (WM) morphometry. We focus on WM tracts, and propose to represent them by their mean lines, to which we associate the attributes derived from high-angular resolution diffusion imaging (HARDI). The definition of the tract mean line derives directly from the geometry of the tract fibres. We determine the fibre point correspondences and impact factors of individual fibres, upon which we estimate average HARDI models along the tract mean lines. This way we obtain a compact tract representation that exploits all the available information, and is at the same time free of the outlier influence and undesired tract edge effects.

Keywords: Tract mean-line, high-angular resolution diffusion imaging, white matter morphometry, constrained Procrustes analysis with point sliding.

1 Introduction

To circumvent the ill-posed problem of the inter-image alignment typically encountered in voxel-based studies of brain white matter (WM) morphometry, we adopt the concept of object-based analysis [1], and define WM entities, such as fibre tracts. In order to assess WM changes on a microscopic scale (e.g., concerning the cyto- and myelo-architectonics) [2], the attributes assigned to fibre tracts should be based on diffusion spectrum imaging or its derived methods, like high-angular resolution diffusion imaging (HARDI). For adequate representation of tracts, these attributes should remain objective, not reflecting, or at worst, reflecting only weakly the effects of deficient image resolution, like partial voluming, that is typically present at tract borders. To satisfy these demands, we put forth the idea of accentuating the information along the tract mean line (similar to [3, 4, 5]), and appropriately weigh the data away from the mean line. This way we lessen the edge effects while taking into consideration all the data present. The mean line that we define derives directly from the tract fibre constellation, that way exploiting the knowledge of the exact geometry of the tract's interior. The tract assigned attributes that we introduce result from HARDI, and thus bear affluent local information. HARDI data are adequately aligned and averaged inside the tract sections perpendicular to the tract mean line. This way the anisotropy estimates are representative of the overall tract volume (while rejecting the outlying points), and are enhanced by sectional averaging.

In order to define the mean line from a bundle of tracked fibres, we need to specify a distance metric that would enable appropriate inter-fibre comparison and approximation of the ensemble average. The fibres resulting from the tracking algorithm [6], could be thought of as samples from a shape distribution around the mean shape. The deviations from the mean shape, at each related point along the fibres are expected to be small, and could be approximated by Gaussians. Together, these properties imply the employment of a shape-based metric and an analysis in the shape-space [7]. We opt for Procrustes analysis [8], similar to [9]. However, we build on the approach of [9] by incorporating certain constraints, and by implicitly allowing for some non-affine transformations to improve the fibre point correspondence.

This paper presents the method to extract the WM fibre-tract mean-line, and to compute the average HARDI, in order to estimate the mean q-balls along the tract mean line. The goal is to setup a framework for robust tract-based WM morphometry through compact WM tract models and diminished partial voluming, while exploiting all the HARDI-based information at hand. The details and conclusions on the methods, experiments and results are given in the text that follows. Note that in this text, the term "tract" does not refer directly to an anatomical tract, but rather to a bundle of fibres that results from a tracking algorithm.

2 Methods

The core technique underpinning this study is Procrustes based shape analysis [10]. It is used to align the tracked fibres, to estimate the tract mean line, and to evaluate the rotations for HARDI data alignment. The overall algorithm flow is as follows. First, we place the soft-landmarks along each fibre. Initially those landmarks are equidistant. After landmark initialization, we reject the outlying fibres by first and last points dispersion, and by fibre point-distance. Then, Procrustes analysis with landmark sliding [8], point weighting, and an additional constraint to assure proper rotations [11] is employed. This results in the tract mean line, as well as the rotations for fibre alignment. The rotations are also used to turn the HARDI data onto the mean line direction. Thus transformed HARDI data are weighted by tracked fibre density, and averaged. The motivation and details for each of the aforementioned steps are given bellow.

2.1 Landmark Placing

In many cases of biomedical images, landmark points cannot be accurately deduced from the data [8]. With the general idea of soft point correspondence between different fibres of the same tract, we initially place the landmarks equidistantly along the fibres. Subsequent Procrustes alignment allows for landmark re-positioning depending on fibre point correspondences, while minimizing the inter-fibre spline energy. The optimal landmark number is determined empirically, and is proportional to the tract mean curvature.

2.2 Outlier Rejection

The probabilistic nature of the tractography algorithm [6] allows for a distribution of the tracked fibres, and thus the final tract definition may admit outliers. We employ filters based on fibres' start/end points dispersion, and "max-fibre distance". This way, we render the distribution of corresponding landmarks across the fibre sufficiently narrow (where the tightness of the distribution refers to linearly matched fibres [8]).

2.3 Constrained Procrustes Analysis with Landmark Sliding

General Procrustes analysis (GPA) [10] acts on a set of equivalent shapes, transforming them in an affine manner to minimize the square distance between the shapes, each of them represented by a set of landmarks. The procedure is iterative and is based on the ordinary Procrustes analysis (OPA) [10]. The initial step is to scale all the shapes (typically to unit size, to assure the symmetry [10]), and to align their centers of mass (commonly by translating them all to zero). Then, at each iteration we loop through the equivalence class, define the pair of shapes as a current shape (A) and the average of all other shapes (B), where A and B are $n \times p$ matrices (n- landmark number, p- space dimension) that encode the coordinates of n landmark points. OPA analysis assumes a least square solution of:

$$min\ arg(R)\ ||A - RB||^2 \qquad (1)$$

where R is the rotation matrix. It can be shown that the solution to (1) results from the singular value decomposition (SVD) UDV^T of A^TB (T is the matrix transpose operator, $UU^T = VV^T = I$, I - identity matrix, $D = diag(d_i)$, $d_1 \geq d_2 \geq ... \geq d_n \geq 0$, I [11]):

$$A^TB = UDV^T \qquad (2)$$

$$R = VU^T \qquad (3)$$

After all the optimal rotations for all the shapes are calculated at each iteration, the shapes are transformed accordingly, and the overall, Generalized Procrustes distance (GPD) is calculated as a sum of all square (Euclidean) distances between each pair of shapes. Iterations are repeated while the difference in two successive iterations is above a predefined threshold, or the maximum number of iterations is reached.

However, GPA can result in some improper rotations if the assumption on the small deviation from the mean shape is violated. To prevent such a degeneracy, we pose an additional constraint on rotation matrices, by inserting a sort of "sign" diagonal matrix, S, into the SVD solution of (3) above [11]:

$$S = \begin{cases} I & \text{if } det(U)det(V) = 1, \\ diag(1,1,...,1,-1) & \text{if } det(U)det(V) = -1 \end{cases} \qquad (4)$$

$$R = VSU^T \qquad (5)$$

The point deviations for the fibre equivalent class can vary along the mean fibre. We want to assure that the points with larger spread will influence less the least square solution for optimal rotations. This is particularly important for certain tract geometries, such as in tracts that end in a "fan" shape. Thus, we insert a weighting matrix into the A^TB term prior to SVD (2,3):

$$A^TWB = UDV^T \qquad (6)$$

The weighting matrix, W, is of a diagonal form, $W = diag(w_i)$, where w_i represent normalized weights inversely proportional to the point standard deviation. Similar SVD weighting was employed in [12], however, the weighting matrix also accounted for the case of landmark cross-correspondence. The improvement obtained by introducing the constraints on proper rotations and point-weights into the unconstrained GPA is illustrated in Fig. 1. Since the unconstrained GPA allows for reflections and assigns an equal importance to all points (irrespective of local landmark distribution across the bundle), the aligned fibres may result in a bundle that is globally not in the same position as the original bundle ("unconstrained" mean line, Fig.1.). This should be avoided, because for the subsequent HARDI averaging (Section 2.4) we need to bring the mean line to the original bundle space and the motion is not known directly. Fibre reflection might provoke a complete perturbation in inter-fibre point correspondences. The constrained GPA ("constrained" mean line, Fig.1.) results in proper inter-fibre point correspondences, and a bundle of aligned fibres that does not change its global position (compared to the original bundle).

While GPA acts as a sort of high-pass filter for shape differences [8], small local variations, like the ones resulting from the landmark location ambiguity, need to be addressed in complement. To accost this issue, with the main goal of resolving the inter-fibre point correspondences, we adopt the approach of Bookstein [8] and allow for a shift in landmark position, while imposing a regularity constraint in a form of 3D *"thin-plate"* spline energy. Landmarks are allowed to slide only along a predefined set of directions that are typically the directions towards neighbouring landmarks along the fibre, or the directions of tangents at landmark points.

The final form of our constrained GPA with landmark sliding is as follows:

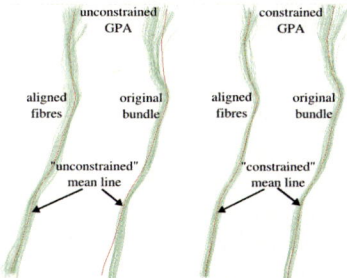

Fig. 1. Comparison between the mean line obtained by unconstrained GPA, and the mean line that resulted from the constrained Procrustes analysis

1. Choose randomly a fibre for the target for the initial linear fibre alignment and landmark relaxation
2. Apply constrained GPA on relaxed fibres
3. Perform landmark relaxation with respect to the mean fibre calculated in 2
4. Repeat 2-3 until convergence.

Typically, we employ ~10 iterations for each GPA step (step 2 above). Steps 2 and 3 are commonly repeated 2-3 times. The mean line is calculated by averaging the corresponding landmarks along the aligned fibres.

2.4 Average HARDI and q-Balls

HARDI averaging is based on the assumption that HARDI signal represents a set of (independent) measurements along the prescribed directions. For each landmark point i of the mean line we defined a thin cylinder C_i with the axis parallel to the tangent at that point and of the radius superior to the maximal tract radius. All tract points p_{ik} (from no matter what fibre f_k inside the tract) that belong to a particular C_i, form a set P_i. The points p_{ik} from P_i belong to different f_k, and we can associate to them the GPA rotations R_k, related to f_k. We use these rotations to turn the HARDI data (using geodesic interpolation [15]) in voxels that correspond (by nearest neighbour interpolation) to the points p_{ik}. Rotated HARDI data corresponding to p_{ik} of P_i are weighted by tracked fibre density [6] in their related voxels and averaged (note that the weights are normalized prior to averaging). This results in the averaged HARDI H_i, at the mean line point i. Different rotations that act on H_i in the same voxel have equal influence in the final H_i averaging. Thus, statistically, for a large number of tracked fibres, rotation of H_i will converge to that determined by the majority of fibres inside the voxel. Weighting by tracked fibre density prioritize HARDI data in more central voxels of the tract, while HARDI data inside edge voxels are assigned very low weights. This way we are able to use all the data, but at the same time substantially decrease the influence of the potential outliers. Consequently, we boost the power to detect and describe anisotropy inside transverse tract sections. We repeat the step of HARDI rotating and averaging for all the mean line points i. Upon this, at each mean line point, mean q-balls were reconstructed from the averaged H_i, by decomposing the signal to the modified spherical harmonics basis, using the algorithm described in [14].

3 Experiments and Results

After estimating the q-balls at every voxel of the diffusion-weighted data (b = 3000s/mm², 200 directions) by Funk-Radon transform [15], a probabilistic fibre tracking algorithm [6] was performed inside the WM to track all the fibres starting at two regions of interest, defined on the entire left and right cortical grey matter surface. Fibres were clustered using the algorithm of [16].

Due to obvious space limitations, we show only a part of the results. In Fig 2, we illustrate the method on two tracts of largely different geometry: a callosal tract, and a cortico-spinal tract (of the same healthy volunteer). The final, averaged q-ball data along the mean lines of the callosal and cortico-spinal tracts are shown in Fig. 2a and b. The data are presented on the background of a RGB map of the principal diffusivities (R-x, G-y, and B-z). Note how the information on of the fibre crossing is preserved at the level of the brainstem (Fig 2. c). Figure 3 depicts the detailed results of the analysis of the generalized fractional anisotropy (GFA) along the left cingulum fascicle for a group of 5 healthy volunteers. We calculated the GFA of the q-ball models along the estimated mean lines, for the cases where we do not match/do match these mean lines by the above described Procrustes method with point sliding, this time *between* subjects. We wanted to assess the impact of line matching with point sliding on GFA group estimates. GFA was linearly interpolated at 15 equidistant points along the mean lines, upon which we averaged the values across the group of

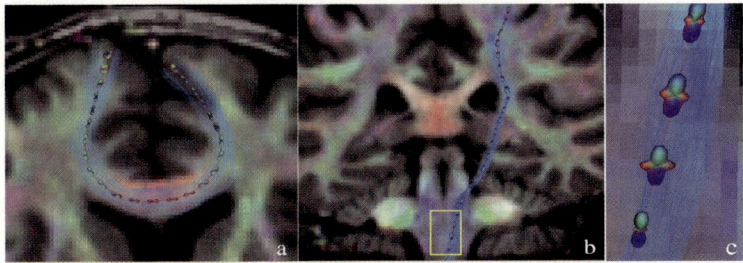

Fig. 2. Mean q-balls superimposed onto the corresponding bundles (blue), and mean-lines (red). (a) Callosal tract. (b) Cortico-spinal tract. (c) The zoom of the yellow region in b.

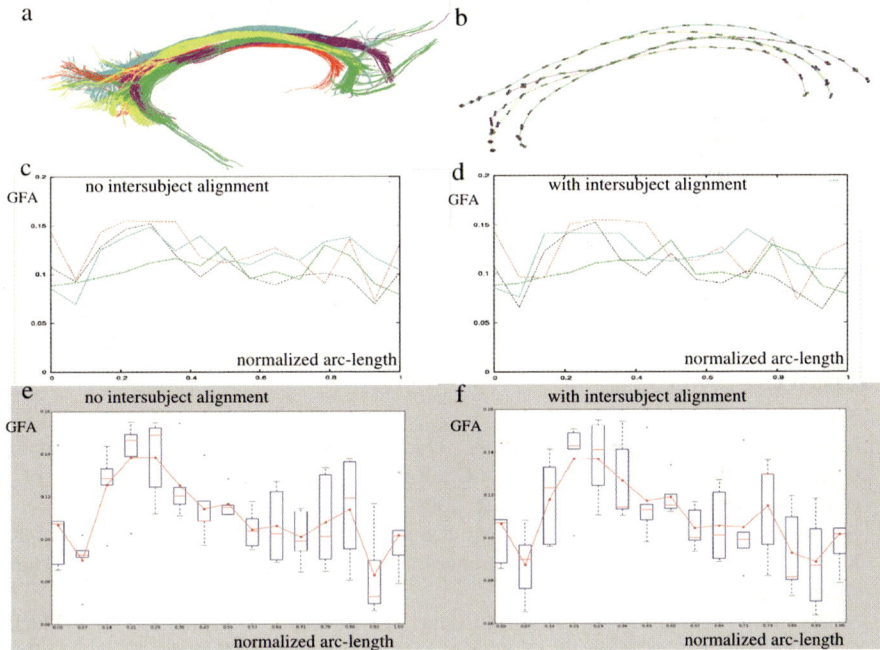

Fig. 3. Comparison of GFA estimates in "matching vs. not matching" the mean lines between subjects tests, using the constrained Procrustes method with point sliding. (a) Unfiltered fibres of the left cingulum fascicle of 5 healthy volunteers (MRIs were linearly aligned). (b) Estimated mean lines and average q-ball models along those lines. (c)-(d) GFA along the mean lines with no "sliding Procrustes" alignment , and with "sliding Procrustes" alignment. (e)-(f) The corresponding box plots of c and d. (Red line connects the mean GFA values, red bar shows the median, and the lower/upper box limits correspond to lower/upper quartiles of the distribution at each point).

subjects. Despite the scarce number of the studied subjects, and for both cases (matching *vs.* not matching the mean lines between subjects), the inter-subject similarity in the pattern of GFA is already noticeable (Fig. 3c and d). For this small group of subjects, the results did not reveal any significant differences in GFA in "*not matching vs. matching*" tests. The idea was that while we cannot pair the first and the last points exactly due to important anatomical variability (howbeit the extreme points are also allowed to slide), point sliding should help us improve the point correspondence for the intermediate points. Although not fully conclusive (due to the small cohort size), the results raise/restate some questions: Should we match the fibres between subjects according to their shape, or rather by the attributes (e.g., GFA) attached to those fibres? How much non-linearity in fibre matching should be allowed for? The future work will comprise similar studies on larger cohorts of healthy volunteers, and with different regularization energies for matching. Hopefully, it will allow us to understand better the aforementioned problems, and to describe the distribution/patterns of GFA (and other HARDI derived attributes) with higher statistical power. This may turn into a valuable descriptor for WM morphometry studies, especially when comparing a healthy population to a population affected by a neurodegenerative or a psychiatric disorder.

4 Conclusions

We presented a method to robustly estimate WM tracts' mean lines, and to define the compact tract attributes derived from HARDI data. Reduced partial voluming and enhanced ability to detect and quantify anisotropy should enable unbiased tract-based WM morphometry. Other attributes could equally be included into the morphometric analysis, such as the attributes derived from the tract geometry.

References

1. Mangin, J.-F., Riviére, D., Cachia, A., Duchesnay, E., Cointepas, Y., Papadopoulos-Orfanos, D., Collins, D.L., Evans, A.C., Régis, J.: Object-based morphometry of the cerebral cortex. IEEE Trans. Med. Imag. 23(8), 968–982 (2004)
2. Ashburner, J., Hutton, C., Frackowiak, R.S.J., Johnsrude, I., Price, C.J., Friston, K.J.: Identifying Global Anatomical Differences: Deformation-Based Morphometry. Human Brain Mapping 6(5), 348–357 (1998)
3. Smith, S.M., Jenkinson, M., Johansen-Berg, H., Rueckert, D., Nichols, T.E., Mackay, C.E., Watkins, K.E., Ciccarelli, O., Cader, M.Z., Matthews, P.M., Behrens, T.E.J.: Tract-based spatial statistics: Voxelwise analysis of multi-subject diffusion data. NeuroImage 31(4), 1487–1505 (2006)
4. Maddah, M., Warfield, S.K., Westin, C.-F., Grimson, W.E.L.: Probabilistic clustering and quantitative analysis of white matter fiber tracts. In: Karssemeijer, N., Lelieveldt, B. (eds.) IPMI 2007. LNCS, vol. 4584, pp. 372–383. Springer, Heidelberg (2007)
5. O'Donnell, L.J., Westin, C.-F., Golby, A.J.: Tract-based morphometry. In: Ayache, N., Ourselin, S., Maeder, A. (eds.) MICCAI 2007, Part II. LNCS, vol. 4792, pp. 160–168. Springer, Heidelberg (2007)
6. Perrin, M., Cointepas, Y., Cachia, A., Poupon, C., Thirion, B., Rivière, D., Cathier, P., El Kouby, V., Constantinesco, A., Le Bihan, D., Mangin, J.-F.: Connectivity-Based Parcellation of the Cortical Mantle Using q-Ball Diffusion Imaging. Int. J. Biomed Imaging (2008)

7. Kendall, D.G.: Shape Manifolds, Procrustean Metrics, and Complex Projective Spaces. Bull. London Math. Soc. 16(2), 81–121 (1984)
8. Bookstein, F.L.: Landmark methods for forms without landmarks: morphometrics of group differences in outline shape. MedIA 1(3), 225–243 (1997)
9. Corouge, I., Fletcher, P.T., Joshi, S., Gouttard, S., Gerig, G.: Fiber tract-oriented statistics for quantitative diffusion tensor MRI analysis. MedI. A 10(5), 786–798 (2006)
10. Mardia, K.V., Dreyden, I.L.: Statistical shape analysis, London (1998)
11. Umeyama, S.: Least-squares estimation of transformation parameters between two point patterns. IEEE Trans. PAMI 13(4), 376–380 (1991)
12. Luo, B., Hancock, E.R.: Matching point-sets using Procrustes alignment and the EM algoritm. In: BMVC, pp. 43–52 (1999)
13. Zhang, F., Goodlett, C., Hancock, E., Gerig, G.: Probabilistic Fiber Tracking Using Particle Filtering. In: Ayache, N., Ourselin, S., Maeder, A. (eds.) MICCAI 2007, Part II. LNCS, vol. 4792, pp. 144–152. Springer, Heidelberg (2007)
14. Descoteaux, M., Angelino, E., Fitzgibbons, S., Deriche, R.: Regularized, Fast and Robust Analytical Q-Ball Imaging. Magn. Res. Med. 58(3), 497–510 (2007)
15. Tuch, D.: Q-ball imaging. Magn. Res. Med. 52, 1358–1372 (2004)
16. El Kouby, V., Cointepas, Y., Poupon, C., Rivière, D., Golestani, N., Poline, J.-B., Mangin, J.-F.: MR diffusion-based inference of a fiber bundle model from a population of subjects. In: Duncan, J.S., Gerig, G. (eds.) MICCAI 2005. LNCS, vol. 3749, pp. 196–204. Springer, Heidelberg (2005)

Noninvasive Functional Imaging of Volumetric Cardiac Electrical Activity: A Human Study on Myocardial Infarction

Linwei Wang[1], Ken C.L. Wong[1], Heye Zhang[2], and Pengcheng Shi[1]

[1] Golisano College of Computing and Information Science
Rochester Institute of Technology, Rochester, NY, USA
maomaowlw@mail.rit.edu
[2] Bioengineering Institute, University of Auckland, Auckland, New Zealand

Abstract. Identification of infarct substrates provides necessary guidance to the prevention and treatment of cardiac arrhythmias. Compared to diagnostic criteria of body surface potentials (BSP) or electrophysiological information on heart surfaces, the underlying volumetric cardiac electrical activity is of more direct clinical relevance in exhibiting patient-specific arrhythmic dynamics and arrhythmogenic substrates. We have developed a paradigm for noninvasive imaging of volumetric myocardial transmembrane potential from BSPs. In this paper, we present a human study for a patient with acute myocardial infarction. Using patient MRI and BSP data, the framework is able to reconstruct details of the complete arrhythmic electrical activity on the 3D myocardium of the patient. Exploring a subset of the results, the extent, centroid and affected segments of the infarct is correctly evaluated, with comparable performance to existent best results. This human study demonstrates the potential of the presented paradigm as a noninvasive functional imaging technique for patient-specific volumetric cardiac electrical activity in practice.

1 Introduction

Arrhythmogenic substrates created by myocardial infarction (MI) lead to a high incidence of lethal ventricular tachycardia and fibrillation. Identification of infarct substrates could significantly improve the prevention and treatment of cardiac arrhythmias. The ablative therapy is a typical example requiring such guidance to destroy or interrupt arrhythmogenic substrates. In current clinical practice, the 12-lead ECG is the most frequently used tool for evaluating MI, though the limitaion in its diagnostic capability has been widely recognized [1].

As an extension to ECG, body surface potential map (BSPM) records potentials from hundreds of electrodes on thorax surface. It provides functional images implying the spatiotemporal dynamics of the underlying cardiac electrical activity. While large efforts have been put to build up BSPM database for arrhythmia identification [2], BSPM is not able to reflect local details of the electrical activity ongoing throughout the 3D myocardium, since each electrode actually only measures a *smoothed integration* of the entire cardiac activity.

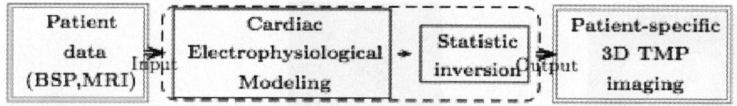

Fig. 1. Noninvasive functional imaging of volumetric cardiac electrical activity

The inverse problem of electrocardiography (IECG) aims at noninvasive reconstruction of cardiac electrical activity from BSPMs. Several recent IECG approaches have been applied to MI evaluation [3,4]. Mostly the solutions are confined to electrophysiological information on heart surfaces, assuming that it contains characteristics associated with infarct substrates [3]. However, to localize intramural arrhythmogenic substrates more directly, reconstruction of volumetric cardiac electrical activity is desired. A heart-model-based approach was reported in simulation experiments to estimate the site and size of MI in 3D myocardium [4]. By deterministically optimizing the heart model, it imposes high requirements on the initial approximation and modeling of the infarct. How these factors would affect the results in real-data experiments remains unknown.

We have presented a model-constrained Bayesian paradigm for noninvasive imaging of volumetric myocardial transmembrane potential (TMP) from BSPMs [5]. Its practical potential has been demonstrated by extensive phantom experiments in cardiac arrhythmia imaging [6]. In this paper, we experiment this paradigm for a human study. With MRI and BSP data collected from a patient with acute MI, volumetric arrhythmic TMP dynamics of this specific subject's heart is noninvasively imaged. The associated MI evaluation is compared to existent works and cardiologists' interpretation of the infarct. This study validates the potential of the paradigm as a noninvasive functional imaging technique for patient-specific volumetric cardiac electrical activity, and demonstrates how a subset of the results is of promising clinical relevance in MI evaluation.

2 Method

2.1 Model-Constrained Bayesian Paradigm for TMP Imaging

The architecture of this noninvasive TMP imaging paradigm is illustrated in Fig 1. To combine general physiological knowledge and patient clinical data with regard to their respective uncertainties, the Bayesian paradigm estimates patient-specific TMPs via statistic inversion. *A priori* physiological knowledge is contained in the cardiac electrophysiological system customized to patient heart-torso structure. It consists of volumetric myocardial TMP activity model for system dynamics and TMP-to-BSP model for system observations. After reformulating the physiological system into a stochastic state space representation with associated model and data errors, data assimilation is utilized to estimate volumetric myocardial TMP dynamics from BSPMs of specific patients [5].

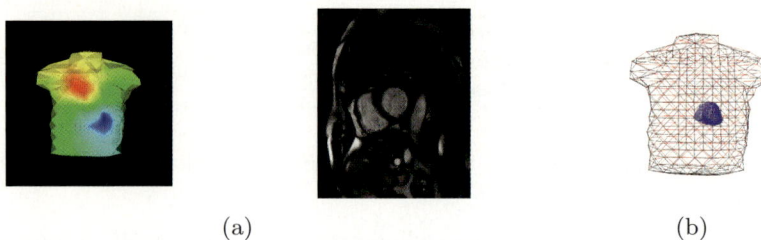

Fig. 2. (a) Input patient data. Left: BSPM at 85ms of ventricular activation. Right: MRI slice. (b) Combined heart-torso model customized from patient-specific MRIs.

2.2 Volumetric Myocaridal TMP Imaging of MI

Experiment data. Fig 2 (a) lists paradigm inputs: MRI and BSP data collected from a patient with acute MI who returned for one-year follow-up MRI [7]. The set of static MRIs contains 9 slices, with 8mm inter-slice spacing and 1.33mm/pixel in-plane resolution. BSPs are recorded from 123 electrodes and interpolated to 370 nodes on the torso surface, each consisting of a single averaged PQRST complex sampled at 2k Hz. Anatomical locations of all electrodes and nodes are available. Reference MI interpretation is obtained from gadolinium enhanced images, evaluating the infarct extent (the percentage of infarcted myocardial mass), centroid (the myocardial segment containing the centroid) and segments containing infarcted tissues.

Model specification. For its ability to balance the model plausibility with inversion feasibility, the family of 2-variable FitzHugh-Nagumo-type models is favorable in IECG approaches. Among different variations, we select the model in [8] because it produces realistic TMP features which are closely related to BSP morphology. Besides, by a flexible control on TMP shapes, it allows an easy description of myocardial electrical heterogeneity and infarcted tissues.

Data processing. By segmenting MRIs slice by slice with hand-tracing, initial triangulated surfaces of thorax tissues are obtained. Because of the independent segmentation of each slice and the relatively low inter-slice imaging resolution, these surfaces are faceted. Surface smoothing is done by a two-stage Gaussian algorithm [9], which is able to reduce the shrinkage effect to keep the overall size and shape-feature of the surfaces. Fig 2 (b) displays the combined heart-torso model for the patient under study. The torso is assumed as a homogeneous conductor and represented with triangulated body surface. The 3D ventricular mass is described by a cloud of meshfree points [5]. Detailed 3D fiber structure is mapped from experimental results of [10] and determines intracellular conductive anisotropy. Transmural electrical heterogeneity is taken into account by associating different TMP shapes with epi-, endo-, and mid-myocardial regions [11] (Fig 3 (a)). In addition, to evaluate MI in a standard terminology, the LV wall is divided into 17 segments by AHA consensus [12] (Fig 3 (b)). Fig 4 displays the simulated normal TMP activation in the patient's ventricles.

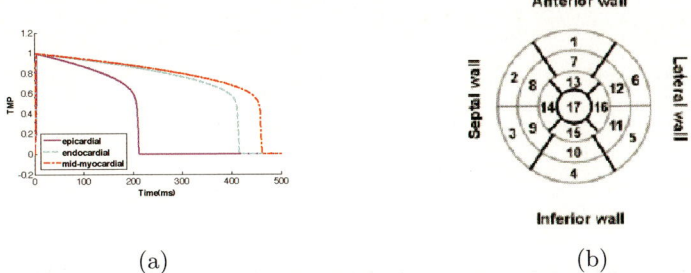

(a)   (b)

Fig. 3. (a) Different TMP shapes in epi-, endo-, mid-myocardial tissues. (b) Schematics of the LV wall divided into 17 segments by AHA consensus (polar map) [12].

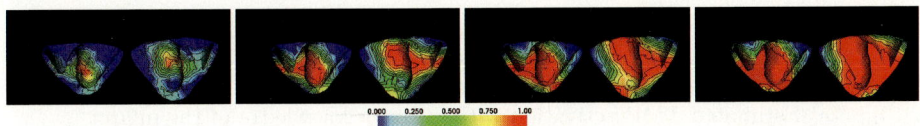

Fig. 4. Simulated normal TMP activation in the specific patient's ventricles. The color encodes TMP values and black contours represent potential ischrones. Left to Right: 35, 64, 78, 89ms after the onset of ventricular activation.

Meanwhile, preprocessing of patient BSP data is necessary to coordinate the real data with the physiological system. Firstly, since only *ventricular* electrical activity is considered at present, we select QRST intervals out of the complete BSP as paradigm input (Fig 5 (a)). Next, the TMP activity model has normalized TMP values, and its temporal interval for discretization is usually one magnitude smaller than BSP sampling interval. BSP data, therefore, go through temproal interpolation and magnitude scaling before being input into the paradigm.

TMP imaging and MI evaluation. In the following, we present a practical TMP imaging scheme composed of progressive iterations. Without using any prior knowledge of the infarct, TMP reconstruction starts with state estimation using models parameterized with standard values. The direct results of TMP estimates approximate local details of patient-specific volumetric cardiac arrhythmic pattern and arrhythmic substrates. Exploring a subset of the estimates, the infarct extent (EP), centroid (CE) and affected segments are evaluated. This approximate knowledge of the infarct is fed back to the paradigm to modify relevant model parameters and improve the 2nd-pass state estimation and MI evaluation. Subsequent passes of feedbacks and estimations iterate in a similar manner until no significant improvements are observed in the results.

Two primary characteristics of infarcted tissues are exhibited in the changes of activation time (AT) and TMP duration (PD), which can be calculated from TMP (Fig 5 (b)). The late AT and reduced PD of the estimates are used as the foremost indicator of infarct substrates. The relative label of AT ($rlAT$) is defined to represent the order in which the myocardium is activated and is

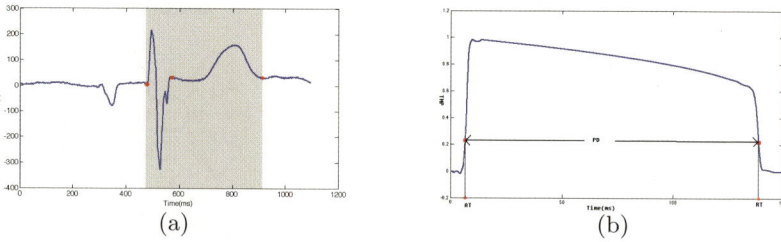

Fig. 5. (a) Complete BSP signal and selected QRST interval (shadowed) used as paradigm inputs. (b) Calculation of AT and PD from TMP. AT is determined by the largest positive derivative, and repolarization time (RT) is when TMP value returns below that at AT. PD = RT − AT.

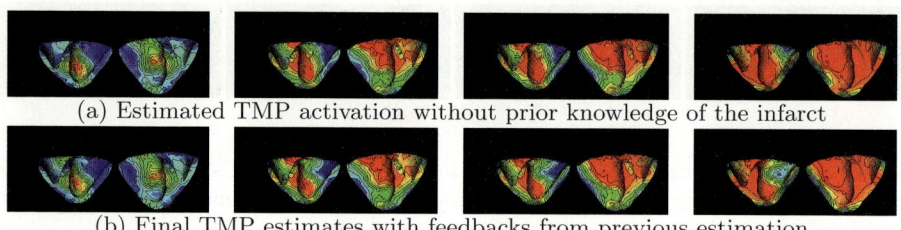

Fig. 6. Volumetric TMP imaging during ventricular activation. The color bar is the same as that in Fig 4. Left to Right: 35, 64, 78, 89ms after ventricular activation onset.

closer to 1 with larger AT. The relative label of PD ($rlPD$) is defined in a similar manner but $rlPD$ is closer to 1 with smaller PD. Infarcted tissues, therefore, would have $rlAT$ and $rlPD$ close to 1 in the estimates. Meanwhile, because the TMP activity model has impacts on the estimates, the discrepancy between model-generated and estimated $rlAT$ and $rlPD$ are used as the secondary infarct indicator and normalized into another two relative indices $rdAT$ and $rdPD$. Naturally, arrhythmogenic substrates would have larger $rdAT$ and/or $rdPD$. Accordingly, a relatively robust metric for infarct identification ($0 \leq M_i \leq 1$) is defined as the weighted summation of $rlAT, rlPD, rdAT$ and $rdPD$.

Generally, the distribution curve of M_i from all meshfree points shows a notable distinction between larger and smaller values. It provides a proper threshold T by which points with $M_i \geq T$ are initially suspected as infarcted. For each segment, the percentage of its suspected infarcted points (p) is calculated. Segments with $p \geq T_s$ and the containing suspected infarcted points are confirmed as infarcted, where T_s is another empirical threshold. By this step, isolated suspected infarcted points are removed. Since M_i actually measures the credibility of a meshfree point being infarcted, it is used to generate the approximate distribution map of the infarct substrate. EP is then calculated as the percentage of infarcted points in all ventricular meshfree points. CE is located as the center of infarcted points weighted by M_i. As we observed, exact values of weights and T, T_s have few impacts on CE localization or infarct identification. A set of empirical values for T, T_s

Table 1. Comparison of MI evaluation results with reference interpretation. SO is the segment overlap between the results and reference interpretation weighted by p.

	Reference Interpretation	Initial results	2nd-pass	3rd-pass
EP	52%	27%	27%	28%
SO	NA	70%	85%	90%
CE	10/11	12	11	11
segments	3-5,9-12,15-16	5-7,11-12,16	5,11-12,16	5,10-12,16

and weights of $rlAT, rdAT, rlPD, rdPD$ ($0.5, 30\%, 0.3, 0.2, 0.3, 0.2$) is used in our following analysis. Future studies would benefit from training or online adjustment of these parameters.

3 Results and Discussions

Results. Expert examinations report the infarct substrate as in inferior-lateral basal-middle LV. Announced as a challenge for MI evaluation, it attracted a variety of efforts [13,14,15]. The best results were obtained from simple ECG analysis without reference to MRIs [13]. The 4th and 5th place out of 6 awarded efforts took IECG approaches, based on aforementioned epicardial-potential-reconstruction [14] and heart-model-optimization [15] respectively. In the following, we will demonstrate the contribution of our paradigm to this problem.

TMP reconstruction starts by state estimation with standard models, and MI evaluation results at previous iteration are fed back to modify model parameters for the following TMP estimation. The results show negligible changes after 3 iterations. Fig 6 (a) lists the initial and final volumetric myocardial TMP estimates. Compared to the simulated normal TMP dynamics (Fig 4), both estimates exhibit distinct arrhythmic activation caused by conduction delay/block in the inferior-lateral basal-middle sections of LV. The final results further improves initial results by additional identification of the inferior infarct substrate.

Quantitative MI evaluation results for all iterations are listed in Table 1. The reference interpretation calculates EP in the segment level ($EP = 9/17 \simeq 52\%$). In comparison, able to differentiate between normal and infarcted tissues within the same segment, our approach usually produces smaller EP than the reference interpretation. Compared to the IECG efforts in the challenge [14,15], the initial results has the same 1-segment deviation in CE but EP and segments identification are largely improved. During the iteration, CE is corrected. EP and identification of affected segments are progressively refined, producing final results comparable to the best in the challenge [13]. The accuracy of TMP estimates is also validated by the closeness between estimates-generated BSPs and the input data (Fig 7). Derived from the final TMP estimates, the ventricular electrical activation time map (Fig 8) clearly indicates the infarct substrate with abnormally large AT. The associated distribution map of the infarct substrate (Fig 8 (b)) also localizes the substrate as around the inferior-lateral basal-middle

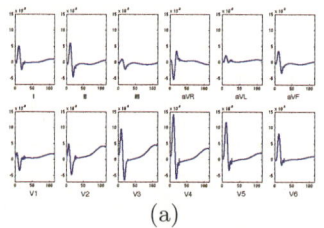 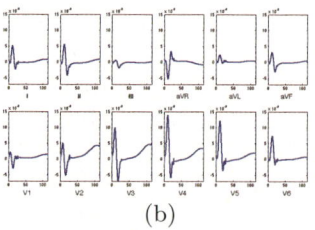

(a)   (b)

Fig. 7. 12-lead ECG. (a): paradigm inputs (processed). (b): generated from final TMP estimates. They are in close accordance with relative root mean squared error as 0.15.

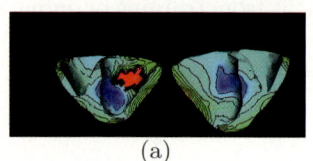 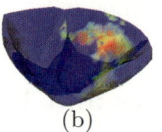

(a)   (b)

Fig. 8. (a) Final ventricular electrical activation time map. The red and blue encodes maximum and minimum time values. Black contours represents time ischrones. (b) Final distribution map of infarct substrate (highlighted areas).

LV wall. In addition, instead of identifying the infarct substrate by segments, the distribution map displays its detailed location in the 3D myocardium.

Discussions. Without any prior knowledge of the infarct, this paradigm is able to produce MI evaluation results comparable to the best existent results [13]. More importantly, it has the advantage of describing complete volumetric myocardial TMP dynamics for the specific patient, from which MI evaluation only utilize a subset of information. When affirmative prior knowledge is unavailable, the presented progressive imaging scheme is practical. In practice, though, it is worthwhile to take advantage of prior knowledge from reliable sources, such as standard ECG diagnostic criteria and cardiac structural images.

In current study, the impact of model assumptions on the estimates are taken into account by considering the discrepancy between models and estimates during MI evaluation. An essential alternative is to reduce the constraining effects of models. By using unknown model parameters, simultaneous estimation of TMP and related myocardial electrophysiological property can modify models in accordance to patient data. Meanwhile, we have developed a data integration paradigm where information in BSPs and structural images are fused together for TMP imaging[16]. Its applicability will be investigated in the human study.

4 Conclusions

This human study demonstrates the potential of the presented paradigm as a noninvasive functional imaging technique for patient-specific volumetric cardiac electrical activity. Its practical value is highlighted by the facts that 1), functional imaging of complete cardiac electrical activity is still a challenging task for current cardiac mapping techniques (noninvasive or invasive); 2), physiological modeling techniques, on the other hand, has the issue of requiring patient-specific knowledge *a prior*. The paradigm has the advantage to noninvasively describe volumetric patient-specific myocardial TMP dynamics. By exploring just a subset of the results, it shows promises in clinical practices such as MI evaluation.

Thorough validation of such technique is very challenging since it requires not only the collection of BSP and structural image of specific subjects, but also complete electrical mapping on the 3D myocardium. The dataset provided in current case is valuable for reasonable validations. In the future, it is desirable to look into the possibility of obtaining 3D cardiac electrical mapping data, and more real-data studies will be performed with regard to various pathologies.

References

1. Mirvis, D.M.: What's wrong with electrocardiography? J. Electrocardiol 31, 313–316 (1998)
2. Kornreich, F., Montague, T.J., Rautaharju, P.M.: Identification of first acute q wave and non-q wave myocardial infarction by multivariate analysis of body surface potential maps. Circ. 84, 2442–2453 (1991)
3. Burnes, J.E., Rudy, Y.: Noninvasive ecg imaging of electrophysiologically abnormal substrates in infarcted hearts: a model study. Circ. 101, 533–540 (2000)
4. Li, G., He, B.: Noninvasive estimatin of myocardial infarction by means of a heart-model-based imaging approach: a simulation study. Med. Biol. Eng. Comput. 42, 128–136 (2004)
5. Wang, L., Zhang, H., Liu, H., Shi, P.: Imaging of 3D cardiac electrical activity: A model-based recovery framework. In: Larsen, R., Nielsen, M., Sporring, J. (eds.) MICCAI 2006. LNCS, vol. 4190, pp. 792–799. Springer, Heidelberg (2006)
6. Wang, L., Zhang, H., Shi, P.: Towards noninvasive 3D imaging of cardiac arrhythmias. In: Sachse, F.B., Seemann, G. (eds.) FIHM 2007. LNCS, vol. 4466, pp. 280–289. Springer, Heidelberg (2007)
7. Goldberger, A.L., et al.: Physiobank, physiotoolkit, and physionet components of a new research resource for complex physiological signals. Cric. 101, 215–220 (2000)
8. Aliev, R.R., Panfilov, A.V.: A simple two-variable model of cardiac excitation. Chaos, Solitions & Fractals 7(3), 293–301 (1996)
9. Taubin, G.: Curve and surface smoothing without shrinkage. In: Proc. ICCV, pp. 825–857 (1995)
10. Nash, M.: Mechanics and Material Properties of the Heart using an Anatomically Accurate Mathematical Model. PhD thesis, Univ. of Auckland, New Zealand (May 1998)
11. Yan, G.X., et al.: Charactetistics and distribution of m cells in arterially perfused canine left ventricular wedge preparations. Circ. 98, 1921–1927 (1998)
12. Cerqueira, M.D., et al.: Standardized myocardial segmentation and nomenclature for tomographic imaging of the heart. Circ. 105, 539–542 (2002)

13. Mneimneh, M.A., Povinelli, R.J.: Rps/gmm approach toward the localization of myocardial infarction. In: Proc. CinC. (2007)
14. Dawoud, F.D.: Using inverse electrocardiography to image myocardial infarction. In: Proc. CinC. (2007)
15. Farina, D.: Model-based approach to the localization of infarction. In: Proc. CinC. (2007)
16. Wang, L., Zhang, H., Wong, K.C., Shi, P.: Idynamic structural-image-guided non-invasive 3d cardiac electrophysiological mapping. In: Proc. ICIP (in press, 2008)

A Slicing-Based Coherence Measure for Clusters of DTI Integral Curves

Çağatay Demiralp[1], Gregory Shakhnarovich[2], Song Zhang[3], and David H. Laidlaw[1]

[1] Brown University
[2] Toyota Technological Institute at Chicago
[3] Mississippi State University

Abstract. We present a slicing-based coherence measure for clusters of DTI integral curves. For a given cluster, we probe samples from the cluster by slicing it with a plane at regularly spaced locations parametrized by curve arc lengths. Then we compute a stability measure based on the spatial relations between the projections of the curve points in individual slices and their change across the slices. We demonstrate its use in refining agglomerative hierarchical clustering results of DTI curves that correspond to neural pathways. Expert evaluation shows that refinement based on our measure can lead to improvement of clustering that is not possible directly by using standard methods.

1 Introduction

Diffusion-Tensor Magnetic Resonance Imaging (DTI) measures the rate of self-diffusion due to the Brownian motion of water molecules in tissues [1]. Integral curves showing paths of fastest diffusion are among the most common information derived from DTI volumes, enabling the exploration of fibrous structures such as brain white matter and muscles non-invasively *in-vivo*. They are generated by tracking the principal eigenvector of the underlying diffusion tensor field in both directions [2] and often visualized as streamlines or variations of streamlines (streamtubes and hyperstreamlines) in 3D [3]. However, these 3D models are generally visually dense making it difficult for experts to ascertain anatomical and functional structures clearly. Therefore, there is a considerable interest in developing effective clustering methods.

In this context, we introduce a measure of coherence for a "hypothesized" cluster of curves. The cluster coherence measure we propose relies on evaluating the stability of further subdivision of the cluster. To this end, we use the configurations at what we call "slices"– cross-sections of the cluster. Each slice is effectively an embedding of the curves into points in two-dimensional space. These points can be clustered using any off-the-shelf clustering algorithm. Each slice therefore provides a "vote" for each pair of curves being together or separate in the overall clustering. Furthermore, assuming reasonable smoothness of the curves, we can assess the temporal coherence of these votes: two adjacent slices carry more weight voting the same way than if their votes are opposite.

We demonstrate our measure's use to improve an agglomerative hierarchical clustering algorithm that has been shown to be working relatively well in clustering integral curves corresponding neurofibers [4]. When our slice-based method detects that a stable split exists in the cluster, it provides a specific partitioning, that can be used as part of a clustering algorithm. Expert evaluation shows that this mechanism may be superior to the standard hierarchical clustering approach. While our primary motivation in designing the slicing-based coherence measure is the task of refining an initial clustering assignment, it can be used for validating clusterings, quantifying connectivity or parametrizing clusters.

In the next section we discuss related work briefly, focusing on clustering methods. We then describe the details of the slice-based coherence measure in Section 3. Its application in improving hierarchical clustering results is described in Section 4, followed by discussion and conclusion in Section 5.

2 Related Work

There have been several clustering methods proposed for DTI curves. All of them are adaptations of some of the well-known clustering methods including fuzzy c-means (a variation of k-means) [5], agglomerative hierarchical clustering [6,7], and spectral clustering [8,9]. An evaluation of the most popular fiber clustering of algorithms can be found in [4]. While we are not aware of any coherence measure specific to DTI integral curves (or 3D curves of any origin, for that matter), we found stability (or confidence) argument for cluster analysis in statistics to be common [10,11,12] and often used to compare and validate clustering methods.

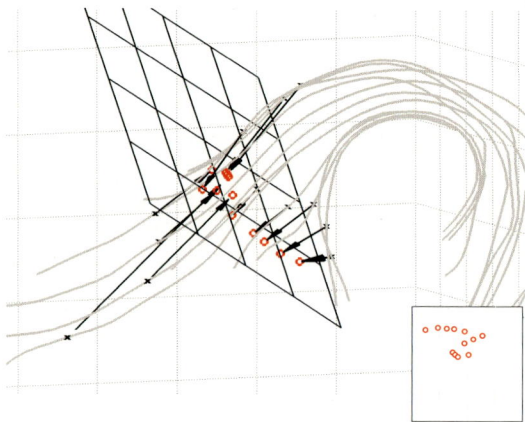

Fig. 1. Illustration: the cluster is sliced using the arc length ratio $\alpha = 0.2$. Crosses (black): points on the curve corresponding to the arc length parameter αS_i. Circles (red): projections on the slicing plane. The bottom-right legend shows the embedding of the curves in the axis-aligned plane of the current slice.

In this context, our notion of stability can be seen as an internal geometric index primarily aiming to quantify the quality of hypothesized individual clusters.

3 Slicing and Cluster Stability

The basic idea of our method is to assess the behavior of curves, that comprise a candidate cluster, relative to each other in a number of cross-sections (slices). A clustering pattern with more than one clusters, consistent over neighboring slices, is found, the cluster is considered incoherent, and split, with the splitting details deduced from the slices. Otherwise, the cluster is considered coherent, and preserved intact. Note that a clustering pattern in our case is a particular number of clusters and cluster membership. Therefore, consistency of a clustering pattern suggests consistency in number of clusters as well as consistency in cluster membership.

3.1 Slicing a Candidate Cluster

Given a cluster of undirected curves $X_1, \ldots, X_N$ in $\mathbb{R}^3$, we first orient the curves (in the sense of assigning start- and end-point designations), in a way that makes orientations consistent within the cluster. This is done by computing the start-to-end vector for each curve and iteratively re-orienting the curves until all the vectors are in the same half-space.

Next we sample each curve uniformly along its path in the following manner. Let S_i be the arc length of the curve X_i; i.e., the curve can be parametrized as $\mathbf{X}(s)$ where s goes from 0 to S_i (arc length parametrization). We take M samples $x_i^{(1)}, \ldots, x_i^{(M)}$ from each curve such that $x_i^{(m)} = X_i(\alpha S_i)$ where $\alpha = \frac{m}{M}$. Note that while the arc length ratio α is the same at the mth sample for all curves, the arc length parameter αS_i will be different for each curve unless the curves have the same arc length. In other words, the arc length distance from the beginning of the curve to $x_i(m)$ will be different for every curve in general.

Now for each m, we have a point set $X^{(m)} = \{x_1^{(m)}, \ldots x_N^{(m)}\}$. Each point set is then projected onto a two-dimensional slicing plane. Intuitively, we would like this plane to be normal to the "cluster tangent" at a given arc length. We estimate this by computing the tangent $\tau_i^{(m)}$ to the i-th curve at $x_i^{(m)}$ and averaging this direction over the curves, to yield $\tau^{(m)}$. The slicing plane is spanned by the columns of the 3×2 matrix $\mathbf{P}_m$ that are set to be orthonormal and orthogonal to $\tau^{(m)}$. Furthermore, we require the plane to pass through the mean location $\mu^{(m)} = \frac{1}{N}\sum_{i=1}^{N} x_i^{(m)}$. The geometry of this construction is illustrated in Figure 1.

This slicing mechanism is motivated by the following intuition. Suppose that the cluster is coherent, i.e. the curves comprising it follow similar paths. In that case, the slicing plane will be close to normal to the tangent of each individual curve, and moreover the points corresponding to the m-th sample will be close in space. On the other hand, if the cluster contains a number of distinct subgroups, there will be two sets of samples, which will be clustered around distinct sub-means. Moreover, in such a case we can expect that projecting those samples onto the slicing plane, orthogonal to the cluster, will emphasize the separation between the subgroups.

Given the m-th slicing plane, we represent the cluster by a set of two-dimensional projections, which we call the "slice", $Y^{(m)} = \{\mathbf{y}_1^{(m)}, \ldots, \mathbf{y}_N^{(m)}\}$:

$$\mathbf{y}_i^{(m)} = \mathbf{P}_m^T (\mathbf{x}_i^{(m)} - \mu^{(m)}) \qquad (1)$$

Before we proceed, we note that an alternative slicing technique could be based on fitting a plane to $X^{(m)}$ using Principal Component Analysis [13]. A straightforward application of this in our experiments has proved inferior to the tangent-based technique described above, due to the effect of outliers. This could be alleviated by using robust PCA; we do not, however, pursue it further in this paper.

3.2 Cluster Co-membership within Slices

We now treat each slice separately. Effectively, each slice is an embedding of the set of curves into two-dimensional space. The set of points in this space can in principle be clustered using any off-the-shelf clustering method. However, we are specifically interested in determining whether there is an "interesting" partition in the slice. Therefore, of most interest to us are methods that allow automatic determination of the number of clusters. We use the Gaussian mixture clustering, accompanied by the Bayesian Information Criterion (BIC) for setting the number of components [14,15].

3.3 Spatial and Temporal Coherence

Once a Gaussian mixture model has been fit to the slice $Y^{(m)}$ for a range of values of k, we select the optimal model based on BIC. With the mixture model, we cluster the data by assigning each point to the component with the highest responsibility (i.e., the highest posterior probability of the point drawn by the associated Gaussian distribution). We will denote the label of $\mathbf{y}_i^{(m)}$ by $c_i^{(m)}$.

There is of course no direct relationship between the cluster labels across slices, since those are assigned arbitrarily. Even if the same partition of the curves to two clusters is reached in two slices, a given set of curves could be labeled 1 in one slice and 2 in the other slice. The information of interest to us is conveyed by the co-membership of a given pair of curves in a particular slice. Specifically, we define $J_{ij}^{(m)}$ such that

$$J_{ij}^{(m)} = \begin{cases} 1 & \text{if } c_i^{(m)} = c_j^{(m)}, \\ 0 & \text{otherwise.} \end{cases} \qquad (2)$$

Intuitively, the m-th slice votes for X_i and X_j being in the same cluster if $J_{ij}^{(m)} = 1$. One could now simply combine the values of this vote across all slices. However, it is possible for a particular pair of curves to be separated by the clustering in a given slice m simply due to the randomized nature of the procedure (placement of slicing plane, random initialization of the EM, etc.) despite genuinely belonging to the same subgroup. If indeed such an accidental result occurs, we expect that it will not persist in the neighboring slices, $m-1$ and $m+1$. This suggests the notion of temporal coherence. We formalize it with the value $T_{ij}^{(m)}$ defined as

$$T_{ij}^{(m)} = \begin{cases} 1 & \text{if } J_{ij}^{(m)} = J_{ij}^{(m-1)} \text{ and } J_{ij}^{(m)} = J_{ij}^{(m+1)}, \\ 0 & \text{otherwise.} \end{cases} \quad (3)$$

Finally, we can now represent the vote of the m-th slice regarding the similarity of curves i and j, weighted by the temporal coherence of that slice (with respect to that pair!):

$$W_{ij}^{(m)} = (1 - J_{ij}^{(m)}) \cdot T_{ij}^{(m)}. \quad (4)$$

$W_{ij}^{(m)}$ takes the value of 0 or 1. When it is 1, it indicates that the m-th slice supports a split where X_i and X_j are separated. $W_{ij}^{(m)}$ with 0 value, on the other hand, does not mean that the slice supports keeping X_i and X_j in the same cluster. It simply means that there is no evidence to the contrary. This may be due to the two curves being separated in the slice (zero co-membership), or the lack of temporal coherence, i.e., the co-membership of i and j being unstable in this slice–or both. This sort of asymmetric reasoning is similar in spirit to the statistical hypothesis testing formalism, in which the null hypothesis is either rejected or not, but never "accepted". In our case, this reflects the notion that not splitting the cluster is the default action.

We are now ready to describe the algorithm for evaluating the coherence of the cluster. Given the set of curves, we calculate a set of M slices, and cluster each of them using the Gaussian mixture clustering, with BIC model selection. We then compute the cluster co-membership values $J_{ij}^{(m)}$ and the temporal coherence $T_{ij}^{(m)}$ for each $m = 1, \ldots, M$ and $i, j = 1, \ldots, N$. This yields for each pair i, j a set of M votes $W_{ij}^{(m)}$. We combine the evidence regarding X_i and X_j across all slices in a single value:

$$W_{ij} = M - \sum_{m=1}^{M} W_{ij}^{(m)}. \quad (5)$$

This provides us with a measure of similarity for each pair of curves, organized in the form of an $N \times N$ matrix $\mathbf{W}$. By default, its diagonal is set to zero. For example, a value of 0 indicates that the two curves are consistently separated in all slices; the value of M indicates that no evidence for separating the two curves is provided by any of the slices. It is important to note that our similarity values are computed in the context of the given cluster, specifically with the objective to evaluate potential splits. This is in contrast to "global" distance measures, that operate on the same scale throughout the data set.

4 Refining Hierarchical Clustering Results

Given initial hypothesized (candidate) clusters as a result of hierarchical clustering, we evaluate the decision of splitting the cluster by applying the spectral clustering algorithm described in [16] to $\mathbf{W}$. Briefly, the algorithm is based on eigendecomposition of the symmetric matrix $\mathbf{D}^{-1/2}\mathbf{W}\mathbf{D}^{-1/2}$, where $\mathbf{D}$ contains the sums of corresponding rows of $\mathbf{W}$ on its main diagonal and zeros everywhere else. When two clusters are requested, the algorithm divides the data according to the sign of the corresponding entries of the $N \times 1$ second largest eigenvector of the matrix above. Note that this can lead to either two clusters, or a single one (if all the entries in the eigenvector are of the same sign).

4.1 Expert Evaluation

In order to assess the utility of our method for a practitioner, we conducted a comparative evaluation study with a domain expert. The fiber tracking data used in our experiments were obtained from DTI brain data sets scanned from four volunteers. We first obtained initial candidate clusters by applying the single linkage hierarchical clustering algorithm, with a distance measure adapted from [3]. Note that the adapted distance measure does not prevents curves with radically different lengths to be in the same cluster. Let $\mathcal{D}$ represent the similarity matrix obtained using this distance measure. We used the cut-off threshold of 3 (set heuristically to produce reasonable cluster sizes). The expert has significant experience with DTI and uses fiber-track models (integral curves) generated from DTI data sets in clinical research regularly. We compared three methods. The first one is our slicing-based method described above; we used $M = 50$ slices for each candidate cluster. The second method applies the single-linkage hierarchical clustering algorithm on $\mathcal{D}$ for the candidate cluster, with the objective of obtaining two sub-clusters. In other words, this method finds the optimal split of the appropriate subtree in the original dendrogram.

The third method applies the spectral clustering algorithm as does our method, but it uses the similarity matrix $\mathcal{D}$.

We displayed 93 cases where at least one of the methods produced a different split to the expert. The expert was shown the results from the three methods side-by-side, and asked to rank them. The evaluation was blind (i.e., the expert was not told which of the methods produced each result). We used a streamtube representation for the curves and juxtaposed clusters with the surface of lateral ventricles (areas of

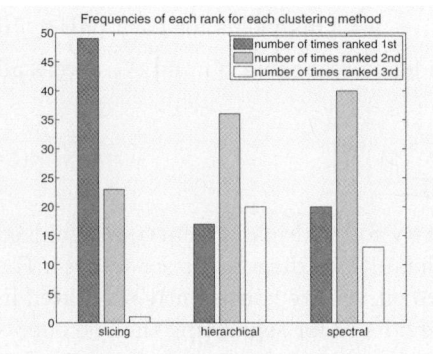

Fig. 2. Ranking frequencies of each clustering method for 93 cases as evaluated by an expert

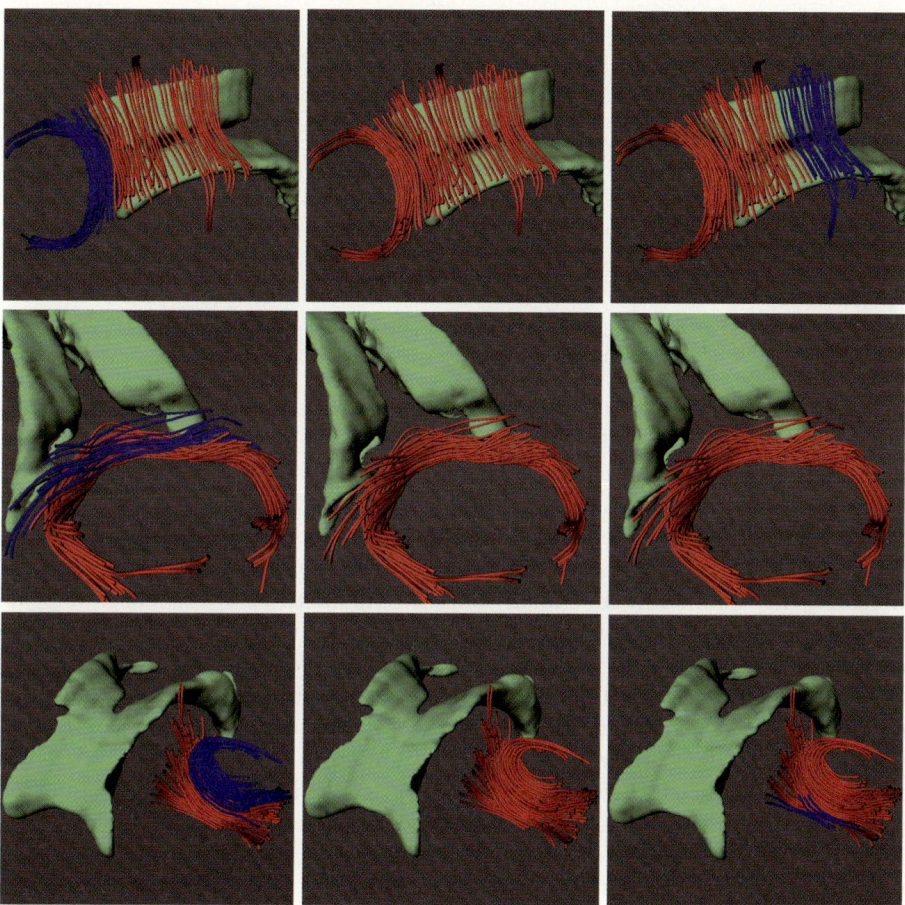

Fig. 3. Examples of clusters where our method was ranked to be the best by the expert. Split, if exists, is visualized by two colors (red and blue). The surface of lateral ventricles (green) provides an anatomical landmark. Left: the slicing-based split. It works well on clusters with curves having high curvatures as well as varying arc lengths. Middle: split based on the dendrogram used in hierarchical clustering. Right: split based on spectral clustering using the distance measure used to obtain the initial candidate clusters.

cerebrospinal fluid in the brain) extracted to provide an anatomical landmark. The expert were able to interactively manipulate the viewpoint, zoom-in and out, and rotate the models. The ranking decisions were based on the following criteria: anatomical correctness (whenever the expert recognized a candidate cluster), anatomical and physiological plausibility, and amount of information conveyed by the resulting clustering. The goal in this scenario is to evaluate whether the resulting clustering decision helps to identify biologically distinct structures in the DTI data.

4.2 Results

Out of 93 cases considered, 20 were ranked as three-way ties (i.e., undecided, equally good, or equally arbitrary). In the remaining 73, the expert ranked our slicing-based method the best method in 49 cases while only in 9 of these cases there was another method ranked the same. Furthermore, our method ranked worse than the other two methods only in one case. We summarize these results in Figure 2. In Figure 3, we show examples where our method produced better results (according to the expert feedback) than the other two methods.

5 Discussion and Conclusions

The main contribution of this paper is the novel coherence measure that is obtained by combining an intuitive geometric idea, slicing, with known statistical machine learning techniques. An important property of our method is its reliance on the context of the cluster in evaluating similarity between curves. The quantities computed in each slice, and across slices, are tied directly to the clustering objective. This is in contrast to the more standard setup in which distances and thresholds are defined in the global context. Our method works reasonably well on clusters with curves having high curvatures and varying arc lengths. While our motivation and the experimental evaluation have been on 3D DTI integral curves, our method generalizes to higher and lower dimensions easily and may apply to curve data in other domains. There is a number of technical aspects that we believe could be improved. Specifically, a more robust slicing and projection method that explicitly down-weights outliers could help reduce uncertainty in the per-slice quantities. Also, while we are not aware of any "gold standard" DTI fiber-track clustering data set, it is still possible to validate our method more quantitatively. The approach taken by Mobert et al. [4] can be a good starting point. A more challenging extension of the idea of slicing that we would like to pursue is to build a semi-parametric generative model for a cluster. Although our primary interest is in the analysis of DTI data, we believe our method is general and can be applied to any domain where data instances are represented by curves or trajectories.

References

1. Basser, P.J., Mattiello, J., LeBihan, D.: Estimation of the effective self-diffusion tensor from the nmr spin echo. Journal of Magnetic Resonance B, 247–254 (1994)
2. Basser, P.J., Pajevic, S., Pierpaoli, C., Duda, J., Aldroubi, A.: In vivo fiber tractography using DT-MRI data. Magnetic Resonance in Medicine 44, 625–632 (2000)
3. Zhang, S., Demiralp, C., Laidlaw, D.H.: Visualizing diffusion tensor MR images using streamtubes and streamsurfaces. IEEE TVCG 9, 454–462 (2003)
4. Moberts, B., Vilanova, A., van Wijk, J.J.: Evaluation of fiber clustering methods for diffusion tensor imaging. In: Procs. of Vis 2005, pp. 65–72 (2005)
5. Shimony, J., Snyder, A., Lori, N., Conturo, T.: Automated fuzzy clustering of neuronal pathways in diffusion tensor tracking. In: Proceedings of ISMRM (2002)

6. Ding, Z., Gore, J.C., Anderson, A.W.: Case study: reconstruction, visualization and quantification of neuronal fiber pathways. In: VIS 2001: Proceedings of the conference on Visualization 2001, pp. 453–456. IEEE Computer Society, Los Alamitos (2001)
7. Corouge, I., Gouttard, S., Gerig, G.: Towards a shape model of white matter fiber bundles using diffusion tensor MRI. In: International Symposium on Biomedical Imaging, pp. 344–347 (2004)
8. Brun, A., Knutsson, H., Park, H.J., Shenton, M., Westin, C.F.: Clustering fiber traces using normalized cuts. In: Barillot, C., Haynor, D.R., Hellier, P. (eds.) MICCAI 2004. LNCS, vol. 3216, pp. 368–375. Springer, Heidelberg (2004)
9. O'Donnell, L., Kubicki, M., Shenton, M.E., Dreusicke, M., Grimson, W.E.L., Westin, C.-F.: A method for clustering white matter fiber tracts. AJNR 27(5) (2006)
10. Breckenridge, J.N.: Replicating cluster analysis: Method, consistency, and validity. Multivariate Behavioral Research 24, 147–161 (1989)
11. Fridlyand, J., Dudoit, S.: Applications of resampling methods to estimate the number of clusters and to improve the accuracy of a clustering method. Technical report, Division of Biostatistics, School of Public Healty, UC Berkeley (2001)
12. Lange, T., Roth, V., Braun, M.L., Buhmann, J.M.: Stability-based validation of clustering solutions. Neural Computation, 1299–1323 (2004)
13. Joliffe, I.T.: Principal Component Analysis, 2nd edn. Springer, Heidelberg (2002)
14. Schwarz, G.: Estimating the dimension of a model. The Annals of Statistics 6, 461–464 (1978)
15. Bishop, C.M.: Pattern Recognition and Machine Learning. Springer, Heidelberg (2006)
16. Ng, A.Y., Jordan, M.I., Weiss, Y.: On spectral clustering: Analysis and an algorithm. In: Neural Information Processing Systems, pp. 849–856. MIT Press, Cambridge (2001)

Brain Fiber Architecture, Genetics, and Intelligence: A High Angular Resolution Diffusion Imaging (HARDI) Study[*]

Ming-Chang Chiang[1], Marina Barysheva[1], Agatha D. Lee[1], Sarah Madsen[1], Andrea D. Klunder[1], Arthur W. Toga[1], Katie L. McMahon[2], Greig I. de Zubicaray[2], Matthew Meredith[2], Margaret J. Wright[3], Anuj Srivastava[4], Nikolay Balov[4], and Paul M. Thompson[1]

[1] Laboratory of Neuro Imaging, Dept. of Neurology, UCLA School of Medicine, Los Angeles, CA
[2] Functional MRI Lab., Centre for Magnetic Resonance, Univ. Queensland, Brisbane, Australia
[3] Queensland Institute of Medical Research, Brisbane, Australia
[4] Dept. of Statistics, Florida State University, Tallahassee, FL

Abstract. We developed an analysis pipeline enabling population studies of HARDI data, and applied it to map genetic influences on fiber architecture in 90 twin subjects. We applied tensor-driven 3D fluid registration to HARDI, resampling the spherical fiber orientation distribution functions (ODFs) in appropriate Riemannian manifolds, after ODF regularization and sharpening. Fitting structural equation models (SEM) from quantitative genetics, we evaluated genetic influences on the Jensen-Shannon divergence (JSD), a novel measure of fiber spatial coherence, and on the generalized fiber anisotropy (GFA; [1]) a measure of fiber integrity. With random-effects regression, we mapped regions where diffusion profiles were highly correlated with subjects' intelligence quotient (IQ). Fiber complexity was predominantly under genetic control, and higher in more highly anisotropic regions; the proportion of genetic versus environmental control varied spatially. Our methods show promise for discovering genes affecting fiber connectivity in the brain.

1 Introduction

Diffusion profiles of brain white-matter fibers are intermediate phenotypes that can be causally related to more basic biological measures, such as genetic variations across subjects, and to more high-order cognitive processes, such as intellectual performance. They serve as a valuable link in the quest to find genes that influence cognition and disease, as fiber integrity may be associated with genetic variation using quantitative genetic modeling, and with cognitive scores (such as intelligence quotient or IQ).

In this paper we analyzed the high angular resolution diffusion imaging (HARDI) data of 90 twin subjects. Studies of identical and fraternal twins – who share all or

---

[*] This work was funded in part by NIH grant R01 HD050735.

half of their genes respectively - are informative for understanding the genetic control of brain structure and function. We measured the regional complexity of diffusion orientation distribution functions (ODF) by applying statistics to high-dimensional HARDI data in appropriate Riemannian manifolds. We visualized associations between diffusion profiles and genetic and environmental factors, and with IQ, by fitting structural equation (SEM) and random-effects regression (RRM) models at each voxel. To our knowledge, these are the first 3D maps of genetic influences on HARDI, and reveal that HARDI signals that are genetically controlled, to some extent, are also correlated with intelligence.

2 Methods

2.1 Subject Description and Image Acquisition

HARDI data were acquired from 22 pairs of monozygotic (MZ; 20 males/24 females; age = 25.1±1.5 years) and 23 pairs of dizygotic twins (DZ; all same-sex pairs; 20 males/26 females; age = 23.5±2.2 years) on a 4T Bruker Medspec MRI scanner using an optimized diffusion tensor sequence [2]. Imaging parameters were: 21 axial slices (5 mm thick), FOV = 23 cm, TR/TE 6090/91.7 ms, 0.5 mm gap, with a 128×100 acquisition matrix. 30 images were acquired: 3 with no diffusion sensitization (i.e., T2-weighted images) and 27 diffusion-weighted images in which the gradient directions were evenly distributed on the hemisphere [2]. The reconstruction matrix was 128×128, yielding a 1.8×1.8 mm^2 in-plane resolution. Total scan time was 3.05 minutes.

2.2 DTI Registration

For each subject, diffusion tensor (DT) images (denoted by D_{ij}, $1 \leq i, j \leq 3$) were computed from the HARDI signals using MedINRIA software (http://www-sop.inria.fr/asclepios/software/MedINRIA). One diagonal component image (D_{11}) was manually stripped of nonbrain tissues, yielding a binary brain extraction mask (cerebellum included). The masked image was then registered to the ICBM53 average brain template with a 12-parameter linear transformation using the software FLIRT [3], and resampled to isotropic voxel resolution (dimension: 128×128×93 voxels, resolution: 1.7×1.7×1.7 mm^3). The resulting transformation parameters were used to rotationally reorient the tensor at each voxel [4], and then affine align the tensor-valued images based on trilinear interpolation of the log-transformed tensors [5]. All affine-registered DT images were then registered to a randomly selected subject's image (a MZ subject), using an inverse-consistent fluid registration algorithm that minimizes the symmetrized Kullback-Leibler divergence (sKL-divergence) of the two tensor-valued images [6].

2.3 HARDI Processing and Registration

Orientation distribution functions (ODF) for water diffusion were computed voxelwise from the HARDI signals using the Funk-Radon Transform (FRT) [1]. We used Descoteaux's method [7], which expands the HARDI signals as a spherical harmonic

(SH) series, simplifying the FRT to a linear matrix operation on the coefficients. To estimate the SH coefficients, we set the order of the SH series to 4, and added a Laplacian smoothing regularizer to reduce the noise level, and also a Laplacian sharpening regularizer to help detect the peaks of the ODF, as in [7]. The estimated ODF was normalized to unit mass, creating a diffusion probability density function (PDF) parameterized by spherical angle.

Images of the diffusion ODFs were registered to the target subject by applying the corresponding DTI mapping (both affine and fluid mappings) in the previous section. To keep the direction of the diffusion ODFs oriented with the direction of the underlying fibers, ODFs were reoriented using the Preservation of Principal Direction (PPD) method [4], where the principal direction of the ODF was determined by principal component analysis [8]. A generalized fractional anisotropy (GFA) map was constructed from the registered ODF ψ [1]:

$$GFA = \sqrt{n\sum_{i=1}^{n}(\psi(\mathbf{u}_i)-\langle\psi\rangle)^2 \Big/ (n-1)\sum_{i=1}^{n}\psi(\mathbf{u}_i)^2} \qquad (1)$$

Here $\mathbf{u}_i$, $1 \leq i \leq n$, are n gradient directions, and $\langle\psi\rangle$ is the mean of the ODF with respect to spherical angle.

Spatial interpolation of HARDI ODFs is a new issue, and is required when the registration mapping falls on non-lattice points. We addressed this by taking the square root of the ODF: the Riemannian manifold for the square root of a PDF is isomorphic to a unit sphere and there are closed form expressions defining the geodesic distance, exponential and inverse exponential mappings [9]. The interpolated square-rooted ODF (sqrt-ODF) ϕ at point (x, y, z) was then constructed by finding the weighted Karcher mean of its 8 diagonal neighbors ϕ_i in 3D at lattice points (x_i, y_i, z_i), which minimizes the square sum of the geodesic distance d:

$$\phi = \arg\min \sum_{i=1}^{8} w_i d(\phi, \phi_i)^2. \qquad (2)$$

Here w_i is the trilinear interpolation weight defined as $w_i = (1-|x-x_i|)(1-|y-y_i|)(1-|z-z_i|)$. The weighted Karcher mean ϕ was computed using a gradient descent approach as in [9].

2.4 Measuring Regional Complexity of Diffusion

We defined the regional complexity of diffusion using the generalized Jensen-Shannon divergence (JSD) [10]. JSD measures the dissimilarity of n probability distributions, given by:

$$JSD_w(\mathbf{p}_1,...,\mathbf{p}_n) = H\left(\sum_{i=1}^{n}w_i\mathbf{p}_i\right) - \sum_{i=1}^{n}w_iH(\mathbf{p}_i). \qquad (3)$$

Here $\mathbf{p}_i = \{p_{ij}, 1 \leq j \leq k | \sum_{j=1}^{k} p_{ij} =1\}$, and $w = \{w_i, 1 \leq i \leq n | \sum_{i=1}^{n} w_i =1\}$. $H(\bullet)$ is the Shannon entropy, defined as $H(\mathbf{p}) = -\sum_{j=1}^{k} p_j \log p_j$. $JSD_w(\mathbf{p}_1,...,\mathbf{p}_n) = 0$ if and only if all $\mathbf{p}_1,..., \mathbf{p}_n$ are equal. The complexity of diffusion at voxel $\mathbf{x}$ was defined as the JSD for the ODF at $\mathbf{x}$ and its contiguous 26 ODFs. We adopted an equal weight of $1/n$ for simplicity.

2.5 Statistical Analysis of Structural Models for Twins

To analyze genetic and environmental correlations in twins, structural equation models (SEM; [11, 12]) can evaluate contributions of additive genetic (A), shared environmental (C) and random environmental (E) components to the covariances of the observed variables (*y*) for MZ and DZ twins, according to the following model:

$$y_j = aA_j + cC_j + eE_j, \qquad (4)$$

where $j = 1$ or 2 for the first or second twin in the same pair. Since A, C, and E are unobservable variables, their weights $\theta = (a, c, e)$ were estimated by comparing the covariance matrix implied by the model, $\Sigma(\theta)$, and the sample covariance matrix of the observed variables, **S**, using maximum-likelihood fitting:

$$F_{ML,\theta} = \log|\Sigma(\theta)| + trace(\Sigma^{-1}(\theta)\mathbf{S}) - \log|\mathbf{S}| - p, \qquad (5)$$

where $p = 2$ is the number of observed variables. Under the null hypothesis that the population covariance matrix of the observed variables equals $\Sigma(\theta)$, and the *n*-sample data *y* are multivariate normal, $T_{ML,\theta} = (n-1)F_{ML,\theta}$ follows a χ^2 distribution with $p(p+1)-t$ degrees of freedom, where *t* is the number of free model parameters. Acceptance of the null hypothesis ($p > 0.05$) indicates a good fit for the model.

Parameter fitting based on the above χ^2 distribution may be biased if the sample data are non-normal. To free SEM from distributional assumptions, we used permutation methods to determine goodness of fit [13]. At each voxel, the GFA or JSD of the diffusion ODFs served as the observed variable, with the subject's age regressed out. We computed $T_{ML,\theta}$ using the Broyden-Fletcher-Goldfarb-Shanno (BFGS) method [14] to minimize F_{ML} in (5) in the original sample, as well as in 2000 permuted samples in which the twin pairs' MZ or DZ labels were randomly shuffled. In each permutation relabeling, four null hypotheses with different θ were evaluated, for fitting the E: $\theta = (e)$, CE: $\theta = (c, e)$, AE: $\theta = (a, e)$, and ACE: $\theta = (a, c, e)$ models, and the *p*-values, p_E, p_{CE}, p_{AE}, and p_{ACE}, were determined separately by comparing $T_{ML,\theta}$ in the true labeling to the permutation distribution. Since the permutation distribution of the χ^2 statistic $T_{ML,\theta}$ may differ from its original distribution, we rescaled the sample data using the Bollen-Stine transformation for each null hypothesis [13]:

$$\mathbf{Z} = \mathbf{Y}\mathbf{S}^{-1/2}\Sigma^{1/2}(\theta). \qquad (6)$$

Here **Y** is an $n \times 2$ matrix of the observed variables for the *n* twin pairs. Matrix square roots were computed by Cholesky factorization. The rows of **Z** instead of **Y** were permuted.

The four permutation *p*-values, p_E, p_{CE}, p_{AE}, and p_{ACE}, were compared at each voxel and the voxel was assigned to one of E, CE, AE, and ACE models if the *p*-value for that model was greater than the other three and also greater than 0.05. Color-coded maps visualized the optimal model fitted at each voxel, with E coded as blue, CE as green, AE as red, and ACE as yellow. For better visualization, we defined "model clusters", i.e. sets of connected (26-neighborhood) voxels where the same model fitted, for each of the four models, and displayed only clusters of more than 10,000 voxels.

2.6 Linkage of Diffusion Anisotropy or Complexity with Cognitive Function

We used random-effects regression models (RRM) [15] to measure correlations between the full-scale intelligence quotient (FSIQ) and GFA or JSD. Ordinary regression methods are inappropriate because observations are clustered within twin pairs, violating the assumption that observations must be statistically independent. In RRM, the lack of independence is addressed by adding a random variable α_i, to incorporate the clustering of the observed variables within the ith pair, into the ordinary regression equations:

$$\mathbf{y}_i = \mathbf{X}_i \beta + \mathbf{1}_i \alpha_i + \varepsilon_i. \qquad (7)$$

Here $\mathbf{y}_i$ = the 2×1 vector of observed variables (GFA or JSD) within the ith pair, β = a $(q+1) \times 1$ vector of unknown regression coefficients, $\mathbf{X}_i$ = a known $2 \times (q+1)$ covariate matrix, $\mathbf{1}_i$ = a 2×1 vector of ones, and ε_i represents the 2×1 error vector. q was set to 1 for subjects' FSIQ score as the covariate. We assumed that α_i and ε_i, and thus $\mathbf{y}_i$, were normally distributed, with $\alpha_i \sim N(0, \sigma_\alpha^2)$, $\varepsilon_i \sim N(0, \sigma^2 \mathbf{I}_2)$, and $\mathbf{y}_i \sim N(\mathbf{X}_i \beta, \sigma_\alpha^2 \mathbf{1}_i \mathbf{1}_i^T + \sigma^2 \mathbf{I}_2)$, where $\mathbf{I}_m$ represents an $m \times m$ identity matrix. Estimation of these unknown parameters (β, σ_α^2, σ^2) was based on maximum marginal likelihood (MML) methods detailed in [15].

We applied RRM to each voxel and tested the significance of the correlations by comparing the full ($\beta = [\beta_0, \beta_{IQ}]^T$; β_0 is a constant) and the reduced ($\beta = \beta_0$) models, which gave a significance P-value based on Wilks' lambda distribution [16]: $\Lambda = |\Sigma_{full}|/|\Sigma_{reduced}| \sim \Lambda(p, vH, vE)$, where Σ is the estimated covariance matrix of $\mathbf{y}_i$. $p = 2$ is the number of subjects in each pair, $vH = 1$ is the difference in the number of parameters between full and reduced models, and $vE = n-q-1$, where n is the number of twin pairs. Overall significance was assessed using the positive false discovery rate (pFDR) method [17]. A pFDR value < 0.05 was considered to be significant.

3 Results

Fig. 1 displays the spatial distribution of the average JSD (averaged across all 90 subjects). The average JSD increases with GFA, suggesting that JSD is sensitive to the complexity of ODFs in major white matter fibers with high diffusion anisotropy, especially in regions where anisotropy values vary over a small spatial neighborhood.

Fig. 2 shows the covariance structure fitting for GFA and JSD maps in the 90 twins. When the AE model fits best, variation in GFA or JSD values is more attributable to genetic influences, i.e., the covariance structures are best accounted for by additive genetic (added effect of genes) and random environmental effects (random experimental error is also lumped into the E term). When the CE model fits best, the variation in the observed measures is more due to environmental influences shared by twins reared in the same family [11]. The full ACE model, where all terms fit at once, could not be fitted for either GFA or JSD. For both GFA and JSD measures, more voxels had AE as the best-fitting model than CE or any other model, indicating that diffusion properties are more genetically influenced than environmentally influenced, in most brain regions.

Brain Fiber Architecture, Genetics, and Intelligence   1065

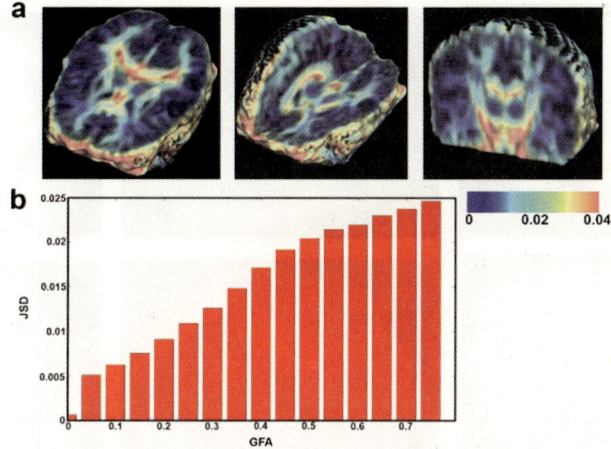

Fig. 1. (**a**) The color-coded map shows that the JSD, a measure of fiber complexity, is greater in regions of high diffusion anisotropy (e.g., the corpus callosum), especially at interfaces between high and low anisotropy. This trend is clear when plotting JSD against the GFA (**b**). This property of JSD is useful because in DTI/HARDI studies, diffusion properties are more informative in highly anisotropic regions, where fiber structures are highly resolved.

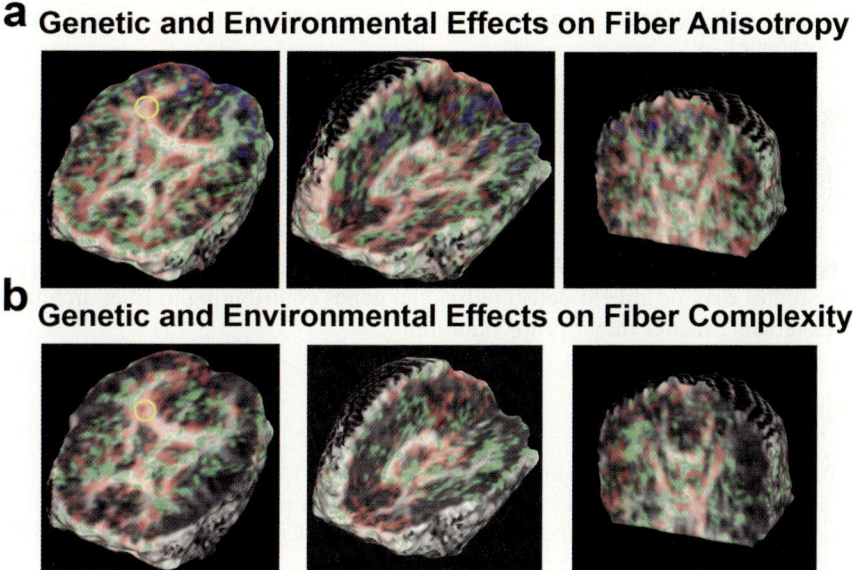

Fig. 2. The color-coded map shows which model fits best for the covariance matrices of (**a**) GFA, a measure of fiber integrity, and (**b**) JSD for fiber complexity, at each voxel. Voxels where the E model fits best are coded as blue, CE as green, and AE as red. For GFA and JSD, major fiber structures, such as the corpus callosum, cingulum, and internal capsules, are optimally fitted using the AE and the CE models. Model fitting is visibly asymmetrical in the cingulum fibers: the AE model fits in the right cingulum (yellow circles in (a) and (b)), while the CE model fits better in the left cingulum.

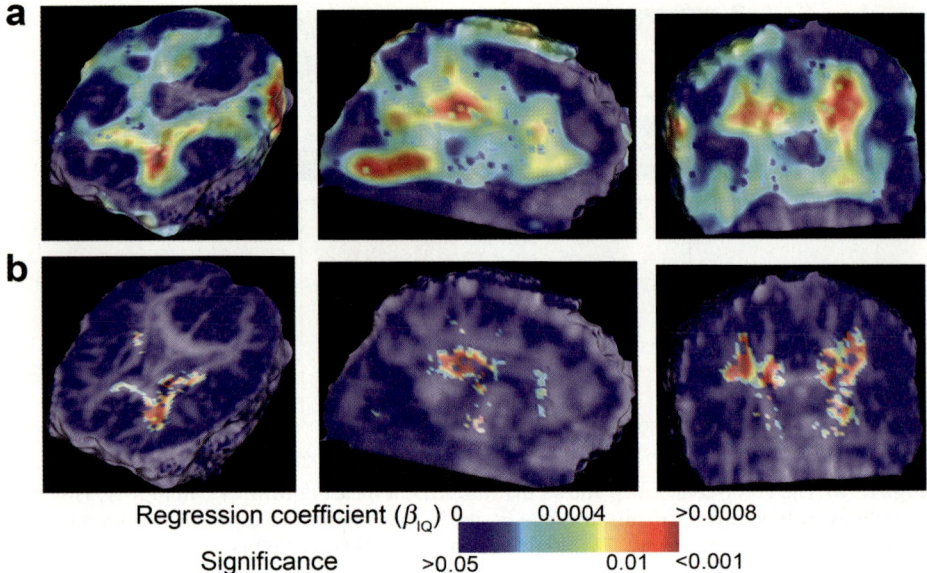

Fig. 3. Correlations of GFA with the FSIQ score based on random-effects regression, visualized as maps of (**a**) regression coefficients (β_{IQ}) and (**b**) *P*-values. Higher diffusion anisotropy is associated with higher IQ in the left anterior region of the *corona radiata*, *cingulum*, and internal capsule.

Fig. 3 shows that GFA is positively correlated with FSIQ scores in the *corona radiata*, corpus callosum and internal capsule (pFDR = 0.04). The correlations of JSD with FSIQ scores were not significant (pFDR = 0.21; figures not shown). Fiber measures were highly genetically controlled, especially in regions of high diffusion anisotropy. We also found that higher diffusion anisotropy is correlated with better intellectual performance in specific WM regions. Based on these measures and algorithms, future studies may be able to detect individual genes contributing to fiber architecture, and relate white matter integrity to cognition.

References

1. Tuch, D.S.: Q-ball imaging. Magn. Reson. Med. 52(6), 1358–1372 (2004)
2. Jones, D.K., Horsfield, M.A., Simmons, A.: Optimal strategies for measuring diffusion in anisotropic systems by magnetic resonance imaging. Magn. Reson. Med. 42(3), 515–525 (1999)
3. Jenkinson, M., Smith, S.: A global optimisation method for robust affine registration of brain images. Med. Image Anal. 5(2), 143–156 (2001)
4. Alexander, D.C., et al.: Spatial transformations of diffusion tensor magnetic resonance. IEEE Transactions on Medical Imaging 20, 1131–1139 (2001)
5. Arsigny, V., et al.: Fast and simple calculus on tensors in the log-Euclidean framework. In: Duncan, J.S., Gerig, G. (eds.) MICCAI 2005. LNCS, vol. 3749, pp. 115–122. Springer, Heidelberg (2005)

6. Chiang, M.C., et al.: Fluid Registration of Diffusion Tensor Images Using Information Theory. IEEE Transactions on Medical Imaging 27, 442–456 (2008)
7. Descoteaux, M., et al.: Regularized, fast, and robust analytical Q-ball imaging. Magn. Reson. Med. 58(3), 497–510 (2007)
8. Chiang, M.-C., et al.: Information-theoretic analysis of brain white matter fiber orientation distribution functions. In: Karssemeijer, N., Lelieveldt, B. (eds.) IPMI 2007. LNCS, vol. 4584, pp. 172–182. Springer, Heidelberg (2007)
9. Srivastava, A., Jermyn, I., Joshi, S.H.: Riemannian Analysis of Probability Density Functions with applications in Vision. In: CVPR 2007, Minneapolis, Minnesota, USA (2007)
10. Lin, J.: Divergence measures based on the Shannon entropy. IEEE Trans. Information Theory 37(1), 145–151 (1991)
11. Neale, M.C., Cardon, L.R.: The NATO Scientific Affairs Division. Methodology for genetic studies of twins and families, vol. xxv, 496 p. Kluwer Academic Publishers, Dordrecht (1992)
12. Schmitt, J.E., et al.: A multivariate analysis of neuroanatomic relationships in a genetically informative pediatric sample. Neuroimage 35(1), 70–82 (2007)
13. Bollen, K.A., Stine, R.A.: Bootstrapping goodness-of-fit measures in structural equation models. Sociological Methods Research 21(2), 205–229 (1992)
14. Press, W.H., et al.: Numerical recipes in C++, 2nd edn., vol. viii, 318 p. Cambridge Univ. Press, Cambridge (2002)
15. Hedeker, D., Gibbons, R.D., Flay, B.R.: Random-effects regression models for clustered data with an example from smoking prevention research. J. Consult. Clin. Psych. 62(4), 757–765 (1994)
16. Rencher, A.C.: Methods of multivariate analysis, 2nd edn. J. Wiley, New York (2002)
17. Storey, J.D.: A direct approach to false discovery rates. J. Roy. Stat. Soc. B 64(3), 479–498 (2002)

Group Statistics of DTI Fiber Bundles Using Spatial Functions of Tensor Measures

Casey B. Goodlett[1,2], P. Thomas Fletcher[1,2], John H. Gilmore[3], and Guido Gerig[1,2]

[1] School of Computing, University of Utah
[2] Scientific Computing and Imaging Institute, University of Utah
[3] Department of Psychiatry, University of North Carolina*

Abstract. We present a framework for hypothesis testing of differences between groups of DTI fiber tracts. An anatomical, tract-oriented coordinate system provides a basis for estimating the distribution of diffusion properties. The parametrization of sampled, smooth functions is normalized across a population using DTI atlas building. Functional data analysis, an extension of multivariate statistics to continuous functions is applied to the problem of hypothesis testing and discrimination. B-spline models of fractional anisotropy (FA) and Frobenius norm measures are analyzed jointly. Plots of the discrimination direction provide a clinical interpretation of the group differences. The methodology is tested on a pediatric study of subjects aged one and two years.

1 Introduction

The diffusion properties of white matter tracts measured by DTI provide a novel and important source of information for group comparison and regression in clinical neuroimaging studies. Significant challenges remain in the development of an automatic framework for testing significance of group differences in a manner which provides clinically relevant results. Previous work has shown the importance of modeling the diffusion properties of a fiber tract as functions sampled by arc length along the axis of the bundle [1,2]. The major challenge in applying this type of analysis is the need for a consistent parametrization of fiber bundles across a large population of images. Deformable registration has been proposed as a method of mapping a population to a reference atlas coordinate system [3,4,5]. Most of the analysis using atlas building has focused on independent voxelwise tests, which can be challenging to interpret and require sophisticated multiple comparison correction. Most studies have also analyzed fractional anisotropy (FA) or mean diffusivity (MD) values independently. We propose to combine the anatomically relevant coordinate system of tract statistics with the

---

* This work is part of the National Alliance for Medical Image Computing (NA-MIC), funded by the National Institutes of Health through Grant U54 EB005149 as well as support from the NIMH Silvio O. Conte Center Grant MH064065. Dr. Fletcher is partially funded through an Autism Speaks Mentor-Based Postdoctoral Fellowship.

population coordinate system provided by atlas building. The combination of the tract coordinate system with atlas building provides an automated, clinically interpretable framework for understanding group differences. The closest related work has been done using nonlinear registration and projection onto a skeleton representation of FA [6]. Another proposed approach uses fiber clustering to compute correspondence across a population [7].

We use deformable registration to estimate and remove shape variability in a population of images. Analysis of shape normalized fiber bundles is performed in an anatomically relevant coordinate system based on fiber tractography. The atlas normalized diffusion measures are treated as a continuous smooth function of arc length, and statistical tests are applied for the joint analysis of the orthogonal FA and Frobenius norm measures. The framework provides a single multivariate hypothesis test between groups eliminating the need for multiple comparison correction and incorporating the joint information of tensor anisotropy and size. Visualization of the linear discriminant provides a clinically meaningful interpretation of the group differences as shown in an example study of pediatric images. Fig. 1 shows an overview of the analysis procedure.

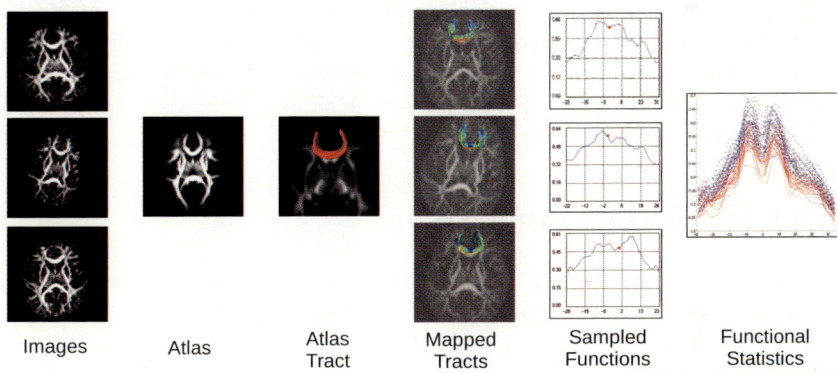

Fig. 1. Schematic overview of the tract analysis procedure

2 Atlas Parametrization and Fiber Extraction

Atlas building based on diffeomorphic registration estimates a set of transformations such that each image in the population can be mapped into the atlas coordinate system. In the DTI atlas building framework, each tensor image I_i is mapped into a common atlas space by a transformation T_i with inverse T_i^{-1} using appropriate measures to account for reorientation and interpolation of tensors. For the study presented here, the procedure of Goodlett *et al.* based on the atlas building procedure of Joshi *et al.* is applied [4,8]. In our framework, images from two groups are combined to produce a single pooled atlas. Our assumption is that the overall topology of the images in the two groups are similar enough to allow all images to be combined into one atlas, but differences may occur in the diffusion properties of fiber tracts. Thus, we use registration to normalize the image shapes and perform statistics on the diffusion properties of the normalized fiber bundles. The set of tensor images are averaged in atlas space to produce an atlas tensor image with improved signal-to-noise ratio (SNR). The average tensor volume allows reliable extraction of tracts even in populations of images with low SNR such as pediatric images. The diffeomorphic transforms guaranteed by the atlas building procedure allow atlas tracts to be mapped back into each individual subject.

Fiber tracts are extracted in the average tensor image using a standard Runge-Kutta streamline integration technique based on the principal eigenvector field. Source and target regions are manually developed to extract each bundle of interest. For each subject, the data within the fiber bundle is modeled as a sampled function of arc length using a method similar to that described in Corouge et al. [1]. The result of the procedure is a set of sampled functions parametrized by arc length $t_j \in [-a, b]$ from the atlas fiber tract. The atlas-normalized parametrization of the curves is possible because of the smooth, invertible nature of the transformations T_i, T_i^{-1}. That is the samples from each subject are obtained by $FA_i(T_i(t_j))$ for each sample point t_j in the atlas tract. A sampled function is created for each tensor scalar measure such as fractional anisotropy, mean diffusivity (MD), Frobenius norm $\|D\|$, etc. For the purpose of this work we chose FA and the Frobenius norm as orthogonal anisotropy and size measures respectively [9]. Fig. 2 shows the sampled curves extracted for the genu fiber bundle for our example study.

3 Functional Data Analysis

Image sampling as well as the fiber tract extraction process create a sampled representation of the fiber bundle diffusion properties. However, there exists a

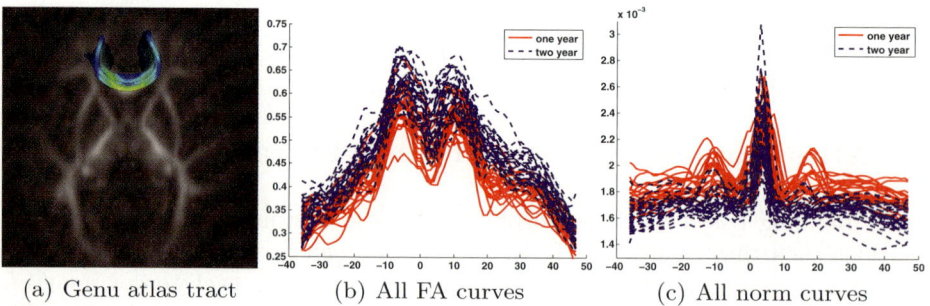

Fig. 2. (a) Genu tract extracted from the tensor atlas colored by FA value. The diffusion values are sampled along the atlas-normalized arc length for each individual in the study for FA and Frobenius norm values. The sampled FA and Frobenius norm functions for the two groups are shown in (b) and (c) respectively. The one year old subjects are the dashed red lines and the two year old subjects are the solid blue lines. The spikes in the center of the Frobenius norm functions are likely partial voluming with the ventricles.

continuous underlying biology which generates these samples. Therefore, statistical analysis of the sampled diffusion functions must account for the underlying continuity and spatial correlation of the samples. We compute statistics of the diffusion curves as an infinite-dimensional extension to multivariate statistics known as functional data analysis [10]. The simplest extensions of ordinary statistics to the functional setting are the sample mean function $\bar{f}(t)$ and the sample variance-covariance function $v(s,t)$, which is the bivariate function given by

$$\bar{f}(t) = \frac{1}{N} \sum_{i=1}^{N} f_i(t), \text{ and } v(s,t) = \frac{1}{N-1} \sum_{i=1}^{N} (f_i(s) - \bar{f}_i(s))(f_i(t) - \bar{f}_i(t)) \quad (1)$$

The diagonal of the function, $v(t,t)$, is the pointwise variance. Hypothesis testing and discriminant analysis of the space of functions has an inherent high dimension low sample size problem, because of the infinite dimensional space of continuous functions. Regularization methods are, therefore, essential in the computation of functional statistics. To enforce regularity, B-spline fitting and functional principal components analysis (PCA) is used for data driven smoothing where the number of retained PCA modes acts as a smoothing parameter.

In order to make computations tractable smooth basis functions are fit to the sampled diffusion curves. B-splines were selected as basis functions due to the nonperiodic nature of the data, the compact support of the B-spline basis, and the ability to enforce derivative continuity. A large number of B-spline bases are first fit to the sampled functions using a least squares approach. The number of basis functions is chosen subjectively to maintain local features while providing some smoothing. Computation of the mean function is computed by the sample mean of the B-spline coefficients. Computation of the variance-covariance function requires accounting for mapping between basis coefficients and function values. Let $f_i(t)$ be the B-spline function fit to the samples from subject i. In matrix notation we express all functions $f_i(t)$ as a matrix of coefficients $\mathbf{C}$ times the basis functions $\boldsymbol{\phi}$

$$\mathbf{f}(t) = \mathbf{C}\boldsymbol{\phi}(t). \quad (2)$$

Similarly, the variance-covariance function of $\mathbf{f}(t)$ can be written as

$$v(s,t) = \frac{1}{N-1} \boldsymbol{\phi}(s)^T \mathbf{C}^T \mathbf{C} \boldsymbol{\phi}(t). \quad (3)$$

Principal component analysis (PCA) of the functions $f_i(t)$ decomposes $v(s,t)$ into the orthogonal unit eigenfunctions $\xi(t)$ which satisfy

$$\int v(s,t)\xi(t)dt = \lambda \xi(s). \quad (4)$$

The B-Spline basis is not orthonormal resulting in a non-symmetric eigenvalue problem to solve (4). As shown in Ramsay and Silverman [10], this minimization can solved by the symmetric eigenvalue problem for the basis coefficients $\mathbf{b}$, with the change of variable $\mathbf{W}^{1/2}\mathbf{u} = \mathbf{b}$ as

$$\mathbf{W}^{1/2}\mathbf{C}^T\mathbf{C}\mathbf{W}^{1/2}\mathbf{u} = \lambda\mathbf{u}, \quad (5)$$

where $\mathbf{W}$ is the matrix of basis function inner products with entries

$$W_{ij} = \int \phi_i(t)\phi_j(j). \tag{6}$$

In our analysis we consider jointly the analysis of FA and tensor norm functions with basis coefficients $\mathbf{C}_1$ and $\mathbf{C}_2$ respectively. We therefore compute PCA from the eigenanalysis of $\boldsymbol{\Sigma}$, where

$$\boldsymbol{\Sigma}_{ij} = \mathbf{W}^{1/2}\mathbf{C}_i^T\mathbf{C}_j\mathbf{W}^{1/2}, \text{ and}$$

$$\boldsymbol{\Sigma} = \begin{bmatrix} \boldsymbol{\Sigma}_{11} & \boldsymbol{\Sigma}_{12} \\ \boldsymbol{\Sigma}_{21} & \boldsymbol{\Sigma}_{22} \end{bmatrix}. \tag{7}$$

Hypothesis testing and discriminant analysis is performed on the projection into the first K PCA modes, where K serves as a smoothing parameter. Let $\mathbf{x}_i$ and $\mathbf{y}_i$ be the projection of the curves from the two population of functions $f_i(t)$ and $g_i(t)$ into the PCA space. In this space the basis mapping has already been incorporated and standard multivariate analysis can be applied. The normal parametric hypothesis test for mean differences is the Hotelling T^2 statistic,

$$T^2 = \frac{n_x n_y}{n_x + n_y}(\bar{\mathbf{x}} - \bar{\mathbf{y}})\mathbf{S}^{-1}(\bar{\mathbf{x}} - \bar{\mathbf{y}})^T \tag{8}$$

where $\mathbf{S}$ is the pooled covariance matrix. In order to relax the normality assumptions associated with the parametric test, we apply a permutation test based on the T^2 statistic to compute the p-value.

The T^2 statistic is proportional to the group mean differences projected on the Fisher linear discriminant (FLD),

$$\boldsymbol{\omega} = \mathbf{S}^{-1}(\bar{\mathbf{x}} - \bar{\mathbf{y}})^T. \tag{9}$$

The linear discriminant, therefore, provides a direction for interpreting the group differences. The coefficients of the discriminant can be expanded into the original function basis so that $FLD(t) = \phi(t)\boldsymbol{\omega}$ is a function whose inner product with the original data provides maximal separation between the groups.

4 Pediatric Data Application and Validation

We have tested the methodology on a study of pediatric DTI images. A population of 22 one year old subjects and 30 two year old subjects were chosen from a database of pediatric DTI. In this example we expected to find large differences between the two groups, and the purpose of this study is to illustrate the methodology rather than to determine clinical results. Each image was acquired with $2x2x2mm^3$ isotropic voxels, 10 repetitions of a six direction protocol, and a b-value of $1000s/mm^2$. We selected as representative fiber bundles the genu of the corpus callosum and the left motor tract. An atlas was computed from the combined set of 52 images, and tractography was performed to extract the two tracts.

Sampled functions of FA and tensor norm parametrized by atlas-normalized arc length were computed in the genu and left motor tracts. For the genu curves, a B-spline basis with 60 basis functions was used to provide preliminary smoothing and smooth curve estimation. For the motor tract, 80 basis functions were used. Functional joint PCA of FA and Frobenius norm was then estimated for the whole population. The number of PCA modes was selected to retain 90% of the total variance. For this study 7 and 11 PCA modes were retained for the genu and motor tracts respectively. The mean function plus the first two principal modes for the genu tract are shown below in Fig. 3.

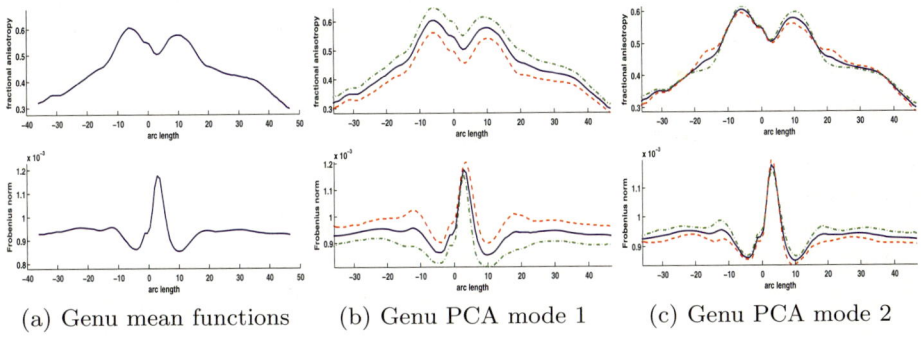

(a) Genu mean functions   (b) Genu PCA mode 1   (c) Genu PCA mode 2

Fig. 3. Visualization of the PCA modes for the joint analysis of FA and Frobenius norm in the genu tract. The (a) mean functions for the combined population are shown with (b) the first and (c) second PCA modes. The first PCA mode accounts for a large percentage of the variability and shows an overall constant change in FA and an anti-correlated constant change in norm.

The Hotelling T^2 statistic was then computed in PCA space. The genu tract test was extremely significant with a T^2 statistic of 133.1 and parametric p-value of 3.3e-8. The motor tract was also extremely significant with T^2 statistic of 93.8 and a parametric p-value of 2.7e-6. In this case there was such a large difference between groups that the permutation test did not result in any permutations with a statistic greater than the original. The p-values are uncommonly low because of the strong differences in the test data and the relatively large sample size. Visualization of the discriminant direction provides an interpretation of the detected differences and is shown in Fig. 4. The discriminant direction for the genu tract shows the difference from one to two year old groups is caused by an overall increase in FA and correlated decrease in Frobenius norm. Furthermore, the increased value of FA in the center of the tract indicates the central region of the tract provides more discriminative power between the two groups. These results are similar to differences which have been found between neonates and one year old subjects in the same tract [11]. The results in the motor tract indicate a similar constant increase in FA across the whole tract, and the Frobenius norm increases towards the inferior region of the tract, and decreases at a specific location in the superior region of the tract.

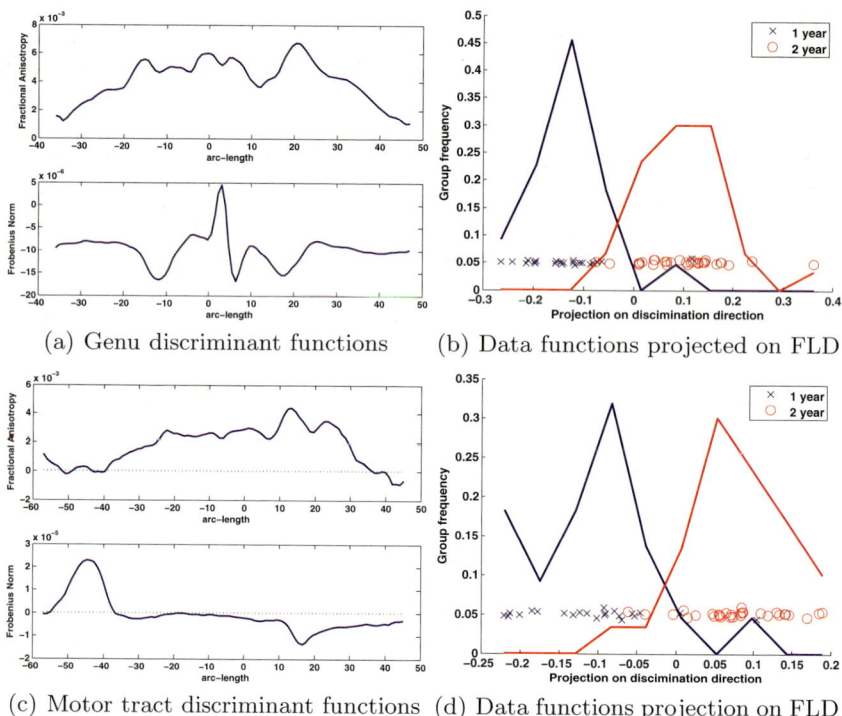

Fig. 4. Linear discriminants from one to two years for the (a) genu and (c) left motor tracts expanded into original functional basis. These are the functions integrated with the original data that maximally separate the groups. In the genu tract the FA values increase from one to two years, and the Frobenius norm values decrease. For the motor tract, the results are similar for FA, but the norm increases at the base of the tract and decreases towards the top. The projection of the (b) genu and (d) motor tract curves onto the discrimination direction shows the strong separation between the groups.

5 Conclusions and Discussion

Computing fiber tract statistics as a function of arc length provides a sensitive mechanism for detecting and understanding changes in fiber tract properties between populations. Our framework avoids the problems of multiple comparison correction by providing a single nonparametric hypothesis test for each fiber bundle. Furthermore, the discrimination information contained within the hypothesis test can be visualized to provide a clinically relevant interpretation of the group differences. The framework presented here is closely related to previous work on shape analysis using PCA, and we intend to explore in more detail how tools from shape analysis can be applied to this problem. We are currently applying the methodology to a study of Schizophrenia in adults.

References

1. Corouge, I., Fletcher, P.T., Joshi, S., Gouttard, S., Gerig, G.: Fiber tract-oriented statistics for quantitative diffusion tensor MRI analysis. Medical Image Analysis 10(5), 786–798 (2006)
2. Fletcher, P.T., Tao, R., Joeng, W.K., Whitaker, R.: A Volumetric Approach to Quantifying Region-to-Region White Matter Connectivity in Diffusion Tensor MRI. In: Karssemeijer, N., Lelieveldt, B. (eds.) IPMI 2007. LNCS, vol. 4584, pp. 346–358. Springer, Heidelberg (2007)
3. Peyrat, J.M., Sermesant, M., Pennec, X., Delingette, H., Xu, C., McVeigh, E., Ayache, N.: A Computational Framework for the Statistical Analysis of Cardiac Diffusion Tensors: Application to a Small Database of Canine Hearts. IEEE Transactions on Medical Imaging 26(11), 1500–1514 (2007)
4. Goodlett, C., Davis, B., Jean, R., Gilmore, J., Gerig, G.: Improved Correspondance for DTI population studies via unbiased atlas building. In: Larsen, R., Nielsen, M., Sporring, J. (eds.) MICCAI 2006. LNCS, vol. 4191, pp. 260–267. Springer, Heidelberg (2006)
5. Zhang, H., Yushkevich, P.A., Rueckert, D., Gee, J.C.: Unbiased white matter atlas construction using diffusion tensor images. In: Ayache, N., Ourselin, S., Maeder, A. (eds.) MICCAI 2007, Part I. LNCS, vol. 4791, pp. 211–218. Springer, Heidelberg (2007)
6. Smith, S.M., Jenkinson, M., Johansen-Berg, H., Rueckert, D., Nichols, T.E., Mackay, C.E., Watkins, K.E., Ciccarelli, O., Cader, M.Z., Matthews, P.M., Behrens, T.E.: Tract-based spatial statistics: Voxelwise analysis of multi-subject diffusion data. NeuroImage 31, 1487–1505 (2006)
7. O'Donnell, L., Westin, C.F., Golby, A.: Tract-Based Morphometry. In: Ayache, N., Ourselin, S., Maeder, A. (eds.) MICCAI 2007, Part II. LNCS, vol. 4792, pp. 161–168. Springer, Heidelberg (2007)
8. Joshi, S., Davis, B., Jomier, M., Gerig, G.: Unbiased diffeomorphic atlas construction for computational anatomy. NeuroImage 23(suppl. 1), S151–S160 (2004)
9. Ennis, D.B., Kindlmann, G.: Orthogonal tensor invariants and the analysis of diffusion tensor magnetic resonance images. Magnetic Resonance in Medicine 55(1), 136–146 (2006)
10. Ramsay, J., Silverman, B.: Functional Data Analysis, 2nd edn. Springer, Heidelberg (2005)
11. Gilmore, J.H., Lin, W., Corouge, I., Vetsa, Y.S., Smith, J.K., Kang, C., Gu, H., Hamer, R.A., Lieberman, J.A., Gerig, G.: Early Postnatal Development of Corpus Callosum and Corticospinal White Matter Assessed with Quantitative Tractography. American Journal of Neuroradiology 28(9), 1789–1795 (2007)

Author Index

Abolmaesumi, Purang   I-76, II-493, II-1032
Abramovitch, Rinat   I-93
Abugharbieh, Rafeef   I-287
Acosta, Oscar   I-253, I-442
Ahmed, Hashim Uddin   I-737
Aja-Fernández, Santiago   II-27
Ali, Wajid   II-587
Alia-Klein, Nelly   I-925
Aljabar, Paul   I-409, II-442
Alkadhi, Hatem   I-170
Allen, Clare   I-737
Allison, Jerry D.   I-866
Alomari, Raja' S.   I-202
Alvino, Christopher   I-367
Anton, Jean-Luc   I-959
Aplas, Alexander   I-67
Apostolova, Liana G.   I-194
Arbel, Tal   II-1023
Armspach, Jean-Paul   II-897
Arridge, Simon   II-425
Ashraf, Haseem   II-863
Assemlal, Haz-Edine   II-70
Assumpcao, Lia   II-458
Atasoy, Selen   I-850
Atkinson, David   I-703, II-948
Aubert-Broche, Berengere   II-180
Augustinack, Jean   I-235
Aukema, Eline   I-535
Avants, Brian B.   I-510, II-766
Awate, Suyash P.   I-559
Axel, Leon   I-331, I-636, I-789, II-289, II-313
Ayache, Nicholas   I-678, I-745, I-754, II-390, II-972
Azzabou, Noura   I-951

Babalola, Kolawole O.   I-401, I-409
Baggerman, Wouter   I-219
Bajka, Michael   II-726
Bakkour, Akram   I-235
Balci, Serdar K.   II-381
Balicki, Marcin   II-543
Balocco, Simone   II-131

Balov, Nikolay   I-1060
Barbagli, Federico   II-847
Bardin, Sabine   II-95
Bardinet, Eric   II-956
Barillot, Christian   II-122, II-171
Barkovich, A. James   I-351
Barmpoutis, Angelos   I-9
Barnes, Nick   I-628
Barnett, Alan S.   II-321
Barratt, Dean   I-737, II-356
Barthel, Andrew   II-855
Barysheva, Marina   I-1060, II-298, II-914
Bashar, Md. Khayrul   II-603
Bathula, Deepti R.   II-246
Bauer, Thomas   II-238
Beechey-Newman, Nicolas   II-356
Behrends, Johannes   II-306
Ben Ayed, Ismail   I-1025
Bender, Frederik   II-668
Benhimane, Selim   I-850, II-526, II-578
Benner, Thomas   I-235
Bergmann, Helmar   II-964
Bernasconi, Andrea   I-645, I-1008
Bernasconi, Neda   I-645, I-1008
Bessho, Masahiko   II-501
Besson, Pierre   I-645, I-1008
Bhattacharjee, Manik   II-956
Birkfellner, Wolfgang   II-964
Bloch, B. Nicolas   I-662
Bloy, Luke   I-1
Blum, Tobias   II-627
Boag, Alexander   I-76
Boctor, Emad   II-458
Boehler, Tobias   II-998
Bonin, Tim   I-815
Bonner, Erik   I-253
Bourgeat, Pierrick   I-253, I-442
Breeuwer, Marcel   I-178
Bresson, Xavier   II-980
Brooks, Rupert   II-1023
Brown, Matthew R.G.   I-359
Brun, Caroline   II-914
Brun, Luc   II-70

Brunner, Gerd   I-144
Bryan, R. Nick   I-620
Bühler, Katja   II-213
Buhmann, Joachim M.   II-1
Bulot, Rémy   I-959
Bunyak, Filiz   I-376
Büther, Florian   II-155

Caan, Matthan   I-535
Camara, Oscar   II-131
Campbell, Jennifer S.W.   I-135
Carlson, Christopher R.   II-847
Carneiro, Gustavo   I-67
Carter, Timothy   II-356
Casero, Ramón   I-527
Castro, Javier Sanchez   II-980
Cates, Joshua   I-477
Cattin, Philippe C.   I-170
Chabrier, Renée   I-211
Chambellan, Dominique   II-255
Chan, Kap Luk   I-51
Chan, Raymond C.   II-61
Chan, Tony F.   I-494, I-585
Chan, Wing-Yin   II-551
Chang, Lin-Ching   II-321
Chappelow, Jonathan   I-653, I-662
Chaudhary, Vipin   I-202
Chefd'hotel, Christophe   II-35, II-205
Chelikani, Sudhakar   I-780
Chen, Jeremy   I-594
Chen, Rong   II-1041
Chen, Ting   I-636, II-313
Chen, Xian   II-742
Chen, Zhe   I-780
Cheng, Mario   I-703
Chiang, Ming-Chang   I-1060, II-298
Chien, Aichi   I-162
Chintalapani, Gouthami   II-871
Chittajallu, Deepak R.   I-144
Chong, Vincent   I-51
Choti, Michael   II-458
Chou, Yi-Yu   II-914
Chui, Yim-Pan   II-52, II-551
Chung, Adrian J.   II-467
Chung, Albert C.S.   II-888, II-1092
Chung, Jae-Hoon   II-750, II-758
Chung, Moo K.   I-999
Ciofolo, Cybèle   I-178, I-186
Clark, James   II-467
Clatz, Olivier   I-975

Clemens, Mark   I-127
Clouchoux, Cédric   I-959
Cointepas, Yann   I-1034
Colchester, Alan   II-1050
Collewet, Christophe   II-339
Collins, D. Louis   II-180, II-1023
Colliot, Olivier   I-645, I-1008
Comaniciu, Dorin   I-67, I-686, I-983, II-230
Comas, Olivier   I-703
Combès, Benoît   I-17
Commean, Paul   I-296
Commowick, Olivier   I-975
Cook, Philip A.   I-305
Cootes, Tim F.   I-401, I-409
Cornellà, Jordi   II-587
Corso, Jason J.   I-202, I-612
Cotin, Stéphane   I-695
Coulon, Olivier   I-959
Coupé, Pierrick   II-171
Cowan, Brett R.   II-880
Cowen, Andrew C.   II-434
Crum, William R.   I-409, II-442
Csoma, Csaba   II-509, II-701
Cuadra, Meritxell Bach   II-980

D'Haese, Pierre-Francois   I-670
Darkner, Sune   I-842
Darzi, Ara   I-425, II-595, II-676
Davatzikos, Christos   I-620, II-905
Dawant, Benoit   I-670
Dawood, Mohammad   II-155
de Bruijne, Marleen   I-934, II-863
de Zubicaray, Greig I.   I-1060, II-298, II-914
Deguchi, Daisuke   II-535
Dehghan, Ehsan   II-660
Del Nido, Pedro J.   I-711
Delingette, Hervé   I-678, II-972
Demiralp, Çağatay   I-1051
Dequidt, Jérémie   I-695
Derbyshire, J. Andrew   II-163
Deriche, Rachid   I-858, II-122
Desbiolles, Lotus   I-170
Descoteaux, Maxime   I-858, II-122
Detre, John A.   I-510
Deverre, Jean-Robert   II-255
Dhandapani, Krishnan   I-866
Dickerson, Bradford C.   I-235
DiMaio, Simon P.   II-701

Ding, Zhaohua   II-1083
Dinov, Ivo   II-147, II-407
Dione, Donald   II-280
Dirksen, Asger   II-863
Dohi, Takeyoshi   I-262
Dojat, Michel   II-1066
Dong, Bin   I-162
Dong, Shuo   II-964
Dormont, Didier   II-956
Duay, Valérie   II-980
Duffy, Frank H.   I-762
Duncan, James S.   II-246, II-450
Duncan, Jim   I-780
Duriez, Christian   I-695
Durrleman, Stanley   II-390

Ecabert, Olivier   II-61
Eckstein, Felix   I-568
Edrei, Yifat   I-93
Edwards, A. David   I-486
Edwards, Philip   I-425, I-720
El-Ba, Ayman   I-322
Eliassaf, Ofer   I-85
Elle, Ole Jakob   II-587
Ellis, Randy   II-493
Elson, Daniel S.   II-222
Emberton, Mark   I-737
Englander, Sarah   I-342
Ennis, Daniel B.   II-814
Ericsson, Anders   I-486
Ersoy, Ilker   I-376
Euler, Ekkehard   II-578
Evans, Alan   I-645

Faisan, Sylvain   I-211
Falk, Robert   I-322
Fang, Tong   I-518
Fenchel, Matthias   I-576
Ferre, Josepa Mauri   II-518
Fessler, Jeffrey A.   I-991
Feußner, Hubertus   II-627
Fichtinger, Gabor   II-458, II-493, II-509, II-636, II-701, II-871
Fieseler, Michael   II-155
Figl, Michael   I-425, I-720
Fillard, Pierre   I-975
Firmin, David   II-79
Fischer, Gregory S.   II-509, II-701
Fischl, Bruce   I-235, I-468, I-745
Fleming, Ioana   II-458, II-543

Fletcher, P. Thomas   I-477, I-1068
Florent, Raoul   II-87
Fonov, Vladimir   II-180
Foran, David J.   I-833
Forbes, Florence   II-1066
Ford, Eric   II-619
Forder, John R.   I-9
Forgacs, Gabor   I-376
Foroughi, Pezhman   II-871
Fortin, Madeleine   II-407
Foskey, Mark   II-830
Fradkin, Maxim   I-178, I-186
Frangi, Alejandro F.   II-131, II-766, II-790
Frank, Gary R.   I-101
Franz, Astrid   I-227
Freiman, Moti   I-85, I-93
Fripp, Jurgen   I-253, I-442
Fritscher, Karl   I-568
Fuchs, Thomas J.   II-1

Galatsanos, Nikolaos   I-43
Gall, Johannes   II-1058
Gao, Yan   I-51
Garbay, Catherine   II-1066
Gassner, Eva   I-686
Gatenby, Chris   II-1083
Gatta, Carlo   II-518
Gee, James C.   I-305, I-510, I-559, II-766
Geiger, Bernhard   II-205
Genega, Elisabeth   I-662
Georgescu, Bogdan   I-686
Gerig, Guido   I-1068, II-263
Ghosh, Aurobrata   I-858
Gibaud, Bernard   I-807
Gilles, Benjamin   II-822
Gilmore, John H.   I-1068
Gimel'farb, Georgy   I-322
Glenn, Orit A.   I-351
Glocker, Ben   II-113
Gobbi, David G.   II-493, II-701
Golbreich, Christine   I-807
Golby, Alexandra J.   II-271
Goldstein, Rita Z.   I-925
Golland, Polina   I-26, I-235, I-468, I-745, I-842, I-1016, II-381
Goodlett, Casey B.   I-1068
Gooya, Ali   I-262
Gorbunova, Vladlena   II-863
Gore, John   II-1083

Goud, Bruno   II-95
Gouttard, Sylvain   II-263
Grabner, Markus   II-652
Grady, Leo   I-153
Grant, P. Ellen   I-468
Grau, Patrick   II-726
Graumann, Rainer   II-578
Green, Amity E.   I-194
Greene, William H.   I-780
Gregori, Giovanni   I-883
Greiner, Russell   I-359
Grimbergen, Kees   I-535
Grimson, W. Eric L.   I-917
Groher, Martin   II-668
Gross, Eitan   I-93
Grossman, Murray   I-510
Gu, Xianfeng   I-585
Guehring, Jens   II-35
Guendel, Lutz   II-205
Guiraudon, Gerard   I-967
Gülsün, M. Akif   I-602
Guo, Lei   I-270
Guo, Weihong   II-939
Gurcan, Metin   II-196
Guttman, Michael A.   II-163

Habas, Piotr A.   I-351
Hacihaliloglu, Ilker   I-287
Hadjidemetriou, Stathis   I-450
Hager, Gregory   II-458, II-543
Hajnal, Joseph V.   II-35
Hämäläinen, Matti   I-26
Hamarneh, Ghassan   I-244, I-459
Hammers, Alexander   I-486
Hamper, Ulrike   II-458
Han, Xiao   II-434
Handa, James   II-543
Hänni, Markus   I-568
Hans, Arne   I-762
Hansen, Michael Sass   II-113
Hara, Kenji   II-742
Hartley, Richard   I-628, II-734
Hasegawa, Yosihnori   II-535
Hashizume, Makoto   II-742
Hata, Nobuhiko   II-701
Hautvast, Gilion   I-178
Hawkes, David   I-703, I-720, I-737, II-356, II-425, II-948
Hazlett, Heather Cody   I-477
Hefny, Mohamed   II-493

Heibel, Tim Hauke   II-668
Heining, Sandro Michael   II-578
Heinrich, Christian   I-43, II-897
Heitz, Fabrice   II-897
Heng, Pheng-Ann   II-551
Heng, Pheng Ann   II-52
Hengg, Clemens   I-568
Hermans, Jeroen   I-393
Herskovits, Edward H.   II-1041
Hibbard, Lyndon S.   II-434
Hill, Derek   II-425
Himeno, Ryutaro   II-560
Hinterleitner, Isabella   II-964
Hladůvka, Jiří   II-213
Ho, Simon S.M.   II-52, II-551
Hobson, Maritza A.   I-101
Hodgson, Antony   I-287
Hojjat, Ali   II-1050
Holland, Trevor   I-322
Hollenstein, Marc   II-726
Honorio, Jean   I-925
Hoogeman, Mischa S.   II-434
Hoole, Phil   II-306
Hori, Masatoshi   I-502
Hornegger, Joachim   I-67
Horvath, Keith A.   II-476
Howe, Robert D.   I-711, II-930
Howland, Dena   I-9
Hu, Mingxing   I-720
Hu, Tom C.-C.   I-866
Hu, Yipeng   I-737
Hua, Jing   II-44
Huang, Feng   II-939
Huang, Junzhou   I-331, II-289
Huang, Rui   II-1083
Huang, Wei   I-51
Huang, Xiaolei   I-331, II-289
Huber, Martin   I-67
Hubert, Xavier   II-255
Huettmann, Gereon   I-815
Hughes, Nicholas P.   II-139
Huntbatch, Andrew   I-892, II-79
Huynh, Toan   I-127

Ide, Jaime   II-1041
Imaizumi, Kazuyoshi   II-535
Ionasec, Razvan Ioan   I-686
Iordachita, Iulian   II-509, II-543, II-619
Irfanoglu, Mustafa Okan   II-1014
Iseki, Hiroshi   II-373

Iwaki, Junichiro   II-501
Iwashita, Yumi   II-742

Jackowski, Marcel   II-280
Jackson, John   I-983
Jassi, Preet   I-459
Jenkinson, Mark   I-409, II-271
Jia, Peifa   II-569
Jiang, Li   II-798
Jiang, Xiaoyi   II-155
Jolly, Marie-Pierre   I-110, I-153
Jones, Doug   I-967
Jones, Gareth   I-442
Jordan, Petr   II-930
Joskowicz, Leo   I-85, I-93
Joung, Sanghyun   II-501
Ju, Tao   I-296

Kagiyama, Yoshiyuki   II-718
Kainz, Bernhard   II-652
Kakadiaris, Ioannis A.   I-144
Kalyanpur, Arjun   I-653
Kambhamettu, Chandra   II-238
Kamon, Hirokazu   II-501
Kanade, Takeo   II-485
Kanterakis, Stathis   I-620
Kanwisher, Nancy   I-1016
Kao, Chiu-Yen   I-384
Kao, Chris   I-670
Karhu, Jari   I-543
Karimaghaloo, Zahra   II-493
Kataoka, Hiroyuki   II-560
Kazanzides, Peter   II-619
Keller, Steve   I-127
Kellman, Peter   II-163
Kennedy, David   I-409
Kenwright, Chris   II-1050
Kerien, Erwan   I-695
Kern, Kyle   II-147
Kervrann, Charles   II-95
Kesner, Samuel B.   I-711
Kettenbach, Joachim   II-964
Kezele, Irina   I-1034
Khairy, Khaled   II-1075
Khamene, Ali   II-668
Khan, Shahid   I-824
Kim, Boklye   I-991
Kim, Hosung   I-1008
Kim, Kio   I-351

Kitasaka, Takayuki   II-535, II-603
Klein, Stefan   II-1006
Klinder, Tobias   I-227
Klunder, Andrea D.   I-1060
Kneser, Reinhard   II-61
Knisely, Jonathan P.S.   I-780
Knopp, Michael   II-1014
Kobayashi, Etsuko   II-373
Koh, Kevin R.   II-222
Koikkalainen, Juha   I-543
Komodakis, Nikos   II-113
Könönen, Mervi   I-543
Konrad, Peter   I-670
Koo, John   II-543
Koolwal, Aditya B.   II-847
Kösters, Thomas   II-155
Kouby, Vincent El   I-1034
Koyama, Tsuyoshi   II-501
Krieger, Axel   II-509
Krishnan, Arun   I-313
Kruger, Jennifer A.   II-750
Krupa, Alexandre   II-339
Kubicki, Marek   I-917
Kupelian, Patrick   II-710
Kurazume, Ryo   II-742
Kurkure, Uday   I-144
Kurtcuoglu, Vartan   II-774
Kutter, Oliver   I-686
Kwok, Ka-Wai   II-676

Ladikos, Alexander   II-526
Lai, Rongjie   II-147
Lai, Zhaoqiang   II-44
Laidlaw, David H.   I-1051
Laissue, Philippe   II-1050
Lam, Hoi Ieng   II-814
Langs, Georg   I-925
Larrabide, Ignacio   II-790
Larsen, Rasmus   I-842
Lashkari, Danial   I-1016
Lassonde, Maryse   II-407
Lee, Agatha D.   I-1060, II-914
Lee, Chi-Hoon   I-359
Lee, Huai-Ping   II-830
Lee, Junghoon   II-636
Lee, Su-Lin   I-892, II-79
Leff, Daniel Richard   II-595
Legoupil, Samuel   II-255
Leinsinger, Gerda L.   II-306
Lekadir, Karim   I-434

Lelong, Pierre   II-87
Lemaitre, Herve   II-321
Lenkinski, Robert   I-662
Leong, Julian   II-595
Leor, Oriol Rodriguez   II-518
Lepiller, Damien   I-678
Leporé, Franco   II-407
Leporé, Natasha   II-407, II-914
Leppert, Ilana   II-180
Lerotic, Mirna   II-467
Levendag, Peter C.   II-434
Li, Bo   II-880
Li, Chunming   I-384, II-1083
Li, Gang   I-270
Li, Houqiang   II-18
Li, Ming   II-476
Li, Shengying   II-280
Li, Shuo   I-1025
Li, Xinshan   II-750
Liang, David H.   II-847
Liao, Hongen   I-262, II-373, II-501
Liao, Shu   II-888
Lieby, Paulette   I-628
Likar, Boštjan   I-762, I-942
Lin, Ming C.   II-830
Link, Thomas   I-568
Linte, Cristian A.   I-967, II-644
Litvin, Andrew   I-367
Liu, Chao   II-684
Liu, Lu   I-296
Liu, Qingshan   I-789
Liu, Tianming   I-270
Liu, Xiaofeng   II-636
Liu, Xinyang   II-407
Liu, Xiuwen   II-407
Lo, Benny   II-104
Lo, Pechin   II-863
Loeckx, Dirk   I-393, II-839
Loew, Murray H.   II-798
Lopez, Alfredo   II-1058
Lorenz, Cristian   I-227
Lorenzen, Peter   I-450
Lötjönen, Jyrki   I-543
Lu, Yingli   I-1025
Lui, Lok Ming   I-494
Lujan, Brandon   I-883

Ma, Burton   II-1032
Machiraju, Raghu   II-1014
Madabhushi, Anant   I-653, I-662, II-330

Maddah, Mahnaz   I-917
Madsen, Ernest L.   I-101
Madsen, Sarah   I-1060
Maeda, Yuki   II-501
Maes, Frederik   I-393, II-839
Magnenat-Thalmann, Nadia   I-119
Mahapatra, Dwarikanath   I-771
Majoie, Charles   I-535
Malcolm, James   II-416
Mangin, Jean-François   I-1034, II-399
Manolidis, Spiros   II-692
Mansor, Sarina   II-139
Manzke, Robert   II-61
Mao, Yu   I-162
Marchal, Maud   I-695
Marenco, Stefano   II-321
Martinez, Oscar   I-883
Maruyama, Takashi   II-373
Matinfar, Mohammad   II-619
Matsumoto, Takuya   II-501
Mattes, Julian   II-1058
Mazilu, Dumitru   II-476
Mazza, Edoardo   II-726
McGregor, Robert   II-782
McMahon, Katie L.   I-1060, II-298, II-914
McVeigh, Elliot R.   II-163
Mebarki, Rafik   II-339
Mechouche, Ammar   I-807
Meeks, Sanford   II-710
Meer, Peter   I-833
Mei, Lin   I-425
Mekada, Yoshito   II-603
Melbourne, Andrew   II-948
Meredith, Matthew   I-1060, II-298, II-914
Metaxas, Dimitris   I-35, I-331, I-636, I-789, II-289, II-313, II-1083
Metz, Coert T.   I-900
Meyer, Carsten   II-61
Meyer, Christophe   I-211
Minkoff, David   I-510
Mio, Washington   II-407
Mitchell, Ben   II-543
Mitsuishi, Mamoru   II-501
Miyazaki, Fumio   II-611
Moch, Holger   II-1
Moghari, Mehdi Hedjazi   II-1032
Mollemans, Wouter   II-839
Möller, Torsten   I-244

Monden, Morito   II-611
Moore, John   I-967, II-644
Moradi, Mehdi   I-76
Morandi, Xavier   I-807, II-1023
Moreno, Guillermo   I-815
Morgan, Dominic   I-737
Mori, Kensaku   II-535, II-603
Morooka, Ken'ichi   II-742
Morra, Jonathan H.   I-194
Morrissey, Sean Patrick   II-171
Mory, Benoit   I-178
Mountney, Peter   II-364
Mousavi, Parvin   I-76
Mueller, Heike   I-815
Mueller, Klaus   II-280
Mueller, Susanne   I-450
Mukherjee, Lopamudra   I-999
Muragaki, Yoshihiro   II-373
Muralidhar, Krishnamurthy   II-782
Murphy, Keelin   II-1006
Murtha, Albert   I-359
Mylonas, George P.   II-347, II-676

Nain, Delphine   I-518
Nakagoe, Hiroaki   II-611
Nakajima, Yoshikazu   II-501
Nakamoto, Masahiko   I-502, II-718
Nakamura, Hironobu   I-502
Nakazawa, Touji   II-501
Nash, Martyn P.   II-750, II-758, II-814
Navab, Nassir   I-686, I-850, II-113, II-526, II-578, II-627, II-668, II-734
Neimat, Joseph   I-670
Nguyen, Nhat   I-127
Ni, Dong   II-52, II-551
Nie, Jingxin   I-270
Nielsen, Mads   II-863
Nielsen, Poul M.F.   II-750, II-758
Niessen, Wiro J.   I-900
Nikou, Christophoros   I-43
Nishikawa, Atsushi   II-611
Niskanen, Eini   I-543
Noble, J. Alison   I-527, II-139
Noblet, Vincent   I-211, II-897
Noda, Shigeho   II-560
Noguchi, Masafumi   II-373
Noonan, David P.   I-850
Nopachai, David   I-296
Nwogu, Ifeoma   I-612

O'keefe, Graeme   I-442
Ohashi, Satoru   II-501
Ohnishi, Isao   II-501
Okada, Toshiyuki   I-502
Okazawa, Shigenobu   II-560
Olgac, Ufuk   II-774
Operto, Grégory   I-959
Orchard, Jeff   II-188
Orihuela-Espina, Felipe   II-595
Osher, Stanley   I-162
Ostermann, Jörn   I-227
Otomaru, Itaru   II-718
Ou, Wanmei   I-26
Ourselin, Sébastien   I-253, I-442, I-703, II-425

Padoy, Nicolas   II-627
Pai, Dinesh K.   II-822
Palaniappan, Kannappan   I-376
Pallavaram, Srivatsan   I-670
Papademetris, Xenophon   I-780, II-246, II-450
Paragios, Nikos   I-925, I-951, II-113, II-255
Park, JinHyeong   I-983, II-230
Passat, Nicolas   I-211
Passenger, Josh   I-703
Patenaude, Brian   I-409
Paulsen, Rasmus R.   I-842
Pécot, Thierry   II-95
Peitgen, Heinz-Otto   II-998
Pendsé, Doug   I-737
Peng, Zhigang   I-313
Pennec, Xavier   I-754, II-390, II-914, II-972
Penney, Graeme   I-720
Perchant, Aymeric   I-754
Pernuš, Franjo   I-762, I-942
Perrin, Muriel   I-1034
Perrot, Matthieu   II-399
Peters, Jochen   II-61
Peters, Terry M.   I-967, II-644
Petrovic, Vlad   I-401
Peyrat, Jean-Marc   II-972
Pfefferbaum, Adolf   I-798
Pierpaoli, Carlo   II-321, II-1014
Pike, G. Bruce   I-135, II-180
Pinel, Philippe   II-399
Pitiot, Alain   II-956
Piven, Joseph   II-263

Pless, Robert I-296
Pluim, Josien P.W. II-1006
Pluta, John I-510
Poignet, Philippe II-684
Poline, Jean-Baptiste II-399
Pollo, Claudio II-980
Pop, Mihaela I-678
Poulikakos, Dimos II-774
Poupon, Cyril I-1034
Poupon, Fabrice I-1034
Poynton, Clare II-271
Prasad, Mithun I-59
Prastawa, Marcel II-263
Pratt, Philip I-720
Prčkovska, Vesna II-9
Prima, Sylvain I-17, II-122, II-171
Prince, Jerry L. II-636
Prior, Fred I-296
Pujol, Oriol II-518
Pullens, W.L.P.M. II-9
Pungavkar, Sona I-653
Purushothaman, Kailas I-780

Qian, Zhen I-789, II-289
Qin, Jing II-551
Qu, Yingge II-52, II-551
Qureshi, Hammad II-196

Raber, David I-296
Radaelli, Alessandro II-790
Rademacher, Martin H. I-798
Radeva, Petia II-518
Rajagopal, Vijay II-758
Rajpoot, Nasir II-196
Ramirez-Manzanares, Alonso I-305
Ramrath, Lukas I-815
Raniga, Parnesh I-442
Rathi, Yogesh II-416
Razavi, Reza II-425
Reddy, Vivek Y. II-61
Reiser, Maximilian F. II-306
Remple, Michael I-670
Restif, Christophe I-35
Reynaud, Emmanuel II-1075
Rhode, Kawal II-425
Richa, Rogério II-684
Rit, Simon I-729
Rivaz, Hassan II-458
Robinson, Emma C. I-486
Roche, Alexis II-956

Roebroeck, Alard F. II-9
Rofsky, Neil I-662
Rohlfing, Torsten I-798
Rohling, Robert I-287
Roland Jr., J. Thomas II-692
Rolland, Jannick P. II-710
Roose, Liesbet II-839
Rosen, Mark I-653, II-330
Rosenfeld, Philip J. I-883
Ross, Ian I-1025
Ross, James C. II-806
Rousseau, Francois I-351
Rowe, Christopher I-442
Rueckert, Daniel I-409, I-425, I-486,
    I-720, II-35, II-442
Ruohonen, Jarmo I-543
Rüther, Matthias II-652

Saad, Ahmed I-244
Sabuncu, Mert R. I-745, I-842, II-381
Saddi, Kinda II-35
Sahu, Mahua I-737
Sakuma, Ichiro I-262, II-373, II-501
Salamero, Jean II-95
Salcudean, Septimiu E. II-660
Salvado, Olivier I-253, I-442
Samaras, Dimitris I-925
Sammet, Steffen II-1014
Samset, Eigil II-587
Santhanam, Anand P. II-710
Sato, Yoshinobu I-502, II-718
Sauerbrei, Eric I-76
Saur, Stefan C. I-170, II-774
Savadjiev, Peter I-135
Saybasili, Haris II-163
Scarzanella, Marco Visentini II-104
Schäfers, Klaus P. II-155
Schaap, Michiel I-900
Scherrer, Benoit II-1066
Scheuering, Michael I-686
Schilling, Andreas I-576
Schmid, Jérôme I-119
Schmugge, Stephen J. I-127
Schnabel, Julia I-409
Schnall, Mitchell I-342
Schoonenberg, Gert II-87
Schubert, Rainer I-568
Schuff, Norbert I-450
Schuler, Benedikt I-568
Schultz, Robert T. I-559, II-246

Schwartzman, David   II-485
Schweikard, Achim   I-815
Seghers, Dieter   I-393
Sekimoto, Mitsugu   II-611
Sela, Yehonatan   I-93
Sermesant, Maxime   I-678, II-972
Sertel, Olcay   II-196
Sfikas, Giorgos   I-43
Shaffer, Teresa   I-322
Shah, Amish   II-710
Shah, Mubarak   I-824
Shaker, Saher B.   I-934
Shakhnarovich, Gregory   I-1051
Shams, Ramtin   II-734
Shanbhag, Dattesh   II-806
Shattuck, David W.   II-298
Shen, Dinggang   I-342, I-417, II-905, II-1041
Shen, Hong   I-367
Shen, Tian   I-331
Sheng, Lin   II-569
Shenton, Martha E.   I-917, II-416
Shi, Jin   I-874
Shi, Pengcheng   I-1042
Shi, Yonggang   II-147, II-407
Shi, Yonghong   I-417
Shimaya, Koji   II-373
Shin, Min C.   I-127
Shmidmayer, Yitzchak   I-93
Shriram, K.S.   I-551
Sicotte, Nancy   II-147
Siddiqi, Kaleem   I-135
Siemens, Robert   I-76
Sigworth, Frederick   II-855
Simaan, Nabil   II-692
Simopoulos, Costas   II-230
Sinacore, David   I-296
Singh, Vikas   I-999
Sinusas, Albert J.   II-450
Slabaugh, Greg   I-518
Smith, Ben   I-244
Smith, Stephen   I-409
Socrate, Simona   II-930
Sofka, Michal   II-989
Song, Danny   II-871
Song, Yixu   II-569
Sonke, Jan-Jakob   I-729
Sosna, Jacob   I-85
Souvenir, Richard   I-127
Sowmya, Arcot   I-59

Špiclin, Žiga   I-762
Srinivasan, Latha   II-35
Srinivasan, Rajagopalan   I-551
Srivastava, Anuj   I-1060
Staib, Lawrence H.   I-780, II-246, II-280
Staring, Marius   II-1006
Steiner, Karl   II-238
Stelzer, Ernst   II-1075
Stewart, Charles V.   II-989
Stoyanov, Danail   II-104, II-347
Studholme, Colin   I-351
Styner, Martin   I-477, II-263
Sudarsky, Sandra   II-205
Suenaga, Yasuhito   II-535, II-603
Suetens, Paul   I-393, II-839
Sugano, Nobuhiko   II-501, II-718
Suhm, Norbert   I-568
Sukno, Federico   II-766
Sun, Hui   II-766
Sun, Mingzhai   I-376
Sun, Quansen   I-384
Sun, Ying   I-771
Suryanarayanan, Srikanth   I-551
Székely, Gábor   I-170, II-782
Szczerba, Dominik   II-782
Sørensen, Lauge   I-934

Tada, Yukio   II-718
Tagare, Hemant D.   I-101, II-246, II-855
Taieb, Yoav   I-85
Takabatake, Hirotsugu   II-535
Takagi, Shu   II-560
Takao, Masaki   II-718
Takiguchi, Shuji   II-611
Tang, Lisa   I-459
Taniguchi, Kazuhiro   II-611
Tannenbaum, Allen   II-416
Tanner, Christine   II-356
Taylor, Chris   I-401
Taylor, Russell H.   II-543, II-871
Taylor, Zeike A.   I-703
Teguh, David N.   II-434
Tek, Hüseyin   I-602
Tempany, Clare M.   II-701
ter Haar Romeny, Bart M.   II-9, II-87
Thesen, Stefan   I-576
Thiemjarus, Surapa   II-222
Thiran, Jean-Philippe   II-980
Thirion, Bertrand   II-399
Thiruvenkadam, Sheshadri   I-494

Thomasson, David   I-594
Thompson, Paul M.   I-194, I-494, I-585, I-1060, II-298, II-407, II-914
Tian, Jie   I-874
Tiwari, Pallavi   II-330
Toga, Arthur W.   I-194, I-1060, II-147, II-298, II-914
Tokuda, Junichi   II-701
Tomasi, Dardo   I-925
Toth, Robert   I-653, I-662
Trébossen, Régine   II-255
Tranquebar, Rekha   II-806
Traub, Joerg   II-578
Tristán-Vega, Antonio   II-27
Trouvé, Alain   II-390
Tschumperlé, David   II-70
Tsechpenakis, Gabriel   I-883
Tu, Zhuowen   I-194
Tucholka, Alan   II-399
Tuzel, Oncel   I-833
Twinning, Carole J.   I-401

Uchida, Seiichi   II-742
Unal, Gozde   I-518

Valibeik, Salman   II-467
Valstar, Michel   I-486
van der Giessen, Alina G.   I-900
van Ginneken, Bram   I-219, II-1006
van Herk, Marcel   I-729
Van Leemput, Koen   I-235
van Rikxoort, Eva M.   I-219
van Vliet, Lucas   I-535
van Walsum, Theo   I-900
Vandermeulen, Dirk   I-393
Vasilyev, Nikolay V.   I-711
Vemuri, Baba C.   I-9
Vercauteren, Tom   I-745, I-754
Verma, Ragini   I-1, I-908, II-905
Vilanova, Anna   II-9
Villemagne, Victor   I-442
Viswanath, Satish   I-662
Voet, Peter   II-434
Vogt, Sebastian   I-686
Volkow, Nora D.   I-925
von Siebenthal, Martin   II-782
Vos, Frans   I-535
Voss, Patrice   II-407
Vrtovec, Tomaž   I-942
Vul, Ed   I-1016

Wachinger, Christian   II-113
Wald, Lawrence L.   I-235
Walker, Lindsay   II-321
Wang, Kaimeng   II-373
Wang, Lei   I-628
Wang, Lejing   II-578
Wang, Li   I-384
Wang, Linwei   I-1042
Wang, Peng   I-908
Wang, Shaojun   I-359
Wang, Vicky Y.   II-814
Wang, Xiaoxu   I-636, II-313
Wang, Yalin   I-494, I-585
Warfield, Simon K.   I-762, I-975
Wedlake, Chris   I-967, II-644
Weese, Jurgen   II-61
Wei, Wei   II-692
Wein, Wolfgang   II-668
Weiner, Michael   I-450
Wells III, William   II-271
Wells, William M.   I-917
Wels, Michael   I-67
Westesson, Per-Lennart   II-306
Westin, Carl-Fredrik   I-279, I-917
Whalen, Stephen   II-271
Whitaker, Ross   I-477
Whitcomb, Louis L.   II-509
Wiest-Daesslé, Nicolas   II-122, II-171
Wiggins, Graham   I-235
Wild, Peter J.   II-1
Wiles, Andrew   II-644
Willoughby, Twyla   II-710
Wilson, Kevin   I-967
Wilson, Roland   II-196
Win, Lawrence   I-559
Wink, Onno   II-87
Wismueller, Axel   II-306
Wolf, Theresa K.   II-434
Wolthaus, Jochem   I-729
Wolz, Robin   I-227
Wong, John   II-619
Wong, Ken C.L.   I-1042
Wong, Stephen T.C.   I-270
Wong, Tien-Tsin   II-52
Wood, Tobias C.   II-222
Wright, Graham A.   I-678
Wright, Margaret J.   I-1060, II-298, II-914
Wu, Jue   II-1092

Author Index

Wu, Minjie II-321
Wübbeling, Frank II-155

Xia, Deshen I-384
Xie, Jun I-824
Xing, Ye I-342
Xu, Chenyang II-972
Xu, Jing II-569
Xu, Min I-874
Xue, Hui II-35
Xue, Zhong I-342

Yalamanchili, Raja P. I-144
Yamada, Yasuo II-611
Yanasak, Nathan I-866
Yang, Guang-Zhong I-434, I-850, I-892,
    II-79, II-104, II-222, II-347, II-364,
    II-467, II-595, II-676
Yang, Jinzhong II-905
Yang, Lin I-833
Yang, Wei I-874
Yang, Xuan II-52
Yao, Jianhua I-594
Yau, Shing-Tung I-585
Ye, Jian I-162
Yeo, B.T. Thomas I-468, I-745
Yeo, Desmond Teck Beng I-991
Yeow, John T.W. II-188
Yokota, Hideo II-560
Yokota, Keita I-502
Yoshikawa, Hideki II-718
Young, Alistair A. II-814, II-880
Yu, Hong I-670

Yu, Peng I-468
Yue, Yong I-101
Yuen, Shelten G. I-711
Yushkevich, Paul A. I-510, I-559, II-766

Zacharaki, Evangelia I. I-620
Zambal, Sebastian II-213
Zeltner, Jochen II-113
Zhai, Weiming II-569
Zhan, Wang II-798
Zhan, Yiqiang I-313
Zhang, Heye I-1042
Zhang, Jian II-692
Zhang, Shaoting I-636
Zhang, Song I-1051
Zhao, Qun I-866
Zhao, Yannan II-569
Zheng, Guoyan II-922
Zheng, Yuanjie II-238
Zhong, Hua II-485
Zhou, Jiayin I-51
Zhou, Luping I-628
Zhou, S. Kevin I-983, II-230
Zhou, Wengang II-18
Zhou, Xiang Sean I-313
Zhou, Xiaobo II-18
Zhu, Yaoyao I-331
Zhu, Yun II-450
Zhuang, Xiahai II-425
Zickler, Todd E. II-930
Ziyan, Ulas I-279
Zuehlsdorff, Sven II-35

Printing: Mercedes-Druck, Berlin
Binding: Stein+Lehmann, Berlin

Lecture Notes in Computer Science

Sublibrary 6: Image Processing, Computer Vision, Pattern Recognition, and Graphics

For information about Vols. 1– 4046
please contact your bookseller or Springer

Vol. 5242: D. Metaxas, L. Axel, G. Fichtinger, G. Székely (Eds.), Medical Image Computing and Computer-Assisted Intervention – MICCAI 2008, Part II. LI, 1111 pages. 2008.

Vol. 5241: D. Metaxas, L. Axel, G. Fichtinger, G. Székely (Eds.), Medical Image Computing and Computer-Assisted Intervention – MICCAI 2008, Part I. LI, 1087 pages. 2008.

Vol. 5197: J. Ruiz-Shulcloper, W.G. Kropatsch (Eds.), Progress in Pattern Recognition, Image Analysis and Applications. XXI, 809 pages. 2008.

Vol. 5188: M. Sebillo, G. Vitiello, G. Schaefer (Eds.), Visual Information Systems. XIV, 340 pages. 2008.

Vol. 5166: A. Butz, B. Fisher, A. Krüger, P. Olivier, M. Christie (Eds.), Smart Graphics. XI, 277 pages. 2008.

Vol. 5158: S.N. Srihari, K. Franke (Eds.), Computational Forensics. IX, 229 pages. 2008.

Vol. 5128: T. Dohi, I. Sakuma, H. Liao (Eds.), Medical Imaging and Augmented Reality. XVI, 441 pages. 2008.

Vol. 5116: E.A. Krupinski (Ed.), Digital Mammography. XXVII, 769 pages. 2008.

Vol. 5112: A. Campilho, M.S. Kamel (Eds.), Image Analysis and Recognition. XXII, 1126 pages. 2008.

Vol. 5099: A. Elmoataz, O. Lezoray, F. Nouboud, D. Mammass (Eds.), Image and Signal Processing. XVI, 625 pages. 2008.

Vol. 5098: F.J. Perales, R.B. Fisher (Eds.), Articulated Motion and Deformable Objects. XIV, 458 pages. 2008.

Vol. 5096: G. Rigoll (Ed.), Pattern Recognition. XIII, 538 pages. 2008.

Vol. 4992: D. Coeurjolly, I. Sivignon, L. Tougne, F. Dupont (Eds.), Discrete Geometry for Computer Imagery. XIII, 554 pages. 2008.

Vol. 4987: X. Gao, H. Müller, M.J. Loomes, R. Comley, S. Luo (Eds.), Medical Imaging and Informatics. XV, 388 pages. 2008.

Vol. 4958: V.E. Brimkov, R.P. Barneva, H.A. Hauptman (Eds.), Combinatorial Image Analysis. XVI, 446 pages. 2008.

Vol. 4931: G. Sommer, R. Klette (Eds.), Robot Vision. XI, 468 pages. 2008.

Vol. 4901: D. Zhang (Ed.), Medical Biometrics. XII, 324 pages. 2007.

Vol. 4889: A. Pasko, V. Adzhiev, P. Comninos (Eds.), Heterogeneous Objects Modelling and Applications. VII, 285 pages. 2008.

Vol. 4844: Y. Yagi, S.B. Kang, I.S. Kweon, H. Zha (Eds.), Computer Vision – ACCV 2007, Part II. XXVIII, 915 pages. 2007.

Vol. 4843: Y. Yagi, S.B. Kang, I.S. Kweon, H. Zha (Eds.), Computer Vision – ACCV 2007, Part I. XXVIII, 969 pages. 2007.

Vol. 4842: G. Bebis, R. Boyle, B. Parvin, D. Koracin, N. Paragios, S.-M. Tanveer, T. Ju, Z. Liu, S. Coquillart, C. Cruz-Neira, T. Müller, T. Malzbender (Eds.), Advances in Visual Computing, Part II. XXXIII, 827 pages. 2007.

Vol. 4841: G. Bebis, R. Boyle, B. Parvin, D. Koracin, N. Paragios, S.-M. Tanveer, T. Ju, Z. Liu, S. Coquillart, C. Cruz-Neira, T. Müller, T. Malzbender (Eds.), Advances in Visual Computing, Part I. XXXIII, 831 pages. 2007.

Vol. 4815: A. Ghosh, R.K. De, S.K. Pal (Eds.), Pattern Recognition and Machine Intelligence. XIX, 677 pages. 2007.

Vol. 4814: A. Elgammal, B. Rosenhahn, R. Klette (Eds.), Human Motion – Understanding, Modeling, Capture and Animation. X, 329 pages. 2007.

Vol. 4792: N. Ayache, S. Ourselin, A. Maeder (Eds.), Medical Image Computing and Computer-Assisted Intervention – MICCAI 2007, Part II. XLVI, 988 pages. 2007.

Vol. 4791: N. Ayache, S. Ourselin, A. Maeder (Eds.), Medical Image Computing and Computer-Assisted Intervention – MICCAI 2007, Part I. XLVI, 1012 pages. 2007.

Vol. 4781: G. Qiu, C. Leung, X.-Y. Xue, R. Laurini (Eds.), Advances in Visual Information Systems. XIII, 582 pages. 2007.

Vol. 4778: S.K. Zhou, W. Zhao, X. Tang, S. Gong (Eds.), Analysis and Modeling of Faces and Gestures. X, 305 pages. 2007.

Vol. 4768: D. Doermann, S. Jaeger (Eds.), Arabic and Chinese Handwriting Recognition. VIII, 279 pages. 2008.

Vol. 4756: L. Rueda, D. Mery, J. Kittler (Eds.), Progress in Pattern Recognition, Image Analysis and Applications. XXI, 989 pages. 2007.

Vol. 4738: A.C.R. Paiva, R. Prada, R.W. Picard (Eds.), Affective Computing and Intelligent Interaction. XVIII, 781 pages. 2007.

Vol. 4729: F. Mele, G. Ramella, S. Santillo, F. Ventriglia (Eds.), Advances in Brain, Vision, and Artificial Intelligence. XVI, 618 pages. 2007.

Vol. 4713: F.A. Hamprecht, C. Schnörr, B. Jähne (Eds.), Pattern Recognition. XIII, 560 pages. 2007.

Vol. 4679: A.L. Yuille, S.-C. Zhu, D. Cremers, Y. Wang (Eds.), Energy Minimization Methods in Computer Vision and Pattern Recognition. XII, 494 pages. 2007.

Vol. 4678: J. Blanc-Talon, W. Philips, D. Popescu, P. Scheunders (Eds.), Advanced Concepts for Intelligent Vision Systems. XXIII, 1100 pages. 2007.

Vol. 4673: W.G. Kropatsch, M. Kampel, A. Hanbury (Eds.), Computer Analysis of Images and Patterns. XX, 1006 pages. 2007.

Vol. 4642: S.-W. Lee, S.Z. Li (Eds.), Advances in Biometrics. XX, 1216 pages. 2007.

Vol. 4633: M.S. Kamel, A. Campilho (Eds.), Image Analysis and Recognition. XII, 1312 pages. 2007.

Vol. 4625: R. Stiefelhagen, R. Bowers, J.G. Fiscus (Eds.), Multimodal Technologies for Perception of Humans. XIII, 556 pages. 2008.

Vol. 4584: N. Karssemeijer, B. Lelieveldt (Eds.), Information Processing in Medical Imaging. XX, 777 pages. 2007.

Vol. 4569: A. Butz, B. Fisher, A. Krüger, P. Olivier, S. Owada (Eds.), Smart Graphics. IX, 237 pages. 2007.

Vol. 4538: F. Escolano, M. Vento (Eds.), Graph-Based Representations in Pattern Recognition. XII, 416 pages. 2007.

Vol. 4522: B.K. Ersbøll, K.S. Pedersen (Eds.), Image Analysis. XVIII, 989 pages. 2007.

Vol. 4485: F. Sgallari, A. Murli, N. Paragios (Eds.), Scale Space and Variational Methods in Computer Vision. XV, 931 pages. 2007.

Vol. 4478: J. Martí, J.M. Benedí, A.M. Mendonça, J. Serrat (Eds.), Pattern Recognition and Image Analysis, Part II. XXVII, 657 pages. 2007.

Vol. 4477: J. Martí, J.M. Benedí, A.M. Mendonça, J. Serrat (Eds.), Pattern Recognition and Image Analysis, Part I. XXVII, 625 pages. 2007.

Vol. 4472: M. Haindl, J. Kittler, F. Roli (Eds.), Multiple Classifier Systems. XI, 524 pages. 2007.

Vol. 4466: F.B. Sachse, G. Seemann (Eds.), Functional Imaging and Modeling of the Heart. XV, 486 pages. 2007.

Vol. 4418: A. Gagalowicz, W. Philips (Eds.), Computer Vision/Computer Graphics Collaboration Techniques. XV, 620 pages. 2007.

Vol. 4417: A. Kerren, A. Ebert, J. Meyer (Eds.), Human-Centered Visualization Environments. XIX, 403 pages. 2007.

Vol. 4391: Y. Stylianou, M. Faundez-Zanuy, A. Esposito (Eds.), Progress in Nonlinear Speech Processing. XII, 269 pages. 2007.

Vol. 4370: P.P. Lévy, B. Le Grand, F. Poulet, M. Soto, L. Darago, L. Toubiana, J.-F. Vibert (Eds.), Pixelization Paradigm. XV, 279 pages. 2007.

Vol. 4358: R. Vidal, A. Heyden, Y. Ma (Eds.), Dynamical Vision. IX, 329 pages. 2007.

Vol. 4338: P.K. Kalra, S. Peleg (Eds.), Computer Vision, Graphics and Image Processing. XV, 965 pages. 2006.

Vol. 4319: L.-W. Chang, W.-N. Lie (Eds.), Advances in Image and Video Technology. XXVI, 1347 pages. 2006.

Vol. 4292: G. Bebis, R. Boyle, B. Parvin, D. Koracin, P. Remagnino, A. Nefian, G. Meenakshisundaram, V. Pascucci, J. Zara, J. Molineros, H. Theisel, T. Malzbender (Eds.), Advances in Visual Computing, Part II. XXXII, 906 pages. 2006.

Vol. 4291: G. Bebis, R. Boyle, B. Parvin, D. Koracin, P. Remagnino, A. Nefian, G. Meenakshisundaram, V. Pascucci, J. Zara, J. Molineros, H. Theisel, T. Malzbender (Eds.), Advances in Visual Computing, Part I. XXXI, 916 pages. 2006.

Vol. 4245: A. Kuba, L.G. Nyúl, K. Palágyi (Eds.), Discrete Geometry for Computer Imagery. XIII, 688 pages. 2006.

Vol. 4241: R.R. Beichel, M. Sonka (Eds.), Computer Vision Approaches to Medical Image Analysis. XI, 262 pages. 2006.

Vol. 4225: J.F. Martínez-Trinidad, J.A. Carrasco Ochoa, J. Kittler (Eds.), Progress in Pattern Recognition, Image Analysis and Applications. XIX, 995 pages. 2006.

Vol. 4191: R. Larsen, M. Nielsen, J. Sporring (Eds.), Medical Image Computing and Computer-Assisted Intervention – MICCAI 2006, Part II. XXXVIII, 981 pages. 2006.

Vol. 4190: R. Larsen, M. Nielsen, J. Sporring (Eds.), Medical Image Computing and Computer-Assisted Intervention – MICCAI 2006, Part I. XXXVIII, 949 pages. 2006.

Vol. 4179: J. Blanc-Talon, W. Philips, D. Popescu, P. Scheunders (Eds.), Advanced Concepts for Intelligent Vision Systems. XXIV, 1224 pages. 2006.

Vol. 4174: K. Franke, K.-R. Müller, B. Nickolay, R. Schäfer (Eds.), Pattern Recognition. XX, 773 pages. 2006.

Vol. 4170: J. Ponce, M. Hebert, C. Schmid, A. Zisserman (Eds.), Toward Category-Level Object Recognition. XI, 618 pages. 2006.

Vol. 4153: N. Zheng, X. Jiang, X. Lan (Eds.), Advances in Machine Vision, Image Processing, and Pattern Analysis. XIII, 506 pages. 2006.

Vol. 4142: A. Campilho, M.S. Kamel (Eds.), Image Analysis and Recognition, Part II. XXVII, 923 pages. 2006.

Vol. 4141: A. Campilho, M.S. Kamel (Eds.), Image Analysis and Recognition, Part I. XXVIII, 939 pages. 2006.

Vol. 4122: R. Stiefelhagen, J.S. Garofolo (Eds.), Multimodal Technologies for Perception of Humans. XII, 360 pages. 2007.

Vol. 4109: D.-Y. Yeung, J.T. Kwok, A. Fred, F. Roli, D. de Ridder (Eds.), Structural, Syntactic, and Statistical Pattern Recognition. XXI, 939 pages. 2006.

Vol. 4091: G.-Z. Yang, T. Jiang, D. Shen, L. Gu, J. Yang (Eds.), Medical Imaging and Augmented Reality. XIII, 399 pages. 2006.

Vol. 4073: A. Butz, B. Fisher, A. Krüger, P. Olivier (Eds.), Smart Graphics. XI, 263 pages. 2006.

Vol. 4069: F.J. Perales, R.B. Fisher (Eds.), Articulated Motion and Deformable Objects. XV, 526 pages. 2006.

Vol. 4057: J.P.W. Pluim, B. Likar, F.A. Gerritsen (Eds.), Biomedical Image Registration. XII, 324 pages. 2006.